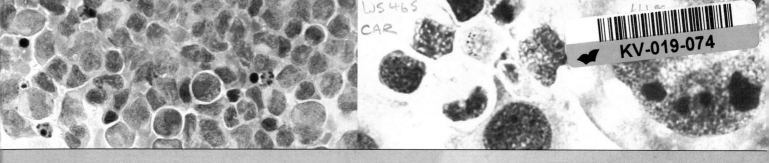

CANCER
in Children and Adolescents

Edited by

William L. Carroll, MD

Julie and Edward J. Minskoff Professor of Pediatrics
Director, New York University Cancer Institute
Chief, Division of Pediatric Hematology and Oncology
Director, Stephen D. Hassenfeld Children's Center for Cancer and Blood Disorders
New York, NY

and

Jonathan L. Finlay, MB, ChB

Professor of Pediatrics, Neurology and Neurosurgery
Keck School of Medicine
University of Southern California
Director, Neural Tumors Program
Children's Center for Cancer and Blood Diseases
Childrens Hospital of Los Angeles
Los Angeles, CA

World Headquarters

Jones and Bartlett Publishers
40 Tall Pine Drive
Sudbury, MA 01776
978-443-5000
info@jbpub.com
www.jbpub.com

Jones and Bartlett Publishers Canada
6339 Ormindale Way
Mississauga, Ontario L5V 1J2
Canada

Jones and Bartlett Publishers International
Barb House, Barb Mews
London W6 7PA
United Kingdom

Jones and Bartlett's books and products are available through most bookstores and online booksellers. To contact Jones and Bartlett Publishers directly, call 800-832-0034, fax 978-443-8000, or visit our website, www.jbpub.com.

Substantial discounts on bulk quantities of Jones and Bartlett's publications are available to corporations, professional associations, and other qualified organizations. For details and specific discount information, contact the special sales department at Jones and Bartlett via the above contact information or send an email to specialsales@jbpub.com.

The authors, editor, and publisher have made every effort to provide accurate information. However, they are not responsible for errors, omissions, or for any outcomes related to the use of the contents of this book and take no responsibility for the use of the products described. Treatments and side effects described in this book may not be applicable to all patients; likewise, some patients may require a dose or experience a side effect that is not described herein. The reader should confer with his or her own physician regarding specific treatments and side effects. Drugs and medical devices are discussed that may have limited availability controlled by the Food and Drug Administration (FDA) for use only in a research study or clinical trial. The drug information presented has been derived from reference sources, recently published data, and pharmaceutical research data. Research, clinical practice, and government regulations often change the accepted standard in this field. When consideration is being given to use of any drug in the clinical setting, the healthcare provider or reader is responsible for determining FDA status of the drug, reading the package insert, reviewing prescribing information for the most up-to-date recommendations on dose, precautions, and contraindications, and determining the appropriate usage for the product. This is especially important in the case of drugs that are new or seldom used.

Production Credits
Executive Publisher: Christopher Davis
Custom Projects Editor: Kathy Richardson
Senior Editorial Assistant: Jessica Acox
Editorial Assistant: Sara Cameron
Production Editor: Daniel Stone / Mike Boblitt
Production Assistant: Laura Almozara
V.P., Manufacturing and Inventory Control: Therese Connell
Composition: DBS
Printing and Binding: Replika Press Pvt. Ltd.
Cover Printing: Replika Press Pvt. Ltd.

Cover Credits
Cover Design: Kristin E. Parker
Cover Image: © Mikael Damkler/Shutterstock, Inc.

Library of Congress Cataloging-in-Publication Data
Cancer in children and adolescents / [edited by] William L. Carroll and Jonathan L. Finlay.
   p.   ;   cm.
   Includes bibliographical references and index.
      ISBN-13: 978-0-7637-3141-0
      ISBN-10: 0-7637-3141-2
   1. Cancer in children.   2. Cancer in adolescence.   I. Carroll, William L. (William Larkin) II. Finlay, Jonathan L.
[DNLM: 1.   Neoplasms.   2.   Adolescent.   3.   Child.   4.   Infant.   QZ 275
C2145 2009]
RC281.C4C365 2009
616.99′400835—dc22

2008005247

6048

Printed in India
13 12 11 10 09   10 9 8 7 6 5 4 3 2 1

In Memoriam

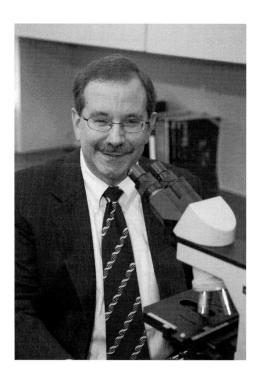

This first edition of *Cancer in Children and Adolescents* is in memory of Dr. Stephen J. Qualman, a leader in the field of pediatric oncology, a close friend and colleague, and a tireless advocate for children affected with cancer.

CONTENTS

CONTRIBUTORS

Editors

William L. Carroll, MD
Julie and Edward J. Minskoff Professor of Pediatrics
Director, New York University Cancer Institute
Chief, Division of Pediatric Hematology and Oncology
Director, Stephen D. Hassenfeld Children's Center for Cancer and
    Blood Disorders
New York, NY

Jonathan L. Finlay, MB, ChB
Professor of Pediatrics, Neurology and Neurosurgery
Keck School of Medicine
University of Southern California
Director, Neural Tumors Program
Children's Center for Cancer & Blood Diseases
Childrens Hospital Los Angeles
Los Angeles, CA

Contributing Authors

Peter C. Adamson, MD
Chief, Division of Clinical Pharmacology and Therapeutics
Director, Experimental Therapeutics in Oncology
The Children's Hospital of Philadelphia
Philadelphia, PA

Sarah W. Alexander, MD
Division of Haematology/Oncology
The Hospital for Sick Children
Toronto, Ontario, Canada

Federico Antillon-Klussman, MD, MMM, PhD
Medical Director, Pediatric Oncology
National Pediatric Oncology Unit
Guatemala City, Guatemala

Robert J. Arceci, MD, PhD
King Fahd Professor of Pediatric Oncology
Professor of Pediatrics, Oncology and the Cellular and Molecular
    Medicine Graduate Program
Kimmel Comprehensive Cancer Center at Johns Hopkins
Baltimore, MD

Mark Bernstein, MD, FRCP(C)
Division of Hematology/Oncology
IWK Health Center
Professor of Pediatrics
Dalhousie University
Halifax, Nova Scotia, Canada

Deepa Bhojwani, MD
Assistant Member, Department of Oncology
St. Jude Children's Research Hospital
Memphis, TN

Stefan Bielack, MD
Professor and Director, Pediatric Oncology / Hematology /
    Immunology
Klinikum Stuttgart
Zentrum für Kinder- und Jugendmedizin - Olgahospital
Stuttgart, Germany

Eric Bouffet, MD
Neuro-oncology Section, Division of Haematology/Oncology
The Hospital for Sick Children
Toronto, Ontario, Canada

Patrick A. Brown, MD
Instructor in Oncology
The Sidney Kimmel Comprehensive Cancer Center
Johns Hopkins University School of Medicine
Baltimore, MD

Mitchell S. Cairo, MD
Chief, Division of Blood and Marrow Transplantation
Professor, Pediatrics, Medicine and Pathology
Morgan Stanley Children's Hospital—New York Presbyterian
Columbia University
New York, NY

Steven C. Clifford, PhD
Senior Lecturer in Molecular Oncology
Northern Institute for Cancer Research
Newcastle University
Newcastle-upon-Tyne, United Kingdom

Susan L. Cohn, MD
Professor and Director, Clinical Services
Department of Pediatrics
Section of Hematology/Oncology
University of Chicago
Chicago, IL

John J. Collins, MD, PhD
Head, Department of Pain Medicine and Palliative Care
The Children's Hospital at Westmead
and
Clinical Associate Professor, Discipline of
    Paediatrics and Child Health
Faculty Medicine
University of Sydney
Sydney, Australia

Timothy P. Cripe, MD, PhD
Professor of Pediatrics, Division of Hematology/Oncology
Cincinnati Children's Hospital Medical Center
University of Cincinnati College of Medicine
Cincinnati, OH

Piotr Czauderna, MD, PhD
Associate Professor, Department of Pediatric Surgery
Institute of Pediatrics
Medical University of Gdansk, Poland

Blanca Diez, MD
Fundacion para la Lucha de las Enfermedades Neurologicas de la
   Infancia (FLENI)
Institute of Neurological Research
Buenos Aires, Argentina

Jeffrey S. Dome, MD
Chief, Division of Oncology
Center for Cancer and Blood Disorders
Children's National Medical Center
Washington, DC

R. Maarten Egeler, MD, PhD
Professor of Pediatrics
Director, Immunology, Hematology, Oncology, Bone Marrow
   Transplantation and Auto-Immune Diseases
Leiden University Medical Center
Leiden, The Netherlands

Sarah Friebert, MD
Director, Division of Palliative Care
Member, Division of Hematology/Oncology
Associate Professor of Pediatrics
Akron Children's Hospital
Akron, OH

J. Russell Geyer
Seattle Children's Hospital
and
University of Washington School of Medicine
Seattle, WA

Roger H. Giller
The Children's Hospital
Department of Hematology/Oncology
Aurora, CO

Lia Gore, MD
Associate Professor of Pediatrics and Medical Oncology
University of Colorado, Denver
and
Director, Experimental Therapeutics Program
The Children's Hospital
Aurora, CO

Richard Gorlick, MD
Department of Pediatrics
Albert Einstein College of Medicine
Division of Hematology-Oncology
The Children's Hospital at Montefiore
New York, NY

Richard Grundy
Professor of Paediatric Neuro-oncology and Cancer Biology
Children's Brain Tumor Research Centre
The Medical School
Queen's Medical Centre
Nottingham, United Kingdom

Paul E. Grundy, MD
Professor and Director of Pediatric Hematology and Oncology
University of Alberta
Edmonton, Alberta, Canada

Stephan A. Grupp, MD, PhD
Director, Stem Cell Biology
Oncology/BMT Program
The Children's Hospital of Philadelphia
and
Associate Professor of Pediatrics
University of Pennsylvania
Phliadelphia, PA

Ria G. Hawks, MS, CNS, CPNP
Division of Pediatric Hematology and Blood and Marrow
   Transplantation
Columbia University
Morgan Stanely Children's Hospital of New York Presbyterian
New York, NY

John A. Heath, MD, PhD
Clinical Associate Professor
University of Melbourne
Melbourne, Victoria
and
Children's Cancer Center
Royal Children's Hospital
Parkville, Victoria, Australia

Thomas C. Hofstra, MD
Associate Professor of Pediatrics
Keck School of Medicine
University of Southern California
Children's Center for Cancer and Blood Diseases
Childrens Hospital Los Angeles
Los Angeles, CA

Scott C. Howard, MD, MSc
Director of Clinical Trials
International Outreach Program
St. Jude Children's Research Hospital
and
Associate Professor
University of Tennessee College of Medicine
Memphis, TN

Stephen P. Hunger, MD
Professor and Ergen Family Chair in Pediatric Cancer
Chief, Section of Pediatric Hematology/Oncology/Bone Marrow
   Transplantation
University of Colorado Denver School of Medicine
Director, Center for Cancer and Blood Disorders
The Children's Hospital
Aurora, CO

Hollie A. Jackson, MD
Assistant Professor of Radiology
Keck School of Medicine
University of Southern California
Director, Nuclear Medicine Program
Department of Radiology
Childrens Hospital Los Angeles
Los Angeles, CA

Regina I. Jakacki, MD
Pediatric Neuro-Oncology Program
Children's Hospital of Pittsburgh
Pittsburgh, PA

Heribert Juergens, MD, PhD
Professor, Department of Pediatric Hematology and Oncology
University Children's Hospital
Muenster, Germany

Nina S. Kadan-Lottick, MD, MSPH, FAAP
Assistant Professor, Department of Pediatrics
Division of Pediatric Hematology/Oncology
Medical Director, Health, Education, Research & Outcomes for
    Survivors of Childhood Cancer Program (HEROS)
Yale University School of Medicine
New Haven, CT

John Kalapurakal, MD
Co-Director, Pediatric Radiation Oncology
Falk Brain Tumor Center
Assistant Professor of Radiology
Children's Memorial Hospital
Chicago, IL

Thomas A. Kaleita, PhD
Department of Psychiatry and Biobehavioral Sciences
Semel Institute for Neuroscience and Human Behavior
The UCLA Neuro-Oncology Program
David Geffen School of Medicine at UCLA
Los Angeles, CA

Howard M. Katzenstein, MD
Aflac Cancer Center and Blood Disorders Service
Emory University
Children's Healthcare of Atlanta
Atlanta, GA

Chantal Kalifa, MD
Department of Pediatric Oncology
Institute Gustave Roussy
Villejuif, France

Stewart J. Kellie, MD
Clinical Associate Professor
University of Sydney
and
Department of Oncology
Children's Hospital at Westmead
Westmead, Sydney, Australia

Kara M. Kelly, MD
Associate Professor of Clinical Pediatrics
Columbia University Medical Center
Division of Pediatric Oncology
and

Morgan Stanley Children's Hospital of New York-Presbyterian
New York, NY

Heinrich Kovar, PhD
Associate Professor
Children's Cancer Research Institute
Vienna, Austria

Mark Krailo, PhD
Department of Preventive Medicine
Keck School of Medicine
University of Southern California
Los Angeles, CA

Elena J. Ladas, MS, RD
Division of Pediatric Oncology
Columbia University
Children's Hospital of New York
New York, NY

Michael P. LaQuaglia, MD
Chief of Pediatric Surgery, Department of Surgery
Memorial Sloan Kettering Cancer Center
New York, NY

Robert S. Lavey, MD, MPH
Center for Radiation Oncology
Brandon, FL

Marcio H. Malogolowkin, MD
Division Head, Hematology-Oncology for Clinical
    Affairs and Clinical Research
Director, Bone and Soft Tissue Tumor Program
Childrens Hospital Los Angeles
Associate Professor of Pediatrics
Keck School Of Medicine
University of Southern California
Los Angeles, CA

Neyssa Marina, MD
Professor of Pediatrics, Division of Pediatric
    Hematology/Oncology
Stanford University Medical Center
Palo Alto, CA

Leo Mascarenhas, MD
Associate Professor of Pediatrics
Keck School of Medicine
University of Southern California
Director-Clinical Trials Office
Children's Center for Cancer and Blood Diseases
Childrens Hospital Los Angeles
Los Angeles, CA

Geoffrey B. McCowage, MD
Pediatric Oncologist
The Children's Hospital at Westmead
Westmead, Sydney, Australia

Thomas W. McLean, MD
Department of Pediatrics
Wake Forest University School of Medicine
Winston-Salem, NC

Anna T. Meadows, MD
Professor of Pediatrics
Medical Director, Cancer Survivorship and Living Well After Cancer
   Program
The Children's Hospital of Philadelphia
Philadelphia, PA

Thomas E. Merchant, DO, PhD
Faculty Member
Division Chief, Radiation Oncology
Department of Radiological Sciences
St. Jude Children's Research Hospital
Memphis, TN

Ann C. Mertens, PhD
Department of Pediatrics
Children's Healthcare of Atlanta/Emory University
Atlanta, GA

William H. Meyer, MD
CMRI Ben Johnson Professor and Section Head
Section of Hematology/Oncology
Department of Pediatrics
University of Oklahoma Health Sciences Center
Oklahoma City, OK

Jeff M. Michalski, MD, MBA
Department of Radiation Oncology
Washington University School of Medicine
St. Louis, MO

Hector L. Monforte, MD
Clinical Associate Professor of Pathology
University of South Florida College of Medicine at Tampa
Department of Anatomic Pathology
All Children's Hospital
St. Petersburg, FL

James Nachman, MD
Professor of Pediatrics
Director, Clinical Programs
University of Chicago Comer Children's Hospital
Chicago, IL

Joseph P. Neglia, MD, MPH
Professor of Pediatrics
Section Chief, Pediatric Hematology and Oncology
Department of Pediatrics
Masonic Cancer Center
University of Minnesota
Minneapolis, MN

Jorge A. Ortega, MD
Emeritus Professor of Pediatrics
Keck School of Medicine
University of Southern California
Children's Center for Cancer and Blood Diseases
Childrens Hospital Los Angeles
Los Angeles, CA

Chintan Parekh, MD
Fellow, Pediatric Hematology-Oncology
Children's Center for Cancer and Blood Diseases
Childrens Hospital Los Angeles
Los Angeles, CA

Michael Paulussen, MD
Department of Paediatric Oncology/Hematology
University Children's Hospital (UKBB)
Basel, Switzerland

Giorgio Perilongo, MD
Division of Haematology-Oncology
Paediatric Neuro-Oncology Program
University-Hospital of Padua
Padua, Italy

Sherrie L. Perkins, MD, PhD
Professor, Department of Pathology
Director, Hematopathology
University of Utah and ARUP Laboratories
Salt Lake City, UT

Elizabeth J. Perlman, MD
Professor of Pathology and Laboratory Medicine
Northwestern University's Feinberg School of Medicine
Head, Division of Pathology and Laboratory Medicine
Children's Memorial Hospital
Chicago, IL

Barry L. Pizer, MBChB, FRCPCH, PhD
Consultant Paediatric Oncologist
Alder Hey Children's Hospital
Liverpool, Merseyside
United Kingdom

Ian F. Pollack, MD, FACS, FAAP
Chief, Pediatric Neurosurgery
Children's Hospital of Pittsburgh
Walter Dandy Professor of Neurosurgery
Vice Chairman for Academic Affairs
Department of Neurological Surgery
Director, UPCI Brain Tumor Program
University of Pittsburgh School of Medicine
Pittsburgh, PA

Janice Post-White, RN, PhD
Complementary and Alternative Medicine
Children's Oncology Group
University of Minnesota School of Nursing
Minneapolis, MN

Michael A. Pulsipher, MD
Director, University of Utah Hospitals and Clinics
   Blood and Marrow Transplant Program
Medical Director, Pediatric Blood and Marrow
   Transplantation at Primary Children's Medical Center
Huntsman Cancer Institute
Assistant Professor, Pediatrics and Hematology
University of Utah School of Medicine
Salk Lake City, UT

Stephen J. Qualman, MD
Professor and Vice Chair, Pediatric Pathology Branch,
   Department of Pathology
The Ohio State University School of Medicine
Director, Center for Childhood Cancer
Pathologist-in-Chief, Department of Laboratory Medicine
Richard M. and M. Elizabeth Ross Endowed Chair in Pediatric
   Research
The Research Institute at Nationwide Children's Hospital
Columbus, OH

John J. Quinn, MD
Professor of Clinical Pediatrics
Keck School of Medicine
University of Southern California
Director of Clinical Oncology
Children's Center for Cancer and Blood Diseases
Childrens Hospital Los Angeles
Los Angeles, CA

Elizabeth A. Raetz, MD
Associate Professor of Pediatrics, Division of Pediatric
    Hematology/Oncology
Department of Pediatrics
New York University Cancer Institute
New York University Langone Medical Center
New York, NY

R. Lor Randall, MD, FACS
Associate Professor
Director of Sarcoma Services
Huntsman Cancer Institute
The University of Utah School of Medicine
Salt Lake City, UT

Gregory H. Reaman, MD
Professor of Pediatrics
The George Washington University
School of Medicine and Health Sciences
Division of Oncology
Children's National Medical Center
and
Chair, Children's Oncology Group
Washington, DC

Gregor S. D. Reid, PhD
Senior Research Associate
Oncology/BMT Program
The Children's Hospital of Philadelphia
Philadelphia, PA

Michael L. Ritchey, MD
Professor of Urology
Mayo Clinic College of Medicine
Scottsdale, Arizona

Joerg Ritter, MD
University Children's Hospital
Department of Pediatric Hematology and Oncology
Muenster, Germany

Carlos Rodriguez-Galindo, MD
Associate Member, Department of Oncology
St. Jude Children's Research Hospital
Memphis, TN

Paul C. Rogers, MD
Professor and Director, Pediatric Oncology
British Columbia Children's Hospital & University of British
    Columbia
Vancouver, Canada

Julie A. Ross
Professor, Department of Pediatrics
University of Minnesota
Minneapolis, MN

Andreas Schuck
Department of Radiotherapy
University Hospital
Muenster, Germany

Kirk R. Schultz, MD
Associate Professor, Department of Pediatrics
Division of Oncology/BMT
University of British Columbia
Vancouver, British Columbia, Canada

Peter J. Shaw, MD
Clinical Associate Professor, BMT Services
Oncology Unit
and
Clinical Associate Professor, Discipline of
    Paediatrics & Child Health
Sydney, Australia

Michael C.G. Stevens, MD
CLIC Professor of Paediatric Oncology
University of Bristol
United Kingdom

Lisa A. Teot, MD
Associate Professor and Staff Pathologist
Children's Hospital of Pittsburgh of UPMC
Pittsburgh, PA

Jeffrey A. Toretsky, MD
Associate Professor, Departments of Oncology and Pediatrics
Lombardi Comprehensive Cancer Center
Georgetown University Hospital
Washington, DC

Sheila Weitzman, MB, BCh
Professor of Pediatrics, Division of Pediatric
    Hematology/Oncology
The Hospital for Sick Children
University of Toronto
Toronto, Ontario, Canada

Keith S. White, MD
Pediatric Radiologist
Salt Lake City, UT

Brigitte C. Widemann, MD
Investigator, Pediatric Oncology Branch
Pharmacology and Experimental Therapeutics Section
National Cancer Institute
Bethesda, MD

Naomi J. Winick, MD
Professor, Pediatric Hematology-Oncology
University of Texas Southwestern Medical Center/Children's
    Medical Center-Dallas Dallas, TX

Johannes E.A. Wolff, MD
Professor, Pediatrics and Biostatistics
MD Anderson Cancer Center
Houston, TX

Serious efforts to treat childhood cancers, with surgery and irradiation, began in the late 19th and early 20th centuries, respectively. The introduction of chemotherapy for the treatment of childhood acute lymphoid leukemia, and other solid cancers, dates back only to the late 1940's and early 1950's, spanning therefore the lives of both editors and many of the contributing authors of this text. In this brief interval of six decades, we have witnessed tremendous improvements in the survival rates for the majority of children affected with cancer. In 2009, it is estimated that in North America and Western Europe, approximately 80% of all children diagnosed this year with cancer will be cured. Furthermore, we have learned over the last couple of decades that such increased survival can, in many cancers, be achieved with fewer substantial and permanent sequelae, due to the ability to restrict or avoid the deleterious effects of radiation therapy and certain chemotherapeutic agents.

In spite of these dramatic advances, many challenges remain; the most significant of these is the plain fact that the progress achieved in treating childhood cancer in the "developed" countries has by no means translated into improvements for the remaining 85% of children globally suffering from cancer.

Even a cure rate of 80% amongst the 'developed' countries is woefully inadequate when one considers that cancer remains the second leading cause of death in children, after the societal ills of accidents, homicide, and suicide. Certain cancers, such as many forms of central nervous system tumors, acute myelogenous leukemia, and advanced neuroblastoma have not benefited to the same degree from the advances made in other tumors. While intensifying therapy has improved outcome overall, many children are likely over-treated and a ceiling of intensity for conventional chemotherapy and radiotherapeutic strategies has been reached for refractory tumors.

However, hope for improved survival now comes from laboratory advances in the past two to three decades, including the revolution in molecular biology that led to the field of cancer genomics. The underlying biological processes that account for malignant transformation are now being revealed on an unprecedented scale. The discovery of imatinib (Gleevec®) for chronic myeloid leukemia and Philadelphia chromosome positive acute lymphoblastic leukemia has ushered in a new era of "targeted therapy," and numerous clinical trials are evaluating other such targeted and/or biological agents in a wide variety of adult and pediatric cancers. Further advances in the definition of cancer stem cells, the contribution of the tumor microenvironment and angiogenesis as well as the impact of host factors (pharmacogenomics) undoubtedly will lead to new targets and the development of new classes of agents that interrupt essential pathways involved in tumor development and maintenance.

Given the complexity and multidisciplinary nature of the subject, we have attempted to compile a very readable textbook of childhood cancer, one that can be tackled with ease from cover to cover to provide the fundamentals of diagnosis and management of cancers that affect children and adolescents. The book is divided into four major sections and starts with overviews of individual disciplines involved in diagnosis and management, including those related to basic biology, followed by descriptions of individual tumor types and finishing with critical advances in supportive and complementary care. The authors have attempted to summarize current understanding of tumor biology, approach to diagnosis, optimal treatment and the price of survival measured in terms of late effects.

We have attempted whenever feasible to provide a truly international flavor to our endeavors, in that many of the chapters are co-authored by recognized specialists from around the world. This is perhaps the singular feature which distinguishes our text uniquely from others currently available. No textbook can be completely all-encompassing, especially in its first edition, and we do apologize if certain rare tumor entities have been neglected in presentation.

This book is dedicated to a number of important people who have influenced our careers. First and foremost our wives, Adriana Maria (JF) and Saba (WLC), provide understanding for our passion and ongoing encouragement. The love of our children, Anna Victoria and Bryan, Brenden, Michelle, Thomas and Will remain a constant joy that surpasses our professional achievements. We are grateful for the inspiration and support of our parents, Minnie and Mark Finlay and Olga and William Carroll and our siblings, Margot Showman and Michael and Peter Carroll.

This book was first suggested by Chris Davis at Jones and Barlett and without his constant encouragement and support it would have never come to fruition. It was a privilege to work with other members of the Jones and Bartlett team—Mike Boblitt, Laura Almozara, and Dan Stone. Finally, Katrina Manzano, Janice Pelt, Venna Raju, and especially Melissa Neligan at New York University, played key roles in organizing the editorial process and communicating with authors. You have our everlasting thanks for your valuable assistance.

We have had the privilege and good fortune of studying under distinguished teachers and mentors including Drs. Jillian Mann, Patricia Morris-Jones, Jeffrey Rosenstock, Richard Hong, Nasrollah Shahidi, Audrey Evans, Giulio D'Angio, Anna Meadows, and Richard O'Reilly; and Drs.

William Schubert, Bertil Glader, Michael Link, Ronald Levy, Alan Schwartz, Teresa Vietti, Stanley Korsmeyer, and Stephen Prescott. Their constant encouragement and occasional warranted admonitions made everything possible. We have been honored by our own students and trainees who continue to teach us through their enthusiasm and intellect. Finally it is with great admiration that we dedicate this book to our heroic patients and their families, who continue to provide us and others with the strength to carry on the crusade against childhood cancer.

Jonathan Finlay
William L. Carroll
Los Angeles and New York City

The Biology and Diagnostic Evaluation of Childhood Cancer

Epidemiology of Cancer in Children

John A. Heath and Julie A. Ross

Cancer is predominantly a disease of aging. Its occurrence in childhood is rare, with a lifetime incidence of less than 0.5%. Despite this rarity, it remains the second most common cause of death, after accidents, in childhood and a significant public health problem in developed countries.[1] In the developing world, challenges for epidemiologists and oncologists alike include the increasing threat of human immunodeficiency virus (HIV)-related tumor epidemics, the high incidence of Burkitt's lymphoma in Africa and the Middle East, and poorly understood case clustering such as is seen with adrenocortical carcinoma in regions of South America.

Over the past three decades, improvements in treatments (surgery, irradiation, and chemotherapy) and supportive care together with the use of large, international collaborative trials have led to dramatic improvements in survival rates for most types of childhood cancer[2] (Figure 1-1). Today, it is estimated that 1 in 900 young adults in the developed world is a cancer survivor.[3] Some of these survivors will suffer significant treatment-related health and psychosocial problems and have a reduced life expectancy.[4] The factors that predispose particular individuals to these health problems are the subject of new and innovative epidemiological research.

Descriptive Epidemiology

The types of cancer seen in children are classified according to the standard International Classification of Childhood Cancer[5] (Table 1-1). The two largest incidence and survival data series, the National Cancer Institute's Surveillance, Epidemiology, and End Results (SEER) Program in the United States and the National Registry of Childhood Tumours in the United Kingdom, give a comprehensive and accurate picture of geographical, racial, gender, and temporal trends in the developed world. Elsewhere, registries are more variable in their quality. Inadequate reporting and documentation of malignancy can lead to problems with data from less-developed countries. Monitoring of incidence rates and distribution of cancer types across the entire world (through collation of these data) are largely the responsibility of the International Union of

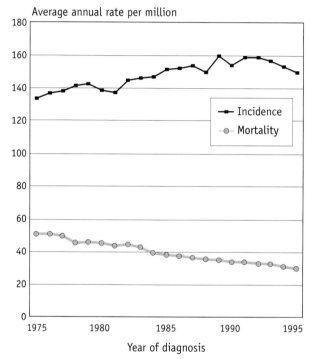

Figure 1-1 Trends in age-adjusted* SEER incidence and US mortality rates for all childhood cancers age <20, all races, both sexes, 1975–95.

Cancer.[6] There has been a suggestion that the incidence rates of childhood cancer have increased over time.[7] In some if not all instances, this may be due to better registration of cases and increased diagnosis due to better imaging. There has also been considerable interest in childhood cancer clusters. To date, no strong evidence to confirm and explain this phenomenon has been presented.

Unlike adult cancer, where carcinomas of the lung, bowel, breast, and prostate predominate, childhood cancers are extremely diverse both in origin and distribution (Figure 1-2). Many solid tumors in children are embryonal neoplasms, the morphology of which resembles that observed during embryogenesis and fetal development. Early age peaks in incidence are a feature of these tumors.

Table 1-1

International Classification of Childhood Cancer (ICCC).

ICCC Group	Morphology	Topography
I Leukemia		
(a) Lymphoid Leukemia		
Excluding ALL	9820,9822-9827,9850	C00.0-C80.9
ALL	9821	C00.0-C80.9
(b) Acute Leukemia		
Excluding AML	9840, 9841, 9864, 9866, 9867, 9891, 9894, 9910	C00.0-C80.9
AML	9861	C00.0-C80.9
(c) Chronic Myeloid Leukemia	9863, 9868	C00.0-C80.9
(d) Other Specified Leukemias	9830, 9842, 9860, 9862, 9870-9890, 9892, 9893, 9900, 9930-9941	C00.0-C80.9
(e) Unspecified Leukemias	9800-9804	C00.0-C80.9
II Lymphomas and Reticuloendothelial Neoplasms		
(a) Hodgkin's disease	9650-9667	C00.0-C80.9
(b) Non-Hodgkin's lymphomas	9591-9595, 9670-9686, 9690-9717, 9723, 9688	C00.0-C80.9
(c) Burkitt's lymphoma	9687	C00.0-C80.9
(d) Miscellaneous lymphoreticular neoplasms	9720, 9731-9764	C00.0-C80.9
(e) Unspecified lymphomas	9590	C00.0-C80.9
III CNS and Miscellaneous Intracranial and Intraspinal Neoplasms		
(a) Ependymoma	9383, 9390-9394	C00.0-C80.9
(b Astrocytoma	9380	C72.3
	9381, 9400-9441	C00.0-C80.9
(c) Primitive neuroectodermal tumors	9470-9473	C00.0-C80.9*
(d) Other gliomas	9380	C70.0-C72.2, C72.4-C72.9
	9382, 9384, 9442-9460, 9481	C00.0-C80.9
(e) Miscellaneous intracranial and intraspinal neoplasms	8270-8281, 8300, 9350-9362, 9480, 9505, 9530-9539	C00.0-C80.9
(f) Unspecified intracranial and intraspinal neoplasms	8000-8004	C70.0-C72.9, C75.1-C75.3
IV Sympathetic Nervous System Tumors		
(a) Neuroblastoma and ganglioneuroblastoma	9490, 9500	C00.0-C80.9
(b) Other sympathetic nervous system tumors	8680, 8693-8710, 9501-9504, 9520-9523	C00.0-C80.9

Table 1-1

International Classification of Childhood Cancer (ICCC) (continued)

ICCC Group	Morphology	Topography
V Retinoblastoma	9510-9512	C00.0-C80.9
VI Renal Tumors		
(a) Wilms' tumor, rhabdoid and clear cell sarcoma	8963	C64.9, C80.9
	8960, 8964	C00.0-C80.9
(b) Renal carcinoma	8010-8041, 8050-8075, 8082, 8120-8122, 8130-8141, 8143, 8155, 8190-8201, 8210, 8211, 8221-8231, 8240, 8241, 8244-8246, 8260-8263, 8290, 8310, 8320, 8323, 8401, 8430, 8440, 8480-8490, 8504, 8510, 8550, 8560-8573	C64.9
	8312	C00.0-C80.9
(c) Unspecified malignant renal tumors	8000-8004	C64.9
VII Hepatic Tumors		
(a) Hepatoblastoma	8970	C00.0-C80.9
(b) Hepatic carcinoma	8010-8041, 8050-8075, 8082, 8120-8122, 8140, 8141, 8143, 8155, 8190-8201, 8210, 8211, 8230, 8231, 8240, 8241, 8244-8246, 8260-8263, 8310, 8320, 8323, 8401, 8430, 8440,8480-8490, 8504, 8510, 8550, 8560-8573	C22.0, 022.1
	8160-8180	C00.0-C80.9
(c) Unspecified malignant hepatic tumors	8000-8004	C22.0, 022.1
VIII Malignant Bone Tumors		
(a) Osteosarcoma	9180-9200	C00.0-C80.9
(b) Chondrosarcoma	9220-9230	C00.0-C80.9
	9231, 9240	C40.0-C41.9
(c) Ewing's sarcoma	9260	C40.0-C41.9, C80.9
	9363, 9364	C40.0-C41.9
(d) Other specified malignant bone tumors	8812, 9250, 9261-9330, 9370	C00.0-C80.9
(e) Unspecified malignant bone tumors	8000-8004, 8800, 8801, 8803, 8804	C40.0-C41.9
IX Soft-Tissue Sarcomas		
(a) Rhabdomyosarcoma and embryonal sarcoma	8900-8920, 8991	C00.0-C80.9
(b) Fibrosarcoma, neuro-fibrosarcoma and other fibromatous neoplasms	8810, 8811, 8813-8833, 9540-9561	C00.0-C80.9
(c) Kaposi's sarcoma	9140	C00.0-C80.9
(d) Other specified soft-tissue sarcomas	8840-8896, 8982, 8990, 9040-9044, 9120-9134, 9150-9170, 9251, 9581	C00.0-C80.9
	8963	C00.0-C63.9, C65.9-C76.8
	9231, 9240, 9363, 9364	C00.0-C39.9, C44.0-C80.9
	9260	C00.0-C39.9, C47.0-C76.8
(e) Unspecified soft-tissue sarcomas	8800-8804	C00.0-C39.9, C44.0-C80.9

Table 1-1

International Classification of Childhood Cancer (ICCC) (continued)

ICCC Group	Morphology	Topography
X Germ-Cell, Trophoblastic and other Gonadal Neoplasms		
(a) Intracranial and intraspinal germ-cell tumors	9060-9102	C70.0-C72.9, C75.1-C75.3
(b) Other and unspecified non-gonadal germ-cell tumors	9060-9102	C00.0-C55.9, C57.0-C61.9, C63.0-C69.9, C73.9-C75.0, C75.4-C80.9
(c) Gonadal germ-cell tumors	9060-9102	C56.9, C62.0-C62.9
(d) Gonadal carcinomas	8010-8041, 8050-8075, 8082, 8120-8122, 8130-8141, 8143, 8155, 8190-8201, 8210, 8211, 8221-8241, 8244-8246, 8260-8263, 8290, 8310, 8320, 8323, 8430, 8440, 8480-8490, 8504, 8510, 8550, 8560-8573	C56.9, C62.0-C62.9
	8380, 8,381, 8441-8473	C00.0-C80.9
(e) Other and unspecified malignant gonadal tumors	8590-8670, 9000	C00.0-C80.9
	8000-8004	C56.9, C62.0-C62.9
XI Carcinomas and other Malignant Epithelial Neoplasms		
(a) Adrenocortical carcinoma	8370-8375	C00.0-C80.9
(b) Thyroid carcinoma	8010-8041, 8050-8075, 8082, 8120-8122, 8130-8141, 8155, 8190, 8200, 8201, 8211, 8230, 8231, 8244-8246, 8260-8263, 8290, 8310, 8320, 8323, 8430, 8440, 8480, 8481, 8500-8573	C73.9
	8330-8350	C00.0-C80.9
(c) Nasopharyngeal carcinoma	8010-8041, 8050-8075, 8082, 8120-8122, 8130-8141, 8155, 8190, 8200, 8201, 8211, 8230, 8231, 8244-8246, 8260-8263, 8290, 8310, 8320, 8323, 8430, 8440, 8480, 8481, 8504, 8510, 8550, 8560-8573	C11.0-C11.9
(d) Malignant melanoma	8720-8780	C00.0-C80.9
(e) Skin carcinoma	8010-8041, 8050-8075, 8082, 8090-8110, 8140, 8143, 8147, 8190, 8200, 8240, 8246, 8247, 8260, 8310, 8320, 8323, 8390-8420, 8430, 8480, 8542, 8560, 8570-8573, 8940	C44.0-C44.9
(f) Other and unspecified carcinomas	8010-8082, 8120-8155, 8190-8263, 8290, 8310, 8314-8323, 8430-8440, 8480-8580, 8940, 8941	C00.0-C10.9, C12.9-C21.8, C23.9-C39.9, C48.0-C48.8, C50.0-C55.9, C57.0-C61.9, C63.0-C63.9, C65.9-C72.9, C75.0-C80.9
XLI Other and Unspecified Malignant Neoplasms		
(a) Other specified malignant tumors	8930, 8933, 8950, 8951, 8971-8981, 9020, 9050-9053, 9110, 9580	C00.0-C80.9
(b) Other unspecified malignant tumors	8000-8004	C00.0-C21.8, C23.9-C39.9, C42.0-C55.9, C57.0-C61.9, C63.0-C63.9, C65.9-C69.9, C73.9-C75.0, C75.4-C80.9

Source: Kramárová E, Stiller CA, Ferlay J, Parkin DM, Draper GJ, Michaelis J, Neglia J, Qureshi S (1996) International Classification of Childhood Cancer 1996. IARC Technical Report No. 29, International Agency for Research of Cancer, Lyon.

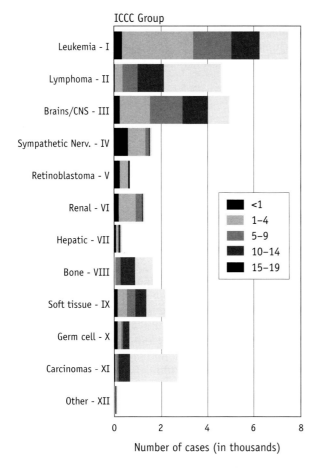

ICCC Group

Legend:
- <1
- 1–4
- 5–9
- 10–14
- 15–19

Number of cases (in thousands)

Figure 1-2 Number of cases of all childhood cancers by ICCC and age group, SEER 1975-95.

In contrast, some childhood cancers are also seen in adults. When seen in children, they tend to be the more aggressive subtypes, with short latent periods and rapid growth cycles.

Tumor Types

The 12 major diagnostic groups in childhood cancer are leukemias, lymphomas, brain tumors, sympathetic nervous system tumors, retinoblastoma, kidney tumors, liver tumors, bone tumors, soft-tissue sarcomas, gonadal and germ-cell tumors, epithelial tumors, and other unspecified tumors.

Leukemias

Acute lymphoblastic leukemia (ALL) is the most common pediatric malignancy, accounting for 75% of all newly diagnosed leukemias and 25% of all cancers in childhood.[8] The frequency, age distribution, and subtypes of ALL show striking geographical variations.[9] It is not clear whether these variations reflect genetic or environmental differences, or both. In the developed world, the peak incidence is between 3 and 4 years, with gender (male to female 1.2:1) and racial (whites to blacks 1.8:1) imbalances.[8] For a small minority of cases, constitutional genetic defects (ataxia telangiectasia, congenital immunodeficiency, Down syndrome) have been linked to an

increased risk of ALL.[10] For the majority of cases however, there appears to be little if any familial risk. Monozygotic twins do have a 2- to 4-fold increased risk of developing ALL, but this is now known to occur through transplacental sharing of the leukemic clone.[11] Acute lymphoblastic leukemia has been linked with *in utero* diagnostic radiation exposure,[12] although due to declining dosage and frequency this is unlikely to be a current risk factor. High birth weight (>4000 grams) has also consistently been associated with about a 2-fold increased risk of ALL.[13] Over the past two decades, there has been great interest in a potential infectious etiology for childhood ALL, due to the notable age peak. It has been hypothesized that lymphoblast proliferation in response to a general infection, particularly later exposure as is often experienced in higher socioeconomic groups and developed countries, may result in an altered immune response and sufficient number of genetic mutations necessary to produce ALL (the Kinlen hypothesis).[14] In contrast to this "nonspecific response" hypothesis, others have postulated that ALL may arise as a rare response to infection by a specific agent, such as a virus.[15]

Unlike ALL, the incidence of acute myeloid leukemia (AML) is highest in infancy and then declines to remain constant throughout childhood with a case ratio of 1:4 compared with ALL.[8] In a small minority of children with AML, congenital syndromes with impaired myelopoiesis (Diamond-Blackfan anemia,[16] Kostmann syndrome),[17] impaired DNA repair mechanisms (Bloom syndrome,[18] Fanconi anemia),[19] or impaired tumor suppression (neurofibromatosis type 1)[20] are identified. Down syndrome is also a risk factor for AML, with the megakaryocytic French-American-British (FAB) M7 subtype being commonly observed in younger patients.[21] Like ALL, AML has also been associated with fetal exposure to *in utero* radiation,[22] and to a lesser extent, high birth weight.[23] Other potential risk factors that appear more consistently with childhood AML compared with ALL include maternal alcohol consumption during pregnancy[24–26] and, similar to adult AML, exposure to pesticides and benzene.[27,28] Secondary AML following exposure to DNA topoisomerase-2 inhibitors (especially epipodophyllotoxins such as etoposide),[29] alkylators,[30] and ionizing radiation[31] account for a small but significant number of cases in childhood.

Lymphomas

Lymphomas account for approximately 15% of all newly diagnosed childhood cancers. Approximately 60% of pediatric lymphomas are non-Hodgkin's lymphoma (NHL), with the remainder being Hodgkin's lymphoma.[8] While the incidence rate of adult NHL appears to have increased over the past few decades,[32] this has not been observed in children. Compared with adults, a narrower spectrum of the more diffuse, aggressive, NHL subtypes is observed in children. The incidence and subtype prevalence also varies markedly across the world. In parts of equatorial Africa, for example, approximately 50% of all childhood cancers are Burkitt's lymphoma.[33] Malaria and perinatal infection with Epstein-Barr virus (EBV), a lymphotropic herpes virus, seem to be independent risk factors in this setting.[34] Elsewhere, childhood Burkitt's lymphomas appears to differ biologically, with less EBV involvement and different chromosomal breakpoints in the characteristic 8;21 (c-myc/Ig) translocation.[35] In the developed world, congenital (ataxia telangiectasia, Wiskott-Aldrich syndrome, X-linked lymphoproliferative disorder) and acquired (acquired immunodeficiency syndrome and post-organ transplant) immune deficiencies are a small but strong risk factor for NHL.[36] Beyond this, very few epidemiology studies have been conducted on childhood NHL. One study from China reported that breastfeeding may be protective,[37] while in the United States a positive association with pesticides in the home was reported.[38]

Hodgkin's lymphoma exhibits a characteristic bimodal age distribution, the first peak occurring in late adolescence/early adult life.[39] Genetic susceptibility may be a contributing factor, as evidenced by a 99-fold higher risk for monozygotic twins[40] and a 7-fold higher risk for siblings.[41] Rates of Hodgkin's lymphoma in younger children are strongly linked to lower socioeconomic status,[42] while adolescent/young adult cases are linked to higher standards of living in childhood[43] and tend to cluster,[44] suggesting that timing of infections may play a key role. The most consistent association with an infection is with EBV.[45]

Brain Tumors

Malignant brain tumors are the leading cause of death and the second most common type of cancer in childhood, accounting for approximately 20% of cases.[8] They are heterogeneous in nature, and include glial tumors (most commonly astrocytomas), primitive neuroectodermal tumors (PNET)/medulloblastomas, and ependymomas. Some tumor types (medulloblastoma, ependymoma) have a higher incidence in males.[46] In a minority of cases, genetic syndromes (ataxia telangiectasia, basal cell nevus/Gorlin syndrome, Li-Fraumeni syndrome (LFS), neurofibromatosis-type 1, Turcot syndrome) impart a clear predisposition to tumorogenesis.[47] Ionizing irradiation, most often therapeutic irradiation nowadays, is also a well-established risk factor.[48] Other environmental exposures, including N-Nitroso compounds found in cured meats[49] and polyomaviruses,[50] remain possible but unproven risk factors for the development of brain tumors.

Sympathetic Nervous System Tumors

Neuroblastoma is a malignant tumor of the sympathetic nervous system, arising from the primitive progenitor cells of the sympathetic ganglia and adrenal medulla, and accounting for 9% of all childhood cancers. The incidence rate is highest in the first year of life and declines rapidly thereafter.[8] Two large studies of screening in newborns for neuroblastoma using urinary catecholamines proved to be ineffective at the population level.[51,52] A number of studies have suggested that environmental factors (paternal occupational exposure to electromagnetic fields; maternal exposure to diuretics; prenatal exposure to phenytoin, phenobarbitol, and alcohol) may increase the risk of neuroblastoma in offspring.[53] There also appears to be an association with congenital, particularly urogenital and cardiac, anomalies.[54]

Retinoblastoma

Retinoblastoma, a malignant tumor of the retina occurring almost exclusively in infants and young children, accounts for approximately 3% of childhood cancers.[8] It was the original tumor modelled by Knudsen to describe the role of a tumor suppressor gene.[55] In approximately 40% of cases (100% bilateral and 10% unilateral), the child carries a germline mutation in one copy of the *RB1* gene. This can be inherited from an affected parent (autosomal dominant with 90% penetrance) or spontaneously acquired. These cases tend to present in the first year of life, have multiple tumors, and carry an increased risk of second nonocular tumors including osteosarcoma, melanoma, and brain tumors.[56] The remaining nonhereditary/sporadic cases are almost always unilateral and tend to present in the second or third year of life. Little is known about the causes of these sporadic retinoblastomas. One recent study from the Netherlands reported that 5 cases of retinoblastoma were conceived through *in vitro* fertilization, resulting in a 7-fold increased risk.[57] This observation will need to be confirmed in additional studies.

Kidney Tumors

Wilms tumor is the most common primary malignant kidney tumor of childhood, accounting for 6% of all childhood cancers.[8] There is a clear racial difference in incidence rates (highest in blacks and lowest in Asian children).[58] The tumor sometimes arises in association with congenital urogenital defects or recognized syndromes (Beckwith-Wiedemann syndrome, hemihypertrophy, Perlman syndrome, Sotos syndrome, WAGR syndrome).[59] The role of parental, particularly paternal, environmental exposures remains controversial.[60]

Liver Tumors

Hepatoblastoma is the most common primary malignant liver tumor of childhood.[8] It occurs with increased frequency in children with Beckwith-Wiedemann syndrome and hemihypertrophy[61] and in families with familial adenomatous polyposis and Gardner syndrome, both heritable conditions associated with defects in the *APC* gene, the development of bowel polyps and a high risk of bowel carcinoma.[62] More recently, interest in the contributions of premature birth and extremely low birth weight has increased.[63] Hepatocellular carcinoma is extremely rare in children, occurring at increased rates in association with chronic hepatitis B infection, particularly in Asian countries.[64]

Bone Tumors

Among children, osteosarcoma accounts for approximately 60% of bone cancers, with Ewing sarcoma accounting for most of the remainder.[8] Osteosarcoma is extremely rare before the age of 5 years and the peak incidence (the second decade of life) coincides with the period of rapid growth around puberty. Despite this, there is no consistent association with taller stature.[65] Radiation exposure[66] and prior treatment of childhood cancer with alkylating agents,[67] and germline mutations of either P53[68] or RB1[69] are all well-documented causal factors.

Ewing sarcoma can occur in bone, soft tissue, or both. Most occur in later childhood/adolescence, with a slight male predominance.[70] These tumors are extremely rare in blacks (both in Africa and the Americas) and in children of Asian origin.[71] Otherwise, no genetic or environmental risk factor has been clearly identified.

Soft-Tissue Sarcomas

Rhabdomyosarcoma is the most common soft-tissue sarcoma in children, with nearly half of cases being diagnosed before the age of 5 years.[8] Genetic syndromes including Beckwith-Wiedemann syndrome, neurofibromatosis type-1, LFS, and Costello syndrome are associated with a small number of rhabdomyosarcoma cases. In other cases, the anatomic location of tumor concords with a major birth defect.[72,73] The largest case-control study to date found an increased risk with parental use of cocaine and marijuana.[74] A few smaller case-control studies have also suggested roles for increased maternal age[75] and pregnancy-related toxemia.[76]

Gonadal and Germ Cell Tumors

Germ cell tumors (GCT) are a heterogeneous group of benign and malignant tumors. They usually arise in the midline, reflecting the migratory pathway of embryonic germ cells. GCT incidence varies considerably across the world, with highest levels reported in Asia.[77] Cryptorchidism is the most clearly defined risk factor, with up to a 10-fold increase in incidence rates of testicular cancer.[78] The roles of estrogen, preterm birth, high birth weight, congenital anomalies, and environmental exposures in the pathogenesis are all under investigation.[79]

Epithelial Tumors

Epithelial cancers are very rare in children. The most common types are adrenocortical carcinoma, nasopharyngeal carcinoma, and thyroid cancers. Adrenocortical carcinoma accounts for 10% of childhood cancers in Li Fraumeni Syndrome families.[73] The incidence of adrenocortical carcinoma in southern Brazil is 10-fold higher than elsewhere[80] and appears to reflect inheritance of a unique p53 mutation.[81] Nasopharyngeal carcinoma in childhood is associated with EBV infection.[82] The most well established risk factor for thyroid cancer is ionizing radiation exposure, both from environmental and therapeutic sources.[83] Other possible contributory factors include female gender, benign thyroid conditions, and certain cancer susceptibility syndromes, such as multiple endocrine neoplasia types I, IIA, and IIB.[84–86]

Other Tumors

Melanoma is rare in children.[8] The primary risk factors include fair skin, ultraviolet light exposure,[87] and numbers of melanocytic and dysplastic nevi.[88] Other types of skin cancers (basal cell and squamous cell carcinoma) are seen in patients with impaired DNA repair mechanisms (Fanconi anemia[19] and xeroderma pigmentosa),[89] nevoid basal cell carcinoma (Gorlin) syndrome,[90] and following organ transplantation with immunosuppression.[91]

Analytical Epidemiology

A framework for considering the etiology of childhood cancer is presented in Figure 1-3. The following sections discuss what is currently known about both genetic and environmental triggers in the process of carcinogenesis.

Genetic Epidemiology

Genetic Predisposition to Cancer and Familial Cancer Syndromes

A congenital or genetic disorder that is known to predispose to the development of cancer can be identified in approximately 10% to 15% of cases (Table 1-2). These usually involve constitutional gene alterations that disrupt normal mechanisms of genomic repair. They are mostly inherited in an autosomal recessive fashion and often associated with failure to thrive, small stature, and congenital anomalies. Examples include ataxia telangiectasia, a gene mutation resulting in chromosomal sensitivity to ionizing irradiation, cerebellar ataxia, telangiectasia, and immune defects that predispose to leukemias,[92] Bloom syndrome, a disorder of genomic instability strongly correlated with the development of solid tumors,[18] Fanconi anemia, a disorder of chromosomal breakage repair that exhibits a wide variety of congenital anomalies, a propensity to develop bone marrow failure and AML, and an increased incidence of solid tumors,[19] and xeroderma pigmentosa, a DNA repair disorder predisposing to the development of skin cancers.[89]

Other hereditary disorders with an increased incidence of neoplasia may involve a constitutional activation of molecular pathways leading to deregulated cellular growth and proliferation. These include Beckwith-Wiedemann syndrome, a complex disorder with alterations to growth regulatory genes (IGF2) on chromosome 11p15 leading to macroglossia; macrosomia; hemihypertrophy; abdominal wall defects; and an increased incidence of Wilms tumor, hepatoblastoma, and other solid tumors;[93] neurofibromatosis type 1 involving a gene mutation on chromosome 17q11 leading to dysregulation of Ras, an important signal transducer that leads to short stature, scoliosis, learning difficulties, and tumors of the nerve sheath, glia, and meninges, and less so leukemias, osteosarcoma, rhabdomyosarcoma and Wilms tumor,[94] and the multiple endocrine neoplasias type 1 and 2.[86]

Still other hereditary disorders reflect an inactivation of tumor suppressor genes. Examples include retinoblastoma (see above), LFS, familial adenomatous polyposis

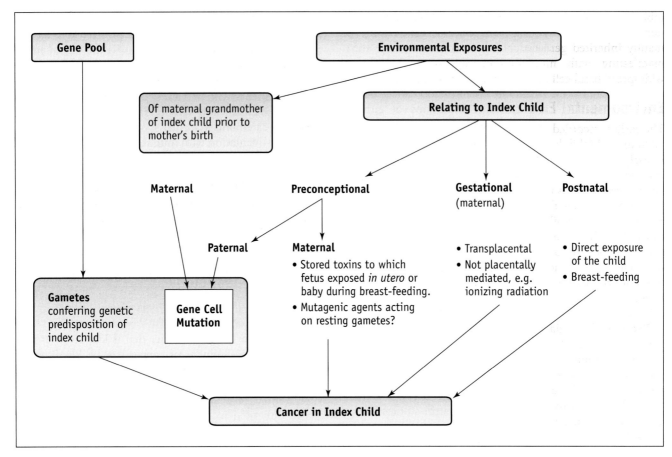

Figure 1-3 A schematic framework for considering etiology of childhood cancer.

Table 1-2

Hereditary syndromes associated with childhood cancers.

Hereditary Syndrome	Childhood Cancer	Implicated Gene
Ataxia-telangiectasia	Leukemia, lymphoma	ATM
Beckwith-Wiedemann	Wilms tumor, hepatoblastoma rhabdomyosarcoma, adrenocortical carcinoma	WT1, WT2
Bloom	Leukemia, skin cancer	?
Familial polyposis coli	Hepatoblastoma, colon carcinoma	FAP
Gorlin's (basal cell nevus syndrome)	Medulloblastoma, skin cancer	PTCH
Li-Fraumeni	Sarcomas, carcinomas	P53
MEN Type 1/2	Endocrine carcinomas	RET
Neurofibromatosis 1	Lymphomas, brain tumors	NF1
Retinoblastoma	Retinoblastoma, sarcomas	RB1

coli (FAP), and Gorlin syndrome. LFS is a familial cancer syndrome defined by a proband case of sarcoma younger than 45 years, a first-degree relative with cancer before 45 years of age, and another first- or second-degree relative in the same lineage with any cancer diagnosed younger than 45 years or with sarcoma at any age.[95] In many cases, an alteration in P53 function as a regulator of transcription of growth regulatory genes can be demonstrated.[96] FAP is an autosomal dominantly inherited germline mutation in the *APC* gene on chromosome 5q21, which manifests as congenital hypertrophy of the retinal pigment epithelium, profuse adenomatous colonic polyposis by the second decade of life, with 90% developing adenocarcinoma without prophylactic colectomy and an increased risk of hepatoblastoma in childhood.[62] Finally, nevoid basal cell carcinoma syndrome (Gorlin syndrome) is an autosomal dominantly inherited germline mutation of the *PTCH* gene, manifesting with multiple developmental anomalies, widespread basal cell carcinomas, and medulloblastoma.[90]

Environmental Epidemiology

The earliest recorded association between an environmental toxin and (childhood) cancer was that of scrotal cancer in early 19th century chimney sweeps.[97] In the intervening two centuries, very little additional information about environmental links to childhood cancers has been clearly established. Given that current evidence shows a clear association of a familial/genetic syndrome and childhood cancer in only a minority of cases, however, other factors such as exposure to carcinogens are likely to be important. The highest incidence at an early age and the cell types of origin strongly suggest that preconceptual, antenatal, and early infancy exposures contribute to cancers in children.

Because of the relative rarity of cases, large prospective studies are almost impossible. Therefore, case-control studies continue to be the basis for most epidemiologic investigations. The challenges of accurate exposure assessment, recall bias, control selection bias, and issues of the heterogeneity of many tumor types continue to limit the conclusions derived from many such case-control studies.

Parental Exposures

Occupational and other environmental exposures of parents might be related to cancer in their offspring. The strongest evidence is for childhood leukemia and paternal exposure to solvents, paints, and employment in motor vehicle–related occupations, and childhood brain tumors and paternal exposure to paints.[98]

Antenatal Exposures

A causal link between the prenatal maternal use of diethylstilbestrol and the development of clear cell adenocarcinoma of the vagina/cervix in offspring has been well established.[99] Another strong historical link between *in utero* radiation exposure and childhood leukemia[12] is established. More recently interest in a possible link between the use of assisted reproductive technologies, genomic imprinting, and the development of embryonal tumors has become a focus of attention.[100] There also appears to be a link between prematurity and early exposure to as yet unidentified environmental toxins in some embryonal tumors.[101]

Childhood Exposures

The most well established environmental factor currently contributing to the incidence of childhood cancer is radiation. While this includes contamination such as experienced by children at Hiroshima and Chernobyl,[102] therapeutic irradiation is by far the most significant contributor. Low-frequency electromagnetic fields emitted by electrical sources such as power transmission lines and cellular telephones have been the source of much conjecture but remain unproven factors to date.[103]

A number of drugs (epipodophyllotoxins such as etoposide and tenoposide;[29] alkylators such as cyclophosphamide and melphalan)[30] are known to increase the risk of certain leukemias, including 11q23, monosomy 7, and 5q-myeloid leukemias.

Exposure to infections is clearly associated with the development of some childhood cancers. For example, EBV infection is linked to the development of Burkitt's lymphoma, Hodgkin's lymphoma, and nasopharyngeal carcinoma.[45] Similarly, the incidence of hepatocellular carcinoma is highest in Asia, where hepatitis B is prevalent.[64] Over the past three decades, infection with HIV has been associated with the development of central nervous system lymphomas and other cancers.[104]

Genetic/Environmental Epidemiology

Ultimately, it is likely that most cancers are the result of an interaction between genes and environment. Thus, there is increasing interest in polymorphisms in genes that relate to the bioactivation and detoxification of a variety of xenobiotics present in food, organic solvents, tobacco smoke, drugs, alcohol, pesticides, and environmental pollutants.[105] This may in part explain why individuals exposed to the same known environmental carcinogen are at different risk of tumor development.

Survival Rates for Childhood Cancers

The age-standardized annual mortality rates for childhood cancers have declined dramatically in the developed world over the past 20 to 30 years (Figure 1-4). With improved surgical and radiation therapy delivery techniques, the institution of novel chemotherapies, better supportive care, and better understanding of prognostic factors through multicenter collaborations, survival rates are now greater than 70% for the most common types of childhood cancers (leukemias, lymphomas, and brain tumors).[3] Nevertheless, metastatic disease still portends a guarded to poor prognosis. Further, there are certain subgroups of children, such as infants with leukemia and high-grade brain tumors, that continue to experience poor survival outcomes.

Epidemiology of Childhood Cancer Survivors

Among the ever-increasing numbers of childhood cancer survivors, approximately 50% will develop significant health-related problems and early mortality.[106] The largest survivor cohort is currently being studied through the Childhood Cancer Survivor Study in the United States.[107] Current investigations include evaluations of predictors of psychological outcomes, health-related behaviors, incidence of second neoplasms, predictors of late-onset organ dysfunction, and cause-specific late mortality. More recently, to strengthen the research scope of the study, collection of buccal cells for DNA extraction has commenced.

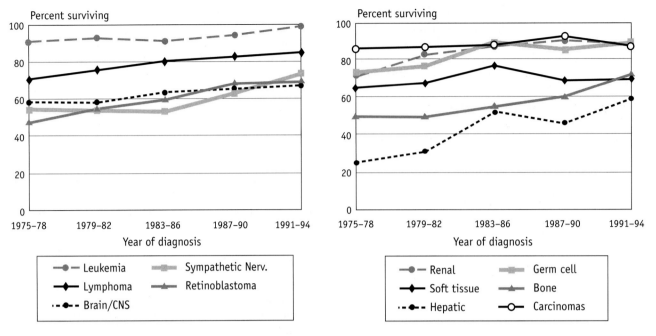

Figure 1-4 Trends in 5-year relative cancer survival rates by ICCC group, age < 20 years, SEER 1975–94.

Future Prospects

Given the rarity of childhood cancer and the lack of simple cause-effect relationships, it is important that large, multinational epidemiology collaborations combined with new strategies are developed. Future considerations include: better methods of case identification in the developing world, greater investigation of cases outside North America and Europe, greater consideration of variation in cancer subtypes, improvements in diagnostic classification, improved methods for exposure assessment, the evaluation of data from molecular biology to generate biologically derived hypotheses, and finally the incorporation of markers of genetic susceptibility into research studies. The possibility of combining large child health cohorts from throughout the world to prospectively examine both genetic and environmental risk factors for the commoner childhood cancers is also an exciting prospect.

References

1. Ries LAG, Smith MA, Gurney JG, et al, eds. Cancer incidence and survival among children and adolescents: United States SEER program 1975–1995; Bethesda, MD: National Cancer Institute, SEER program. 1999. NIH pub. no. 99–4649.
2. Brenner H. Up-to-date survival curves of children with cancer by period analysis. *Br J Cancer.* 2003;88:1693–1697.
3. Bleyer WA. The US Paediatric Cancer Clinical Trials programmes: international implications and the way forward. *Eur J Cancer.* 1997;33:1439–1447.
4. Schwartz CL. Late effects of treatment in long-term survivors of cancer. *Cancer Treat Rev.* 1995;21:355–366.
5. Kramarova E, Stiller CA. The international classification of childhood cancer. *Int J Cancer.* 1996;68:759–765.
6. Parkin DM, Stiller CA, Draper GJ, et al, eds. International incidence of childhood cancer. Lyon: WHO, IARC. 1988. Scientific publication no. 87.
7. Gurney JG, Severson RK, Davis S, et al. Incidence of cancer in children in the United States. *Cancer.* 1995;75:2186.
8. Little J. Epidemiology of childhood cancer. Lyon: WHO, IARC. 1999. Scientific publication no. 149.
9. Greaves MF, Colman SM, Beard MEJ, et al. Geographical distribution of acute lymphoblastic leukaemia subtypes: second report of the Collaborative Group Study. *Leukemia.* 1993;7:27.
10. Pui CH. Acute leukemia in children. *N Engl J Med.* 1995;332:1618.
11. Hartley SE, Sainsbury SE. Acute leukaemia and the same chromosome abnormality in monozygotic twins. *Human Genetics.* 1981;58:408–410.
12. Doll R, Wakeford R. Risk of childhood cancer from fetal irradiation. *Br J Radiol.* 1997;70:130–139.
13. Hjalgrim LL, Westergaard T, Rostgaard K, et al. Birth weight as a risk factor for childhood leukemia: a meta-analysis of 18 epidemiologic studies. *Am J Epidemiol.* 2003;158:724–735.
14. Kinlen LJ, Clarke K, Hudson C. Evidence from population mixing in British new towns 1946–85 of an infective basis for childhood leukaemia. *Lancet.* 1990;336:577–582.
15. Schlehofer B, Blettner M, Geletneky K, et al. Sero-epidemiological analysis of the risk of viral infections for childhood leukaemia. *Int J Cancer.* 1996;65:584–590.
16. Willig TN, Gazda H, Sieff CA. Diamond-Blackfan anemia. *Curr Opin Hematol.* 2000;7:85–94.
17. Rosen RB, Kang SJA. Congenital agranulocytosis terminating in acute myelomonocytic leukemia. *J Pediatr.* 1979;94:406.
18. Amor-Gueret M. Bloom syndrome, genomic instability and cancer: the SOS-like hypothesis. *Cancer Lett.* June 8, 2005, Epub.
19. Tischkowitz MD, Hodgson SV. Fanconi anaemia. *J Med Genet.* 2003;40:1–10.
20. Bader JL, Miller RW. Neurofibromatosis and childhood leukemia. *J Pediatr.* 1978;92:925.
21. Rosner F, Lee SL. Down's syndrome and acute leukemia: myeloblastic or lymphoblastic? *Am J Med.* 1972;53:203.
22. Ross JA, Potter JD, Shu XO, et al. Epidemiology of childhood leukemia, with a focus on infants. *Epidemiol Rev.* 1994;16:243–272.
23. Hjalgrim LL, Rostgaard K, Hjalgrim H, et al. Birth weight and risk for childhood leukemia in Denmark, Sweden, Norway, and Iceland. *J Natl Cancer Inst.* 2004;96:1549–1556.
24. Severson RK, Buckley JD, Woods WG, et al. Cigarette smoking and alcohol consumption by parents of children with acute myeloid leukemia: an analysis within morphological subgroups—a report from the Children's Cancer Group. *Cancer Epidemiol Biomarkers Prev.* 1993;2:433–439.
25. Shu XO, Ross JA, Pendergrass TW, et al. Parental alcohol consumption, cigarette smoking, and risk of infant leukemia: a Children's Cancer Group study. *J Natl Cancer Inst.* 1996;88:24–31.
26. van Duijn CM, van Steensel-Moll HA, Coebergh JW, van Zanen GE. Risk factors for childhood acute non-lymphocytic leukemia: an association with maternal alcohol consumption during pregnancy? *Cancer Epidemiol Biomarkers Prev.* 1994;3:457–460.
27. Shu XO, Gao YT, Brinton LA, et al. A population-based case-control study of childhood leukemia in Shanghai. *Cancer.* 1988;62:635–644.
28. Buckley JD, Robison LL, Swotinsky R, et al. Occupational exposures of parents of children with acute nonlymphocytic leukemia: a report from the Children's Cancer Study Group. *Cancer Res.* 1989;49:4030–4037.
29. Pui CH, Ribeiro R, Hancock M, et al. Acute myeloid leukemia in children treated with epipodophyllotoxins for acute lymphoblastic leukemia. *N Engl J Med.* 1991;325:1682.

30. Tucker MA, Meadows AT, Boice JD, et al. Leukemia after therapy with alkylating agents for childhood cancer. *J Natl Cancer Inst.* 1987;78:459.
31. Shimizu Y, Schull WJ, Kato H. Cancer risk among atomic bomb survivors: The RERF life span study. *JAMA.* 1990;264:601.
32. Rabkin CS, Devesa SS, Zahm SH, Gail MH. Increasing incidence of non-Hodgkin's lymphoma. *Semin Hematol.* 1993;30:286–296.
33. Magrath IT. African Burkitt's lymphoma: history, biology, clinical features, and treatment. *Am J Ped Hem Onc.* 1991;13:222–246.
34. de-The G, Geser A, Day NE, et al. Epidemiological evidence for causal relationship between Epstein-Barr virus and Burkitt's lymphoma from Ugandan prospective study. *Nature.* 1978;274:756–761.
35. Gutierrez MI, Bhatia K, Barriga F, et al. Molecular epidemiology of Burkitt's lymphoma from South America: differences in breakpoint location and Epstein-Barr virus association from tumors in other world regions. *Blood.* 1992;79:3261–3266.
36. Filipovich AH, Mathur A, Kamat D, Shapiro RS. Primary immunodeficiencies: genetic risk factors for lymphoma. *Cancer Res.* 1992;52(suppl 19):5465s–5467s.
37. Shu XO, Clemens J, Zheng W, et al. Infant breastfeeding and the risk of childhood lymphoma and leukaemia. *Int J Epidemiol.* 1995;24:27–32.
38. Buckley JD, Meadows AT, Kadin M, et al. Pesticide exposures in children with non-Hodgkin lymphoma. *Cancer.* 2000;89:2315–2321.
39. Grufferman SL, Delzell E. Epidemiology of Hodgkin's disease. *Epidemiol Rev.* 1984;6:76.
40. Mack TM, Cozen W, Shibata DK, et al. Concordance for Hodgkin's disease in identical twins suggesting genetic susceptibility to the young adult form of the disease. *N Engl J Med.* 1995;332:413–418.
41. Grufferman S, Cole P, Smith PG, et al. Hodgkin's disease in siblings. *N Engl J Med.* 1977;296:248–250.
42. Guthenson NM, Shapiro DS. Social class risk factors among children with Hodgkin's disease. *Int J Cancer.* 1982;30:433–435.
43. Gutensohn NM. Social class and age at diagnosis of Hodgkin's disease: new epidemiologic evidence for the "two-disease" hypothesis. *Cancer Treat Rep.* 1982;66:689–695.
44. Greenberg RS, Grufferman S, Cole P. An evaluation of space-time clustering in Hodgkin's disease. *J Chronic Dis.* 1983;36:257–262.
45. Hjalgrim H, Askling J, Sorensen P, et al. Risk of Hodgkin's disease and other cancers after infectious mononucleosis. *J Natl Cancer Inst.* 2000;92:1522–1528.
46. Preston-Martin S, Mack WJ. Neoplasms of the nervous system. In: Schottenfeld D, Fraumeni JF, eds. *Cancer Epidemiology and Prevention.* New York, NY: Oxford University Press; 1996;1231–1281.
47. Bondy ML, Lustbader ED, Buffler PA, et al. Genetic epidemiology of childhood brain tumours. *Genet Epidemiol.* 1992;8:253–267.
48. Ron E, Modan B, Boice JD, et al. Tumours of the brain and nervous system after radiotherapy in childhood. *N Engl J Med.* 1988;319:1033–1039.
49. Preston-Martin S, Yu MC, Benton B, Henderson BE. N Nitroso compounds and childhood brain tumours: a case-control study. *Cancer Res.* 1982;42:5240–5425.
50. Krynska B, Del Valle L, Croul S, et al. Detection of human neurotropic JC virus DNA sequence and expression of the viral oncogenic protein in pediatric medulloblastomas. *Proc Natl Acad Sci USA.* 1999;96:1519–1524.
51. Woods WG, Gao RN, Shuster JJ, et al. Screening of infants and mortality due to neuroblastoma. *N Engl J Med.* 2002;346:1041–1046.
52. Schilling FH, Spix C, Berthold F, et al. Neuroblastoma screening at one year of age. *N Engl J Med.* 2002;346:1047–1053.
53. Neglia JP, Smithson WA, Gunderson P, et al. Prenatal and perinatal risk factors for neuroblastoma: a case-control study. *Cancer.* 1988;61:2202–2206.
54. Menegaux F, Olshan AF, Reitnauer PJ, et al. Positive association between congenital anomalies and risk of neuroblastoma. *Pediatr Blood Cancer.* November 16, 2004, Epub.
55. Knudson AJ. Mutation and cancer: statistical study of retinoblastoma. *Proc Natl Acad Sci USA.* 1971;68:820–827.
56. Eng C, Li FP, Abramson DH, et al. Mortality from second tumours among long-term survivors of retinoblastoma. *J Natl Cancer Inst.* 1993;85:1121–1128.
57. Moll AC, Imhof SM, Cruysberg JR, et al. Incidence of retinoblastoma in children born after in-vitro fertilisation. *Lancet.* 2003;361:309–310.
58. Kramer S, Meadows AT, Jarrett P. Racial variation in incidence of Wilms' tumour: relationship to congenital anomalies. *Med Pediatr Oncol.* 1984;12:401–405.
59. Miller R, Fraumeni JJ, Manning M. Association of Wilms' tumor with aniridia, hemihypertrophy and other congenital malformations. *N Engl J Med.* 1964;270:922–927.
60. Sharpe CR, Fraco EL, de Camargo B, et al. Parental exposures to pesticides and risk of Wilms' tumor in Brazil. *Am J Epidemiol.* 1997;141:210–217.
61. DeBaun MR, Tucker MA. Risk of cancer during the first four years of life in children from the Beckwith-Wiedemann syndrome registry. *J Pediatr.* 1998;132:398–400.
62. Giardiello FM, Offerhaus GJ, Krush AJ, et al. Risk of hepatoblastoma in familial adenomatous polyposis. *J Pediatr.* 119:766–768.
63. Kapfer SA, Petruzzi MJ, Caty MG. Hepatoblastoma in low birth weight infants: an institutional review. *Pediatr Surg Int.* 2001;20:753–756.
64. Chang MH, Chen CJ, Lai MS, et al. Universal hepatitis B vaccination in Taiwan and the incidence of hepatocellular carcinoma in children. Taiwan Childhood Hepatoma Study Group. *N Engl J Med.* 1997;366:1855–1859.
65. Buckley JD, Pendergrass TW, Buckley CM, et al. Epidemiology of osteosarcoma and Ewing's sarcoma in childhood: a study of 305 cases from the Children's Cancer Group. *Cancer.* 1998;83:1440–1448.
66. Freeman C, Gledhill R, Chevalier L, et al. Osteogenic sarcoma following treatment with megavoltage radiation and chemotherapy for bone tumors in children. *Med Pediatr Oncol.* 1980;8:375–382.
67. Hawkins MM, Wilson LMK, Burton HS, et al. Radiotherapy, alkylating agents, and risk of bone cancer after childhood cancer. *J Natl Cancer Inst.* 1996;88:270–278.
68. Malkin D, Jolly KW, Barbier N, et al. Germline mutations of the p53 tumor-suppressor gene in children and young adults with second malignant neoplasms. *N Engl J Med.* 1992;326:1309–1315.
69. Abramson DH, Ellsworth RM, Kitchin D, Tung G. Second nonocular tumors in retinoblastoma survivors. *Ophthalmology.* 1984;91:1351–1355.
70. Valery PC, McWhirter W, Sleigh A, et al. A national case-control study of Ewing's sarcoma family of tumors. *Int J Cancer.* 2003;105:825–830.
71. Parkin DM, Stiller CA, Nectoux J. International variations in the incidence of childhood bone tumours. *Int J Cancer.* 1993;53:371–376.
72. Yang P, Grufferman S, Khoury MJ, et al. Association of childhood rhabdomyosarcoma with neurofibromatosis type 1 and birth defects. *Genet Epidemiol.* 1995;12:467–474.
73. Li FP, Fraumeni JF Jr, Mulvihill JJ, et al. A cancer family syndrome in twenty-four kindreds. *Cancer Res.* 1988;48:5358–5362.
74. Grufferman S, Schwartz AG, Ruymann FB, Maurer HM. Parents' use of cocaine and marijuana and increased risk of rhabdomyosarcoma in their children. *Cancer Causes Control.* 1993;4:217–224.
75. Grufferman S, Wang HH, Delong ER, et al. Environmental factors in the etiology of rhabdomyosarcoma in childhood. *J Natl Cancer Inst.* 1982;68:107–113.
76. Hartley AL, Birch JM, McKinney PA, et al. The Inter-Regional Epidemiological Study of Childhood Cancer (IRESCC): case control study of children with bone and soft tissue sarcomas. *Br J Cancer.* 1988;58:838–842.
77. Dehner LP. Gonadal and extragonadal germ cell neoplasia of childhood. *Hum Pathol.* 1983;14:493–511.
78. Strader CH, Weiss NS, Daling JR, et al. Cryptorchidism, orchiopexy, and the risk of testicular cancer. *Am J Epidemiol.* 1988;127:1013–1018.
79. Shu XO, Nesbit ME, Buckley JD, et al. An exploratory analysis of risk factors for childhood malignant germ-cell tumors; report from the Children's Cancer Group (Canada, United States). *Cancer Causes Control.* 1995;6:187–198.
80. Sandrini R, Ribeiro RC, DeLacerda L. Childhood adrenocortical tumors. *J Clin Endocrinol Metab.* 1997;82:2027–2031.
81. Ribeiro RC, Sandrini F, Figueiredo B, et al. An inherited p53 mutation that contributes in a tissue specific manner to pediatric adrenal cortical carcinoma. *Proc Natl Acad Sci USA.* 2001;98:9330–9335.
82. Yang XR, Diehl S, Pfeiffer R, et al. Evaluation of risk factors for nasopharyngeal carcinoma in high-risk nasopharyngeal carcinoma families in Taiwan. *Cancer Epidemiol Biomarkers Prev.* 2005;14:900–905.
83. Fraker DL. Radiation exposure and other factors that predispose to human thyroid neoplasia. *Surg Clin North Am.* 1995;3:365–375.
84. McClollan DR, Francis GL. Thyroid cancer in children, pregnant women, and patients with Graves' disease. *Endocrin Metab Clin North Am.* 1996;25:27–47.
85. Geirger JD, Thompson NW. Thyroid tumors in children. *Otolaryngol Clin North Am.* 1996;29:711–719.
86. Brandi ML, Gagel RF, Angeli A, et al. Guidelines for diagnosis and therapy of MEN type 1 and type 2. *J Clin Endocrinol Metab.* 2001;86:5658–5671.
87. Strouse JJ, Fears TR, Tucker MA, Wayne AS. Pediatric melanoma: risk factor and survival analysis of the Surveillance, Epidemiology and End Results database. *J Clin Oncol.* 2005;23:4735–4741.
88. Rager EL, Bridgeford EP, Ollila DW. Cutaneous melanoma: update on prevention, screening, diagnosis, and treatment. *Am Fam Physician.* 2005;72:269–276.
89. Kraemer KH, Lee MM, Scotto J. DNA repair protects against cutaneous and internal neoplasia: evidence from xeroderma pigmentosum. *Carcinogenesis.* 1984;5:511–514.
90. Shanley S, Ratcliffe J, Hockey A, et al. Nevoid basal cell carcinoma syndrome: review of 118 affected individuals. *Am J Med Genet.* 1994;50:282–290.
91. Fortina AB, Piaserico S, Alaibac M, et al. Skin disorders in patients transplanted in childhood. *Transpl Int.* 2005;18:360–365.
92. Taylor AM, Metcalfe JA, Thick J, Mak YF. Leukemia and lymphoma in ataxia telangiectasis. *Blood.* 1996;8:423–438.
93. Wiedemann HR. Tumours and hemihypertrophy associated with Wiedemann-Beckwith syndrome. *Eur J Pediatr.* 1983;141:129.
94. North KN. Neurofibramatosis 1 in childhood. *Semin Pediatr Neurol.* 1998;5:231–242.
95. Li FP, Fraumeni JF Jr. Soft-tissue sarcomas, breast cancer, and other neoplasms: a familial syndrome? *Ann Intern Med.* 1969;71:747–752.
96. Malkin D, Li FP, Strong LC, et al. Germline p53 mutations in a familial syndrome of breast cancer, sarcomas and other neoplasms. *Science.* 1990;250:1233–1238.
97. Hall EJ. From chimney sweeps to astronauts: cancer risks in the work place: the 1998 Lauriston Taylor lecture. *Health Phys.* 1998;75:357–366.

98. Colt JS, Blair A. Parental occupational exposures and risk of childhood cancer. *Environ Health Perspect.* 1998;106:909–925.
99. Herbst AI, Ulfeder H. Poskanzer DC. Clear-cell adenocarcinoma of the genital tract in young females. *N Engl J Med.* 1971;284:878–881.
100. Lightfoot T, Bunch K, Ansell P, Murphy M. Ovulation induction, assisted conception and childhood cancer. *Eur J Cancer.* 2005;41:715–724.
101. Spector LG, Feusner JH, Ross JA. Hepatoblastoma and low birth weight. *Pediatr Blood Cancer.* 2004;43:706.
102. Kazakov VS, Demidchik EP, Astakhova LN. Thyroid cancer after Chernobyl. *Nature.* 1992;359:21.
103. Feychting M, Ahlbom A, Kheifets L. EMF and health. *Annu Rev Public Health.* 2005;26:165–189.
104. Kest H, Brogly S, McSherry G, et al. Malignancy in perinatally human immunodeficiency virus-infected children in the United States. *Pediatr Infect Dis J.* 2005;24:237–242.
105. Canalle R, Burim RV, Tone LG, Takahashi CS. Genetic polymorphisms and susceptibility to childhood acute lymphoblastic leukemia. *Environ Mol Mutagen.* 2004;43:100–109.
106. Hudson MM, Mertens AC, Yasui Y, et al. Health status of adult long-term survivors of childhood cancer: a report from the Childhood Cancer Survivor Study. *JAMA.* 2003;290:1583–1592.
107. Robison LL, Mertens AC, Boice JD, et al. Study design and cohort characteristics of the Childhood Cancer Survivor Study: a multi-institutional collaborative project. *Med Pediatr Oncol.* 2004;38:229–239.

Childhood Cancer in the Developing World

Deepa Bhojwani, Federico Antillon-Klussman, and Scott C. Howard

Introduction

In many ways, childhood cancer is similar in low-income countries (LIC), middle-income countries (MIC), and high-income countries (HIC), as defined in Table 2-1; in most cases the types of malignancies, treatment protocols used, and response to therapy are identical. The major differences in outcome result from poverty and dramatic disparities in access to health care. This leads to late or incorrect diagnosis, a high rate of abandonment of therapy, and excess death from toxicity. Eighty percent of the world's children live in LIC and MIC where about 208,000 children develop cancer each year, of whom only an estimated 25% are diagnosed, treated, and cured. Many never arrive at tertiary care centers,[1] some who do arrive are not correctly diagnosed, many more refuse treatment or abandon therapy after a short time,[2] and many succumb to comorbidities such as death from infection, malnutrition, or other toxicities while in remission.[3,4] These conditions make it extremely difficult if not impossible to achieve the 75% to 79% 5-year event-free survival (EFS) seen in children with cancer in HIC.[5-7] In this chapter we review some of the causes of the large differences in outcome in LIC versus HIC and highlight global, regional, and local efforts to improve childhood cancer care in a sustainable way for the benefit of children worldwide.

Global Initiatives

Childhood cancer has not been a high priority for health care systems in LIC and MIC, which focus on infectious diseases and other acute illnesses. Recently, however, advocacy and knowledge dissemination by international professional organizations and special interest working groups has resulted in the development of strategies to improve care of children with cancer in limited resource settings.

Advocacy by Professional Organizations

The International Society of Pediatric Oncology (SIOP) generated the "Montevideo Document" more than a decade ago[8] to bring attention to the global impact of childhood cancer. This document stressed the need for specialized pediatric oncology centers to provide free basic care to all children with cancer as a step toward fulfilling the United Nations' Convention on the Rights of the Child. It urged governments and financial bodies to initiate programs for pediatric oncology care in resource-poor countries and committed to mobilizing resources to foster international cooperation. The International Acute Lymphoblastic Leukemia Group (also known as the Ponte Di Legno working group) is a collaboration of major acute lymphoblastic leukemia (ALL) study groups and institutions. In December 2003, the group issued

Table 2-1

Definitions of low-, middle-, and high-income countries.

Term	Abbreviation	Definition (Gross national income per capita)*
Low-income country	LIC	US $905 or less
Middle-income country	MIC	US $906 to $11,115
Lower middle-income country	LMIC	US $906 to $3,595
Upper middle-income country	UMIC	US $3,596 to $11,115
High-income country	HIC	More than US $11,116

*Gross national income per capita measured in 2006 (World Bank; http://siteresources.worldbank.org/DATASTATISTICS/Resources/CLASS.XLS).

a position paper urging agencies such as the World Health Organization (WHO) to "recognize that the care of children with ALL (and other curable cancers) is essential."[9] Their recommendations included supporting centers where children are treated according to "essential protocols" and advocated a price policy for drugs used in these protocols to make them both affordable and accessible. The position paper was followed by a published list of drugs considered essential for childhood cancer care in developing countries.[10]

Nonprofit organizations, such as the International Union Against Cancer (UICC) and the International Network for Cancer Treatment and Research, focus primarily on cancer control, especially the disparities between high- and low-income countries. They have successfully brought together world leaders and established networks to promote and sponsor international collaborations. In partnership with Sanofi-Aventis, UICC launched its biennial World Cancer Campaign in 2005 with a focus on childhood cancer under the theme "My child matters." Over the next 2 years, 26 local projects in 16 LIC and MIC were funded with seed grants (up to 50,000 euros/year) on the basis of feasibility, potential benefits, sustainability, and their potential to serve as models for other countries.[11,12] These projects include the development of a palliative care unit in Bangladesh, early detection campaigns for retinoblastoma in Indonesia, creation of regional satellite clinics in Honduras to reduce abandonment, and many others that demonstrate that focused efforts to improve childhood cancer care are feasible and can have high impact.[3,13] It is anticipated that local governments, professionals, and the public will be motivated to continue and expand these demonstration projects to build stronger programs that serve larger numbers.

Policy Promulgation by Development Organizations

In May 2005, the 58th World Health Assembly (WHA) approved for the first time a resolution on cancer prevention and control.[14] Though childhood cancers constitute only 2% to 3% of the global burden, the resolution urged national health authorities to consider "disseminated cancers that have potential of being cured or the patient's life being prolonged considerably (such as acute leukemia in childhood)" as an objective in their cancer control programs. A joint WHO-United Nations Children's Fund consultation meeting was held in August 2006 to address the lack of availability of essential medicines for children. Among other concerns it was recognized that there is a lack of current and appropriate WHO guidelines for pediatric oncology and palliative care.[15] Thus, the 60th WHA adopted a "Better Medicines for Children" initiative and urged prioritization of access to essential drugs for children.[16] Consequently, in June 2007 a subcommittee on the selection and use of essential medicines was established. The initial draft of the first model list for children included 18 cytotoxic agents, but the section on "Antineoplastics, immunosuppressives and medicines used in palliative care" is expected to undergo a special review at the next subcommittee meeting. Refinement of this list of essential medications is hoped to provide easier access to countries with limited resources.

Subspecialty Institutional Efforts

Twinning Programs

Twinning programs, ie, long-term, multifaceted partnerships between institutions in HIC and LIC, have been described as one of the most successful approaches to improve care in LIC.[17] This kind of collaboration facilitates education, transfer of technology, consultation of difficult cases, pathology review, development of standardized treatment clinical guidelines to be applied in the different scarce resource settings encountered around the world, and in some cases economic resources that serve as seed money to start a program. Several twinning programs have been operating for many years, one of the earliest being the partnership between La Mascota Hospital in Nicaragua and collaborators in Monza, Italy, initiated in 1986.[18] The International Outreach Program (IOP) from St. Jude Children's Research Hospital (SJCRH) has developed programs in Central America, South America, the Middle East, China, Singapore, the Philippines, Russia, and Morocco.[14] Other successful partnerships have also been developed by various groups worldwide.[2,19]

Infrastructure Development

In addition to twinning between two individual centers, notable efforts have been made by institutions in HIC to benefit several aspects of childhood cancer care in multiple LIC and MIC. An excellent example is the Internet resource Cure4kids (www.Cure4Kids.org) developed by Quintana and collaborators at SJCRH.[20] This free Web-based program offers more than 1000 seminars and conferences in several languages, a digital library, and Oncopedia (a collection of special cases with the opportunity for real-time educational exchange focused on specific cases in LIC). The most important aspect of Cure4Kids is that it provides a software platform for live, simultaneous communication between several distant centers and investigators. This technology is used for discussion of protocols and difficult clinical cases, for review of outcomes, and to address administrative issues between twinning partners. As of December 2007, approximately 120 online meetings are held monthly with several hundred participants from 27 countries.

Another freely available vital resource is the Pediatric Oncology Networked Database (POND, www.Pond4kids.org).[21–23] It is well established that a data management program is essential to optimize care because it allows frequent assessment of outcomes and documentation of the effectiveness of interventions. POND is a multilingual (English, Spanish, French, Portuguese, and Chinese), secure, online database designed for quality improvement projects and clinical research in LIC. It is provided at no cost and includes a tumor registry, cancer-specific information, detailed nutritional status data, psychosocial and socioeconomic information, and treatment protocols.

POND can also generate Kaplan-Meier curves and perform other basic statistical analyses. Additional analytic support is provided by the Monza International School of Pediatric Hematology and Oncology (MISPHO) and the Pediatric Oncology Group of Ontario (POGO).[21,23-26] It is currently used in more than 20 countries and serves as one component in data management programs that help clinicians identify, quantify, and address local problems, such as abandonment of treatment and toxicity of various treatment regimens. Secure sharing of anonymous patient information with collaborators is also permitted, thus facilitating multicenter comparison and collaboration.

Special-Interest Groups and Private Organizations

Besides the professional, governmental, and nongovernmental organizations mentioned above, parent support groups play a key role to address the needs of children with cancer.[24] The International Confederation of Childhood Cancer Parent Organizations (ICCCPO) is a worldwide network composed of more than 100 parent organizations from 60 countries. ICCCPO meets in conjunction with SIOP annual conferences and has increased public awareness of childhood cancer worldwide. One important result of their efforts has been promotion of the annual International Childhood Cancer Day.[27] Media coverage and fund-raising activities commemorate this event held on February 15 each year.

Pharma-initiated projects like the Novartis "Glivec International Patient Assistance Program," which supplies imatinib free to patients with chronic myeloid leukemia in low-income countries, should be commended.[28] As of August 2005, this well-sustained program has worked through the health care complexities in 81 countries to benefit more than 14 000 patients. In addition to free access to imatinib, their direct-to-patient model also supports patient education, monitoring, and follow up. In the not-for-profit sector, the International Dispensary Organization based in Amsterdam supplies essential medications, including chemotherapy and medical supplies to developing countries at low costs (www.idafoundation.org). The National Children's Cancer Society (NCCS, www.children-cancer.org) coordinates the distribution of donated pharmaceuticals, medical supplies, equipment, and supportive-care products wherever in the world they are most needed. Since its inception in 1993, the global outreach program of the NCCS has distributed more than $190 million in donated medical products to 54 facilities in 35 countries around the world. Donated materials are shipped to member sites in LIC free of charge.

Regional Initiatives

A snapshot of regional conditions and updates provided here are grouped by continent. Though the general barriers to providing adequate care are common, it is clear that local needs and challenges vary, even in distinct regions within individual countries.

Africa

A few nations (eg, Egypt, South Africa) have relatively better facilities than the majority of nations in the rest of Africa. Delayed diagnoses and abandonment remain fundamental problems accounting for the very poor overall survival. Specialized pediatric oncology units are few, though larger general hospitals care for the common childhood cancers. For example, at the Principal Hospital in Dakar, Senegal, the cure rate for all malignant diseases was 50% for the 23 children that completed therapy; however, only 23 of 130 children completed therapy, thus only 10% of the entire cohort was cured.[29]

Since Burkitt's lymphoma and Wilm's tumor (both highly curable) are the most common tumors seen in African children, initial efforts have focused on improving survival for these two entities. The Burkitt-Malawi project sponsored by SIOP is a significant undertaking; through successive trials, the survival rates have increased to 50% with the use of an inexpensive protocol (less than 50 Euros/patient) with reduced toxicities.[30]

The French African Pediatric Oncology Group is a collaborative effort established in 2000 comprising 11 pediatric oncology programs in 9 countries in French-speaking Africa. The group documented a 2-year EFS of 69.7% for Wilms' tumor and 65.2% for Burkitt's lymphoma.[31] Although these pilot studies excluded patients who presented in a poor general condition and those with very high risk features, they have paved the way for successive trials that will impact more children and more cancers in Africa.

Asia

The relative proportion of the world population represented by China and India translates to approximately 80 000 children diagnosed with cancer every year in these two countries alone (3 times the number in the United States and Europe combined). Although China and India are considered MIC, they struggle with limited health care infrastructure in the public sector, inconsistent access to specialized care, and prohibitive costs of treatment. It is estimated that only 10% of Chinese children with cancer receive protocol-based therapy with curative intent.[32] Intra-China twinning programs such as the one between the Prince of Wales Hospital in Hong Kong and the Guangzhou Leukemia Study Group (a consortium of seven large hospitals in Guangzhou province) have recently demonstrated improved cure rates and low toxicities for childhood ALL.[33]

Cancer care in India depends entirely on a patient's socioeconomic status. Little or no care is available to the 60% of the population that lives in extreme poverty (a monthly family income of $50 or less), some care is available to the middle-class families that earn approximately $200/month (35% of the population), and modern treatment is available to the 5% of families with sufficient resources.[34] Pediatric cancer units (PCU) provide appropriate care in major cities, but 80% of the population in India lives in rural areas and thus does not have access to these academic medical centers. Although many patients find their way to the tertiary care centers, the expense of travel and living away from home cannot be sustained for the duration of therapy, so the family abandons care. To address this problem of poor access, the Pediatric Hematology Oncology chapter of the Indian Academy of Pediatrics has adopted the shared care model, in which some of the functions of the PCU (eg, follow-up, maintenance chemotherapy) are shifted to the local community pediatrician.[35] The Indian National Training Program in practical pediatric oncology was initiated in 1997 to train willing pediatricians to provide shared care; zonal workshops are held regularly, and approximately 1000 pediatricians have been trained to improve their diagnostic and therapeutic skills in pediatric oncology.

The high cost of effective chemotherapeutic and supportive care drugs has led to the development of innovative local regimens. Dr. Mamman Chandy's group from Vellore, India, has demonstrated the effectiveness of single agent arsenic trioxide for newly diagnosed acute promyelocytic leukemia (APML) in pediatric patients who could not afford all-trans rentinoic acid and chemotherapy.[36] Results were excellent at a median follow-up of 30 months, with overall survival at 91% and relapse-free survival at 81%. This regimen was well tolerated, was easy to administer, and cost less than 15% of the cost of conventional therapy in the same setting. Long-term follow-up will determine whether this regimen would benefit other patients with APL, not just those with limited monetary resources.

Latin America

For 20 years, international collaborations and cooperative group efforts have been the hallmark of Central and South America. In 1999, the Latin American Society for Pediatric Oncology generated the "Margarita Statement," an adaptation of the Montevideo document, which applied specifically to Latin American countries.[37] The proposed strategies included adoption of feasible treatment protocols, establishment of specialized centers, multidisciplinary teams, cooperative groups, and implementation of specific programs to reduce abandonment rates.

An exceptionally successful international collaboration was the establishment of MISPHO in 1996.[26] MISPHO has promoted the improvement of pediatric oncology and hematology in the majority of countries in Central and South America. These courses supported the development of treatment guidelines/protocols, infrastructure development, and most important, the creation of the Asociación Hematología Oncología Pediátrica Centro Americana (AHOPCA, Central American Association of Pediatric Hematology and Oncology).[23] In addition, POGO is intimately involved with AHOPCA and has led to the promotion of several programs such as the education and salary support of data managers for local cancer registries and outcome analysis.[22] Another example is the implementation of comprehensive nutritional assessment of all newly diagnosed pediatric cancer patients in Central America and longitudinal evaluation of those with ALL.[38]

The Road Ahead

Many strategies to improve cancer care have been successfully implemented in LIC and MIC, and many of these can be reproduced in other settings, especially where cultural and socioeconomic factors are similar. Components of a successful childhood cancer program are illustrated in Figure 2-1. These include acknowledgment of the existence and importance of the problem by government and private organizations, directives by national and international policy makers specific to childhood cancer, a strong fund-raising organization, trained personnel who implement uniform treatment regimens adapted to local conditions, and international collaboration. A program developed in Guatemala illustrates what can be accomplished.

The Guatemala National Pediatric Cancer Program: A Model of Childhood Cancer Care in Low-Income Countries

In Guatemala, the most populous country in Central America, 56% of the population lives on less than US $2 per day, and there are significant obstacles to obtaining optimal childhood cancer care. In spite of these obstacles, Guatemalan children have benefited from the stepwise improvements detailed here that resulted from development of the Guatemala National Pediatric Cancer Program, which is committed to deliver high-quality cancer care to all children of Guatemala, regardless of their ability to pay.

Needs Assessment
The first step to improve care for pediatric cancer patients was to assess the current care and outcomes candidly. In

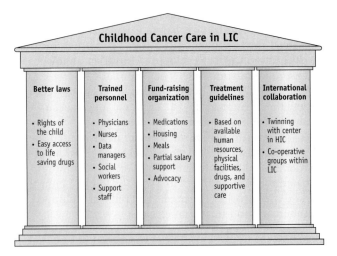

Figure 2-1 Foundation for optimal childhood cancer care in low income countries. These elements should be considered vital while building successful childhood cancer programs. Many of these have been addressed in the Guatemala program as described in the text.

Source: Courtesy of St. Jude Children's Research Hospital (www.Cure4Kids.org).

1996 a 5-year retrospective study was conducted on the outcomes of pediatric patients diagnosed with cancer from 1990 to 1995 and treated at the two existing public tertiary care hospitals in Guatemala City.[39] Between the two institutions, 100 patients were diagnosed per year, the abandonment rate was 42%, and the 2-year EFS was 28%. At that time the expected annual incidence of pediatric cancer according to the Guatemala population was approximately 600 cases. Therefore, only 1 in 6 pediatric patients with cancer were being diagnosed and treated, and EFS for treated patients was much lower than international standards. Diagnostic tools such as flow cytometry, molecular pathology to detect leukemic translocations, and immunohistochemical stains for the classification of solid tumors were not available. Chemotherapy was not given at full intensity due to the lack of adequate supportive measures such as treatment of severe infections and blood bank support.

Mobilization of the Community and International Collaborators

The second step was the creation of a not-for-profit organization with the responsibility of designing an initial strategic plan for establishing a medical care program for children with cancer, raising funds to maintain the cancer program, and establishing international cooperative liaisons. A site visit from the leadership of the IOP of SJCRH, the involvement of local medical and nonmedical leaders and the participation of the Guatemalan government through the Ministry of Health and Social Welfare created a foundation on which to build. The establishment of a local foundation, Fundación Ayúdame a Vivir (AYUVI, "Help me to live," www.ayuvi.org.gt), in May 1997 led to several important successes: (1) passage of a law in December 1998 that created the Unidad Nacional de Oncología Pediátrica (UNOP, National Pediatric Cancer Unit) as the single center for providing conventional cancer treatment to children in collaboration with the Ministry of Health, (2) the signing of a collaboration agreement with the IOP of SJCRH, (3) the opening of a free-standing pediatric cancer hospital adjacent to the Roosevelt Hospital in April 2000, and (4) development of AYUVI into a professional foundation successful in both advocacy and fund-raising. Indeed, at initiation of the program in 1998, the budget of UNOP was initially almost entirely composed of funds from SJCRH, whereas in 2007 SJCRH support represented less than 5% of this budget (Figure 2-2). UNOP expenditures by category for 2007 are shown in Table 2-2.

Focus on Fundamentals

The philosophy of UNOP is based on four fundamentals: (1) correct diagnosis and staging of pediatric cancer in order to provide appropriate curative or palliative care, (2) education of health professionals and the public about childhood cancer, (3) clinical research that addresses local problems, and (4) community involvement. The guidelines for pediatric cancer centers of the American Aca-

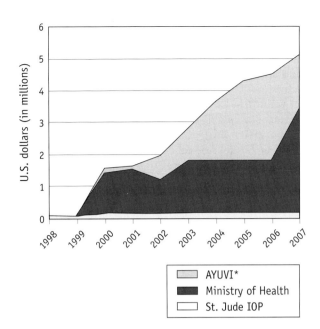

Figure 2-2   Funding sources for the operational budget of the Guatemala National Pediatric Cancer Program. The annual contribution of the 3 funding sources to the total budget is shown in this graph. The program was initiated by seed funds from the St. Jude International Outreach Program (IOP). Support soon followed from the Guatemala Ministry of Health and the local nongovernmental, nonprofit foundation Ayúdame a Vivir (AYUVI). IOP funds currently compose less than 5% of the total budget.

*AYUVI's fund-raising includes corporate funding and other sources.
Source: Courtesy of St. Jude Children's Research Hospital (www.Cure4Kids.org).

Table 2-2

Budgeted expenses of the National Pediatric Oncology Unit of Guatemala for 2007.

Category	Budget (US dollars)
Personnel	2,041,145
Drugs	1,423,619
Medical and surgical supplies	257,167
Blood bank	289,294
Clinical laboratory reagents	207,141
Imaging	177,628
Patient food services	94,893
Radiotherapy	86,868
Pathology	86,867
Laundry	38,961
Other	209,857
Total	4,913,440

demic of Pediatrics served as a blueprint for establishing UNOP.[40] Since the opening of UNOP a local, well-designed cancer registry has been in place. Other key components, including an adequate number of well-trained personnel, improved physical facilities, and access to pediatric intensive care were instituted during the first few years of operation.[41]

Improved Accuracy of Diagnosis

The improvement of diagnostic techniques is of utmost importance. For example, technology transfer for immunophenotyping is one of the successful initiatives that benefited not only patients from Guatemala but also from other countries in Central America.[42,43] The flow cytometry laboratory was established in 1998. Initially, all results were reviewed in Dr. Dario Campana's reference laboratory at SJCRH. As local personnel developed experience, the need for consultation has decreased to less than 1% of cases. The cost of immunophenotyping is US $230 per sample when performed in Guatemala, and correct risk stratification of children with acute leukemia using flow cytometry is highly cost effective. Similarly, for accurate diagnoses of solid tumors, the anatomic pathologist received 4 weeks of training at SJCRH for the application and interpretation of immunocytochemistry techniques, with ongoing support for consultations and real-time review of difficult cases.

Access to Care and Prevention of Abandonment

Each month 25 new cases of pediatric malignancies are diagnosed, which represents 45% of the expected pediatric cancer incidence in Guatemala. The various cancers treated are shown in Figure 2-3. Thirty-five percent of patients with solid tumors have metastatic disease at diagnosis. Although abandonment of treatment has decreased substantially from the 42% rate in the late 1990s, 3% of patients/families still refuse to initiate treatment and another 15.6% abandon prior to completion of treatment. Recently the introduction of a more aggressive program to

prevent abandonment that includes low-cost housing for patients from out of town, subsidized meals, detailed social work assessment, intense family education, and a system to contact patients who miss appointments has decreased the abandonment rate to less than 5% in 2007.

Partnerships with the Private Sector and Nongovernmental Organizations

Acquiring sufficient resources for sustained maintenance of pediatric cancer programs in developing countries is essential. Health care budgets allocated by governments are often insufficient to provide even basic services like water sanitation, nutrition, vaccination, primary health care services, and maternal health, and rarely provide for pediatric cancer care. Local foundations must partner with the private sector to fund treatment. For example, for the past 7 years, AYUVI in Guatemala has raised US $2,000,000 per year by collaborating with corporate donors including restaurants, beverage companies, banks, and technology firms to conduct a raffle. Other non-government organizations, like Ciudad de Guatemala Rotary Club, have promoted a yearly mini-marathon, the Arco Iris (rainbow) race. This initiative raises US $100,000 per year. These are only two of many creative ideas to raise funds.

Education and Training

Continued education is a critical need for health care professionals working in developing countries. Standard training approaches in the setting of twinning programs require knowledge of the language of the host country, time investments, and travel expenditure. Primary local training of personnel supplemented by training in a developed country may be feasible. A 3-year fellowship training program in pediatric oncology with the joint effort of UNOP and the School of Medicine of the Universidad Francisco Marroquín has recently been implemented in Guatemala. The fellows learn English and Italian in order to rotate for a 3-month period in SJCRH and also a 3-month period in Monza, Italy, with Dr. Giuseppe Masera. This program receives a grant from the National Cancer Institute providing the fellows with a stipend that covers basic costs of living, books, and one medical meeting per year. Training of subspecialty nurses has long been recognized as important to provide quality cancer care. The International Training Center for Pediatric Oncology Nurses in El Salvador was established by the IOP in 1998 and utilizes a teach-the-teacher approach.[44] Performance indicators show high retention rates and improved nursing practices achieved at relatively low cost. A subsequent strategy is the appointment of a local bilingual nursing educator at each partner center.

April 2000 to October 2007 (N=2100)

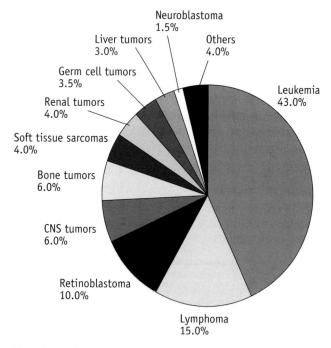

Figure 2-3 Distribution of cancer diagnoses at UNOP, Guatemala. As in developing countries, leukemias and lymphomas constitute the majority of childhood cancers seen in Guatemala. A higher incidence of retinoblastoma and a lower incidence of central nervous system tumors and neuroblastoma are observed.

Pediatric Cancer Research Is a Global Enterprise

Providing adequate care for children with cancer in countries with limited resources is an enormous challenge. Obstacles include fatalism, financial constraints, limited drug availability, lack of trained personnel, lack of salary support for trained personnel, understaffing, inadequate parental education, abandonment, and lack of rapidly available general pediatric, emergency, and intensive care services. Despite these barriers, development of PCUs with active treatment and clinical research programs is necessary for progress. Studies of childhood cancer in different regions, including LIC, MIC, and HIC, can improve outcomes by promoting early diagnosis and identifying biologic differences that may require different therapeutic strategies. Studies in LIC can also identify specific causes of treatment failure so that quality improvement initiatives can focus on these causes. Outcomes in HIC can improve through studies of tumor biology and collaborative clinical trials. Geographic differences in incidence may suggest unique genetic or environmental exposures.[45–47] For example, APML occurs more frequently in Latin Americans.[48] The distribution of the breakpoint site of the *PML* gene also differs in these patients compared to non-Hispanic Caucasians.[49] Retinoblastoma has a high incidence in Honduras, and many patients present with disease at an advanced stage.[13] Mobilization of the community and international collaborators led to development of screening programs to promote early diagnosis, improvements in treatment, collaborative studies of tumor biology with scientists at SJCRH, and a multinational clinical trial of therapy for retinoblastoma in Central America.[13,21] Since patients with extraocular extension of retinoblastoma are often incurable in both HIC and LIC, new treatment strategies are needed for them. However, clinical trials of new agents or combinations will not be feasible if performed only in HIC, where fewer than 1000 children are diagnosed with retinoblastoma each year and fewer than 50 have extraocular disease. The participation of centers in LIC will be critical.

Conclusions

Curing childhood cancer is a global responsibility. Although 80% of children with cancer in HIC are cured, cure rates still must improve another 20%, and reduction of acute and late toxicities remains an area of active research. In LIC and MIC, the first step toward progress is an accurate assessment of the current local situation, development of country-specific interventions, and careful documentation of what succeeds and what fails, so that cure rates can increase from current levels to the 80% achieved in HIC.

Despite many hurdles, the Guatemala program and others have demonstrated that a systematic approach, mobilization of the community, and international cooperation can make a significant and lasting impact. This impact not only improves and extends the lives of children treated in specific centers, but also creates infrastructure for collaborative research that ultimately can improve outcomes for all patients.

References

1. Howard S, Metzger ML, Wilimas J, et al. Childhood cancer epidemiology in low-income countries. *Cancer.* In press.
2. Veerman AJ, Sutaryo S. Twinning: a rewarding scenario for development of oncology services in transitional countries. *Pediatr Blood Cancer.* 2005;45(2):103–106.
3. Howard SC, Pedrosa M, Lins M, et al. Establishment of a pediatric oncology program and outcomes of childhood acute lymphoblastic leukemia in a resource-poor area. *JAMA.* 2004;291(20):2471–2475.
4. Metzger ML, Howard SC, Fu LC, et al. Outcome of childhood acute lymphoblastic leukaemia in resource-poor countries. *Lancet.* 2003;362(9385):706–708.
5. Jemal A, Siegel R, Ward E, Murray T, Xu J, Thun MJ. Cancer statistics, 2007. *CA Cancer J Clin.* 2007;57(1):43–66.
6. Gatta G, Capocaccia R, Stiller C, Kaatsch P, Berrino F, Terenziani M. Childhood cancer survival trends in Europe: a EUROCARE Working Group study. *J Clin Oncol.* 2005;23(16):3742–3751.
7. Pui CH, Evans WE. Treatment of acute lymphoblastic leukemia. *N Engl J Med.* 2006;354(2):166–178.
8. The Montevideo Document. SIOP News: The International Society of Pediatric Oncology; Pediatric Oncology in Low-Income Countries. October 1995.
9. Pui CH, Schrappe M, Masera G, et al. Ponte di Legno Working Group: statement on the right of children with leukemia to have full access to essential treatment and report on the Sixth International Childhood Acute Lymphoblastic Leukemia Workshop. *Leukemia.* 2004;18(6):1043–1053.
10. Barr RD, Sala A, Wiernikowski J, et al. A formulary for pediatric oncology in developing countries. *Pediatr Blood Cancer.* 2005;44(5):433–435.
11. Burton A. The UICC My Child Matters initiative awards: combating cancer in children in the developing world. *Lancet Oncol.* 2006;7(1):13–14.
12. Burton A. UICC *My Child Matters* awards: 2006 winners. *Lancet Oncol.* 2007;8(2):99.
13. Leander C, Fu LC, Pena A, et al. Impact of an education program on late diagnosis of retinoblastoma in Honduras. *Pediatr Blood Cancer.* 2007;49(6):817–819.
14. Resolution on Cancer Control. *World Health Assembly.* 2005;58:22.
15. Joint WHO-UNICEF Expert Consultation on Paediatric Essential Medicines. (http://www.who.int/medicines/publications/UNICEFconsultation.pdf). Published 2006. Accessed April 4, 2008.
16. Better Medicines for Children. Sixtieth World Health Assembly: Agenda Item 12.18. (http://www.who.int/gb/ebwha/pdf_files/WHA60/A60_R20-en.pdf) Published 2007. Accessed April 4, 2008.
17. Pui CH, Ribeiro RC. International collaboration on childhood leukemia. *Int J Hematol.* 2003;78(5):383–389.
18. Masera G, Baez F, Biondi A, et al. North-South twinning in paediatric haemato-oncology: the La Mascota programme, Nicaragua. *Lancet.* 1998;352(9144):1923–1926.
19. Qaddoumi I, Musharbash A, Elayyan M, et al. Closing the survival gap: implementation of medulloblastoma protocols in a low-income country through a twinning program. *Int J Cancer.* 2007.
20. Quintana Y, Nambayan A, Ribeiro R, Bowers L, Shuler A, O'Brien R. Cure4Kids—building online learning and collaboration networks. *AMIA Annu Symp Proc.* 2003:978.
21. Howard SC, Ortiz R, Baez LF, et al. Protocol-based treatment for children with cancer in low income countries in Latin America: a report on the recent meetings of the Monza International School of Pediatric Hematology/Oncology (MISPHO)—part II. *Pediatr Blood Cancer.* 2007;48(4):486–490.
22. Ayoub L, Fu L, Pena A, et al. Implementation of a data management program in a pediatric cancer unit in a low income country. *Pediatr Blood Cancer.* 2007;49(1):23–27.
23. Howard SC, Marinoni M, Castillo L, et al. Improving outcomes for children with cancer in low-income countries in Latin America: a report on the recent meetings of the Monza International School of Pediatric Hematology/Oncology (MISPHO)-Part I. *Pediatr Blood Cancer.* 2007;48(3):364–369.
24. Naafs-Wilstra M, Barr R, Greenberg C, et al. Pediatric oncology in developing countries: development of an alliance of stakeholders. *Med Pediatr Oncol.* 2001;36(2):305–309.
25. Barr RD, Ribeiro RC, Agarwal BR, Masera G, Hesseling PB, Magrath I. Pediatric oncology in countries with limited resources. In: PA Pizzo, DG Poplack, eds. *Principles and Practice of Pediatric Oncology.* Philadelphia, PA: Lippincott, Williams and Wilkins; 2006:1604–1616.
26. Sala A, Barr RD, Masera G. A survey of resources and activities in the MISPHO family of institutions in Latin America: a comparison of two eras. *Pediatr Blood Cancer.* 2004;43(7):758–764.
27. Saul H. International childhood cancer day. *Eur J Cancer.* 2003;39(6):710.
28. Lassarat S, Jootar S. Ongoing challenges of a global international patient assistance program. *Ann Oncol.* 2006;17(Suppl 8):viii43–viii46.
29. Ka AS, Imbert P, Moreira C, et al. Epidemiology and prognosis of childhood cancers in Dakar, Senegal. *Med Trop (Mars).* 2003;63(4-5):521–526.
30. Hesseling P, Molyneux E, McCormick PA, et al. High frequency cyclophosphamide plus intrathecal methotrexate in endemic Burkitt lymphoma. analysis of multicenter trial in Malawi, Cameroon, and Ghana. *Pediatr Blood Cancer.* 2005;45(4):412–413.
31. Harif M, Barsaoul S, Benchekroun S, et al. Treatment of childhood cancer in Africa: preliminary results of the French-African paediatric oncology group. *Arch Pediatr.* 2005;12(6):851–853.
32. Ribeiro RC, Pui CH. Saving the children—improving childhood cancer treatment in developing countries. *N Engl J Med.* 2005;352(21):2158–2160.
33. Fang J, Li CK, Huang SL, et al. The first collaborative childhood acute lymphoblastic leukemia (ALL) study in South China: 3 years experience. *Pediatr Blood Cancer.* 2006;47(4):452.

34. Chandy M. An approach to the management of leukemia in the developing world. *Clin Lab Haematol.* 2006;28(3):147–153.

35. Agarwal B. Pediatric hematology and oncology in India. *Pediatr Blood Cancer.* 2007;49(4):397.

36. George B, Mathews V, Poonkuzhali B, Shaji RV, Srivastava A, Chandy M. Treatment of children with newly diagnosed acute promyelocytic leukemia with arsenic trioxide: a single center experience. *Leukemia.* 2004;18(10):1587–1590.

37. Marchevsky DS. Margarita Statement, Sociedad Latinoamericana de Oncologia Pediatrica (SLAOP): Latin American Society of Pediatric Oncology. *Med Pediatr Oncol.* 2001;37(4):405–406.

38. Sala A, Antillon F, Pencharz P, Barr R. Nutritional status in children with cancer: a report from the AHOPCA Workshop held in Guatemala City, August 31–September 5, 2004. *Pediatr Blood Cancer.* 2005;45(2):230–236.

39. Luna-Fineman S, Slowing K, Valverde P, Antillon F, Challinor J. Pediatric cancer in Guatemala: a retrospective study [Abstract] *Med Pediatr Oncol.* 1997;229:553.

40. Corrigan JJ, Feig SA. Guidelines for pediatric cancer centers. *Pediatrics.* 2004;113(6):1833–1835.

41. Luna-Fineman S, Antillon-Klussman F, Valverde-Gonzales P, Challinor J, Ribeiro R, Wilimas J. Unit in Guatemala [Abstract]. *Med Pediatr Oncol.* 2002;39:399.

42. Lorenzana R, Coustan-Smith E, Antillon F, Ribeiro RC, Campana D. Simple methods for the rapid exchange of flow cytometric data between remote centers. *Leukemia.* 2000;14(2):336–337.

43. Howard SC, Campana D, Coustan-Smith E, et al. Development of a regional flow cytometry center for diagnosis of childhood leukemia in Central America. *Leukemia.* 2005;19(3):323–325.

44. Wilimas JA, Donahue N, Chammas G, Fouladi M, Bowers LJ, Ribeiro RC. Training subspecialty nurses in developing countries: methods, outcome, and cost. *Med Pediatr Oncol.* 2003;41(2):136–140.

45. Miller RW. Geographical and ethnic differences in the occurrence of childhood cancer. *IARC Sci Publ.* 1988(87):3–7.

46. Miller RW. Epidemiologic evidence for genetic variability in the frequency of cancer: ethnic differences. *Basic Life Sci.* 1988;43:65–70.

47. Parkin DM, Kramarova E, Draper GJ, Masuyer E, Michaelis J, Neglia J. International incidence of childhood cancer. Vol. 2. Lyon, France: International Agency for Cancer Research. 1998:1–391.

48. Ribeiro RC, Rego E. Management of APL in developing countries: epidemiology, challenges and opportunities for international collaboration. *Hematol Am Soc Hematol Educ Program.* 2006:162–168.

49. Douer D, Santillana S, Ramezani L, et al. Acute promyelocytic leukaemia in patients originating in Latin America is associated with an increased frequency of the bcr1 subtype of the PML/RARalpha fusion gene. *Br J Haematol.* 2003;122(4):563–570.

Molecular Oncology and Translational Therapy

Lia Gore and Stephen P. Hunger

Introduction and Overview

A major biomedical advance of the past quarter century has been the identification and characterization of genes involved in the pathogenesis of human cancer through detailed molecular investigations of specimens derived from cancer patients. These studies reveal that cancer is the phenotypic manifestation of cumulative mutations in oncogenes and/or tumor suppressor genes (TSGs). These advances have provided fundamental insights into the normal processes of cell growth, differentiation, and death, with critical implications for patient diagnosis and treatment. Development, evaluation, and incorporation of new molecularly targeted therapies into treatment regimens for children with cancer are anticipated to be a major focus of pediatric oncology over the next few decades.

The Nature of Oncogenes and Tumor Suppressor Genes

Most, and likely all, cancers contain mutations in a number of different oncogenes/TSGs by the time they become clinically evident. Mathematical models predict that the vast majority of cancers require 6 to 8 different mutations to develop, which is quite consistent with genetic analyses of primary cancers.[1,2] In some cases, mutations are present in the germline DNA of a patient who develops cancer; the prototype being hereditary *RB* gene mutations in retinoblastoma;[3] however, most cancers result from mutations that are acquired in somatic cells. The causes of these somatic mutations remain obscure. This is particularly evident in childhood cancers, where there is little likelihood that environmental factors or host lifestyle issues (ie, cigarette smoking, alcohol consumption, diet, etc) play a significant role in etiology.

Different types of mutations, with different functional consequences, occur in oncogenes and TSGs. Oncogene mutations cause a gain-of-function and are dominant, genetically and functionally, promoting transformation even though the normal protein from the wild type allele is still expressed. In contrast, TSG mutations generally inactivate the protein product and are typically both genetically and functionally recessive; the remaining wild type allele continues to produce a normal protein that can carry out necessary cellular functions. In general, both alleles of a TSG must be inactivated to alter cell growth significantly. Frequently each allele is inactivated by a different mechanism; for example, point mutation of one allele and deletion of the other. In some instances, TSG mutations may act in a "dominant-negative" manner and exert their phenotype even in the presence of a nonmutated wild type allele or there may be a gene dosage effect such that the amount of protein produced from one allele is suboptimal when compared to that produced from two alleles.

Mechanisms of Oncogene Activation and TSG Inactivation

Oncogenes can be activated by several different mechanisms, as illustrated in Figure 3-1. Point mutations are the result of an alteration in a single nucleotide at the DNA level that changes one amino acid in the protein product of that gene. For example, activating point mutations in the *RAS* oncogene occur in many human cancers, including juvenile myelomonocytic leukemia.[4]

Oncogenes can also be activated by overexpression of the native protein. In neuroblastoma, the N-myc protein is overexpressed due to amplification of the *MYCN* gene.[5] In leukemias, oncogenes are frequently activated by chromosome translocations that relocate an oncogene into the vicinity of active regulatory elements of another gene, frequently one of the immunoglobulin (*Ig*) or T-cell receptor (*TCR*) genes, causing dysregulated expression of a structurally intact protein.[6] Translocations in B-lineage leukemias/lymphomas often involve chromosome bands 14q32 (heavy chain gene, *IgH*), 2q12 (light chain gene, *Igκ*), or 22q11 (light chain gene, *Igλ*), while T-lineage malignancies involve 14q11 (*TCRδ* or *TCRα*) or 7q35 (*TCRβ*). For example, *c-MYC* is involved in translocations with each of the three *Ig* loci, at least one of the *TCR* genes, and at least one other gene.[7] In Burkitt's lym-

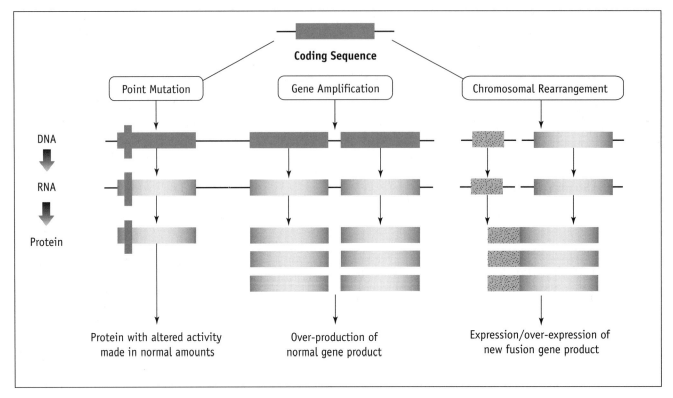

Figure 3-1 Mechanisms of oncogene activation.

phoma or leukemia, the t(8;14)(q24;q32) juxtaposes *c-MYC* with the *IgH* regulatory elements and results in dysregulated high-level expression of *c-MYC*. Myc is a transcription factor that turns on expression of target genes resulting in entry into S phase, decreased growth factor requirements, and escape from normal regulation of cell cycle progression.[7]

Another class of chromosome translocation that occurs frequently in pediatric leukemias and mesenchymal-derived sarcomas are those that create fusion genes encoding chimeric proteins that possess novel structural and functional properties not present in the parental wild type proteins. This class of translocation typically affects transcription factors, often fusing a DNA binding and/or protein oligomerization domain from one protein with effector domains, such as a transcriptional activation domain, from another protein. Translocations of this class typically occur in introns of each gene; exons of the two genes are then joined together during mRNA splicing. Creation of a functional chimera generally requires that the joined exons from each gene are in the same reading frame.[8] Examples include *E2A* fusion proteins in acute lymphoblastic leukemia (ALL) and *EWS* fusion proteins in Ewing sarcoma and related tumors.[9,10] The fusion genes and their mRNA products are extremely useful for molecular diagnosis, while the novel proteins they encode can provide excellent targets for therapeutic intervention.

Inactivation of TSGs can also occur via several different mechanisms. Missense mutations in *TP53* generate mutant p53 proteins that are impaired in important transcriptional and cell cycle–regulatory functions.[11] Another common mode of TSG inactivation is through gene deletion. Two functionally related genes that are located within approximately 25 kilobases of one another on chromosome 9, *p16^INK4A* and *p15^INK4b*, have been identified as the target of deletions in a wide variety of malignancies, including ALL.[12–14] These genes encode proteins of approximately 16 (p16INK4a) and 15 (p15INK4b) kilodaltons that are members of a large family of cyclin-dependent kinase inhibitors, which interact with specific cyclin-dependent protein kinase/cyclin complexes and negatively regulate cell cycle progression. Inactivation of these genes leads to dysregulated progression through the cell cycle. Many other TSGs involved in the development of human cancers have been discovered via identification of recurrent chromosome deletions in tumors, definition of the minimum common deleted segment, and targeted analyses of genes located within this segment.[15]

Specific Mutations Occur Nonrandomly and Are Tightly Associated with Distinct Cancers and Subtypes of Cancer

Many cytogenetic and molecular abnormalities are tightly associated with distinct clinical subtypes of disease with important prognostic or therapeutic implications. Striking examples of this in leukemia include the almost universal occurrence of the t(15;17)(q22;q21) and *PML-RARα* fusion in acute promyelocytic leukemia (APML) and the t(9;22)(q34;q11) and *BCR-ABL* fusion in chronic myelogenous leukemia (CML).[16,17] Tight links between specific molecular abnormalities and subtypes of disease also occur in childhood sarcomas. The *EWS* gene was first identified by virtue of its fusion to the human homologue of the murine *FLI-1* gene by the t(11;22)(q24;q12) in Ewing sarcoma.[18] Subsequently, a variety of different *EWS* fusion genes created by distinct chromosome translocations have been described in Ewing sarcoma family tumors, extraskeletal myxoid chondrosarcoma, desmoplastic small round cell tumor, melanoma of soft parts, myxoid liposarcoma, and other undifferentiated small round cell tumors[10] (see Table 3-1). Indeed the identification of a specific molecular defect is now a very accurate and efficient way by which the so-called small, round, blue cell tumors of childhood can be diagnosed and characterized.[19] Moreover, recent use of both antibodies and small molecule inhibitors of the insulin-like growth factor type I receptor (IGF1R) have shown significant promise in *EWS*-fusion gene tumors, and in Ewing sarcoma particularly. This is another striking example of how knowledge of the specific molecular abnormality in a given tumor can lead to the development of a clinically successful targeted therapy. Phase II studies of IGF1R targeted agents are progressing quickly.

Risk-Directed Therapy and Molecular/Cytogenetic Abnormalities

Molecular and/or cytogenetic abnormalities present in childhood cancer can identify patients with identical clinical characteristics that have very different risks of relapse. This information can then be used in risk-adapted therapy. Prominent examples of this are provided by childhood ALL and neuroblastoma.

In ALL, contemporary strategies for risk group stratification rely heavily on the presence or absence of specific cytogenetic abnormalities in the leukemic clone, including translocations and changes in chromosome number. Patients with t(9;22) or the Philadelphia chromosome (Ph[1]) and *BCR-ABL* fusion, and those with t(12;21) and *TEL-AML1* fusion or favorable chromosome trisomies, constitute two opposite ends of the spectrum but may have identical clinical features. Only a small minority of patients with Philadelphia chromosome-positive ALL are cured with conventional chemotherapy.[20] For this reason, many centers and cooperative groups perform reverse

Table 3-1

Selected common, nonrandom, recurrent chromosomal translocations in childhood malignancies.

Chromosomal Translocation	Fusion Gene	Disease Phenotype
t(15;17)(q22;q11-21)	PML-RARa	Acute promyelocytic leukemia, M3
t(8;21)(q22;q22)	AML-ETO	Acute myelogenous leukemia, M2
inv(16)(p13;q22), del(16)(q22), or t(16;16)(p13;q22)	CBFβ-MYH11	Acute myelogenous leukemia, M4Eo
t(9;11)(p21-22;q23)	MLL-AF9	Acute myelogenous leukemia, M5
t(9;22)(q34;q11)	BCR-ABL	"Philadelphia chromosome positive" CML and ALL
t(4;11)(q21;q23)	MLL-AF4	Infant acute leukemia
t(1;19)(q23;p13)	E2A-PBX1	Precursor B-ALL
t(12;21)(p12;q22)	TEL-AML1	Precursor B ALL
t(8;14)(q24;q32)	IgH-MYC	Burkitt's Leukemia/Lymphoma
t(2;8)(p12;q24)	Igκ-MYC	Burkitt's Leukemia/Lymphoma
t(8;22)(q24;q11)	Igλ-MYC	Burkitt's Leukemia/Lymphoma
t(8;14)(q24;q11)	TCRα-MYC	T-cell ALL
t(1;7)(p32;q35)	TCRβ-TAL1	T-cell ALL
t(10;14)(q24;q11)	TCRβ-HOX11	T-cell ALL
t(1;14)(p32;q11)	TCRδ-TAL1	T-cell ALL
t(2;13)(q35-37;q14)	PAX3-FKHR	Rhabdomyosarcoma, alveolar
t(1;13)(p36;q14)	PAX7-FKHR	Rhabdomyosarcoma, alveolar
t(11;22)(q24;q12)	EWS-FLI1	Ewing Sarcoma/PNET
t(11;22)(p13;q12)	EWS-WT1	Desmoplastic small round cell tumor

transcription-polymerase chain reaction for the *BCR-ABL* fusion mRNA in all patients with ALL at the time of diagnosis. When it is detected, patients are offered alternative therapies including high-dose chemotherapy and stem cell transplant. New studies are also investigating the combination of intensive chemotherapy with targeted Abl kinase inhibitors, including imatinib mesylate,[21] dasatinib, and nilotinib. In contrast, 40% to 50% of children younger than 10 years of age with ALL will have either favorable chromosome trisomies or *TEL-AML1* fusion; these children have a particularly good prognosis with modern chemotherapy and may have cure rates over 90%.[22] Many contemporary ALL clinical trials use the presence of either of these features in treatment stratification algorithms. However, it is critical to realize that the Philadelphia chromosome-positive and the *TEL-AML1*⁺ or favorable trisomy groups are not homogeneous. Some *BCR-ABL*⁺ patients will be cured with chemotherapy, while some *TEL-AML1*⁺/favorable trisomy patients will relapse. An ongoing challenge is to dissect the heterogeneity that exists even within molecularly defined groups at the extremes of the prognostic spectrum. Measures of early treatment response as assessed by minimal residual disease are increasingly in routine use, and there are emerging data to suggest that gene expression profiles may also provide critical data to complement risk stratification algorithms.[23–25]

In neuroblastoma, highly divergent clinical outcomes are also seen in patients with different clinical and biologic features. While age and stage of disease are important predictors of outcome, biologic characteristics can be incorporated to generate a more refined and powerful algorithm for risk group stratification and treatment assignment.[5] Patients with the best prognosis are those whose tumors have hyperdiploid karyotypes, favorable histology, and lack the high-risk genetic features outlined below. These patients are typically young and have low-stage disease. They can be cured with relatively modest chemotherapy, and some investigators advocate they be treated initially with surgery alone, reserving chemotherapy for the subset that relapse.[26] The patients with the worst prognosis are those with structural chromosome changes, especially *MYCN* amplification and/or unfavorable histology. These patients have a poor outcome, even with very intensive therapy. However, the high-risk patients in particular benefit from aggressive treatment strategies such as high-dose chemo/radiotherapy with autologous stem cell support.[27] As in ALL, ongoing studies seek to identify additional characteristics to refine risk group stratification.

Another example of how specific molecular/cytogenetic lesions can determine outcome and influence therapy is provided by *PAX-FKHR* fusion genes in alveolar rhabdomyosarcoma (ARMS). A substantial majority of cases of ARMS contain either a t(2;13)(q35;q14) that fuses *PAX3* to *FKHR* (*forkhead*), or a t(1;13)(p35;q14) that joins *PAX7* to *FKHR*.[28] Both fusion genes encode chimeric transcription factors that include the DNA-binding domains specified by *PAX3* or *PAX7* fused to a transcriptional activation domain from FKHR and display similar effects on transcriptional regulation *in vitro*. However, there is a substantial difference in treatment outcome for ARMS patients associated with these different fusion genes. While there was no significant difference in outcome associated with the different *FKHR* fusion genes among patients with localized ARMS, patients with metastatic ARMS associated with *PAX7-FKHR* fusion had a 75% 4-year overall survival rate as compared to 8% for patients with similar tumors that contained *PAX3-FKHR*.[29] Thus, treatment strategies for patients with metastatic ARMS may differ based on the subtype of *PAX-FKHR* fusion gene present in the tumor.

Molecularly Targeted Therapies

Although it is important to use the presence or absence of specific molecular lesions to diagnose patients and stratify their therapy based on the risk of treatment success or failure, a more ambitious aim is to develop therapies targeted at the fundamental genetic alterations that differentiate cancer from normal cells ("molecularly targeted therapy"). This goal has been realized for some cancers over the past decade, and developmental therapeutics has become one of the most exciting areas of modern cancer biology and therapy. Numerous molecularly targeted agents are in, or will soon enter, clinical testing and it is critical to understand how they are developed and evaluated. Two of the most successful molecularly targeted therapies are imatinib mesylate in CML, and all-trans retinoic acid (ATRA) in APML. While both agents act directly on fundamental alterations caused by chromosome translocations, they were identified and tested in very different ways: imatinib by careful and rational design, and ATRA substantially through serendipity.

Imatinib was developed based on an understanding of how *BCR-ABL* caused leukemia. *BCR-ABL* encodes a protein tyrosine kinase (PTK) that activates downstream signaling cascades by phosphorylating critical tyrosine residues in other proteins (see Druker[30] for a comprehensive review of *BCR-ABL* biology and the development of imatinib). *In vitro* models were developed in which expression of *BCR-ABL* led to cell transformation. In contrast, mutant constructs in which the kinase function of *BCR-ABL* was inactivated were not transforming, establishing that the PTK activity of *BCR-ABL* was critical for transformation. Based on this understanding, it was hypothesized that small molecule drugs that inhibited adenosine triphosphate binding of *BCR-ABL* might inhibit its PTK activity. Large libraries of chemical compounds were screened to identify a lead compound that inhibited *BCR-ABL* kinase activity. Using rational design, an optimized compound (STI 571) was identified that specifically inhibited the Abl class of PTKs, with little effect against other classes of PTKs. This drug, imatinib, was then formulated for optimal oral absorption and first tested in Phase I trials in humans in 1998. Imatinib rapidly demonstrated remarkable clinical activity and received Food and Drug Administration (FDA) approval in 2001 for the treatment of CML. Although the treatment of CML has been revolutionized in a very short period of time, major questions remain. It is improbable that monotherapy will cure most patients with CML, but it is very likely that imatinib and the next generations of Abl small molecule inhibitors will be a major component of effective treatment regimens for this disease. Indeed, mechanisms of imatinib resistance in CML have been identified, including *BCR-ABL* gene amplification and development of point mutations in the binding pocket of Abl domain that alter affinity for imatinib.[31] Fulfilling the promise of rational treatment design, second-generation Abl tyrosine kinase inhibitors have been developed that are more potent than imatinib and can inhibit most, but not all, *BCR-ABL* point mutations.[32] Rapid testing of these agents led to FDA approval of dasatinib and nilotinib in 2006.[33,34]

In contrast to imatinib mesylate in CML, ATRA was integrated into APML therapy based on empiric observations of clinical activity prior to identification of the genetic cause of APML. The molecular mechanism of action was only later understood. Investigations in Shanghai of the potential role of inducers of differentiation in the treatment of leukemia culminated in the observation in 1988 that treatment with ATRA resulted in complete remissions without marrow hypoplasia in both relapsed and newly diagnosed APML patients.[35] This effect was termed "differentiation therapy." Although this observation was certainly noteworthy, it generated much more widespread interest when the t(15;17), present in almost all patients with APML, was shown to involve the gene that encodes the retinoic acid receptor alpha (RARα) in 1990 (see Melnick and Licht for a comprehensive review of PML-RARα and ATRA).[36] This observation accelerated clinical testing of ATRA in patients with APML, and it rapidly became apparent that ATRA alone could induce remission in almost 90% of APML patients and that combination therapy of ATRA plus chemotherapy was dramatically better than chemotherapy alone.[37] Parallel developments in the laboratory revealed that PML-RARα blocks myeloid differentiation by acting as a repressor of critical target genes that are normally activated by physiologic levels of ATRA, and that pharmacologic doses of ATRA overcome this differentiation block in APML.

For other molecularly targeted therapies to impact patient outcome, a number of steps must be taken. It will be necessary to identify suitable targets, begin preclinical development and optimization of agents, prioritize these for testing in early-phase single-agent trials, discover and/or develop techniques to assess the effect on specific targets, and evaluate the therapeutic contribution of the new agent when it is integrated into existing "standard of care" treatment regimens. For a more complete discussion of how new agents are tested in childhood cancer, see Chapter 7 (Fundamentals of Cancer Chemotherapy). The remainder of this chapter will focus on a description of general principles in the field of molecular oncology and how they are integrated into design and evaluation of data derived from contemporary clinical trials.

Oncogene Addiction: Target Identification and Patient Selection

Because cancers have mutations in multiple genes, targeted therapy is likely to be most effective when an agent inhibits a specific abnormality that is critical to tumor growth and/or survival, particularly a sentinel lesion that is an initiating or very early step in oncogenesis. At its essence, the concept of "oncogene addiction" posits that the more dependent on a genetic lesion a tumor cell is, the more effective an inhibitor of this abnormality will be.[38] In chronic-phase CML, *BCR-ABL* fulfills all of these criteria; thus Abl kinase inhibitors are highly effective treatment for CML in chronic phase. In contrast, although *BCR-ABL* plays a critical role in the pathogenesis of Ph+ ALL, there are more genetic lesions in Ph+ ALL than are present in chronic-phase CML. Thus, unlike CML, Abl kinase inhibitors are not effective long-term monotherapy for Ph+ ALL, although they appear to increase the effectiveness of combination chemotherapy regimens significantly.

Even if an agent can inhibit the target with great efficiency, one may not see the clinical response produced by imatinib in CML or by ATRA in APML. *BCR-ABL* and PML-RARα are likely to be exceptions in another critical respect: expression of these mutant proteins defines the disease. A patient without *BCR-ABL* expression does not have true CML, and one without PML-RARα (or one of the rare variant RARα fusion proteins) expression does not have true APML. Most cancers are not so sharply defined by molecular abnormalities, and therefore targeted agents might be effective only in specific, molecularly defined subsets of the clinical disease. An excellent example is provided by recent studies of gefitinib, a rationally designed small molecule PTK inhibitor targeted against the epidermal growth factor receptor (EGFR) in non–small cell lung cancer (NSCLC). Despite EGFR overexpression in a high percentage of NSCLCs, Phase I trials showed that only 10% to 20% of patients with chemotherapy-refractory NSCLC responded to gefitinib, and Phase III trials found no benefit to the addition of gefitinib to standard chemotherapy regimens. However, subsequent molecular studies revealed that a substantial majority of the patients who responded to gefitinib had tumors with activating mutations in the *EGFR*, which were not observed in patients who did not respond to this agent.[39,40] Thus, gefitinib may play a critical role in the treatment of those 10% to 20% of patients with NSCLC that have *EGFR* mutations, but it is of little utility in the remaining 80% to 90%.

A new paradigm for development and testing of cancer therapies is emerging, that of cross-platform target identification. First, basic laboratory studies must characterize the sentinel molecular lesions that are present in a specific subtype of cancer. Next, one must develop and refine targeted therapies that can inhibit the activity of the protein products of these sentinel lesions. To determine if these targeted therapies improve outcome for the disease (through improved cure rates and/or cures with fewer long- and short-term side effects), they must be tested in the right subsets of patients, those with tumors that are dependent upon, ideally addicted to, the molecular target.

Apoptosis as a Therapeutic Target

Mutated tyrosine kinases are ideal therapeutic targets, but it is likely that most cancers do not contain kinase domain mutations. Fortunately, this does not mean that targeted therapy is not an option in such tumors. There are other common pathways that are critical to oncogenesis and therefore may serve as important therapeutic targets. One example is the process of apoptosis, the progressive, organized sequence of programmed cell death critical for normal development. To maintain homeostasis, there must be a precise balance between forces that promote cell growth and those that control senescence and cell death. For several decades, the field of molecular oncology was focused on oncogenes that promoted growth. The importance of dysregulated cell death in oncogenesis was first appreciated in the early 1990s when it was discovered that *BCL2*, an oncogene of previously unknown function discovered by virtue of its involvement in the t(14;18) in follicular lymphoma, was a homolog of *ced9*, a gene that inhibited apoptosis in the worm *C. elegans*. Following this discovery, it quickly became apparent that alterations in the pathways that regulate apoptosis were present in a variety of human cancers.

In this regard, the process of apoptosis is an important potential therapeutic target in human cancer. *BCL2* is an obvious potential target; oblimersen sodium, an antisense oligonucleotide that down-regulates *BCL2* expression, is being tested in clinical trials for a variety of tumor types. While definitive trials have not yet been completed, it appears that this agent might be most effective as a potentiator of chemotherapy and/or radiation, not as a single agent. There are a variety of other proteins involved in regulation of apoptosis that are attractive potential therapeutic targets. The caspase family of cysteine proteases plays a critical role in the regulation of apoptosis. Caspases are activated in response to inflammation, cell stress and injury, and DNA damage. Once initiated, pro-apoptotic caspases activate downstream effector proteins that subsequently lead to cell shrinkage, membrane contraction, and DNA fragmentation, the hallmarks of apoptosis. For example, relevant to pediatric oncology, the protein kinase Akt inhibits the pro-apoptotic molecule Bad by direct phosphorylation and prevents expression of another pro-apoptotic molecule Bim by the phosphorylation and inhibition of the FKHR transcription factors active in ARMS. Figure 3-2 demonstrates a simplified overview of the apoptosis pathway, and selected relevant molecules.

Genomics in Pediatric Oncology

Until the late 1990s, most studies of human tumor specimens were targeted analyses focused on analyzing the role of one specific, or a small number of, candidate genes. Several technological advances paved the way for large-scale, unbiased examinations of the human genome in cancer. First were efforts to sequence the entire human genome that were begun in the early to mid-1990s and completed in 2003. The second was development of new DNA chip technologies that allow the analysis of literally hundreds of thousands of genes in a single experiment. Several competing strategies were developed in parallel, but oligonucleotide-based technologies have become the standard. To create a DNA chip or an array, tens of thousands of short, 25 to 45 base pair, DNA probes (oligonucleotides) are robotically spotted on a coated quartz surface. Test RNA or DNA is then labeled with a fluorescent dye and hybridized (allowed to bond) to the probes. Following washing to eliminate nonspecific binding, the chips are visualized under light of a specific wavelength to determine which probes have been bound by the sample, and the intensity of the binding. Using this technology, one can examine gene expression, differential splicing of different genes, the presence/absence of specific mutations or polymorphisms (naturally occurring variations in gene sequence).

Microarray technologies have revolutionized modern cancer research and are becoming an integral part of cancer treatment, drug development, and clinical trials. Several examples follow that illustrate these emerging trends.

Gene Expression Profiles

Using gene expression arrays, one can examine the expression of tens of thousands of genes in a single experiment. Chips available in 2006 allow analysis of more than 50,000 transcripts derived from almost 40,000 individual genes. Golub and colleagues first reported in 1999 proof of principle experiments that demonstrated the ability to use expression profiles (crude by today's standards) to distinguish between acute lymphoid leukemia and acute myeloid leukemia.[41] New analytic techniques have been developed to deal with the enormous volume of data derived from expression profile experiments. In general, two broad classes of analysis are performed. Unsupervised analysis is used to compare the expression profiles of multiple different specimens and group them into classes based on intrinsic biologic properties that dictate patterns of gene expression. In contrast, supervised analysis seeks to identify patterns of gene expression that can be used to characterize specimens more accurately. For example, supervised analysis can be used to attempt to identify patterns of gene expression that correlate with relapse vs freedom from relapse on a cohort with known outcome. This class predictor must then be validated on an independent sample set. If confirmed, a class predictor could

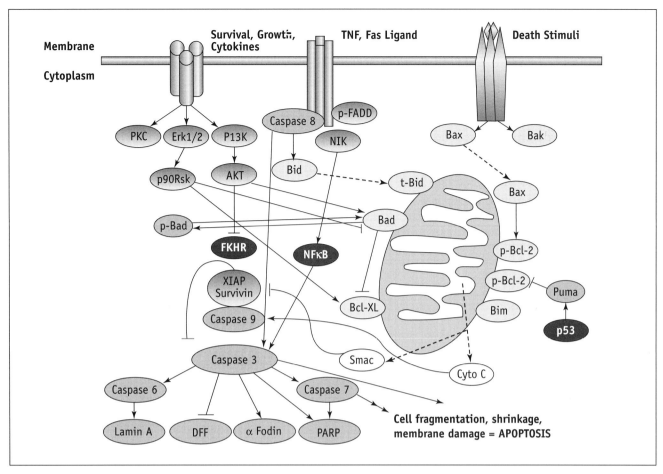

Figure 3-2 Pathways relevant to apoptosis and induction of programmed cell death.

be used to identify whether or not a newly diagnosed patient is likely to relapse.

Although these technologies are not yet used routinely to select therapy in pediatric oncology, they are in some adult tumors. For example, it is clear that adjuvant chemotherapy is beneficial for women with breast cancer. However, not all patients benefit equally. Breast cancer patients whose tumors have "poor outcome" expression profiles have a relatively high risk of relapse and derive significant clinical benefit from treatment with adjuvant chemotherapy. In contrast, patients whose tumors have good outcome expression profiles have a low risk of relapse. For these patients, there is no benefit derived from adjuvant chemotherapy. It has now become common practice to use the gene expression profile of about 20 genes, selected from tens of thousands initially examined on arrays, to select which women with breast cancer receive adjuvant chemotherapy and which do not. Similar situations exist in pediatric oncology. We know from historical experience that subsets of patients with Wilms' tumor and osteosarcoma can be cured with surgery alone; perhaps in the future we will be able to identify these patients via expression profiles and spare them the toxicities of chemotherapy. Similarly, about 40% to 45% of children with a late bone marrow relapse of ALL (36+ months from initial diagnosis) can be cured with chemotherapy. It

would be ideal to identify these patients at the time of relapse and focus novel treatment and transplant strategies on the remaining patients that will not be cured with today's chemotherapy regimens.

Single Nucleotide Polymorphisms

The gene expression profiles discussed in the prior section focused on characterizing differences in gene expression among tumor cells derived from different patients. It is likely that intrinsic differences in host characteristics also have a major influence on the disease biology and the outcome of cancer therapy. Many of these differences are due to polymorphisms, differences in the coding sequence of individual genes that occur commonly in our genomes. Individual host polymorphisms have been analyzed using a candidate gene approach to attempt to predict response to treatment in patients with cancer, and to predict which patients will/will not develop toxicity. An excellent example is provided by differences in the enzyme thiopurine methyltransferase (TPMT), which inactivates 6-thioguanine and 6-mercaptopurine via methylation. Approximately 10% of the population has one hypofunctional TPMT allele, and 0.3% has two hypofunctional alleles. The latter homozygous-deficient patients have severe toxicity with thiopurines used in therapy of ALL. Thus, testing for TPMT genetic variations may help to guide therapy of children with ALL. Analogous to gene expression profiles, one can use chip technology to analyze tens of thousands of single nucleotide polymorphisms in one experiment. Analysis of large numbers of patients treated for cancer with well-annotated clinical details has the potential to identify patients at high or low risk of various toxicities. Why do some patients develop secondary leukemia, or antracycline-induced cardiotoxicity, or osteonecrosis? It is reasonable to expect that genetic variation in drug metabolism and other features may play a major role in the occurrence of these uncommon, yet clinically extremely important, toxicities. Ongoing studies should facilitate much better elucidation of risk assessment.

The expected long-term result of these genomic technologies is a move toward personalized cancer treatment, whereby host and tumor characteristics are used to group patients into different risk categories, select specific therapies (targeted or not), and predict who is at high risk for specific uncommon toxicities.

Novel Trial Designs and Assessments for New Agents

Until recently, most chemotherapy agents that were developed were cytotoxic and had significant potential toxicities. Thus, it was critical to identify a dose with an acceptable therapeutic index of activity versus toxicity. The established traditional pathway for evaluation of new drugs in patients with cancer dictated that Phase I studies be performed first to determine the maximally tolerated dose (MTD) and dose-limiting toxicity. The next step was a single-agent Phase II trial, in which the activity of the agent is tested against different tumor types. In subsequent Phase III trials, the agent was compared with standard therapy, often by integrating it into complex, multiagent chemotherapy regimens.

New molecularly targeted agents challenge this drug development paradigm. The concentration at which a given agent causes toxicity may be significantly higher than the concentration at which it exerts its biologic effects against the relevant oncogenic target. Instead of, or in addition to, determining an MTD in Phase I trials, it will be critical to find a "biologically efficacious dose" or "biologically optimal dose" at which a targeted protein or enzyme is optimally down-regulated or inhibited. Significant escalation above this dose may not be necessary, a major departure from the paradigm of dose escalation that has proved so effective in many cancers. Rather than focusing on disease stabilization or response as measured by blood counts or imaging studies, surrogate measures must be found to evaluate an agent's ability to modulate the target. Because leukemia cells can be readily obtained from peripheral blood in many patients and bone marrow sampling is a minimally invasive, easy to perform, and standard procedure, evaluation of impact is relatively simple. In solid tumors, repeat biopsies are more invasive, impart a greater risk to the patient, and are not an accepted part of response evaluation. Nonetheless, tumor sampling will likely be critical for the accurate assessment of target modulation. Investigators are challenged to develop mechanisms for determining target modulation that are consistent with relevant considerations regarding ethics, patient safety, and comfort. These challenges are particularly acute when the patient is a child.

Many new agents may have cytostatic rather than cytotoxic effects. Agents that cause rapid cell kill are expected to lead to brisk tumor shrinkage, making response assessment relatively straightforward. Conversely, if an agent targets a more slowly evolving pathway that regulates cell growth and/or survival, the time it takes to see an effect might be substantially longer. As such, the pace of disease progression with a given agent or the tempo of response to an agent may provide good insight into the role and timing that agent should play in combination therapy regimens. Rapid early acceleration of disease after treatment with a particular agent means either it is less effective than one that causes slower progression, or it should be combined with another agent or agents that can slow the disease progression until the biologic effects of the slower-acting agent can emerge. It is critical to define trial endpoints carefully so that agents that might be very effective in combination therapy are not discarded because they do not show convincing response as single agents.

As new molecularly targeted agents are combined with more traditional cytotoxic agents, it is important to consider the schedule of administration with care. Ideally, combination therapy leads to additive or synergistic killing, but it can also result in antagonism if the combinations and sequence are wrong. A good example is provided by first-generation FLT3 (FMS-like-tyrosine kinase-3) inhibitors now in clinical trials. Activating FLT3 mutations occur commonly in AML and are associated with an adverse treatment outcome.[42] Lestaurtinib, a FLT3 inhibitor, is a potent inducer of apoptosis of cell lines and primary AML samples with mutant FLT3. It displays synergism when administered simultaneously or immediately following standard chemotherapy drugs used to treat AML but is antagonistic when given before the cytotoxic agents.[43]

New and existing technologies will play a key role in trial design and response assessment. In leukemia, molecular and flow cytometry studies can identify subclinical levels of minimal residual disease at a sensitivity of 1 leukemia cell in 10^4 to 10^6 normal cells. Assessment of MRD is becoming an important component of contemporary risk stratification algorithms. This technology also has great potential to predict response to novel agents and long-term outcome much more rapidly than standard markers. Since many molecularly targeted therapies have minimal toxicity, it is hoped that they can be integrated into existing chemotherapy regimens to improve patient outcome. The new generation of clinical trials for relapsed ALL is adding novel agents to well-tested existing multi-agent chemotherapy backbones. While many potential agents are available, it is likely that only a few will move to frontline trials for newly diagnosed patients. Because the chemotherapy backbone produces remission in a substantial majority of patients, it is unlikely that the percentage of patients to achieve remission will be a clinical useful tool in this setting, given the limited number of patients. Thus, we must develop mechanisms to rapidly assess and compare the activity of different agents. Reduction of disease burden as assessed by MRD levels present during the first few months of therapy will be necessary to prioritize agents for future study in newly diagnosed patients.

New methodologies are also needed to assess how pediatric solid tumors respond to targeted therapies, particularly those that are cytostatic and therefore may not lead to tumor regression. While Ewing sarcoma and rhabdomyosarcoma have fusion genes that can be used as markers for MRD assessment, other mechanisms are needed to assess the majority of tumors that lack such markers. Fortunately the area of functional imaging is evolving rapidly and new technologies including functional nuclear magnetic resonance imaging, spectroscopy, and positron emission tomography are available to assess tumor metabolic activity and growth. Significant efforts are now devoted to integrating functional imaging into the assessment of new molecularly targeted therapies in patients with solid tumors.[44]

Summary and Conclusions

Knowledge about the biology of pediatric cancers now plays an integral part in how patients are diagnosed, classified into risk groups, and assigned to different therapies. Proof that molecularly targeted therapies can have major clinical impact has radically altered concepts of new drug development and testing. Because the majority of pediatric leukemias and many pediatric solid tumors, unlike their adult counterparts, have well-defined chromosomal translocations that produce novel proteins, targeted therapies may be more effective in patients with these better-characterized, more biologically homogeneous cell populations. The challenge at present is to identify those patients who can benefit from molecular therapies and to "customize" these treatments most effectively. Clinical trial design must keep pace with the rapidly evolving strategies and targets to rapidly determine which agents should be developed further while maximizing the potential benefit to patients.

References

1. Renan MJ. How many mutations are required for tumorigenesis? Implications from human cancer data. Mol Carcinog. 1993;7:139–146.
2. Fearon ER, Vogelstein B. A genetic model for colorectal tumorigenesis. Cell. 1990;61:759–767.
3. Friend SH, Bernards R, Rogelj S, et al. A human DNA segment with properties of the gene that predisposes to retinoblastoma and osteosarcoma. Nature. 1986;323:643–646.
4. Niemeyer CM, Kratz C. Juvenile myelomonocytic leukemia. Curr Oncol Rep. 2003;5:510 515.
5. Brodeur GM. Neuroblastoma: biological insights into a clinical enigma. Nat Rev Cancer. 2003;3:203–216.
6. Look AT. Oncogenic transcription factors in the human acute leukemias. Science. 1997;278:1059–1064.
7. Kuppers R, Dalla-Favera R. Mechanisms of chromosomal translocations in B cell lymphomas. Oncogene. 2001;20:5580–5594.
8. Hunger SP, Brown R, Cleary ML. DNA-binding and transcriptional regulatory properties of hepatic leukemia factor (HLF) and the t(17;19) acute lymphoblastic leukemia chimera E2A-HLF. Mol Cell Biol. 1994;14:5986–5996.
9. Hunger SP. Chromosomal translocations involving the E2A gene in acute lymphoblastic leukemia: clinical features and molecular pathogenesis. Blood. 1996;87:1211–1224.
10. Burchill SA. Ewing's sarcoma: diagnostic, prognostic, and therapeutic implications of molecular abnormalities. J Clin Pathol. 2003;56:96–102.
11. Imamura J, Miyoshi I, Koeffler HP. p53 in hematologic malignancies. Blood. 1994;84:2412–2421.
12. Kamb A, Gruis NA, Weaver-Feldhaus J, et al. A cell cycle regulator potentially involved in genesis of many tumor types [see comments]. Science. 1994;264:436–440.
13. Nobori T, Miura K, Wu DJ, Lois A, Takabayashi K, Carson DA. Deletions of the cyclin-dependent kinase-4 inhibitor gene in multiple human cancers. Nature. 1994;368:753–756.
14. Drexler HG. Review of alterations of the cyclin-dependent kinase inhibitor INK4 family genes p15, p16, p18 and p19 in human leukemia-lymphoma cells. Leukemia. 1998;12:845–859.
15. Presneau N, Manderson EN, Tonin PN. The quest for a tumor suppressor gene phenotype. Curr Mol Med. 2003;3:605–629.
16. Sawyers CL. Chronic myeloid leukemia. N Engl J Med. 1999;340:1330–1340.
17. Sirulnik A, Melnick A, Zelent A, Licht JD. Molecular pathogenesis of acute promyelocytic leukaemia and APL variants. Best Pract Res Clin Haematol. 2003;16:387–408.
18. Delattre O, Zucman J, Plougastel B, et al. Gene fusion with an ETS DNA-binding domain caused by chromosome translocation in human tumours. Nature. 1992;359:162–165.
19. Bennicelli JL, Barr FG. Chromosomal translocations and sarcomas. Curr Opin Oncol. 2002;14:412–419.
20. Arico M, Valsecchi MG, Camitta B, et al. Outcome of treatment in children with Philadelphia chromosome-positive acute lymphoblastic leukemia. N Engl J Med. 2000;342:998–1006.
21. Kebriaei P, Larson RA. Progress and challenges in the therapy of adult acute lymphoblastic leukemia. Curr Opin Hematol. 2003;10:284–289.
22. Pui CH, Gaynon PS, Boyett JM, et al. Outcome of treatment in childhood acute lymphoblastic leukaemia with rearrangements of the 11q23 chromosomal region. Lancet. 2002;359:1909–1915.
23. Gaynon PS, Crotty ML, Sather HN, et al. Expression of BCR-ABL, E2A-PBX1, and MLL-AF4 fusion transcripts in newly diagnosed children with acute lymphoblastic leukemia: a Children's Cancer Group initiative. Leuk Lymphoma. 1997;26:57–65.
24. Moos PJ, Raetz EA, Carlson MA, et al. Identification of gene expression profiles that segregate patients with childhood leukemia. Clin Cancer Res. 2002;8:3118–3130.
25. Yeoh EJ, Ross ME, Shurtleff SA, et al. Classification, subtype discovery, and prediction of outcome in pediatric acute lymphoblastic leukemia by gene expression profiling. Cancer Cell. 2002;1:133–143.
26. Kushner BH, Cheung NK, LaQuaglia MP, et al. Survival from locally invasive or widespread neuroblastoma without cytotoxic therapy. J Clin Oncol. 1996;14:373–381.
27. Maris JM, Matthay KK. Molecular biology of neuroblastoma. J Clin Oncol. 1999;17:2264–2279.
28. Xia SJ, Barr FG. Chromosome translocations in sarcomas and the emergence of oncogenic transcription factors. Eur J Cancer. 2005;41:2513–2527.
29. Sorensen PH, Lynch JC, Qualman SJ, et al. PAX3-FKHR and PAX7-FKHR gene fusions are prognostic indicators in alveolar rhabdomyosarcoma: a report from the children's oncology group. J Clin Oncol. 2002;20:2672–2679.
30. Druker BJ. Imatinib as a paradigm of targeted therapies. Adv Cancer Res. 2004;91:1–30.
31. Shah NP, Nicoll JM, Nagar B, et al. Multiple BCR-ABL kinase domain mutations confer polyclonal resistance to the tyrosine kinase inhibitor imatinib (STI571) in chronic phase and blast crisis chronic myeloid leukemia. Cancer Cell. 2002;2:117–125.
32. Shah NP, Tran C, Lee FY, Chen P, Norris D, Sawyers CL. Overriding imatinib resistance with a novel ABL kinase inhibitor. Science. 2004;305:399–401.
33. Talpaz M, Shah NP, Kantarjian H, et al. Dasatinib in imatinib-resistant Philadelphia chromosome-positive leukemias. N Engl J Med. 2006;354:2531–2541.
34. Kantarjian HM, Talpaz M, Giles F, O'Brien S, Cortes J. New insights into the pathophysiology of chronic myeloid leukemia and imatinib resistance. Ann Intern Med. 2006;145:913–923.
35. Huang ME, Yu-chen Y, Shu-rong C, et al. Use of all-trans retinoic acid in the treatment of acute promyelocytic leukemia. Blood. 1988;72:567–572.
36. Melnick A, Licht JD. Deconstructing a disease: RARalpha, its fusion partners, and their roles in the pathogenesis of acute promyelocytic leukemia. Blood. 1999;93:3167–3215.

37. Tallman MS, Andersen JW, Schiffer CA, et al. All-trans-retinoic acid in acute promyelocytic leukemia. *N Engl J Med.* 1997;337:1021–1028.

38. Weinstein IB. Cancer. Addiction to oncogenes—the Achilles heel of cancer. *Science.* 2002;297:63–64.

39. Lynch DK, Winata SC, Lyons RJ, et al. A Cortactin-CD2-associated protein (CD2AP) complex provides a novel link between epidermal growth factor receptor endocytosis and the actin cytoskeleton. *J Biol Chem.* 2003;278:21805–21813.

40. Paez JG, Janne PA, Lee JC, et al. EGFR mutations in lung cancer: correlation with clinical response to gefitinib therapy. *Science.* 2004;304:1497–1500.

41. Golub TR, Slonim DK, Tamayo P, et al. Molecular classification of cancer: class discovery and class prediction by gene expression monitoring. *Science.* 1999;286:531–537.

42. Levis M, Small D. FLT3: It does matter in leukemia. *Leukemia.* 2003;17:1738–1752.

43. Levis M, Pham R, Smith BD, Small D. In vitro studies of a FLT3 inhibitor combined with chemotherapy: sequence of administration is important to achieve synergistic cytotoxic effects. *Blood.* 2004;104:1145–1150.

44. Hammond LA, Denis L, Salman U, Jerabek P, Thomas CR, Jr., Kuhn JG. Positron emission tomography (PET): expanding the horizons of oncology drug development. *Invest New Drugs.* 2003;21:309–340.

Tumor Immunology and Immunotherapy

Gregor S. D. Reid, Stephan A. Grupp, and Kirk R. Schultz

Introduction

Chemotherapy and irradiation are well established as therapies for pediatric malignancies and have led to highly successful outcomes, with survival rates of approximately 75% to 80%.[1] However, these approaches are not universally successful, with several malignancies remaining refractory to primary therapy or recurring after initial response. While the development of novel therapeutic agents that target apoptotic and proliferation pathways in malignant cells is a major area of investigation, other facets of the interaction between the host environment and the malignant cell present possible opportunities for intervention. One such interaction is between the cancer cell and the host immune system. Thus, approaches to manipulate the host immune environment are attractive options to control disease. Unfortunately, while the hypothesis has generated great interest for decades, it has produced only mixed results. Factors limiting the success of immune therapies include (a) inability of immune therapy to treat bulk disease; (b) only partial understanding of the components of the immune system that exert antitumor activity; and (c) a limited understanding of the endogenous characteristics of tumor cells that influence sensitivity to immune mechanisms. Important advances in each of these areas have been made in the past few years that may provide the foundation for the development of a new generation of immune-based treatments. Here we will review the progress in our understanding of the interactions between pediatric cancer cells and the immune system, and identify the areas that show the most promise for effective clinical application.

Principles of Immune Therapy for Pediatric Malignancy

The immune system is composed of a myriad of different cell types, each with its own specific role to play. Traditionally separated into two distinct systems, the innate (macrophages, granulocytes, and natural killer cells) and the adaptive (T and B cells), it has become increasingly apparent that a full immune response requires contribu-

tions from cells in both these compartments. This is as true for immune responses against tumor cells as it is for those against infectious agents. Antitumor activity has been attributed to α/β T cell receptor (TcR) expressing T cells, γ/δ TcR expressing T cells, B cells (through antibody production), macrophages, dendritic cells, neutrophils (through antibody-dependent cell-mediated cytotoxicity), natural killer (NK) cells, and NK-T cells. From this array of cellular tools, a substantial body of research suggests that α/β T cells and NK cells have the greatest potential for use in treatment of pediatric cancer. Although T cells and NK cells share similar cytotoxic mechanisms, they utilize very different strategies to identify their targets. Because the development of any successful immune therapy using these effector cells will require efficient targeting to the tumor cell, a brief overview of the recognition and activation strategies of T cells and NK cells is given below.

T cell recognition is mediated by the TcR, whose clonal specificity is the result of somatic DNA rearrangement.[2] T cells recognize major histocompatibility complex (MHC) molecules expressed on the surface of antigen-presenting cells (APC) or target cells.[3] MHC Class I molecules (HLA-A,-B,-C) are expressed by most nucleated cells, and are recognized by CD8+ T cells, primarily the cytotoxic T cells (CTL). Expression of MHC Class II molecules (HLA-DP,-DQ,-DR), the ligands for CD4+ T cells, is primarily restricted to hematopoietic APC. While the ubiquitous expression of MHC Class I renders it the relevant T cell targeting molecule for most cancers, it is apparent that for sustained CTL activity and the generation of immunological memory, CD4 T responses directed at MHC Class II antigens are required.[4] Because most cancer cells, with the exception of hematologic malignancies, do not generally express MHC Class II, activation of CD4+ tumor-specific T cells requires presentation of tumor epitopes by so-called professional APC. These APC, primarily dendritic cells, possess the ability to take up exogenous antigens and present them in the context of MHC antigens along with the necessary costimulatory signals to activate T cells.

Both MHC Class I and Class II complexes present short peptides to the TcR.[5,6] Recognition of these peptides, derived by proteolytic digestion of primarily endogenous (MHC Class I) or exogenous (MHC Class II) proteins, provides a critical first activation signal to the T cell.[7] TcR engagement, however, is not sufficient to induce primary T cell activation. Full activation requires that TcR stimulation be accompanied by signaling through other receptors on the T cell.[8,9] A key step in the primary activation of T cells is the interaction between CD40 ligand, up-regulated on T cells after TcR ligation, with CD40 on the APC.[10] Signaling through CD40 leads to the increased expression of costimulatory molecules by APC that bind counter receptors on the T cell, delivering the second signal required for full activation. The best-known costimulatory molecules are CD80 (formerly B7-1) and CD86 (formerly B7-2), members of the B7 family.[11] However, in recent years it has been appreciated that additional costimulatory molecules, primarily members of the B7 and TNF/TNFR families, impact also on the strength and duration of T cell responses, as well as on memory development and inhibition of responses (Figure 4-1).[11,12]

The strict requirement for TcR ligation with simultaneous stimulation through coreceptors effectively limits the number of cells that are capable of activating naive T cells. These "professional" APC are primarily the dendritic cells. Most tumor cells are incapable of primary T cell activation because they lack at least one of the necessary components, most commonly costimulatory molecule

expression. If primary TCR engagement occurs in the absence of satisfactory costimulation, no T cell activation occurs and this can lead instead to T cell anergy, a state in which the T cell is rendered unresponsive to future encounters with its specific peptide ligand.[9,13] The inefficient presentation of antigen to T cells by cancer cells is thought to be one of the key mechanisms undermining antitumor immune responses. Because tumor cells do not express suitable costimulatory molecules, cross-presentation of tumor-derived MHC Class I antigens by APC is often necessary to induce a primary immune response.[14] In this process, proteins or peptides released by dying tumor cells are taken up, processed, and presented in the MHC Class I binding groove by the APC.

Although the successful activation of T cells leads to the deployment of their effector functions, all T cell responses are not the same. Two primary types of T cell response have been defined by their cytokine production profiles.[15] T cell helper 1 (Th1) responses, characterized by the production of interferon-gamma (IFN-γ) and IL-2, mediate cellular immunity. Th2 responses, producing IL-4 and IL-5, are associated with humoral responses. Consistent with the importance of CTL in antitumor activity, Th1 immune responses have been shown in many studies to exert the most effective immune control of cancer. The development of a Th1 or Th2 response is influenced by a variety of factors, including amount of antigen, costimulatory molecule expression, and the cytokine milieu.[16] The generation of effective immune therapy against pediatric cancer will likely require optimizing conditions that favor the generation of Th1 responses. A third type of T cell response that can shape antitumor activity is that dominated by regulatory T (T_{REG}) cells. T_{REG} cells serve to inhibit the responses of other immune cells, thus dampening overall responses. Although an understanding of the precise role and mechanism of action of these cells in controlling cancer immune responses is incomplete, it is clear that they exert a significant influence over spontaneous and induced antitumor immune activity.[17,18]

NK cells do not express a clonal receptor but rather integrate the balance of signals received through a panel of activating and inhibitory receptors to determine the outcome of interactions with target cells.[19] The primary inhibitory receptors expressed by human NK cells that down regulate NK responses are the members of the killer cell immunoglobulin-like receptor (KIR) family, which recognize HLA-A, HLA-B, and HLA-C alleles on target cells. In contrast to the TcR, this recognition is peptide independent. Signaling through the cytoplasmic ITIM domain of KIR account for the "missing self" model of NK cell activation,[20] in which autologous cells that have down-regulated expression of MHC Class I molecules are killed by NK cells because they cannot engage the inhibitory KIR on the surface of the NK cells. This is an important element of immune surveillance against tumors. The activating receptors expressed on NK cells, including some KIRs, NKp30, NKp44, NKp46, and

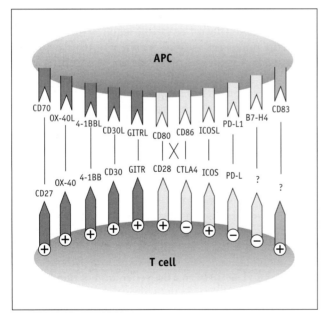

Figure 4-1 Costimulatory molecule interactions in T cell activation. T cell activation, acquisition of effector properties, and generation of immunological memory are influenced by a multitude of molecular interactions occurring at the APC/T cell interface. Several of the key primary and secondary interactions are mediated by members of the TNF/TNFR and B7 families of costimulatory molecules. Positive costimulation is indicated by [+], while inhibition is indicated by [−], although it should be noted that the nature of the signal can vary in different settings.

NKG2D, engage a number of receptors expressed on virally infected and malignant cells. However, the outcome of this signaling is influenced by the simultaneous signals being provided through the KIR and other inhibitory receptors.

Once activated, T cells and NK cells are capable of killing their targets via the perforin/granzyme or TNF pathways of cytotoxicity.[21] In the case of previously activated T cells, binding of the TcR to its specific ligand on the target cell does not require simultaneous costimulatory molecule signaling to induce cytotoxic activity. In this setting, the expression of only those accessory molecules, such as ICAM-1 and LFA-1, necessary for the formation of a functional immunological synapse is required.[22] Given the readiness of activated T cells and NK cells to kill their targets, it is apparent that the primary obstacle to successful immune therapy is achieving a sufficient level of specific effector cell activation. A clear demonstration of the significant antitumor activity that can be exerted by a fully activated immune response is provided by the clinical responses achieved with hematopoietic stem cell transplantation (HSCT) in pediatric cancer patients as described below.

Hematopoietic Stem Cell Transplantation as a Model for Immunotherapy of Pediatric Cancer

Hematopoietic stem cell transplantation (HSCT) is the only established cell-mediated immune therapy for pediatric cancer. It is now widely recognized that an important therapeutic mechanism of HSCT is the antitumor response of transplanted donor immune cells, in addition to effects provided by the high-dose chemotherapy and irradiation employed prior to transplant. The antileukemia immune activity exerted in the transplant setting was first noted by the correlation of graft-versus-host disease (GVHD) with reduced relapse rates.[23] This immune activity is known as the graft-versus-tumor (GVT) or graft-versus-leukemia (GVL) effect and is distinct from but often coincident with GVHD. The GVL effect in children was first described in acute lymphoblastic leukemia (ALL) when the presence of chronic GVHD was associated with a lower relapse rate,[24] and it has been further supported by the comparison of the relapse rates associated with donors with different degrees of immunological mismatch.[25–31] Although acute myeloid leukemia (AML) is a less frequent indication for allogeneic BMT in children, HLA-identical matched HSCT achieves good responses due to a strong GVL effect, especially in first complete remission.[32] GVL effects have also been demonstrated for both juvenile myelomonocytic leukemia[33,34] and myelodysplastic syndrome.[35] There are few data to support an allogeneic T cell response for pediatric lymphoma and Hodgkin disease after transplantation.[36,37]

Graft-versus-tumor effects have also been generated against nonhematological malignancies. Allogeneic HSCT has been used as a therapeutic approach for sarcomas in limited settings, but at the present time offers little benefit for Ewing sarcoma[38–40] or rhabdomyosarcoma.[40–42] Although early studies showed control of pulmonary metastases in osteogenic sarcoma patients by allogeneic HSCT,[43] these findings have not been confirmed by any follow-up studies. Similar to that in adults, an allogeneic effect in pediatric patients with metastatic malignant melanoma that received allogeneic HSCT has been reported.[44] There is evidence that a recurrent ependymoma regressed in a patient that received allogeneic HSCT for leukemia and had chronic GVHD.[45] A durable remission was also achieved after allogeneic HSCT for a patient with metastatic medulloblastoma.[46]

Evidence of a role for T cells in GVL/GVT activity was obtained by comparison of outcomes between patients receiving T cell depleted versus unmanipulated grafts[47] and is further supported in pediatric patients by the correlation of chronic GVHD, primarily a T cell-mediated disease, with reduced relapse rates.[48–50] There has been extensive investigation into the nature of these responding T cells, which are primarily α/β TcR+,[51] and this has culminated in the identification of specific target epitopes recognized by T cells mediating GVT effects.[52,53] These minor histocompatibility (MiHC) antigens, such as HA-1 and HA-2, may provide a potentially powerful tool for enhancing GVT responses against a variety of tumors.[54] A role for NK cells in GVT reactions has also been well documented.[51] The clearest evidence of their importance, however, came with the recent application of haploidentical transplantation based on KIR mismatches.[55,56] In this setting, donors are selected on the basis of KIR expression that would permit NK activity in the graft-versus-host, but not host-versus-graft, direction (Figure 4-2). By eliminating the influence of inhibitory KIR signaling to the donor-derived NK cells, this strategy has enhanced GVL activity, without increasing GVHD, in a number of transplantation studies. Consistent with the original observation of GVL activity against different leukemia types, prevention of relapse by haploidentical transplantation was achieved more effectively for AML patients than for ALL patients. A recent modification of the method to predict KIR mismatch, however, has shown that significant NK activity can be generated against KIR-mismatched pediatric ALL.[57]

Donor lymphocyte infusion (DLI) after HSCT has been shown to significantly augment immune activity against some cancers.[58] The application of this approach has been less effective against pediatric leukemia.[59,60] However, the identification of MiHC targets in GVL that result from differences in antigenic peptide presentation between the MHC-matched donor and recipient,[52,53] the development of improved ex vivo expansion of antigen-specific T cells,[61,62] and an improved understanding of the optimal timing of DLI[63,64] may soon generate successes for the infusion of large numbers of cancer-specific donor T cells into pediatric transplant recipients. Preclinical testing of this strategy has shown that human ALL cells can be eradicated in vivo using ALL-specific CTL in the Non-Obese Diabetic/Severe Combined Immune Deficient mouse model.[65] Further support

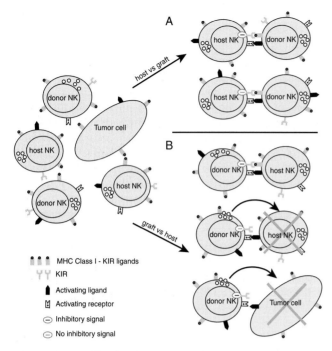

Figure 4-2 NK cell activity in a KIR mismatched transplant setting. (A) Host-vs-graft direction: all KIR on host NK cells are engaged by MHC Class I complexes on donor cells. The negative signal delivered through the bound KIR overrides the signal delivered via the activation receptor, and as a result there is no NK-mediated killing of donor cells. (B) Graft-vs-host direction: a subset of donor NK cells expresses a KIR for which the relevant MHC Class I is absent from host cells. This subset of NK cells receives no negative signal to inhibit the signal delivered through the activation receptor. The resultant killing of host lymphocytes enhances graft survival, while the killing of tumor cells contributes to the GVT effect.

for this approach is provided by the control of viral and virus-associated disease in the post-HSCT setting achieved by the adoptive transfer of antigen-specific T cells.[66,67] The transfer of CTL reactive against latency type-III Epstein-Barr virus (EBV) antigens is now established as an approach for posttransplant lymphoproliferative disease (PTLD).[67] In addition, recent reports of successful adoptive therapy for EBV-associated nasopharyngeal carcinoma indicate that this approach may be applicable to other EBV-related malignancies.[68] It is interesting to note that there has been extensive speculation that some pediatric cancers have a viral etiology.[69–71] The results obtained for EBV-related malignancies suggest that should a viral component of carcinogenesis be identified, adoptive transfer of virus-specific T cells may provide a strong therapeutic benefit.

Pediatric Cancer as a Target for Immune Therapy

Identifying the best targets for T cell immune therapy is a difficult task. The optimal targets or peptide epitopes may be derived from any one, or more, of a substantial number of proteins aberrantly expressed by the malignant cells. Although central and peripheral tolerance mechanisms may cause many potential peptide epitopes to be unsuitable or inefficient targets,[72–74] recent progress has been made in the areas of T cell activation and expansion,[61,62] the use of genomics and proteomics for epitope identification,[75] and understanding and overcoming tolerance.[76]

The array of potential protein targets in pediatric cancer mirrors those recognized in adult malignancy. These include overexpressed proteins (eg, WT1 in leukemia),[77–79] ectopically expressed differentiation antigens (eg, PAX3 in rhabdomyosarcoma),[80] and mutated proteins.[81] One potential source of mutated protein antigens that occurs with far greater frequency in pediatric cancer are the chimeric fusion proteins resulting from chromosomal translocations. The breakpoint region of these proteins represents a tumor-specific target whose expression is required for the transformed phenotype, a situation that may reduce the likelihood of antigen escape variants emerging. Epitopes derived from the breakpoints of several translocation-generated proteins, including ETV6-AML1 and BCR-ABL, have been shown to act as targets for T cell responses.[82–86]

It has recently been shown in studies of identical twins with concordant leukemia that common pediatric chromosomal translocations, involving Mixed Lineage Leukemia fusions, ETV6-AML1, and AML1-ETO, occur predominantly in utero.[87–93] The frequency of fusion-positive cells within individuals indicates that clonal expansion has taken place, suggesting that the preleukemic cells are capable of self-renewal.[94] In some relapsed ETV6-AML1 patients, the leukemic clone present at relapse appears to have been derived from a common preleukemic stem cell that was unaffected by treatment of the initial leukemia.[95,96] These findings have significant implications for the treatment and management of pediatric leukemia because they suggest that treatments that can be directed against the fusion gene may be more effective for preventing relapse than those targeted only to overtly leukemic cells. In this regard, it is encouraging that T cells capable of recognizing the ETV6-AML1 fusion breakpoint peptide can be isolated from pediatric ALL patients, indicating that tolerance through clonal deletion of T cells specific for this peptide has not occurred.[86]

Immune Escape of Pediatric Cancer

The development of cancer can be viewed hypothetically as a failure of immune surveillance to prevent clonal outgrowth of malignant cells, and mechanisms that may contribute to the evasion of host responses by pediatric tumor cells have been identified.[81] These mechanisms include extremely rapid growth (particularly in acute leukemia),[97] loss of MHC Class I antigen presentation (commonly observed in neuroblastoma),[98] down-regulation of costimulatory molecule expression (prevalent in leukemia and lymphoma),[99,100] resistance to cytotoxic mechanisms (observed for NK killing of leukemia),[101,102] and blockade of NK cell activating receptors (described in neuroblastoma).[103] In addition, pediatric cancer patients often display systemic immune defects, such as dysregulated APC function or high levels of immunosuppressive cytokines that are often directly caused by the cancer.[81,104–106] It is widely believed that development of these immune-evasive tumor phenotypes is the direct result of selection by the immune system and renders pediatric cancer a challenging environment in which to generate effective immune therapy.

The outgrowth of variants of the original tumor cell that are not as immunogenic to the immune system results in so-called tumor editing by the immune system[107] and has profound implications for pediatric cancer immune therapy. The specificity and complexity of the protection gained from these phenotypic changes is revealed clearly using neuroblastoma as an example.[108] MHC Class I expression is frequently down-regulated on neuroblastoma cells. Although this event serves to inhibit killing by CTL, as discussed earlier it should also render neuroblastoma cells susceptible to NK cytotoxicity, and indeed this has been confirmed in vitro.[109] However, neuroblastoma cells release soluble forms of the NK cell activating receptor ligands. This leads to down-regulation of activating receptors expressed by NK cells and reduces NK cell cytotoxicity.[103] This demonstrates that neuroblastoma, likely through immune-driven clonal selection, has acquired specific protection from cytotoxicity mediated by T cells and NK cells, two primary mediators of immune therapy. For this reason, immune therapies must be able to exert a significantly greater and ideally wider-ranging antitumor activity to prevent further escape by the tumor cells.

Strategies to Augment Pediatric Tumor-Specific Immune Activity

Several distinct approaches have been taken in the attempt to enhance the generation of T cell responses against pediatric cancers (Table 4-1). One approach is to identify specific peptide targets or epitopes that mediate tumor-specific killing. This approach has been used to identify MiHC antigens involved in the GVT effect after HSCT,[52,53] and to select peptides from a variety of tumor-specific and -associated proteins, including fusion breakpoint region peptides.[83–86,110–112] Once identified, peptide antigens can then be used to induce specific T cell responses in a number of ways, including their presentation by adoptively transferred APC or directly by vaccination. One large study used tumor-specific peptide pulsed onto peripheral blood mononuclear cells as vaccines with IL-2 in rhabdomyosarcoma and Ewing sarcoma but showed no response in advanced disease.[113] Powerful new molecular biology techniques have provided the means to streamline the process of identifying optimal epitopes, and many more candidates are likely to be identified in the next few years.[75] The ability to accurately predict the best candidates in stringent preclinical testing will be critical to the success of this approach.

A second approach to generating specific T cells involves the manipulation of tumor cells to render them more efficient as APC. An advantage of this approach is that it requires no knowledge of suitable leukemia antigens, because the cancer cell will present a full complement of peptides to the responding T cell population. This approach involves the introduction of a variety of cytokine and costimulatory molecule genes into numerous cancer cell types. For example, neuroblastoma cells engineered to express IL-2 have been shown to induce immunologic and to a lesser extent clinical responses against tumor cells.[114,115] A similar approach with lymphotactin and IL-2 secreting allogeneic neuroblastoma cells was able to induce a Th2 type response with IL-4 and IL-5 production, tumor-reactive antibodies, and NK activity.[116] The most promising results have been obtained using tumor cells expressing GM-CSF and CD80 or CD86.[117–122] An alternative strategy to up-regulate costimulatory molecules is through ligation of CD40, an antigen expressed on many leukemia cells.[123] In vitro cross-linking of CD40 leads to increased expression of several costimulatory molecules, including CD80, facilitating the generation of ALL-specific T cells from patient blood and bone marrow.[124–127] Promising early clinical trial results using ALL blasts mixed with fibroblasts expressing CD40 ligand and IL-2 have recently been reported for high-risk pediatric ALL.[128] The use of DNA oligonucleotides containing unmethylated CpG motifs, which mimic the "danger signal" of bacterial DNA, have also recently been shown to increase costimulatory molecule expression on leukemia cells and enhance antitumor T cell activity in vitro.[129]

A third approach to generate antitumor immune responses involves the presentation of leukemia-specific peptide antigens to T cells by professional APC such as dendritic cells. This approach circumvents any APC deficiencies present in the cancer cells. Moreover, when lysates of the tumor cells are used to provide a large number of tumor-derived proteins and peptides, knowledge of the peptide antigen's identity may not be required. This approach was demonstrated to induce antitumor immune activity in children with relapsed solid tumors using patient-derived dendritic cells pulsed with tumor cell lysates.[130] A similar strategy has been employed against gliomas[131] and leukemia.[132] Fusion of dendritic cells with tumor cells has also been used to induce immune activity in children with glioma, with no adverse effects and some immunologic responses induced.[133] A variation on this approach that has recently provided promising results in a neuroblastoma model is the transduction of APC with RNA purified from tumor cells.[134–136] The expression of tumor RNA by the APC, either dendritic cells or activated B cells, leads to the efficient presentation of tumor epitopes to the specific T cells.

Each of the above approaches to generating T cells specific for pediatric cancer cells can be applied to either the *ex vivo* expansion of tumor-specific T cell populations for

Table 4-1

Approaches to generating in vivo anti-cancer adaptive responses.

Approach	Advantages	Disadvantages
Cancer-specific protein or peptide subunit vaccine	Applicable to all patients with suitable MHC Amenable to mass production Ease of multiple administrations	Difficult to identify appropriate targets Limited by immune deficiencies of patient More sensitive to loss of antigen expression
Tumor pulsed APC	Does not require prior antigen identification Presents full array of peptide antigens Circumvents patient APC deficiencies	Patient specific and labor intensive May be limited by tolerance induced by tumor
Tumor cells modified as APC	Does not require prior antigen identification Presents full array of peptide antigens Large number of cells can be generated for multiple administrations	May be limited by lack of MHC expression May not exert full APC activity May be limited by tolerance induced by tumor

adoptive transfer or as the basis of vaccination protocols for the *in vivo* generation of antitumor activity. Although vaccine development remains the more attractive therapeutic approach, the timing of such therapy may be problematic.[137] Adoptive transfer bypasses the immune deficiencies, such as loss of dendritic cell function or treatment-induced immune suppression, that are often observed in cancer patients and that may impede the generation of endogenous immune responses in response to vaccination. An alternative approach to developing tumor-reactive T cells for adoptive transfer is the generation of T cells engineered to express chimeric receptors for proteins present on the surface of tumor cells.[138] These chimeric receptors are composed of an extracellular immunoglobulin variable region that recognizes a protein present on the tumor cell surface (eg, CD19 on leukemia cells) and a cytoplasmic signaling domain (eg, CD3 zeta chain) that mediates an activation signal when the immunoglobulin region binds to its target. Tumor-associated proteins have been developed as targets for several pediatric malignancies, including neuroblastoma, leukemia, lymphoma, rhabdomyosarcoma, and glioblastoma multiforme.[139–144] Binding of these receptors to their targets generates signaling within the T cell that is sufficient to achieve full activation and effector function. One significant advantage of such redirected cytotoxic cells is that they are not MHC restricted and so are insensitive to the loss of MHC antigen presentation frequently observed on pediatric tumors, and they may thus provide an ideal complement to the use of traditionally targeted T cells to prevent the outgrowth of tumor escape variants.

Strategies to augment NK cell-mediated killing of tumor cells have generally involved providing additional stimulation to activate these cells. Most often this approach has utilized IL-2, also a potent growth factor for T cells, to generate highly cytotoxic lymphokine activated killer (LAK) cells.[145] Although LAK cells generated *in vivo* or *ex vivo* have shown enhanced killing of pediatric cancer cells,[146] the results of clinical trials have been generally disappointing.[147–149] While the response to IL-2 post autologous transplant may be dependent on sufficient immune reconstitution,[150] IL-2 in combination with interferon-alpha has successfully induced immune response against lymphoma in this setting.[151] Recently the use of IL-12 and IL-15 has been shown to further augment LAK cell killing.[152–153] In another approach to augment NK cell antitumor activity, the development of NK cells expressing chimeric receptors similar to those described for T cells has shown encouraging preclinical results for pediatric leukemia.[154–155] Lastly, the generation of large numbers of KIR-mismatched donor NK cells for adoptive transfer after haploidentical transplant has been achieved, suggesting that further applications of this technique will soon be available.[156]

Monoclonal Antibody Therapy

One approach to immune therapy that bypasses the need for effector cell activation and targeting is the use of monoclonal antibodies (mAb), one of the most developed immune-based approaches to treatment of adult and pediatric malignancies. The therapeutic mechanism of action of these antibodies is mediated by complement-mediated tumor lysis or antibody-dependent cellular cytotoxicity (ADCC).[157] Alternatively, antibodies that are linked to a cytotoxic agent or radioisotope can be used to deliver an apoptotic signal directly to tumor cells.[158] The pediatric malignancy most evaluated for the effectiveness of mAb

Table 4-2

NCI-sponsored trials using monoclonal antibody therapy for pediatric cancers in 2007.

Antibody	Target	Indication	Phase
Trastuzumab (Herceptin)	Her2	osteosarcoma	II
Alemtuzumab (Campath-1H)	CD52	ALL	II
Gemtuzumab (Mylotarg)	CD33	AML	III
Epratuzumab	CD22	ALL, NHL	II
Ibritumomab tiuxetan (Zevalin)	CD20	NHL	I
Rituximab (Rituxan)	CD20	ALL, NHL	II
Bevacizumab (Avastin)	VEGF	solid tumors	I
Daclizumab (Zenapax)	IL-2R	T cell leukemia/Lymphoma	II
Lexatumumab	TRAIL-R2	solid tumors	I
ch14.18	GD2	neuroblastoma	III
hu14.18-IL2	GD2	neuroblastoma	II
BL22 immunotoxin	CD22	ALL, NHL	I

therapy is neuroblastoma, where antibodies targeting the disialoganglioside GD2 can induce temporary responses in chemotherapy-resistant neuroblastoma, although no improvement in overall therapeutic outcome has been demonstrated.[159-161] Approaches to increase ADCC by activating NK cell effectors with IL-2 also have some promise.[162] Interestingly, failure of monoclonal antibody treatment does not appear to correlate to loss of GD2 antigen expression on the cell surface, suggesting alternative etiologies for treatment failure.[163] Monoclonal antibody therapy is currently being investigated for several pediatric malignancies in addition to neuroblastoma. A list of antibodies currently being evaluated in National Cancer Institute-sponsored clinical trials is shown in Table 4-2. To date, none has had a high enough level of success to be adopted as standard therapy, except for PTLD therapy by anti-CD20 monoclonal antibody.[164]

Challenges for the Development of Immune Therapy Studies

The development of immune therapeutic trials to evaluate efficacy presents a number of logistical challenges. Immune therapy appears to have its greatest effect when the following conditions exist: (a) when only a minimal amount of malignant cells are present; (b) when functional immune effector populations are present in adequate numbers; and (c) when tumor cells express sufficient antigen to be recognized by immune effector cells. Novel approaches are needed to meet the challenges presented by these requirements. Ongoing neuroblastoma treatment trials provide an illustrative example of how state-of-the-art techniques are being applied to immune therapy for pediatric cancer.

The standard of care for neuroblastoma, including consolidation with autologous stem cell transplantation (SCT), produces a 3-year event-free survival of less than 40%.

More recently, there has been an attempt to improve on these results using the strategy of intensifying the consolidation phase with 2 or more cycles of SCT or high-dose chemotherapy with stem cell support. This approach was initially tried using bone marrow as a stem cell source, but was associated with an unacceptable 24% rate of treatment-related mortality.[165] However, the use of peripheral blood stem cells (PBSC) has allowed more rapid clinical recovery from transplant, and several groups have tested tandem SCT supported by PBSC in neuroblastoma.[166-169]

Recovery of cellular immune function after conventional SCT is slow, however, and recovery in patients after tandem SCT is even slower. In a larger (N=138) patient experience of SCT in neuroblastoma, at least four patients experienced EBV lymphoproliferative disease (EBV-LPD) and one patient died of this complication. EBV-LPD is described in the setting of autologous SCT, but it is an uncommon complication.[170-173] This experience indicates that tandem SCT produces profound deficits in functional cellular immunity. Possible causes of this include intensive induction with high doses of cyclophosphamide, intensive consolidation with further immune suppression, plus the inherent T cell depletion that is provided by CD34 selection.[170,174] Here we reach a major challenge in considering immunotherapy for chemotherapy-responsive diseases. Almost certainly, cellular immunotherapy has the best chance of working when the disease burden is lowest, which is at the point of minimal residual disease reached directly after SCT. In contrast, immunotherapeutic approaches might be significantly limited by the period of very low T cell numbers and function that occur for months after such procedures.

In order to address this concern and to provide a foundation for antitumor vaccination in the setting of post-SCT minimal residual disease, a study testing T cell infusions after tandem SCT is now in progress. This study uses the tandem transplant backbone and adds T cell collection by pheresis at diagnosis. These T cells undergo

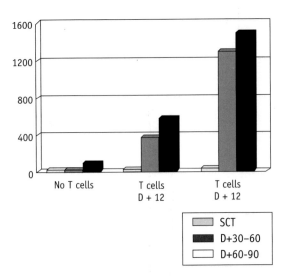

Figure 4-3 Impact of costimulated T cell infusions (T cell augmentation) on CD4+ T cell recovery in children undergoing tandem SCT for neuroblastoma. Absolute number of CD4+ cells in the peripheral blood were determined by flow cytometry at the times indicated, except at the time of SCT, where absolute lymphocyte counts approaching 0 allowed measurement of CD4+ cells in very few patients, and the ALC is presented.

costimulated expansion using the anti-CD3/anti-CD28 system developed by Carl June and colleagues.[175–178] This approach is now called T cell augmentation. Preliminary experience with T cell augmentation shows a significant impact of costimulated T cell infusion on CD4+ cell reconstitution (Figure 4-3). There is also preliminary indication that earlier T cell augmentation (d+2 after PBSC infusion as opposed to d+12) may improve expansion and result in even more robust CD4+ cell reconstitution.[178]

Conclusion

Although immune therapy is relatively unproven, considerable promise now exists for its development against pediatric malignancies. Significant progress has been made in identifying the components of the immune system that exert antitumor activity, and technological advances now provide the means to translate this knowledge into practical clinical treatments. Although it remains to be seen which, if any, of the developing approaches will attain integration into standard treatment protocols, there is much reason to be optimistic that future successes will indeed be achieved.

References

1. Reaman GH. Pediatric cancer research from past successes through collaboration to future transdisciplinary research. *J Pediatr Oncol Nurs.* 2004;21:123–127.
2. Davis MM, Bjorkman PJ. T-cell antigen receptor genes and T-cell. *Nature.* 1988. 334:395–402.
3. Matis LA. The molecular basis of T-cell specificity. *Annu Rev Immunol.* 1990;8:65–82.
4. Bennett SR, Carbone FR, Karamalis F, Miller JF, Heath WR. Induction of a CD8+ cytotoxic T lymphocyte response by cross-priming requires cognate CD4+ T cell help. *J Exp Med.* 1997;186(1):65–70.
5. York IA, Rock KL. Antigen processing and presentation by the class I major histocompatibility complex. *Annu Rev Immunol.* 1996;14:369–396.
6. Cresswell P. Assembly, transport, and function of MHC class II molecules. *Annu Rev Immunol.* 1994;12:259–293.
7. Trombetta ES, Mellman I. Cell biology of antigen processing in vitro and in vivo. *Annu Rev Immunol.* 2005;23:975–1028.
8. Bretscher P, Cohn M. A theory of self-nonself discrimination. *Science.* 1970. 169:1042–1049.
9. Schwartz RH. A cell culture model for T lymphocyte clonal anergy. *Science.* 1990;248:1349–1356.
10. Diehl L, Den Boer AT, van der Voort EI, Melief CJ, Offringa R, Toes RE. The role of CD40 in peripheral T cell tolerance and immunity. *J Mol Med.* 2000; 78:363–371.
11. Greenwald RJ, Freeman GJ, Sharpe AH. The B7 family revisited. *Annu Rev Immunol.* 2005;23:515–548.
12. Watts TH. TNF/TNFR family members in costimulation of T cell responses. *Annu Rev Immunol.* 2005;23:23–68.
13. Appleman LJ, Boussiotis VA. T cell anergy and costimulation. *Immunol Rev.* 2003;192:161–180.
14. Heath WR, Carbone FR. Cross-presentation, dendritic cells, tolerance and immunity. *Annu Rev Immunol.* 2001;19:47–64.
15. Mosmann TR, Sad S. The expanding universe of T-cell subsets: Th1, Th2 and more. *Immunol Today.* 1996;17:138–146.
16. Constant SL, Bottomly K. Induction of Th1 and Th2 CD4+ T cell responses: the alternative approaches. *Annu Rev Immunol.* 1997;15:297–322.
17. Zou W. Regulatory T cells, tumour immunity and immunotherapy. *Nat Rev Immunol.* 2006;6:295–307.
18. Baecher-Allan C, Anderson DE. Immune regulation in tumor-bearing hosts. *Curr Opin Immunol.* 2006;18:214–219.
19. Lanier LL. NK cell receptors. *Annu Rev Immunol.* 1998;16:359–393.
20. Ljunggren HG, Karre K. In search of the "missing self": MHC molecules and NK cell recognition. *Immunol Today.* 1990;11:237–244.
21. Young JD, Liu CC, Persechini PM, Cohn ZA. Perforin-dependent and -independent pathways of cytotoxicity mediated by lymphocytes. *Immunol Rev.* 1988;103:161–202.
22. Montoya MC, Sancho D, Vicente-Manzanares M, Sanchez-Madrid F. Cell adhesion and polarity during immune interactions. *Immunol Rev.* 2002;186: 68–82.
23. Weiden PL, Sullivan KM, Flournoy N, Storb R, Thomas ED. Antileukemic effect of chronic graft-versus-host disease: contribution to improved survival after allogeneic marrow transplantation. *N Engl J Med.* 1981;304:1529–1533.
24. Sanders JE, Flournoy N, Thomas ED, et al. Marrow transplant experience in children with acute lymphoblastic leukemia: an analysis of factors associated with survival, relapse, and graft-versus-host disease. *Med Pediatr Oncol.* 1985;13:165–172.
25. Marmont AM, Horowitz MM, Gale RP, et al. T-cell depletion of HLA-identical transplants in leukemia. *Blood.* 1991;78:2120–2130.
26. Rocha V, Cornish J, Sievers EL, et al. Comparison of outcomes of unrelated bone marrow and umbilical cord blood transplants in children with acute leukemia. *Blood.* 2001;97:2962–2971.
27. Horowitz MM, Gale RP, Sondel PM, et al. Graft-versus-leukemia reactions after bone marrow transplantation. *Blood.* 1990;75:555–562.
28. Ringden O, Labopin M, Gorin NC, et al. Is there a graft-versus-leukaemia effect in the absence of graft-versus-host disease in patients undergoing bone marrow transplantation for acute leukaemia? *Br J Haematol.* 2000;111: 1130–1137.
29. Barrett AJ, Ringden O, Zhang MJ, et al. Effect of nucleated marrow cell dose on relapse and survival in identical twin bone marrow transplants for leukemia. *Blood.* 2000;95:3323–3327.
30. Weisdorf D, Bishop M, Dharan B, et al. Autologous versus allogeneic unrelated donor transplantation for acute lymphoblastic leukemia: comparative toxicity and outcomes. *Biol Blood Marrow Transplant.* 2002;8:213–220.
31. Bunin N, Carston M, Wall D, et al. Unrelated marrow transplantation for children with acute lymphoblastic leukemia in second remission. *Blood.* 2002;99:3151–3157.
32. Neudorf S, Sanders J, Kobrinsky N, et al. Allogeneic bone marrow transplantation for children with acute myelocytic leukemia in first remission demonstrates a role for graft versus leukemia in the maintenance of disease-free survival. *Blood.* 2004;103(10):3655–3661.
33. Korthof ET, Snijder PP, de Graaff AA, et al. Allogeneic bone marrow transplantation for juvenile myelomonocytic leukemia: a single center experience of 23 patients. *Bone Marrow Transplant.* 2005;35(5):455–461.
34. Pulsipher MA, Adams RH, Asch J, Petersen FB. Successful treatment of JMML relapsed after unrelated allogeneic transplant with cytoreduction followed by DLI and interferon-alpha: evidence for a graft-versus-leukemia effect in non-monosomy-7 JMML. *Bone Marrow Transplant.* 2004;33(1):113–115.
35. Bader P, Stoll K, Huber S, et al. Characterization of lineage-specific chimaerism in patients with acute leukaemia and myelodysplastic syndrome after allogeneic stem cell transplantation before and after relapse. *Br J Haematol.* 2000;108(4):761–768.
36. Levine JE, Harris RE, Loberiza FR Jr, et al. Lymphoma Study Writing Committee, International Bone Marrow Transplant Registry and Autologous Blood and Marrow Transplant Registry. A comparison of allogeneic and autologous bone marrow transplantation for lymphoblastic lymphoma. *Blood.* 2003;101(7):2476–2482.
37. Bierman PJ, Sweetenham JW, Loberiza FR Jr, et al. Syngeneic hematopoietic stem-cell transplantation for non-Hodgkin's lymphoma: a comparison with allogeneic and autologous transplantation—The Lymphoma Working Com-

mittee of the International Bone Marrow Transplant Registry and the European Group for Blood and Marrow Transplantation. *J Clin Oncol.* 2003; 21(20):3744–3753.

38. Frohlich B, Ahrens S, Burdach S, et al. High-dosage chemotherapy in primary metastasized and relapsed Ewing's sarcoma. *Klin Padiatr.* 1999;211(4):284–290.

39. Burdach S, van Kaick B, Laws HJ, et al. Allogeneic and autologous stem-cell transplantation in advanced Ewing tumors. *Ann Oncol.* 2000;11(11):1451–1462.

40. Pedrazzoli P, Da Prada GA, Giorgiani G, et al. Allogeneic blood stem cell transplantation after a reduced-intensity, preparative regimen: a pilot study in patients with refractory malignancies. *Cancer.* 2002;94(9):2409–2415.

41. Chan KW, Rogers PC, Fryer CJ. Breast metastases after bone marrow transplantation for rhabdomyosarcoma. *Bone Marrow Transplant.* 1991;7(2):171–172.

42. Misawa A, Hosoi H, Tsuchiya K, Iehara T, Sawada T, Sugimoto T. Regression of refractory rhabdomyosarcoma after allogeneic stem-cell transplantation. *Pediatr Hematol Oncol.* 2003;20(2):151–155.

43. Esartia PT, Deichman GI, Kluchareva TE, Matveeva VA, Uvarova EN, Trapesnikov NN. Allogenic bone-marrow transfusion suppresses development of lung metastases in osteogenic sarcoma patients after radical surgery. *Int J Cancer.* 1993;54(6):907–910.

44. Kasow KA, Handgretinger R, Krasin MJ, Pappo AS, Leung W. Possible allogeneic graft-versus-tumor effect in childhood melanoma. *J Pediatr Hematol Oncol.* 2003;25(12):982–986.

45. Tanaka M, Shibui S, Kobayashi Y, Nomura K, Nakanishi Y. A graft-versus-tumor effect in a patient with ependymoma who received an allogenic bone marrow transplant for therapy-related leukemia. Case report. *J Neurosurg.* 2002;97(2):474–476.

46. Lundberg JH, Weissman DE, Beatty PA, Ash RC. Treatment of recurrent metastatic medulloblastoma with intensive chemotherapy and allogeneic bone marrow transplantation. *J Neurooncol.* 1992;13(2):151–155.

47. Horowitz MM, Gale RP, Sondel PM, et al. Graft-versus-leukemia reactions after bone marrow transplantation. *Blood.* 1990;75:555–562.

48. Uzunel M, Mattsson J, Jaksch M, Remberger M, Ringden O. The significance of graft-versus-host disease and pretransplantation minimal residual disease status to outcome after allogeneic stem cell transplantation in patients with acute lymphoblastic leukemia. *Blood.* 2001;98:1982–1984.

49. Gustafsson Jernberg A, Remberger M, Ringden O, Winiarski J. Graft-versus-leukaemia effect in children: chronic GVHD has a significant impact on relapse and survival. *Bone Marrow Transplant.* 2003;31:175–181.

50. Nordlander A, Mattsson J, Ringden O, et al. Graft-versus-host disease is associated with a lower relapse incidence after hematopoietic stem cell transplantation in patients with acute lymphoblastic leukemia. *Biol Blood Marrow Transplant.* 2004;10(3):195–203.

51. Barrett AJ. Mechanisms of the graft-versus-leukemia reaction. *Stem Cells.* 1997;15:248–258.

52. Warren EH, Greenberg PD, Riddell SR. Cytotoxic T-lymphocyte-defined human minor histocompatibility antigens with a restricted tissue distribution. *Blood.* 1998;91:2197–2207.

53. Dolstra H, Fredrix H, Preijers F, et al. Recognition of a B cell leukemia-associated minor histocompatibility antigen by CTL. *J Immunol.* 1997;158:560–565.

54. Falkenburg JH, van de Corput L, Marijt EW, Willemze R. Minor histocompatibility antigens in human stem cell transplantation. *Exp Hematol.* 2003;31:743–751.

55. Ruggeri L, Capanni M, Urbani E, et al. Effectiveness of donor natural killer cell alloreactivity in mismatched hematopoietic transplants. *Science.* 2002; 295:2097–2100.

56. Ruggeri L, Capanni M, Casucci M, et al. Role of natural killer cell alloreactivity in HLA-mismatched hematopoietic stem cell transplantation. *Blood.* 1999; 94:333–339.

57. Leung W, Iyengar R, Turner V. Determinants of antileukemia effects of allogeneic NK cells. *J Immunol.* 2004;172:644–650.

58. Kolb HJ, Schmid C, Barrett AJ, Schendel DJ. Graft-versus-leukemia reactions in allogeneic chimeras. *Blood.* 2004;103:767–776.

59. Collins RH Jr, Goldstein S, Giralt S, et al. Donor leukocyte infusions in acute lymphocytic leukemia. *Bone Marrow Transplant.* 2000;26(5):511.

60. Kolb HJ, Schattenberg A, Goldman JM, et al. Graft-versus-leukemia effect of donor lymphocyte transfusions in marrow grafted patients. *Blood.* 1995;86:2041–2050.

61. Vonderheide RH, June CH. A translational bridge to cancer immunotherapy: exploiting costimulation and target antigens for active and passive T cell immunotherapy. *Immunol Res.* 2003;27:341–356.

62. Cardoso AA, Seamon MJ, Afonso HM, et al. Ex vivo generation of human anti-pre-B leukemia-specific autologous cytolytic T cells. *Blood.* 1997;90(2):549–561.

63. Gorczynska E, Turkiewicz D, Toporski J, et al. Prompt initiation of immunotherapy in children with an increasing number of autologous cells after allogeneic HCT can induce complete donor-type chimerism: a report of 14 children. *Bone Marrow Transplant.* 2004;33:211–217.

64. Bader P, Kreyenberg H, Hoelle W, et al. Increasing mixed chimerism is an important prognostic factor for unfavorable outcome in children with acute

lymphoblastic leukemia after allogeneic stem-cell transplantation: possible role for pre-emptive immunotherapy? *J Clin Oncol.* 2004;22:1696–1705.

65. Hambach L, Nijmeijer BA, Aghai Z, et al. Human cytotoxic T lymphocytes specific for a single minor histocompatibility antigen HA-1 are effective against human lymphoblastic leukaemia in NOD/SCID mice. *Leukemia.* 2006;20:371–374.

66. Gottschalk S, Heslop HE, Rooney CM. Adoptive immunotherapy for EBV-associated malignancies. *Leuk Lymphoma.* 2005;46:1–10.

67. Straathof KC, Bollard CM, Rooney CM, Heslop HE. Immunotherapy for Epstein-Barr virus-associated cancers in children. *Oncologist.* 2003;8:83–98.

68. Straathof KC, Bollard CM, Popat U, et al. Treatment of nasopharyngeal carcinoma with Epstein-Barr virus-specific T lymphocytes. *Blood.* 2005;105:1898–1904.

69. McNally RJ, Eden TO. An infectious aetiology for childhood acute leukaemia: a review of the evidence. *Br J Haematol.* 2004;127:243–263.

70. Greaves M. Pre-natal origins of childhood leukemia. *Rev Clin Exp Hematol.* 2003;7:233–245.

71. Smith M. Considerations on a possible viral etiology for B-precursor acute lymphoblastic leukemia of childhood. *J Immunother.* 1997;20:89–100.

72. Arnold B. Levels of peripheral T cell tolerance. *Transpl Immunol.* 2002;10:109–114.

73. Kyewski B, Klein L. A central role for central tolerance. *Annu Rev Immunol.* 2006;24:571–606.

74. Pardoll D. Does the immune system see tumors as foreign or self? *Annu Rev Immunol.* 2003;21:807–839.

75. Maia S, Haining WN, Ansen S, et al. Gene expression profiling identifies BAX-delta as a novel tumor antigen in acute lymphoblastic leukemia. *Cancer Res.* 2005;65:10050–10058.

76. Mapara MY, Sykes M. Tolerance and cancer: mechanisms of tumor evasion and strategies for breaking tolerance. *J Clin Oncol.* 2004;22:1136–1151.

77. Siehl JM, Reinwald M, Heufelder K, Menssen HD, Keilholz U, Thiel E. Expression of Wilms' tumor gene 1 at different stages of acute myeloid leukemia and analysis of its major splice variants. *Ann Hematol.* 2004;83(12):745–750.

78. Lapillonne H, Renneville A, Auvrignon A, et al. High WT1 expression after induction therapy predicts high risk of relapse and death in pediatric acute myeloid leukemia. *J Clin Oncol.* 2006;24(10):1507–1515.

79. Cilloni D, Gottardi E, Saglio G. WT1 overexpression in acute myeloid leukemia and myelodysplastic syndromes. *Methods Mol Med.* 2006;125:199–211.

80. Epstein JA, Lam P, Jepeal L, Maas RL, Shapiro DN. Pax3 inhibits myogenic differentiation of cultured myoblast cells. *J Biol Chem.* 1995;270(20):11719–11722.

81. Rousseau RF, Brenner MK. Vaccine therapies for pediatric malignancies. *Cancer J.* 2005;11(4):331–339.

82. Mackall CL, Helman LJ. Targeting pediatric malignancies for T cell-mediated immune responses. *Curr Oncol Rep.* 2000;2:539–546.

83. Chen W, Peace DJ, Rovira DK, You SG, Cheever MA. T-cell immunity to the joining region of p210BCR-ABL protein. *Proc Natl Acad Sci USA.* 1992;89:1468.

84. Pawelec G, Max H, Halder T, et al. BCR/ABL leukemia oncogene fusion peptides selectively bind to certain HLA-DR alleles and can be recognized by T cells found at low frequency in the repertoire of normal donors. *Blood.* 1996; 88:2118.

85. Gambacorti-Passerini C, Grignani F, Arienti F, Pandolfi PP, Pelicci PG, Parmiani G. Human CD4 lymphocytes specifically recognize a peptide representing the fusion region of the hybrid protein pml/RAR alpha present in acute promyelocytic leukemia cells. *Blood.* 1993;81:1369.

86. Yotnda P, Garcia F, Peuchmaur M, et al. Cytotoxic T cell response against the chimeric ETV6-AML1 protein in childhood acute lymphoblastic leukemia. *J Clin Invest.* 1998;102:455–462.

87. Ford AM, Ridge SA, Cabrera ME, et al. In utero rearrangements in the trithorax-related oncogene in infant leukaemias. *Nature.* 1993;363:358–360.

88. Ford AM, Bennett CA, Price CM, Bruin MC, Van Wering ER, Greaves M. Fetal origins of the TEL-AML1 fusion gene in identical twins with leukemia. *Proc Natl Acad Sci USA.* 1998;95:4584–4588.

89. Wiemels JL, Ford AM, Van Wering ER, Postma A, Greaves M. Protracted and variable latency of acute lymphoblastic leukemia after TEL-AML1 gene fusion in utero. *Blood.* 1999;94:1057–1062.

90. Gale KB, Ford AM, Repp R, et al. Backtracking leukemia to birth: identification of clonotypic gene fusion sequences in neonatal blood spots. *Proc Natl Acad Sci USA.* 1997;94:13950–13954.

91. Wiemels JL, Cazzaniga G, Daniotti M, et al. Prenatal origin of acute lymphoblastic leukaemia in children. *Lancet.* 1999;354:1499–1503.

92. Wiemels JL, Xiao Z, Buffler PA, et al. In utero origin of t(8;21) AML1-ETO translocations in childhood acute myeloid leukemia. *Blood.* 2002;99:3801–3805.

93. Hjalgrim LL, Madsen HO, Melbye M, et al. Presence of clone-specific markers at birth in children with acute lymphoblastic leukaemia. *Br J Cancer.* 2002;87:994–999.

94. Mori H, Colman SM, Xiao Z, et al. Chromosome translocations and covert leukemic clones are generated during normal fetal development. *Proc Natl Acad Sci USA.* 2002;99:8242–8247.

95. Ford AM, Fasching K, Panzer-Grumayer ER, Koenig M, Haas OA, Greaves MF. Origins of "late" relapse in childhood acute lymphoblastic leukemia with TEL-AML1 fusion genes. *Blood.* 2001;98:558–564.

96. Konrad M, Metzler M, Panzer S, et al. Late relapses evolve from slow-responding subclones in t(12;21) positive acute lymphoblastic leukemia: evidence for the persistence of a preleukemic clone. *Blood.* 2003;101: 3635–3640.

97. Nijmeijer BA, van Schie ML, Verzaal P, Willemze R, Falkenburg JH. Responses to donor lymphocyte infusion for acute lymphoblastic leukemia may be determined by both qualitative and quantitative limitations of antileukemic T-cell responses as observed in an animal model for human leukemia. *Exp Hematol.* 2005;33(10):1172–1181.

98. Raffaghello L, Prigione I, Bocca P, et al. Multiple defects of the antigen-processing machinery components in human neuroblastoma: immunotherapeutic implications. *Oncogene.* 2005;24:4634–4644.

99. Alessandri AJ, Reid GS, Bader SA, Massing BG, Sorensen PH, Schultz KR. ETV6 (TEL)-AML1 pre-B acute lymphoblastic leukaemia cells are associated with a distinct antigen-presenting phenotype. *Br J Haematol.* 2002;116: 266–272.

100. Cardoso AA, Schultze JL, Boussiotis VA, et al. Pre-B acute lymphoblastic leukemia cells may induce T-cell anergy to alloantigen. *Blood.* 1996;88:41–48.

101. Reid GS, Bharya S, Klingemann HG, Schultz KR. Differential killing of pre-B acute lymphoblastic leukaemia cells by activated NK cells and the NK-92 ci cell line. *Clin Exp Immunol.* 2002;129:265–271.

102. Romanski A, Bug G, Becker S, et al. Mechanisms of resistance to natural killer cell-mediated cytotoxicity in acute lymphoblastic leukemia. *Exp Hematol.* 2005;33:344–352.

103. Raffaghello L, Prigione I, Airoldi I, et al. Downregulation and/or release of NKG2D ligands as immune evasion strategy of human neuroblastoma. *Neoplasia.* 2004;6(5):558–568.

104. Redlinger RE Jr, Mailliard RB, Barksdale EM Jr. Neuroblastoma and dendritic cell function. *Semin Pediatr Surg.* 2004;13:61–71.

105. Maecker B, Mougiakakos D, Zimmermann M, et al. Dendritic cell deficiencies in pediatric acute lymphoblastic leukemia patients. *Leukemia.* 2006;20:645–649.

106. Weller M, Fontana A. The failure of current immunotherapy for malignant glioma. Tumor-derived TGF-beta, T-cell apoptosis, and the immune privilege of the brain. *Brain Res Rev.* 1995;21(2):128–151.

107. Dunn GP, Old LJ, Schreiber RD. The three Es of cancer immunoediting. *Annu Rev Immunol.* 2004;22:329–360.

108. Raffaghello L, Prigione I, Airoldi I, et al. Mechanisms of immune evasion of human neuroblastoma. *Cancer Lett.* 2005;228(1–2):155–161.

109. Sivori S, Parolini S, Marcenaro E, et al. Involvement of natural cytotoxicity receptors in human natural killer cell-mediated lysis of neuroblastoma and glioblastoma cell lines. *J Neuroimmunol.* 2000. 107:220–225.

110. Van Driessche A, Gao L, Stauss HJ, et al. Antigen-specific cellular immunotherapy of leukemia. *Leukemia.* 2005;19:1863–1871.

111. Rosenfeld C, Cheever MA, Gaiger A. WT1 in acute leukemia, chronic myelogenous leukemia and myelodysplastic syndrome: therapeutic potential of WT1 targeted therapies. *Leukemia.* 2003;17:1301–1312.

112. van den Broeke LT, Pendleton CD, Mackall C, Helman LJ, Berzofsky JA. Identification and epitope enhancement of a PAX-FKHR fusion protein breakpoint epitope in alveolar rhabdomyosarcoma cells created by a tumorigenic chromosomal translocation inducing CTL capable of lysing human tumors. *Cancer Res.* 2006;66:1818–1823.

113. Dagher R, Long LM, Read EJ, et al. Pilot trial of tumor-specific peptide vaccination and continuous infusion interleukin-2 in patients with recurrent Ewing sarcoma and alveolar rhabdomyosarcoma: an inter-institute NIH study. *Med Pediatr Oncol.* 2002;38(3):158–164.

114. Bowman L, Grossmann M, Rill D, et al. IL-2 adenovector-transduced autologous tumor cells induce antitumor immune responses in patients with neuroblastoma. *Blood.* 1998;92(6):1941–1949.

115. Bowman LC, Grossmann M, Rill D, et al. Interleukin-2 gene-modified allogeneic tumor cells for treatment of relapsed neuroblastoma. *Hum Gene Ther.* 1998;9(9):1303–1311.

116. Rousseau RF, Haight AE, Hirschmann-Jax C, et al. Local and systemic effects of an allogeneic tumor cell vaccine combining transgenic human lymphotactin with interleukin-2 in patients with advanced or refractory neuroblastoma. *Blood.* 2003;101(5):1718–1726.

117. Cignetti A, Guarini A, Carbone A, et al. Transduction of the IL2 gene into human acute leukemia cells: induction of tumor rejection without modifying cell proliferation and IL2 receptor expression. *J Natl Cancer Inst.* 1994;86: 785–791.

118. Parney IF, Farr-Jones MA, Kane K, Chang LJ, Petruk KC. Human autologous in vitro models of glioma immunogene therapy using B7-2, GM-CSF, and IL12. *Can J Neurol Sci.* 2002;29:267–275.

119. Yoshida H, Tanabe M, Miyauchi M, et al. Induced immunity by expression of interleukin-2 or GM-CSF gene in murine neuroblastoma cells can generate antitumor response to established tumors. *Cancer Gene Ther.* 1999;6:395–401.

120. Stripecke R, Skelton DC, Pattengale PK, Shimada H, Kohn DB. Combination of CD80 and granulocyte-macrophage colony-stimulating factor coexpression by a leukemia cell vaccine: preclinical studies in a murine model recapitulating Philadelphia chromosome-positive acute lymphoblastic leukemia. *Hum Gene Ther.* 1999;10(13):2109–2122.

121. Vereecque R, Buffenoir G, Preudhomme C, et al. Gene transfer of GM-CSF, CD80 and CD154 cDNA enhances survival in a murine model of acute leukemia with persistence of a minimal residual disease. *Gene Ther.* 2000;7: 1312–1316.

122. Stripecke R, Cardoso AA, Pepper KA, et al. Lentiviral vectors for efficient delivery of CD80 and granulocyte-macrophage-colony-stimulating factor in human acute lymphoblastic leukemia and acute myeloid leukemia cells to induce antileukemic immune responses. *Blood.* 2000;96:1317–1326.

123. D'Amico G, Marin V, Biondi A, Bonamino MH. Potential use of CD40 ligand for immunotherapy of childhood B-cell precursor acute lymphoblastic leukaemia. *Best Pract Res Clin Haematol.* 2004;17:465–477.

124. Cardoso AA, Seamon MJ, Afonso HM, et al. Ex vivo generation of human anti-pre-B leukemia-specific autologous cytolytic T cells. *Blood.* 1997;90: 549–561.

125. Schultze JL, Anderson KC, Gilleece MH, Gribben JG, Nadler LM. A pilot study of combined immunotherapy with autologous adoptive tumour-specific T-cell transfer, vaccination with CD40-activated malignant B cells and interleukin 2. *Br J Haematol.* 2001;113:455–460.

126. Todisco E, Gaipa G, Biagi E, et al. CD40 ligand-stimulated B cell precursor leukemic cells el cit interferon-gamma production by autologous bone marrow T cells in childhood acute lymphoblastic leukemia. *Leukemia.* 2002;16: 2046–2054.

127. D'Amico G, Vulcano M, Bugarin C, et al. CD40 activation of BCP-ALL cells generates IL-10-producing, IL-12-defective APCs that induce allogeneic T-cell anergy. *Blood.* 2004;104:744–751.

128. Rousseau RF, Biagi E, Dutour A, et al. Immunotherapy of high-risk acute leukemia with a recipient (autologous) vaccine expressing transgenic human CD40L and IL-2 after chemotherapy and allogeneic stem cell transplantation. *Blood.* 2006;107(4):1332–1341.

129. Reid GS, She K, Terrett L, et al. CpG stimulation of precursor B lineage acute lymphoblastic leukemia induces a distinct change in costimulatory molecule expression and shifts allogeneic T cells towards a Th1 response. *Blood.* 2005;105:3641–3647.

130. Geiger J, Hutchinson R, Hohenkirk L, McKenna E, Chang A, Mule J. Treatment of solid tumours in children with tumour-lysate-pulsed dendritic cells. *Lancet.* 2000;356(9236):1163–1165.

131. De Vleeschouwer S, Van Calenbergh F, Demaerel P, et al. Transient local response and persistent tumor control in a child with recurrent malignant glioma: treatment with combination therapy including dendritic cell therapy. Case report. *J Neurosurg.* 2004;100(5)(Suppl Pediatrics):492–497.

132. Montagna D, Maccario R, Montini E, et al. Generation and ex vivo expansion of cytotoxic T lymphocytes directed toward different types of leukemia or myelodysplastic cells using both HLA-matched and partially matched donors. *Exp Hematol.* 2003;31:1031–1038.

133. Kikuchi T, Akasaki Y, Abe T, et al. Vaccination of glioma patients with fusions of dendritic and glioma cells and recombinant human interleukin 12. *J Immunother.* 2004;27(6):452–459.

134. Jarnjak-Jankovic S, Pettersen RD, Saeboe-Larssen S, Wesenberg F, Olafsen MR, Gaudernack G. Preclinical evaluation of autologous dendritic cells transfected with mRNA or loaded with apoptotic cells for immunotherapy of high-risk neuroblastoma. *Cancer Gene Ther.* 2005;12:699–707.

135. Coughlin CM, Vance BA, Grupp SA, Vonderheide RH. RNA-transfected CD40-activated B cells induce functional T-cell responses against viral and tumor antigen targets: implications for pediatric immunotherapy. *Blood.* 2004;103:2046–2054.

136. Caruso DA, Orme LM, Neale AM, et al. Results of a phase 1 study utilizing monocyte-derived dendritic cells pulsed with tumor RNA in children and young adults with brain cancer. *Neuro Oncol.* 2004;6:236–246.

137. Haining WN, Cardoso AA, Keczkemethy HL, et al. Failure to define window of time for autologous tumor vaccination in patients with newly diagnosed or relapsed acute lymphoblastic leukemia. *Exp Hematol.* 2005;33:286–294.

138. Rossig C, Brenner MK. Chimeric T-cell receptors for the targeting of cancer cells. *Acta Haematol.* 2003;110:154–159.

139. Rossig C, Bollard CM, Nuchtern JG, Merchant DA, Brenner MK. Targeting of G(D2)-positive tumor cells by human T lymphocytes engineered to express chimeric T-cell receptor genes. *Int J Cancer.* 2001;94:228–236.

140. Jensen MC, Cooper LJ, Wu AM, Forman SJ, Raubitschek A. Engineered CD20-specific primary human cytotoxic T lymphocytes for targeting B-cell malignancy. *Cytotherapy.* 2003;5:131–138.

141. Kahlon KS, Brown C, Cooper LJ, Raubitschek A, Forman SJ, Jensen MC. Specific recognition and killing of glioblastoma multiforme by interleukin 13-zetakine redirected cytolytic T cells. *Cancer Res.* 2004;64(24):9160–9166.

142. Cooper LJ, Al-Kadhimi Z, Serrano LM, et al. Enhanced antilymphoma efficacy of CD19-redirected influenza MP1-specific CTLs by cotransfer of T cells modified to present influenza MP1. *Blood.* 2005;105:1622–1631.

143. Zhang T, Lemoi BA, Sentman CL. Chimeric NK-receptor-bearing T cells mediate antitumor immunotherapy. *Blood.* 2005;106:1544–1551.

144. Gattenlohner S, Marx A, Markfort B, et al. Rhabdomyosarcoma lysis by T cells expressing a human autoantibody-based chimeric receptor targeting the fetal acetylcholine receptor. *Cancer Res.* 2006;66:24–28.

145. Rosenberg SA, Lotze MT. Cancer immunotherapy using Interleukin-2 and Interleukin-2-activated lymphocytes. *Annu Rev Immunol.* 1986;4:681–709.

146. Parrado A, Rodriguez-Fernandez JM, Casares S, et al. Generation of LAK cells in vitro in patients with acute leukemia. *Leukemia.* 1993;7:1344–1348.

147. Messina C, Zambello R, Rossetti F, et al. Interleukin-2 before and/or after autologous bone marrow transplantation for pediatric acute leukemia patients. *Bone Marrow Transplant.* 1996;17:729–735.
148. Maraninchi D, Vey N, Viens P, Stoppa AM, et al. A phase II study of interleukin-2 in 49 patients with relapsed or refractory acute leukemia. *Leuk Lymphoma.* 1998;31:343–349.
149. Bauer M, Reaman GH, Hank JA, et al. A phase II trial of human recombinant interleukin-2 administered as a 4-day continuous infusion for children with refractory neuroblastoma, non-Hodgkin's lymphoma, sarcoma, renal cell carcinoma, and malignant melanoma. A Children's Cancer Group study. *Cancer.* 1995;75(12):2959–2965.
150. Bonig H, Laws HJ, Wundes A, et al. In vivo cytokine responses to interleukin-2 immunotherapy after autologous stem cell transplantation in children with solid tumors. *Bone Marrow Transplant.* 2000;26(1):91–96.
151. Nagler A, Ackerstein A, Or R, Naparstek E, Slavin S. Immunotherapy with recombinant human interleukin-2 and recombinant interferon-alpha in lymphoma patients postautologous marrow or stem cell transplantation. *Blood.* 1997;89(11):3951–3959.
152. Torelli GF, Guarini A, Maggio R, et al. Expansion of natural killer cells with lytic activity against autologous blasts from adult and pediatric acute lymphoid leukemia patients in complete hematologic remission. *Haematologica.* 2005;90:785–792.
153. Gruber TA, Skelton DC, Kohn DB. Recombinant murine interleukin-12 elicits potent antileukemic immune responses in a murine model of Philadelphia chromosome-positive acute lymphoblastic leukemia. *Cancer Gene Ther.* 2005;12:818–824.
154. Schirrmann T, Pecher G. Specific targeting of CD33(+) leukemia cells by a natural killer cell line modified with a chimeric receptor. *Leuk Res.* 2005;29:301–306.
155. Imai C, Iwamoto S, Campana D. Genetic modification of primary natural killer cells overcomes inhibitory signals and induces specific killing of leukemic cells. *Blood.* 2005;106:376–383.
156. Koehl U, Esser R, Zimmermann S, et al. Ex vivo expansion of highly purified NK cells for immunotherapy after haploidentical stem cell transplantation in children. *Klin Padiatr.* 2005;217(6):345–350.
157. Schaedel O, Reiter Y. Antibodies and their fragments as anti-cancer agents. *Curr Pharm Des.* 2006;12(3):363–378.
158. Modak S, Cheung NK. Antibody-based targeted radiation to pediatric tumors. *J Nucl Med.* 2005;46(Suppl 1):157S–63S.
159. Yu AL, Uttenreuther-Fischer MM, Huang CS, et al. Phase I trial of a human-mouse chimeric anti-disialoganglioside monoclonal antibody ch14.18 in patients with refractory neuroblastoma and osteosarcoma. *J Clin Oncol.* 1998;16(6):2169–2180.
160. Simon T, Hero B, Faldum A. Consolidation treatment with chimeric anti-GD2-antibody ch14.18 in children older than 1 year with metastatic neuroblastoma. *J Clin Oncol.* 2004;22:17:3549–3557.
161. Simon T, Hero B, Faldum A. Infants with stage 4 neuroblastoma: the impact of the chimeric anti-GD2-antibody ch14.18 consolidation therapy. *Klin Padiatr.* 2005;217(3):147–152.
162. Hank JA, Surfus J, Gan J, et al. Treatment of neuroblastoma patients with antiganglioside GD2 antibody plus interleukin-2 induces antibody-dependent cellular cytotoxicity against neuroblastoma detected *in vitro. J Immunother.* 1994;15(1):29–37.
163. Kramer K, Gerald WL, Kushner BH, Larson SM, Hameed M, Cheung NK. Disialoganglioside G(D2) loss following monoclonal antibody therapy is rare in neuroblastoma. *Clin Cancer Res.* 1998;4(9):2135–2139.
164. Pescovitz MD. The use of rituximab, anti-CD20 monoclonal antibody, in pediatric transplantation. *Pediatr Transplant.* 2004;8(1):9–21.
165. Philip T, Ladenstein R, Zucker JM, et al. Double megatherapy and autologous bone marrow transplantation for advanced neuroblastoma: the LMCE2 Study. *Br J Cancer.* 1993;67:119–127.
166. Grupp SA, Stern JW, Bunin N, et al. Rapid-sequence tandem transplant for children with high-risk neuroblastoma. *Med Pediatr Oncol.* 2000;35(6):696–700.
167. Grupp SA, Stern JW, Bunin N, et al. Tandem high-dose therapy in rapid sequence for children with high-risk neuroblastoma. *J Clin Oncol.* 2000;18:2567–2575.
168. Kletzel M, Katzenstein HM, Haut PR, et al. Treatment of high-risk neuroblastoma with triple-tandem high-dose therapy and stem-cell rescue: results of the Chicago Pilot II Study. *J Clin Oncol.* 2002;20:2284–2292.
169. Sung KW, Yoo KH, Chung EH, et al. Successive double high-dose chemotherapy with peripheral blood stem cell rescue collected during a single leukapheresis round in patients with high-risk pediatric solid tumors: a pilot study in a single center. *Bone Marrow Transplant.* 2003;31(6):447–452.
170. Kanold J, Yakouben K, Tchirkov A, et al. Long-term results of CD34(+) cell transplantation in children with neuroblastoma. *Med Pediatr Oncol.* 2000;35(1):1–7.
171. Peniket AJ, Perry AR, Williams CD, et al. A case of EBV-associated lymphoproliferative disease following high-dose therapy and CD34-purified autologous peripheral blood progenitor cell transplantation. *Bone Marrow Transplant.* 1998;22:307–309.
172. Heath JA, Broxson EH, Jr, Dole MG, et al. Epstein-Barr virus-associated lymphoma in a child undergoing an autologous stem cell rescue. *J Pediatr Hematol Oncol.* 2002;24:160–163.
173. Lones MA, Kirov I, Said JW, et al. Post-transplant lymphoproliferative disorder after autologous stem cell transplantation in a pediatric patient. *Bone Marrow Transplant.* 2000;26:1021–1024.
174. Powell JL, Bunin NJ, Callahan C, et al. An unexpectedly high incidence of Epstein-Barr virus lymphoproliferative disease after CD34+ selected autologous peripheral blood stem cell transplant in neuroblastoma. *Bone Marrow Transplant.* 2004;33(6):651–657.
175. Levine BL, Bernstein WB, Aronson NE, et al. Adoptive transfer of costimulated CD4+ T cells induces expansion of peripheral T cells and decreased CCR5 expression in HIV infection. *Nature Med.* 2002:8:47–53.
176. Laport GG, Levine BL, Stadtmauer EA, et al. Adoptive transfer of costimulated T cells induces lymphocytosis in patients with relapsed/refractory non-Hodgkin lymphoma following CD34+-selected hematopoietic cell transplantation. *Blood.* 2003;102(6):2004–2013.
177. Porter DL, Levine BL, Bunin N, et al. A phase 1 trial of donor lymphocyte infusions expanded and activated ex vivo via CD3/CD28 costimulation. *Blood.* 2006;107(4):1325–1331.
178. Rapoport AP, Stadtmauer EA, Aqui N, et al. Restoration of immunity in lymphopenic individuals with cancer by vaccination and adoptive T-cell transfer. *Nature Med.* 2005;11(11):1230–1237.

Pathological Evaluation of Childhood Cancer

Sherrie L. Perkins and Stephen J. Qualman

Introduction

Pediatric malignancies present with diagnostic challenges due to their multiple differences with adult malignancies[1] as enumerated below:

- Pediatric tumors are rare, with only 6000 to 7000 new cases a year.[2]
- Organ systems involved by primarily pediatric neoplasms (hematopoietic, neural, soft tissue) commonly differ sharply from those involved in adults (lung, prostate, colon, and so on).
- Pediatric tumors have a relatively undifferentiated (embryonal) character (so-called small blue cell tumors). They are more often sarcomatous in nature and are rarely carcinomas.
- A close relationship between abnormal development (teratogenesis) and tumor induction (oncogenesis) is seen in pediatric tumors.
- Many childhood tumors are associated with specific genetic and chromosomal defects.

- Multicentric tumors (multiple sites) are common in childhood.
- Many benign lesions of childhood mimic malignancy based on exaggerated mitotic activity.
- Pediatric malignancies are often detected incidentally or accidentally, with little ability to screen for their occurrence—making prevention difficult.
- Prognosis in childhood cancer is often influenced by age at diagnosis (younger is usually better). The age of occurrence of common pediatric malignancies can be measured in pentads (Table 5-1).

This chapter will discuss the diagnostic challenges inherent in the pathologic identification of pediatric malignancies. The chapter will be divided between nonhematolymphoid (or "solid") tumors of childhood and hematolymphoid (or "liquid") tumors of childhood. This approach is based in part on the fact that hematolymphoid tumors account for almost 50% of new cases of childhood malignancies annually;[2] of the nonhematolymphoid tumors of childhood—nearly one-third are central nervous system

Table 5-1

Common pediatric malignancies by age of diagnosis (pentads).

Diagnosis	<5 years	<10 years	<15 years
Leukemia	X	X	
Non-Hodgkin Lymphoma		X	
Hodgkin Lymphoma			X
Central Nervous System	X	X	
Neuroblastoma	X	X	
Nephroblastoma (Wilms tumor)	X		
Retinoblastoma	X	X	
Hepatic	X (hepatoblastoma)	X (carcinoma)	X (carcinoma)
Soft Tissue	X (rhabdomyosarcoma)	X	X
Germ Cell	X (teratoma)		
Bone		X (Ewing)	X (osteosarcoma)

(CNS) or brain tumors; nearly another one-third are the so-called blastomas of childhood (neuroblastoma, nephroblastoma or Wilms tumor (WT), rhabdomyosarcoma (RMS), retinoblastoma, hepatoblastoma); with the final one-third including a miscellany of tumors, particularly bone tumors. An example of the mix of malignancies accrued annually by a major children's hospital, reflecting the trends noted above, is illustrated in Table 5-2.

This chapter will emphasize the morphologic details of diagnosis for these broad tumor groups. Because of similar morphologic appearances, pediatric tumor diagnosis may require ancillary studies such as immunophenotyping by flow cytometry or immunohistochemistry,[3,4] or molecular genetic analysis.[5,6] In addition, extensive work in the area of pediatric neoplasia has identified many prognostic factors that can be identified by immunophenotyping or molecular genetic studies.[6,7,8] An important role for the pathologist in the workup of a suspected pediatric tumor is in making a proper diagnosis as well as collecting appropriate and adequate tissue for ancillary testing.

Morphologic Analysis

Most pediatric biopsies come to the pathologist in a fresh state to allow for tissue allocation to ensure that proper testing may be undertaken. It is important that the pathologist be aware of a suspected diagnosis of neoplasia and possible clinical differential diagnoses to ensure that all of the appropriate testing is done. Often the suspected tumor diagnosis will be confirmed by performance of a frozen section of the tissue submitted to confirm that a neoplasm is present. Although frozen section is often not sufficient to make a definitive diagnosis, it will help to direct the handling of the tissue to ensure that appropriate testing can be undertaken.[9]

Morphology provides the keystone for diagnosis of pediatric neoplasia. This requires that adequate tissue be sampled to allow for proper morphologic analysis.[10] In pediatric neoplasia, most diagnoses will require tissue sampling either by biopsy (excisional or incisional) or needle core biopsy. It should be noted that often cytologic analysis may not be definitive and require subsequent biopsy to confirm a suspected diagnosis. Because of the ancillary testing that may be required, the pathologist and the surgeon or other personnel performing the biopsy must work together to ensure that adequate tissue is collected to meet all needs.[10] This requires that sufficient tumor be present without extensive necrosis. Electron microscopic study of glutaraldehyde-fixed, plastic-embedded tumor specimens still may play a definitive ultrastructural role in diagnostic confirmation. This is often done in combination with the other ancillary techniques described below.

Ancillary Laboratory Techniques

Immunohistochemistry

By use of immunophenotypic analysis, a diagnosis of a specific tumor type may often be made. In most cases using fixed tissue this will be done by immunohistochemical staining on tissue slides. The fixative of choice is 10% neutral-buffered formalin. Immunohistochemical staining involves use of a specific antibody that will recognize a given antigenic epitope on a tumor cell. Use of panels of antibodies and observation of the staining patterns generated by those antibodies will help to allow a diagnosis to be made.

Flow Cytometry

Immunophenotyping may also be done on fresh tissues using flow cytometry.[4,11] This is most useful in the hema-

---

Table 5-2

Cases of pediatric malignancy (n=138 total) accession by Columbus Children's Cancer Registry in 2002.

Tumor	Percent Incidence
Leukemia	28.0
ALL (27 cases)	
AML (5 cases)	
Other (6 cases)	
Lymphoma	9.0
Hodgkin (5 cases)	
Other (7 cases)	
Central Nervous System	28.0
Supratentorial (14 cases)	
Infratentorial (20 case)	
Spinal cord (5 cases)	
Neuroblastoma	6.5
Renal	3.0
Wilms (4 cases)	
Other (1 case)	
Hepatic	3.0
Retinoblastoma	5.0
Soft Tissue	8.0
Rhabdomyosarcoma (4 cases)	
Other (7 cases)	
Bone	8.0
Osteosarcoma (9 cases)	
Ewing sarcoma (2 cases)	
Germ Cell	2.0
Gonadal/ovary (2 cases)	
Gonadal/testis (2 cases)	

tolymphoid neoplasms where the cells are not adherent, allowing for a single cell suspension to be easily obtained. Flow cytometry allows for the measurement of numerous cell properties including cell size, organelle complexity, and antigenic expression. Using this approach, a specific fluorescently labeled antibody will bind to the cell if a specific antigen epitope is present. The cells are then passed through a flow cytometric instrument and analyzed by a laser light source. The presence of flow cytometers that can analyze up to 4 or 6 different fluorochrome stains allows for integration of multiple antigenic signals simultaneously.[12] Measurement of total tumor DNA content (ploidy state) by flow cytometry can be achieved using a nuclear fluorescent dye such as propidium iodide.

Cytogenetics

Many pediatric neoplasms also have specific cytogenetic and molecular findings that impart additional diagnostic as well as prognostic information.[5,6] Cytogenetics, or the study of chromosomes, requires fresh samples that contain malignant cells. Bone marrows (usually 1–2 ml), blood (approximately 10 ml) or a tissue sample (usually 0.2-0.5 mm³) can be studied. Conventional cytogenetic approaches are useful in that they provide the ability to view the entire chromosomal component by analysis of a chromosomal spread.[13,14] This allows identification of many abnormalities and is particularly useful in demonstrating complex cytogenetic abnormalities;[15] however, abnormalities may not be detected if the tumor cells fail to grow.

Fluorescent in situ Hybridization

Molecular testing using fluorescent in situ hybridization (FISH) is another cytogenetic approach that is often utilized in pediatric neoplasia.[6,16–19] FISH technology uses specific, fluorescently labeled probes to identify specific chromosomal abnormalities. This approach is useful because it is much more rapid, requiring only 24 to 48 hours compared with 5 to 7 days for conventional cytogenetics and may be performed on interphase nuclei on touch preparations or tissue sections. However, FISH technology will identify only those abnormalities for which the specific probe is created.[20] In some cases, FISH approaches are more sensitive than conventional cytogenetics where conventional cytogenetics often misses specific chromosomal anomalies in conventional preparations.[16,21]

Molecular Genetic Tests

Molecular testing for specific molecular and cytogenetic abnormalities is also becoming much more common in pediatric tumors.[6,7,21] Several molecular tests have been developed using either Southern Blot analysis (requiring fresh or frozen tissue) or reverse transcription polymerase chain reaction (RT-PCR), (which can use fresh, frozen, or sometimes fixed tissue).[22] The sensitivity of molecular testing is very high, and it has the ability to detect very small numbers of cells harboring a specific defect.[7] This is particularly useful in monitoring of minimal residual dis-

ease.[23,24] As with FISH analysis described above, molecular testing will test only for a specific abnormality. Molecular testing (RT-PCR) often requires 24 to 48 hours as compared with the longer turnaround time for conventional cytogenetics. In addition, many molecular tests may be more sensitive than conventional cytogenetics (similar to the situation with FISH technologies) in identifying some abnormalities.[7,21]

Classification of Solid (Nonhematolymphoid) Tumors

Many solid tumors of childhood (neuroblastoma, Ewing sarcoma (ES), rhabdomyosarcoma, nephroblastoma, etc) including lymphomas (see later in this chapter) can assume a relatively undifferentiated "small blue cell" appearance (Figure 5-1) with high cellularity, relatively uniform nuclei, and scant cytoplasm; hence, ancillary testing is of considerable value. This is especially true of detection of molecular genetic markers[6] (deletion of tumor suppressor genes, presence of fusion genes, amplification of oncogenes) that can add significant diagnostic and prognostic information (Table 5-3). Both morphologic and molecular genetic features of pediatric solid tumors will be emphasized in the following discussion, along with results of other ancillary studies.

Central Nervous System Tumors

Brain tumors are the most common solid tumors of childhood and the second most common pediatric malignancy overall, after leukemia.[25] Unlike brain tumors in adults, a significant proportion of those occurring in children are associated with an excellent prognosis.[25] The most frequent types are astrocytoma, medulloblastoma, and ependymoma. A larger proportion of brain tumors occur in the posterior fossa in children as opposed to adults. Therapeutic efforts include surgery, radiotherapy, and chemotherapy. In large part, this still produces less than desirable results,

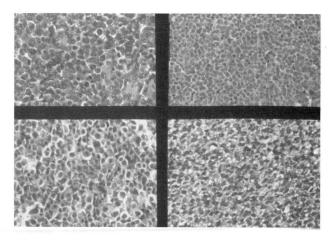

Figure 5-1 Small blue cell tumors of childhood. Note the similar embryonal appearance of four different such tumors (clockwise from upper left: rhabdomyosarcoma, lymphoblastic lymphoma, neuroblastoma, and nephroblastoma, or Wilms tumor). 200X, hematoxylin and eosin stain. **See Plate 1 for color image.**

Table 5-3

Molecular genetics of pediatric solid (non-hematolymphoid) tumors.

Tumor	Suppressor Gene (location)	Fusion Gene (location)	Oncogene (location)
Neuroblastoma	Unknown (1p36 +/− extension to 1p32)	Unknown t(1p36;17q)	MYCN (2p24)
Nephroblastoma (Wilms)	WT-1 (11p13) Unknown (11p15)		
Rhabdomyosarcoma -Alveolar		PAX3/FKHR t(2;13)	MYCN (2p24)
-Embryonal	Unknown (11p15) p53 (17p12-13)	PAX7/FKHR t(1;13)	
Ewing/PNET		EWS/FLI1 t(11;22) EWS/ERG t(21;22)	
Retinoblastoma	Rb-1 (11p13)		

although pilocytic astrocytoma of the cerebellum can be associated with long-term disease-free survival.

Despite improvement in imaging techniques in the past decade, the final tumor diagnosis still depends on the interpretation of the histologic features of the tumor. As alluded to above, almost 90% of pediatric CNS tumors fall into one of four categories: astrocytoma, ependymoma, craniopharyngioma, and primitive neuroectodermal tumor (PNET) (including medulloblastoma in the posterior fossa). The remaining more than 10% of less-frequent tumors include germ cell, choroid plexus, and subependymal giant cell tumors. Categorization of brain tumors and prediction of their behavior cannot rely on conventional histology alone but encompasses important advances in immunohistochemistry and molecular biology.[26] The World Health Organization (WHO) classification can be applied to brain tumors in childhood to provide a framework for diagnosis, which is beyond the scope of this chapter.[27]

Neuroblastoma

Neuroblastoma[28] is a tumor composed of primitive to differentiated neuroblasts and/or ganglion cells (Figure 5-2A and B). The tumor typically arises within the first several years of life and most frequently involves the region of the adrenal glands or the paraspinal sympathetic ganglia. Many factors are important in prognosis, among them being tumor stage, patient age, tumor site, histopathological classification, ploidy, serum ferritin, urinary catecholamine metabolite lev-

els, MYCN oncogene copy number (oncogene amplification), and tumor ploidy state. MYCN amplification has shown some correlation with the presence of double minute chromosomes or homogeneously staining regions on cytogenetic analysis (Figure 5-2C) (refer to Table 5-3).

The International Neuroblastoma Pathology Classification[29] distinguishes favorable histology (FH) and unfavorable histology (UH) groups. Tumors in the FH group fall within a framework of age-linked maturational sequence from poorly differentiated and < 1.5 years of age at diagnosis to differentiating neuroblastoma and < 5 years old, to ganglioneuroblastoma, intermixed at any age to ganglioneuroma at any age. The neuroblastoma tumors in this FH group should also have a low mitotic karyorrhectic index (MKI) (nuclear mitosis or debris) and be ≥ 1.5 years and < 5 years old at diagnosis or an intermediate MKI and < 1.5 years old at diagnosis. By contrast, tumors in the UH group have immature histologies for patient's age and include undifferentiated (at any age), poorly differentiated and ≥ 1.5 years old, and all subtypes of neuroblastoma diagnosed at ≥ 5 years old. Among neuroblastoma tumors, those with a high MKI (any age) or an intermediate MKI at ≥ 1.5 years old also are qualified as UH. Ganglioneuroblastoma, intermixed, and ganglioneuroma are classifed into the FH group regardless of the patient age, although they are usually diagnosed in older children. Ganglioneuroblastoma, nodular can be divided into two subsets, favorable and unfavorable, by applying the same criteria of age-linked histopathological evaluation to the nodular component.

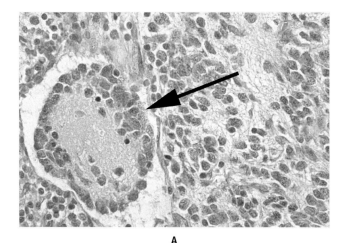

A

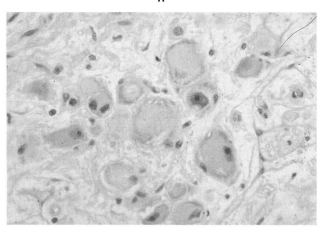

B

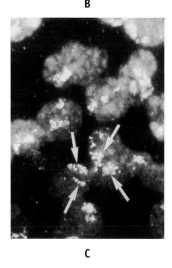

C

Figure 5-2 (A) Homer Wright rosette (arrow) in neuroblastoma. 400X, hematoxylin and eosin stain. (B) Ganglion cell differentiation in neuroblastoma. 400X, hematoxylin and eosin stain. (C) Homogenously staining regions with MYCN amplification (arrows) in neuroblastoma. 200X, FISH. **See Plates 2-4 for color images.**

The vast majority of *MYCN* amplified tumors[30,31] are of the *undifferentiated* or *poorly differentiated* subtype of neuroblastoma with markedly increased MKI, classified as UH, and have a very poor prognosis. Four biologically and prognostically distinct subsets (percentage of cases) are defined by histopathology and *MYCN* status: they are FH and nonamplified *MYCN* (58.2%, excellent prognosis), FH and amplified *MYCN* (1.3%, unknown prognosis), UH and nonamplified *MYCN* (23.6%, poor prognosis), and UH and amplified *MYCN* (16.9%, extremely poor prognosis). Ploidy analysis may also be prognostically significant in neuroblastoma as measured by flow cytometry, but only in infant cases.

Nephroblastoma (Wilms Tumor)

Wilms tumor[32] is the most common pediatric renal tumor, with a peak age of occurrence in the range of 2 to 4 years. Less common pediatric renal tumors include clear cell sarcoma of kidney, malignant rhabdoid tumor, and congenital mesoblastic nephroma, which are beyond the scope of this chapter but are detailed elsewhere.[32]

More than 30% of Wilms nephrectomy specimens contain nephrogenic rests. Samples of native kidney with areas containing more pale than the usual parenchyma may reveal incidental nephrogenic rests (NR) (Figure 5-3A). Nephrogenic rests have important implications concerning the risk of contralateral WT development and may have other syndromatic implications. At least 1 random section of kidney and possibly more may be taken to detect NRs microscopically. The presence of multiple or diffusely distributed NRs is termed *nephroblastomatosis*. Two fundamental categories of NRs are recognized: intralobar (ILNR) and perilobar (PLNR). In addition to increased risk of tumor arising in the contralateral kidney, ILNR and PLNR have specific genetic implications (noted below). The topographic and microscopic distinction of PLNR and ILNR have been well described elsewhere.[33]

No single cytogenetic or molecular abnormality has been consistently abnormal in WT or its host (Table 5-3), but constitutional deletions of the *WT-1* tumor suppressor gene at 11p13 often predispose the patient to development of Wilms tumors. The deletion or mutation of this gene characterizes both WAGR syndrome (WT, aniridia, genitourinary anomalies, and mental retardation) and Denys-Drash syndrome. Intralobar nephrogenic rests are associated with WAGR and Denys-Drash syndrome. Perilobar nephrogenic rests are associated with Beckwith-Weidemann syndrome, Perlman syndrome, and hemihypertrophy.[33]

Microscopically, WT has a variable appearance ranging from the classic triphasic mixture of tubules, blastema, and stroma (Figure 5-3B) to monophasic tumors such as purely blastemal WT. Once a tumor is diagnosed as WT, it is necessary to determine whether it is of favorable histopathology, or if anaplasia is present. Although anaplasia is present in only 4% of all cases, it characterizes unfavorable histopathology and a poor outcome. Anaplasia in WT is characterized by the presence of abnormal multipolar mitotic figures and enlarged hyperchromatic nuclei 3-fold or more the size of neighboring nuclei of the same cell type (Figure 5-3C). Whether the anaplasia that is present occurs only focally in a tumor or whether it is diffuse or multifocal has recently been recognized as important with regard to prognosis. Therefore, it is now

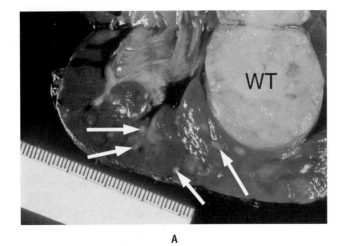

A

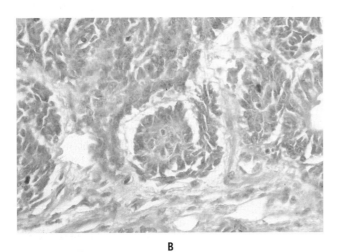

B

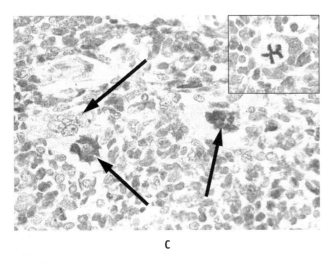

C

Figure 5-3   (A) Gross photograph of cut section of Wilms tumor (WT) in kidney, with associated nephrogenic rests (arrows). (B) Favorable histopathology nephroblastoma or Wilms tumor with triphasic histology, including tubular and glomeruloid structures. 400X hematoxylin and eosin stain. (C) Unfavorable histopathology in nephroblastoma or Wilms tumor. Both nuclei (arrows) and mitotic figures (inset) can be three to four times the size of their neighboring cellular counterparts. 200X, hematoxylin and eosin stain. **See Plates 5 and 6 for color images of (B) and (C).**

necessary to document the location of each section taken on a "tumor map," and this should be done for all WTs, because it is impossible to predict beforehand which tumors will show anaplasia.[32]

Soft-Tissue Sarcomas (Rhabdomyosarcoma)

Rhabdomyosarcoma[34] is the most common soft-tissue sarcoma of childhood, occurring at an average age of 4.5 years. It is a sarcoma with skeletal muscle differentiation (Figure 5-4A) and a predilection for certain sites, including the genitourinary tract, head and neck (including the orbit), biliary tract, and paratesticular region, and is predominantly of the embryonal type at these sites. Many RMS are poorly differentiated, and immunohistochemistry is often essential to establishing the diagnosis, particularly on small biopsies,[34] and particularly for the intranuclear transcription factors MyoD1 and myogenin. Prognosis depends largely on location (paratesticular and orbital tumors do relatively well), stage and group (which translates into resectability of the tumor). The only cur-

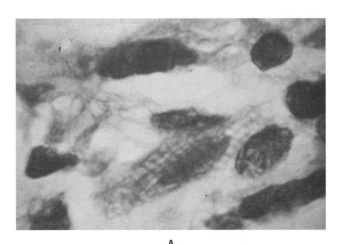

A

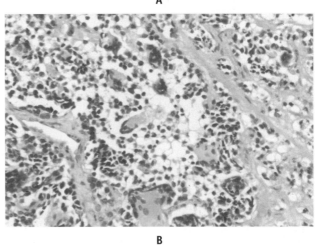

B

Figure 5-4   (A) Rhabdomyoblast showing skeletal muscle differentiation (contractile elements or cross striations) defining the malignancy as rhabdomyosarcoma at the light microscopic level. 630X, hematoxylin and eosin stain. (B) Classical alveolar rhabdomyosarcoma (unfavorable histopathology) with cystic, cleft-like (or alveolar) spaces and associated tumor giant cells. 200X, hematoxylin and eosin stain. **See Plates 7 and 8 for color images.**

rent officially recognized unfavorable histologic feature is the alveolar subtype of RMS (ARMS),[35] which can be either classic alveolar (Figure 5-4B) or the so-called solid variant and occurs most frequently on the extremities of older children. Anaplasia (large bizarre nuclei and mitoses, as also described in WT) may also have a worse prognosis and is currently being studied prospectively in Children's Oncology Group clinical trials.[35]

The presence of t(1;13) (*PAX7-FKHR*) and t(2;13) (*PAX3-FKHR*) is strongly correlated with the ARMS (Table 5-3). The *PAX3-FKHR* fusion gene is more prevalent. Recent data indicate that when gene fusion status is compared in patients with metastatic disease at diagnosis, a striking difference in outcome is seen between *PAX3-FKHR* and *PAX7-FKHR* (estimated 4-year overall survival of 75% for *PAX7-FKHR*, and 8% for *PAX3-FKHR*; p = 0.002).[22] These translocations may be found in as much as 85% of ARMS cases.[22]

Germ Cell Tumors

Pediatric germ cell tumors occur in multiple sites. The most common location in the newborn is the sacrococcygeal teratoma.[1] For any sacrococcygeal teratoma, one must document the presence of the tip of the coccyx in the specimen, which usually will be present as a small irregular lump of cartilage on the capsule of the tumor (this may contain residual malignant elements that should be resected). Other frequent sites in childhood include the ovary, testis, mediastinum, and region of the pineal and pituitary glands. These tumors are typically midline. Teratomas may be mature or immature (Figure 5-5A). The significance of immature somatic elements within a teratoma varies with the age and location of the tumor, but in an extragonadal site in an infant it is generally not unfavorable. The histopathologic appearances of germ cell tumors are diverse and beyond the scope of this chapter. They range from mature or immature teratoma to fully malignant patterns, including yolk sac tumor, germinoma,

and choriocarcinoma. Perhaps the most important caveat is to thoroughly sample and carefully evaluate any teratoma, especially an immature one, for the presence of even minor foci of a malignant germ cell pattern. The most frequent malignant germ cell component[36] is endodermal sinus tumor (yolk sac carcinoma) (Figure 5-5B), which is often associated with an elevated serum *AFP*. Choriocarcinoma is rare in children.

Bone Tumors

Osteosarcoma

Osteosarcoma is the most common primary malignant tumor of bone in children and adolescents.[37] It is characterized histologically by malignant osteoid (bone matrix) production by the sarcoma. Some 70% of cases are diagnosed before the age of 20, but only 10% under the age of 10, indicating the marked propensity for the second decade of life. The long bones of the extremities are by far the most common site, but this tumor can involve other sites as well, including the jaw.

Histologic evaluation of the resection specimen, following a period of preoperative chemotherapy, has taken on considerable importance recently.[37] The total cross-sectional area of tumor on a representative sagittal slice of the tumor should be submitted, along with sections of the epiphyseal plate, joint space, uninvolved marrow, any areas radiologically suggestive of skip lesions, and/or other relevant margins or unique features of the case. The extent of preoperative tumor necrosis has been found to correlate with the likelihood of continued postoperative tumor-free survival;[38] ablation of 95% or more of the tumor is considered a positive response (Table 5-4).

Ewing Sarcoma

Ewing sarcoma is a small, undifferentiated "round cell" tumor of childhood[39] that most frequently involves the

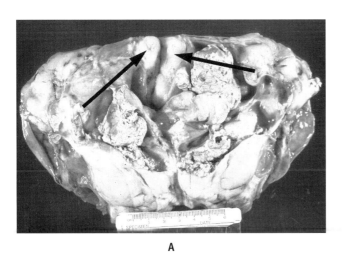

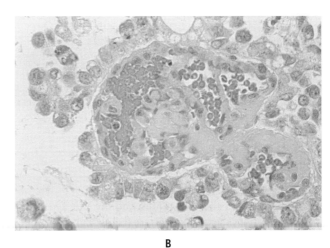

| A | B |

Figure 5-5 (A) Gross photograph of opened cystic teratoma with mature somatic elements including hair and sebaceous material. Solid areas of tumor (arrows) should be heavily sampled to detect immature or malignant germ cell elements. (B) Yolk sac carcinoma (with Schiller-Duvall structure), a typical occult malignant germ cell tumor that may be found focally in an otherwise benign cystic teratoma as in 5A. 400X, hematoxylin and eosin stain. **See Plate 9 for color image of (B).**

Table 5-4

Histologic grading of tumor necrosis[38]

Grade	Viable Tumor Remaining	5-Year Event-Free Survival*
I	All (no chemotherapy effect)	49%
IIA	>50% viable tumor	64%
IIB	5%-50% viable tumor	
III	Only scattered foci viable (<5%)	86%
IV	No viable tumor, despite extensive sampling	91%

*Glasser DB, Lane JM, Huvos AG, Marcove RC, Rosen G. Survival, prognosis, and therapeutic response in osteogenic sarcoma. The Memorial Hospital experience. *Cancer.* 1992, Feb. 1;69(3):698–708. American Cancer Society.

long bones of the (lower) extremities but can involve the pelvis and spine (Figure 5-6A). It can even occur as a primary soft-tissue sarcoma, where it is often called either extraosseous ES or PNET. Ewing sarcoma of bone affects a somewhat younger population than osteosarcoma, with a peak affected age between 10 and 15 years. The most important predictor of outcome is tumor site. Complete resection is very important in the control of this tumor, and sites such as the pelvis, where the tumor is often difficult to resect and frequently of advanced stage or size at diagnosis, are associated with a poor prognosis.

Microscopically, a uniform population of small to intermediate-size monotonous nuclei (Figure 5-6B) with cytoplasmic glycogen (in well-fixed material) characterize ES with focal areas of neuroectodermal differentiation (eg, Homer-Wright rosettes) sometimes seen. In the restricted setting of a pediatric small blue cell tumor, membrane staining for CD99 (Figure 5-6C) is a useful marker for tumors of the ES/PNET group, although CD99 is also prominently expressed by lymphoblastic lymphomas and in a cytoplasmic pattern in some cells of RMS, so it should always be used as part of a panel of markers.[39]

The presence (Table 5-3) of t(11;22) (*EWS-FLI1*) and t(21;22) (*EWS-ERG*) is strongly correlated with the specific diagnosis of PNET/ES. The most common gene fusion is the *EWS-FLI1* (90% to 95% of patients) (Figure 5-6D). Recent investigations[40] suggest that different types of *EWS-FLI1* fusions (type 1 versus type 2) may have prognostic implications; patients with type 1 fusions (in which *EWS* exons 1-7 link with *FLI1* exons 6-9) fare better than patients with type 2 fusions (involving other sites within the relevant genes). This relationship remains under active investigation.

Liver Tumors

The histopathological features of hepatocellular carcinomas overlap with those of adults and are not a point of discussion in this text, but they are detailed elsewhere.[4]

Hepatoblastoma

Hepatoblastoma, the principal malignant tumor affecting the pediatric liver, is overwhelmingly a tumor of the first 3 years of life. It is a rare tumor, accounting for only about 1% of pediatric tumors. Completeness of resection—ie, stage—remains the most important prognostic predictor at this point (Figure 5-7A).[41]

The epithelial elements of hepatoblastoma are fairly easily recognized as resembling the hepatocytes of fetal liver (Figure 5-7B) and distinguished from hepatocellular carcinoma by the small size of the tumor cells, which are smaller than normal hepatocytes (rather than larger, as in hepatocellular carcinoma), and by the lesser degree of atypia present. Hepatoblastoma may be mixed, containing diverse and sometimes heterologous stromal elements, such as bone or cartilage, as well as the epithelial elements. The pure fetal type of hepatoblastoma (Figure 5-7B) (lacking in an embryonal or sarcomatous component) appears to have a better prognosis when completely resected (stage I).[42]

Retinoblastoma

Retinoblastoma is the most common malignant eye tumor of childhood.[1] The median age at presentation is two years, although the tumor may be present at birth. Untreated, the tumors are usually fatal, but early treatment that may include chemotherapy, radiotherapy, and/or enucleation (Figure 5-8A) now produces survival as a rule. Pathologic features with prognostic significance for survival include the following: invasion of optic nerve, particularly if tumor is present at the surgical margin (most important feature); invasion of sclera; invasion of choroid; tumor size; basophilic staining of tumor vessels; seeding of vitreous; degree of differentiation; involvement of anterior segment; and growth pattern.[43]

Typical histologic features (Figure 5-8B) include cells with large, basophilic nuclei and scant cytoplasm. Mitoses are generally frequent. Calcification and necrosis are common with sleeves of viable cells typically surrounding blood vessels (pseudorosettes). Apoptotic cells may be seen. The extent of differentiation may be judged based on the presence and type of rosettes. Homer-Wright rosettes similar to those seen in neuroblastoma or medulloblastoma may be seen and are not a sign of significant differentiation. Flexner-Wintersteiner rosettes (with true lumina) are evidence of higher differentiation. Fleurettes are considered the most differentiated form of rosette found in the tumor.[43]

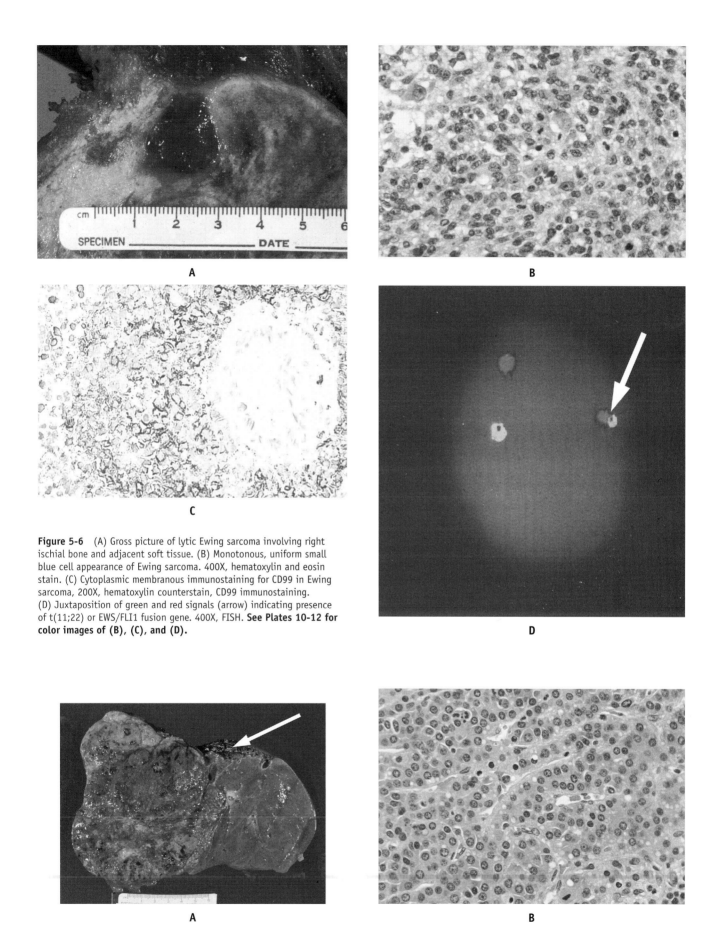

Figure 5-6 (A) Gross picture of lytic Ewing sarcoma involving right ischial bone and adjacent soft tissue. (B) Monotonous, uniform small blue cell appearance of Ewing sarcoma. 400X, hematoxylin and eosin stain. (C) Cytoplasmic membranous immunostaining for CD99 in Ewing sarcoma, 200X, hematoxylin counterstain, CD99 immunostaining. (D) Juxtaposition of green and red signals (arrow) indicating presence of t(11;22) or EWS/FLI1 fusion gene. 400X, FISH. **See Plates 10-12 for color images of (B), (C), and (D).**

Figure 5-7 (A) Gross photograph of hepatoblastoma; note adjacent inked margin (arrow); correct staging is critical to correct prognostication in this malignancy. (B) Hepatoblastoma, fetal subtype. 400X, hematoxylin and eosin stain. **See Plate 13 for color image of (B).**

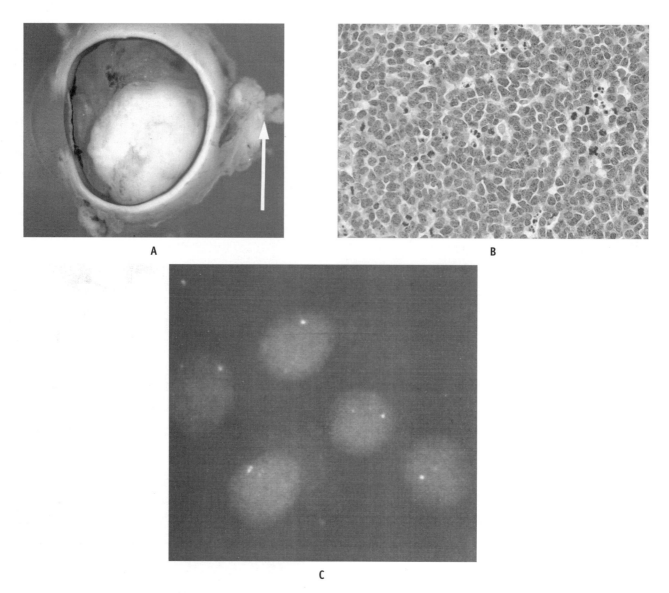

Figure 5-8 (A) Gross photograph of enucleation of retinoblastoma. Accuracy of gross examination and sampling, including optic nerve margin (arrow), is critical to proper staging and treatment. (B) Retinoblastoma in many areas can have an embryonal or undifferentiated small blue cell appearance. 400X, hematoxylin and eosin stain. (C) In familial cases, *RB1* deletions may be seen in associated somatic tissues such as white blood cells. 400x, hematoxylin and eosin stain. **See Plates 14 and 15 for color images of (B) and (C).**

Approximately 60% to 70% of tumors are associated with a germline mutation in the *RB1* gene (Table 5-3) (Figure 5-8C) and are heritable. The remaining 30% to 40% of the tumors develop sporadically and have somatic *RB1* gene mutations.[1,43] Genetic studies may be requested on neoplastic tissue and should be harvested prior to fixation.[43] Once tissue is harvested for genetic studies, the globe can be fixed prior to completing macroscopic and microscopic examination.

Classification of Hematolymphoid Tumors

Work on the biology of hematologic neoplasms has led to increased understanding of the pathogenesis of many hematolymphoid tumors including non-Hodgkin lym-phomas (NHL), acute lymphoid and myeloid leukemias, and Hodgkin lymphoma (HL). Recent classification systems, such as the REAL (Revised European and American Lymphoma)[44] or the WHO classifications,[45] incorporate morphologic, immunophenotypic, and molecular characteristics into definition of each disease entity. This inclusion is in direct contrast with earlier classification systems[46] that made use only of morphologic or cytochemical staining characteristics. It is anticipated that use of defined immunophenotypic or molecular/cytogenetic data in diagnosis of specific entities will help lead to more objective diagnostic criteria and should help to create more uniform disease categories and diagnoses. Specific criteria for diagnosis will be further outlined for each disease category below.

Lymphomas

Non-Hodgkin Lymphoma

Non-Hodgkin lymphomas make up approximately 10% of all childhood cancers and are a diverse collection of malignant neoplasms of lymphoreticular cells.[47] Pediatric NHL includes a diverse group of neoplasms that derive from both mature and immature (blastic) cells of both B-cell and T-cell origin. These neoplasms in children are widely diverse but in general are intermediate- to high-grade (clinically aggressive) tumors, in direct contrast to the fact that in adults, more than two-thirds of the tumors are indolent, low-grade malignancies.[48] Pediatric NHL also appears very different from adult lymphomas in that all of the tumors are diffuse neoplasms, and follicular (nodular) lymphomas are exceedingly rare.[48] Similarly, the immunophenotypic subclassification of pediatric NHL shows marked differences from adult NHL. Pediatric NHLs are almost evenly split between B- and T-cell neoplasms, whereas T-cell neoplasms make up less than 10% of adult NHL. Pediatric NHL also has many more lesions that are derived from blast-like or precursor B- or T-cells than are seen in adults.[10,48] There are four major pathologic subtypes of pediatric NHL: Burkitt lymphomas (BL), diffuse large B-cell lymphoma (DLBCL), lymphoblastic lymphomas (LBL), and anaplastic large cell lymphoma (ALCL) (Table 5-5).

Burkitt Lymphomas

The sporadic form of BL also tends to involve extranodal sites but is more common in the gastrointestinal tract, particularly in the ileocecal area, as well as in kidneys and ovaries.[49,50] BL accounts for 40% to 50% of pediatric NHL in nonendemic areas. Morphologically, BL are characterized by intermediate-sized homogeneous cells with round to oval nuclei with multiple, variably prominent basophilic nucleoli (Figure 5-9A). The cells have a modest amount of somewhat basophilic cytoplasm, which will appear vacuolated, due to lipid droplets, on cytologic preparations (Figure 5-9B). The tumor has very high mitotic activity, and tissue sections will often show a "starry sky" appearance that results from tingible body macrophages scattered among the malignant lymphoid cells (Figure 5-9C).[45] It should be noted that the "starry sky" appearance is not specific for BL, but it can be seen in any rapidly dividing NHL.[10]

The BLs also include a second histologic subtype that has previously been termed non-Burkitt or Burkitt-like lymphoma.[51] These tumors have also been termed as high-grade mature B-cell lymphomas in the REAL classification[44] or atypical BL in the most current WHO classification.[45] They are characterized by more cellular pleomorphism, variable nuclear irregularities, and variable numbers of nucleoli that may be more prominent than are typically seen in BL. It should be noted that these two entities are more clinically alike than different, and the value of making

---

Table 5-5

Most frequent subtypes of pediatric NHL.

Histologic Subtypes	% Pediatric NHL	Common Presentation	Immunophenotype Paraffin	Flow
Burkitt and atypical Burkitt lymphoma	40%	Extranodal	CD79a+, CD20+, CD22, CD10+, CD10+, TdT−	CD19+, CD20+, CD10+, monoclonal cell surface Ig
Precursor (lymphoblastic) lymphoma	30%	LN, mediastinal mass (T-cell) LN, skin (B-cell)	90%-precursor T CD2+/−, CD3−/+, CD5+/−, TdT+	Variable expression CD2, CD4, CD5, CD7 and CD8, TdT+, usually lack cell surfaceCD3
			10% precursor B CD19+, CD10+, TdT+	CD19+, CD20−, CD10+, TdT+
Diffuse large B-cell lymphoma	20%	LN, mediastinum	CD79a+, CD20+, CD22+, CD10+/−	CD19+, CD20+, CD10+/−, monoclonal cell surface Ig
Anaplastic large cell lymphoma	10%	LN, skin, extranodal	80-90% − T-cell CD2+, CD3−/+, CD5+/−, CD7−/+, CD43+, TIA-1+, CD30+, ALK-1+, EMA+	CD2+/−, CD3−/+, CD4+, CD5+/−, CD7−/+, CD8−, CD30+
			10-20% null cell CD45+, CD30+, ALK-1+	CD30+, CD45+

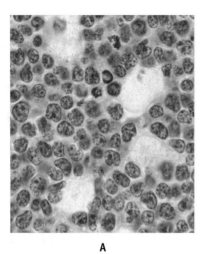

A

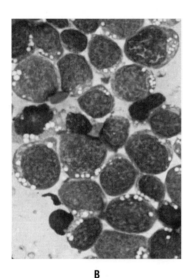

B

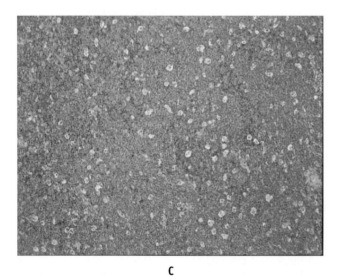

C

Figure 5-9 (A) Burkitt lymphoma showing relatively monomorphous population with high mitotic rate and tingible body macrophages. 400X, hematoxylin and eosin stain. (B) Burkitt lymphoma showing vacuolation of the cytoplasm and monomorphic nuclear appearance. 1000X oil, Wright's stain. (C) Burkitt lymphoma, low power showing multiple tingible body macrophages, giving rise to the starry sky morphology. 100X, hematoxylin and eosin stain. **See Plates 16-18 for color images.**

this distinction in pediatric NHL, other than for descriptive purposes, has not been conclusively demonstrated.

Immunophenotypic features of both the Burkitt and atypical Burkitt lymphomas are nearly identical (Table 5-5). Both are composed of mature B-cells that express cell surface CD19, CD20, CD22, CD10, and cell surface immunoglobulin. Usually the immunoglobulin is IgM heavy chain with light chain restriction.[10,49] The atypical Burkitt or Burkitt-like tumors tend to have more variability in cell surface antigen expression with variable CD10 or expression of cell surface IgG.[52]

Cytogenetic analysis of BL will demonstrate characteristic translocations involving the *C-MYC* oncogene locus on chromosome 8 in most cases,[53] and the WHO classification requires demonstration of a *C-MYC* translocation in order to make a definitive diagnosis of BL.[45] The predominant cytogenetic aberration that is seen is t(8;14)(q24;q32), which is seen in approximately 80% of BL cases. The remaining 20% of cases demonstrate alternative translocations including a t(2;8)(p11;q24) or t(8;22)(q24;q11).[54]

Diffuse Large B-Cell Lymphoma

Diffuse large B-cell lymphoma makes up approximately 20% of pediatric NHL.[48,55] DLBCL tends to occur in slightly older age groups and is the most common histology of lymphomas seen in children older than 5 years of age and teenagers. DLBCL tends to occur as a single site of disease, with mediastinal and abdominal primary sites being most common.[44,55,56] Nodal disease is very common, in contrast to BL. DLBCL is the most common subtype of lymphoma associated with immunodeficiency (inherited or iatrogenic) seen in childhood.[55,57]

DLBCL may display a variety of morphologic appearances including tumors composed of large noncleaved cells, large cleaved cells, polylobated cells, and immunoblastic cells (exhibiting a single prominent eosinophilic nucleolus) (Figure 5-10). The neoplastic lymphoid cells are large and

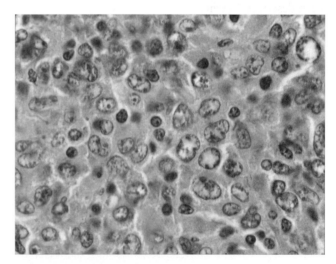

Figure 5-10 Diffuse large B-cell lymphoma showing large neoplastic lymphoid cells with nuclei that are greater than 2 to 3 times the size of a small lymphocyte with relatively abundant eosinophilic cytoplasm. 400X, hematoxylin and eosin stain. **See Plate 19 for color image.**

have a nucleus that is at least the size of a tissue histiocyte or twice the size of a small, reactive lymphocyte. The cytoplasm may vary in abundance but is always significantly more prominent than that seen in BL or LBL. The overall growth pattern is diffuse.[10,44,45] In more recent classifications such as the WHO and REAL classifications, all DLBCLs are considered to be of similar aggressiveness without a significant impact imparted by histologic subtype.[44,45]

Immunophenotypic analysis of DLBCL (Table 5-5) will show that it has a mature B-cell phenotype with expression of cell surface immunoglobulins and B-cell specific lineage markers such as CD19, CD20, CD22, and CD79a.[10,45,58] There are no specific, recurrent characteristic cytogenetic abnormalities associated with DLBCL in children and adolescents.[59]

Anaplastic Large Cell Lymphoma

Anaplastic large cell lymphoma is the most common mature T-cell lymphoma that is seen in children and makes up approximately 10% of pediatric NHL and approximately 30% to 40% of the large cell lymphomas seen in the pediatric population.[10,48,55] It is often associated with lymphadenopathy in combination with extranodal disease most commonly involving the skin, bone, and soft tissue.[60] CNS involvement is more commonly seen in children than in adults.[61] Patients are most commonly male and older than 10 years of age. Most patients will present with advanced (stage III or IV) disease.[60,62]

There are several morphologic subtypes of ALCL that have been described in the literature. So-called classic ALCL has a predominance of tumor cells that are large, pleomorphic, and often multinucleated. Often these cells contain eccentric horseshoe-shaped nuclei with abundant clear to basophilic cytoplasm with an area of eosinophilia near the nucleus (termed "hallmark cells") (Figure 5-11A). These large hallmark cells may resemble Reed-Sternberg cells, although they typically do not have as prominent nucleoli. A small-cell variant of ALCL has also been described in which the cells are more monomorphic and show minimal cytologic variation (Figure 5-11B). In some cases, there may be a prominent histiocytic component accompanying the tumor, which has been termed the lymphohistiocytic variant of ALCL.[61,63] The classical variant makes up approximately 75% of pediatric ALCL, whereas the lymphohistiocytic and small-cell variants compose approximately 10% of tumors.

Anaplastic large cell lymphoma is defined as having tumor cells that express the CD30 (Ki-1) antigen in virtually all tumor cells (Figure 5-12A). The majority of tumors will have a T-cell phenotype when tested with a sufficient number of T-cell antigens (Table 5-5).[45] Particularly in pediatric ALCL, expression of ALK (anaplastic lymphoma kinase) protein by immunohistochemistry is extremely common (Figure 5-12B). Anaplastic lymphoma kinase staining has been strongly associated with systemic disease and is characteristically absent in primary cutaneous ALCL.[64–66] Cytogenetic and molecular analyses will almost uniformly demonstrate characteristic genetic alterations involving the ALK gene locus on chromosome 2 (Figure 5-13).[67,68]

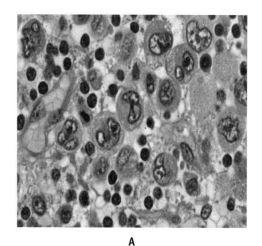

A

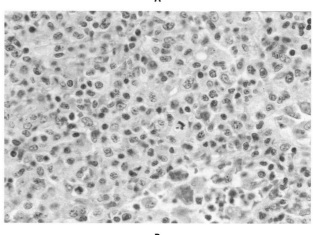

B

Figure 5-11 (A) Anaplastic large cell lymphoma, classic type, showing a proliferation of large anaplastic cells that are horseshoe-shaped and multinucleated with abundant, slightly basophilic cytoplasm. 400X, H&E. (B) Anaplastic large cell lymphoma, small cell variant, showing a smaller atypical neoplastic proliferation of T-cells that are small to intermediate in size and show evidence of vascular invasion. This tumor stained positively with both CD30 and ALK-1. 200X, hematoxylin and eosin stain. **See Plates 20 and 21 for color images.**

Lymphoblastic Lymphoma

Lymphoblastic lymphoma is part of the spectrum of the precursor of blast cell neoplasms seen in children. These neoplasms may present as disseminated bone marrow and blood disease (acute lymphoblastic leukemia, or ALL), or as tissue masses (LBL). Definitions that have been used therapeutically require < 25% bone marrow blasts as well as tissue masses for a process to be identified as a LBL.[10,47] However, current WHO classification notes that this represents a spectrum of precursor lymphoid cell disease and many new therapeutic regimes treat LBL similarly to ALL.[45] Lymphoblastic lymphomas represent about 30% of lymphomas in children but compose < 10% of those NHL seen in adults.[48] As noted above, these immature lymphoid neoplasms frequently have both lymphomatous and leukemic components, making designation as a lymphoma somewhat arbitrary. Whereas precursor B-cell disease usually presents as ALL, most lymphomatous presentations are of

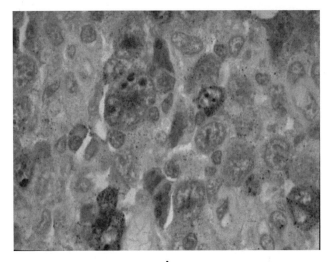

A

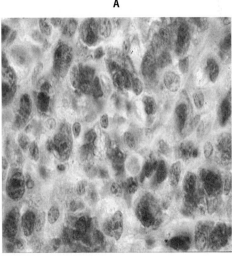

B

Figure 5-12 (A) CD30 staining in anaplastic large cell lymphoma showing typical strong staining in a cytoplasmic and Golgi pattern in the neoplastic cells. 1000X oil, hematoxylin counterstain, CD30 immunostaining. (B) ALK-1 in an anaplastic large cell lymphoma that carries the t(2;5) translocation showing the typical nuclear and cytoplasmic staining pattern seen with that translocation. 400X, hematoxylin counterstain ALK-1 immunostaining. **See Plates 22 and 23 for color images.**

precursor T-cell derivation.[10,45] Precursor T-cell LBL tends to present as mediastinal or upper torso nodal masses, whereas precursor B-cell LBL is more likely to present in skin, soft tissue, bone, tonsil, or as a single peripheral lymph node.[69]

Characteristically, LBL may show diffuse or partial effacement of nodal architecture. Particularly in precursor T-cell LBL, the neoplastic cells may infiltrate in an interfollicular zone with sparing of benign, reactive follicles.[10] Lymphoblastic lymphomas are often rapidly dividing neoplasms with a high mitotic rate, and there may be tingible body macrophages present creating a "starry sky" appearance similar to that seen in BL.[10] By cytology the neoplastic cells are indistinguishable from the blasts seen in ALL. The cells will have immature blast-like appearance with fine ("dusty") chromatin and inconspicuous or absent nucleoli. The cytoplasm is scanty and ranges from pale to basophilic

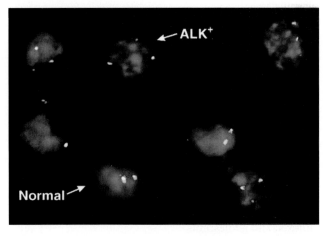

Figure 5-13 FISH analysis for the ALK translocation in anaplastic large cell lymphoma showing breakapart of the yellow fusion signal when a translocation is present giving rise to separate red and green signals. 1000X, FISH. **See Plate 24 for color image.**

in color (Figure 5-14).[44,45] It should be noted that cytoplasmic vacuoles may occasionally be seen in precursor lymphoblastic lesions and are not specific for BL.[10] Particularly in precursor T-cell disease, the cells may have irregular nuclear contours with multiple in-foldings. Precursor B-cell neoplasms tend to have more rounded and smooth contours. Cytochemical studies may show strong, focal cytoplasmic acid phosphatase reactivity. Terminal deoxytidyl nuclear transferase (TdT) will also be positive.[45]

The immunophenotype of precursor T-LBL will display a cortical thymocyte immunophenotype, usually reflecting middle to late stages of differentiation (Tables 5-4 and 5-5). Precursor B-LBL most often displays an early pre B- or pre B-phenotype (Tables 5-5 and 5-6). Specific flow cytometric markers are particularly useful in separating B-lymphoid, T-lymphoid, and myeloid leukemic lineages (Table 5-7).

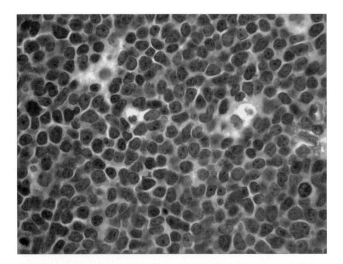

Figure 5-14 Precursor T lymphoblastic lymphoma showing monomorphic infiltrate of neoplastic cells with fine chromatin, minimal cytoplasm and slightly irregular nuclear contours. 400X, hematoxylin and eosin stain. **See Plate 25 for color image.**

Table 5-6

Common antigen expression patterns of the precursor lymphoblastic neoplasms.

				B-cell					
	CD19	**CD20**	**CD22**	**CD24**	**CD10**	**CD34**	**Tdt**	**HLA-DR**	**SIg**
B-Precursor ALL	+	−/+	−	+	+/−	+	+	+	−
Pre-B ALL	+	+/−	−/+	+	+	+	+/−	+	−
B-ALL	+	+	+	+	+/−	−	−	+	+

					T-Cell						
	CD1	**CD2**	**CD3**	**CD4**	**CD5**	**CD7**	**CD8**	**CD10**	**CD34**	**Tdt**	**HLA-DR**
T-ALL	+	+	+ (C)	+	+	+	+	+/−	−/+	+	−/+

Abbreviations: SIg = surface immunoglobulin, C = usually cytoplasmic, + = positive, +/− = often positive, −/+ = occasionally positive, − = negative

Table 5-7

Flow cytometric markers useful in defining leukemic lineage.

	B-lymphoid	T-lymphoid	Myeloid
Most specific	CytCD79a*	CD3(M/cyt)	MPO
	Cyt IgM	Anti-TCR	
	CytCD22		
Intermediate specificity	CD19	CD2	CD117
	CD20	CD5	CD13
	CD10	CD8	CD33
		CD10	CD65
Low specificity	TdT	TdT	CD14
	CD24	CD7	CD15
			CD64

*CD79a may also be expressed in some cases of precursor T lymphoblastic leukemia/lymphoma.

Cyt = cytoplasmic   M = Membrane   MPO = myeloperoxidase

Hodgkin Lymphoma

Hodgkin lymphoma makes up approximately 5% to 10% of childhood cancers in the United States and is more commonly seen in males.[70–71] In developing countries, HL is seen more commonly in younger children than in more advanced Western countries.[72] This epidemiology has suggested that there may be an environmental factor, possibly infectious in nature, that is involved in disease pathogenesis. Epstein-Barr viral DNA has been shown in tissues of HL and is localized to the Reed-Sternberg cells of patients.[73] It is uncertain whether Epstein-Barr virus has a direct role in the pathogenesis of the disease or if it is a secondary marker.

The WHO classification of HL divides the disease into two predominant subtypes, classical Hodgkin lymphoma (CHL) and nodular lymphocyte predominant Hodgkin lymphoma (NLPHL) (Table 5-8).[45] These two subtypes are primarily separated based on the identification of the neoplastic R-S cells and variants.[72,74]

Classical Hodgkin Lymphoma

Classical Hodgkin lymphoma is characterized by architectural effacement of lymph nodes by a mixed inflammatory infiltrate that contains R-S cells and R-S variants. The mixed infiltrate contains small lymphocytes, macrophages, plasma cells, eosinophils, neutrophils, and fibroblasts. The

Table 5-8

WHO classification of Hodgkin lymphoma.

Disease	Neoplastic Cell
Nodular lymphocyte predominant Hodgkin lymphoma	L & H cell
Classical Hodgkin lymphoma	Reed-Sternberg cell
Nodular sclerosis classical Hodgkin lymphoma	Reed-Sternberg cell
Mixed cellularity classical Hodgkin lymphoma	Reed-Sternberg cell
Lymphocyte-rich classical Hodgkin lymphoma	Reed-Sternberg cell
Lymphocyte-depleted classical Hodgkin lymphoma	Reed-Sternberg cell

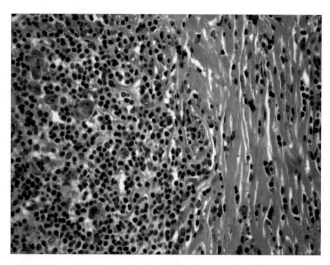

Figure 5-16 Nodular sclerosis classical Hodgkin lymphoma. This shows the nodular appearance of a classical Hodgkin lymphoma of the nodular sclerosis subtype. There are broad bands of collegen fibrosis separating nodules that are composed of a mixture of reactive cells with numerous Reed-Sternberg cells and variants. 200X, hematoxylin and eosin stain. **See Plate 27 for color image.**

neoplastic R-S cells and R-S variants are usually outnumbered by the inflammatory host response.[72,74] The R-S cells are large cells with bilobed or multilobed nuclei and prominent eosinophilic nucleoli (Figure 5-15).

The subtypes of CHL that are recognized by the WHO classification include nodular sclerosis, mixed cellularity, lymphocyte-rich, and lymphocyte depletion CHL.[45] In the pediatric population, nodular sclerosis is by far the most common subtype of CHL observed. The mixed cellularity subtype of CHL is relatively rare in the pediatric population when compared with older adults, and it is most commonly seen in children less than 10 years of age whereas the nodular sclerosing subtype is more prominent in the teenage age group.[70]

Nodular sclerosis CHL is characterized by extensive collagen band formation and a predominance of single nuclear R-S cell variants that show significant cytoplasmic retraction when fixed in formalin (Figure 5-16). This causes a characteristic of appearance of a cell sitting within an empty space called a lacunar cell.

Immunophenotypic analysis of all subtypes of CHL will show similar findings (Table 5-9). The R-S cell is characteristically positive with CD30 (Ki-1) and CD15 (Leu-M1), although up to 20% of CHL may lack expression of CD15 in paraffin sections. The R-S cells are negative for leukocyte common antigen or CD45. Usually the R-S cells are negative for T- and B-cell markers, although approximately 20% of classical Hodgkin disease will show expression of CD20.[72,74] In contrast with NHL, the R-S cells will have inconsistent expression of CD20 with only a proportion of the cells being positive.[72,75]

Cytogenetic analysis of CHL shows karyotypes that are abnormal and clonal in up to 82% of cases.[76,77] However, there is no consistent recurring karyotypic abnormality that is characteristic of CHL.[71,76,78]

Nodular Lymphocyte Predominant Hodgkin Lymphoma

A biologically separate category of HL is NLPHL. This type of HL is relatively rare, making up approximately 5% of HL in adults series and between 10% and 20% in most pediatric series.[71,79] There is a strong male predominance and most cases present at low stage (I or II) at diagnosis. Involvement is usually in peripheral lymph nodes, particularly in the axillary and cervical regions. Mediastinal lymphadenopathy is extremely rare.[79,80]

Nodular lymphocyte predominant Hodgkin lymphoma is defined by the presence of R-S variants that are termed L&H (lymphocyte and histiocyte) cells and a host response that is predominantly lymphocytic with

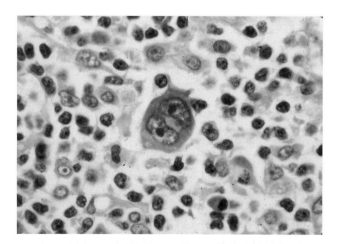

Figure 5-15 Reed-Sternberg cell from classical Hodgkin lymphoma showing the typical binuclear Reed-Sternberg cell with prominent eosinophilic nucleoli that are the neoplastic cell in classical Hodgkin lymphoma. 1000X, hematoxylin and eosin stain. **See Plate 26 for color image.**

admixed macrophages. The L&H cells are somewhat larger than typical small lymphocytes and show a characteristic lobulated or distinctly indented nucleus that has caused them to be called "popcorn cells" (Figure 5-17). The numbers of L&H cells are variable, ranging from scattered single cells to small clusters or sheets. Classic R-S cells are extremely rare or not seen, and are therefore not required for diagnosis. In contrast to CHL, plasma cells, eosinophils, and fibrosis are not present.[80]

Unlike in CHL, the L&H variants in NLPHL have a distinctive and consistent B-cell phenotype (Table 5-9) with expression of CD19, CD20, CD22, and CD79a.[74] The reactive lymphocytes that are admixed with the L&H cells are predominantly polyclonal B-lymphocytes.

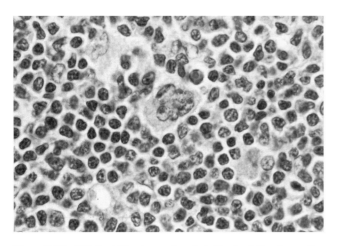

Figure 5-17 L&H Reed-Sternberg cell variant. The Reed-Sternberg cell variant that is seen in nodular lymphocyte predominant Hodgkin lymphoma with the classical multilobated nucleus, giving rise to the "popcorn cell." 1000X, hematoxylin and eosin stain. **See Plate 28 for color image.**

Acute Lymphoblastic Leukemia

Acute lymphoblastic leukemia is a malignant neoplasm deriving from precursor lymphoid cells of either B or T phenotype. Approximately 80% of the childhood acute leukemias are ALL and there is significant overlap in clinical presentation with the lymphoblastic lymphomas. Recognition of this overlap has led to current classifications, such as the WHO classification, to recognize these as acute lymphoblastic leukemia/lymphoma.[45] Definition of leukemia is based on demonstrating an excess of 25% or more lymphoblasts in the marrow. When there are < 25% lymphoblasts in the marrow and mass lesions, the designation of lymphoblastic lymphoma is preferred.[81] Acute lymphoblastic leukemia is defined as being either derived from precursor B-cells or precursor T-cells as determined by immunophenotype (see Tables 5-5, 5-6, 5-7). A leukemic presentation is far more common with the precursor B phenotype, which represents 80% to 85% of pediatric ALL.[82]

Clinically, patients with ALL will present with bone marrow insufficiency or failure due to extensive bone marrow infiltration by the neoplastic cells. This gives rise to resultant blood cytopenias including anemia, thrombocytopenia, and neutropenia. White blood cell counts may be low or normal in many cases of pediatric ALL,[81,83,84] and lower blood white blood cell counts are associated with a better prognosis.[85] Acute lymphoblastic leukemia may also present with a high white count and many peripheral blasts at presentation, most commonly in precursor T-ALL.[86] Extramedullary manifestations may also be seen including lymphadenopathy, hepatosplenomegaly, and tissue infiltration.[81,84] The CNS, and in male patients the testes, may also be involved and may be sanctuary sites where blasts may persist despite therapy.[82,83]

Morphologic diagnosis of ALL requires identification of lymphoblasts[45,81] (Figure 5-18A and B). These blast cells are primitive precursors lacking many features of differentiation. The French-American-British classification

Table 5-9

Immunophenotype of Reed-Sternberg cells and variants in Hodgkin lymphoma.

	Classical Hodgkin lymphoma	Nodular LP Hodgkin lymphoma
CD30	+	−/+
CD45	−	+
CD20	−/+	+
CD15	+/−	−
CD43	−	−
Vimentin	+	−/+
EBV (LMP)	+/−	−
ALK Protein	−	−

+ = Positive   − = negative   +/− = often positive   −/+ = usually negative   LP = lymphocyte predominant

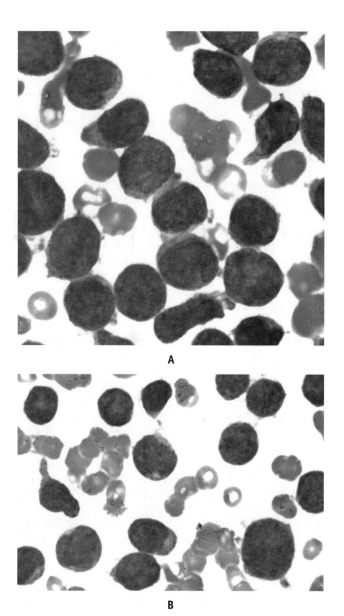

Figure 5-18 (A) L1 lymphoid blast. These lymphoid blasts show relatively little morphologic diversity and have a low nuclear: cytoplasmic ratio with minimal cytoplasm and relatively smooth nuclear contours. 1000X, Wright's stain. (B) L2 lymphoid blast. These lymphoid blasts show more diversity in nuclear size and shape with variation from small L1 type blasts to larger blasts with more abundant cytoplasm and somewhat irregular nuclear contours. 1000X, Wright's stain. **See Plates 29 and 30 for color images.**

identified specific morphologic subtypes of lymphoblasts in ALL (Table 5-10).[87]

It should be noted that there is no cytochemical profile that is diagnostic of ALL. All of the cytochemical patterns found in ALL may overlap with other types of leukemia and emphasize the need for appropriate immunophenotypic studies[81,88] (Tables 5-5, 5-6, 5-7).

Immunophenotyping allows distinction of ALL derived from either precursor B-cells from precursor T-cells (Tables 5-6, 5-7).[4,81] Furthermore, specific expression of B-cell antigens allows for evaluation of the degree of differentiation of precursor B lineage lymphoblasts, a feature that has been

associated with specific clinical and genetic findings.[4,81,85] Flow cytometric techniques provide the most easily utilized means for assigning both lineage and stage of maturation in ALL. Blast cell DNA content (aneuploidy) may also be measured by using flow cytometric techniques.[4]

Cytogenetic abnormalities in precursor B-ALL include both numerical abnormalities and reciprocal translocations.[89,90] Cytogenetics findings are considered prognostically important and may be used to modify treatment.[14,91,92] Good prognostic groups include hyperdiploidy (containing between 51 and 65 chromosomes or a flow cytometric DNA content of 1.16 to 1.6) or identification of a t(12;21)(p12;q22).[14,90,92,93] Cytogenetic findings associated with a poor prognosis include t(9;22)(q34;q11.2) or *BCR/ABL-1* translocation.[14,90,92,93] Another poor prognostic cytogenetic finding is a demonstration of rearrangement of the MLL (mixed lineage leukemia) gene at 11q23, particularly a t(4;11), which is strongly associated with early precursor B-ALL that is characteristically CD10 negative[90,95] and seen in infants.[96] The t(1;19)(q23;p13.3) translocation and hypodiploidy are also associated with a poor prognosis.

In contrast to precursor B-ALL, precursor T-ALL is relatively rare, making up only about 15% of pediatric ALL.[83] The precursor T-lymphoblastic lesions most commonly present as lymphomas, with the mediastinal presentation being the most frequent.[10] Precursor T-ALL is more common in adolescents and occurs more frequently in males than in females. Precursor T-ALL typically presents with a high peripheral blast count and leukemia tissue infiltrates, including lymphadenopathy and mediastinal masses.

Approximately one-third of cases of T-ALL will show chromosomal translocations.[14,17,90,93] Approximately half of these are involving the alpha and delta T-cell receptor loci at 14q11, the T-cell beta locus at 7q34, and the T-cell receptor gamma locus at 7p14-15 with a variety of partner genes.[90]

Pediatric Myeloid Malignancies

Myeloid malignancies are characterized by clonal expansions by a hematopoietic precursor of the myeloid, erythroid, or megakaryocytic cell lineages. Myeloid malignancies are much more frequently seen in adults than in children, although some disease entities, such as juvenile myelomonocytic leukemia (JMML), are limited to the pediatric age group.[97] The myeloid malignancies include chronic myeloproliferative disorders (CMD), myelodysplastic syndromes (MDS), myeloproliferative/myelodysplastic disorders, and acute myeloid leukemias (AML).[45]

Pediatric Chronic Myeloproliferative Disorders

Chronic myeloproliferative disorders, as defined by the WHO classification, include chronic myelogenous leukemia (CML), chronic neurophilic leukemia, chronic eosinophilic leukemia, the hypereosinophilic syndromes, polycythemia vera, chronic idiopathic myeloid fibrosis, essential thrombocythemia, and chronic myeloproliferative disease unclassifi-

Table 5-10

FAB morphologic classification of lymphoid blasts.

Cytologic Features	L1	L2
Cell size	Small	Large, heterogeneous
Nuclear chromatin	Homogeneous in any one case	Variable, heterogeneous in any one case
Nuclear features	Smooth, contour, occasional clefting or indentation	Irregular, clefting and indentation common
Nucleoli	Not visible, or small and inconspicuous	One or more present, often large
Amount of cytoplasm	Scanty	Variable, often moderately abundant
Basophilia of cytoplasm	Slight or moderate, rarely intense	Variable, deep in some
Cytoplasmic vacuolization	Variable	Variable

able. Most CMDs are typically seen in adults, and with the exception of CML are extremely rare in children.[97,98] All CMDs are due to a clonal proliferation of an abnormal stem cell that causes overproduction of one or more hematopoietic cell lines, leading to polycythemia, leukocytosis, and/or thrombocytosis.[97,99] One other disease of childhood, transient myeloproliferative disorder of newborns, particularly those with trisomy 21, is also considered to be a myeloproliferative disorder.[100,101]

Chronic myelogenous leukemia is a clonal stem cell neoplasm that leads to excessive proliferation of the myeloid series.[102,103] It is consistently associated with a specific cytogenetic abnormality, the Philadelphia chromosome or t(9;22)(q34;q11).[104] This causes a resultant *BCR/ABL-1* fusion gene that is associated with a striking neutrophilia of the blood and granulocytic hyperplasia in the bone marrow.[105,106] Although CML is predominantly a disease of adults, approximately 9% of cases of CML occur in the pediatric age group. This disorder usually affects adolescents, but CML has also been reported in younger children.[103,107] Patients with CML usually present with nonspecific symptoms such as fatigue, bleeding, malaise, and weight loss or symptoms attributable to marked splenomegaly. The blood often has extremely high white blood cell counts, and children are more likely to have symptoms of hyperleukocytosis.[102,103,107]

Immunophenotypic analysis of patients with CML shows no distinctive abnormalities. Flow cytometry analysis of either blood or bone marrow will show a myeloid predominance with normal expression of myeloid markers. There will often be evidence of a shift to immaturity with a small increase in blasts.[97,108]

Chronic myelogenous leukemia is genetically defined by the presence of the specific Philadelphia chromosome or t(9;22)(q34;q11).[103] This abnormality is demonstrable by conventional cytogenetics as well as FISH.[14,105] This cytogenetic abnormality will lead to production of a *BCR/ABL* fusion protein with tyrosine kinase activity. Without therapy, many patients will proceed on to development of acute leukemia that may be either myeloid or lymphoid derivation.[97,102,103]

An apparent myeloid proliferative disorder that is unique and confined to the pediatric population is the transient myeloproliferative disorder (TMD) usually seen in neonates with Down syndrome (trisomy 21).[109,110] The most common hematologic manifestation of TMD is transient leukocytosis with a markedly increased white blood cell count that may exceed 50,000/mm^3. The blood smear will show a spectrum of myeloid differentiation including morphologically normal neutrophils, although up to 50% of the circulating cells may be blasts. These blasts include myeloblasts but may have a predominance of megakaryoblasts and erythroblasts. Platelets are often abnormal, with enlarged platelets and circulating megakaryocytes or megakaryocytic fragments. Hemoglobin levels and platelet counts are variable but are usually within normal limits. In TMD there will be spontaneous resolution of all blood and bone marrow abnormalities within 1 to 2 months.[111] Molecular analysis of patients with TMD has shown the myeloid proliferation to be clonal and associated with mutations involving the X-linked GATA-1 transcription factor.[112] It is uncertain what drives the transient appearance of blasts and the ultimate resolution of this disorder.[101] However, patients with TMD are at an increased risk for subsequent development of acute leukemia, often megakaryoblastic leukemia, within 6 to 12 months after experiencing TMD.[111,113,114]

Myelodysplastic Syndrome

Myelodysplastic syndromes are clonal disorders of multipotential hematopoietic stem cells that are characterized by blood cytopenias, bone marrow hypercellularity, and ineffective hematopoiesis.[45] Most MDSs are associated with an increase in development of AML. Myelodysplastic syndromes occur far less commonly in children than in adults, and most children with MDS will have an associated congenital abnormality or possible toxic exposure, including prior tumor therapy with alkylating agents or radiation.[115–117]

Myelodysplastic syndrome is much more likely to develop in children with certain genetic disorders. Children with trisomy 21 often develop MDS before progression to acute leukemia.[118] This may be associated with increased reticulin fibrosis.[119] Cytogenetic analysis often shows acquisition of additional karyotypic abnormalities, such as trisomy 8.[120] Neurofibromatosis type I is also associated with an increase in MDS, often associated with monosomy 7.[121,122] Patients with MDS and neurofibromatosis type I are usually older than those patients typically described with the infantile monosomy 7 syndrome (described below).[123] Myelodysplastic syndrome is also seen in patients with Fanconi anemia, an abnormality with increased susceptibility to chromosomal damage. In patients with Fanconi anemia, development of dysplastic changes often precedes development of acute leukemia.[124]

The clinical course of MDS in children is progressive cytopenias, often culminating in the development of acute leukemia.[125] Bone marrow transplantation appears to be the most effective therapy option, and chemotherapy is usually ineffective in young patients.[125]

Myelodysplastic/Myeloproliferative Diseases

The myelodysplastic/myeloproliferative diseases are clonal hematopoietic neoplasms that have some clinical, laboratory, or morphologic findings that have features of both MDS and CMD. The WHO recognizes several entities in the myelodysplastic/myeloproliferative disorders but only one is seen with any frequency in the pediatric population, JMML,[98,125] which is characterized by proliferation of granulocytic and monocytic precursors with associated dysplasia in the erythroid and megakaryocytic lines[97,98] (Figure 5-19). JMML is thought to arise from an abnormality affecting a bone marrow stem cell with multilineage potential.[126] The major diagnostic criteria for JMML (Table 5-11) include a peripheral blood monocytosis ($>1 \times 10^9$ liter), blasts (including promonocytes) are less than 20% of the white blood cells in the blood and

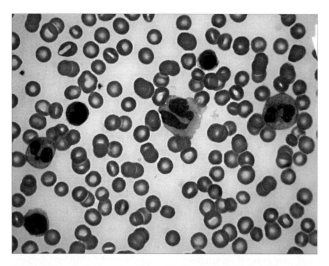

Figure 5-19 Peripheral blood in JMML. The peripheral blood of this child shows a monocytosis with circulating nucleated red blood cells and dyspoietic changes in the neutrophils including abnormal segmentation and granulation of neutrophils. Platelets also appear hypogranular. 1000X, Wright's stain. **See Plate 31 for color image.**

Table 5-11
Diagnostic criteria for JMML.

1. Peripheral blood monocytosis $>1 \times 10^9$/L
2. Blasts + promonocytes are $<20\%$ of the WBCs in the blood
3. Blasts + promonocytes are $<20\%$ of marrow cells
4. No Philadelphia chromosome, t(9;22) or *BCR/ABL* fusion gene
5. Plus two or more of the following:
   Hemoglobin F increased for age
   Immature granulocytes in the peripheral blood
   WBC count $>10 \times 10^9$/L
   Clonal chromosomal abnormality (eg, may be monosomy 7)
   GM-CSF hypersensitivity of myeloid progenitors in vitro

nucleated bone marrow cells, no evidence of a *BCR/ABL-1* fusion gene or Philadelphia chromosome. Minor criteria include increased hemoglobin F for the patient's age, myeloid shift to immaturity in the peripheral blood, elevated white blood cell count ($>10 \times 10^9$ liter), clonal chromosomal abnormalities including monosomy 7 and increased sensitivity to GM-CSF by myeloid progenitors in vitro.[45] Juvenile myelomonocytic leukemia is the most frequently seen MDS/MPD seen in patients less than 14 years of age.[98] The age of diagnosis can range from one month to early adolescence, but most cases occur in children less than 3 years of age. Boys are affected approximately twice as frequently as girls, and there is a strong association with clinical diagnosis of neurofibromatosis, type I.[98,125]

Genetic analysis of patients with JMML shows no evidence of a Philadelphia chromosome or *BCR/ABL-1* fusion gene.[126] Cytogenetic abnormalities, most commonly monosomy 7, occur in 30% to 40% of patients but are not specific for JMML.[98,125,126] The clinical course is variable, but approximately 30% of patients will show rapid progression. Patients <1 year of age and children >2 years of age have a worse prognosis, as do patients with very low platelet counts or increased hemoglobin F levels at the time of diagnosis.[125] Most patients will die from organ failure due to leukemic infiltration.[127] Approximately 10% to 20% of patients may evolve to acute leukemia.[117]

Acute Myeloid Leukemia

Acute myeloid leukemia is a clonal expansion of myeloid blasts. This disease is less frequently seen in children than adults, and makes up approximately 20% of pediatric acute leukemias, with approximately 5.2 cases per 1 million children under the age of 15. Males and females are equally affected. The incidence of AML is increased during the first year of life and then declines, with a second incidence peak seen in adolescence.[96] The majority of children with AML have no preceding risk factors. There has been an association with genetic disorders (including Fanconi anemia, Kostmann syndrome, Down syndrome, neurofibromatosis type I), previous exposure to carcinogens, previous chemotherapy, or radiation exposure. Often patients with the above predisposing conditions will have preceding MDS before the development of AML.[101] Children with posttherapeutic AML often present within three years, after exposure to therapy with alkylating agents.[128] Children may also develop posttherapeutic AML in a shorter time frame after exposure to topoisomerase II inhibitors with AML occurring months to years after exposure. The topoisomerase II inhibitor associated therapy-related AML appears to be related more to the frequency of exposure than to the accumulated dose and is often associated with translocation of chromosome 11q23 (Figure 5-20), t(8;21) or t(15;15), and inv(16) in over half of cases.[93,94,129]

Classification of AML under the WHO classification calls for the AML to be separated on the basis of immunophenotypic (Table 5-7), cytochemical, and morphologic as well as genetic abnormalities. Patients with specific cytogenetic abnormalities, associated multilineage dysplasia or therapy-related AML, need to be separated from those that do not have the above features.[45] Initial diagnosis of AML is based on morphological, cytochemical, and immunophenotypic analysis in determining the punitive cell of origin for the AML.[130] The bone marrow aspirate and biopsy should have greater than 20% blasts or there should be an extramedullary mass that is composed of myeloblasts.[45,131] These will be placed into the AML, not otherwise categorized.[45] Definition of the subtype of AML is based on the morphologic appearance of the blasts, the percentage of myeloblasts or monoblasts, as well as cytochemical staining characteristics with myeloperoxidase, Sudan black B, or nonspecific esterase stains.[132] The acute megakaryoblastic leukemias and the acute minimally differentiated myeloid leukemias may require immunophenotypic analysis (Table 5-7) for definitive diagnosis because they lack specific cytochemical staining profiles.[133] The categories of acute myeloid leukemia not otherwise categorized are presented in Table 5-12.

Two types of AML occur more frequently in children, acute monoblastic leukemia (Figure 5-20) and acute megakaryoblastic leukemia.[134] Monoblastic leukemia (Figure 5-20) is often associated with tissue infiltrates, and initial diagnosis may be made on materials other than blood and bone marrow (and the tissue-based disease may precede marrow disease by months). Monoblastic leukemias are characterized by relatively undifferentiated blasts with round nuclear contours and somewhat basophilic cytoplasm or monocytoid blasts with irregular (kidney-shaped) nuclei and abundant clear to basophilic cytoplasm. They will stain brightly with nonspecific esterase and express monocytic antigens (CD13, CD14, and CD4).[132] Cytogenetic studies are heterogeneous, with no recurrent abnormality described.[13] Megakaryoblastic leukemias are also increased in children, particularly those with Down syndrome (and are especially frequent in patients with preceding TMD).[133] Megakaryoblastic leukemias have blasts that range from undifferentiated blasts to blasts that have granular cytoplasm and resemble atypical megakaryocytes with platelet budding.[133] The megakaryoblasts have no distinctive cytochemical staining patterns and may require electron microscopy to identify platelet peroxidase activity.[135] Flow cytometry will demonstrate megakaryocytic antigens, such as CD41 and CD61, and is very useful in making the diagnosis.[136] Molecular studies will identify mutations in the GATA-1 transcription factor gene, leading to decreased or abnormal GATA-1 synthesis, in many of the patients with Down syndrome and leukemia.[114] These mutations are similar to those identified in TMD, suggesting a pathophysiologic link between these entities.[114] Cytogenetics will usually show complex abnormalities in addition to the trisomy 21.[137]

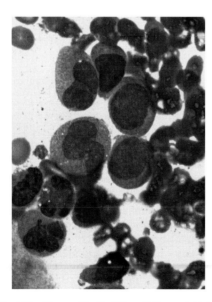

Figure 5-20 AML with monoblastic differentiation and 11q23 abnormality. This AML showed strong NSE positivity and monoblastic markers by flow cytometry. Cytogenetics showed 11q23 abnormality. 1000X, Wright's stain. **See Plate 32 for color image.**

Table 5-12
WHO classification of acute myeloid leukemias (NOS).
Acute myeloid leukemias minimally differentiated
Acute myeloid leukemias without maturation
Acute myeloid leukemias with maturation
Acute myelomonocytic leukemias
Acute monoblastic and monocytic leukemias
Acute erythroid leukemias
Acute megakaryoblastic leukemias
Acute basophilic leukemias
Acute panmyelosis with myelofibrosis
Myeloid sarcoma

Summary

Pediatric cancers involve a broad variety of neoplastic processes involving many organ systems. Many of these entities, such as neuroblastoma or JMML, are unique to children and are not seen commonly in adults. Furthermore, many diseases that are seen in both adults and children, such as ALL, appear to have different pathogenetic mechanisms in the pediatric population. For example, pediatric ALL is a relatively common neoplasm in children that is highly treatable whereas in adults it is rare, with a poor prognosis, and demonstrates a different spectrum of cytogenetic and molecular findings than are commonly seen in children.[90,92,93] Further investigation into the molecular and genetic underpinnings of pediatric cancers through a variety of new technologies, such as gene microarray analysis[138-141] and comparative genomic hybridization techniques,[142-144] should help to further elucidate the molecular pathophysiology of pediatric cancers and help us to understand their biology. With additional understanding of biology it is anticipated that we will develop better ability to diagnose pediatric cancers accurately, determine prognosis, and eventually discover targeted disease-specific therapies that will further enhance our ability to effectively treat and cure these disorders.

References

1. Maitra, A, Kumar V. Genetic and pediatric diseases. In: Kumar V, Cotran R, Robbins S, eds. *Robbins Basic Pathology*. 7th ed. Philadelphia, PA: Saunders; 2003:252–257.
2. Young JL, et al. Cancer incidence, survival and mortality for children younger than age 15 years. *Cancer*. 1986:598–602.
3. Tubbs R, Sheibani K. Immunohistology of lymphoproliferative disorders. *Semin Diagn Pathol*. 1984;1:272–284.
4. Weir EG, Borowitz MJ. Flow cytometry in the diagnosis of acute leukemia. *Semin Hematol*. 2001;38(2):124–138.
5. Armes J, Southey M, et al. Molecular analysis in the diagnosis of pediatric lymphomas. *Pediatr Pathol Lab Med*. 1996;16:435–449.
6. Thorner PS, Squire JA. Molecular genetics in the diagnosis and prognosis of solid pediatric tumors. *Pediatr Develop Pathol*. 1998;1:337–365.
7. Goldsby R, Carroll W. The molecular biology of pediatric lymphomas. *J Pediatr Hematol Oncol*. 1998;20:282–296.
8. Hayashi Y. The molecular genetics of recurring chromosome abnormalities in acute myeloid leukemia. *Semin Hematol*. 2000;37(4):368–380.
9. Solomon AC, Kossev PM. Frozen sections in hematopathology. *Semin Diagn Pathol*. 2002;19(4):255–262.
10. Perkins SL. Work-up and diagnosis of pediatric non-Hodgkin's lymphomas. *Pediatr Dev Pathol*. 2000;3(4):374–390.
11. Weisberger J, Wu CD, et al. (2000). Differential diagnosis of malignant lymphomas and related disorders by specific pattern of expression of immunophenotypic markers revealed by multiparameter flow cytometry (Review). *Int J Oncol*. 17(6):1165–1177.
12. Patrick CW. Clinical flow cytometry: milestones along the pathway of progress. *MLO Med Lab Obs*. 2002;34(9):10–11,14–16;20–21.
13. Swansbury J. Cytogenetic and genetic studies in solid tumors: background. *Methods Mol Biol*. 2003;220:125–133.
14. Swansbury J. Cytogenetic studies in hematologic malignancies: an overview. *Methods Mol Biol*. 2003;220:9–22.
15. Mrozek K, Heinonen K, et al. Clinical importance of cytogenetics in acute myeloid leukaemia. *Best Pract Res Clin Haematol*. 2001;14(1):19–47.
16. Glassman AB. Chromosomal abnormalities in acute leukemias. *Clin Lab Med*. 2000;20(1):39–48.
17. Harrison CJ. The genetics of childhood acute lymphoblastic leukaemia. *Baillieres Best Pract Res Clin Haematol*. 2000;13(3):427–439.
18. Raimondi SC. Fluorescence in situ hybridization: molecular probes for diagnosis of pediatric neoplastic diseases. *Cancer Invest*. 2000;18(2):135–147.
19. Kebriaei P, Anastasi J, et al. Acute lymphoblastic leukaemia: diagnosis and classification. *Best Pract Res Clin Haematol*. 2002;15(4):597–621.
20. Szeles A. Fluorescence in situ hybridization (FISH) in the molecular cytogenetics of cancer. *Acta Microbiol Immunol Hung*. 2002;49(1):69–80.
21. Seiter K. Diagnosis and management of core-binding factor leukemias. *Curr Hematol Rep*. 2003;2(1):78–85.
22. Qualman SJ, Morotti RA. Risk assignment in pediatric soft-tissue sarcomas: an evolving molecular classification. *Curr Oncol Rep*. 2002;4:123–130.
23. Potter MN. The detection of minimal residual disease in acute lymphoblastic leukemia. *Blood Rev*. 1992;6:68–82.
24. Sharp JG, Chan WC. Detection and relevance of minimal disease in lymphomas. *Cancer Metastasis Rev*. 1999;18(1):127–142.
25. Becker LE. The nervous system. In: Stecker JT, Dehner LP, eds. *Pediatric Pathology*. 2nd ed. Philadelphia, PA: Lippincott, Williams and Wilkins; 2001:285–397.
26. Kleihues P, Cavance WK. *Pathology and Genetics: Tumors of the Nervous System*. Lyon, France: International Agency for Research on Cancer; 2000:215–242.
27. Kleihues P, Berger PC, Scheithuer BW. *World Health Organization: International Histological Classification of Tumors of the Central Nervous System*. 2nd ed. World Health Organization. Lyon, France, 1993.
28. Qualman SJ, Bowen J, Fitzgibbons PL, Cohn SL, Shimada H. Protocol for the examination of specimens from patients with neuroblastoma and related neuroblastic tumors. *Arch Pathol Lab Med*. 129:874–883, 2005.
29. Shimada H, et al. The International Pathology Classification (Shimada system). *Cancer*. 1999;86:364–372.
30. Shimada H, et al. Identification of subsets of neuroblastoma, combined histopathologic and N-myc analysis. *J Natl Cancer Inst*. 1995;87:1470–1476.
31. Goto S, et al. Histopathological (International Neuroblastoma Pathology Classification) and MYCN status in patients with peripheral neuroblastic tumors. *Cancer*. 2001;92:2699–2708.
32. Qualman SJ, Bowen J, Amin MB, Srigley JR, Grundy PE, Perlman EJ. Protocol for the examination of specimens from patients with Wilms tumor (nephroblastoma) or other renal tumors of childhood. *Arch Pathol Lab Med*. 2003;127:1280–1289.
33. Beckwith JB. Nephrogenic rests and the pathogenesis of Wilms tumor: developmental and clinical considerations. *Am J Med Genet*. 1998;79:268–273.
34. Qualman SJ, Bowen J, Parham DM, Branton PA, Meyer WH. Protocol for the examination of specimens from patients (children and young adults) with rhabdomyosarcoma. *Arch Pathol Lab Med*. 2003;127:1290–1297.
35. Qualman SJ, Coffin CM, Newton WA, et al. Intergroup Rhabdomyosarcoma Study: update for pathologists. *Pediatr Dev Pathol*. 1998;1:550–561.
36. Burns DK. The male genital system. In: Kumar V, Cotran R, Robbins S, eds. *Robbins Basic Pathology*. 7th ed. Philadelphia, PA: Saunders; 2003:660–664.
37. Dehner LP, O'Sullivan MJ, Strauss BL, Wold LE, McAllister WH. Skeletal system: congenital, developmental and acquired disorders. In: Stocker JT, Dehner LP, eds. *Pediatric Pathology*. 2nd ed. Philadelphia, PA: Lippincott, Williams & Wilkins; 2001:1340–1345.
38. Huvos AG, Rosen G, Marcove RC. Primary osteogenic sarcoma: pathologic aspects in 20 patients after treatment with chemotherapy en bloc resection and prosthetic bone replacement. *Arch Pathol Lab Med*. 1977;1001:14–18.
39. Carpentieri DF, Qualman SJ, Bowen J, Krausz T, Marchevsky A, Dickman PS. Protocol for the examination of specimens from pediatric and adult patients with osseous and extraosseous ewing sarcoma family of tumors, including peripheral primitive neuroectodermal tumor and ewing sarcoma. *Arch Pathol Lab Med*. 129:866–873, 2005.
40. De Alava E, Kawai A, Healey JH, et al. EWS-FLI1 fusion transcript structure is an independent determinant of prognosis in Ewing's sarcoma. *J Clin Oncol*. 1998;16:1248–1255.
41. Stocker JT, Husain AN, Dehner LP, Chandra RS. The liver, gallbladder and biliary tract. In: Stocker JT, Dehner LP, eds. *Pediatric Pathology*. 2nd ed. Philadelphia, PA: Lippincott, Williams & Wilkins; 2001:763–775.
42. Tomlinson GE, Finegold MJ. Tumors of the liver. In: Pizzo PA, Poplack DG, eds. *Pediatric Pathology*. 2nd ed. Philadelphia, PA: Lippincott, Williams & Wilkins; 2001:763–775.
43. Page DL, Brown HH. Retinoblastoma. In: Compton C, ed. *Reporting on Specimens: Case Summaries and Background Documentation*. Northfield, IL: College of American Pathologists; 2003:1–21.
44. Harris NL, ES Jaffe, et al. A revised European-American classification of lymphoid neoplasms: a proposal from the International Lymphoma Study Group. *Blood*. 1994;84(5):1361–1392.
45. Jaffe ES, Harris NL, Stein H, Vardiman JW, eds. *Pathology and Genetics: Tumours of Haematopoietic and Lymphoid Tissues*. Washington, DC: IARC Press; 2001.
46. Rappaport H. *Tumors of the Hematopoietic System*. Washington, DC: US Armed Forces Institute of Pathology; 1966.
47. Cairo MS, Ratees E, et al. *Non-Hodgkin's lymphoma in children*. In: Kufe D, Pollack RE, Weishelbaum RR, et al., eds., *Cancer Medicine*. 6th ed. London: BC Decker; 2003:2337–2348.
48. Sandlund JT, Downing JR, et al. Non-Hodgkin's lymphoma in childhood. *NEJM*. 1996;334:1238–1248.
49. Magrath IT. *Small Noncleaved Cell Lymphomas (Burkitt and Burkitt-like Lymphomas)*, 2nd ed. New York, NY: Arnold; 1997:781–811.
50. Diebold JJE, et al. *Burkitt Lymphoma*. Lyon, France: IARC Press; 2001.
51. The Non-Hodgkin's Lymphoma Pathologic Classification Project. The National Cancer Institute sponsored study of classification of non-Hodgkin's lymphomas: summary and description of Working Formulation for clinical usage. *Cancer*. 1982;49:2112–2135.
52. Spina D, Leoncini L, et al. Cellular kinetic and phenotypic heterogeneity in and among Burkitt's and Burkitt-like lymphomas. *J Pathol*. 1997;182:145–150.

53. Sanger, W. Primary (8q24) and secondary chromosome abnormalities (1q, 6q, 13q, & 17p) are similar in pediatric Burkitt lymphoma/Burkitt leukemia & Burkitt-like lymphoma: A report of the International Pediatric B-cell Non-Hodgkin Lymphoma Study. *Blood*. 2003;102(11):845a.

54. Nowell P, Croce C. Chromosome translocations and oncogenes in human lymphoid tumors. *Am J Clin Pathol*. 1990;94:229–237.

55. Cairo MS, Sposto R, et al. Childhood and adolescent large-cell lymphoma (LCL): a review of the Children's Cancer Group experience. *Am J Hematol*. 2003;72(1):53–63.

56. Cairo MS. Current advances and future strategies of B large cell lymphoma in children and adolescents. *Proc Am Soc Oncol*. 2002;21:512–519.

57. Preciado MV, Fallo A, et al. Epstein Barr virus-associated lymphoma in HIV-infected children. *Pathol Res Pract*. 2002;198(5):327–332.

58. Perkins S, Kjeldsberg C. Immunophenotyping of lymphomas and leukemias in paraffin-embedded tissues. *Am J Clin Pathol*. 1993;99:362–372.

59. Heerema N. Chromosomal abnormalities of pediatric (ped) and adult diffuse large B-cell lymphoma (DLBCL) differ and may reflect potential differences in oncogenesis. *Blood*. 2003;102(11):373a.

60. Alessandri AJ, Pritchard SL, et al. A population-based study of pediatric anaplastic large cell lymphoma. *Cancer*. 2002;94(7):1830–1835.

61. Kinney MC, Kadin ME. The pathologic and clinical spectrum of anaplastic large cell lymphoma and correlation with ALK gene dysregulation. *Am J Clin Pathol*. 1999;111(1)(suppl 1):S56–S67.

62. Massimino M, Gasparini M, et al. Ki-1 (CD30) anaplastic large-cell lymphoma in children. *Ann Oncol*. 1995;6(9):915–920.

63. Kadin M. Anaplastic large cell lymphoma and its morphologic variants. *Cancer Surv*. 1997;30:77–86.

64. Oertel J, Huhn D. Immunocytochemical methods in haematology and oncology. *J Cancer Res Clin Oncol*. 2000;126(8):425–440.

65. Brugieres L, Deley MC, et al. CD30(+) anaplastic large-cell lymphoma in children: analysis of 82 patients enrolled in two consecutive studies of the French Society of Pediatric Oncology. *Blood*. 1998;92(10):3591–3598.

66. Pulford K, Lamant L, et al. Detection of anaplastic lymphoma kinase (ALK) and nucleolar protein nucleophosmin (NPM)-ALK proteins in normal and neoplastic cells with the monoclonal antibody ALK1. *Blood*. 1997;89(4):1394–1404.

67. Ladanyi M. The NPM/ALK gene fusion in the pathogenesis of anaplastic large cell lymphoma. *Cancer Surv*. 1997;30:59–75.

68. Drexler HG, Gignac SM, et al. Pathobiology of NPM-ALK and variant fusion genes in anaplastic large cell lymphoma and other lymphomas. *Leukemia*. 2000;14(9):1533–1559.

69. Thomas DA, Kantarjian HM. Lymphoblastic lymphoma. *Hematol Oncol Clin North Am*. 2001;15(1):51–95, vi.

70. Potter R. Paediatric Hodgkin's disease. *Eur J Cancer*. 1999;35(10):1466–1476.

71. Diehl V, Josting A. Hodgkin's disease. *Cancer J*. 2000;6(suppl 2): S150–S158.

72. Harris NL. The many faces of Hodgkin's disease around the world: what have we learned from its pathology? *Ann Oncol*. 1998;9(suppl 5):S45–S56

73. Axdorph U, Porwit-MacDonald A, et al. Epstein-Barr virus expression in Hodgkin's disease in relation to patient characteristics, serum factors and blood lymphocyte function. *Br J Cancer*. 1999;81(7):1182–1187.

74. Pileri SA, Ascani S, et al. (2002). Hodgkin's lymphoma: the pathologist's viewpoint. *J Clin Pathol*. 55(3):162–176.

75. Chan WC. The Reed-Sternberg cell in classical Hodgkin's disease. *Hematol Oncol*. 2001;19(1):1–17.

76. Atkin NB. Cytogenetics of Hodgkin's disease. *Cytogenet Cell Genet*. 1998; 80(1–4):23–27.

77. Zander T, Wiedenmann S, et al. Prognostic factors in Hodgkin's lymphoma. *Ann Oncol*. 2002;13(suppl 1):67–74.

78. Yung L, Linch D. Hodgkin's lymphoma. *Lancet*. 2003;361(9361):943–951.

79. Ekstrand BC, Horning SJ. Lymphocyte predominant Hodgkin's disease. *Curr Oncol Rep*. 2002;4(5):424–433.

80. Pellegrino B, Terrier-Lacombe MJ, et al. Lymphocyte-predominant Hodgkin's lymphoma in children: therapeutic abstention after initial lymph node resection—a Study of the French Society of Pediatric Oncology. *J Clin Oncol*. 2003;21(15):2948–2952.

81. Lai R, Hirsch-Ginsberg CF, et al. Pathologic diagnosis of acute lymphocytic leukemia. *Hematol Oncol Clin North Am*. 2000;14(6):1209–1235.

82. Hoelzer D, Gokbuget N, et al. Acute lymphoblastic leukemia. *Hematology (Am Soc Hematol Educ Program)*. 2002;162–192.

83. Pui CH. Acute lymphoblastic leukemia in children. *Curr Opin Oncol*. 2000;12(1):3–12.

84. Chessells JM. Pitfalls in the diagnosis of childhood leukaemia. *Br J Haematol*. 2001;114(3):506–511.

85. Friedmann AM, Weinstein HJ. The role of prognostic features in the treatment of childhood acute lymphoblastic leukemia. *Oncologist*. 2000;5(4):321–328.

86. Goldberg JM, Silverman LB, et al. Childhood T-cell acute lymphoblastic leukemia: the Dana-Farber Cancer Institute acute lymphoblastic leukemia consortium experience. *J Clin Oncol*. 2003;21(19):3616–3622.

87. Bennett J, Catovsky D, et al. Proposals for the classification of acute leukemias. French-American-British (FAB) Cooperative Group. *Br J Hematol*. 1976;33:451–458.

88. Behm FG. Morphologic and cytochemical characteristics of childhood lymphoblastic leukemia. *Hematol Oncol Clin North Am*. 1990;4(4):715–741.

89. McKenna RW, Washington LT, et al. Immunophenotypic analysis of hematogones (B-lymphocyte precursors) in 662 consecutive bone marrow specimens by 4-color flow cytometry. *Blood*. 2001;98(8):2498–2507.

90. Harrison CJ, Foroni L. Cytogenetics and molecular genetics of acute lymphoblastic leukemia. *Rev Clin Exp Hematol*. 2002;6(2):91–113.

91. Krajinovic M, Labuda D, et al. Childhood acute lymphoblastic leukemia: genetic determinants of susceptibility and disease outcome. *Rev Environ Health*. 2001;16(4):263–279.

92. Chen Z, Sandberg AA. Molecular cytogenetic aspects of hematological malignancies: clinical implications. *Am J Med Genet*. 2002;115(3):130–141.

93. Harrison CJ. The detection and significance of chromosomal abnormalities in childhood acute lymphoblastic leukaemia. *Blood Rev*. 2001;15(1):49–59.

94. Bartolo C, Viswanatha DS. Molecular diagnosis in pediatric acute leukemias. *Clin Lab Med*. 2000;20(1):139–182, x.

95. Consolini R, Legitimo A, et al. Clinical relevance of CD10 expression in childhood ALL. The Italian Association for Pediatric Hematology and Oncology (AIEOP). *Haematologica*. 1998;83(11):967–973.

96. Isaacs H Jr. Fetal and neonatal leukemia. *J Pediatr Hematol Oncol*. 2003;25(5):348–361.

97. George TI, Arber DA. Pathology of the myeloproliferative diseases. *Hematol Oncol Clin North Am*. 2003;17(5):1101–1127.

98. Hasle H, Niemeyer CM, et al. A pediatric approach to the WHO classification of myelodysplastic and myeloproliferative diseases. *Leukemia*. 2003;17(2):277–282.

99. Michiels JJ, Thiele J. Clinical and pathological criteria for the diagnosis of essential thrombocythemia, polycythemia vera, and idiopathic myelofibrosis (agnogenic myeloid metaplasia). *Int J Hematol*. 2002;76(2):133–145.

100. Zipursky A, Brown E, et al. Leukemia and/or myeloproliferative syndrome in neonates with Down syndrome. *Semin Perinatol*. 1997;21(1):97–101.

101. Arceci RJ. Down syndrome, transient myeloproliferative syndrome, and leukemia: bridging development and neoplasia. *J Pediatr Hematol Oncol*. 2002;24(1):9–13.

102. O'Dwyer ME. Chronic myelogenous leukemia. *Curr Opin Oncol*. 2003; 15(1):10–15.

103. Silver RT. Chronic myeloid leukemia. *Hematol Oncol Clin North Am*. 2003;17(5):1159–1173, vi-vii.

104. Adeyinka A, Dewald GW. Cytogenetics of chronic myeloproliferative disorders and related myelodysplastic syndromes. *Hematol Oncol Clin North Am*. 2003;17(5):1129–1149.

105. Barnes DJ, Melo JV. Cytogenetic and molecular genetic aspects of chronic myeloid leukaemia. *Acta Haematol*. 2002;108(4):180–202.

106. Pane F, Intrieri M, et al. BCR/ABL genes and leukemic phenotype: from molecular mechanisms to clinical correlations. *Oncogene*. 2002;21(56): 8652–8667.

107. Castro-Malaspina H, Schaison G, et al. Philadelphia chromosome-positive chronic myelocytic leukemia in children. *Cancer*. 1983;52:721–727.

108. Spivak JL. Diagnosis of the myeloproliferative disorders: resolving phenotypic mimicry. *Semin Hematol*. 2003;40(1)(Suppl 1):1–5.

109. Gamis AS, Hilden JM. Transient myeloproliferative disorder, a disorder with too few data and many unanswered questions: does it contain an important piece of the puzzle to understanding hematopoiesis and acute myelogenous leukemia? *J Pediatr Hematol Oncol*. 2002;24(1):2–5.

110. Taub JW, Ravindranath Y. Down syndrome and the transient myeloproliferative disorder: why is it transient? *J Pediatr Hematol Oncol*. 2002;24(1):6–8.

111. Zipursky A, Brown EJ, et al. Transient myeloproliferative disorder (transient leukemia) and hematologic manifestations of Down syndrome. *Clin Lab Med*. 1999;19(1):157–167, vii.

112. Xu G, Nagano M, et al. Frequent mutations in the GATA-1 gene in the transient myeloproliferative disorder of Down syndrome. *Blood*. 2003;102(8): 2960–2968.

113. Zipursky A. Transient leukaemia—a benign form of leukaemia in newborn infants with trisomy 21. *Br J Haematol*. 2003;120(6):930–938.

114. Gurbuxani S, Vyas P, et al. Recent insights into the mechanisms of myeloid leukemogenesis in Down syndrome. *Blood*. 2004;103(2):399–406.

115. Luna-Fineman S, Shannon KM, et al. Myelodysplastic and myeloproliferative disorders of childhood: a study of 167 patients. *Blood*. 1999;93(2):459–466.

116. Alter BP, Caruso JP, et al. Fanconi anemia: myelodysplasia as a predictor of outcome. *Cancer Genet Cytogenet*. 2000;117(2):125–131.

117. Novitzky N. Myelodysplastic syndromes in children. A critical review of the clinical manifestations and management. *Am J Hematol*. 2000;63(4):212–222.

118. Creutzig U, Ritter J, et al. Myelodysplasia and acute myelogenous leukemia in Down's syndrome: a report of 40 children of the AML-BFM Study Group. *Leukemia*. 1996;10(11):1677–1686.

119. Zipursky A, Thorner P, et al. Myelodysplasia and acute megakaryoblastic leukemia in Down's syndrome. *Leuk Res*. 1994;18:163–171.

120. Hayashi Y, Eguchi M, et al. Cytogenetic findings and clinical features in acute leukemia and transient myeloproliferative disorder in Down's syndrome. *Blood*. 1988;72:15–23.

121. Miles DK, Freedman MH, et al. Patterns of hematopoietic lineage involvement in children with neurofibromatosis type 1 and malignant myeloid disorders. *Blood*. 1996;88:4314–4320.

122. Side L, Taylor B, et al. Homozygous inactivation of the *NF1* gene in bone marrow cells from children with neurofibromatosis type 1 and malignant myeloid disorders. *N Engl J Med*. 1997;336:1713–1720.

123. Maris JM, Weirsma SR, et al. Monosomy 7 myelodysplastic syndrome and other second malignant neoplasms in children with neurofibromatosis type 1. *Cancer.* 1997;79:1438–1436.

124. Alter BP. Fanconi's anemia and malignancies. *Am J Hematol.* 1996;53:99–110.

125. Passmore SJ, Chessells JM, et al. Paediatric myelodysplastic syndromes and juvenile myelomonocytic leukaemia in the UK: a population-based study of incidence and survival. *Br J Haematol.* 2003;121(5):758–767.

126. Hall GW. Cytogenetic and molecular genetic aspects of childhood myeloproliferative/myelodysplastic disorders. *Acta Haematol.* 2002;108(4):171–179.

127. Woods WG, Barnard DR, et al. Prospective study of 90 children requiring treatment for juvenile myelomonocytic leukemia or myelodysplastic syndrome: a report from the Children's Cancer Group. *J Clin Oncol.* 2002;20(2):434–440.

128. Downing JR, Shannon KM. Acute leukemia: a pediatric perspective. *Cancer Cell.* 2002;2(6):437–445.

129. Leone G, Voso MT, et al. Therapy related leukemias: susceptibility, prevention and treatment. *Leuk Lymphoma.* 2001;41(3–4):255–276.

130. Schumacher HR, Alvares CJ, et al. Acute leukemia. *Clin Lab Med.* 2002;22(1):153–192, vii.

131. Reinhardt D, Creutzig U. Isolated myelosarcoma in children—update and review. *Leuk Lymphoma.* 2002;43(3):565–574.

132. Arber DA. Realistic pathologic classification of acute myeloid leukemias. *Am J Clin Pathol.* 2001;115(4):552–560.

133. Paredes-Aguilera R, Romero-Guzman L, et al. Biology, clinical, and hematologic features of acute megakaryoblastic leukemia in children. *Am J Hematol.* 2003;73(2):71–80.

134. Ravindranath Y. Recent advances in pediatric acute lymphoblastic and myeloid leukemia. *Curr Opin Oncol.* 2003;15(1):23–35.

135. Klobusicka M. Reliability and limitations of cytochemistry in diagnosis of acute myeloid leukemia. (Mini-review). *Neoplasma.* 2000;47(6):329–334.

136. Hrusak O, Porwit-MacDonald A. Antigen expression patterns reflecting genotype of acute leukemias. *Leukemia.* 2002;16(7):1233–1258.

137. Schoch C, Haferlach T. Cytogenetics in acute myeloid leukemia. *Curr Oncol Rep.* 2002;4(5):390–397.

138. Heerema NA, Bernheim A, Lim MS, et al. State of the art and future needs in cytogenetic/molecular genetics/arrays in childhood lymphoma: summary report of workshop at the First International Symposium on childhood and adolescent non-Hodgkin lymphoma, April 9, 2003, New York City, NY. *Pediatr Blood Cancer.* 2005;45(5):616–622.

139. Schramm A, Schulte JH, Klein-Hitpass L, et al. Prediction of clinical outcome and biological characterization of neuroblastoma by expression profiling. *Oncogene.* 2005;24(53):7902–7912.

140. Ferrando AA, Look AT. DNA microarrays in the diagnosis and management of acute lymphoblastic leukemia. *Int J Hematol.* 2004;80(5):395–400.

141. Ross ME, Mahfouz R, Onciu M, et al. Gene expression profiling of pediatric acute myelogenous leukemia. *Blood.* 2004;104(12):3679–3687.

142. Rossi MR, Conroy J, McQuaid D, Nowak NJ, Rutka JT, Cowell JK. Array CGH analysis of pediatric medulloblastomas. *Genes Chromosomes Cancer.* 2006;45(3):290–303.

143. Yoshimoto M, de Toledo SR, da Silva NS, et al. Comparative genomic hybridization analysis of pediatric adamantinomatous craniopharyngiomas and a review of the literature. *J Neurosurg.* 2004;101(1)(Suppl):85–90.

144. Dhen QR, Bilke S, Khan J. High-resolution cDNA microarray-based comparative genomic hybridization analysis in neuroblastoma. *Cancer Lett.* 2005;228(1–2):71–81.

Imaging Techniques in Pediatric Oncology

Keith S. White

Introduction

Medical imaging provides a fundamental supportive role in diagnosing and managing the child with cancer. Imaging is used extensively to screen for, diagnose, and stage cancer. In addition, once the patient begins therapy, imaging is used to assess treatment response, detect recurrence, and identify complications of therapy. Over the course of a cancer patient's treatment, large numbers of imaging studies are performed, resulting in a large aggregate cost and significant potential risk. Appropriate selection of imaging studies is, therefore, essential in the management of these patients.

In this chapter, the application of imaging techniques to diagnosis and treatment in pediatric oncology will be discussed, with specific focus on reviewing the indications, risks, and limitations of the different imaging modalities. Particular focus will be made of the potential oncogenic effects of ionizing radiation and suggestions made as to how these effects can be minimized.

Health Effects of Ionizing Radiation

The short- and long-term health effects of the tragic exposure of large numbers of people to radiation caused by the bombing of Hiroshima and Nagasaki continues to be an area of ongoing investigation. New data are emerging suggesting that long-term effects of low-level radiation may not be as negligible as originally thought. In the past, the oncogenic potential of low-level exposure of ionizing radiation used in medical imaging was thought to be too low to measure. However, recent publications have challenged this notion and heightened concerns that exposure of infants and young children to doses of ionizing radiation generated with computed tomography (CT) may significantly increase their risk of late onset of cancer.[1,2]

It is now known that the oncogenic potential of ionizing radiation is inversely proportional to age. The younger a child is at the time of exposure, the greater the risk that he or she will develop cancer. This oncogenic effect manifests itself as an increased incidence of latent cancer occurring in adulthood. The tumor types are those that are common to the adult population (carcinomas, lymphomas, etc). Consequently, it has taken more than 50 years to quantify the increased incidence of adult onset cancer occurring in these persons exposed to radiation as infants and young children.

Data also indicate that the risk of latent cancer development is roughly linearly related to the dose of exposure. Although there is concern for all imaging modalities that use radiation, this concern is highest for CT and fluoroscopy.

There is ongoing controversy over the magnitude of these risks with considerable debate that is likely to continue for some time. Despite the controversy over the magnitude of the risk, it is clear that every effort should be made to prudently manage the exposure of infants and young children to ionizing radiation, especially CT. The CT exam is frequently a very valuable diagnostic tool and as such is being used with increasing frequency with a growing number of clinical indications. Many pediatric oncology patients undergo serial CT examinations and cancer risk is incremental so that each additional exam adds to their cumulative risk of developing cancer.

Methods of dose reduction are actively being developed and taught.[3,4] Institutions that feature imaging services for pediatric patients are frequently more conscious of the latent health effects of ionizing radiation and use CT scanning protocols tailored to the small size of the patient.[5] Children imaged in adult facilities may be at risk to be scanned with adult protocols, thereby exposing the patient to a much higher dosage of radiation than is needed to create a diagnostic image.

The Society for Pediatric Radiology is working actively to educate physicians on this issue and is promoting the as low as reasonably achievable principle.[6] This principle teaches that radiation dose should be reduced by eliminating unnecessary exams, replacing CT with ultrasound (US) or magnetic resonance imaging (MRI) where appropriate, and decreasing the dosage of ionizing radiation for CT to as low a level as will yield diagnostic images.

Technical Considerations
Radiography

Since Wilhelm Conrad Roentgen generated the first radiograph of his wife's hand, radiography has been the primary imaging modality in radiology. Although many new imaging modalities have emerged, more radiographic examinations are performed annually than any other imaging modality.

Radiography provides a rapid, excellent screening examination of body parts with high inherent contrast such as the chest and bones. This is because radiography has very high spatial resolution (ability to distinguish two small, adjacent, high-contrast objects, primarily manifested as image sharpness). But, because radiography is a projectional (as opposed to tomographic or cross-sectional) modality, this benefit is not fully realized. Overlap of structures often produces complex image patterns that may obscure pertinent findings.

An even greater limitation of radiography is its relatively low-contrast resolution (ability to distinguish adjacent structures of similar density). Nonetheless, radiography does provide adequate visualization in high-contrast areas such as the chest and skeleton to be a valuable screening examination in these regions.

Radiation exposures from conventional radiography are relatively low. However, the large aggregate number of exposures that can occur over a lifetime can be significant. Consequently, care must be taken to ensure that there is a clear indication for each radiographic exam that is ordered.

Fluoroscopy

Fluoroscopy allows real-time dynamic radiographic imaging of the body. Spatial resolution is less than with conventional radiography, and the limitations caused by overlap and relatively poor contrast resolution previously described for radiography are also inherent limitations with this modality. The dynamic aspect of fluoroscopic imaging is the feature that gives this modality its greatest value. Enteric contrast agents such as barium sulfate or water-soluble iodine-based agents are used extensively in the evaluation of the gastrointestinal (GI) system.

The continuous flow of x-ray energy results in potentially high radiation exposures from these procedures. Radiation dose from these studies can be greatly reduced when performed by radiologists specifically trained and experienced in pediatric fluoroscopy. Modern fluoroscopy equipment can be configured to provide excellent image quality with a marked reduction in radiation dose as compared with older equipment.[7,8]

Oncology patients frequently undergo fluoroscopy exams to evaluate GI function or as a guide to interventional procedures, but there is no significant primary role for this modality in primary diagnosis and staging of malignancies.

Ultrasound

Ultrasound provides real time imaging without ionizing radiation. Cross-sectional images are generated real-time as a transducer is passed over the body. The transducer serves both to transmit sound into the body and to receive the sound waves that are reflected back as sound traveling through the body strikes soft-tissue interfaces.

Image contrast is provided by variations in the reflectivity of soft-tissue interfaces. Ultrasound is an excellent modality for evaluating soft-tissue structures such as the neck, liver, spleen, kidneys, uterus, and ovaries. Cystic or fluid-containing structures including the bladder are also imaged with high fidelity. Because of the very high reflectivity of gas interfaces such as air and bone, the United States has limited application to areas of the body shielded by bone or surrounded by lung or gas-filled bowel.

Because as sound strikes a moving reflector its frequency is shifted in proportion to the speed of the traveling reflector, US can be used to detect and map velocities of moving blood. Doppler US is used primarily to evaluate patency of arteries and veins but can also be used in evaluating flow characteristics of tumors and detecting distortions in blood flow caused by increasing resistance to flow in the solid organs.

Ultrasound has a primary role in screening for tumor but because of its inherent limitations is only considered an adjunct to staging. It is an excellent modality for verification of abdominal and pelvic masses, evaluation of the urinary tract for masses or obstruction, assessing for tumor invasion of the inferior vena cava (IVC), documenting patency of venous structures, and evaluating pleural and abdominal fluid collections.

Computed Tomography

Computed tomography is a primary modality used in diagnosing and staging cancer. This modality generates tomographic or cross-sectional images of the body by rotating a fan beam of radiation around the patient and simultaneously detecting the radiation passing through the body with a radiation detector system. The data acquired are then reconstructed using advanced mathematical computation to form cross-sectional images.

Spiral or helical scanners allow data collection to occur continuously, with no requirement that the table be stopped and advanced to the next scan location while the gantry changes directions. The gantry (which includes the radiation fan beam and detectors) rotates continuously around the patient as the table smoothly advances the patient through the beam. This technique results in faster scan speeds and can potentially be used to reduce radiation dosage by increasing the table translation speed relative to the gantry rotation speed. The ratio of translation speed to rotation speed is called pitch. As pitch increases, overall scan speed decreases, radiation dose decreases, but image quality slightly degrades. Increasing pitch is an excellent means of decreasing effective radiation exposure without significantly impacting image quality.[9]

The latest generation of CT scanners has added the feature of multiple detector rows. These multislice scanners allow more than one slice of data to be acquired per rotation. Consequently, very rapid scanning can be performed and very thin slices can be acquired. It is now possible to perform "isotropic" imaging where the slice thickness is 0.6 mm, allowing for reconstruction of data in any plane without loss of resolution. Multislice scanning has greatly increased the quality of 3-dimensional CT imaging including CT angiography. These gains need to be balanced against radiation dose because increased radiation doses of approximately 27% can be expected.[10]

The primary advantage of CT over radiography is the elimination of overlap of structures. Poor soft-tissue contrast is a problem that can be mitigated by using oral and intravenous (IV) contrast agents. Patients with renal insufficiency or contrast allergies requiring IV contrast should, where possible, undergo US or MRI examinations instead of CT. Patients with contrast allergies who must have CT should be pretreated with steroids prior to receiving IV contrast. Significant idiosyncratic contrast reactions are rare. Allergic reactions to non-ionic contrast media are less than to ionic media.[11] Although the risk of reaction is low, it is preferable to use non-ionic media in all pediatric patients.

Areas of high inherent contrast such as lung and bone do not generally require contrast administration. For imaging of the neck, mediastinum, abdomen, and pelvis, IV contrast material should usually be used. Oral contrast is strongly encouraged for all CT imaging of the abdomen and pelvis.

Computed tomography is an excellent modality for diagnosing and performing local staging of intrathoracic, intra-abdominal, and pelvic malignancies. Evaluation for lymphadenopathy, hepatic metastasis, and pulmonary parenchymal metastasis is achieved with high fidelity. Computed tomography is also used in diagnosing infectious complications such as abdominal abscess and pneumonia.

Magnetic Resonance Imaging

Magnetic resonance imaging generates tomographic images of the body using radio frequency waves and a strong magnetic field. Due to the large amount of hydrogen in the body, proton imaging is used. The MRI imaging space has a large static magnetic field (usually 1.5 or 3.0 Tesla). Imaging is achieved by exposing the body to radiofrequency pulses. Spatial variation in proton density and local chemical composition of tissues yields images with excellent soft-tissue contrast.

A variety of imaging parameters can be varied to modify the soft-tissue contrast, scan quality, and scan time. A detailed description of these parameters is beyond the scope of this publication, but several excellent primers on MRI physics are available.[12–14] Parameters can be selected to optimally display anatomy, highlight increased water content, demonstrate abnormalities in proton diffusion, and demonstrate blood flow. Techniques are available to diminish signal from specific tissue types such as fat. This is particularly helpful in T1-weighted imaging of areas surrounded by fat where it would otherwise be very difficult to differentiate bright signal caused by contrast enhancement from the bright signal of fat.

Using these various scan parameters, excellent soft-tissue contrast can be achieved. While spatial resolution of MRI is less than that of CT, there is generally a much higher contrast resolution than with CT. Axial, sagittal, coronal, and oblique scan planes can be generated directly. Because of the longer imaging times, motion is more problematic with MRI than with CT. Sedation is generally required for patients under 8 years of age. Despite the availability of techniques to mitigate the effects of cardiac and respiratory motion, image degradation caused by motion can be a significant problem in imaging the chest and abdomen.

Gadolinium is a paramagnetic contrast agent for intravascular use. It is used extensively in MRI imaging of the central nervous system (CNS), allowing for imaging of blood-brain barrier breakdown. Gadolinium is also a useful adjunct in evaluating the enhancement pattern of non-CNS solid tumors. Magnetic resonance imaging angiography is frequently enhanced with gadolinium to produce highest-quality images.

Magnetic resonance imaging spectroscopy is a technique used to investigate the biochemical constituents within a selected volume. With this technique, the focus is not on imaging anatomy. Rather, a volume of interest is selected and the relative concentrations of biochemical constituents within the volume are displayed as an overlapping integration of the spectra produced by the individual constituents. Classic patterns of spectra have been described for tumor, ischemia, abscess, etc. Differentiation of benign processes from tumor can be achieved.[15–18] Early results suggest that automated spectra analysis may be used to define tumor histology preoperatively.[17] Proton spectroscopy and diffusion-weighted imaging appear to be complementary methods that can be used in combination to differentiate and grade CNS tumors.[19]

New MRI techniques are being developed to map brain anatomy and function as a presurgical planning tool. This is particularly important in tumors that involve the motor strip, speech areas, or other eloquent areas. Functional MRI, cortical mapping, and diffusion tensor imaging are methods that are in the process of development.[20,21]

Magnetic resonance imaging is the primary imaging modality for diagnosis, staging, and follow-up of CNS neoplasms. The extent of musculoskeletal neoplasms is also best assessed with this modality. Tumors of the abdomen and chest can also be imaged, and in some cases MRI can be used instead of CT in evaluation of these tumors.

Nuclear Medicine

Nuclear medicine provides images that depict the spatial distribution of radioactive tracers that have been bound to an agent molecule and injected into the body. The radioactive tracer is essentially a tag that accompanies the carrier molecule. Useful images are acquired by binding the tracer to a carrier that has meaningful physiological activity. Agents are available for imaging metabolic activity in bone, liver function and excretion, renal function and excretion, inflammatory responses, macrophage ingestion, blood pool distribution, and direct tumor uptake.

Several radioactive tracers are commonly available. They vary with regard to mode of emission (beta versus alpha versus positron emission), half-life, photon energies (hence imaging efficiency), and biochemical binding properties. Conventional gamma camera systems are used to image alpha and beta emitters such as technetium, gallium, thallium, indium, and radioactive iodine. Positron emitters such as fluorodeoxyglucose (FDG) are imaged with positron emission tomography (PET) scanning equipment.[22,23]

Conventional gamma camera imaging generates projectional or planar images. Tomographic images can be acquired by using the single photo emission computed tomography (SPECT) imaging capabilities of most contemporary nuclear medicine systems. This imaging is useful to spatially define overlapping areas of uptake in areas of high tracer concentration. PET scans can be displayed in projectional or tomographic formats. Software applications to perform image fusion (combining tomographic nuclear medicine images with either CT or MRI) can now be performed with PET-CT scanners in which both imaging modalities are housed in the same unit. These images provide both high anatomic detail and the physiologic information inherent with PET.[24]

Nuclear medicine studies are used extensively in pediatric oncology[25] and are part of imaging protocols for most solid tumors. Bone scans are used extensively to screen for metastatic disease. Whole-body and SPECT gallium scans are used in primary diagnosis and follow-up of Hodgkin and non-Hodgkin lymphoma. Thallium has potential utility as a surrogate marker of tumor kill in a variety of sarcomas. Metaiodobenzylguanidine (MIBG) is a useful agent for staging and treatment of neuroblastoma. Fluorodeoxyglucose PET scanning is becoming a valuable technique in staging lymphomas, brain tumors, osteosarcoma,[26] and a variety of other tumors.

Tumor Imaging

Central Nervous System Neoplasms

Screening and Primary Tumor Evaluation
Although CT is frequently the first modality used in diagnosing CNS neoplasms, MRI is more sensitive and generally provides greater anatomic detail than does CT. Anatomic definition and extent of tumor are well defined. Avid enhancement, especially when observed with dynamic gadolinium-enhanced imaging, correlates with high tumor grade.[27–30] Due to its availability and decreased expense relative to those of MRI, CT is frequently used as a screening test in patients with headache, uncomplicated seizure, vomiting, diffuse weakness, etc.[31] If findings indicative of neoplasm are encountered, the patient should undergo MRI for definitive diagnosis and staging.

Patients with underlying genetic diseases such as neurofibromatosis and tuberous sclerosis can also be screened with MRI.[32]

Although CT is superior to MRI in evaluation of calcification, skull erosion, or other effects of tumor on bony structures, this advantage is usually of little clinical relevance and is generally not considered of sufficient importance to merit routine use of CT in evaluating all brain tumors. In selected cases where the relationships of tumors to bone are important in surgical planning (such as skull-base tumors), high-resolution CT should be performed.[33]

The primary modality used in evaluating intracranial and intraspinal CNS neoplasia is gadolinium-enhanced MRI.[34–38] Preliminary T1 and T2 sequences are obtained followed by gadolinium-enhanced T1 sequences in multiple planes. Diffusion-weighted imaging, spectroscopy, diffusion tensor imaging, and functional MRI are useful adjuncts in selected cases that require greater anatomic and functional definition.[39] For example, tumors in or near the motor strip or speech areas can be better defined with these techniques to aid in surgical planning.[21]

Several factors that determine the differential diagnosis of CNS neoplasms include: patient age, site of tumor, growth pattern of tumor, enhancement pattern, presence or absence of associated cysts, and presence of associated findings indicated by associated disease processes such as tuberous sclerosis or neurofibromatosis. Typical examples of solid intraspinal and intracranial CNS tumors are illustrated in Figures 6-1, 6-2, 6-3, 6-4, and 6-5.

Staging
Magnetic resonance imaging not only provides excellent definition of the primary tumor, but it is also the preferred staging modality for identifying metastatic disease. Gadolinium enhancement is essential in identifying areas of nodular or linear leptomeningeal enhancement indica-

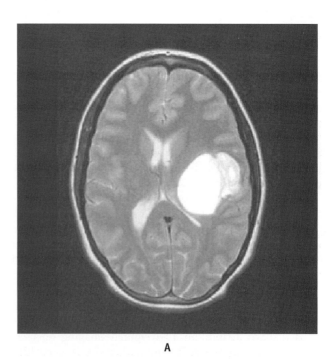

A

Figure 6-1 (A) Seventeen-year-old female with astrocytoma. Axial T2-weighted MRI demonstrating left hemispheric mass with solid and cystic components.

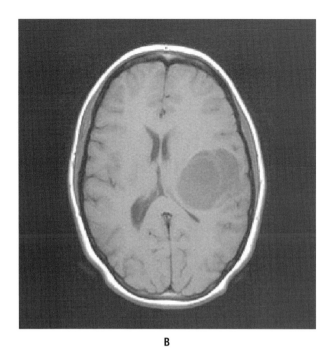

B

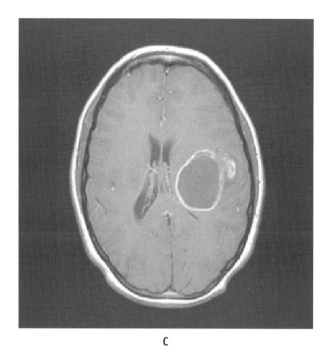

C

Figure 6-1 (*continued*) (B) Seventeen-year-old female with astrocytoma. Axial T1-weighted MRI without gadolinium shows low T1 signal within the mass. Mass effect on adjacent ventricle is moderate. (C) Seventeen-year-old female with astrocytoma. Axial T1-weighted gadolinium-enhanced MRI demonstrates a thin linear wall of enhancement around the periphery of the mass.

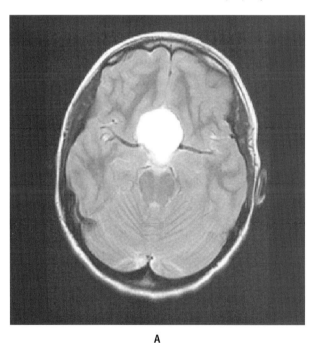

A

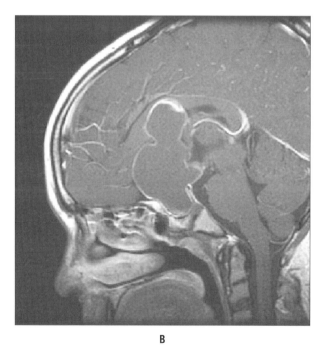

B

Figure 6-2 (A) Fourteen-year-old male with craniopharyngioma. Axial T2-weighted MRI demonstrates uniformly bright T2 signal within a peri-sellar mass. The mass displaces adjacent internal carotid artery branches. (B) Fourteen-year-old male with craniopharyngioma. Sagittal T1-weighted MRI obtained with gadolinium enhancement demonstrates a thin rim of peripheral enhancement at the margin of the mass. The mass extends inferiorly into the sella and superiorly into the 3rd ventricle. The optic chiasm cannot be identified.

tive of metastatic disease.[37] There is little role for conventional or CT myelography in evaluating for spinal metastatic disease. Metastatic disease outside of the CNS is so rare that additional routine staging procedures are not recommended.

Treatment Response and Follow-Up

There is controversy on whether follow-up imaging improves long-term survival in patients with high-grade brain tumors.[40] When imaging follow-up is used, MRI is the modality of choice in assessing treatment response

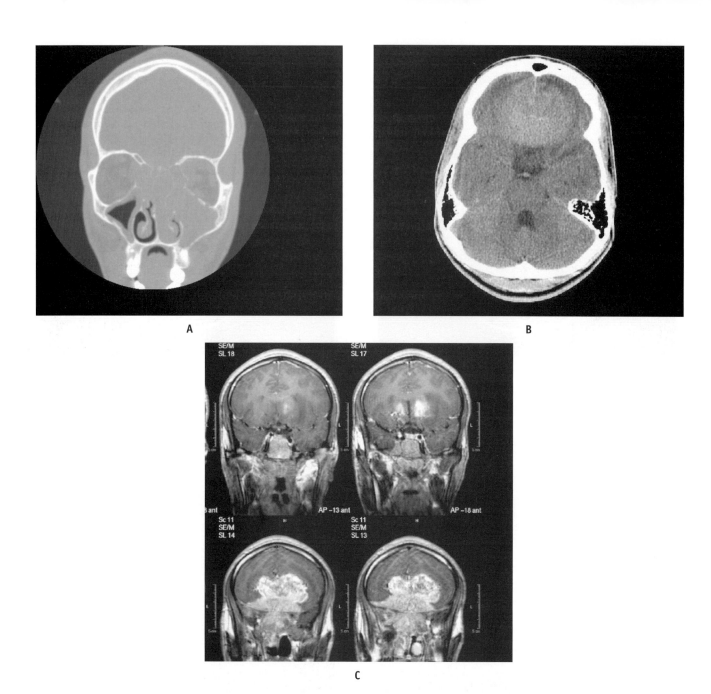

Figure 6-3 (A) Fourteen-year-old with olfactory neuroblastoma. Coronal CT demonstrates complete opacification of the left maxillary and bilateral ethmoid sinuses with expansion and destruction of bone. (B) Fourteen-year-old with olfactory neuroblastoma. Axial nonenhanced CT shows a high attenuation mass extending superiorly from the region of the cribiform plate to involve both frontal lobes. (C) Fourteen-year-old with olfactory neuroblastoma. Coronal T1 gadolinium-enhanced MRI demonstrates very large, heterogeneously enhancing mass extending into the frontal lobes superiorly and paranasal sinuses inferiorly.

and in surveillance for the development of late metastatic disease. Because there is an expected gadolinium enhancement effect that occurs in response to postsurgical inflammation, immediate post-resection gadolinium-enhanced MRI should be performed in the first 48 hours following tumor resection to evaluate for the presence of residual tumor.

Some tumors that are treated with chemotherapy and/or radiation therapy will have unusual patterns of nodular and bulky enhancement that will be indeterminate for residual tumor. Specifically, it may be very difficult to differentiate

residual viable tumor from inflammatory response to tumor necrosis. In these cases, MRI spectroscopy or FDG PET scanning are useful adjuncts.[41–44]

Lymphoma

Screening and Primary Tumor Evaluation
Chest radiography is frequently the first modality to identify an intrathoracic lymphoma. The chest radiograph is a convenient and inexpensive means of screening for disease and subsequently evaluating gross response in fol-

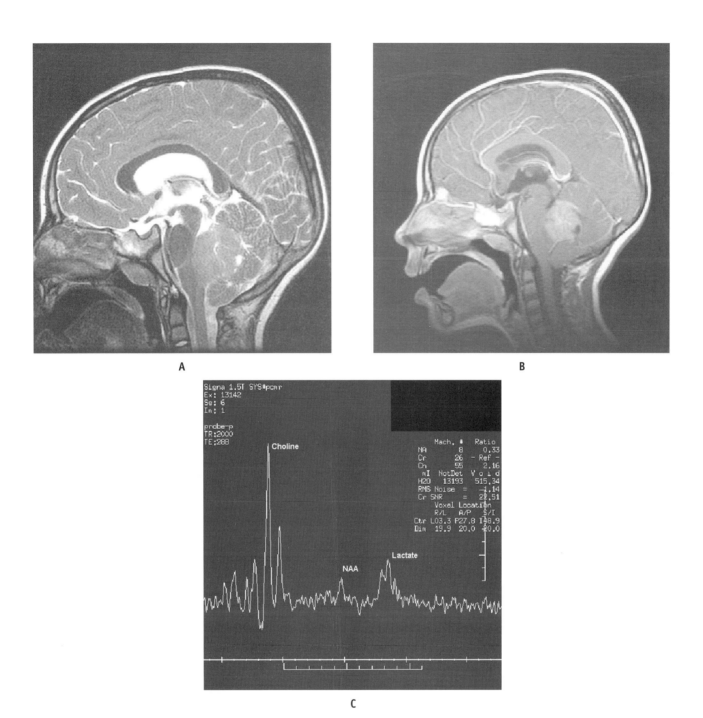

Figure 6-4 (A) Eight-year-old with PNET/medulloblastoma. Sagittal T2-weighted MRI demonstrates a mass in the 4th ventricle with slightly increased T2 signal relative to normal brain. (B) Eight year old with PNET/ medulloblastoma: Sagittal T1 weighted MRI post gadolinium shows avid enhancement of this well-circumscribed mass. (C) Eight-year-old with PNET/medulloblastoma. Single voxel PRESS technique MR spectroscopy shows absence of N-acetyl aspartate, a marker of neuronal integrity at 2.0 ppm; marked elevation of choline, a marker of cell wall breakdown at 3.2 ppm; and presence of lactate, indicating anaerobic metabolism at 1.3 ppm. This spectral pattern is typical of a malignant tumor.

low-up. Although the presence of the mass is clearly defined, radiography is not sufficient to define the extent of disease and is much less sensitive than CT or MRI in identifying areas of lymphadenopathy.

Contrast-enhanced CT is the primary modality used in evaluation of primary tumors in the chest, neck, and abdomen. Oral contrast should be administered for all abdominal and pelvic exams unless contraindicated. MRI can also be used but because of increased expense, the

greater need for sedation, image degradation by motion, and less availability, it has a subsidiary role to CT. Because intra-intestinal fluid will be bright on T2-weighted sequences and oral MRI contrast agents are not routinely used, bowel can present a significant problem in evaluation of the abdomen.

Because the lymphomas are essentially systemic tumors, the differentiation between primary and secondary tumor is blurred and evaluation of the primary mass is

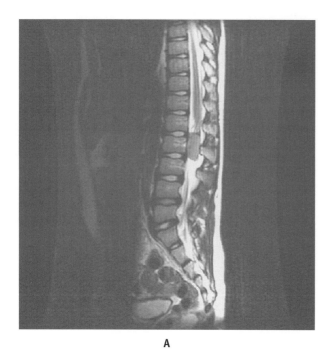 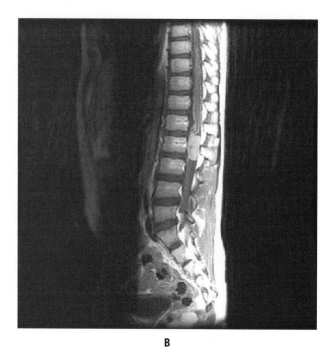

A   B

Figure 6-5 (A) Six-year-old male with spinal myxopapillary ependymoma. Sagittal T2-weighted MRI demonstrates a well-circumscribed intradural, extramedullary mass at the level of the conus medullaris. (B) Six-year-old male with spinal myxopapillary ependymoma. Sagittal T1-weighted MRI post gadolinium shows uniform enhancement of the mass. Note that the mass fills the neural canal at this level and compresses and displaces adjacent nerve roots.

discussed in the staging section below. The concepts discussed generally apply to Hodgkin and non-Hodgkin lymphoma unless otherwise designated.

Staging

Patients with lymphoma should undergo cross-sectional imaging of the chest, abdomen, and pelvis with either CT or MRI. For the reasons listed above, CT is the preferred modality. If there are abnormal lymph nodes palpable in the neck, the neck should also be imaged. All areas of tumor involvement should be identified for subsequent follow-up. Largest aggregates of tumor should be measured according to protocol to allow response tracking.

The differentiation between malignant and nonmalignant lymph nodes is a particular problem in pediatrics because of the prevalence of reactive and inflammatory lymphadenopathy (especially in the neck) and the lack of good measurement standards for maximal nodal diameter. The presence of lymphadenopathy must be considered with the clinical context to determine the likelihood of neoplastic involvement. As a general rule, nodes larger than 1.5 cm in diameter should be considered suspicious for malignancy.

In evaluation of the chest, the presence of an anterior mediastinal mass is the typical pattern for lymphoblastic lymphoma. Differentiation of the normal or hypertrophic thymus from malignancy can be problematic even for experienced pediatric radiologists.[45] Classically, the thymus is a soft organ compliant to adjacent structures with no mass effect. The normal thymus is homogeneous and devoid of calcification. Gross enlargement of the thymus, mass effect, presence of heterogeneity, nodularity, calcifi-

cation, associated lymphadenopathy, or cyst formation increases likelihood of malignancy.

Contrast-enhanced CT gives excellent definition of the neck, chest, abdomen, and pelvis. Where patient motion is limited by either sedation or voluntary cooperation and adequate technical parameters have been used, all areas of macroscopic disease can be detected.

Gallium and PET scanning have an important role in staging for both Hodgkin and non-Hodgkin lymphoma.[46–48] There is a wider experience with gallium scanning in Hodgkin lymphoma, but new Children's Oncology Group imaging protocols for non-Hodgkin lymphomas include gallium and/or FDG PET scanning as well. These studies give a whole-body map of increased metabolic activity typical of lymphomas. Areas of equivocal disease seen with CT can be confirmed with gallium and/or FDG PET. These scans will serve as reference points for posttreatment scans that are vital in treatment response evaluation. Because gallium and FDG PET scans give a global evaluation of the body, including potential sites of osseous metastatic disease, bone scanning is no longer recommended. Typical examples of Hodgkin and non-Hodgkin lymphoma imaging are shown in Figures 6-6, 6-7, 6-8, and 6-9.

Treatment Response and Follow-Up

Areas of disease diagnosed on initial staging should be periodically reevaluated with CT (or MRI). If gallium or FDG PET scans were initially positive, they should be repeated periodically as well. Many patients with lymphoma will have residual masses in areas of bulk tumor on follow-up.[49,50] This is particularly true for nodular sclerosing Hodgkin disease. Smaller areas of disease will usually nor-

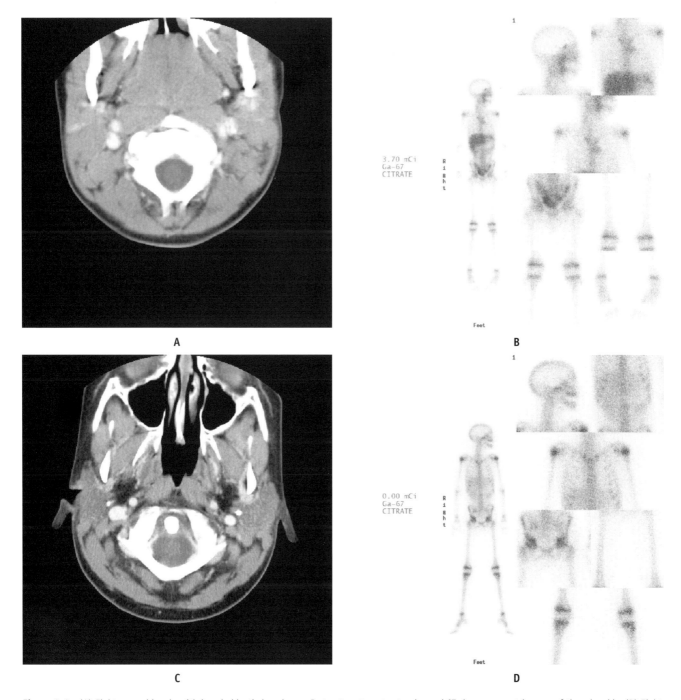

A

B

C

D

Figure 6-6 (A) Eight-year-old male with lymphoblastic lymphoma. Pretreatment contrast-enhanced CT shows concentric mass of the adenoids. (B) Eight-year-old male with lymphoblastic lymphoma. Pretreatment gallium scan demonstrates increased tracer uptake in the nasopharynx, neck, and superior mediastinum. (C) Eight-year-old male with lymphoblastic lymphoma. Posttreatment neck CT shows resolution of adenoidal mass. (D) Eight-year-old male with lymphoblastic lymphoma. Posttreatment gallium scan demonstrates normal tracer distribution.

malize. In response to therapy, masses typically decrease in size, become better defined, at first become lower in attenuation then subsequently denser. Ultimately, they may calcify. Treatment protocols stratify patients based on the size reduction determined on follow-up scans. Consistent, accurate measurements must therefore be made. This process is greatly facilitated by using consistent scan parameters such as slice thickness on serial scans.

Gallium and FDG PET are particularly valuable in assessing residual masses for evidence of viable tumor.[51–54] Where the initial tumor was avid for the tracer, activity within a residual mass is likely indicative of continuing tumor viability. Conversely, the resolution of abnormal tracer uptake is evidence for complete tumor kill despite the presence of residual mass. Equivocal masses can be either followed on subsequent studies or biopsied for confirmation.

Thymic rebound is a problem that frequently causes confusion.[55] As the patient recovers from chemotherapy, the thymus will frequently become transiently enlarged and metabolically active. Consequently, slight enlargement of the gland will be seen with CT and the activity

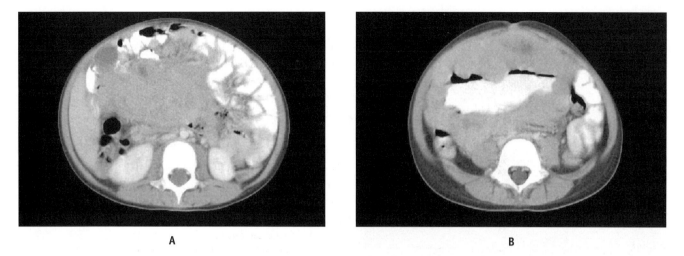

Figure 6-7 (A) Four-year-old male with abdominal Burkitt lymphoma. Contrast-enhanced CT demonstrates large confluent aggregate of lymph nodes at the base of the small-bowel mesentery. (B) Four-year-old male with abdominal Burkitt lymphoma. CT at lower level demonstrates marked thickening of the wall and dilation of the lumen of the cecum characteristic of colonic involvement with Burkitt lymphoma.

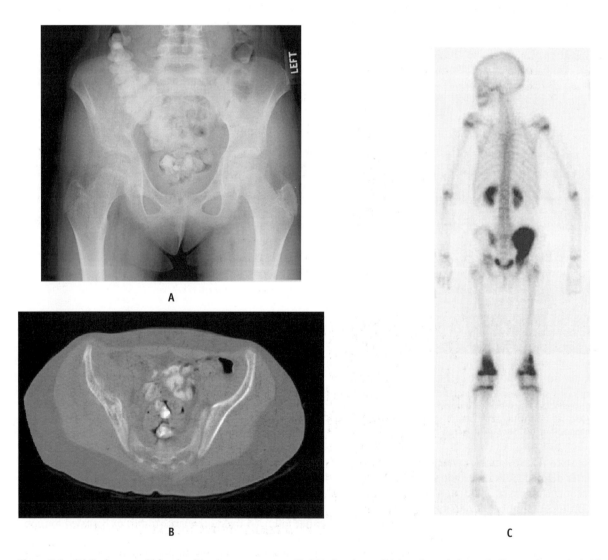

Figure 6-8 (A) Twelve-year-old female with primary osseous non-Hodgkin lymphoma. Pelvic radiograph demonstrating poorly marginated lytic lesion of the right iliac bone with associated periosteal new-bone formation. (B) Twelve-year-old female with primary osseous non-Hodgkin lymphoma. Bone window form pelvic CT demonstrates permeative destruction of the iliac bone with associated concentric soft-tissue mass. (C) Twelve-year-old female with primary osseous non-Hodgkin lymphoma. Bone scan demonstrates marked diffuse increase in tracer uptake in the right iliac bone. Other areas of abnormal uptake including the distal femoral metaphysis indicate systemic disease.

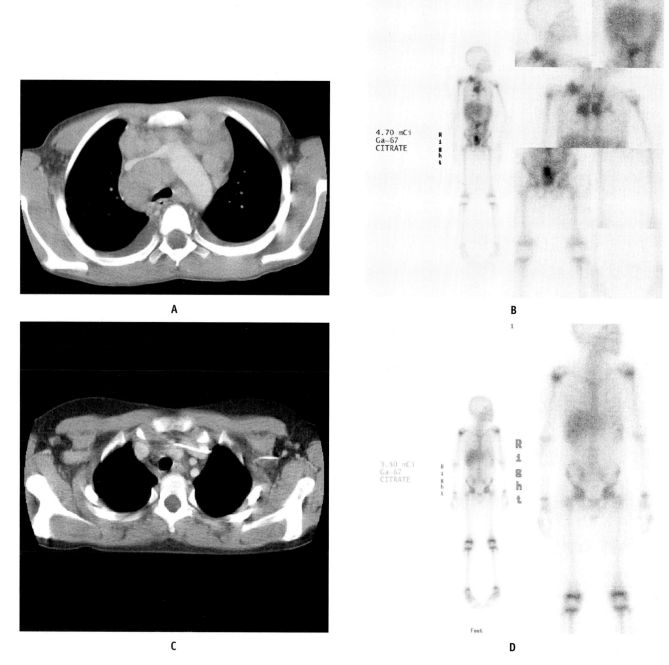

Figure 6-9 (A) Fifteen-year-old male with Hodgkin lymphoma. Pretreatment axial CT at the level of the aortic arch demonstrates extensive lymphadenopathy with prevascular and peritracheal nodes. (B) Fifteen-year-old male with Hodgkin lymphoma. Pretreatment gallium scan shows abnormal uptake in right supraclavicular and mediastinal regions. (C) Fifteen-year-old male with Hodgkin lymphoma. Posttreatment chest CT shows resolution of lymphadenopathy. (D) Fifteen-year-old male with Hodgkin lymphoma. Posttreatment gallium scan demonstrates normal tracer distribution.

within the gland as defined with gallium or PET will likewise increase. The enlargement and increased activity are confined to the gland. There are no known imaging modalities to definitively distinguish between thymic rebound and progressive tumor. Identification of these findings in the appropriate clinical context is usually sufficient to justify further follow-up rather than biopsy. In patients where the changes occur in an unsuitable context or are accompanied by other evidence for disease progression, biopsy is recommended.

Neuroblastoma

Screening and Primary Tumor Evaluation

Ultrasound is a primary imaging modality used in screening patients with a suspected intra-abdominal mass. Differentiation between hydronephrosis, cysts, organomegaly, and solid tumors is readily performed. Although this modality can provide an approximate estimate of the extent of disease, it is considered inadequate for staging, and further imaging of the primary tumor with MRI or CT is required.[56]

Because neuroblastoma arises in the posterior mediastinum and retroperitoneum, motion-related artifacts caused by respiratory or peristaltic motion are not a major problem with MRI. The local extent of the primary tumor is well demonstrated with MRI or CT.[57,58] MRI allows superior definition of the intraspinal extension of tumor, but CT is a better modality for detecting pulmonary metastatic disease. Aside from these limitations, both CT and MRI demonstrate the extent of disease with high fidelity. Selection between CT and MRI is made on a case-by-case basis depending on availability, need for sedation, concern about radiation, need to evaluate the spine and lungs, and cost. Many groups have replaced CT with MRI in primary evaluation.[59,60]

Sensitivity and specificity are improved by combining MRI with MIBG.[61]

When CT is used, oral and IV contrast should be administered. Neuroblastoma has an aggressive growth pattern that classically encases the major retroperitoneal vessels. Extension into the neural canal is common. When present, this feature is best imaged with gadolinium-enhanced MRI. Relationship of the primary tumor to critical anatomic structures is important to surgical planning. Although most patients will undergo biopsy, neoadjuvant chemotherapy, and delayed resection, some patients will be candidates for early primary resection based on imaging findings. Typical examples of neuroblastoma imaging are provided in Figures 6-10, 6-11, and 6-12.

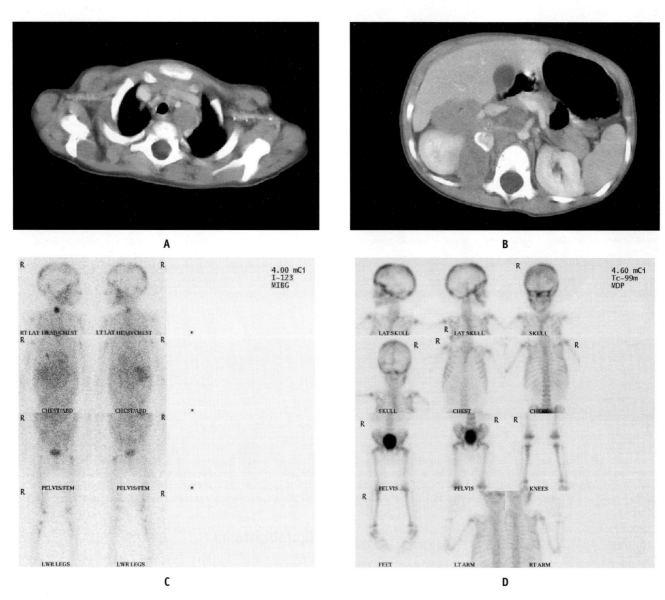

Figure 6-10 (A) Two-year-old male with stage IV neuroblastoma. Contrast-enhanced chest CT shows metastatic lymphadenopathy in left superior mediastinum. (B) Two-year-old male with stage IV neuroblastoma. Abdominal CT with contrast demonstrates a large primary tumor in right adrenal with metastatic lymphadenopathy encasing the aorta, right renal artery, superior mesenteric artery, and inferior vena cava. Note typical pattern of calcification. (C) Two-year-old male with stage IV neuroblastoma. Whole body MIBG scan shows abnormal uptake in skull, multiple metaphyseal regions of long bones, upper chest, and right mid-abdomen. (D) Two-year-old male with stage IV neuroblastoma. Bone scan demonstrates diffusely increased uptake of tracer with patchy areas of activity in the skull, ribs, and spine. Metaphysis of long bones demonstrates increased activity disrupting the normal sharp line of uptake that would be expected at the physis.

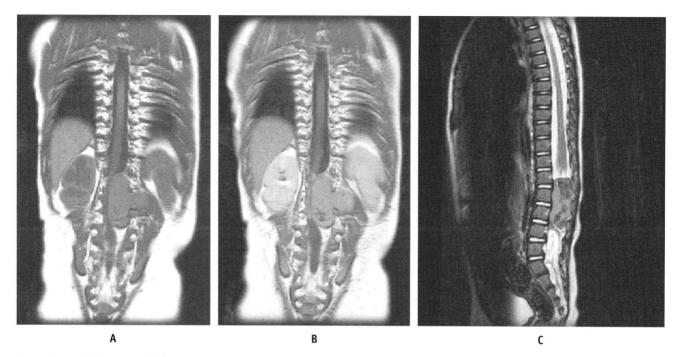

Figure 6-11 (A) Seven-month-old male with intraspinal extension of neuroblastoma. Coronal T1-weighted MRI shows typical "dumbbell" lesion with marked intraspinal component compressing the conus and nerve roots. (B) Seven-month-old male with intraspinal extension of neuroblastoma. Post gadolinium-enhanced T1-weighted lesion shows uniform enhancement of the intraspinal mass. (C) Seven-month-old male with intraspinal extension of neuroblastoma. Nonenhanced T2-weighted sequence demonstrates obliteration of arachnoid fluid space at the level of the mass. Heterogeneous signal including dark T2 signal suggests calcification.

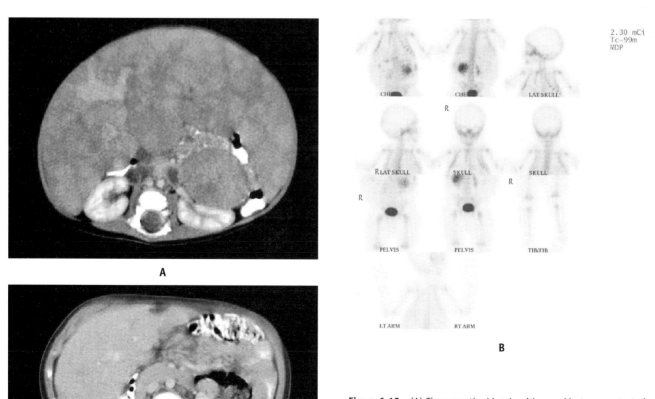

Figure 6-12 (A) Three-month-old male with neuroblastoma, metastatic to bone and liver. Pretreatment contrast-enhanced CT demonstrates left adrenal primary with massive, diffuse hepatic metastatic disease. (B) Three-month-old male with neuroblastoma, metastatic to bone and liver. Bone scan demonstrates diffusely increased tracer uptake throughout the skeleton. (C) Three-month-old male with neuroblastoma, metastatic to bone and liver. Posttreatment CT shows marked response. Liver demonstrates irregular margins with linear areas of scarring.

Staging

Evaluation of the primary tumor should include additional scanning to cover the chest, abdomen, and pelvis. This can be performed with either CT or MRI.[62] Pulmonary parenchymal metastases are best evaluated with chest CT. Because of the extensive range of metastatic disease possible with neuroblastoma, assessment of bone, lung, and soft-tissue windows is important with CT.

Evaluation of distant skeletal metastatic disease is most readily accomplished with bone scan. Rather than identifying specific discreet foci of increased uptake, some patients with diffuse bone metastasis will have symmetrically increased metaphyseal uptake of tracer that will cause the discrete increased uptake of the physis normally detected on bone scan to be blurred.

Radionuclide imaging with iodine-123 or iodine-131 MIBG is a powerful tool in staging neuroblastoma.[63] This agent is a guanethidine analog and accumulates in sympathetic adrenergic tissues. MIBG scans are positive in approximately 90% of neuroblastoma patients at diagnosis. When correlated with MRI or CT, MIBG imaging increases specificity and sensitivity for sites of disease including nodal, bone, bone marrow, and lung metastasis. SPECT images should be acquired to improve spatial resolution. MIBG cannot fully replace bone scan to evaluate skeletal metastasis.[64] There is ongoing investigation regarding use of fast MRI as a sole imaging modality in staging of neuroblastoma and other small round cell tumors.[65]

Treatment Response and Follow-Up

Periodic evaluation of the primary tumor as well as sites of previously documented disease should be performed with CT or MRI. Tumors that are avid for MIBG may also be followed with serial MIBG scans.

Treated areas of disease will show decreasing bulk, improved margination, and decreasing vascular encasement. Previously unresectable lesions may become more circumscribed and allow attempt at resection. Initially, the lesions may become low attenuation due to necrosis. Increasing dystrophic calcification frequently develops in response to tumor necrosis.

Residual soft-tissue masses are presumed to represent residual tumor. This is especially true for lesions that continue to exhibit MIBG avidity. It is not possible to distinguish between ganglioneuroma, bland treated tumor, and residual viable neuroblastoma using MRI or CT alone.

Wilms Tumor

Screening and Primary Tumor Evaluation

Patients with nephroblastomatosis, or syndromes such as Beckwith-Wiedemann syndrome that have associations with the development of Wilms tumor should undergo screening examinations with ultrasonography.[66] Although CT and MRI are more sensitive modalities in detecting nephrogenic rests and Wilms tumors, US is a convenient exam that does not require sedation nor use radiation.[67,68] As with neuroblastoma, US is frequently used as a screening exam for the detection of an intra-abdominal mass.

Computed tomography is the primary imaging modality used to diagnose and stage Wilms tumor.[69] Oral and IV contrast are used with imaging of the entire abdomen and pelvis. Invasion of the renal vein and IVC is an important finding that can be diagnosed with CT. In cases where there is incomplete or equivocal evaluation of the IVC, US or MRI can be useful adjuncts in identifying intravascular extension of tumor. Examples of Wilms tumor are shown in Figures 6-13, 6-14, and 6-15.

Staging

Patients with Wilms tumor should have CT scans of the abdomen and pelvis. Computed tomography alone does not, however, appear to provide accurate staging as compared with surgical staging.[70] Evaluation of the contralateral kidney is important in identifying associated nephroblastomatosis and synchronous bilateral disease. Patients should be evaluated for nodal metastasis and liver lesions. Because osseous metastatic disease is rare in Wilms tumor, bone scans are not required. Pulmonary parenchymal metastasis are best evaluated with CT. The value of chest screening with CT versus use of radiography is, however, controversial.[71,72] Because intrathoracic lymphadenopathy is rare, IV contrast is not needed.

Treatment Response and Follow-Up

In most cases of Wilms tumor, primary tumor resection and chemotherapy will be sufficient to completely remove the primary tumor and treat metastatic disease. Although CT continues to be used in follow-up at some centers, US should be considered as a screen for intra-abdominal recurrence of Wilms tumor because it avoids the risks of radiation exposure and is less expensive. The role of chest CT in follow-up of Wilms tumor continues to be controversial. There is no doubt that CT is more sensitive than chest radiography. However, the very favorable response to chemotherapy may indicate that failure to detect small metastatic nodules may not have clinically significant effect on outcome in many patients.

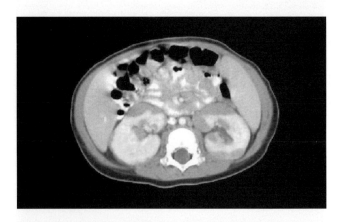

Figure 6-13 Eight-month-old female with nephroblastomatosis. Contrast-enhanced CT shows bilateral peripheral plaques of nonenhancing tissue characteristic of nephroblatomatosis.

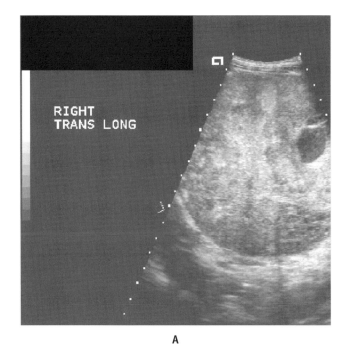

A

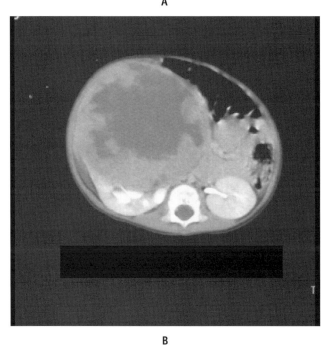

B

Figure 6-14 (A) Twenty-month-old female with stage I Wilms tumor. Abdominal ultrasound confirms the presence of a heterogeneously echogenic mass in the right kidney. (B) Twenty-month-old female with stage I Wilms tumor. Contrast-enhanced CT shows typical rounded, noninfiltrative growth pattern of a large Wilms tumor. The central area of low attenuation is characteristic of necrosis.

Bone and Soft-Tissue Sarcomas

Screening and Primary Tumor Evaluation

Primary bone tumors are often first diagnosed radiographically, and radiography is an excellent modality for evaluation of primary bone lesions. Characteristics of malignant lesions include ill-defined margins, aggressive periosteal new bone formation, typical location, an accompanying

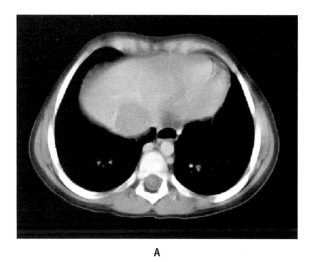

A

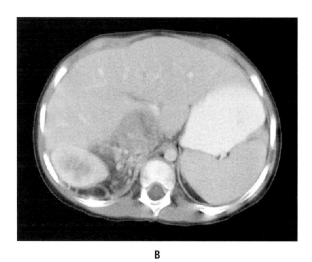

B

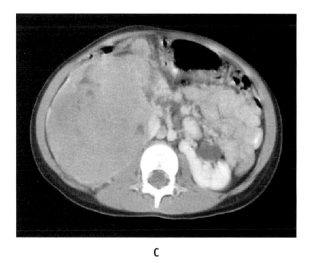

C

Figure 6-15 (A) Four-year-old male with intracaval extension of Wilms tumor. Contrast-enhanced CT shows low attenuation mass expanding the intrahepatic inferior vena cava. (B) Four-year-old male with intracaval extension of Wilms tumor. CT image just superior to the right renal vein shows extensive vascular collateralization. (C) Four-year-old male with intracaval extension of Wilms tumor. Large primary renal tumor nearly replaces renal parenchyma. A small, rounded metastatic lymph node is identified anterior to the tumor.

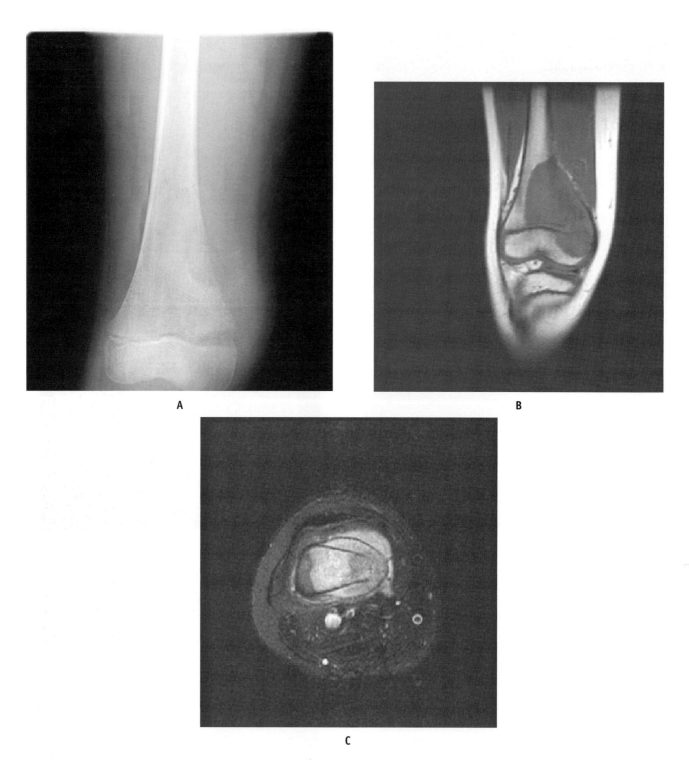

Figure 6-16 (A) Seven-year-old male with osteosarcoma of the distal right femur. Radiograph of the right knee demonstrates poorly marginated destructive lesion of the femoral metaphysis. (B) Seven-year-old male with osteosarcoma of the distal right femur. T1-weighted MRI shows sharply demarcated intramedullary extension of tumor. Note that the tumor crosses the physis to the epiphysis. (C) Seven-year-old male with osteosarcoma of the distal right femur. Axial T2-weighted MRI demonstrates that the tumor extends through the cortex, elevates the periosteum, and breaks through the periosteum into the adjacent soft tissues.

soft-tissue mass, and malignant pattern of calcification within the tumor.

Bone lesions that have a sharp demarcation between normal and abnormal tissue are more often benign than malignant, although there are exceptions to this rule. The margin of a benign lesion typically has a sharp sclerotic line. Ill-defined diffusely infiltrative lesions are classic for small round blue cell processes (most of which are malignant tumors). Osteomyelitis and eosinophylic granuloma are two benign processes that can be indistinguishable from malignant tumors radiographically.

Although destruction of bone architecture and nature of the calcified tumor matrix are best defined with CT, MRI provides much greater soft-tissue contrast and is

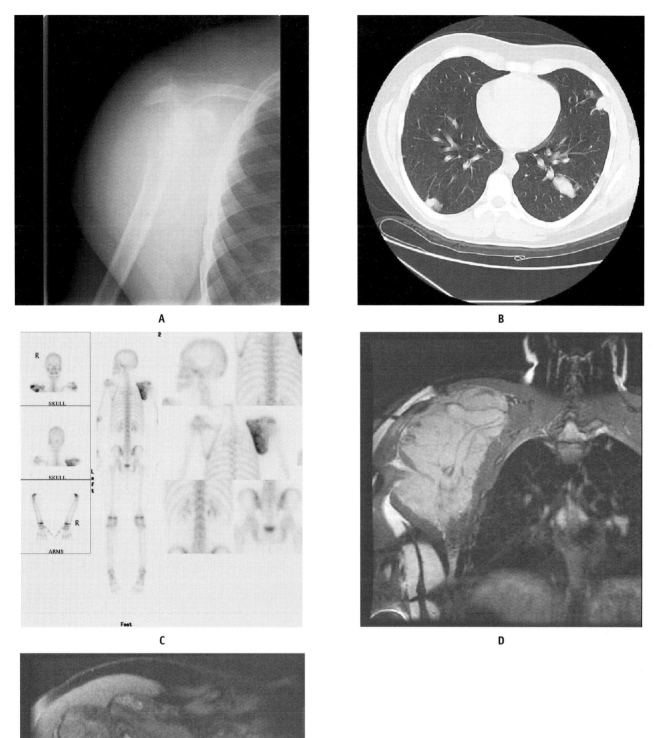

A

B

C

D

E

Figure 6-17 (A) Fifteen-year-old male with scapular Ewing sarcoma. Frontal view of the right shoulder shows diffuse expansion of the scapula with demineralization. Large associated soft tissue mass is also seen. (B) Fifteen-year-old male with scapular Ewing sarcoma. Chest CT without contrast demonstrates multiple metastatic pulmonary nodules. (C) Fifteen-year-old male with scapular Ewing sarcoma. Bone scan shows markedly increased tracer uptake in the scapula with no evidence for distant metastatic bone lesions. (D) Fifteen-year-old male with scapular Ewing sarcoma. Pretreatment fat-saturated proton-density MRI in the coronal plan demonstrates the very large soft-tissue mass concentrically expanding from the scapula. The ghost of scapular cortex is identified within the mass. (E) Fifteen-year-old male with scapular Ewing sarcoma. Posttreatment fat-saturated proton density MRI in the axial plane shows marked reduction in tumor volume. Remaining tissue has increasing signal consistent with increasing tumor edema.

therefore the preferred modality for initial evaluation of a musculoskeletal mass.[73,74] Localized extension of disease including the relationship of the tumor to the physis, epiphysis, joint space, neurovascular structures, and marrow cavity are demonstrated with clarity. Nonosseous soft-tissue sarcomas are also best imaged with MRI.[75] Gadolinium enhancement is an important method, especially for imaging extraosseous components of the tumor. Figures 6-16 and 6-17 show typical examples of bone sarcomas. Soft-tissue sarcomas are illustrated in Figures 6-18 and 6-19.

Staging

Magnetic resonance imaging should be performed in the region of the mass lesion to define the local extent of disease.[76,77] Because of the possibility of multiple lesions within a single bone, the entire affected bone should be evaluated. The use of gadolinium enhancement and fat-saturated sequences will usually allow differentiation of peritumoral edema from tumor. Regional lymphadenopathy should be evaluated as well, but in the absence of palpable lymphadenopathy, imaging of node bearing areas outside of the field of the tumor need not be performed.

The lungs should be screened for pulmonary parenchymal metastasis with CT. Contrast does not generally need to be given. Fluorodeoxyglucose PET scans are being used in some centers in screening for distant osseous metastasis, but there is evidence that bone scan is better in osteogenic sarcoma.[78] In most centers, bone scans will be used to evaluate for osseous metastasis.

Treatment Response and Follow-Up

Most bone sarcomas are treated with neoadjuvant chemotherapy followed by limb-sparing surgery. Patients should be evaluated for therapeutic response and to identify disease progression (including the development or progression of pulmonary or bone metastasis). Follow-up MRI exams usually demonstrate a decrease in tumor bulk,[79] decreased peritumoral edema, and sharper definition of tumor margins. Serial chest CT demonstrates the chemotherapy response of pulmonary metastasis.

Fluorodeoxyglucose PET shows promise as a means of detecting recurrent sarcoma.[80–82] This is especially true in cases in which equivocal findings are present on MRI.[83] Dynamic enhanced MRI has shown promise as a means of predicting tumor kill, and along with other methods including decreasing tumor bulk and decreasing FDG, PET activity can be used to assess tumor kill in vivo.[84–86]

Leukemia

Imaging generally has only a supportive role in patients with leukemia. Despite the fact that leukemia is the most commonly encountered pediatric neoplasm and that imaging studies are frequently abnormal, the primary diagnosis is not made with imaging and imaging does not have any major role in staging or defining response to therapy.

Due to the systemic distribution of leukemic cells, imaging findings of leukemia are occasionally encoun-

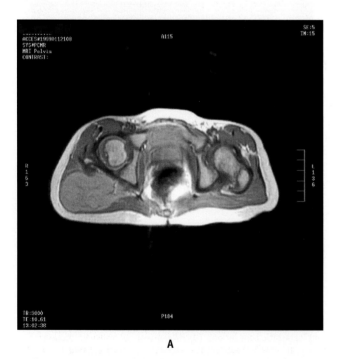

A

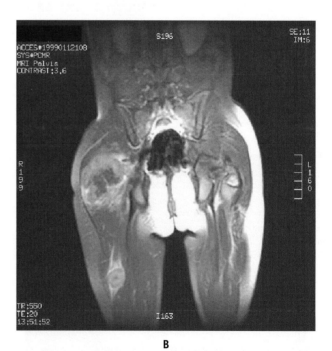

B

Figure 6-18   (A) Four-year-old female with extremity rhabdomyosarcoma. T1-weighted MRI without contrast shows a rounded, well-circumscribed soft-tissue mass in the right gluteal musculature. (B) Four-year-old female with extremity rhabdomyosarcoma. Coronal T1-weighted MRI following gadolinium administration demonstrates heterogeneous enhancement of the gluteal mass with a central area of nonenhancement suggesting necrosis. A second mass is also identified more inferiorly in the lateral thigh musculature.

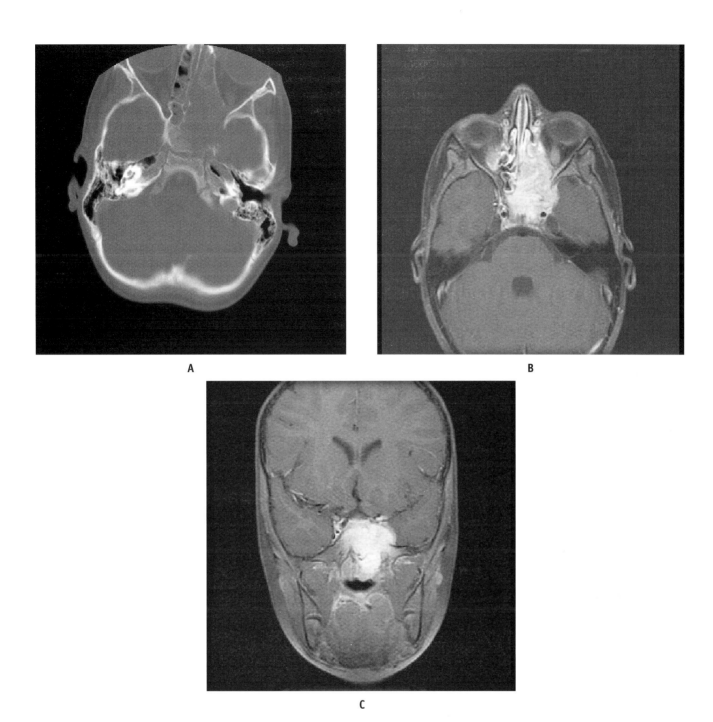

Figure 6-19 (A) Five-year-old male with paramenigeal rhabdomyosarcoma. Axial maxillofacial CT shows demineralization and bone destruction in the skull base with associated opacification of the ethmoid sinuses. The medial wall of the middle cranial fossa has been destroyed by this tumor. (B) Five-year-old male with paramenigeal rhabdomyosarcoma. Axial and coronal fat-saturated T1-weighted images acquired following gadolinium demonstrate avid enhancement of this skull-base tumor. Involvement of the skull base and sinuses is clearly shown. (C) Extension of tumor into the middle cranial fossa with mass effect on the medial aspect of the temporal lobe is well demonstrated.

tered in all organ systems. The most commonly encountered abnormalities are detected on skeletal or chest radiographs.

Patients undergoing skeletal radiography for bone pain may have focal areas of demineralization of poorly marginated bone destruction. Lucent metaphyseal bands, periosteal new bone formation, or frank bone destruction are possible manifestations. These findings are most typi-

cally present at the junction of the diaphysis and metaphysis of long bones. Associated findings can be demonstrated on bone scan.[87] Chest radiographic findings that may indicate leukemia include cardiomegaly, lymphadenopathy, pleural effusion, and pulmonary parenchymal consolidation.

Occasionally, leukemia may present as a focal soft-tissue mass.[88] Most typically, this mass is in the head and neck region, but these so-called chloromas can be encountered throughout the body. Computed tomography and MRI are the preferred modalities in evaluation of these focal mass lesions.

Complications of Therapy

Imaging support is vital to assessment of potential therapeutic complications of cancer therapy. Although the possible complications are widespread, several issues are repeatedly encountered. As with primary diagnosis, there is a balance that must be achieved between screening with the most sensitive and specific modalities and minimizing cost and risk of sedation and radiation exposure.

Pneumonia in the Immune-Compromised Host

Evaluation of the chest in the patient with fever and neutropenia is a daily event in tertiary cancer centers. The spectrum of disease includes the common bacterial and viral pathogens and expands to include other opportunistic agents, including aspergillis and other fungal agents, pneumocystis carinii, cytomegalovirus, septic emboli, legionella, and other rare bacterial pathogens. Correlation of the clinical setting including time course of disease, type of immune suppression, and exposures is critical in evaluation of chest radiographic findings.[89]

Chest radiographic findings are usually nonspecific. In some settings (cavitary nodules, classical lobar consolidation, etc) specific diagnosis can be suggested. Despite its limitations, chest radiography is the firstline imaging modality in evaluation of these patients. Patients with typical radiographic features of pneumonia can be appropriately treated.

Chest CT is a more sensitive and specific modality than chest radiography. Up to 20% more pneumonias are detected with CT as compared with chest radiography. Additionally, pneumonias are detected about 5 days earlier with CT than with radiography. Thin-section CT has been shown to have the highest sensitivity and specificity in this setting.[90] However, thin-section CT can be difficult to perform in children with rapid respiratory rates. Patients with noninfectious causes of tachypnea and hypoxia such as hypersensitivity pneumonitis, pulmonary hemorrhage, and pulmonary edema can also be evaluated with CT. The imaging appearance coupled with the time course of disease will frequently differentiate these processes.

In patients with high clinical indications of pulmonary infection, CT should be performed even in the absence of chest radiographic findings. Patients with chest radiographic abnormalities in which a more detailed assessment of probable pathogens, detection of emphysema or abscess, or in whom localization for biopsy is required should undergo CT.

Abdominal Abscess and Neutropenic Enteritis

Abdominal complications of neutropenia are common. Radiography is nonspecific and is useful in detecting obstruction and perforation. However, it has an otherwise very limited role in evaluation for neutropenic enteritis or intra-abdominal abscess.

Ultrasound is frequently used as a screening test to detect intra-abdominal fluid collections. In some series, it has been an effective means of primary screening for neutropenic enteritis.[91,92] Abdominal and pelvic abscesses can also be identified. However, the limitations of resolution, obscuration of images by overlying bowel gas, and lack of specificity make CT the modality of choice in evaluation of the abdomen for changes of neutropenic enteritis or abscess. Evaluation of the liver, spleen, and kidneys for evidence of fungal infection is also more sensitive and specific with CT than US.

Ultrasound should be considered in ongoing follow-up examinations of patients undergoing treatment for known fungal infections, abscesses, or neutropenic enteritis. If the specific areas of involvement can be visualized, US selection over CT will obviate the radiation exposure that multiple serial CT exams would incur.

Bone Infarctions and Osteomyelitis

Radiography is a convenient and effective way of assessing bone for a variety of pathologic conditions including osteomyelitis and bone infarction. Unfortunately, in order for changes to be detected, there must be a significant alteration in bone mineralization, which requires time for osteoblastic or osteoclastic activity to occur. Therefore, early changes of bone infection and infarction can be missed by radiography alone. Nonetheless, radiography should be the first imaging procedure performed in assessment of these conditions.

Bone scan is an excellent means of assessing for osteomyelitis. The so-called 3-phase bone scan is preferred. Localization of activity in the bone is a finding that makes osteomyelitis likely. In problematic cases, MRI can be a very useful modality in assessing infection.[93,94] Marrow edema, fluid collections, abnormal marrow enhancement, and periosteal edema are indicative of osteomyelitis. The presence of marrow edema is a strong indicator for infection.

In patients with suspected bone infarction, both skeletal scintigraphy and MRI are used as modalities to confirm the diagnosis.[95,96] Because scintigraphy can demonstrate either increased or decreased tracer uptake (depending on the phase of infarction), results can be confusing. Magnetic resonance imaging has the advantage over bone scan of being both sensitive for marrow changes and showing typical patterns that are specific for infarction. The phases of bone repair are clearly shown with MRI.

Brain Injury

Central nervous system complications of cancer therapy include hemorrhage, stroke,[97] and direct toxic effects with leukoencephalopathy. Hemorrhagic complications can be imaged with either CT or MRI. Computed tomography is more readily available and is an excellent screening exam for intracranial hemorrhage.

The evaluation of stroke is best performed with MRI. Although CT can be useful in identifying areas of brain edema, MRI is a much more sensitive exam in detecting the early changes of stroke.[98,99] T2-weighted sequences clearly demonstrate the typical pattern of gray and white matter edema. Even before T2 changes become apparent, diffusion-weighted sequences can detect diffusion restriction typical of stroke.

Early white matter toxicity from methotrexate and other chemotherapeutic agents can be best detected with MRI.[100] Localizing areas of white matter edema (especially in the frontal lobes) are typical. In patients that go on to develop more widespread changes with white matter volume loss, MRI and CT will demonstrate decrease in white matter volume with associated ventricular dilatation and prominence of sulci.

Venous Thrombosis

Venous thrombosis is a frequent and challenging problem in supportive care of patients with cancer. Presence of hypercoagulable states, immobility, and extensive use of indwelling venous catheters make venous thrombosis a very common problem. Ultrasound has largely replaced venography in evaluation of the venous system for clots. Color-flow Doppler is used to verify patency and identify collateral drainage. In the extremities, compression of venous structures is also used to differentiate hypoechoic clot from a normally distended vein. Serial US examinations for diagnosis of recurrent thrombosis and follow-up of treatment response are expensive, frequently difficult to interpret, and not generally indicated.[101]

Veins of the thigh, upper arm, neck, and chest can usually be seen with excellent fidelity using US. Occasionally there can be difficulty seeing the venous system due to large body habitus or because of small insonation windows in the chest. Indirect signs of central venous thrombosis such as loss of cardiac pulsitility and respiratory variation can be helpful secondary signs with US. In ambiguous or complicated cases, MR venography is an excellent means of assessing venous patency.[102] The reproducibility of this technique and its decreased dependence on the operator make it a better modality in following treatment response or evaluating chronic/recurrent thrombosis.

References

1. Brenner DJ, Elliston EC, Hall EJ, et al. Estimated risks of radiation-induced fatal cancer from pediatric CT. *Am J Roentgenol.* 2001;176:289–296.
2. Hall E. Lessons we have learned from our children: cancer risks from diagnostic radiology. *Pediatr Radiol.* 2002;32(10):700–706.
3. Frush D. Strategies of dose reduction. *Pediatr Radiol.* 2002;32(4):293–297.
4. Frush D, Donnelly L, Rosen N. Computed tomography and radiation risks: what pediatric health care providers should know. *Pediatrics.* 2003;112(4):951–957.
5. Paterson A, Frush DP, Donnelly LF. Helical CT of the body: are settings adjusted for pediatric patients? *Am J Roentgenol.* 2001;176:297–301.
6. Slovis T. Introduction to seminar in radiation dose reduction. *Pediatr Radiol.* 2002;32(10):707–708,751–754.
7. Brown P, Thomas RD, Silberberg PJ, Johnson LM. Optimization of a fluoroscope to reduce radiation exposure in pediatric imaging. *Pediatr Radiol.* 2000;30(4):229–235.
8. Lederman HM, Khademian ZP, Felice M, Hurh PJ. Dose reduction fluoroscopy in pediatrics. *Pediatr Radiol.* 2002;32(12):844–848.
9. Sahani D, Saini S, D'souza RV, O'Neill MJ, et al. Comparison between low (3:1) and high (6:1) pitch for routine abdominal/pelvic imaging with multislice computed tomography. *J Comput Assist Tomogr.* 2003;27(2):105–109.
10. Thornton FJ, Paulson EK, Yoshizumi TT, Frush DP, et al. Single versus multidetector row CT: comparison of radiation doses and dose profiles. *Acad Radiol.* 2003;10(4):379–385.
11. Cochran S, Bomyea K, Sayre J. Trends in adverse events after IV administration of contrast media. *Am J Roentgenol.* 2001;176(6):1385–1388.
12. Cercignani M, Horsfield M. The physical basis of diffusion-weighted MRI. *J Neurol Sci.* 2001;186(suppl 1):S11–S14.
13. Pipe J. Basic spin physics. *Magn Reson Imaging Clin North Am.* 1999;7(4):607–627.
14. Luypaert R, Boujraf S, Sourbron S, Osteaux M, et al. Diffusion and perfusion MRI: basic physics. *Eur J Radiol.* 2001;38(1):19–27.
15. Burtscher I, Holtas S. Proton magnetic resonance spectroscopy in brain tumours: clinical applications. *Neuroradiology.* 2001;43(5):345–352.
16. Murphy M, Loosemore A, Clifton AG, Howe FA, et al. The contribution of proton magnetic resonance spectroscopy (1HMRS) to clinical brain tumour diagnosis. *Br J Neurosurg.* 2002;16(4):329–334.
17. Tate AR, Majós C, Moreno A, Howe FA, et al. Automated classification of short echo time in in vivo 1H brain tumor spectra: a multicenter study. *Magn Reson Med.* 2003;49(1):29–36.
18. Nadal Desbarats L, Herlidou S, de Marco G, Gondry-Jouet C, et al. Differential MRI diagnosis between brain abscesses and necrotic or cystic brain tumors using the apparent diffusion coefficient and normalized diffusion-weighted images. *Magn Reson Imaging.* 2003;21(6):645–650.
19. Bulakbasi N, Kocaoglu M, Ors F, Tayfun C, et al. Combination of single-voxel proton MR spectroscopy and apparent diffusion coefficient calculation in the evaluation of common brain tumors. *Am J Neuroradiol.* 2003;24(2):225–233.
20. Gupta N, Berger M. Brain mapping for hemispheric tumors in children. *Pediatr Neurosurg.* 2003;38(6):302–306.
21. Tummala RP, Chu RM, Liu H, Truwit CL, et al. Application of diffusion tensor imaging to magnetic-resonance-guided brain tumor resection. *Pediatr Neurosurg.* 2003;39(1):39–43.
22. Hustinx R, Benard F, Alavi A. Whole-body FDG-PET imaging in the management of patients with cancer. *Semin Nucl Med.* 2002;32(1):35–46.
23. Kostakoglu L, Agress H, Goldsmith S. Clinical role of FDG PET in evaluation of cancer patients. *Radiographics.* 2003;23(2):315–40; quiz 533.
24. Israel O, Keidar Z, Iosilevsky G, Bettman L, et al. The fusion of anatomic and physiologic imaging in the management of patients with cancer. *Semin Nucl Med.* 2001;31(3):191–205.
25. Eary J. Nuclear medicine in cancer diagnosis. *Lancet.* 1999;354(9181):853–857.
26. Brenner W, Bohuslavizki K, Eary J. PET imaging of osteosarcoma. *J Nucl Med.* 2003;44(6):930–942.
27. Roberts HC, Roberts TP, Bollen AW, Ley S, et al. Correlation of microvascular permeability derived from dynamic contrast-enhanced MR imaging with histologic grade and tumor labeling index: a study in human brain tumors. *Acad Radiol.* 2001;8(5):384–391.
28. Roberts HC, Roberts TP, Brasch RC, Dillon WP, et al. Quantitative measurement of microvascular permeability in human brain tumors achieved using dynamic contrast-enhanced MR imaging: correlation with histologic grade. *Am J Neuroradiol.* 2000;21(5):891–899.
29. Tynninen O, Aronen HJ, Ruhala M, Paetau A, et al. MRI enhancement and microvascular density in gliomas. Correlation with tumor cell proliferation. *Invest Radiol.* 1999;34(6):427–434.
30. Lüdemann L, Grieger W, Wurm R, Budzisch M, et al. Comparison of dynamic contrast-enhanced MRI with WHO tumor grading for gliomas. *Eur Radiol.* 2001;11(7):1231–1241.
31. Medina L, Kuntz K, Pomeroy S. Children with headache suspected of having a brain tumor: a cost-effectiveness analysis of diagnostic strategies. *Pediatrics.* 2001;108(2):255–263.
32. Kandt R. Tuberous sclerosis complex and neurofibromatosis type 1: the two most common neurocutaneous diseases. *Neurol Clin.* 2003;21(4):983–1004.
33. Durden D, Williams D. Radiology of skull base neoplasms. *Otolaryngol Clin North Am.* 2001;34(6):1043–64, vii.
34. Poussaint T. Magnetic resonance imaging of pediatric brain tumors: state of the art. *Top Magn Reson Imaging.* 2001;12(6):411–433.
35. Luh G, Bird C. Imaging of brain tumors in the pediatric population. *Neuroimaging Clin North Am.* 1999;9(4):691–716.
36. Griffiths P. A protocol for imaging paediatric brain tumours. United Kingdom Children's Cancer Study Group (UKCCSG) and Societe Francaise D'Oncologie Pediatrique (SFOP) Panelists. *Clin Oncol (R Coll Radiol).* 1999;11(5):290–294.
37. Fouladi M, Gajjar A, Boyett JM, Walter AW, et al. Comparison of CSF cytology and spinal magnetic resonance imaging in the detection of leptomeningeal disease in pediatric medulloblastoma or primitive neuroectodermal tumor. *J Clin Oncol.* 1999;17(10):3234–3237.
38. Sevick R, Wallace C. MR imaging of neoplasms of the lumbar spine. *Magn Reson Imaging Clin North Am.* 1999;7(3):539–553,ix.
39. Tzika AA, Zarifi MK, Goumnerova L, Astrakas LG, et al. Neuroimaging in pediatric brain tumors: Gd-DTPA-enhanced, hemodynamic, and diffusion MR imaging compared with MR spectroscopic imaging. *Am J Neuroradiol.* 2002;23(2):322–333.
40. Korones DN, Butterfield R, Meyers SP, Constine LS. The role of surveillance magnetic resonance imaging (MRI) scanning in detecting recurrent brain tumors in asymptomatic children. *J Neurooncol.* 2001;53(1):33–38.
41. Rock JP, Hearshen D, Scarpace L, Croteau D, et al. Correlations between magnetic resonance spectroscopy and image-guided histopathology, with special attention to radiation necrosis. *Neurosurgery.* 2002;51(4):912–919; discussion 919–920.

42. Schlemmer HP, Bachert P, Henze M, Buslei R, et al. Differentiation of radiation necrosis from tumor progression using proton magnetic resonance spectroscopy. *Neuroradiology.* 2002;44(3):216–222.

43. Chao ST, Suh JH, Raja S, Lee SY, et al. The sensitivity and specificity of FDG PET in distinguishing recurrent brain tumor from radionecrosis in patients treated with stereotactic radiosurgery. *Int J Cancer.* 2001;96(3):191–197.

44. Wong T, van der Westhuizen GJ, Coleman RE. Positron emission tomography imaging of brain tumors. *Neuroimaging Clin North Am.* 2002;12(4):615–626.

45. St Amour TE, Siegel MJ, Glazer HS, Nadel SN. CT appearances of the normal and abnormal thymus in childhood. *J Comput Assist Tomogr.* 1987;11(4):645–650.

46. McLaughlin AF, Magee MA, Greenough R, Allman KC, et al. Current role of gallium scanning in the management of lymphoma. *Eur J Nucl Med.* 1990. 16(8–10):755–771.

47. Front D, Bar-Shalom R, Epelbaum R, Haim N, et al. Early detection of lymphoma recurrence with gallium-67 scintigraphy. *J Nucl Med.* 1993. 34(12):2101–2104.

48. Montravers F, McNamara D, Landman-Parker J, Grahek D, et al. [(18)F]FDG in childhood lymphoma: clinical utility and impact on management. *Eur J Nucl Med Mol Imaging.* 2002;29(9):1155–1165.

49. Karmazyn B, Ash S, Goshen Y, Yaniv I, et al. Significance of residual abdominal masses in children with abdominal Burkitt's lymphoma. *Pediatr Radiol.* 2001;31(11):801–805.

50. White K. Thoracic imaging of pediatric lymphomas. *J Thorac Imaging.* 2001;16(4):224–237.

51. Front D, Bar-Shalom R, Mor M, Haim N, et al. Hodgkin disease: prediction of outcome with 67Ga scintigraphy after one cycle of chemotherapy. *Radiology.* 1999;210(2):487–491.

52. Front D, Ben-Haim S, Israel O, Epelbaum R, et al. Lymphoma: predictive value of Ga-67 scintigraphy after treatment. *Radiology.* 1992;182(2):359–363.

53. Spaepen K, Stroobants S, Dupont P, Van Steenweghen S, et al. Prognostic value of positron emission tomography (PET) with fluorine-18 fluorodeoxyglucose ([18F]FDG) after first-line chemotherapy in non-Hodgkin's lymphoma: is [18F]FDG-PET a valid alternative to conventional diagnostic methods? *J Clin Oncol.* 2001;19(2):414–419.

54. Spaepen K, Stroobants S, Dupont P, Vandenberghe P, et al. Prognostic value of pretransplantation positron emission tomography using fluorine 18-fluorodeoxyglucose in patients with aggressive lymphoma treated with high-dose chemotherapy and stem cell transplantation. *Blood.* 2003;102(1):53–59.

55. Cohen M, Hill CA, Cangir A, Sullivan MP. Thymic rebound after treatment of childhood tumors. *Am J Roentgenol.* 1980. 135(1):151–156.

56. Hugosson C, Nyman R, Jorulf H, McDonald P, et al. Imaging of abdominal neuroblastoma in children. *Acta Radiol.* 1999;40(5):534–542.

57. Siegel MJ, Ishwaran H, Fletcher BD, Meyer JS, et al. Staging of neuroblastoma at imaging: report of the radiology diagnostic oncology group. *Radiology.* 2002;223(1):168–175.

58. Meyer J, Harty M, Khademian Z. Imaging of neuroblastoma and Wilms' tumor. *Magn Reson Imaging Clin North Am.* 2002;10(2):275–302.

59. Uhl M, Altehoefer C, Kontny U, Il'yasov K, et al. MRI-diffusion imaging of neuroblastomas: first results and correlation to histology. *Eur Radiol.* 2002;12(9):2335–2338.

60. Sofka CM, Semelka RC, Kelekis NL, Worawattanakul S, et al. Magnetic resonance imaging of neuroblastoma using current techniques. *Magn Reson Imaging.* 1999;17(2):193–198.

61. Pfluger T, Schmied C, Porn U, Leinsinger G, et al. Integrated imaging using MRI and 123I metaiodobenzylguanidine scintigraphy to improve sensitivity and specificity in the diagnosis of pediatric neuroblastoma. *Am J Roentgenol.* 2003;181(4):1115–1124.

62. Leonidas J. MR imaging in the assessment of staging of neuroblastoma. *Radiology.* 2003;226(1):285;285–286.

63. Hahn K, Charron M, Shulkin B. Role of MR imaging and iodine 123 MIBG scintigraphy in staging of pediatric neuroblastoma. *Radiology.* 2003;227(3):908;908–909.

64. Perel Y, Conway J, Kletzel M, Goldman J, et al. Clinical impact and prognostic value of metaiodobenzylguanidine imaging in children with metastatic neuroblastoma. *J Pediatr Hematol Oncol.* 1999;21(1):13–18.

65. Mazumdar A, Siegel MJ, Narra V, Luchtman-Jones L, et al. Whole-body fast inversion recovery MR imaging of small cell neoplasms in pediatric patients: a pilot study. *Am J Roentgenol.* 2002;179(5):1261–1266.

66. McNeil DE, Brown M, Ching A, DeBaun MR, et al. Screening for Wilms tumor and hepatoblastoma in children with Beckwith-Wiedemann syndromes: a cost-effective model. *Med Pediatr Oncol.* 2001;37(4):349–356.

67. Lowe LH, Isuani BH, Heller RM, Stein SM, et al. Pediatric renal masses: Wilms tumor and beyond. *Radiographics.* 2000;20(6):1585–1603.

68. Choyke PL, Siegel MJ, Craft AW, Green DM, et al. Screening for Wilms tumor in children with Beckwith-Wiedemann syndrome or idiopathic hemihypertrophy. *Med Pediatr Oncol.* 1999;32(3):196–200.

69. Goske M, Mitchell C, Reslan W. Imaging of patients with Wilms' tumor. *Semin Urol Oncol.* 1999;17(1):11–20.

70. Gow KW, Roberts IF, Jamieson DH, Bray H, et al. Local staging of Wilms' tumor: Computerized tomography correlation with histological findings. *J Pediatr Surg.* 2000;35(5):677–679.

71. Wootton-Gorges SL, Albano EA, Riggs JM, Ihrke H, et al. Chest radiography versus chest CT in the evaluation for pulmonary metastases in patients with Wilms' tumor: a retrospective review. *Pediatr Radiol.* 2000;30(8):533-537; discussion 537–539.

72. Owens CM, Veys PA, Pritchard J, Levitt G, et al. Role of chest computed tomography at diagnosis in the management of Wilms' tumor: a study by the United Kingdom Children's Cancer Study Group. *J Clin Oncol.* 2002;20(12):2768–2773.

73. Davies A. Imaging in skeletal paediatric oncology. *Eur J Radiol.* 2001;37(2):79–94.

74. Siegel M. Magnetic resonance imaging of musculoskeletal soft tissue masses. *Radiol Clin North Am.* 2001;39(4):701–720.

75. Mahboubi S. Magnetic resonance imaging of soft-tissue tumors in children. *Top Magn Reson Imaging.* 2002;13(4):263–275.

76. Elias DA, White LM, Simpson DJ, Kandel RA, et al. Osseous invasion by soft-tissue sarcoma: assessment with MR imaging. *Radiology.* 2003;229(1):145–152.

77. Kim EE, Valenzuela RF, Kumar AJ, Raney RB, et al. Imaging and clinical spectrum of rhabdomyosarcoma in children. *Clin Imaging.* 2000;24(5):257–262.

78. Franzius C, Sciuk J, Daldrup-Link HE, Jürgens H, et al. FDG-PET for detection of osseous metastases from malignant primary bone tumours: comparison with bone scintigraphy. *Eur J Nucl Med.* 2000;27(9):1305–1311.

79. Abudu A, Davies AM, Pynsent PB, Mangham DC, et al. Tumour volume as a predictor of necrosis after chemotherapy in Ewing's sarcoma. *J Bone Joint Surg Br.* 1999;81(2):317–322.

80. Bredella M, Caputo G, Steinbach L. Value of FDG positron emission tomography in conjunction with MR imaging for evaluating therapy response in patients with musculoskeletal sarcomas. *Am J Roentgenol.* 2002;179(5):1145–1150.

81. Johnson GR, Zhuang H, Khan J, Chiang SB, et al. Roles of positron emission tomography with fluorine-18-deoxyglucose in the detection of local recurrent and distant metastatic sarcoma. *Clin Nucl Med.* 2003;28(10):815–820.

82. Dyke JP, Panicek DM, Healey JH, Meyers PA, et al. Osteogenic and Ewing sarcomas: estimation of necrotic fraction during induction chemotherapy with dynamic contrast-enhanced MR imaging. *Radiology.* 2003;228(1):271–278.

83. Kaste SC, Hill A, Conley L, Shidler TJ, et al. Magnetic resonance imaging after incomplete resection of soft tissue sarcoma. *Clin Orthop Relat Res.* 2002 Apr;(397):204–211.

84. Miller SL, Hoffer FA, Reddick WE, Wu S, et al. Tumor volume or dynamic contrast-enhanced MRI for prediction of clinical outcome of Ewing sarcoma family of tumors. *Pediatr Radiol.* 2001;31(7):518–523.

85. Reddick W, Taylor J, Fletcher B. Dynamic MR imaging (DEMRI) of microcirculation in bone sarcoma. *J Magn Reson Imaging.* 1999;10(3):277–285.

86. Hawkins DS, Rajendran JG, Conrad EU 3rd, Bruckner JD, et al. Evaluation of chemotherapy response in pediatric bone sarcomas by [F-18]-fluorodeoxy-D-glucose positron emission tomography. *Cancer.* 2002;94(12):3277–3284.

87. Shalaby-Rana E, Majd M. (99m)Tc-MDP scintigraphic findings in children with leukemia: value of early and delayed whole-body imaging. *J Nucl Med.* 2001;42(6):878–883.

88. Guermazi A, Feger C, Rousselot P, Merad M, et al. Granulocytic sarcoma (chloroma): imaging findings in adults and children. *Am J Roentgenol.* 2002;178(2):319–325.

89. Oh Y, Effmann E, Godwin J. Pulmonary infections in immunocompromised hosts: the importance of correlating the conventional radiologic appearance with the clinical setting. *Radiology.* 2000;217(3):647–656.

90. Seely J, Effmann E, Muller N. High-resolution CT of pediatric lung disease: imaging findings. *Am J Roentgenol.* 1997;168(5):1269–1275.

91. Hagiwara S, Togano T, Kajiwara K, Otake H, et al. Role of ultrasonography in diagnosis of neutropenic enteritis: a study of 4 cases. *Rinsho Ketsueki.* 2001;42(2):81–88.

92. Gorschlüter M, Marklein G, Höfling K, Clarenbach R, et al. Abdominal infections in patients with acute leukaemia: a prospective study applying ultrasonography and microbiology. *Br J Haematol.* 2002;117(2):351–358.

93. Santiago RC, Gimenez C, McCarthy K. Imaging of osteomyelitis and musculoskeletal soft tissue infections: current concepts. *Rheum Dis Clin North Am.* 2003;29(1):89–109.

94. Sammak B, Abd El Bagi M, Al Shahed M, Hamilton D, et al. Osteomyelitis: a review of currently used imaging techniques. *Eur Radiol.* 1999;9(5):894–900.

95. DeSmet AA, Dalinka MK, Alazraki N, Berquist TH, et al. Diagnostic imaging of avascular necrosis of the hip. American College of Radiology. ACR Appropriateness Criteria. *Radiology.* 2000;215(suppl):247–254.

96. Ribeiro RC, Fletcher BD, Kennedy W, Harrison PL, et al. Magnetic resonance imaging detection of avascular necrosis of the bone in children receiving intensive prednisone therapy for acute lymphoblastic leukemia or non-Hodgkin lymphoma. *Leukemia.* 2001;15(6):891–897.

97. Rogers L. Cerebrovascular complications in cancer patients. *Neurol Clin.* 2003;21(1):167–192.

98. Provenzale JM, Jahan R, Naidich TP, Fox AJ. Assessment of the patient with hyperacute stroke: imaging and therapy. *Radiology.* 2003;229(2):347–359.

99. Saur D, Kucinski T, Grzyska U, Eckert B, et al. Sensitivity and interrater agreement of CT and diffusion-weighted MR imaging in hyperacute stroke. *Am J Neuroradiol.* 2003;24(5):878–885.

100. Oka M, Terae S, Kobayashi R, Sawamura Y, et al. MRI in methotrexate-related leukoencephalopathy: Disseminated necrotising leukoencephalopathy in comparison with mild leukoencephalopathy. *Neuroradiology.* 2003;45(7):493–497.

101. Perone N, Bounameaux H, Perrier A. Comparison of four strategies for diagnosing deep vein thrombosis: a cost-effectiveness analysis. *Am J Med.* 2001;110(1):33–40.

102. Shankar KR, Abernethy LJ, Das KS, Roche CJ, et al. Magnetic resonance venography in assessing venous patency after multiple venous catheters. *J Pediatr Surg.* 2002;37(2):175–179.

Principles of Cancer Therapy in Children

Fundamentals of Cancer Chemotherapy

Brigitte C. Widemann and Peter C. Adamson

Introduction

Since the institution of chemotherapy for childhood cancers in the late 1940s, there has been steady improvement in the survival of children with solid and hematologic malignancies, such that prolonged disease-free survival is achievable for the majority of affected children. This chapter will review the principles of the chemotherapeutic treatment of childhood cancer that have been the cornerstone of improved clinical outcome. The source, mechanism of action, pharmacokinetics, and toxicities of anticancer agents commonly used in pediatrics, as well as agents commonly used to ameliorate chemotherapy-related toxicities, will be reviewed. The mechanisms of drug resistance, drug interactions, and recent advances in the development of more targeted therapies will be highlighted.

Principles of Cancer Chemotherapy

The commonly used anticancer drugs are nonselective cytotoxins that interfere with metabolic pathways or vital macromolecules critical to both normal and malignant cells. As a result, toxicities from these drugs occur frequently and are often severe. A drug regimen is usually selected according to the histology of the tumor and the extent of the disease. Patients receive the standard, fixed doses of drugs adjusted for body weight or surface area. Both the starting dose and subsequent modifications in the dose or schedule are based only on clinical toxicities, rather than on whether a therapeutic plasma drug concentration has been achieved.

Several important principles of childhood cancer treatment derived from clinical observations over the years have resulted in improved clinical outcome.[1] The approach to treatment is a *multimodality approach*, which optimally combines systemic therapy through administration of chemotherapy and local therapy through surgery and/or radiation therapy. Systemic treatment with chemotherapy works best when a combination of several agents (*combination chemotherapy*) is used as opposed to administering a sequence of single agents. This was first appreciated in the treatment of acute lymphoblastic leukemia (ALL). Although up to 60% of children with ALL treated with a single agent went into complete remission, nearly all patients experienced a relapse within 6 to 9 months despite continuation of treatment with the same drug. Long-term remissions and cures were realized only with institution of combination therapy incorporating the most active single agents.[2] Table 7-1 provides examples of improved outcome with the use of combination chemotherapy for a number of childhood cancers.[3]

Most anticancer drugs have a steep dose response curve such that small increments in the dose can significantly influence the therapeutic efficacy of a drug. Administration of each chemotherapy agent at the maximally tolerated dose at high dose intensity (defined as the amount of drug administered per unit of time -mg/m^2/week) correlates with decreased relapse rates in pediatric cancers.[1] Chemotherapy has been used most successfully when used in the *adjuvant setting;* that is, in patients with no evidence of residual disease following local therapy with surgery or radiation therapy for the primary tumor.[4] Prior to the use of adjuvant chemotherapy, 80% to 95% of children with localized solid tumors treated with local therapy alone developed recurrent distant disease. In the setting of localized tumors, adjuvant chemotherapy improves outcome by controlling systemic microscopic disease. Ideally, adjuvant chemotherapy should begin as soon as possible, because delays in chemotherapy to allow for recovery from local radiation therapy or surgery may adversely affect the outcome. Adjuvant chemotherapy has been demonstrated to be efficacious for the most common pediatric cancers (see Table 7-1).

The initial administration of chemotherapy prior to definitive local therapy, called primary or *neoadjuvant* chemotherapy, may also improve local control of the primary tumor as well as providing earlier therapy for micrometastatic disease. There are limited studies that have explored the benefits of neoadjuvant vs adjuvant chemotherapy for childhood solid tumors. One randomized study in patients with nonmetastatic osteosarcoma could not demonstrate a survival advantage with neoadjuvant chemotherapy.[5] However, as neoadjuvant chemotherapy appears to improve the ability to completely resect larger localized tumors, it is now considered standard

Table 7-1

Beneficial effects of adjuvant chemotherapy on survival of patients with common forms of childhood cancer.

Tumor	Adjuvant Therapy	Survival (%) Without Adjuvant Chemotherapy	Survival (%) With Adjuvant Chemotherapy
Wilms tumor	vincristine, dactinomycin, ± doxorubicin	40	90
Ewing sarcoma	vincristine, dactinomycin, cyclophosphamide	5	50–60
Lymphomas	CHOP, COMP, LSA₂-L₂	< 10	50–90
Rhabdomyosarcoma	vincristine, dactinomycin, cyclophosphamide	10–20	65
Osteosarcoma	HDMTX, doxorubicin, cisplatin, BCD	15	65
Astrocytoma	prednisone, vincristine, lomustine	20	45

C, cyclophosphamide; H, doxorubicin; O, vincristine; P, prednisone; HDMTX, high-dose methotrexate; B, bleomycin; D, dactinomycin; LSA$_2$-L$_2$, 10-drug regimen.

From Berg SL, Grissel DL, DeLaney TF, Balis FM. Principles of treatment of pediatric solid tumors. *Pediatr Clin North Am.* 1991;38:249.

treatment for osteosarcomas and many other pediatric solid tumors. Unfortunately, although neoadjuvant chemotherapy has dramatically improved survival for children with localized solid tumors, the impact for children with metastatic disease at diagnosis has been modest at best, because the large majority of such children ultimately succumb to their disease.

Clinical Pharmacology of Anticancer Drugs

In order to administer chemotherapy agents safely in the setting of multimodality treatment, in-depth knowledge of the clinical pharmacology of these agents is required. Anticancer drugs have the lowest therapeutic index of any class of drugs and predictably produce significant, and at times life-threatening, toxicities. Considering that many patients have no detectable disease when they receive chemotherapy (ie, are in remission), the treatment in the short term can be worse than the disease. It cannot be overemphasized, however, that even small reductions in the doses of these agents or short delays in therapy can increase the risk for recurrence of disease. The risks of toxicities from therapy must therefore be balanced with the risk of tumor recurrence from inadequate treatment.

Source and Mechanism of Action of Anticancer Drugs

Anticancer drugs can be divided into synthetic agents (eg, alkylating agents, antimetabolites) and natural products extracted or isolated from plants or microorganisms (eg, topoisomerase inhibitors, tubulin-binding agents). Although natural products have complex chemical structures, the chemical structure of most synthetic drugs is simpler. Most commonly used anticancer drugs can be grouped into 4 broad categories based on their mechanism of action: alkylating agents, antimetabolites, topoisomerase inhibitors, and tubulin-binding agents (Table 7-2). Within each category there are subgroups of chemically related agents (analogs), such as nitrogen mustards, platinum analogs, anthracyclines, epidophyllotoxins, and vinca alkaloids that share many characteristics but also have pharmacologic properties that make them distinct from their chemically similar relatives. An understanding of the mechanism of drug action is useful in predicting which drug combination may produce additive or synergistic antitumor effects. In addition, a drug's schedule of administration may be influenced by its mechanism of action.

Most anticancer drugs produce their effect by interfering with the synthesis or function of DNA and RNA (Figure 7-1). The largest class of anticancer drugs, the alkylating agents, are chemically reactive compounds that damage DNA by forming covalent bonds to and cross-linking nucleobases (Figure 7-2). These reactions are nonspecific, and the alkylating agent can attack any nucleophilic group it comes in contact with, but it is the reaction with DNA that primarily underlies the cytotoxic effect.

The antimetabolites are close structural analogs of the nucleoside precursors of DNA and RNA or analogs of cofactors involved in the synthesis of these building blocks, and they either deplete precursors or are incorporated into DNA or RNA as fraudulent substrates (Figure 7-3). Antimetabolites are inhibitory only during S phase in the cell cycle and thus produce greater cytotoxicity when administered on a continuous or protracted schedule. The most widely used antimetabolite in pediatric oncology is methotrexate (MTX). Methotrexate, a structural analog of folic acid, enters cells via the

Table 7-2

Pharmacologic properties of commonly used anticancer drugs.

Drug	Route*	Dose/m²	Schedule†	Toxicities‡	Antitumor spectrum
Alkylating agentsΩ					
Nitrogen mustards					
Melphalan	IV	140–220 mg	single dose (BMT)	M, N&V; mucositis & diarrhea (HD)	rhabdomyosarcoma, sarcomas, neuroblastoma, leukemias
Cyclophosphamide[1,2]	IV	250–1800 mg	daily × 1–4 d, q 21–28 d	M, N&V, A, cystitis, water retention, cardiac (HD)	lymphomas, leukemias, sarcomas, neuroblastoma
	PO	100–300 mg	daily		
Ifosfamide[1,2]	IV	1600–2400 mg	daily × 5, q 21–28 d	M, N&V, A, cystitis, NT, renal, cardiac (HD)	sarcomas, germ cell
Nitrosoureas					
Carmustine (BCNU)	IV	200–250 mg	single dose, q 4–6 wk	M, N&V, renal, & pulmonary	brain tumors, lymphoma, Hodgkin disease
Lomustine (CCNU)	PO	100–150 mg	single dose, q 4–6 wk	M, N&V, renal, & pulmonary	brain tumors, lymphoma, Hodgkin disease
Platinum analogs					
Cisplatin	IV	50–200 mg	over 4–6 h, q 21–28 d	M (mild), N&V, A, renal, NT, ototoxicity, HSR	testicular and other germ cell tumors, brain tumors, osteosarcoma, neuroblastoma
	IV	20–40 mg	daily × 5, q 21–28 d		
Carboplatin	IV	400–600 mg	single dose or daily × 2, q 28 d	M (Plt), N&V, A	brain tumors, germ cell tumors, neuroblastoma, sarcomas
Busulfan	PO	1.8 mg	daily	M, A, pulmonary; N&V, mucositis, NT, hepatic (HD)	CML; leukemias (BMT)
	PO	37.5 mg	q 6 h for 4 d (BMT)		
Temozolomide	PO	200 mg	daily × 5, q 28 d	M, N&V	brain tumors
Procarbazine[2]	PO	100 mg	daily for 10–14 d	M, N&V, NT, rash, mucositis	Hodgkin disease, brain tumors
Dacarbazine[2]	IV	250 mg	daily × 5, q 21–28 d	M (mild), N&V, flulike syndrome, hepatic	neuroblastoma, sarcomas, Hodgkin disease

(continued)

Table 7-2 (continued)

Pharmacologic properties of commonly used anticancer drugs.

Drug	Route*	Dose/m²	Schedule†	Toxicities‡	Antitumor spectrum
Antimetabolites					
Antifolates					
Methotrexate	PO, IM, SC	7.5–30 mg	weekly or biweekly	M (mild), mucositis, rash, hepatic; renal, NT (HD)	leukemia, lymphoma, osteosarcoma
	IV	10–33,000 mg	bolus or CI (6–42 h)		
Purine analogs					
Mercaptopurine[3,4]	PO	75–100 mg	daily	M, hepatic, mucositis	leukemia (ALL, CML)
Thioguanine[3,4]	PO	75–100 mg	daily × 5–7	M, N&V, mucositis, hepatic (VOD)	leukemia (ALL, AML)
	PO	40–60 mg	daily		
Fludarabine phosphate	IV	25 mg	daily × 5	M, opportunistic infections, neurotoxicity (high dose)	leukemia (AML, CLL), indolent lymphomas
Pyrimidine analogs					
Cytarabine[4]	IV, SC	100–200 mg	q 12 h or CI for 5–7 d	M, N&V, mucositis, GI, flulike syndrome; NT, ocular, skin (HD)	leukemia, lymphoma
	IV	3000 mg	q 12 h for 4–8 doses		
Fluorouracil[4]	IV	500 mg	single or daily × 5	M (bolus), mucositis, N&V, diarrhea, skin, NT, ocular, cardiac	carcinomas, hepatic tumors
	IV	800–1200 mg	CI (24–120 h)		
Topoisomerase II Inhibitors					
Antitumor antibiotics					
Doxorubicin[5]	IV	45–75 mg	single, q 21 d	M, mucositis, N&V, A, diarrhea, vesicant, cardiac (acute, chronic)	leukemia (ALL, ANL), lymphomas, most solid tumors
	IV	20–30 mg	weekly		
	IV	45–90 mg	CI (24–96 h)		
Daunomycin[5]	IV	30–45 mg	daily × 3 or weekly	M, mucositis, N&V, diarrhea, A, vesicant, cardiac (acute, chronic)	leukemia (ALL, ANL), lymphomas
Idarubicin[5]	IV	10–15 mg	daily or weekly × 3	M, mucositis, N&V, diarrhea, A, vesicant, cardiac (acute, chronic)	leukemia (ALL, ANL), lymphomas
	PO	30–40 mg	daily × 3		
Mitoxantrone	IV	8–12 mg	daily × 3–5 d	M, mucositis, N&V, A, bluish color to urine, veins, sclerae, nails	leukemia (ALL, ANL), lymphomas

(continued)

Table 7-2 (continued)

Pharmacologic properties of commonly used anticancer drugs.

Drug	Route*	Dose/m²	Schedule†	Toxicities‡	Antitumor spectrum
Topoisomerase II Inhibitors					
Antitumor antibiotics					
Bleomycin	IV, IM, SC	10–20 units	weekly	lung, skin, fever, mucositis, alopecia, hypersensitivity, Raynaud, N&V	lymphoma, testicular and other germ cell
Dactinomycin	IV	0.45 mg (15 μg/kg)	daily × 5, q 3–6 wk	M, N&V, A, mucositis, vesicant, hepatic (VOD)	Wilms tumor, sarcomas
	IV	1.35–1.8 mg (45–60 μg/kg)	single dose q 3–6 wk		
Epidophyllotoxins⁶					
Etoposide⁶	IV / PO	60–120 mg / 50 mg	daily × 3–5, q 3–6 wk / daily × 21 d q 4 wk	M, A, N&V, mucositis, mild NT, hypotension, HSR, secondary leukemia; diarrhea (PO)	leukemias (ALL, ANL), lymphomas, neuroblastoma, sarcomas, brain tumors
Topoisomerase I Inhibitors					
Topotecan	IV	1.4–4.5 mg	daily × 5, q 3 wk	M, diarrhea, mucositis, N & V, A, rash, hepatic	neuroblastoma, rhabdomyosarcoma
Irinotecan	IV / IV	50 mg / 125 mg	daily × 5, q 3 wk / weekly × 4 q 6 wk	M, diarrhea, N &V, A, hepatic, dehydration, ileus	rhabdomyosarcoma
Tubulin binders					
Vinca alkaloics⁶					
Vincristine	IV	1.0–1.5 mg (max, 2.0 mg)	weekly × 3–6	NT, A, SIADH, hypotension, vesicant	leukemia (ALL), lymphomas, most solid tumors
Vinblastine	IV	3.5–6.0 mg	weekly × 3–6	M, A, mucositis, mild NT, vesicant	histiocytosis, Hodgkin, testicular
Vinorelbine	IV	30 mg	weekly	M, mild NT, A, vesicant	?
Taxanes⁶					
Docetaxel	IV	100–125 mg	q 3 wk	M, HSR, A, NT, rash, edema, mucositis	?
Paclitaxel	IV	135–250 mg	CI for 3 or 24 h, q 3 wk	M, HSR, A, NT, mucositis, cardiac, EtOH (alcohol) poisoning	?

(continued)

Table 7-2 (continued)

Pharmacologic properties of commonly used anticancer drugs.

Drug	Route*	Dose/m²	Schedule†	Toxicities‡	Antitumor spectrum
MISCELLANEOUS					
Prednisone	PO	40 mg	daily	protean	leukemia, lymphomas
Prednisolone	PO, IV	40 mg	daily	protean	leukemia, lymphomas
Dexamethasone	PO, IV, IM	6 mg	daily	protean	leukemia, lymphomas, brain tumors
Native asparaginase	IV, IM	6000–25,000 IU	3 times per wk	HSR, coagulopathy, pancreatitis, hepatic, NT	leukemia (ALL), lymphoma
PEG-asparaginase	IV, IM	2500 IU	every 1–4 wks	HSR, coagulopathy, pancreatitis, hepatic, NT	leukemia (ALL), lymphoma
Molecularly targeted agents					
All-*trans*-retinoic acid	PO	45 mg	daily for induction daily × 7 days q 28 d for maintenance	retinoic acid syndrome, pseudotumor cerebri, cheilitis, conjunctivitis, dry skin, ↑ triglycerides	acute promyelocytic leukemia
Imatinib mesylate	PO	340 mg	daily	N&V, fatigue, headache, GI, hepatic, M	Ph + CML

*IV, intravenous; Q = every; PO, oral; IM, intramuscular; SC, subcutaneous.

†d, day; wk, week; h, hour; CI, continuous infusion; BMT, bone marrow transplant.

‡M, myelosuppression; N&V, nausea and vomiting; A, alopecia; NT, neurotoxicity; GI, gastrointestinal toxicity; HD, high dose; HSR, hypersensitivity reaction(s).

¹Oxazaphosphorines.

²Prodrug, which requires hepatic biotransformation before expressing alkylating activity.

³Thipopurines.

⁴Prodrugs, which require activation within the target cell for activity.

⁵Anthracyclines.

⁶Plant products.

Adapted from: Balis A, Blaney S, Holcenberg J. General principles of chemotherapy. In: Pizzo P, Poplack D, eds. *Principles and Practice of Pediatric Oncology*. 4th ed. Philadelphia: Lippincott Williams & Wilkins; 2002.

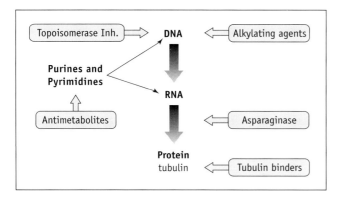

Figure 7-1 Site of action of the commonly used anticancer drugs.

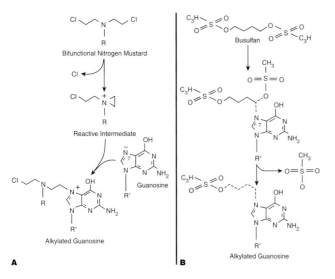

A   **B**

Figure 7-2 Alkylation of DNA: The bifunctional nitrogen mustards illustrate the S_N1 type of alkylation: A reactive intermediate is spontaneously formed that then rapidly reacts with a nucleophilic group (the N^7 position of guanine). Formation of the reactive intermediate is the rate-limiting step, thus the reaction exhibits first-order kinetics. The second bischlorethyl group can react with another nucleobase or protein and a crosslink is formed. Busulfan exemplifies an S_N2 reaction, characterized by a bimolecular displacement. The methyl sulfonate group on either end is displaced by the nucleophilic group on guanine. The reaction follows second-order kinetics because it is dependent on the concentration of alkylating agent and the nucleophile.

Source: Principles and Practice of Pediatric Oncology, Fourth Edition, General Principles of Chemotherapy: Frank Balis, John Holcenberg, Susan Blaney, Lippincott Williams & Wilkins 2002.

reduced folate carrier and undergoes polyglutamation resulting in MTX retention in cells for prolonged periods of time. Methotrexate primarily inhibits dihydrofolate reductase depleting cells of the active (reduced) form of folates, tetrahydrofolate. Methotrexate polyglutamates also inhibit thymidylate synthase and other enzymes involved in the purine biosynthetic pathway.

The topoisomerases are primary targets for a number of agents, including the antitumor antibiotics (anthracyclines, actinomycin) and the epipodophyllotoxins (etoposide and teniposide). Topoisomerases orchestrate the topology of DNA, creating and religating single- (topoiso-

merase I) or double- (topoisomerase II) stranded breaks in the DNA that allow for uncoiling and strand passage. Inhibitors convert topoisomerases into physiologic poisons by blocking religation, resulting in protein-associated DNA strand breaks.[6–8]

Tubulin, the precursor of microtubules, is another major target of cancer chemotherapy. Microtubules are highly dynamic proteins made up of repeating alpha-beta tubulin heterodimers that join end to end into protofilaments. An important role of microtubules is the formation of the mitotic spindle, which is essential for cell replication. Other functions of microtubules include effects on cell support, shape, and structure, and movement of the cell and of organelles within the cell. The vinca alkaloids and taxanes inhibit tubulin by blocking microtubule polymerization and depolymerization, respectively (Figure 7-4).

With a better understanding of the molecular pathogenesis of cancer, the development of more selective and potentially less toxic drugs designed to interfere with critical steps in tumor pathogenesis has become a primary focus of drug development. The first successful example of targeting therapy to the pathogenetic molecular lesion (*molecularly targeted agent*), although discovered empirically, is the use of all-trans retinoic acid for the treatment of acute promyelocytic leukemia (APML).[9] The disease-specific cytogenetic abnormality that characterizes APML is a balanced, reciprocal translocation between chromosomes 15 and 17 (t15;17), resulting in disruption of the promyelocytic (*PML*) gene on chromosome 15 and the retinoic acid receptor-alpha (*RARα*) gene on chromosome 17. This leads to production of the fusion gene *PML-RARα*, and the resulting fusion protein blocks the differentiation of myeloid cells leading to accumulation of abnormal promyelocytes in the bone marrow. This is caused by the association of *PML-RARα* with the nuclear corepressor/histone-deacetylase complex, which blocks the transcription of myeloid differentiation genes. All-trans retinoic acid induces myeloid cell differentiation by binding to *PML-RARα*, producing a dissociation of the nuclear corepressor/histone-deacetylase complex. All-trans retinoic acid has become part of the standard remission induction and maintenance therapy for children and adults with APML.[10]

A more recent and dramatic example is the development of imatinib mesylate (Gleevec, STI-571) for the treatment of Philadelphia chromosome positive (Ph+) chronic myelogenous leukemia (CML).[11,12] Imatinib mesylate is a protein-tyrosine kinase inhibitor that inhibits the Bcr-Abl tyrosine kinase, the constitutive abnormal tyrosine kinase created by the Philadelphia chromosome abnormality in CML. Imatinib is well tolerated when dosed orally daily, has produced hematologic remissions in most patients with Ph+ CML, and is now approved by the Food and Drug Administration for the treatment of Ph+ CML in children and adults. Because the underlying molecular defect for most cancers does not encode for an enzyme (eg, a tyrosine kinase), considerable challenges lie ahead in the development of targeted therapies.

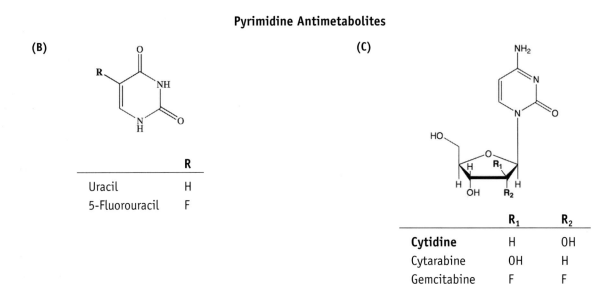

(A)

	R₁	R₂
Folic Acid	OH	H
Methotrexate	NH₂	CH₃

Pyrimidine Antimetabolites

(B)

	R
Uracil	H
5-Fluorouracil	F

(C)

	R₁	R₂
Cytidine	H	OH
Cytarabine	OH	H
Gemcitabine	F	F

Purine Antimetabolites

Thiopurines

(D)

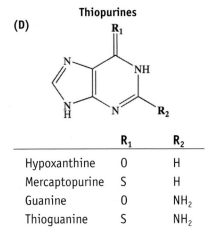

	R₁	R₂
Hypoxanthine	O	H
Mercaptopurine	S	H
Guanine	O	NH₂
Thioguanine	S	NH₂

Figure 7-3 Chemical structures of commonly used antimetabolites compared with structures of corresponding endogenous compounds of which they are analogs: (A) Folate antimetabolites. (B) Pyrimidine antimetabolites with uracil. (C) Pyrimidine antimetabolites with cytidine. (D) Purine antimetabolites-thiopurines.

Source: Principles and Practice of Pediatric Oncology, Fourth Edition, General Principles of Chemotherapy: Frank Balis, John Holcenberg, Susan Blaney, Lippincott Williams and Wilkins 2002.

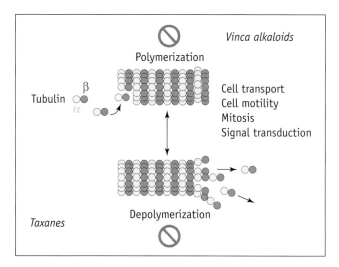

Figure 7-4 Mechanism of action of tubulin-binding agents: Microtubules are made up of repeating alpha-beta tubulin heterodimers that join end to end into protofilaments. Thirteen parallel protofilaments form the microtubule. Microtubules have multiple functions and are essential for survival of all eukaryotic cells. Vinca alkaloids and taxanes block microtubules by opposing mechanisms.

Pharmacokinetics

The discipline of pharmacokinetics deals with the quantitative aspects of drug disposition, including drug absorption, distribution, metabolism (biotransformation), and excretion. Pharmacokinetic parameters are important in determining the proper dose, schedule, and route of administration for these agents (Table 7-3). In addition, knowledge of the route of elimination is required for rational dose adjustments in patients with organ (especially hepatic or renal) dysfunction (Table 7-4).

Pharmacokinetic studies have revealed substantial interpatient variability in drug disposition and systemic drug exposure with most anticancer drugs after intravenous and oral administration.[13] Assuming that the drug effect is most closely related to systemic drug exposure, these differences in drug disposition could account for the variability in toxicities and response noted with most combination chemotherapy regimens employing standardized doses of individual agents.[14] Interpatient variability in drug disposition is further amplified in children. Age-related developmental changes in body composition and excretory organ function, variation in rate of metabolism, and excretion of drug by the kidneys or liver and variation in the extent of drug-protein binding contribute to the variability.[13]

For most anticancer agents therapeutic drug monitoring is not available or practicable, and adjustments in the dose and schedule of chemotherapy needed to achieve this balance must therefore be made empirically. The dose, schedules of administration, toxicities, and spectrum of antitumor activity of commonly used anticancer drugs are shown in Table 7-2.

Table 7-3

Pharmacokinetic terms.

Term	Common Abbreviation	Units	Definition
Clearance	Cl	volume/time (ml/min)	Used to quantify rate of drug elimination, expressed as volume of plasma cleared of drug per unit of time
Half-life	$T_{1/2}$	time (h)	Time required to reduce drug concentration by 50%. Plasma drug disappearance many times has multiple phases (distributive, terminal, or elimination phase)
Area under the curve	AUC	Conc.x time ($\mu M \cdot h$)	Measure of drug exposure; area under the plasma concentration time curve
Volume of distribution	V_d; Vd_{ss}	Volume (L)	Relates plasma concentration to total amount of drug in the body (ie, volume required to dissolve the total amount of drug to give the final concentration found in plasma); a property of the drug rather than a real volume
Bioavailability	F	Fraction (%)	Rate of extent of drug absorption; frequently fraction of dose absorbed when administered by some route other than intravenous
Biotransformation	–	–	Enzymatic metabolism of drug, may result in activation of a prodrug, conversion to other biologically active metabolites, or inactivation of drug

Adapted from: Balis A, Blaney S, Holcenberg J. General principles of chemotherapy. In: Pizzo P, Poplack D, eds. *Principles and Practice of Pediatric Oncology.* 4th ed. Philadelphia: Lippincott Williams & Wilkins; 2002.

Table 7-4

Route of drug elimination for commonly used anticancer drugs.

Alkylating agents:

Nitrogen mustard	Rapid spontaneous chemical decomposition (hydrolysis)
Cyclophosphamide and ifosfamide	Hepatic biotransformation, renal excretion minor route
Cisplatin	Rapid spontaneous decomposition (hydrolysis) and renal excretion
Carboplatin	Renal excretion and spontaneous chemical decomposition
Dacarbazine	Renal excretion (50% of dose) and biotransformation

Antimetabolites:

Methotrexate	Renal excretion; hepatic biotransformation minor route
Mercaptopurine	Hepatic biotransformation (oxidation to thiouric acid by xanthine oxidase)
Cytarabine	Biotransformation (deamination to ara-U by cytidine deaminase)
Fluorouracil	Biotransformation (reduction of the pyrimidine ring followed by ring opening), DPD

Topoisomerase II inhibitors:

Anthracyclines	Hepatic biotransformation and biliary excretion
Dactinomycin	Renal and biliary excretion; biotransformation
Etoposide	Biotransformation and renal excretion (30% to 40%)
Teniposide	Biotransformation and renal excretion (10%)

Tubulin binders:

Vinca alkaloids	Biliary excretion, hepatic biotransformation; renal excretion minor route
Paclitaxel	Hepatic biotransformation

Miscellaneous:

Corticosteroids	Hepatic biotransformation
L-asparaginase	Biotransformation

Absorption

To produce an effect, agents administered orally must first be absorbed into the systemic circulation. Limitations to absorption include degradation of the drug in the intestinal lumen, inability to pass through the gastrointestinal mucosa, and presystemic metabolism in the gastrointestinal epithelium or liver. Only a few anticancer agents are currently administered orally to children. Oral methotrexate and 6-mercaptopurine (6-MP) are the backbone of standard maintenance therapy for childhood ALL. The *bioavailability* of oral methotrexate is highly variable, with 23% to 95% of the dose absorbed.[15] The bioavailability of oral 6-MP is limited because of extensive first-pass (presystemic) metabolism in the liver and gastrointestinal mucosa by the enzyme xanthine oxidase, which converts 6-MP to the inactive metabolite 6-thiouric acid. This results in absorption of less than 20% of the administered 6-MP dose.[15] Corticosteroids are also routinely administered by the oral route in children with ALL, but fortunately prednisone and dexamethasone have near complete bioavailability (>80%).

Oral administration of busulfan is an important component of bone marrow transplant preparative regimens.

Busulfan is rapidly absorbed and has a bioavailability of 70%.[16] Busulfan clearance, however, is more rapid in children than in adults.[17] The reason for this is not lower bioavailability but enhanced glutathione conjugation (primary route of elimination) in enterocytes of young children.[17,18] Busulfan plasma concentrations in the transplant setting have been shown to be predictive for hepatic toxicity and graft rejection, and therapeutic drug monitoring has been successfully used to maintain plasma busulfan levels in a safe and effective range.[19]

Distribution

Distribution of a drug involves its reversible transfer from the circulation to the various tissues, organs, or fluid-containing compartments in the body, as well as to tumor. Direct measurement of drug concentrations in tissues and tumor is usually not feasible in humans and can be estimated only from the rate of plasma drug disappearance using pharmacokinetic modeling.

Following administration of high doses of systemic MTX (>1 g/m^2), retention of MTX in large extravascular fluid collections (pleural fluid, ascites, etc) can result in enhanced toxicity from slow release of drug and prolonged exposure to toxic drug levels.[20] Drainage of the fluid collection and leucovorin rescue guided by measured plasma MTX concentrations help circumvent the risk of excessive toxicities.

Both the anthracyclines and the vinca alkaloids are extensively tissue bound. As a result, following administration the plasma disappearance of drug during the distributive phase is extremely rapid (alpha half-life is <10 minutes). The extensive binding is also responsible for the very large volume of distribution (approximately 1000 L/m²) and the prolonged terminal half-life (approximately 24 hours), resulting from slow release of drug from tissue sites.[21,22]

Metabolism

The most important determinant of variability in anticancer drug pharmacokinetics is the rate of drug metabolism. Drug-metabolizing enzymes are divided into two groups based on the type of reaction they catalyze. Phase I reactions (eg, oxidation, hydrolysis, reduction, and demethylation) introduce or expose a functional group on the drug and usually diminish the drug's pharmacologic activity, but some drugs, such as cyclophosphamide, ifosfamide, and certain antimetabolites, require a metabolic activation step for antitumor activity (Table 7-2). Phase II conjugation reactions covalently link a highly polar conjugate (eg, glucuronic acid, sulfate, glutathione, amino acids, or acetate) to the functional group created by the phase I reaction. The conjugated drugs are highly polar, usually devoid of pharmacologic activity, and rapidly excreted.

The cytochrome P450 (CYP) superfamily of enzymes catalyze oxidation and demethylation reactions for a wide spectrum of drugs and xenobiotics.[23,24] The CYP enzymes have very broad and overlapping substrate specificity and are categorized into families and subfamilies according to their amino acid sequence similarity. CYP3A4 is the most abundant P450 enzyme in the liver and is involved in the metabolism of the largest fraction of drugs. CYP genes are genetically polymorphic, and certain polymorphisms can significantly impact drug metabolism.[25] Pharmacogenetic variation in the level of expression of non-P450 drug-metabolizing enzymes has also been described as an important determinant of toxicity and possible outcome for a number of anticancer drugs including mercaptopurine, fluorouracil, and irinotecan.[26]

The alkylating agents ifosfamide and cyclophosphamide undergo extensive metabolism after their activation by hydroxylation of the 4-carbon position. Although these steps are qualitatively identical, there are quantitative differences. Dechlorethylation, for example, accounts for only 10% of the metabolism of cyclophosphamide, but up to 50% of ifosfamide is dechlorethylated, which results in greater production of the potentially toxic by-product chloracetaldehyde compared with cyclophosphamide.[27]

The antimetabolites are generally metabolized along the same degradative pathways as their endogenous counterparts. Cytarabine is rapidly deaminated to the inactive metabolite uridine arabinoside by the ubiquitous enzyme cytidine deaminase. Similarly, 6-MP and 5-fluorouracil are catabolized through normal purine and pyrimidine degradative pathways to inactive metabolites. 6-MP also undergoes S-methylation catalyzed by thiopurine methyltransferase (TMPT). Thiopurine methyltransferase activity is controlled by a common genetic polymorphism.[28] One in 300 patients has very low TMPT activity and as a result is extremely sensitive to thiopurines (6-MP, thioguanine) in that even a short course of therapy can result in profound myelosuppression.[29] For fluorouracil, inherited partial deficiency of the catabolic enzyme dihydropyrimidine dehydrogenase in 1% to 3% of the population has been associated with severe toxicity.[30]

The primary metabolites of the anthracyclines are the corresponding alcohols (eg, adriamycinol, daunomycinol, idarubicinol),[22] which retain cytotoxic activity to a variable extent. The anthracyclines can undergo chemical reduction through several enzymatically catalyzed pathways or by interaction with oxymyoglobin in the heart, yielding free radical intermediates. Transfer of an electron from these unstable radicals to molecular oxygen yields superoxide radicals that can generate hydrogen peroxide and hydroxyl radicals, which can cause oxidative damage to cellular macromolecules. The anthracyclines can also be conjugated with a sulfate or glucuronide group as a further detoxification step.

The epipodophyllotoxins are also extensively metabolized, and some metabolites retain cytotoxic activity, but the details of the metabolic pathways have not been fully elucidated.[31]

Elimination

Anticancer drugs are eliminated from the body by renal or biliary excretion, by biotransformation to an inactive metabolite, or as a result of spontaneous chemical decomposition (see Table 7-4). The rate of drug elimination (*clearance*) determines the duration of systemic exposure to a drug. Because the cytotoxic effects of these agents are proportional to the duration of systemic exposure, delayed elimination of an anticancer drug can lead to a marked exacerbation of its toxic effects.

Chemically reactive agents like nitrogen mustard are eliminated primarily through spontaneous chemical decomposition to inactive intermediates and are therefore not dependent on normal hepatic or renal function for their elimination.[32,33] Similarly, cisplatin in its active, unbound form also undergoes aquation followed by formation of covalent bonds to plasma or tissue proteins.[34] Once bound to proteins, the drug is inactive. The active platinum species are also excreted by the kidneys, and approximately 25% of the dose is eliminated by this route. The cisplatin dose is routinely modified in patients with renal dysfunction, in part because cisplatin is nephrotoxic and renal function could be further impaired.

High-dose MTX infusions (≥1 g/m² with leucovorin rescue) are used in the treatment of ALL, lymphoma, and osteosarcoma.[20,35] Pharmacokinetic drug monitoring is a routine component of high-dose MTX regimens. Methotrexate is excreted primarily by the kidneys (70% to 90% of the dose), undergoing glomerular filtration and both tubular secretion and reabsorption. In patients with renal dysfunction, MTX clearance is delayed, which can result in significant and potentially life-threatening toxicities even after a relatively low dose of the drug. Serum creatinine or creatinine clearance should be measured before administration of high doses of MTX to ensure adequate renal function, and serum MTX concentration and renal function should be monitored during and after the dose because high doses of MTX can be nephrotoxic. In patients with delayed drug clearance, leucovorin rescue should be promptly adjusted based on plasma MTX concentrations and continued until the plasma MTX concentration falls below 0.05 μmol/L. In patients with known renal dysfunction, the use of MTX should be avoided.

The anthracyclines are eliminated primarily by hepatic biotransformation and biliary excretion, and delayed clearance of adriamycin and enhanced toxicity was observed in early studies of both adults and children with hepatic dysfunction.[22] Current recommendation is that dose reduction be performed in patients with multiple liver-function test abnormalities or direct bilirubin elevations greater than 2.0 mg/dl.

The closely related epipodophyllotoxin analogs etoposide and teniposide are both extensively metabolized, but renal excretion accounts for 30% to 40% of the total systemic clearance of etoposide, but only 10% of teniposide clearance. This difference probably reflects the difference in the degree of protein binding of the two drugs (95% for etoposide, >99% for teniposide).[31] It is therefore recommended that etoposide doses should be reduced in patients with renal dysfunction, but dose modification may not be necessary in those with abnormal liver function tests.

Toxicity of Anticancer Drugs

The mechanism of action of anticancer drugs is not selective to cancer cells. In general, actively dividing normal host tissues such as hematopoietic precursors, mucosal epithelial cells, and hair follicle cells are the most susceptible to toxic effects of chemotherapy,[36] and pediatric oncologists spend considerable effort in managing these toxicities.

Toxicities are categorized according to the time of onset after therapy and their reversibility. They are quantified using grading systems such as the World Health Organization's or the National Cancer Institute's Common Toxicity Criteria. *Acute* side effects occur in the immediate post therapy period (within days to weeks) and are usually reversible, while *long-term* toxicities may have a delayed onset or are irreversible. A number of acute toxicities are common to most of the anticancer drugs including myelosuppression, nausea and vomiting, oro-intestinal mucositis, and hepatotoxicity. In addition, many drugs have unique acute or long-term toxicities (Table 7-5, Table 7-2).

Some *common acute toxicities* such as nausea and vomiting and alopecia occur frequently but are generally not *dose limiting*. However, they can cause significant discomfort or have emotional impact. Hepatic toxicity, usually in the form of elevations in liver function tests, also occurs commonly but tends to be rapidly reversible with most agents and usually does not lead to dose modifications.

Myelosuppression is the most common *dose-limiting toxicity* of anticancer agents. Depression of the white cell count, specifically the granulocyte count with a nadir at 10 to 14 days after chemotherapy, markedly increases the risk of life-threatening infections. Thrombocytopenia and anemia are usually less severe and can be corrected with transfusions or with administration of erythropoietin (anemia). Filgrastim (granulocyte colony-stimulating factor), a glycoprotein hormone, stimulates proliferation of bone marrow progenitor cells and enhances the production and differentiation of neutrophil precursors. Filgrastim has been approved for use in chemotherapy-induced neutropenia, and when administered immediately following a course of myelosuppressive chemotherapy, it shortens the duration of severe neutropenia.[37]

Considerable effort has been devoted to developing agents that can attenuate toxicities of anticancer drugs.[33,38] These rescue agents have improved the safety of therapy and alleviated drug-related symptoms, and have also been used to further intensify the dosing of anticancer agents. Examples of some successful methods to alleviate toxicity without interfering with the anticancer effects of drugs are shown in Table 7-6.

Unique toxicities of anticancer agents include cyclophosphamide- and ifosfamide-induced *hemorrhagic cystitis* (incidence 5% to 10% for cyclophsophamide, 20% to 40% for ifosfamide), caused by the exposure of the bladder wall to active metabolites concentrated in the urine.[33] Mesna^2-mercaptoethane sulfonate, a sulfhydryl scavenging agent, can react with and rapidly inactivate these metabolites.[39] When administered intravenously, mesna is rapidly auto-oxidized to dimesna in plasma and circulates in this inactive form. Therefore, mesna does not inhibit the antitumor effect of the oxazaphosphorines. Mesna is rapidly eliminated by the kidney, and as it passes through the renal tubule it is converted back to its active, free-sulfhydryl form. It thus exists in the active form only at the site of action—in the urine.

Nephrotoxicity: Oxazaphosphorines are nephrotoxic, and with increasing cumulative doses, ifosfamide is associated with proximal renal tubular dysfunction, resembling Fanconi syndrome, which can lead to rickets in young children.[40] Cumulative renal toxicity (decreased glomerular filtration rate and electrolyte disturbances) is a common toxicity of cisplatin.[34] Hydration, hypertonic saline, and amifostine have been used to lessen these toxicities. Methotrexate nephrotoxicity infrequently occurs with high-dose therapy ($\geq$1 g/m^2) and is caused either by precipitation of MTX and its metabolite, 7-hydroxymethotrexate, in acidic urine or by direct toxic effects of the drug on the renal tubule.[20] Vigorous intravenous hydration and alkalinization of the urine are used routinely to prevent drug precipitation. Delayed MTX excretion can

Table 7-5

Toxicities of commonly used anticancer drugs.

Acute Toxicities	
Toxicity	**Chemotherapy Drug**
Cardiotoxicity	Anthracyclines
Hemorrhagic cystitis	Ozazaphosphorines
Fanconi syndrome	Ifosfamide
Peripheral neuropathy	Vinca alkaloids, cisplatin
Coagulopathy	Asparaginase
Ototoxicity	Cisplatin
Nephrotoxicity	Methotrexate, cisplatin
Leukencephalopathy	Methotrexate
Vesicant	Nitrogen mustard, anthracyclines, dactinomycin, vinca alkaloids

Long-Term Toxicities	
Toxicity	**Chemotherapy Drug**
Avascular necrosis	Steroids
Azoospermia, amenorrhea, infertility	Cyclophosphamide, nitrosoureas, procarbazine
Cardiomyopathy	Anthracyclines, cyclophosphamide, dacarbazine, actinomycin, bleomycin
Pulmonary fibrosis	BCNU, cyclophosphamide, melphalan, busulfan, bleomycin
Second malignancies	Cyclophosphamide, nitrosoureas, etoposide
Hepatitis or fibrosis	Methotrexate
Osteoporosis	Steroids

Table 7-6

Agents commonly used to attenuate toxicity of anticancer agents.

Toxicity	Rescue Agent
Myelosuppression	Cytokines: filgrastim, peg-filgrastim Bone marrow or stem cell reinfusion Erythropoietin
Nausea and vomiting	Antiemetics
Hemorrhagic cystitis	Mesna
Nephrotoxicity	Amifostine, chlorouresis
Cardiotoxicity	Dexrazoxane
Myelosuppression/mucositis (methotrexate)	Leucovorin, carboxypeptidase-G_2

markedly enhance the drug's other toxicities, and a prompt increase in the dose of the rescue agent leucovorin in proportion to plasma MTX concentrations is critical to ameliorate MTX associated toxicities.[35] Carboxypeptidase-G_2 is a recombinant bacterial enzyme that rapidly hydrolyzes MTX to inactive metabolites.[41]

Cardiac toxicity: The anthracyclines can produce both acute and chronic cumulative cardiac toxicity.[22] The acute form is characterized by arrhythmias, conduction abnor-malities, and an acute drop in left ventricular function. In general, the acute asymptomatic cardiac effects are transient and do not prevent the further use of anthracyclines.

The more characteristic cardiomyopathy from anthracyclines is related to the cumulative dose of the drug. The incidence of congestive heart failure rises sharply at cumulative doses greater than 550 mg/m², but more sensitive measures of cardiac function demonstrate that myocardial damage accumulates steadily with the dose.

Myocardial damage may be the result of anthracycline-induced free radical formation within the myocardial cell. The risk of an anthracycline-induced cardiomyopathy is increased in patients who have received prior or concurrent mediastinal irradiation, in patients receiving concomitant cyclophosphamide or mitomycin C, in children, especially those under 5 years of age, and in patients receiving a high anthracycline dose rate (more than 50 mg/m² per dose). Careful monitoring of cardiac function in patients receiving anthracyclines with echocardiogram or radionuclide cineangiography is imperative. Measures used to circumvent the cardiomyopathy include limiting the total cumulative lifetime dose of anthracycline to less than 450 mg/m² (even lower in patients receiving mediastinal radiation), administration of doxorubicin by prolonged (not bolus) intravenous infusion, developing less-cardiotoxic anthracycline derivatives, and the development of compounds that block the effects of anthracyclines on the heart. The most promising cardioprotective drug is the chelating agent dexrazoxane. Intracellularly, dexrazoxane is hydrolyzed to a compound that resembles ethylenediaminetetraacetic acid and acts as an iron chelator.[22] By depleting intracellular iron pools, dexrazoxane lowers the risk of cumulative cardiotoxicity caused by the anthracyclines in adults[42] and children.[43,44]

Neurologic toxicity: A wide range of neurologic complications are associated with administration of chemotherapy.[45] Because neurotoxicity can be cumulative with no rescue agents available, regular clinical observations are important to detect onset of toxicity. Peripheral sensory and motor neuropathy is the dose-limiting toxicity for vincristine.[21] Manifestations include loss of deep tendon reflexes, neuritic pain (muscular cramping and jaw pain), paresthesias, wrist and foot drop, and paralytic ileus or urinary retention. Cisplatin also causes a cumulative symmetrical neuropathy and cumulative high-frequency hearing loss.

High-dose cytarabine 3 g/m², when administered on a protracted schedule (every 12 hours for 12 doses), can cause severe cerebellar dysfunction in up to 20% of patients.[46] Early symptoms include ataxia, dysarthria, nystagmus, and somnolence with progression to dementia and coma. Cytarabine administration should be immediately withdrawn with evidence of nystagmus or ataxia. Limiting administration to 4 doses significantly decreases the risk of developing cerebellar toxicity.

Methotrexate neurotoxicity can be acute (lethargy, disorientation, seizures), subacute (transient stroke-like syndrome with hemiparesis, aphasia, dysarthria, seizures, and altered consciousness), or delayed (leukoencephalopathy), which is characterized by progressive dementia, spasticity, seizures, and coma.[20] The risk of leukoencephalopathy is greater in patients who received cranial radiation. Ifosfamide-induced neurotoxicity includes somnolence, mental status changes, motor disturbance, and seizures.[33] This toxicity has been attributed to the formation of the toxic metabolite chloracetaldehyde and is many times reversible.

Extravasation of anticancer drugs that are vesicants (Table 7-5) into subcutaneous tissue or dermis can result in severe local tissue damage and deep ulcerations, heal very slowly, and are difficult to skin graft. Ice packs, local injection of corticosteroids, and sodium bicarbonate may ameliorate this tissue damage, but careful administration of these agents is the best preventive measure.

Long-Term Toxicity

The long-term adverse effects of cancer chemotherapy on growth, development, neurologic, neuropsychological, and reproductive function, as well as possible permanent organ damage and carcinogenic and teratogenic effects are of particular concern in children because of the high cure rates and the long life spans of successfully treated patients (Table 7-5). Consequently, careful long-term clinical evaluation for these effects is critically important for childhood cancer survivors.[47]

Gonadal toxicity: Azoospermia is a common acute toxicity in male patients of all ages, but recovery has been observed with long-term follow-up, especially in those treated when they were prepubertal. Patients treated during puberty or as adults who received high cumulative doses of alkylating agents (>10 grams of cyclophosphamide) appear to be at greatest risk of being infertile. Ovarian function may also be affected by cytotoxic chemotherapy, and, as in males, alkylating agents appear to be the most toxic. Combination chemotherapy can result in amenorrhea in patients treated after menarche, but menses usually return following the completion of therapy. Although current evidence suggests that alkylating agents are primarily responsible for gonadal toxicity in patients treated with combination chemotherapy, adriamycin, procarbazine, cytarabine, and vinblastine have also been implicated.

Carcinogenesis: There is an increased incidence of second tumors, primarily leukemia, in long-term survivors of cancer who have been treated with chemotherapy.[48] Clinical or experimental evidence has implicated the alkylating agents and the antitumor antibiotics as potent carcinogens, presumably related to their mutagenic capabilities. A distinctive form of secondary leukemia, characterized by a short latency period (median time to presentation 30 months), chromosomal translocation involving chromosome band 11q23, and M4 or M5 FAB morphologic subtype, occurs in patients receiving epidophyllotoxins.[49] The risk of secondary tumors increases with the use of radiation therapy.

Anticancer Drug Resistance

Drug resistance is the primary cause of treatment failure in the childhood cancers. The development of most forms of drug resistance has a genetic basis. The genetic instabil-

Table 7-7

Mechanisms of drug resistance.

Mechanisms	Examples	Drug Affected
Drug-specific mechanisms		
↓* Drug uptake into cells	↓ Folic acid transporter	Methotrexate
↓ Drug activation	↓ Deoxycytidine kinase	Cytarabine
↑* Drug catabolism	↑ Aldehyde oxidase	Cyclophosphamide metabolites metabolites
↑ Altered affinity of target	Tubulin alteration	Vincristine/taxanes
↑ Competitive substrates	↑ Dihydrofolate reductase	Methotrexate
	↑ Asparagine synthase	L-asparaginase
Multidrug resistance mechanisms		
↓ Drug accumulation	↑ P-glycoprotein (*mdr*)	Natural products
↑ Drug detoxification	↑ Glutathione transferase	Alkylating agents
or altered affinity of target	Topoisomerases	Topo I and II inhibitors
↑ DNA repair	↑ AGT	Alkylating agents
↓ Apoptosis	↑ Blc-2 expression	All classes of agents

*↓ = decreased; ↑ = increased (compared with normal cells).

Adapted from: Balis A, Blaney S, Holcenberg J. General principles of chemotherapy. In: Pizzo P, Poplack D, eds. *Principles and Practice of Pediatric Oncology*. 4th ed. Philadelphia: Lippincott Williams & Wilkins; 2002

ity of tumor cells results in spontaneous generation of drug-resistant clones as a consequence of mutation, deletion, gene amplification, translocation, or chromosomal rearrangement.[50] Genetically based or biochemical changes in cancer cells can produce anticancer drug resistance that is specific to a single agent or a class of agents, or provides protection from a broad range of anticancer drugs. The latter form of resistance is termed *multidrug resistance* (MDR) (Table 7-7). The best-studied example of MDR is associated with decreased intracellular drug accumulation and an increase in a plasma membrane, adenosine triphosphate-dependent drug efflux pump, such as P-glycoprotein (P-gp), or the family of multidrug resistance proteins.[51,52] P-gp and the mdr-1 gene that encodes for it are expressed in a variety of human tumor tissues, but also in normal human tissues, and P-gp appears to be responsible for excretion of toxic compounds from these normal cells. This example of MDR includes a group of drugs, which are primarily natural products, including the anthracyclines, vinca alkaloids, dactinomycin, and the epipodophyllotoxins. P-gp expression in some tumors has been associated with worse outcome, and multiple research efforts have been undertaken to develop agents capable of reversing multidrug resistance caused by P-gp. Although initially tested agents proved too toxic and nonspecific, more recently tumor-specific, potent, and nontoxic inhibitors of P-gp have been developed.[52] These agents are currently undergoing testing in early clinical trials and may allow to test the potential benefit of these agents in outcome for patients with P-gp expressing tumors.

Drug Interactions

In addition to being administered in combination regimens, anticancer drugs are also administered with multiple agents used to alleviate the side effects of chemotherapy or the underlying cancer, introducing a significant risk of drug interactions. Little information is available concerning drug interactions involving the anticancer drugs either with each other or with other classes of drugs, and as routine therapeutic drug monitoring of anticancer drugs is not performed, possible drug interactions may not be recognized.

A classic example of a drug interaction in cancer therapy is the interaction between 6-MP, an analog of hypoxanthine, and allopurinol, an inhibitor of xanthine oxidase. When mercaptopurine is coadministered with allopurinol, the fraction of the dose absorbed increases 5-fold.[53] Therefore, an oral dose of 6-MP should be reduced by 75% when administered concurrently with allopurinol.

Methotrexate is eliminated by tubular excretion and glomerular filtration. Thus, coadministration of drugs that compete for tubular secretion, such as salicylates, penicillin, or nonsteroidal anti-inflammatory drugs, can enhance MTX toxicity by competitively inhibiting its secretion. In addition, nephrotoxic drugs, like cisplatin or the aminoglycosides, can also indirectly delay MTX excretion by impairing renal function.

Many drugs that are administered concomitantly with chemotherapy may have an effect on drug clearance through induction or inhibition of drug-metabolizing enzymes, particularly those in the P-450 system. For example, phenytoin and phenobarbital induce these enzymes, resulting in increased clearance and decreased exposure to chemotherapeutic agents administered at "standard doses."

Interactions between certain anticancer drugs—for example, adriamycin, dactinomycin, or vincristine—and radiation therapy can increase the risk and severity of toxicities from either modality.

Central Nervous System Pharmacology

Brain tumors are the most common type of solid tumors in children, and the meninges are common sites of metastatic spread for pediatric malignancies, such as ALL and the non-Hodgkin lymphomas. The blood-brain barrier limits the central nervous system (CNS) penetration of most systemically administered anticancer drugs and provides a pharmacologic sanctuary for these tumors. Most anticancer drugs penetrate poorly into the cerebrospinal fluid (CSF) (Table 7-8). The most common pharmacologic approaches utilized to overcome poor CNS penetration include intrathecal chemotherapy and administration of high doses of systemic chemotherapy.

Intrathecal chemotherapy is used primarily for prevention and treatment of meningeal leukemia and lymphoma. Very high drug concentrations can be achieved in the CSF and meninges with small intrathecal drug doses and minimal systemic drug exposure and toxicity.

Limitations to intrathecal chemotherapy include nonuniform drug distribution, limited number of agents available for intrathecal injection (methotrexate, cytarabine, thiotepa), local neurotoxicities such as arachnoidi-

Table 7-8

Cerebrospinal fluid penetration of commonly used anticancer agents.

Drug	CSF:Plasma (%)
Cyclophosphamide	15 (active 4-OH-CP)
Ifosfamide	15 (active 4-OH-IF)
Thiotepa	>95
Temozolomide	30
Cisplatin	7
Carboplatin	30
Methotrexate	1–3
Mercaptoputine	25
Cytarabine	20–40
Doxorubicin	<5
Vincristine	<5
Etoposide	<10
Topotecan	30

tis, procedural pain, and inconvenience. For example, drug exposure in the ventricle following an intralumbar dose of methotrexate is only 10% of that in the lumbar CSF. In addition, 10% of intralumbar injections are ineffective because of leakage of the drug into the epidural space or surrounding tissues.[54] Direct intraventricular administration of chemotherapy after surgical implantation of a subcutaneous Ommaya reservoir is less painful, allows for better drug distribution, and permits more frequent injections of smaller doses of chemotherapy, resulting in greater drug exposure with smaller peak CSF concentrations, and thus less toxicity and enhanced efficacy.[55,56] Intrathecal MTX is a mainstay in the treatment and prevention of meningeal leukemia and lymphoma. The dose of intrathecal MTX is not based on the body surface area because of the poor correlation between CNS extracellular fluid volume and body surface area. Instead, a pharmacokinetically derived dosing schedule based on age is used, and it has been demonstrated to be less neurotoxic and more efficacious.[57]

Neurotoxicity from intrathecal MTX includes acute chemical arachnoiditis, characterized by headache, nuchal rigidity, vomiting, fever, and CSF pleocytosis. A subacute encephalopathy, which may present with paresis of the extremities, cranial nerve palsies, ataxia, visual impairment, seizures, and even coma, has been associated with elevated CSF drug levels. Necrotizing leukoencephalopathy, presenting in the form of progressive dementia, spastic paralysis, seizures, and coma, appears months to years following intrathecal MTX and has been associated with large, cumulative doses of both intrathecal MTX and cranial radiation.

The inadvertent administration of excessive intrathecal doses of MTX (≥ 100 mg) can produce fatal reactions.[58] Treatment includes immediate CSF drainage and ventriculolumbar perfusion.[59] Intrathecal instillation of carboxypeptidase-G_2, which rapidly hydrolyzes MTX to inactive metabolites, is available on an investigational basis.[60]

Intrathecal cytarabine is also effective in the treatment and prevention of meningeal leukemia and is often administered in combination with MTX and hydrocortisone ("triple intrathecal chemotherapy"). Intrathecal cytarabine may be associated with chemical arachnoiditis, similar to that observed with MTX. Seizures and transient paraplegia have also been reported.

High-dose systemic chemotherapy. Limited CNS penetration of some systemically administered agents can be overcome by administering high doses of these drugs systemically. In addition, when administered by continuous intravenous infusion, CSF drug levels can be maintained for a prolonged period. This approach has been used successfully with MTX and cytarabine. Administration of high doses of MTX (≥ 5 g/m^2) followed by leucovorin rescue can produce therapeutic concentrations of MTX within the CSF, despite the fact that the CSF-to-plasma ratio of MTX is only 3%. This strategy has been used successfully in the prevention and treatment of meningeal leukemia. High-dose intravenous cytarabine (3 gm/m^2

dose every 12 hours) has also produced remissions in patients with overt meningeal leukemia. In contrast to high-dose MTX, this approach is associated with significant systemic toxicity (myelosuppression), which limits its applicability.

Future Perspectives

Despite the advances made in the treatment of childhood cancer, approximately 1 of every 5 children continues to die from their disease. Moreover, all children endure varying degrees of acute and sometimes chronic toxicities. Reasons for treatment failures include de novo or acquired drug resistance, inadequate drug delivery, and administration of the wrong agent or the wrong dose. An increased understanding of the pharmacologic basis for treatment failure may ultimately improve therapy. Identification of the mechanisms of drug resistance at a molecular level may lead to the development of effective reversal agents. Optimizing the dosing of anticancer drugs based on patient-specific characteristics (adaptive dosing) and on measured plasma drug concentrations (therapeutic drug monitoring) may result in improved safety and effectiveness. Finally, with a greater understanding of the molecular pathogenesis of malignant transformation, the development of more-selective (targeted) and less-toxic cancer agents is becoming a primary focus of anticancer drug development.

References

1. Balis F, Holcenberg J, Blaney S. General principles of chemotherapy. In: Pizzo P, Poplack D, eds. Principles and Practice of Pediatric Oncology. Philadelphia, PA: Lippincott Williams & Wilkins; 2002:237–308.
2. Poplack DG, Reaman G. Acute lymphoblastic leukemia in childhood. Pediatr Clin North Am. 1988;35(4):903–932.
3. Berg SL, Grisell DL, DeLaney TF, Balis FM. Principles of treatment of pediatric solid tumors. Pediatr Clin North Am. 1991;38(2):249–267.
4. Dawson JW, Taylor I. Principles of adjuvant therapy. Br J Hosp Med. 1995;54(6):249–254.
5. Goorin AM, Schwartzentruber DJ, Devidas M, et al. Presurgical chemotherapy compared with immediate surgery and adjuvant chemotherapy for nonmetastatic osteosarcoma: Pediatric Oncology Group Study POG-8651. J Clin Oncol. 2003;21(8):1574–1580.
6. Bomgaars L, Berg SL, Blaney SM. The development of camptothecin analogs in childhood cancers. Oncologist. 2001;6(6):506–516.
7. Takimoto C, Arbuck S. Topoisomerase I targeting agents: the camptothecins. In: Chabner B, Longo D, eds. Cancer Chemotherapy and Biotherapy. Philadelphia, PA: Lippincott Williams & Wilkins. 2001;579–646.
8. Pommier Y, Goldwasser F, Strumberg D. Topoisomerase II inhibitors: epidophyllotoxins, acridines, ellipticines, and bisdioxopiperazines. In: Chabner B, Longo D, eds. Cancer Chemotherapy and Biotherapy. Philadelphia, PA: Lippincott Williams & Wilkins. 2001:538–578.
9. Tallman MS. Acute promyelocytic leukemia as a paradigm for targeted therapy. Semin Hematol. 2004;41(2)(suppl 4):27–32.
10. de Botton S, Coiteux V, Chevret S, Rayon C, Vilmer E, Sanz M, et al. Outcome of childhood acute promyelocytic leukemia with all-trans-retinoic acid and chemotherapy. J Clin Oncol. 2004;22(8):1404–1412.
11. Druker BJ. Imatinib as a paradigm of targeted therapies. Adv Cancer Res. 2004;91:1–30.
12. Champagne MA, Capdeville R, Krailo M, et al. Imatinib mesylate (STI571) for treatment of children with Philadelphia chromosome-positive leukemia: results from a Children's Oncology Group Phase I study. Blood. 2004;104(9):2655–2660.
13. Chabot GG. Factors involved in clinical pharmacology variability in oncology [review]. Anticancer Res. 1994;14(6A):2269–2272.
14. Kobayashi K, Ratain MJ. Individualizing dosing of cancer chemotherapy. Semin Oncol. 1993;20(1):30–42.
15. Balis FM, Holcenberg JS, Poplack DG, et al. Pharmacokinetics and pharmacodynamics of oral methotrexate and mercaptopurine in children with lower risk acute lymphoblastic leukemia: a joint Children's Cancer Group and Pediatric Oncology branch study. Blood. 1998;92(10):3569–3577.
16. Hassan M, Ljungman P, Bolme P, et al. Busulfan bioavailability. Blood. 1994;84(7):2144–2150.
17. Gibbs JP, Murray G, Risler L, Chien JY, Dev R, Slattery JT. Age-dependent tetrahydrothiophenium ion formation in young children and adults receiving high-dose busulfan. Cancer Res. 1997;57(24):5509–5516.
18. Gibbs JP, Liacouras CA, Baldassano RN, Slattery JT. Up-regulation of glutathione S-transferase activity in enterocytes of young children. Drug Metab Dispos. 1999;27(12):1466–1469.
19. Slattery JT, Risler LJ. Therapeutic monitoring of busulfan in hematopoietic stem cell transplantation. Ther Drug Monit. 1998;20(5):543–549.
20. Messmann R, Allegra C. Antifolates. In: Chabner B, Longo D, eds. Cancer Chemotherapy and Biotherapy. Philadelphia, PA: Lippincott Williams & Wilkins. 2001:139–184.
21. Leveque D, Jehl F, Montail H. Vinblastine, vincristine and vinorelbine. In: Grochow L, Ames M, eds. A Clinician's Guide to Chemotherapy, Pharmacokinetics, and Pharmacodynamics. Baltimore, MD: Williams & Wilkins. 1998:459–470.
22. Doroshow J. Anthracyclines and anthracenediones. In: Chabner B, Longo D, eds. Cancer Chemotherapy and Biotherapy. Philadelphia, PA: Lippincott Williams & Wilkins. 2001:500–537.
23. Oesterheld JR. A review of developmental aspects of cytochrome P450. J Child Adolesc Psychopharmacol. 1998;8(3):161–174.
24. Glue P, Clement RP. Cytochrome P450 enzymes and drug metabolism—basic concepts and methods of assessment. Cell Mol Neurobiol. 1999;19(3):309–323.
25. van der Weide J, Steijns LS. Cytochrome P450 enzyme system: genetic polymorphisms and impact on clinical pharmacology. Ann Clin Biochem. 1999;36(Pt 6):722–729.
26. Innocenti F, Ratain MJ. Update on pharmacogenetics in cancer chemotherapy. Eur J Cancer. 2002;38(5):639–644.
27. Fleming RA. An overview of cyclophosphamide and ifosfamide pharmacology. Pharmacotherapy. 1997;17(5)(Pt 2):146S–154S.
28. Lennard L, Lilleyman JS, Van Loon J, Weinshilboum RM. Genetic variation in response to 6-mercaptopurine for childhood acute lymphoblastic leukaemia. Lancet. 1990;336(8709):225–259.
29. Relling MV, Hancock ML, Rivera GK, et al. Mercaptopurine therapy intolerance and heterozygosity at the thiopurine S-methyltransferase gene locus. J Natl Cancer Inst. 1999;91(23):2001–2008.
30. Johnson MR, Diasio RB. Importance of dihydropyrimidine dehydrogenase (DPD) deficiency in patients exhibiting toxicity following treatment with 5-fluorouracil. Adv Enzyme Regul. 2001;41:151–157.
31. McLeod H, Evans W. Epidophyllotoxins. In: Grochow L, Ames M, eds. A Clinician's Guide to Chemotherapy, Pharmacokinetics, and Pharmacodynamics. Baltimore, MD: Williams & Wilkins. 1998:259–287.
32. Friedman H, Averbuch S, Kurtzberg J. Nonclassical alkylating agents. In: Chabner B, Longo D, eds. Cancer Chemotherapy and Biotherapy. Philadelphia, PA: Lippincott Williams & Wilkins. 2001:415–446.
33. Tew K, Colvin M, Chaner B. Alkylating agents. In: Chabner B, Longo D, eds. Cancer Chemotherapy and Biotherapy. Philadelphia, PA: Lippincott Williams & Wilkins. 2001:373–415.
34. Reed E. Cisplatin and analogs. In: Chabner B, Longo DL, eds. Cancer Chemotherapy and Biotherapy. Philadelphia, PA: Lippincott Williams & Wilkins. 2001:447–465.
35. Bleyer W. The clinical pharmacology of methotrexate. Cancer Res. 1978;41:36–51.
36. Lowenthal RM, Eaton K. Toxicity of chemotherapy. Hematol Oncol Clin North Am. 1996;10(4):967–990.
37. Ozer H, Armitage JO, Bennett CL, et al. 2000 update of recommendations for the use of hematopoietic colony-stimulating factors: evidence-based, clinical practice guidelines. American Society of Clinical Oncology Growth Factors Expert Panel. J Clin Oncol. 2000;18(20):3558–3585.
38. Zagonel V, Rupolo M, Pinto A. Active protection from chemotherapy toxicity. Crit Rev Oncol Hematol. 1998;27(2):125–127.
39. Links M, Lewis C. Chemoprotectants: a review of their clinical pharmacology and therapeutic efficacy. Drugs. 1999;57(3):293–308.
40. Skinner R, Pearson AD, English MW, et al. Risk factors for ifosfamide nephrotoxicity in children. Lancet. 1996;348(9027):578–580.
41. Widemann BC, Balis FM, Murphy RF, et al. Carboxypeptidase-G2, thymidine, and leucovorin rescue in cancer patients with methotrexate-induced renal dysfunction. J Clin Oncol. 1997;15(5):2125–2134.
42. Speyer JL, Green MD, Kramer E, et al. Protective effect of the bispiperazinedione ICRF-187 against doxorubicin-induced cardiac toxicity in women with advanced breast cancer. N Engl J Med. 1988;319(12):745–752.
43. Wexler LH. Ameliorating anthracycline cardiotoxicity in children with cancer: clinical trials with dexrazoxane. Semin Oncol. 1998;25(4)(suppl 10):86–92.
44. Lipshultz SE, Rifai N, Dalton VM, et al. The effect of dexrazoxane on myocardial injury in doxorubicin-treated children with acute lymphoblastic leukemia. N Engl J Med. 2004;351(2):145–153.
45. Tuxen MK, Hansen SW. Neurotoxicity secondary to antineoplastic drugs. Cancer Treat Rev. 1994;20(2):191–214.
46. Garcia-Carbonero R, Ryan D, Chabner B. Cytidine analogs. In: Chabner B, Longo D, eds. Cancer Chemotherapy and Biotherapy. Philadelphia, PA: Lippincott Williams & Wilkins. 2001:265–294.

47. Dreyer Z, Blatt J, Bleyer A. Late effects of childhood cancer and its treatment. In: Pizzo P, Poplack D, eds. *Principles and Practice of Pediatric Oncology.* Philadelphia, PA: Lippincott Williams & Wilkins; 2002:1431–1461.
48. Neglia JP, Friedman DL, Yasui Y, et al. Second malignant neoplasms in five-year survivors of childhood cancer: childhood cancer survivor study. *J Natl Cancer Inst.* 2001;93(8):618–629.
49. Smith MA, Rubinstein L, Ungerleider RS. Therapy-related acute myeloid leukemia following treatment with epipodophyllotoxins: estimating the risks. *Med Pediatr Oncol.* 1994;23(2):86–98.
50. Goldie J. Drug resistance in cancer: a perspective. *Cancer Metastasis Rev.* 2001;20(1–2):63–68.
51. Bradshaw D, Arceci R. Clinical relevance of transmembrane drug efflux as a mechanism of multidrug resistance. *J Clin Oncol.* 1998;16:3674–3690.
52. Gottesman M, Fojo T, Bates S. Multidrug resistance in cancer: role of ATP-dependent transporters. *Nature Rev.* 2002;2:48–58.
53. Zimm S, Collins JM, O'Neill D, Chabner BA, Poplack DG. Inhibition of first-pass metabolism in cancer chemotherapy: interaction of 6-mercaptopurine and allopurinol. *Clin Pharmacol Ther.* 1983;34(6):810–817.
54. Shapiro WR, Young DF, Mehta BM. Methotrexate: distribution in cerebrospinal fluid after intravenous, ventricular and lumbar injections. *N Engl J Med.* 1975;293(4):161–166.
55. Bleyer WA, Poplack DG. Intraventricular versus intralumbar methotrexate for central-nervous-system leukemia: prolonged remission with the Ommaya reservoir. *Med Pediatr Oncol.* 1979;6(3):207–213.
56. Moser AM, Adamson PC, Gillespie AJ, Poplack DG, Balis FM. Intraventricular concentration times time (C × T) methotrexate and cytarabine for patients with recurrent meningeal leukemia and lymphoma. *Cancer.* 1999;85(2):511–516.
57. Bleyer WA, Coccia PF, Sather HN, et al. Reduction in central nervous system leukemia with a pharmacokinetically derived intrathecal methotrexate dosage regimen. *J Clin Oncol.* 1983;1(5):317–325.
58. Ettinger LJ. Pharmacokinetics and biochemical effects of a fatal intrathecal methotrexate overdose. *Cancer.* 1982;50(3):444–450.
59. Poplack DG. Massive intrathecal overdose: "check the label twice!" *N Engl J Med.* 1984;311(6):400–402.
60. Widemann BC, Balis FM, Shalabi A, et al. Treatment of accidental intrathecal methotrexate overdose with intrathecal carboxypeptidase G2. *J Natl Cancer Inst.* 2004;96(20):1557–1559.

The Surgical Management of Pediatric Tumors

Michael P. LaQuaglia

Introduction

Each pediatric solid tumor is an entity unto itself with differing genetics, biology, anatomic location of the primary site and sites of metastases, staging, treatment, and prognosis. Because of this disparity, it is impossible to cite a broad overall surgical approach except to say that most nonhematopoietic solid tumors should be removed with certain important exceptions like rhabdomyosarcoma of the genitourinary system in small infants and toddlers. Therefore, this chapter is divided into sections based on the histopathology of the primary tumor and describes the initial approach to biopsy, surgical elements of staging, and the performance of definitive resection of the primary tumor. There is also a brief commentary on the role of metastatectomy in each section. The surgical principles guiding operative intervention for each system are enumerated in the beginning of the section.

Vascular Access

Surgical Principles:

1. Vascular access devices should provide safe and easy infusion of chemotherapeutic agents, blood products, antibiotics, parenteral nutrition, and other agents.
2. These devices should also allow for convenient blood sampling.
3. Techniques of placement should minimize the risk of dislodgement and surgically acquired infection.

Before speaking about specific tumor systems, it is worthwhile to discuss the role and technique of vascular access in pediatric oncology. This topic is crucial to the successful treatment of almost all children with cancer. Vascular access can be defined as central venous cannulation using either externally exiting or implanted devices. These devices are commonly constructed of plastics, silicone rubber tubing, and in some cases titanium. They are commonly placed through a jugular (internal, external, common facial vein), or subclavian approach. Basilic or cephalic vein peripherally inserted central venous catheter

placement is also done, although this requires a rather long length of catheter with a relatively small lumen in small children and is therefore not as effective, although supported by at least 1 pediatric study.[1] Femoral placement may be required when the upper extremity veins are occluded by thrombus or externally compressed by tumor, as may occur with lymphomas of the mediastinum. Techniques of tunneled external catheter, implanted port, and femoral placement are well described in the literature.

Vascular-access device-related complications are related to catheter placement (acute) or occur after the catheter has been in place (long term). Examples of complications related to catheter placement including malposition, pneumothorax, hemothorax, chylothorax, arterial cannulation, hemorrhage, failure of catheter placement, and cardiac dysrhythmias. In one study, the pneumothorax rate was 1.9% while hemothoraces occurred in 1% of cases.[2] Insertion failure, hemorrhage, and malposition together occur in about 1% of patients.[3]

Long-term catheter-related complications include infections, thromboses, and various mechanical failures like catheter breakage and port extrusions. Figure 8-1 shows an instance of catheter breakage, and Table 8-1 lists studies of catheter complications emphasizing bloodborne infectious complications. As is evident, most analyses associate an increased infection rate with younger children and the use of externally exiting catheters. This favors the use of implanted devices when feasible. However, needle dislodgement and local skin breakdown may occur when ports are cannulated for periods exceeding 1 week. In this cohort of patients, externally exiting catheters may be required. This is often true of patients in the first month after bone marrow or stem cell transplant. It should also be noted that when implanted devices do become infected, a surgical procedure is required for removal compared with bedside removal of externally exiting catheters.

Thrombosis may occur inside the catheter lumen and caused occlusion in 6.8% of patients in a large series of adults.[3] It may also develop in the venous system through which the catheter runs, resulting in a deep-vein thrombosis. It is estimated that the latter condition occurs in 12% to 50% of children with indwelling catheters but is subclinical in most instances.[9,10] Long-term catheter

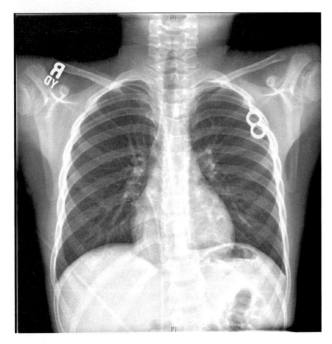

Figure 8-1 This catheter detached from the mediport reservoir and required retrieval in interventional radiology.

breakage, leakage, or displacement occurs in roughly 11% of patients.[3] Catheter or deep-vein thrombosis generally requires device removal and anticoagulation. Breakage, leakage, and displacement require catheter replacement.

In summary, a functional vascular access device is indispensable for the treatment of most pediatric solid tumor patients. Implanted ports are associated with a lower rate of systemic sepsis and are favored for patients who do not require long periods of port cannulation.

Neuroblastoma

Surgical Principles: The surgical approach to patients with neuroblastoma depends on risk status.

1. Low-risk patients: Complete gross resection of the primary tumor before proceeding with chemotherapy, when feasible, and without sacrificing of major organs like the kidney and spleen.
2. Intermediate-risk patients: Complete gross resection of the primary tumor and involved loco-regional lymphatics either before or after systemic chemotherapy. Patients deemed unresectable by imaging studies should undergo a course of neoadjuvant chemotherapy and attempted resection per protocol. If complete resection is not feasible after chemotherapy, at least 50% of the primary tumor mass should be removed. This approach should be taken only after chemotherapy and when complete removal is associated with undue risk or would require organ loss or damage.
3. High-risk patients: All high-risk patients should receive neoadjuvant chemotherapy prior to attempted resection as per protocol. The ultimate goal is complete gross resection of the primary tumor and involved loco-regional lymphatics. Every attempt at an organ-preserving resection should be made. The time-decay of tumor volume by cycle of chemotherapy is illustrated in Figure 8-2.
4. The surgeon must ensure that every time a neuroblastoma is resected or biopsied, adequate samples of viable tumor (1–2 cm^3) are properly preserved (snap frozen) and forwarded to the appropriate laboratories for biological studies that impact on prognosis and stratification of therapy.

Much progress has been made in the treatment of neuroblastoma in the past 20 years. Perhaps the greatest

Table 8-1
Chart of Catheter Infection

Author	Catheter Days	Infection Rate	Determinants of Infection
La Quaglia[4]	78,159	40% catheters 25% ports	Age < 7yrs. (+) Port (−)
Abbas[5]	41,382	25% (all catheters)	Young age (+) Protocol (increased with intensity) Port (−) (p = 0.056)
Cesaro[6]	19,328	65% catheters	Age < 4.6yrs (+)
Adler[7]	92,561	40% ports	Port (−) Stem cell transplant (+)
Fratino[8]	107,012	40% (no ports)	Single lumen catheter (−) Age < 6 yrs (+) Solid tumor (+)

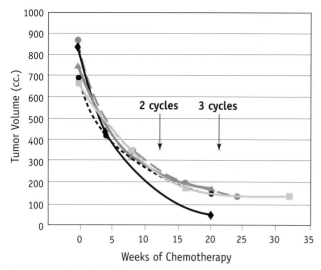

Figure 8-2 Time-decay of neuroblastoma tumor volume with chemotherapy.

advance has been the identification of risk status based on age, stage, and biological variables, which has almost eliminated the need for radiotherapy in all but high-risk patients and eliminated or reduced the intensity of chemotherapy in low-risk patients. The present risk stratification is discussed elsewhere.

Neuroblastoma can arise anywhere along the sympathetic chain from neck to pelvis. Consequently, surgical technique is directed toward the individual anatomic site of the primary tumor. It is almost never possible to obtain a clear microscopic margin, and dissection proceeds along the pseudocapsule of the tumor. It is acceptable and often necessary to remove the tumor in segments, especially near vital structures. Tumor division over vessels like the renal and superior mesenteric arteries allows these to be visualized and protected. The use of titanium surgical clips is also advocated strongly to improve hemostasis and lymphostasis and to identify involved areas for subsequent radiotherapy.

Initial Biopsy

Initial tumor biopsy is extremely important in determining biological aggressiveness, as discussed earlier. The surgeon should obtain at least 1 cm³ of viable tumor tissue (more if possible) and should look for grayish fleshy areas to obtain the biopsy because viable tumor is often present in such sites. Finally, the biopsy incision should be oriented along the direction of the incision used for complete resection and subsequently incorporated in the mass that is removed at the time of definitive surgery.

Often the mass is enclosed by a pseudocapsule, and this can be used to advantage to control bleeding. The surgeon cauterizes a circular area of the pseudocapsule using either bipolar or unipolar electrocautery. The capsule is then opened, and pituitary rongeurs, readily obtainable in most operating rooms, are used to remove pieces of the tumor. Multiple biopsies are taken and the accumulated

volume should be equal to or greater than 1 cm³. Central line placement and staging bone marrow aspirations and biopsies can be conveniently done at the same time.

Cervical Lesions

Extension of the tumor into the thoracic inlet must be determined prior to surgery because the exposure is different for these tumors. Most pure cervical lesions have favorable histologic characteristics, a good pseudocapsule, and occur in patients less than 1 year of age at diagnosis. Very large lesions may require partial or complete division of the sternocleidomastoid muscle. Grossly involved jugulodigastric lymph nodes should be removed in a systematic way using a modified neck dissection technique. Parents should be forewarned that removal of cervical lesions usually results in Horner syndrome. Surgical technique is illustrated in Figure 8-3.

Cervicothoracic Lesions

Tumors that are primary to the neck or chest may extend into and through the thoracic inlet. The best surgical exposure for lesions in this area is a cervicothoracic incision. The sternum is then divided either completely or down to the fourth interspace and then extended laterally. The anesthesiologist must be reminded that nerve stimulation is necessary when dissecting close to the brachial plexus to safeguard against injury.

Mediastinal Tumors

Most mediastinal tumors can be approached through a posterolateral thoracotomy. The blood supply to these lesions is usually derived from perforating vessels off the

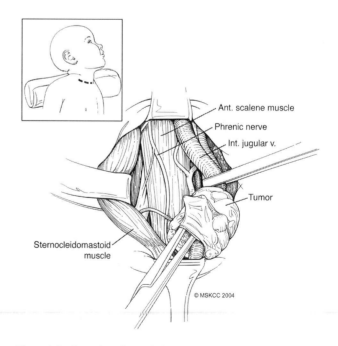

Figure 8-3 Resection of a cervical neuroblastoma. A Horner syndrome is unavoidable.

thoracic aorta. These vessels should be identified and securely clipped or ligated prior to dissection of the main tumor. Mediastinal tumors also insinuate into the intercostal spaces so that identification of the underlying internal intercostal muscles is required for complete dissection. Titanium clips should be liberally used on fibrolymphatic tissues to prevent chylothorax. Injury to the thoracic duct behind the carina is a frequent cause of this complication as well. The positioning and technique are illustrated in Figure 8-4.

Lesions in the Upper Abdomen and Retroperitoneum

Seventy-five percent of high-risk neuroblastomas are primary to the adrenal gland and often involve regional lymph nodes in the ipsilateral, para-aortic, or pericaval chains as well as interaortocaval lymph nodes. Adequate vascular control and retroperitoneal exposure is best obtained using an ipsilateral thoracoabdominal incision with midline extension for lesions extending into the lower abdomen (Figure 8-5).

On the left side a visceral roll of the spleen and pancreatic tail will expose the retroperitoneum and supracoeliac aorta. This allows identification and control of the coeliac axis superior mesenteric artery. The tumor is "unwrapped" from around any encased vessels and removed. This process is illustrated in Figure 8-6, which shows the renal vessels being cleared.

A right-sided thoracoabdominal exposure is focused on control of the supra- and infrarenal vena cava. The cava is identified just below the liver, and dissection proceeds

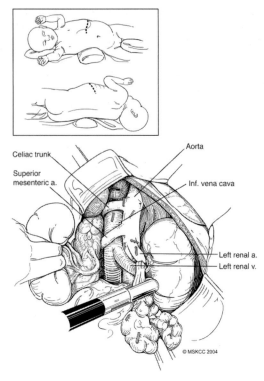

Figure 8-5 Thoracoabdominal approach to an upper abdominal neuroblastoma.

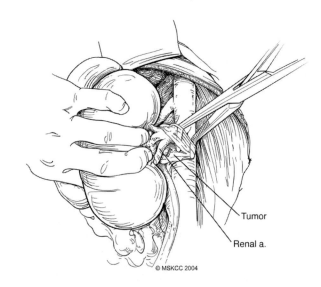

Figure 8-6 Renal hilar dissection.

along its right lateral wall. It is usually best to identify the right renal vein and then move superiorly. The Trendelenburg position may reduce the pressure in the vena cava as well as the chance of air embolism.

Pelvic Tumors

Pelvic tumors usually have favorable biological characteristics but are complicated by encasement of iliac vessels or

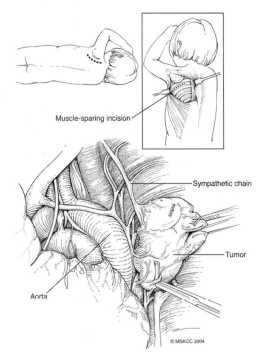

Figure 8-4 Resection of a mediastinal neuroblastoma.

infiltration of the lumbosacral plexus. A low midline incision down to the pubic symphysis gives good exposure and allows control of the distal aorta and vena cava (Figure 8-7). Both lower extremities should be prepped into the field and covered with clear plastic so that nerve stimulation may be done. The ipsilateral internal iliac vessels may be hopelessly encased and can be ligated and resected with the specimen. Foot drop may occur after resection of large pelvic lesions and should be discussed with the family preoperatively. It can be avoided by frequent nerve stimulation and acceptance of a small amount of residual tumor surrounding major nerves of the lumbosacral plexus.

Wilms Tumor

Surgical Principles:

1. In North America, complete resection of the primary tumor is done at the time of diagnosis.* For renal primaries, this requires radical nephrectomy. Ipsilateral adrenalectomy is not required, per se, but should be done if there is any adherence to the tumor. Extrarenal Wilms tumors should be widely resected and regional lymph nodes biopsied. This may require bowel or ureteral resection.

2. Exceptions to primary nephrectomy include bilateral Wilms tumors, those arising in a solitary kidney, and tumors with extensive vascular invasion,

---

*In Europe, almost all patients receive chemotherapy prior to resection.

usually with extension into the retrohepatic vena cava or right atrium. In these cases, neoadjuvant chemotherapy should be given followed by resection. Another exception may be cases of retroperitoneal-contained rupture in which peritoneal contamination would result from initial resection.

3. For right-sided tumors perinephric, pericaval, and interaortocaval lymph nodes should be biopsied. Perinephric, para-aortic, and interaortocaval nodes should be biopsied with left-sided tumors.

4. It is no longer necessary to visualize and palpate the contralateral kidney when it is normal using computerized axial tomography (CAT) with intravenous contrast. However, a thorough evaluation of the peritoneal cavity, including the liver, should be done and suspicious areas biopsied.

The treatment of Wilms tumor is a great success story in pediatric oncology. The 16-year relapse-free survivals of stages I, II/III, and IV favorable histology Wilms tumors were reported at >90%, 85%, and 77%, respectively, for NWTS-3.[11] The surgical contribution to this improvement in survival hinges on the excellent local control associated with complete microscopic resection of the primary tumor without rupture and spillage.[12] The surgeon also makes an essential contribution to staging and the decision to give external beam radiation by sampling regional lymph nodes and performing a thorough exploration of the peritoneal cavity and retroperitoneum. The technique of resection is depicted in Figure 8-8.

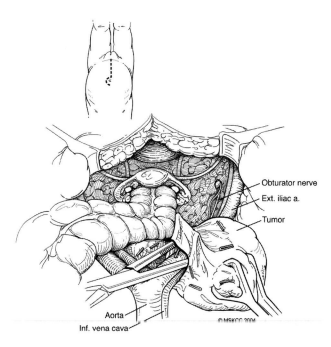

Figure 8-7 Resection of a pelvic neuroblastoma.

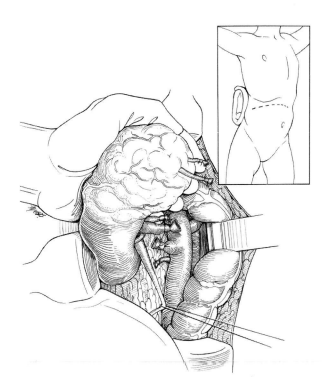

Figure 8-8 Resection of a Wilms tumor.

Intravascular Extension

Intravascular extension of Wilms tumor is an indication for neoadjuvant chemotherapy. In a report from the National Wilms Tumor Study (NWTS), 39 of 49 intravascular tumors regressed with chemotherapy including 7 out of 12 with atrial extension.[13] In the same study there was only one instance of embolization during chemotherapy and the surgical complication rate associated with primary resection without chemotherapy was 26% compared with 13.2% in patients receiving neoadjuvant treatment. In another study of 17 children with cavoatrial extension, similar use of presurgical chemotherapy resulted in tumor regression.[14] Intracaval extension was shown to increase the rate of surgical complications in Wilms tumor.[15] In summary, embolization of intracaval or intra-atrial Wilms tumors rarely occurs with chemotherapy. Tumor regression using chemotherapy with resultant reduction in surgical morbidity and complexity is observed.

Bilateral Wilms Tumor

The overall survival rate of patients who have synchronous bilateral Wilms tumor has been reported to range from 69% to 76%.[16,17] Because of the danger of debilitating loss of renal function, it is acceptable to administer preoperative chemotherapy based on the results of an initial exploration and biopsy. After tumor shrinkage, a second-look procedure and nephron-sparing renal resection can be performed. Using this strategy, survival rates have been achieved that are equivalent to the more traditional approach. The latter involves an initial nephrectomy of the most heavily involved kidney, followed by chemotherapy, and then re-exploration. The frequency of end-stage renal disease is higher in patients with bilateral Wilms tumor. Patients with unilateral disease and without an underlying syndrome have a cumulated incidence of end-stage renal disease of 0.6% compared with 12% for those with bilateral tumors.[18] The presence of the Denys-Drash or WAGR syndromes, genitourinary anomalies, or hypospadias or cryptorchidism also increases the rate of end-stage renal failure with higher rates for all categories when the tumors are bilateral.

Patients with bilateral Wilms tumors are no longer biopsied prior to resection when the diagnosis seems evident from imaging studies.

Preoperative Rupture

Preoperative rupture may be free into the peritoneal cavity or confined to the retroperitoneum by Gerota fascia or the peritoneum itself. With freely ruptured tumors total abdominal radiation will be required. In the case of retroperitoneally contained ruptures, preoperative chemotherapy may allow a subsequent complete resection without spillage. This will obviate the need for total abdominal radiation.

Extrarenal Wilms Tumor

Wilms tumors can arise from areas other than the kidney, but this is extremely rare. The most common site is the retroperitoneum, followed by the pelvis and inguinal canal. They have been reported in the testis, ovary, thorax, lumbosacral, and subcutaneous areas. Therapy should be guided by the same principles used for primary renal Wilms tumor, and complete excision with negative microscopic margins is the goal of resection. Prognosis is similar to primary renal tumors on a stage-by-stage basis. In a report from the NWTS, 7 of 8 patients with extrarenal Wilms tumor had favorable histology while the 8th had teratomatous elements.[19] Seven of the 8 were disease-free at a median of 34.3 months.

Technique of Resection

All abdominal Wilms tumors should be approached transperitoneally through an anterior and not a flank incision. The risk of surgical complications is significantly increased when either a flank or paramedian incision is used.[15] Some authors have suggested early ligation of the ipsilateral renal vein as a first step. However, this is sometimes very difficult with a large tumor and may also result in venous engorgement of the involved kidney with subsequent increased bleeding. If the ipsilateral artery and vein can both be controlled early, then ligation can proceed followed by mobilization. If access to the renal vessels is difficult, it is usually better to mobilize the kidney including the perinephric fat and Gerota fascia. If the tumor arises from the upper pole or is adherent to the adrenal gland in any way, it is better to mobilize and remove that structure as well. Once the kidney is mobilized, the renal artery can be identified posteriorly in the hilus. It should be securely ligated with at least two ligatures or a ligature and suture-ligature placed proximally. The vein can then also be ligated and divided. The ureter is dissected and divided as far in the pelvis as possible. Any remaining fibrolymphatic attachments are then cut and the specimen delivered. Ligation of lymphatics with sutures or clips may reduce the chance of lymphatic ascites.[20] All obviously involved regional lymph nodes should be removed. The surgeon should make sure to biopsy perinephric, interaortocaval, and either pericaval nodes for right-sided tumors, or para-aortic for left-sided. A thorough peritoneal exploration with removal of obvious metastatic deposits and biopsy of suspicious areas should be done.

Soft-Tissue Sarcomas

In childhood, soft-tissue sarcomas are divided into rhabdomyosarcoma and nonrhabdomyomatous soft-tissue sarcomas. Rhabdomyosarcoma is the most common soft-tissue sarcoma, and primary tumors can be anatomically distributed throughout the body. The second most common soft-tissue sarcoma in childhood and adolescence is synovial sarcoma, which, although it can affect truncal sites and even the head and neck, usually arises in an extremity. Fibrosarcoma does occur in childhood and adolescence but must be distinguished from fibromatosis and desmoid tumor. Liposarcoma, leiomyosarcoma, malignant fibrous histiocytoma, gastrointestinal stromal tumor, angiosarcoma, alveolar soft part sarcoma, epithelioid sarcoma, and ever more uncommon varieties can occur but are relatively rare. Osteogenic and Ewing sarcoma are primary bone tumors in most cases.

Surgical Principles:

1. For rhabdomyosarcoma, the surgical approach is determined by the anatomic location of the primary tumor. Fresh tissue should always be sent for molecular genetics to identify the alveolar subtype.
   a. Head and neck lesions require an initial diagnostic biopsy. Resection, if it is possible, is reserved for special circumstances like poor response to chemotherapy and radiation, or recurrence.
   b. Genitourinary lesions also require only an initial diagnostic biopsy.

Rhabdomyosarcoma

Rhabdomyosarcoma are ubiquitously distributed throughout the body. Furthermore, the anatomic site of the primary tumor is a determinant of prognostic risk. Therefore, the following discussion is site-dependent.

Head and Neck: Rhabdomyosarcoma in this region can occur in the orbit, infratemporal fossa, nasopharynx, hypopharynx, middle ear, and other areas. Orbital sites in young children have a favorable outlook, but this is not true of older children. Parameningeal involvement is associated with a worsened outcome. The role of surgery is biopsy to establish the diagnosis.[21] There is a high frequency of regional nodal involvement in head and neck rhabdomyosarcoma, and regional node sampling may be important in determination of risk status.[22] Resection of localized and anatomically accessible tumors may allow a reduction in radiation dosage with equivalent cure.[23] Skull-base surgery or maxillectomy is sometimes used for localized recurrent tumors.

Bladder and Bladder-Prostate: In patients with bladder or bladder-prostate rhabdomyosarcoma, the diagnosis can usually be established by transperineal or transrectal core needle biopsy. Cystoscopic biopsy is usually not feasible because of effacement of the bladder and reduced visibility. In addition, it is difficult to stop bleeding through the small cystoscopes required in children. A urine sample for cytology should be sent. The effects of neoadjuvant chemotherapy and radiotherapy are assessed by imaging studies and repeat cystoscopy and biopsy. Cystectomy is reserved for refractory or recurrent tumors.[24] Partial cystectomy, when anatomically feasible, is effective and preserves bladder function.[25] Newer techniques of urinary

reconstruction involving catheterizable stomas may add to the patient's quality of life.

Paratesticular Rhabdomyosarcoma: Paratesticular rhabdomyosarcoma is treated by ipsilateral radical inguinal orchiectomy. Patients who are older than 10 years of age should also undergo ipsilateral, nerve-sparing retroperitoneal lymph node dissection.[26] Children younger than 10 years do not need retroperitoneal node dissection. If positive retroperitoneal lymph nodes are identified, radiotherapy is given. If a previous transscrotal biopsy has occurred, the surgical approach is complicated. Hemiscrotectomy can be performed in continuity with ipsilateral inguinal orchiectomy. However, this makes subsequent placement of a testicular prosthesis very difficult. Another approach is the use of scrotal radiation. To avoid or minimize radiation damage to the contralateral testicle, it can be temporarily transposed into the groin.

Extremity Rhabdomyosarcoma. Small-extremity rhabdomyosarcomas can usually be completely excised at diagnosis. Larger tumors that invade bone or nerves, or lesions with distant metastases or positive regional lymph nodes, are usually treated with neoadjuvant chemotherapy. In this situation, a diagnostic biopsy should be obtained through a small incision or core needle biopsy. Imaging of the lesion prior to surgery should always be done.

Hepatic Tumors

Surgical Principles:

1. Complete resection of malignant hepatic tumors is essential for long-term survival.
2. Anatomic resection with ligation of feeding and draining vessels using the schema of Couinaud is required in most cases.

Workup of a Hepatic Mass in Childhood

Patients presenting with a suspected hepatic mass first undergo a history and physical examination. Blood work should include a complete blood count, liver function tests, coagulation studies, and tumor markers. Tumor markers include a serum α-fetoprotein and β-human chorionic gonadotropin. Doppler ultrasonography is done to determine whether a mass is cystic or solid, determine the patency of the portal and hepatic veins and vena cava, and identify satellite lesions. At present, magnetic resonance imaging provides the greatest amount of information concerning both the lesion and surrounding veins and bile ducts. If a malignant tumor is suspected, thoracic CAT is done to identify metastases. A tissue diagnosis is mandatory if malignancy is suspected after the workup. Percutaneous needle core or aspiration biopsy is useful for hepatoblastomas but may not be definitive in the case of hepatocellular carcinoma. Staging is based on the SIOPEL "pretext" schema (Figure 8-9).

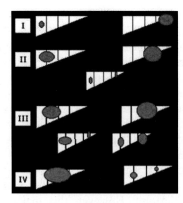

Figure 8-9 SIOPEL "pretext" staging system. Stage I, 3 adjoining sectors free of tumor; Stage II, 2 sectors free; Stage III, 1 sector free; Stage IV, no sectors free.

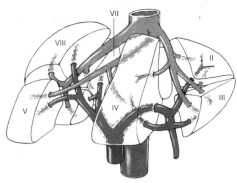

Functional division

Figure 8-10 Couinaud hepatic segments.

The schema of hepatic anatomy most useful for the surgeon is based on the work of Couinaud (Figure 8-10). The portal and hepatic veins subdivide the liver into 8 segments. Segment 1, the caudate lobe, is considered separate from the others because of its unique vascular supply. After resection, there is a rapid recovery to the normal hepatic volume for age despite administration of chemotherapy, or even a history of total hepatic radiation therapy.

Surgical Techniques
Right Hepatic Lobectomy

The patient is positioned supine and a bilateral subcostal incision created. This is then extended superiorly in the midline to expose the confluence of the hepatic veins. Once resectability has been confirmed, the liver is mobilized by dividing the triangular and falciform ligaments. The hilus is then approached and the right hepatic artery and right portal vein ligated. The small, unnamed hepatic veins extending from the posterior right lobe directly into the cava are then divided. The main right hepatic vein is then ligated and divided. The hepatoduodenal ligament is then clamped (Pringle maneuver) and the hepatic substance divided. Clips are used on smaller venous radicles or bile ducts, but large structures are suture-ligated. The last structure to be cut is the main right hepatic duct, and

this should be done as far from the bifurcation as possible to prevent injury to the left hepatic duct or common bile duct. A drain is rarely required.

Left Hepatic Lobectomy

The incision and exposure are the same as for a right-sided resection, and the left hepatic artery and left portal vein are ligated first. The sinus venosus is opened to expose the retrohepatic vena cava, and the space between the vena cava and the confluence of the middle and left hepatic veins is developed. This confluence is then securely ligated. A Pringle maneuver is carried out and the hepatic substance divided.

Complex Hepatic Resections

Extended right or left hepatic resections are feasible and may be required in selected circumstances. Central hepatic resection for small lesions in segments IV, V, and VIII is also used.[27,28]

Summary

The optimal approach to the surgical management of pediatric tumors requires detailed knowledge of their natural history including propensity for invasion and sites of metastasis, their unique biology and the need to get appropriate material for sophisticated laboratory studies, as well as an appreciation of the role of chemotherapy and radiation to plan the need and timing of biopsy vs. resection. Effective surgical procedures for pediatric tumors are complex and differ substantially from those associated with tumors that occur in adults. Immediate referral to an experienced pediatric surgeon who functions as part of a multidisciplinary team is essential to ensure the best outcome.

References

1. Knue M, et al. The efficacy and safety of blood sampling through peripherally inserted central catheter devices in children. *J Infus Nurs.* 2005;28(1):30–35.
2. Casado-Flores J, et al. Complications of central venous catheterization in critically ill children. *Pediatr Crit Care Med.* 2001;2(1):57–62.
3. Schwarz RE, Coit DG, Groeger JS. Transcutaneously tunneled central venous lines in cancer patients: an analysis of device-related morbidity factors based on prospective data collection. *Ann Surg Oncol.* 2000;7(6):441–449.
4. La Quaglia MP, et al. A prospective analysis of vascular access device-related infections in children. *J Pediatr Surg.* 1992;27(7):840–842.
5. Abbas AA, et al. Factors influencing central line infections in children with acute lymphoblastic leukemia: results of a single institutional study. *Pediatr Blood Cancer.* 2004;42(4):325–331.
6. Cesaro S, et al. A prospective survey on incidence and outcome of Broviac/Hickman catheter-related complications in pediatric patients affected by hematological and oncological diseases. *Ann Hematol.* 2004;83(3):183–188.
7. Adler A, et al. Infectious complications of implantable ports and Hickman catheters in paediatric haematology-oncology patients. *J Hosp Infect.* 2005.
8. Fratino G, et al. Central venous catheter-related complications in children with oncological/hematological diseases: an observational study of 418 devices. *Ann Oncol.* 2005;16(4):648–654.
9. Journeycake JM, Buchanan GR. Thrombotic complications of central venous catheters in children. *Curr Opin Hematol.* 2003;10(5):369–374.

10. Wilimas JA, et al. Late vascular occlusion of central lines in pediatric malignancies. *Pediatrics*. 1998;101(2):E7.

11. Green DM. The treatment of stages I-IV favorable histology Wilms' tumor. *J Clin Oncol*. 2004;22(8):1366–1372.

12. Shamberger RC, et al. Surgery-related factors and local recurrence of Wilms tumor in National Wilms Tumor Study 4. *Ann Surg*. 1999;229(2):292–297.

13. Shamberger RC, et al. Intravascular extension of Wilms tumor. *Ann Surg*. 2001;234(1):116–121.

14. Akyuz C, et al. Cavoatrial tumor extension in children with Wilms tumor: a retrospective review of 17 children in a single center. *J Pediatr Hematol Oncol*. 2005. 27(5):267–269.

15. Ritchey ML, et al. Surgical complications after primary nephrectomy for Wilms' tumor: report from the National Wilms' Tumor Study Group. *J Am Coll Surg*. 2001;192(1):63–68; quiz 146.

16. Blute ML, et al. Bilateral Wilms tumor. *J Urol*. 1987;138(4 Pt 2):968–973.

17. Kumar R, Fitzgerald R, Breatnach F. Conservative surgical management of bilateral Wilms tumor: results of the United Kingdom Children's Cancer Study Group. *J Urol*. 1998;160(4):1450–1453.

18. Breslow NE, et al. End stage renal disease in patients with Wilms tumor: results from the National Wilms Tumor Study Group and the United States Renal Data System. *J Urol*. 2005;174(5):1972–1975.

19. Andrews PE, Kelalis PP, Haase GM. Extrarenal Wilms' tumor: results of the National Wilms' Tumor Study. *J Pediatr Surg*. 1992;27(9):1181–1184.

20. Weiser AC, et al. Chylous ascites following surgical treatment for Wilms tumor. *J Urol*. 2003;170(4,Pt 2):1667–1669; discussion 1669.

21. Raney RB, et al. Treatment of children and adolescents with localized parameningeal sarcoma: experience of the Intergroup Rhabdomyosarcoma Study Group protocols IRS-II through -IV, 1978–1997. *Med Pediatr Oncol*. 2002; 38(1):22–32.

22. Kraus DH, et al. Pediatric rhabdomyosarcoma of the head and neck. *Am J Surg*. 1997;174(5):556–560.

23. Daya H, et al. Pediatric rhabdomyosarcoma of the head and neck: is there a place for surgical management? *Arch Otolaryngol Head Neck Surg*. 2000; 126(4):468–472.

24. Lobe TE, et al. The argument for conservative, delayed surgery in the management of prostatic rhabdomyosarcoma. *J Pediatr Surg*. 1996;31(8):1084–1087.

25. Hays DM, et al. Children with vesical rhabdomyosarcoma (RMS) treated by partial cystectomy with neoadjuvant or adjuvant chemotherapy, with or without radiotherapy. A report from the Intergroup Rhabdomyosarcoma Study (IRS) Committee. *J Pediatr Hematol Oncol*. 1995;17(1):46–52.

26. Ferrari A, et al. Paratesticular rhabdomyosarcoma: report from the Italian and German Cooperative Group. *J Clin Oncol*. 2002;20(2):449–455.

27. Glick RD, et al. Extended left hepatectomy (left hepatic trisegmentectomy) in childhood. *J Pediatr Surg*. 2000;35(2):303–307; discussion 308.

28. La Quaglia MP, Shorter NA, Blumgart LH. Central hepatic resection for pediatric tumors. *J Pediatr Surg*. 2002;37(7):986–989.

Fundamentals of Pediatric Radiation Oncology

Robert S. Lavey

Introduction

Radiation therapy has been a mainstay in the treatment of cancer since the initial clinical use of x-rays in 1896. Continuous refinements in the delivery of radiation over the ensuing 110 years have focused on improving its efficacy against tumors and decreasing its untoward effects on normal tissues. Radiation is currently used to treat volumes ranging from a few millimeters to the entire body in patients of all ages. Radiation therapy has a role in the treatment of a wide spectrum of benign disorders as well as malignancies. More than half of all cancer patients undergo irradiation with either curative or palliative intent.

Radiation therapy is usually used as a local or regional treatment. This is because the function of several critical organs, particularly the bone marrow, lungs, kidneys, and liver, is permanently impaired by the dose of radiation required to control most solid tumors. Because the most radiosensitive vital organ is the bone marrow, the entire body can be irradiated to a myeloablative dose followed by salvage with bone marrow or stem cell transplantation. The sensitivity of tumors to radiation varies considerably by histology, but all tumor and normal cells will die after exposure to a sufficiently large dose of radiation. The radiation dose utilized for therapy is determined after consideration of the number of viable tumor cells that must be sterilized and the radiosensitivity of both the tumor cells and normal tissues in the immediate vicinity of the tumor. The radiation dose prescribed is often less than optimal for control of the tumor so as to avoid causing severe chronic morbidity due to normal tissue injury. Radiation oncologists are more accepting of temporary, acute morbidities, such as mucositis and skin desquamation, than of late-developing, life-altering complications such as spinal cord myelopathy and renal failure. Radiation dose prescriptions are standardized because the dose-limiting chronic complications are not associated with acute radiation or chemotherapy tolerance and there are no reliable predictors of late effects. Due to our inability to predict which patients will be more tolerant of high doses of radiation, the number of radiation fractions and total radiation dose are generally determined prior to the start of the radiation therapy course and not altered regardless of acute tolerance of the treatment. The efficacy of radiation with curative intent is assessed by long-term (in years) loco-regional tumor control, progression-free survival, and overall survival rather than response rates. Regrowth of a tumor within the targeted radiation volume at any time after irradiation is usually considered a failure of radiation therapy. The efficacy of radiation with palliative intent is assessed by the degree and duration of relief of symptoms.

The role of radiation therapy in treatment of a patient is determined by the patient's age and physical condition and the tumor type, stage, location, invasiveness, and response to other therapies. Radiation is used primarily to achieve or maintain loco-regional tumor control. It may be selected prior to surgery in order to make resection more feasible (eg, for soft-tissue sarcomas), following surgery to eliminate residual disease when wide surgical margins have not been obtained (eg, brain tumors), or instead of surgery when complete resection is not feasible or would yield functionally or cosmetically unacceptable outcomes (eg, nasopharyngeal carcinoma, orbital rhabdomyosarcoma, pelvic Ewing sarcoma, Hodgkin lymphoma). Radiation therapy is currently used preceding (eg, primitive neuroectodermal tumor), concurrent with (eg, sarcomas), following (eg, neuroblastoma), or without (eg, ependymoma) chemotherapy.

Reduction in the use of radiation therapy has been a major trend in pediatric oncology over the past several decades. As more effective chemotherapy regimens with lower probabilities of life-altering chronic morbidity than radiation therapy are developed, radiation is being given as primary treatment to fewer pediatric patients. Among patients given radiation therapy, a common objective of clinical research protocols is to demonstrate that the radiation dose or volume irradiated can be reduced without compromising progression-free or overall survival. Among the late-developing morbidities pediatric oncologists seek to avoid by minimizing radiation exposure are second malignancies, cognitive deficits, diminished bone growth, infertility, and cardiovascular disease. Recent advances in diagnostic imaging and radiation therapy technology to be discussed later in this chapter, including 3-dimensional treatment planning, image fusion, stereotactic positioning, intensity-modulated radiation therapy (IMRT), and particle therapy, have reduced the radiation dose delivered to normal tissues in the region of the tumor. These techniques have been demonstrated to reduce radiation-induced acute complications and some chronic morbidities. Additional follow-up on large numbers of patients will be required to determine whether these techniques decrease the incidence of second malignancy and cognitive and organ dysfunction. Because of the advances in radiation techniques, previously published studies probably overestimate the incidence and severity of both acute and chronic side effects in current radiation patients.

Cellular Effects of Radiation

Measurement of Radiation

Radiation therapy deposits energy in the form of photons (eg, x-rays, gamma rays) or particles (eg, electrons, protons, alpha or beta particles, carbon ions, neutrons) in the tissues through which the radiation beam travels. The quantity of energy deposited per unit mass of tissue is the radiation dose, expressed in *gray* (Gy) or *centigray* (cGy). The name *gray* was chosen to honor the British radiobiologist L. H. Gray. One Gy indicates 1 joule of radiation energy deposited per kilogram of tissue. With the introduction of the International System, the Gy replaced the *rad* as the unit of radiation dose. One Gy is equal to 100 cGy or 100 rad. Photons and protons transfer their energy to orbiting electrons of biologic molecules, resulting in the release of fast electrons. The fast electrons produced either in tissue or in a radiation therapy machine have a significant biological effect when they change the structure of nuclear DNA either directly or through the action of hydroxyl radicals created by transferring kinetic energy to water molecules in the cell nucleus. Neutrons, alpha particles, and carbon ions have greater mass and carry greater energy than electrons. The density of ionization events they produce per unit path length is greater than that of photons, protons, and electrons (high *linear energy transfer*), causing a greater biological effect per unit of energy deposited (high *relative biologic effectiveness*). While protons, like photons and electrons, are a low linear energy transfer (LET) form of radiation, their LET increases by approximately 10% in the targeted tissue at the end of their path (the *Bragg peak*).

Action of Radiation

The mechanisms of cell killing by ionizing radiation continue to be under active investigation and appear more varied and complex than previously thought. The primary mechanism by which radiation kills cells is by producing free radicals and breaks in nuclear DNA.[1] A break in corresponding regions of each DNA strand (a "double-strand" break) prevents cellular replication and induces apoptosis.[2] The number of double-strand breaks correlates with the radiation dose administered and the LET of the radiation. After an initial rapid phase lasting 10 to 20 minutes, the process of double-strand break repair contin-

ues slowly for several hours. Human cancer cell lines vary in both the number of double-strand breaks induced by a given dose of radiation and their ability to rejoin the breaks. The survival of cells after irradiation correlates with their efficacy at rejoining double-strand breaks. In addition to damaging DNA, radiation induces a wide range of cellular responses. Multiple stress-response signaling pathways that induce apoptosis (eg, sphingomyelin-ceramide) are activated by irradiation.[3] Irradiation also leads to the expression of proteins that promote cell survival, including early growth response 1, tumor necrosis factor-alpha, epidermal growth factor receptors, and c-Jun.[4–6]

Modalities of Radiation

Several environmental and chemical factors influence the probability of a cell surviving a given radiation dose. The best characterized and strongest modulator of radiation sensitivity is the oxygenation status of the cell.[7] Approximately 3 times as much low-LET radiation is required to kill a given proportion of tumor cells in vivo when the tumor is hypoxic (oxygen concentration = 0.2%) than when it is well oxygenated (oxygen concentration > 2%). The efficacy of high-LET forms of radiation is less affected by oxygen concentration, due to the high density of DNA breaks they induce.[8] Oxygen molecules are hypothesized to sensitize cells by binding to the free radicals created by radiation, thereby making the radiation-induced DNA changes permanent. In the absence of oxygen, the free radicals are likely to recombine with free electrons and return to their original state.

Tumor cells tend to be hypoxic due to the paucity and abnormality of tumor vasculature, whereas normal cells are well oxygenated. Radiation damages the blood vessels within tumors, further starving tumor cells of oxygen and nutrients. This may be an additional pathway of tumor cell killing by radiation. A wide variety of measures have been investigated, and some are routinely used clinically, to overcome the relative radiation resistance conferred to tumor cells by hypoxia. Red blood cell transfusions are commonly given to patients with a hemoglobin concentration under 10 g/dL to increase the oxygen-carrying capacity of their blood. Dozens of studies have found an association between patients' hemoglobin level at the start or end of radiation therapy and control of their tumor.[9] Other methods of increasing oxygen delivery to the tumor that have been evaluated clinically in adults, but not children, include breathing carbogen, a mixture of 95% oxygen and 5% carbon dioxide, during irradiation, placing the patient in a hyperbaric oxygen chamber at 3 atmospheres of oxygen immediately prior to radiation,[10] and administering an oxygenmimetic compound, such as misonidazole or nimorazole, prior to radiation treatments.[11] An alternate approach is to administer an agent that preferentially kills hypoxic cells, such as tirapazamine or mitomycin-C.[12] None of these procedures has been unequivocally demonstrated to improve tumor control by radiation therapy in either adults or children.

Fractionation Schedules

Fractionation is the division of the prescribed radiation dose into multiple equally sized fractions. Radiation therapy is generally delivered once daily, 5 days per week. One of the rationales for fractionation is to take advantage of improved oxygenation of the surviving cells as the course of therapy proceeds.[13] Other reasons for fractionation of the radiation course are to irradiate surviving cells at more sensitive phases of their cell[14] cycle and to allow normal cells to repair from radiation-induced DNA damage. The half time of sublethal DNA damage repair is approximately 4 hours; thus repair is essentially complete before the next day's radiation dose is given. The value of fractionation was demonstrated in a randomized trial of total body irradiation prior to bone marrow transplantation for acute nonlymphoblastic leukemia. The survival rate was significantly higher after 12 Gy given in 6 daily fractions than after 10 Gy given in a single fraction, due to fewer deaths due to pneumonitis and other normal tissue complications. The efficacy of the 2 regimens in controlling leukemia was equivalent.[15] Fractionation preferentially spares the function of late-responding normal tissues (eg, brain and lung) to a greater extent than of tumors and acutely responding normal tissues (eg, skin and mucosa), because late-responding tissues undergo mitosis less frequently and are less likely to be in the radiosensitive Gap-2 (G_2) and mitotic (M) phases of the cell cycle.[16]

Whereas tumor cell reoxygenation and redistribution to more radiosensitive phases of the cell cycle are processes that act in favor of radiation fractionation, proliferation in between fractions does not. Tumors often decrease their doubling time during the weeks of radiation therapy, a process termed *accelerated repopulation*.[17] Accelerated repopulation of rapidly dividing tumors during the 24 hours between fractions balances the cell-killing effect of approximately 60 cGy of each radiation dose. Repopulation is responsible for the decrease in tumor-control rate associated with prolongation of the duration of the radiation course. The decrease in loco-regional tumor control has been estimated to be 1% to 2% per day for squamous cell carcinomas of the upper aerodigestive tract and uterine cervix.[18,19] It is for this reason that radiation oncologists generally seek to avoid breaks in the treatment schedule and starting therapy just prior to a weekend.

To balance the factors favoring a smaller daily radiation fractional dose (tumor reoxygenation and cell cycle redistribution, and normal tissue DNA repair) with the factor favoring a larger fractional dose (tumor repopulation), a radiation dose of 180 or 200 cGy given once daily is generally used. Late-responding normal tissues (eg, brain, spinal cord, liver) are more sensitive to fraction size than are most tumor and early-responding normal tissues (eg, skin, mucosa). For particularly radiosensitive tumors such as leukemia, lymphoma, and Wilms tumor, daily doses as small as 150 cGy are often used to minimize adverse radiation effects on the normal brain and gastrointestinal tissues. If radiation is given twice daily in order to decrease the overall treatment time, the radiation dose per fraction must be decreased to 100 to 125 cGy (*hyperfractionation*), and fractions should be separated by a minimum of 6 hours for acute normal tissue toxicity (mucositis and dermatitis) to be manageable. The decrease in fraction size increases the tolerance of late-responding normal tissues, permitting escalation of the total radiation dose. Administering radiation twice daily to an escalated dose increases tumor control in adult squamous cell carcinomas of the upper aerodigestive tract[20,21] but was found to have no effect in multi-institutional randomized trials of pediatric patients with diffuse brainstem glioma, primitive neuroectodermal tumor, or rhabdomyosarcoma.[22,23]

Hypofractionation, the delivery of the radiation therapy course in a lesser number of larger-than-standard sized fractions (eg, 250-500 cGy), is commonly used for the palliation of symptoms. It decreases the number of visits the patient must make to the radiation therapy clinic and may hasten the relief of symptoms. Clinical situations in which hypofractionation is commonly used include symptomatic metastases to bone or brain or compression of spinal cord, trachea, or superior vena cava. The cumulative radiation dose must be substantially reduced when the dose per fraction is increased to avoid exceeding late-responding normal tissue tolerance levels. The required reduction may result in a lower probability of long-term tumor control. This generally limits the use of hypofractionation to patients with a short life expectancy, radiosensitive tumor, need for immediate tumor response, and/or strong reason to minimize the number of patient visits.

Modalities of Radiation Therapy

Photon and Electron Beams

More than 95% of radiation treatments to children are delivered as a radiation beam emitted from a source outside the patient's body, termed external or *teletherapy* (meaning "at a distance" therapy). The earliest machines whose beams were of sufficient energy to deposit as much radiation into a deep-seated tumor as to superficial tissues contained a radioactive Cobalt-60 source with a maximum emitted gamma ray energy of 1.3 million volts (MV). As the energy of a gamma or photon beam increases, the dose given to the skin surface decreases and the dose deposited deeper in the body increases. To increase the dose given to internal tumors in relation to superficial normal tissues, Cobalt-60 machines were replaced starting in the 1960s by linear accelerators generating photon beams of maximum energy of 4 million to 25 MV. The energy of diagnostic x-rays, in comparison, is in the range of 0.1 MV. The vast majority of radiation therapy is now given using linear accelerators. Inside the accelerator, electrons are emitted from a heated cathode, accelerated by a microwave-generated electric field to 99% of the velocity of light, and directed to strike either a thin scattering foil or a thick high-density metal (usually tungsten) target. When the scattering foil is placed in the path of the electron beam, a broad beam of uniform energy electrons is directed to the patient. Most linear accelerators permit the operator a choice of 5 or 6 electron energies, ranging from 4 million to 20 million electron volts (MeV). The energy of an electron field is denoted in MeV to indicate the near-uniform energy of electrons at the indicated level. In contrast, a photon field contains photons having a wide range of energies up to the level indicated by the MV denotation. When the thick metal target is in place, the collision of the accelerated electrons with the target produces a shower of photons in all directions. Those photons traveling along the desired path to the patient are allowed to exit the accelerator unimpeded. At least 99.9% percent of the photons traveling in other directions are absorbed by thick lead shielding in the head of the linear accelerator. The other 0.1% may enter unintended areas of the patient's body as "head leakage." A thin lead shield of the type used to block low-energy diagnostic x-ray beams is insufficient to absorb the megavoltage photons generated by the linear accelerator. To provide significant protecting a lead body shield would need to be several centimeters thick, rendering such a device impractical.

An electron beam, which dissipates within centimeters of the patient's body surface, may be selected to treat superficial tumors (eg, testicular tumors and skin cancer) in order to spare underlying normal tissues. Low-energy electron beams (up to 6 MeV) are used for tumors that extend to a depth of no more than 1 centimeter from the surface. Tissues 3 or more centimeters deep to the surface receive less than one-tenth the dose delivered to the tumor. A very high-energy electron beam (20 MeV) can treat tumors that extend through soft tissues up to 6 centimeters deep to the body surface. Tissues 10 or more centimeters deep to the surface receive less than 15% of the dose delivered to tissues at a depth of between 1 and 4 centimeters. The depth of electron penetration is reduced in high-density tissues (eg, metal prostheses and bone) and increased in low-density tissues (eg, lung).

High-energy photon beams deliver less dosage to the skin surface, are less affected by tissue density, and have a lesser rate of dose fall-off beyond their maximum depth-dose than electrons. A 6 MV photon beam delivers its maximum dose approximately 1.5 centimeters beneath the skin surface with an approximately 3% decrement in dose for each centimeter in soft tissue depth beyond 1.5 centimeters. The dose to the skin surface is less than 25% of the dose at 1.5 centimeters' depth. An 18 MV photon beam delivers even less dose to the skin and its maximum dose is at approximately 4 centimeters beneath the surface, with an approximately 2% decrement in dose for each centimeter beyond 4 centimeters. Although minimizing skin dose is usually desirable to reduce acute erythema and desquamation, photon beams of 15 to 25 MV maximum energy may underdose tumor cells situated within 3 centimeters of the skin surface and give unnecessary dose to normal tissues beyond the deepest (by penetration) and widest (by scatter) extents of the tumor. Because of their small body size, children are generally treated with maximum photon energies of 6 to 10 MV. If a high dose to both the skin and tissues at depth is desired (eg, a surgical scar that may be contaminated with tumor cells), a bolus

material having radiation absorption properties identical to the desired thickness of subcutaneous tissue is placed on the targeted skin during photon irradiation, bringing the maximum dose to the skin surface.

In order to avoid irradiating normal tissues outside the targeted volume, the size and shape of the electron or photon beam is made to conform to the target. The beam size is defined by high-density lead collimators within the linear accelerator and high-density metal blocks or collimators fixed to the accelerator head and positioned in the path of the radiation beam. Using these devices, the radiation beam can be customized to any shape.

The radiation beam can be oriented at almost any angle relative to the patient. This permits the radiation oncologist to select a beam direction that reaches the tumor without entering or exiting through a radiosensitive normal tissue (eg, kidney or lens of the eye) and to utilize multiple radiation beams that intersect in the target volume but not in normal tissues. A tumor located deep within the body would receive a lower radiation dose than normal tissues in the path of a single beam in transit to the tumor, but it can be made to receive a higher radiation dose than normal tissues when multiple beams following different paths are utilized. Although any number of radiation beams can be selected, most commonly a set of 2 to 9 beams is used in each treatment session. The radiation beam direction is defined by the position of the linear accelerator gantry, which can rotate in a full circle around the patient, and the treatment couch on which the patient lies, which pivots in a half-circle perpendicular to the plane of the gantry rotation (Figure 9-1). The isocenter of rotation for the various beams is generally located within the target volume.

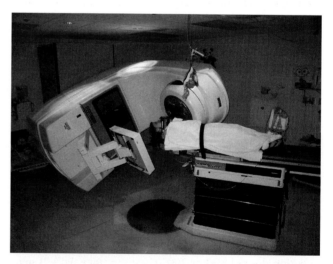

Figure 9-1 The radiation therapy treatment room. Patient is lying supine on the treatment couch in a stereotactic head immobilization device for treatment of a localized brain glioma using 8 noncoplanar radiation beams. For this beam, the accelerator gantry is rotated 65 degrees from vertical, and the couch is rotated 28 degrees from perpendicular to the gantry. The photon beam travels in a straight path from the head of the accelerator through the patient's brain tumor. The digital x-ray imaging array is positioned in the exit path of the beam to record the location of the beam path in relation to the patient's cranial bony anatomy (portal image).

Stereotactic Treatment

Stereotactic radiosurgery describes a complete course of radiation therapy given to a small volume as a single large dose while the patient is immobilized in a rigid frame that is fixed to the treatment couch or floor. The patient is positioned for treatment-planning computed tomography (CT) and radiosurgery treatment using a coordinate system based on fiducial markers on the head frame. The treatment fields are designed based on CT images showing the spatial relationship between the target lesion and fiducial markers. Magnetic resonance imaging (MRI) and/or angiography studies are usually fused with the CT images to better define the target. The term *radiosurgery* is used because the complete radiation course is delivered in a single session, reminiscent of a surgical procedure. It is generally reserved for intracranial lesions, because their position does not change in relation to the cranium and the cranium is readily fixed to the stereotactic frame, using pins that penetrate through the scalp into the outer table of the skull. The frame is fixed in place prior to the treatment-planning imaging studies and remains on the patient until the radiation therapy session is completed. Repositioning of the patient in relation to the coordinate system is accurate to within tenths of a millimeter. The trunk, in contrast, is more difficult to fix to the treatment couch and its contents move in relation to the skeleton with respiration and intestinal and bladder content.

Radiosurgery can be delivered using either a linear accelerator or a Gamma Knife, a hemispheric or toric array of 201 radioactive Cobalt-60 sources embedded in a helmet-shaped structure surrounding the patient's head. The 201 gamma beams are between 4 and 18 millimeters in diameter and are all focused at a single point, the treatment *isocenter* (Figure 9-2). Linear accelerator-based radiosurgery is generally delivered while the accelerator gantry is rotating in a set of between 3 and 6 noncoplanar arcs around the center of the lesion. The circular beams are between 4 and 40 millimeters in diameter. Either delivery method produces a high, inhomogeneous dose to the target volume with a steep fall-off

in dose over a 1 to 3 millimeter rim of normal tissues surrounding the target. Because the volume of normal tissues receiving a lethal radiation dose increases exponentially with increasing size of the target, stereotactic radiosurgery is generally reserved for the treatment of small (generally less than 3 centimeters in greatest diameter), radiographically distinct, noninvasive intracranial lesions such as acoustic neuromas, meningiomas, benign astrocytomas, brain metastases, and arteriovenous malformations. It has also been used in children with malignant tumors to deliver a focal "boost" dose of radiation at the end of a course of fractionated radiation and as sole treatment of tumors that recurred locally following fractionated radiotherapy. The combination of small target volume, lack of critical normal tissue within the target, and precision of positioning permits delivery of a minimum target dose of 12 to 20 Gy, 7 to 11 times the standard fractionated dose, in a single treatment session.

Stereotactic radiotherapy refers to a fractionated course of radiation in which the patient is positioned for treatment using an absolute reference system based on fixed fiducial markers attached to a custom-molded, relocatable immobilization device. Unlike stereotactic radiosurgery, the device does not remain fixed to the patient throughout the course of treatment planning and delivery. Stereotactic radiotherapy can be utilized to treat any size target in head, neck, or trunk. The device may be fitted to the patient's upper dentition and hard palate for a tumor in the head or to the spine for a tumor in the trunk to produce daily repositioning accuracy within 1 to 2 millimeters. Position in a mold shaped to the patient's external contour is less accurate. The course of stereotactic radiotherapy can range from 5 to 35 sessions utilizing radiation fractions of 1.8 to 5 Gy each. The radiation beam configuration and fraction size may be identical for stereotactic and nonstereotactic radiotherapy. The difference is that nonstereotactic radiation therapy uses the patient's own anatomy for positioning, rather than a coordinate system independent of the patient. Stereotactic positioning is generally more accurate, permitting the radiation fields to encompass a small margin of normal tissue surrounding the tumor.

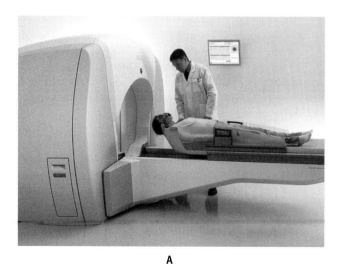

A

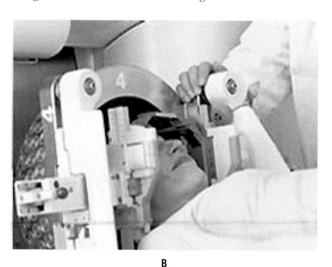

B

Figure 9-2 Gamma Knife radiosurgery. A rigid metal frame (A) is secured to the patient's skull by 4 metal pins. The frame is fixed to the treatment couch (B) in the position that locates the target at the isocenter of the hemispheric array of radioactive Cobalt-60 sources.

Particle Beam Therapy

There is emerging interest in charged particle (eg, protons, carbon ions) beams in place of photon or electron beams for radiation therapy. Approximately 25 clinical facilities dedicated to charged particle radiation therapy opened in several European countries and South Africa, and multiple locations opened in the United States and Japan between 1990 and 2007. The great majority, including all of those in North America, deliver proton therapy. The only operational carbon ion therapy facilities are located in Japan, Germany, and Italy. The proliferation of charged particle facilities has been limited by cost and space requirements. High-energy protons are generated by a synchrotron or cyclotron approximately 20 feet in diameter. Carbon ions are generated by a synchrotron approximately 60 feet in diameter. A proton facility costs approximately 10 times as much to build (well over US $100 million) and twice as much per patient to operate as a comparable photon facility. A carbon ion facility costs approximately 30% more to construct, although less per patient to operate, than a proton facility.

The dose distribution characteristics of charged particles for deep-seated tumors are superior to those of photons or electrons, resulting in a smaller "integral" (overall) radiation dose to the patient's body. This is of particular import in children, because charged particle treatment may therefore cause fewer second malignancies than photon treatment has in the past. Whereas the maximum energy deposition by photons and electrons is within 5 cm of the skin surface, it can be at any specified depth up to 25 cm with protons or carbon ions. The depth at which concentrated radiation deposition occurs (the *Bragg peak*) is determined by the velocity of the charged particle beam, which can be modified by varying either the beam energy or the thickness of absorbent material it passes through before entering the patient. The range of the Bragg peak can also be readily modulated ("spread out") to match the thickness of any target by passing the ion particle beams through an absorber of variable thickness. As the range of the Bragg peak is widened, the difference in dose the target, and the tissues the beam passes through on its path to the target, is reduced. The transit of particles stops at the end of the Bragg peak, resulting in a rapid decrement of radiation dose to zero within 1 centimeter beyond the target, in contrast to the gradual linear decrease in dose deposition of a photon beam beyond its maximum depth dose. This characteristic is particularly beneficial for treatment of the spine or spinal cord, because it avoids irradiation of the organs anterior to the target, including the gastrointestinal tract, liver, heart, and mediastinum.

For a typical tumor treated by protons, the entry dose at the skin surface is approximately one-third less than the dose given to the target, gradually rises to 100% throughout the target depth, then drops to 0 within 1 centimeter beyond the target.

The physical dose distribution of carbon ion beams is even better than that of proton beams. The heavier carbon particles scatter less than protons in the sideways and forward directions, resulting in a dose gradient outside the path 3 times steeper than protons. As a result, the integral radiation dose given to normal tissues by carbon ions is approximately one-half that given by protons.

The biologic effect on cells of proton irradiation is equivalent to photon or electron irradiation. Whereas protons have no biologic advantage over conventional forms of radiation, higher atomic number ions such as carbon deposit their energy far more densely within the target tissue (high *linear energy transfer*), producing direct, concentrated damage to the DNA that is beyond the capacity of the cell to repair.[24] The concentrated DNA damage causes the tumor cell to undergo apoptosis and death regardless of being hypoxic or in a relatively radioresistant phase of the cell cycle.

The safety and efficacy of proton beam therapy have been demonstrated for craniospinal irradiation, retinoblastoma, and several benign and malignant intracranial and base-of-skull tumors in children.[25,26] The proton beam has therefore become an accepted modality of radiation therapy, along with photon beams, on most Children's Oncology Group protocols. Standard quality assurance guidelines for proton treatment, comparable to those long in use for photon treatment, are under development in 2007 by special task forces of the United States National Cancer Institute and the American Association of Physicists in Medicine. Although carbon ions have significant biologic and physical advantages over both photon and proton beams, they have not yet come into common clinical use. Because carbon ions have higher LET than photons, electrons, or protons, innovative carbon hypofractionation schedules need to be piloted with careful monitoring of tumor response and normal tissue tolerance in order to determine the optimal use of carbon for a variety of tumor types.

Total body irradiation (TBI) is often given in conjunction with myeloablative chemotherapy immediately prior to bone marrow transplantation for children and adults with very high risk or recurrent leukemia or lymphoma. The bone marrow is the most sensitive vital organ to radiation. Thus, a radiation dose can be delivered that eliminates all the bone marrow stem cells with only a small risk of destroying the function of any other organs. The dose of TBI that can be safely administered is limited by the tolerance of the lungs and kidneys. Although TBI doses within lung and kidney tolerance limits are highly effective against leukemia and lymphoma cells, they are insufficient to be useful against metastatic solid tumors. The TBI dose tolerance is increased by more than 50% when the dose is fractionated and the dose rate is below 10 cGy per minute. These measures have been found to increase relapse-free and overall survival rates while decreasing morbidity.[15,27] Total body irradiation is generally administered 2 or 3 times daily in order to shorten the time between the start of irradiation and bone marrow transplantation without increasing the fraction size and resultant morbidity. Total body irradiation techniques and fractionation schedules vary widely. Generally, a total dose between 12 and 15 Gy is delivered in 6 to 10 fractions of 1.5 to 2.0 Gy each at a dose rate of 5 to 10 cGy per minute. A minimum interval of 6 hours should elapse between fractions to permit normal cells to repair radiation damage to their DNA. In order to provide a homogeneous (within 10% of the prescribed) dose throughout the body, 2 opposing beams entering from either the anterior and posterior or the right and left lateral surfaces and dose compensators for the lungs and narrow portions of the body are used.

The Radiation Therapy Planning Process

Target Volumes

Prior to the delivery of an external beam radiation treatment, the targeted volume to be irradiated, the radiation dose and fractionation schedule, and the size, shape, and path of the radiation beam(s) to be utilized must be determined. The radiation beams are designed to encompass all of the tumor cells in the region while minimizing significant functional damage to normal tissues. Physical examination, operative findings, and imaging studies are used to define the identifiable extent of tumor cell collections, termed the *gross tumor volume* (GTV). The *clinical target volume* (CTV) includes the GTV in addition to areas of suspected tumor cell spread through infiltration of adjacent bone or soft tissues, lymph nodes, or cerebrospinal fluid. If the radiation therapy destroys all tumor cells within the CTV, loco-regional control of the tumor should result. Because the geographic position of the CTV within the patient may change with time (due to breathing, bladder filling, cardiac and gastrointestinal motion, etc), the patient may shift position during the treatment, the skin or fiducial markers used to position

the patient may move in relation to the internal tissues, and the laser beams and positioning markers used to position the patient daily have a finite width, the final volume targeted (the *planning target volume*, or PTV) must include a margin surrounding the CTV. The extent of the margin is generally between 2 and 10 millimeters, depending on the anatomic location of the CTV, reproducibility of patient setup, and degree of patient immobilization. Because of less target movement and better immobilization, the margin around intracranial tumors is generally less than that around chest or abdominal tumors.

Immobilization Devices

Custom devices are often constructed to reproducibly position the patient throughout the series of treatments and minimize patient movement during each treatment, especially if the margin between the CTV and PTV is small and obliquely angled beams are used. A wide variety of immobilization devices are used at different facilities. For tumors in the head or neck, the patient generally lies supine on a headrest supporting the posterior neck and occiput. The preformed plastic headrests used in the past have been replaced for precision treatment by a custom-molded cast or vacuum-molded bag filled with polystyrene beads. The head is most accurately positioned using a rigid frame attached to the skull or teeth, alveolar ridge, and hard palate, or a custom thermoplastic shell (Figure 9-3). A thermoplastic mask shaped to the skin overlying the facial structures is widely used but less accurate. The trunk and extremities may be immobilized in a

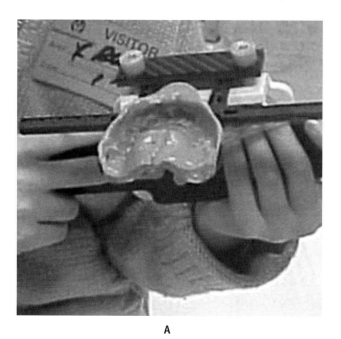

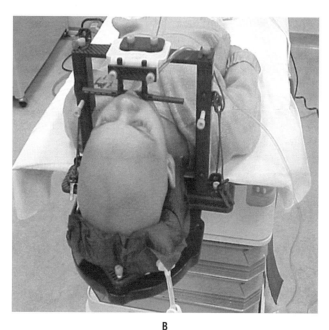

A   B

Figure 9-3 Reproducible immobilization of the head. (A) An impression is made of the patient's maxillary teeth and hard palate. (B) A bag filled with polystyrene beads is molded around the back of the patient's head and neck, the air is suctioned out of the bag, then the air valve is clamped to maintain the molded shape. With the patient lying in the headrest bag, the mouthpiece is then inserted. The mouthpiece is then fixed to the stereotactic localization system in a position that is airtight and comfortable. The mouthpiece remains screwed into the horizontal bar of the stereotactic system in this position for reproducibility of the head position throughout the course of treatment. The vertical bars of the system are attached to specific points of the treatment couch using pegs.

custom foam cradle or vacuum-molded bag filled with polystyrene beads (Figure 9-4). All of the devices are attached to a specified point on the treatment couch using rigid pegs to ensure reproducible positioning. For thoracic tumors, an active breathing control device and respiratory "gating" may be used. With this technique, the delivery of radiation is timed, or "gated," to occur periodically while the patient is holding his breath in inspiration so that the target is in the location at which the treatment was planned whenever the radiation beam is on.

Sedation

A radiation therapy session generally lasts between 10 and 45 minutes, depending on the complexity of the patient setup and beam arrangement and the number of radiation targets. Regulations require the patient to be in the radiation therapy room alone while the radiation beam is on. This can be a frightening experience, and deep sedation is usually required to prevent movement during irradiation in children under 5 years old for simple setups and under 8 years old when treatment time is prolonged or complex immobilization devices are used. Intravenous sedation with a short-acting agent such as propofol is preferable to a longer-acting one, which is more difficult to modulate and reverse in the case of oral agents. The patient intravenously sedated for therapy is usually able to eat and be discharged from medical monitoring within 1 hour of the radiation treatment. The sedative can be administered once or even twice daily throughout the course of radiation therapy without untoward effects. Because the child must have an empty stomach for sedation to be safely administered, treatment in the early morning is advisable to permit unrestricted oral intake throughout the remainder of the day. The rare patient undergoing a prolonged course of twice daily sedation should be considered for intravenous hydration and nutritional supplementation to make up for the limited hours of oral intake following

afternoon treatment. Sedation is not needed for most children over 8 years old, because the procedure is not uncomfortable unless the patient has preexisting pain related to the tumor or surgery.

Radiation Field Planning

Simple radiation beam arrangements (a single or 2 opposing beams) may be planned based on the internal bony anatomy visible using a fluoroscopic ("conventional") radiation simulation machine, or *simulator*. The geometry and movements of the simulator, gantry, and couch are identical to those of the linear accelerator, but the simulator produces x-rays in the kilovoltage diagnostic rather than the megavoltage therapeutic energy range. A conventional simulator produces 2-dimensional radiographs that show the location of the center and borders of the radiation field in relation to the patient's skeletal anatomy. A CT-simulator is similar but produces a 3-dimensional display of the tumor, soft tissues, and bones. During the simulation process, the treatment couch and gantry positions, patient position on the treatment couch, and treatment field size are determined. If a stereotactic positioning system is not used, temporary ink or permanent tattoo marks are made on the patient's skin to indicate how the patient should be positioned and where the radiation beam(s) should be directed. The marks on the patient indicate how the patient should be positioned during treatment in relation to laser beams 0.5 to 1.0 mm wide emanating from fixed points in the walls and ceiling of the treatment room and the light field emanating from the head of the treatment machine. When the patient is immobilized in a stereotactic device, positioning is accomplished using digital coordinates indicating the location of the device and/or alignment of the device with the laser beams (Figure 9-5). The point of intersection of the three laser beams is the isocenter, about which the machine gantry rotates and is usually the center of the

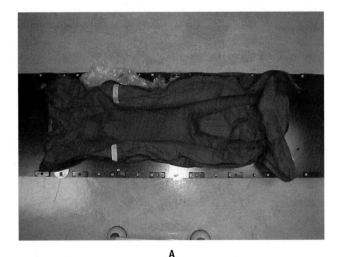

A

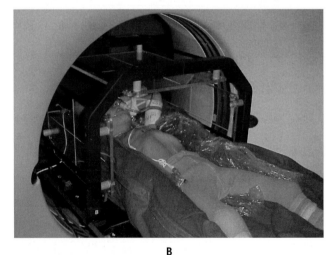

B

Figure 9-4 (A) Reproducible immobilization of the body. A bag filled with polystyrene beads is molded around the entire body or the body part to be treated. The air is suctioned out of the bag, then the air valve is clamped to maintain the molded shape. (B) The bag is fixed to specific points of the treatment couch during treatment using pegs.

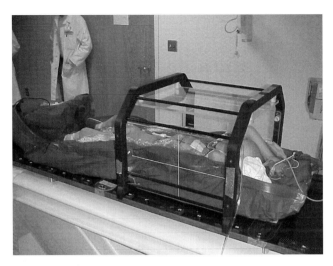

Figure 9-5 Patient positioning using laser alignment of a stereotactic body immobilization system. The immobilization device is shown in position for the treatment-planning CT scan. The 0.5-mm-thick white lines etched into the sides and top of the stereotactic positioning box are aligned with the 3 lasers prior to the treatment-planning CT scan and each radiation treatment. The fiducial markers seen on CT images and used to determine the couch coordinates during treatment are metal BBs that are 1 mm in diameter embedded at 4-cm intervals along the white lines.

target volume. X-ray, CT, or ultrasound images can be taken immediately prior to each treatment to assess whether the radiation beams will be traveling in the desired path through the patient. These *portal images* are compared with those produced during simulation or computer-based treatment planning. The patient or treatment couch position is then adjusted as necessary to match the planned beam pathway. Portal images are taken at least once weekly throughout the treatment course to ensure that the radiation beams are passing through the intended tissues.

Conformal therapy is radiation treatment given using multiple radiation beams, each of which is custom-shaped or intensity-modulated to create a dose distribution that conforms to the target as defined by GTV contours drawn on multiple slices from a "treatment-planning" CT study that is performed with the patient immobilized in the treatment position using custom-made devices. Computed tomography slices are generally taken at intervals of 2 to 3 millimeters, and the GTV and any normal tissues of interest are manually contoured on each slice in which they appear. A CT scan is the basis for treatment planning rather than an MRI scan or positron emission tomography (PET) scan because it produces an undistorted 3-dimensional representation of the stereotactic immobilization system, skin surface, and internal anatomy and indicates the electron density of the patient's internal organs. The electron density information is essential for accurate calculation of absorption of the radiation beam. Magnetic resonance imaging images contain some geographic distortion and do not provide electron density information.

In addition to the GTV, normal tissues are contoured so that their radiation dose can be calculated and minimized. Many tumors (eg, central nervous system tumors and extremity sarcomas) are better delineated on MRI than CT scan. In addition, radiation therapy may follow surgical resection and/or chemotherapy treatment of a tumor for which irradiation of the pretreatment volume is desired. In either situation, it is helpful to utilize image registration software that transforms the coordinate system of a prior MRI, PET, single-photon emission computed tomography, or CT scan to match that of the treatment-planning CT study. The prior study is then overlaid on the treatment-planning study using image fusion software so that the target volume can be outlined most accurately. The radiation oncologist, together with the radiation physicist and/or dosimetrist, contours the GTV and normal tissues of interest on each image of the treatment-planning CT. After the GTV has been fully contoured, the treatment planning software expands the GTV 3-dimensionally by the specified number of millimeters to create the CTV and PTV.

The next step in the conformal therapy process is to select the energy, number, and direction of the beams to be used. Each modern linear accelerator has a defined set of 1 to 3 photon and 5 to 6 electron energies from which to choose. Electrons or low-energy (6-10 MV) photons are advantageous for the treatment of tumors in children and thin adults and for superficially located targets in large patients because they provide maximum dose to target areas close to the skin surface and less radiation dose than high-energy photons to normal tissues in the exit path of the radiation beam. High-energy (16-25 MV) photons underdose tissues within 3 cm of their entry point in relation to deeper tissues. The choice of beam number and directions is unlimited. A comparison of the dose distribution obtained in treating an adrenal neuroblastoma with 6 MV photons using 1 beam, 2 oblique opposing beams, 8 conformal beams, and the same 8 beams using IMRT is shown in Figure 9-6. A comparison of the dose distribution obtained in treating a supratentorial primitive neuroectodermal tumor with 6 MV photons using opposing lateral beams, 8 conformal beams, and the same 8 beams using IMRT is shown in Figure 9-7. Using one beam, the target receives a lower dose than do normal tissues (eg, vertebral body and spinal cord) in the beam path. With 2 opposing beams, the dose is nearly homogenous throughout the beam path, with normal tissues receiving approximately the same dose as the target. Using a higher number of nonopposing beams whose isocenter is in the target volume permits preferential irradiation of the target with sparing of the surrounding organs. The same conformal beam arrangement spares normal tissues to a greater extent when IMRT is incorporated.

Tumors located in the trunk and extremities are typically treated with all beams traveling through the axial plane. Brain tumors, in contrast, are readily treated using beams whose pathways to the tumor transverse multiple planes. The "noncoplanar" beam arrangement is feasible because the head is spatially separated from the rest of the

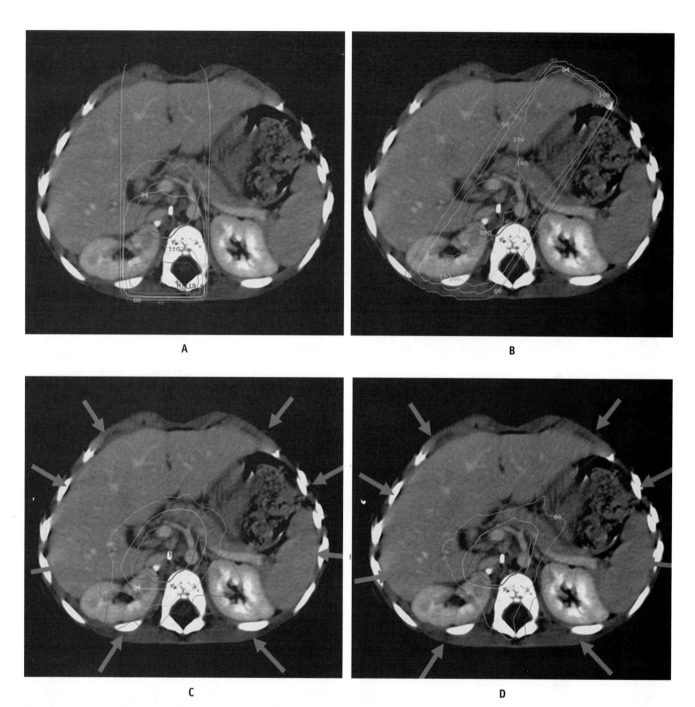

Figure 9-6 Comparison of treatment plans for a right adrenal neuroblastoma. The planning target volume (PTV) is in red (see Plate 33). The 94, 60, and 40 isodose surfaces (IDS) are shown in each illustration. (A) Single posterior beam. The dose is highest 1 to 2 cm from the posterior body surface and decreases gradually as the beam travels anteriorly. The PTV is encompassed by the 86 IDS, whereas the spinal cord is encompassed by the 115 IDS. Forty-six percent of the right kidney also receives a higher dose than the PTV and is within the 94 IDS. The maximum dose at this axial level is 119, 38% higher than the minimum dose to the PTV. (B) Two opposing oblique beams. The beams are angled obliquely to reduce the proportion of the liver and left kidney receiving a significant dose compared with what they would receive from straight anterior and posterior beams. The obliquity increases the proportion of the right kidney receiving a high dose, however. The dose is fairly homogeneous throughout the beam path. The 94 IDS encompasses the PTV, 87% of the right kidney, and 14% of the liver. The maximum dose is deposited in normal tissues rather than the PTV, and is 107 at this axial level. (C) Eight coplanar non-IMRT (3-dimensional conformal) beams. The 94 IDS encompasses and conforms to the shape of the PTV. The 60 IDS encompasses 10 to 14 mm of normal tissue surrounding the PTV, including less than 1% of the left kidney, 9% of the liver, and 42% of the right kidney. The 40 IDS encompasses 26% of the left kidney, 20% of the liver, and 89% of the right kidney. Unlike the single-beam and opposing-beam plans, the maximum radiation dose (99 at this axial level) is within the PTV. (D) Eight coplanar IMRT beams. The 94 IDS encompasses the PTV. The liver and right kidney receive lower doses than with the other plans. The 60 IDS encompasses none of the left kidney, 7% of the liver, and 20% of the right kidney. The 40 IDS encompasses 2% of the left kidney, 15% of the liver, and 30% of the right kidney. Typical of IMRT plans, the dose is less homogeneous within the PTV (maximum dose on this axial level 105) than in the 8-beam non-IMRT plan. **See Plate 33 for color image.**

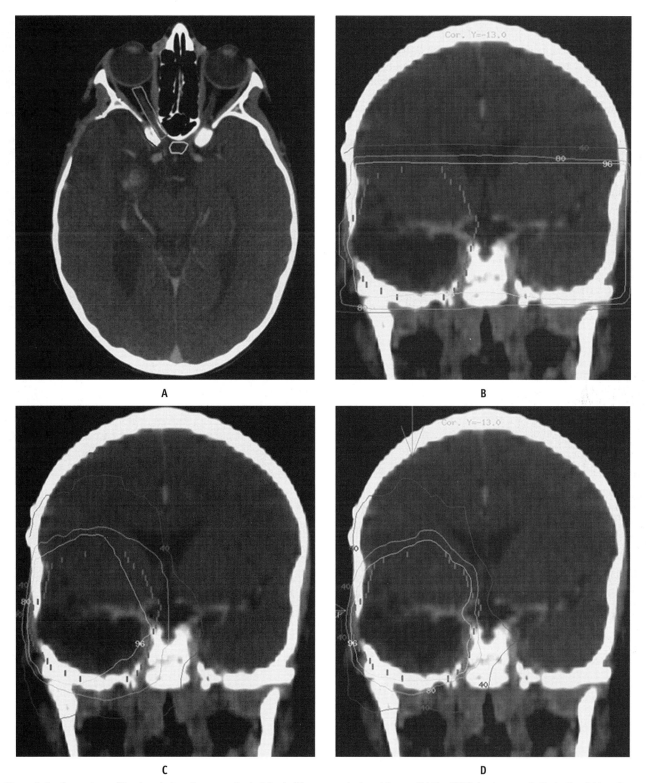

A

B

C

D

Figure 9-7 Comparison of treatment plans for a supratentorial primitive neuroectodermal tumor. (A) The GTV is in close proximity to the right optic nerve (outlined in red) and optic chiasm (outlined in orange). In illustrations B-D, the margins of the PTV are indicated by red dashes and the 96, 80, and 40 IDSs are shown (see Plate 34). (B) Two opposing lateral beams. The dose to the contralateral side of the brain, bilateral optic nerves, and optic chiasm is equal to the dose (minimum of 96) to the PTV. Maximum dose is 105. (C) Eight noncoplanar non-IMRT (3-dimensional conformal) beams. To avoid exceeding the tolerance dose of the optic chiasm and right optic nerve, the superior-medial and inferior-medial portions of the PTV must be underdosed and are not encompassed by the 96 IDS. The optic chiasm, right optic nerve, and pituitary gland are within the 80 IDS. In contrast to the opposing lateral beam plan, almost all of the right cerebral hemisphere is spared from receiving high-dose radiation and is outside the 40 IDS. Maximum dose is 104. (D) Eight noncoplanar IMRT beams. The same 8 beams shown in Figure 9-6C produce isodose surfaces that conform to the PTV and exclude the optic chiasm, right optic nerve, and pituitary gland better when IMRT is used. The 96 IDS encompasses the entire PTV except where it overlaps the optic chiasm and distal optic nerve. The optic chiasm, right optic nerve, and pituitary gland are mostly outside the 80 IDS. The volume of normal brain within the 80 and 40 IDSs is smaller than in the non-IMRT plan in Figure 9-6C. Maximum dose is 106. **See Plate 34 for color image.**

body and desirable because it decreases the overlap of beam paths outside the PTV. The dose distributions obtained with conformal 8-beam IMRT coplanar and non-coplanar plans are compared in Figure 9-8, demonstrating the lower doses to normal brain parenchyma achieved with the noncoplanar beam arrangement. More beams and noncoplanar beams decrease the volume of normal tissues receiving a high radiation dose, in exchange for increasing the normal tissue volume receiving relatively low radiation doses. Although decreasing the radiation dose diminishes the incidence and severity of most normal tissue toxicities, giving a moderate dose to a larger volume may result in a higher incidence of radiation-induced second malignancies. The IMRT technique

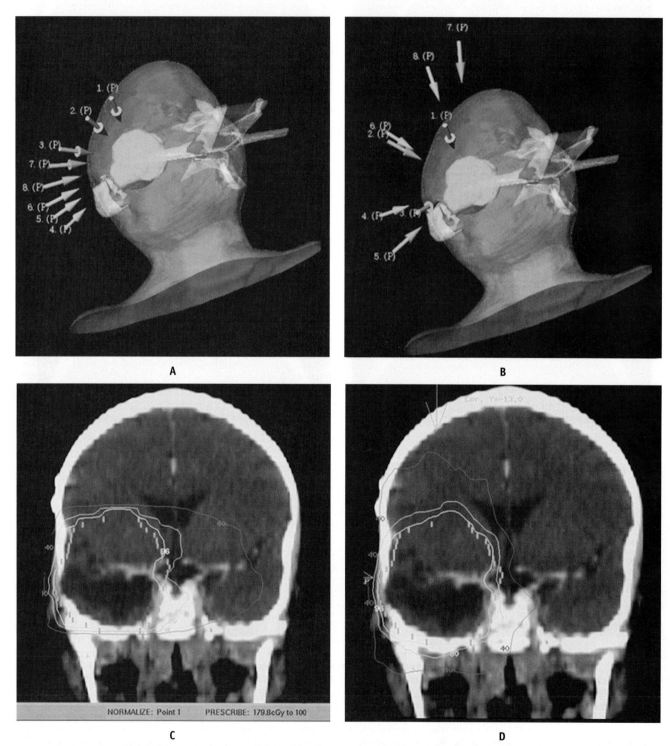

Figure 9-8 Comparison of coplanar and noncoplanar IMRT treatment plans for the supratentorial primitive neuroectodermal tumor in Figure 9-7. A and B show 3-dimensional reconstructions of the PTV in red and the patient's head and neck with the immobilization mouthpiece in place in brown. The green arrows indicate the central axes of the 8 radiation beams in a coplanar (A) and noncoplanar (B) plan (see Plate 35). The isodose distribution of the coplanar plan is shown in C, and that of the noncoplanar plan is shown in D. The noncoplanar plan provides equal coverage of the PTV with greater dose homogeneity (maximum dose 106 vs 110) and less dosage to the optic nerves, optic chiasm, pituitary, and contralateral side of the brain. **See Plate 35 for color image.**

requires the radiation beam to be on longer than other techniques, significantly raising the "integral" dose delivered to normal tissues through leakage of radiation through the linear accelerator head and multileaf collimator. Careful monitoring over decades will be required to determine whether multibeam, noncoplanar, and IMRT therapy increase the risk for a second malignancy arising in normal tissues exposed to a low radiation dose.

The radiation beams are usually custom-shaped to match the shape of the target volume and minimize the dose to normal tissues. The desired shape of the beam can be drawn on 2-dimensional film or digital radiographs generated by the conventional radiation simulator. Beam shaping in 3 dimensions for non-IMRT conformal therapy is accomplished using "virtual simulation" software into which CT-based 3-dimensional reconstructions of the PTV and relevant normal tissues are visualized from the perspective of the radiation beam (*beam's-eye view*). The beam contour is drawn to encompass the PTV while excluding normal tissues. Whether designed in 2 or 3 dimensions, the beam is shaped as it exits the linear accelerator head using high-density metal approximately 8 centimeters thick. Most modern accelerators are equipped with a *multileaf collimator* consisting of numerous (usually 120) tungsten leaves that are electronically positioned to block the photon beam in areas outside the designated beam shape (Figure 9-9). For electron beams and accelerators not equipped with a multileaf collimator, a set of custom-shaped lead-alloy blocks are manually molded for each beam and fixed onto a Lucite tray that is mounted on the accelerator head in the path of the beam. Beam shapes are not drawn for IMRT treatments, because the treatment planning

software creates a continuously changing beam shape defined by the moving leaves of the multileaf collimator in order to better concentrate the radiation dose within the target volume.

In non-IMRT treatment planning, the planner decides on the energy and number of radiation beams to be used, then chooses a direction, size, shape, and relative weighting for each beam. The weighting is the proportion of the total dose that is delivered by that particular beam. For treatments incorporating only a single or 2 opposing beams, a simple point calculation of the resultant dose along the central axis of the beam at a specified depth is then performed based on the beam energy, radiation field size, and tissue depth. To create a 3-dimensional plan, the planner inputs all the beam parameters into the treatment planning software, which then calculates the resulting distribution of radiation dose in the tumor and all normal tissues imaged in the treatment-planning CT scan. The software displays the absolute or relative radiation doses as isodose curves overlaid on 2-dimensional CT images and 3-dimensional anatomic reconstructions of the patient. The dose distributions in the target volume and organs of interest are also displayed graphically by dose-volume histograms, which plot the percentage of the target or organ receiving any specified dose. The planner then evaluates how well the inputted plan achieves the objective of distributing the desired dose uniformly within the PTV while avoiding radiation-induced damage to the surrounding normal tissues. If the radiation dose distribution is judged suboptimal, the planner inputs an alternate plan with a different number, direction, shape, and/or relative weighting of beams. Additional plan modifications are made and tested based on comparison of the resulting isodose distributions. Through this iterative process, called *forward planning*, the plan is honed until a satisfactory dose distribution is achieved.

Intensity-modulated radiation therapy is a sophisticated type of conformal therapy in which the radiation beam shape changes while the beam is on, resulting in the delivery of arbitrarily varying intensities of radiation across the beam. In contrast, unwedged non-IMRT radiation beams deliver a nearly uniform intensity of radiation throughout the beam area. Intensity-modulated radiation therapy systems became commercially available in the United States in 1996 and are increasingly popular for the treatment of a variety of childhood as well as adult tumors because they can reduce the radiation dose to normal tissues outside the target volume compared with other conformal techniques. Intensity-modulated radiation therapy can also be used to match the intensity of radiation delivered to different regions of the target volume to the concentration of tumor cells within each region. One use of this *simultaneous integrated boost* technique is to deliver a high radiation dose to areas of gross tumor identified on imaging studies while simultaneously delivering a moderate dose to suspected areas of microscopic disease spread (eg, regional lymph nodes or ventricles).

The process of planning for IMRT, called *reverse planning*, makes use of the analytic, not just calculating, capa-

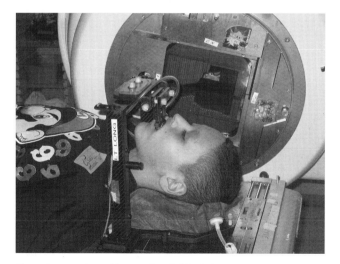

Figure 9-9 Patient with acute lymphoblastic leukemia positioned for whole-cranial irradiation. The leaves of the multileaf collimator block the lateral radiation beam in the areas outside of the desired beam path, shielding the patient's anterior eyes, nose, mouth, and anterior and posterior neck, including the thyroid gland, larynx, and mucosa of the aerodigestive tract, from radiation. The unblocked portion of the radiation beam matches the position and shape of the patient's cranium and upper cervical spinal cord.

bilities of the computer. Similar to forward planning, the planner inputs the energy, number, and directions of the radiation beams to be used. Instead of choosing the shape and weighting of the beams, however, the planner inputs the desired radiation dose distribution within the target volume and organs of interest and the relative importance of achieving the desired distribution within each organ. Through an iterative process, the computer-based algorithm then designs a radiation intensity pattern for each beam that cumulatively achieves the closest possible approximation to the requested dose distribution. This is made possible by computer control of the movement of the multileaf collimator while the radiation beam is on such that a different amount of radiation is transmitted through every area of the radiation beam. In effect, each radiation beam is broken up into hundreds of beamlets, each carrying a different radiation intensity.

In the forward process used for non-IMRT conformal therapy planning, the planner inputs all the radiation beam parameters, and the computer calculates the resultant dose distribution. In the inverse process used for IMRT planning, the planner inputs the desired dose distribution and the computer determines a set of beamlet intensities that will most closely produce that distribution. Either 3-dimensional planning process is a *virtual simulation*, in which the radiation treatment is designed using a volumetric image of the patient in treatment position. After the geometric isocenter of the radiation beams is determined, orthogonal (usually anterior-posterior and lateral) digitally reconstructed radiographs showing beam's-eye views of the patient's bony anatomy in relation to the isocenter are generated. These radiographs, reconstructed from the treatment-planning CT images, are used like conventional simulator radiographs to compare with portal images taken during the course of treatment to ensure proper patient positioning.

Brachytherapy

Brachytherapy (meaning "close" therapy) refers to treatment using small radioactive sources that are placed within or close to the tumor. It has been used to treat human cancers since the discovery of Radium-226 in 1898. Radioactive sources are unstable isotopes (eg, Palladium-103, Ruthenium-106, Iodine-125, Cesium-137, Iridium-192) that decay to a stable state by the spontaneous emission of particles or photons of characteristic energies. The sources are encapsulated in individual cylindrical or seed-shaped metal carriers for treatment. Brachytherapy concentrates the radiation dose within the tumor to a far greater extent than does teletherapy. Whereas teletherapy beams, including protons and carbon ions, deposit significant amounts of radiation in all the normal tissues along their pathway to the tumor, brachytherapy sources emit their radiation from within or in close proximity to the tumor. The radiation dose to tissues decreases exponentially as the distance from the source increases. This relationship ensures that the tumor in which a source is implanted will receive a far higher

radiation dose than the surrounding tissues. The volume effectively irradiated by a source is dependent on the energies emitted by the isotope's radioactive decay process. Brachytherapy radiation dissipates rapidly within millimeters to centimeters from the source, because the emitted energies (generally less than 1 MeV) are far lower than megavoltage teletherapy rays.

A specific isotope is selected for a particular brachytherapy application based on the desired volume and duration of treatment. When the target volume extends only millimeters from the source, an isotope that emits low-energy radiation is chosen. The effectively irradiated volume can be expanded by using additional sources and/or higher-energy isotopes. Brachytherapy can be delivered at either a high dose rate (approximately 200 cGy per minute) for a period of minutes or a low dose rate (approximately 1 cGy per minute) over a period of 1 to 5 days. Isotopes that have a rapid disintegration rate (short half-life), such as Iodine-125, may either be removed from the patient after the desired radiation dose has been delivered (as in an episcleral plaque for retinoblastoma, Figure 9-10) or remain in the target tissue permanently (as in the prostate gland).

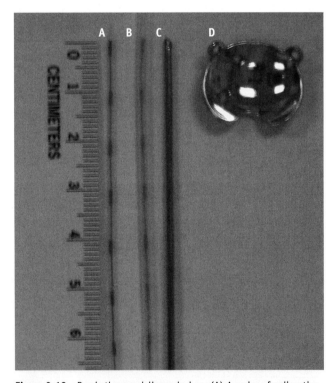

Figure 9-10 Brachytherapy delivery devices. (A) A series of radioactive Iridium-192 seeds spaced 1 cm apart in a flexible plastic strand. (B) The Iridium-192 strand threaded inside a flexible, hollow plastic catheter for implantation in the body. (C) A hollow, sharp-tipped rigid metal probe that can penetrate connective tissue and tumors. A strand of radioactive seeds is then threaded through the probe into the target volume. The probe is then retracted, leaving the radioactive strand in place. (D) An episcleral plaque for Ruthenium-106 treatment of retinoblastoma. The concave shape conforms to the outer surface of the sclera. The plaque is sutured in place through the 2 eyelets extending from the 11 o'clock and 1 o'clock positions.

High-dose-rate treatments are typically done on an outpatient basis and have the advantage of patient convenience. Low-dose-rate brachytherapy provides the biologic advantage of treating mitotically active tumor cells while they are in the radiosensitive phases of their cell cycle.

Most locations in the body may be considered for brachytherapy treatment. Tumors close to the body surface, such as retinoblastoma, can be treated with radioactive seeds embedded in a surface mold shaped to conform to the sclera. More deeply seated tumors such as soft-tissue sarcomas may be treated using *interstitial brachytherapy*, in which radioactive sources are permanently implanted or thin, hollow plastic catheters are temporarily implanted within the tumor. If catheters are implanted, a string of radioactive sources are later threaded through the catheter for the desired period of irradiation, after which both the string of sources and the catheters are removed. Tumors within or close to natural body cavities (eg, the vagina, uterus, rectum, or trachea) or surgical cavities (eg, following resection of a brain or breast tumor) may be treated using *intracavitary brachytherapy*, in which radioactive sources or fluid is inserted temporarily into the cavity.

The childhood tumor most commonly treated with brachytherapy is localized retinoblastoma, which is a small, discrete tumor located close to the body surface. The use of brachytherapy for other childhood tumors is limited by target volume size and location. The sources must be able to be positioned so as to deliver an effective radiation dose to the entire volume suspected of containing malignant cells without causing serious toxicity to critical normal tissues in the area. Radiation is delivered at a far faster rate by brachytherapy than teletherapy, overwhelming the capacity of normal cells to repair damage to their DNA. The extremely high radiation dose and dose rate adjacent to a brachytherapy source contraindicate placement next to a major nerve or blood vessel. Sources are not readily placed within bone and those adjacent to bone can cause osteoradionecrosis. Most tumors that would be suitable for brachytherapy are surgically resected instead, because resection is generally the first treatment option for local control. Placement of interstitial brachytherapy catheters intraoperatively may be considered to sterilize microscopic residual disease at a contaminated resection margin. Interstitial brachytherapy has been used with good results for selected pediatric soft-tissue sarcomas. Localized recurrences of nasopharyngeal carcinoma in teenagers have been controlled with intracavitary brachytherapy.

Acknowledgment

Arthur Olch, PhD, provided many contributions, including developing the treatment plans shown in Figures 9-6 through 9-8.

References

1. Elkind MM, Whitmore GF. *The Radiobiology of Cultured Mammalian Cells.* New York: Gordon & Breach; 1967.
2. Kemp CJ, Sun S, Gurley KE. p 53 induction and apoptosis in response to radio- and chemotherapy in vivo is tumor-type-dependent. *Cancer Res.* 2001;61:327.
3. Belka C, Jendrossek V, Pruschy M, et al. Apoptosis-modulating agents in combination with radiotherapy-current status and outlook. *Int J Radiat Oncol Biol Phys.* 2004;58:542–554.
4. Hallahan DE, Sukhatme VP, Sherman ML, et al. Protein kinase C mediates x-ray inducibility of nuclear signal transducers EGRI and JUN. *Proc Natl Acad Sci USA.* 1991;88:2156.
5. Sherman ML, Datta R, Hallahan DE, et al. Tumor necrosis factor gene expression is transcriptionally and post-transcriptionally regulated by ionizing radiation in human myeloid leukemic cells and peripheral blood monocytes. *J Clin Invest.* 1991;87:1794.
6. Sherman ML, Datta R, Hallahan DE, et al. Ionizing radiation regulates expression of the *c-jun* proto-oncogene. *Proc Natl Acad Sci USA.* 1990;87:5663.
7. Littbrand B, Revesz L. The effect of oxygen on cellular survival and recovery after radiation. *Br J Radiol.* 1969;42:914.
8. Barendsen G. Responses of cultured cells, tumors and normal tissues to radiations of different linear energy transfer. *Curr Top Radiat Res.* 1968;4:295.
9. Clarke H, Pallister CJ. The impact of anaemia on outcome in cancer. *Clin Lab Haematol.* 2005;27:1–13.
10. Dische S: What have we learnt form hyperbaric oxygen? *Radiother Oncol.* 1991;20(suppl 1):71.
11. Overgaard J, Hansen HS, Overgaard M, et al. A randomized doubleblind phase III study of nimorazole as a hypoxic radiosensitizer of primary radiotherapy in supraglottic larynx and pharynx carcinoma. Results of the Danish Head and Neck Cancer Study (DAHANCA) Protocol 5-85. *Radiother Oncol.* 1998;46:135.
12. Denny WA, Wilson WR. Tirapazamine: a bioreductive anticancer drug that exploits tumor hypoxia. *Expert Opin Investig Drugs.* 2000;9:2889.
13. Mayr NA, Yuh WT, Oberley LW, et al. Serial changes in tumor oxygenation during the early phase of radiation therapy in cervical cancer: are we quantitating hypoxia change? *Int J Radiat Oncol Biol Phys.* 2001;49:282.
14. Withers HR. Cell cycle redistribution as a factor in multi-fraction irradiation. *Radiology.* 1975;114:199.
15. Thomas ED, Clift RA, Hersman J, et al. Marrow transplantation for acute nonlymphoblastic leukemic in first remission using fractionated or single-dose irradiation. *Int J Radiat Oncol Biol Phys.* 1982;8:817–821.
16. Withers HR, Thames HD, Peters LJ. Differences in the fractionation response of acute and late-responding tissues. In: Karcher KH, Kogelnik HD, Reinartz G, eds. *Progress in radio-oncology II.* New York: Raven, 1982;287–296.
17. Betzen SM. Repopulation in radiation oncology: Perspectives of clinical research. *Int J Radiat Biol.* 2003;79:581–585.
18. Kearne TJ, Fyles A, O'Sullivan B, et al. The effect of treatment duration on local control of squamous carcinoma of the tonsil and carcinoma of the cervix. *Semin Radiat Oncol.* 1992;2:26.
19. Fowler JF, Lindstrom MJ. Loss of local control with prolongation in radiotherapy. *Int J Radiat Oncol Biol Phys.* 1992;23:457.
20. Horior JC, LeFur R, Nguyen T, et al. Hyperfractionation versus conventional fractionation in oropharyngeal carcinoma: Final analysis of a randomized trial of the EORTC cooperative group of radiotherapy. *Radiother Oncol.* 1992;25:231–241B.
21. Fu KK, Pajak TF, Trotti A, et al. A Radiation Therapy Oncology Group (RTOG) Phase III randomized study to compare hyperfractionation and two variants of accelerated fractionation to standard fractionation radiotherapy for head and neck squamous cell carcinomas: First report of RTOG 9003. *Int J Radiat Oncol Biol Phys.* 2000;48:7–16.
22. Marcus KJ, Dutton SC, Barnes P, et al. A phase I trial of etanidazole and hyperfractionated radiotherapy in children with diffuse brainstem glioma. *Int J Radiat Oncol Biol Phys.* 2003;55:1182–1185.
23. Freeman CR, Bourgouin PM, Sanford RA, et al. Long-term survivors of childhood brain stem gliomas treated with hyperfractionated radiotherapy. Clinical characteristics and treatment related toxicities. The Pediatric Oncology Group. *Cancer.* 1996;77:555–562.
24. Barendsen GW. Response of cultured cells, tumours, and normal tissues to radiations of different linear energy transfer. *Curr Top Radiat Res.* 1968;4:293.
25. St Clair WH, Adams JA, Bues M, et al. Advantage of protons compared to conventional x-ray or IMRT in the treatment of a pediatric patient with medulloblastoma. *Int J Radiat Oncol Bio Phys.* 2004;58:727–734.
26. Kirsch DG, Tarbell NJ. New technologies in radiation therapy for pediatric brain tumors: The rationale for proton radiation therapy. *Pediatr Blood Cancer.* 2004;42:461–464.
27. Depledge MH, Barrett A. Dose-rate dependence of lung damage after total body irradiation in mice. *Int J Radiat Biol Relat Stud Phys Chem Med.* 1982;41:325–334.

The Role of Autologous and Allogeneic Hematopoietic Cell Transplantation in Pediatric Cancer Therapy

Michael A. Pulsipher and Peter J. Shaw

Introduction: History and Rationale

Blood marrow or hematopoietic cell transplantation (BMT or HCT) describes the procedure of giving cells (hematopoietic progenitor or stem cells, HPC or HSC) that can reconstitute the hematopoietic system of a patient. For the first 30 years of this procedure, cells used were invariably obtained from the bone marrow (BM), but in the past decade HPCs have also been obtained from the peripheral blood or umbilical cord blood. The earliest BM transplants failed, with no engraftment in the first 200 transplants reported by 1970[1] except in the case of identical twins.[2] During the 1960s and early 1970s, recognition of human leukocyte antigens (HLA) led to dramatically improved engraftment and BM reconstitution in recipients receiving HLA-matched HPCs.

At the same time, chemotherapy and radiotherapy used to control cancer, particularly in leukemia, produced toxicity to the normal BM (myelotoxicity) that was dose limiting. Commonly, chemotherapeutic agents or irradiation have a dose–response effect that continues at doses above those that cause severe marrow toxicity. Where other organ toxicity does not limit the dose, the dose can be escalated if HPCs are used to rescue the patient from the myelotoxicity of the high-dose therapy.

Hematopoietic cell transplantation is currently used in 3 clinical scenarios: (1) treatment of malignancies, (2) replacement or modulation of an absent or poorly functioning hematopoietic or immune system, and (3) treatment of genetic diseases in which expression of the affected gene product in circulating hematopoietic cells alone is adequate to produce a clinically meaningful result. This chapter will focus on the role of HCT in pediatric cancer care.

Two major transplant approaches are currently in use: autologous (patient HPCs) and allogeneic (related or unrelated donor HPCs). Autologous approaches treat cancer by exposing patients to mega-dose therapy with the intent of overcoming resistance in tumor cells, followed by infusion of the patient's previously stored HPCs. Allogeneic approaches may involve high-dose therapy as well, but because of immunologic differences between the donor and recipient, an additional graft-versus-tumor (GvT) or graft-versus-leukemia (GvL) treatment effect can occur. Although autologous approaches are associated with less toxicity, many malignancies are resistant to mega-dose therapy alone and/or involve the BM, thus requiring allogeneic approaches for optimal outcome.

Human Leukocyte Antigen Matching and Hematopoietic Progenitor Cell Sources

Essential to successful allogeneic HCT is appropriate matching of loci in the major histocompatibility complex located on chromosome 6 called human leukocyte antigens (see Figure 10-1). Human leukocyte antigen class I (A, B, C, etc) and class II (DRB1, DQB1, etc) alleles are highly polymorphic, making matching of unrelated donors a challenge for some patients, especially those of certain racial groups (eg, African Americans, Hispanics). Because full siblings of cancer patients have a 25% chance of being HLA matched, they have been the preferred source of allogeneic HPCs. Early serologic techniques of HLA assessment defined a number of HLA antigens, but more precise DNA methodologies have shown HLA allele-level mismatches in up to 40% of serologic HLA antigen matches. These differences have been found to be clinically relevant, and most centers now perform DNA-based allele-level HLA typing on unrelated donors. Current levels of matching for unrelated allogeneic marrow transplantation result in better outcomes when at least 7 of the 8 HLA-A, -B, -C, and -DRB1 antigens are matched between the donor and the recipient at the allele level (termed a 7/8 or 8/8 match).[3] Although several large studies have shown that DRB1 antigen mismatches are associated with increased graft-versus-host disease (GVHD) and mortality,[4] some small studies have suggested that mismatches at 2 other class II antigens, DQB1 and DPB1, may be associated with more severe GVHD.[5,6] Although matching for the DQB1 and DPB1 class II antigens is not performed by all centers, when HLA-A, -B, -C, -DRB1, and -DQB1 are assessed, the result is termed a 10/10 match. The addition of matching for DPB1 is termed a 12/12 match.

If a fully or near fully HLA-matched family member is not available, 2 other commonly used HPC sources are unrelated donors or unrelated umbilical cord blood.

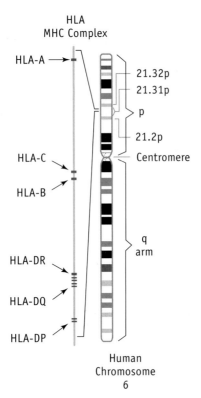

HLA
MHC Complex

HLA-A

21.32p
21.31p

p

21.2p

Centromere

HLA-C

HLA-B

q
arm

HLA-DR

HLA-DQ

HLA-DP

Human
Chromosome
6

Figure 10-1 Human leukocyte antigens.

Unrelated adult donors can give standard BM (via aspiration of the posterior iliac crests) or peripheral blood stem cells (PBSC) obtained by stimulation of the donor BM by cytokines (eg, G-CSF), resulting in increased numbers of HPC in the circulation, followed by leukapheresis. Unrelated cord blood has resulted in successful transplantation with less stringent HLA matching requirements, allowing recipients without an HLA-matched donor the opportunity to undergo transplantation.[7,8] Each source of HPC has advantages and challenges, and careful consideration of clinical circumstances is required to determine the best source for a given patient (see Table 10-1).

Special Considerations for Hospitalized Hematopoietic Cell Transplantation Patients

Patients undergoing myeloablative HCT procedures resemble those receiving intensive chemotherapy induction regimens (acute myeloid leukemia [AML] induction, acute lymphoblastic leukemia [ALL] reinduction after relapse). Major care issues include prevention and treatment of nausea, treatment of febrile neutropenia and infections, painful mucositis and poor nutrition, organ damage secondary to therapy or infection, and transfusion support. Chemotherapy and radiation given for HCT-preparative regimens result in toxicities that must be carefully addressed. Almost all myeloablative chemotherapy regimens are highly emetogenic and require maximal symptom control. Fluid balance and electrolytes need to be monitored closely, because many of the drugs require aggressive fluid regimens and can cause significant renal impairment or syndrome of inappropriate antidiuretic hormone secretion. Table 10-2 outlines special considerations necessary when giving agents commonly found in transplant-preparative regimens.

Graft-Versus-Host Disease

Immunologic differences between donor and patient HLA proteins and other important minor HLAs can initiate an immune response of either the recipient white blood cells (WBCs) against the graft (resulting in rejection) or the graft WBCs against the recipient (resulting in GVHD). Intense immune suppression of the patient during the transplant preparative regimen significantly decreases the number of viable T-cells in the recipient, decreasing the risk of rejection. T-cells from the donor are necessary for engraftment, but too much T-cell activity leads to excessive GVHD. An approach to prevention of GVHD (termed "GVHD prophylaxis") using medications such as cycloporine or methotrexate, or graft manipulation such as T-cell depletion, is essential to successful transplantation. A balance of enough donor T-cell

Table 10-1				
Hematopoietic progenitor cell sources: Advantages and disadvantages.				
	Related BM	**Unrelated BM**	**RD&UD PBSC**	**Unrelated CB**
Advantages	• Rapid acquisition • Least GVHD • Rapid immune recovery	• More GvL • Moderate immune recovery	• More GvL • Less early TRM due to rapid immune recovery	• Rapid acquisition • More GvL • Donor is available for >90% of patients
Disadvantages	• Less GvL • Higher relapse	• Slow acquisition • More GVHD than RD • Higher TRM	• Slow acquisition • More chronic GVHD than BM	• Higher early TRM due to slow immune recovery • Higher rate of rejection

Table 10-2

Preparative regimen concerns specific to given agents.

Agent	Major Toxicities/Effects/Special Considerations
Total Body Irradiation	• Improved outcomes in lymphoid and high-risk disease. • Can reach sites chemotherapy cannot (CNS, testes) and is not cell-cycle dependent. • Myeloablative at standard doses used for TBI (typically 1200 to 1440 cGy). • Further dose escalation limited by GI toxicity. • Nausea and vomiting occur frequently. • Transplant doses increase risk of hemorrhagic cystitis, which may be decreased with MESNA and hydration.
Cyclophosphamide	• Transplant doses of 120 mg/kg (combined with TBI or busulfan) are usually well tolerated. • Higher doses may cause cardiac toxicity, with reported congestive cardiac failure and myocardial necrosis. Protocols using 200 mg/kg usually recommend close observation of cardiac function and fluid balance. • Is excreted in sweat and urine and can cause skin toxicity. Some recommend catheterization; most use frequent voiding and/or barrier creams.

Busulfan	• Achieves high CNS levels and increases risk of seizures: anticonvulsant prophylaxis with phenytoin or benzodiazepines is generally performed.
	• Liver toxicity/VOD risk can be decreased by:
	  1. Use of intravenous line, careful monitoring of drug levels.
	  2. Allowing time for the liver to recover between busulfan and other agents.

Thiotepa	• Good CNS penetration, used frequently for brain tumors. Can cause CNS toxicity. • Can produce significant skin toxicity; frequent bathing required.
Melphalan	• Nephrotoxic—needs aggressive hydration; avoid concomitant nephrotoxins and watch for third spacing. • Unstable—infusion should be completed within 60 minutes of reconstitution.

Carboplatin	• Patients may develop renal impairment during the course of therapy, affecting clearance of further doses of carboplatin and melphalan. Attempts to reduce the risk of severe toxicity as a result of this include:
	  • Adjusting doses according to GFR pre-BMT.
	  • Making serial estimates of GFR during the days of chemotherapy.
	  • Reducing or eliminating doses of other nephrotoxins.

activity to facilitate engraftment and a GvT effect without causing significant GVHD is optimal.

Graft-versus-host disease occurs when tissue damage associated with chemotherapy, radiation, or infection combine with major or minor histocompatibility differences between the graft and the recipient resulting in increased levels of inflammatory cytokines (IL-1, IL-2, tumor necrosis factor, γ-interferon).[9] Reduced-intensity preparative regimens have resulted in decreased rates of GVHD but generally have higher rates of relapse. Elimination of T cells from the graft also markedly decreases the incidence of GVHD; however, this intense immune suppression leads to increased infection, rejection, relapse, and Epstein-Barr virus (EBV) lymphoproliferative disorders. Because outcomes of T-depleted approaches are equivalent or inferior to T-cell-containing regimens, most centers continue to use T-cell-containing HPCs.

Early after transplantation, the most common form of GVHD is termed "acute" and presents with skin rash, gastrointestinal symptoms (measured by volume of diarrhea), and/or liver dysfunction (measured by bilirubin level). Grading systems have been developed (see Table 10-3), and overall grades of III-IV have been associated with an increased risk of transplant-related mortality (TRM). Acute GVHD occurs in spite of prophylactic medications in 20% to 60% of allogeneic transplants, depending on the degree of HLA matching, type of stem cell source, and approach taken. When acute GVHD occurs, patients are usually already on cyclosporine or tacrolimus therapy. If symptoms are significant, additional immunosuppressive

Table 10-3

Modified Glucksberg staging criteria for acute graft-versus-host disease.

Stage	Skin	Liver (bilirubin)	Gut (stool output/day)
0	No GVHD rash	< 2 mg/dL	Adult: < 500 ml/day Child: < 10 ml/kg/day
1	Maculopapular rash < 25% BSA	2-3 mg/dL	Adult: 500-999 ml/day Child: 10-19.9 ml/kg/day *Or persistent nausea, vomiting, or anorexia, with a positive upper GI biopsy.*
2	Maculopapular rash 25-50% BSA	3.1-6 mg/dL	Adult: 1000-1500 ml/day Child: 20-30 ml/kg/day
3	Maculopapular rash > 50% BSA	6.1-15 mg/dL	Adult: > 1500 ml/day Child: > 30 ml/kg/day
4	Generalized erythroderma plus bullous formation and desquamation > 5% BSA	> 15 mg/dl	Severe abdominal pain with or without ileus, or grossly bloody stool (regardless of stool volume).

Overall clinical grade (based on the highest stage obtained):

Grade 0: No stage I-IV of any organ

Grade I: Stage I-II skin and no liver or gut involvement

Grade II: Stage III skin, or stage 1 liver involvement, or stage I GI

Grade III: Stage 0-III skin, with stage II-III liver, or stage II-III GI

Grade IV: Stage IV skin, liver, or GI involvement

---

agents such as prednisolone (2 mg/kg/day, higher doses for patients already on steroids) are added to control symptoms. Once symptoms are controlled, careful weaning of immune suppression occurs over several months. If patients do not respond to prednisone, they are termed "steroid refractory," and treatment with a number of different agents (mycophenolate mofetil, etanercept, pentostatin, infliximab, antithymocyte globulin, daclizumab, extracorporeal photopheresis) can be attempted. The best second-line agents have not been established, but ongoing trials are currently comparing second-line approaches and adding agents along with prednisone to improve initial responses. Patients with steroid-refractory acute GVHD are at high risk for fatality due to infection or organ failure. Although acute GVHD has traditionally been thought to occur only in the first 100 days after transplant, recently the use of PBSCs, reduced-intensity regimens, and donor lymphocyte infusions has resulted in delayed forms of acute GVHD, occurring generally in the first 6 months after transplantation.

Chronic GVHD (cGVHD) presents as early as 2 months after allogeneic transplant with a wide variety of clinical symptoms (see Table 10-4). Chronic GVHD syndromes other than limited cGVHD require long-term therapy with immune suppressive agents. Most treatment plans include prednisone and/or calcineurin inhibitors (cyclosporine or tacrolimus), but a variety of agents targeted at T- and recently B-cells have been employed (mycophenolate mofetil, sirolimus, pentostatin, extracorporeal photopheresis, antithymocyte globulin, rituximab). Treatment of cGHVD focuses on establishing a low toxicity profile while controlling symptoms. Although abrupt cessation of immune suppressive agents can lead to GVHD exacerbations, slow weaning of immune suppression results in immune tolerance in most patients.[10,11] Because GVHD causes poor immune function, and therapy with immune suppressive agents exacerbates this condition, patients remain at high risk for opportunistic infection during therapy and for several months after completion of therapy.[12]

Posttransplant Infectious Risks

Bacterial infections tend to occur the first few weeks after transplant during the neutropenic phase when mucosal barriers are damaged from the conditioning regimen. Fungal infections are important to identify early because they are now amenable to a variety of powerful antifungal therapies. Patients with chronic GVHD during therapy are at very high risk of acquisition of invasive fungal infections. Antifungal prophylaxis is vital and must be tailored to the patient's underlying immune status. Pneumocystis infection can occur in all patients post-BMT, autologous and allogeneic, and prophylaxis is mandatory.

Table 10-4

Manifestations of chronic GVHD. (from BMT CTN MOP Sept. 2005)

Organ System	Definite Manifestations of Chronic GVHD	Possible Manifestations of Chronic GVHD
Skin	Scleroderma (superficial or fasciitis), lichen planus, vitiligo, scarring alopecia, hyperkeratosis pilaris, contractures from skin immobility, nail bed dysplasia	Eczematoid rash, dry skin, maculopapular rash, hyperpigmentation, hair loss
Mucous membranes	Lichen planus, noninfectious ulcers, corneal erosions/noninfectious conjunctivitis	Xerostomia, keratoconjunctivitis sicca
GI tract	Esophageal strictures, steatorrhea	Anorexia, malabsorption, weight loss, diarrhea, abdominal pain
Liver	None	Elevation of alkaline phosphatase, transaminitis, cholangitis, hyperbilirubinemia
GU	Vaginal structure, lichen planus	Noninfectious vaginitis, vaginal atrophy
Musculoskeletal/Serosa	Nonseptic arthritis, myositis, myasthenia, polyserositis, contractures from joint immobilization	Arthralgia
Hematologic	None	Thrombocytopenia, eosinophilia, autoimmune cytopenias
Lung	Bronchiolitis obliterans	Bronchiolitis obliterans with organizing pneumonia, interstitial pneumonitis

In the general oncology population, herpes simplex virus and varicella zoster virus infections are seen often, but cytomegalovirus (CMV) only occasionally and EBV rarely. After HCT, CMV infection has been a major cause of morbidity and mortality. Effective drugs to treat and prevent CMV are available; therefore, careful prevention of infection transmission by using CMV-negative blood products for CMV-negative patients and monitoring by frequent testing of CMV by antigen screening or polymerase chain reaction methods followed by preemptive therapy with ganciclovir is standard practice after allogeneic HCT. EBV can cause lympho-proliferative disease, but this is rare, generally associated with intensive, multidrug GVHD therapy or T-cell-depleted HCT.

Late bacterial infections can occur in patients who have central lines in place or patients with significant chronic GVHD. These patients are susceptible to infection with encapsulated organisms, particularly pneumococcus. Despite reimmunization these patients can sometimes develop significant infections, and continued prophylaxis is recommended until one has documented a serological response to immunizations. Occasionally, postallogeneic HCT patients can become functionally asplenic, and antibiotic prophylaxis is recommended. Patients should remain on infection prophylaxis (eg, *Pneumocystic jiroveci* pneumonia prophylaxis) until immune recovery. Time to immune recovery varies, but ranges from 3 to 9 months after autologous HCT and 9 to 24 months after allogeneic HCT without GVHD. Patients with active chronic GVHD may have persistent immunosuppression for years. Many centers monitor T-cell subset recovery post-BMT as a guide to infection risk.

Late Effects After Hematopoetic Cell Transplantation

Three broad categories of late effects can occur after transplant: (1) endocrine issues (gonadal failure, delayed puberty, hypothyroidism, osteoporosis, etc), (2) secondary malignancies, and (3) neurocognitive dysfunction (see Table 10-5). Risks of these late complications vary tremendously based upon age at transplant, choice of preparative regimen, and prior therapy. Younger children (< 3 years old) are thought to be more at risk for growth failure or cognitive challenges using total body irradiation (TBI) regimens, prompting development of chemotherapy regimens targeting this younger group. Some groups claim less relapse and acceptable long-term toxicities in infants treated with TBI.[13] Growth hormone deficiency, hypothyroidism, and pubertal delay occur in a portion of children after transplant, with increased risks in those who received additional central nervous system (CNS) irradiation or single-fraction TBI.[14] Infertility occurs in the large majority of children after standard-intensity TBI or

Table 10-5

Late effects associated with hematopoietic cell transplantation.

Endocrine-Related Effects	Secondary Malignancies	Neurocognitive Effects
Infertility/hypogonadism	tAML/tMDS	Impaired memory
Hypothyroidism	EBV+LPD/Lymphoma	Shortened attention span
Pubertal delay	Solid tumors	Defects in verbal fluency
Osteoporosis (related to long-term steroid use)		Decreased in visual-motor processing skills and in some IQ tests (in patients where additional cranial radiation was performed)
Growth failure		

busulfan-based myeloablative transplants; however, most children will have normal sexual development and fertility after receiving cytoxan alone as a preparative regimen for aplastic anemia.[15] Secondary AML/myelodysplastic syndrome (MDS) occurs more frequently after autologous transplantation in heavily pretreated patients. Secondary lymphomas occur most often after allogeneic transplant in the context of intense immune suppression, and solid tumors occur late, with oral carcinomas being associated with GVHD.[16] Reduced-intensity regimens may decrease complications such as infertility, but only if pretransplant therapy has not already resulted in this side effect.

Hematopoetic Cell Transplantation Approaches to Specific Pediatric Cancers

Acute Lymphoblastic Leukemia

Intensive, risk-based chemotherapy approaches cure more than 80% of children with ALL.[17–19] Studies have identified several risk factors associated with poor outcome that can be identified at presentation and after relapse.[20] Although both allogeneic and autologous transplantation approaches have been used in selected high-risk patient populations, a number of studies have failed to show an advantage of autologous approaches over intensive chemotherapy. The discussion below will therefore focus on allogeneic transplantation. Recent studies have confirmed the superiority of TBI over chemotherapy-based preparative regimens in ALL.[21,22] Although some groups prefer non–TBI-based regimens for infants due to concerns about late effects, fractionated TBI between 12 and 1440 centigray is considered an essential part of ALL transplantation.

Indications for Allogeneic Transplantation in First Remission Acute Lymphoblastic Leukemia

Newly diagnosed children with ALL presenting with high-risk cytogenetic abnormalities (Ph+, hypodiploid [< 44 chromosomes], and t(4;11) failing to achieve an M1 marrow by day 14) have been noted to have poor outcomes with chemotherapy, making consideration of HCT appropriate. CR1 transplantation has been shown to be benefi-

cial for Ph+ patients, with long-term survival outcomes exceeding 60%.[23] The recent introduction of imatinib mesylate and second-generation tyrosine kinase inhibitors such as dasatinib may alter chemotherapy outcomes for a portion of Ph+ ALL patients, but currently, CR1 transplantation of Ph+ ALL patients is appropriate therapy.

Other high-risk characteristics prompting early consideration of HCT include primary induction failure (PIF) and infant ALL. When children do not obtain a remission with initial therapy (PIF), chemotherapy outcomes have been uniformly dismal. Hematopoietic cell transplantation can salvage a portion of these children if they obtain a subsequent remission, but if they go to transplant without obtaining a remission, < 10% will be cured.[24] Although infants presenting with leukemia have traditionally been classified as very high risk and thus eligible for transplant, intensified chemotherapy and risk classification has resulted in successful treatment of many of these children.[25] A key risk factor is the presence of a translocation associated with the MLL gene (11q23). Other high-risk characteristics include infants less than 6 months of age or infants presenting with high white counts. Transplantation has been reported to result in cure in up to 75% of infants in CR1 in single-institution studies and just under 60% in registry studies.[13,26] Current data from the Children's Oncology Group (COG) using intensive chemotherapy approaches show survival outcomes nearing or exceeding 60% for all infant groups except MLL-rearranged infants less than 3 months, obviating the need for CR1 HCT in these groups.[25] Younger MLL+ infants have survival rates less than 20%, and transplantation of infants in this very high risk group who achieve a remission and have a donor may be of benefit, because registry data show survival rates in the 50% to 60% range.[26]

Indications for Allogeneic Transplantation in Second- or Subsequent-Remission Acute Lymphoblastic Leukemia

The prognosis of high-risk relapsed ALL in pediatric patients is poor with long-term survival less than 20%. High-risk features for BM relapse include T-lineage, Ph+, or early occurrence (< 36 months from diagnosis). All patients with a second or subsequent relapse are also considered high risk, because the chance of cure with chemotherapy alone is remote. An intermediate risk group has been defined (B-lineage late BM [=36 months] and very early isolated extramedullary relapses [<18 months]) in which long-term survival with intensive chemotherapeutic approaches cures more than 35% of relapsed children.[27–29]

Hematopoietic cell transplantation has been used extensively for the treatment of relapsed ALL. Several studies have shown a survival benefit as salvage therapy for high-risk relapsed ALL patients compared with aggressive chemotherapy.[30–38] Matched sibling transplantation has been shown to offer a favorable outcome compared with chemotherapy in intermediate-risk patients,[30,31,33,36,38] although a recent retrospective registry study showed similar outcomes between chemotherapy and transplant approaches.[22] Several studies have demonstrated equivalent outcome between related donor and unrelated donor approaches, noting more GVHD-related morbidity and less relapse with unrelated donor sources.[26,39]

Although center practice may vary, several large cooperative groups, including the COG, recommend transplantation with any stem cell source for high-risk relapsed patients. Intermediate-risk patients with sibling donors are also offered transplantation as an alternative to chemotherapeutic approaches.

Acute Myeloid Leukemia

Hematopoietic cell transplantation has always played a major role in treatment of AML, but the timing and type of HCT continues to change as transplant and chemotherapy approaches improve. Acute myeloid leukemia is the only disease for which large, well-conducted studies have compared allogeneic, autologous, and chemotherapeutic approaches. Several studies have randomized patients according to the presence of a matched sibling donor, as typified by the UK Medical Research Council (MRC) AML10 study. Four courses of intensive induction/consolidation were followed by a matched sibling allograft, autograft, or no further therapy. A simple prognostic index was derived; good risk was those with favorable cytogenetics (inv(16); t(8;21), t(15;17)), poor risk those not achieving partial remission after course 1 or with Monosomy 5 or 7 or del(5q), etc, and standard risk forming the rest. Not only did good-risk patients have the best disease-free survival (59% at 7 years) compared with standard (54%) or poor risk (32%), but they also had the best 3-year survival from relapse (61% vs 17% or 0%).[40] In this study, presence of a matched sibling donor was not associated with a improved outcome, as TRM offset the reduced rate of relapse. Similarly, although an autograft was associated with a reduced relapse rate compared with chemotherapy, the benefit was offset by a higher salvage rate in relapsing patients who had not had a preceding autograft.

Lack of benefit from an autologous transplant was also seen in the Children's Cancer Group study CCG-2891,[41] and a systematic review and metaanalysis confirmed the lack of benefit of autologous BMT and the superior disease control of an allogeneic BMT.[42] Children's Cancer Group study 2891 showed an overall improvement in disease-free and event-free survival (EFS) for those undergoing allogeneic matched sibling BMT in CR1, and this result was confirmed by the metaanalysis (MRC AML10 data included). There is international agreement that patients with t(15;17) do not need a transplant in first remission. The US data were unable to confirm the benefit in survival for the t(8;21) and inv (16) groups seen by the MRC, mainly because the numbers were small. Current studies exclude patients with favorable cytogenetics from matched sibling BMT in CR1; however, this recommendation is not based upon prospective data.

It is hoped that, as in ALL, incorporation of more refined risk stratification up front will allow better identification of patients whose leukemia is destined to relapse, allowing a donor to be identified early and HCT in CR1. It is generally agreed that after relapse, patients should be offered allogeneic transplantation. A portion of late relapses may be salvaged with autologous HCT, but this has not been the preferred approach of the pediatric transplant community.

For AML, the 2 main conditioning regimens used are busulfan/cytoxan (BuCy) and cytoxan/total body irradiation (Cy-TBI), but studies that have compared them for AML are in adults. The BuCy regimen has been associated with more veno-occlusive disease (VOD), hemorrhagic cystitis, and alopecia but a reduced incidence of cataracts in the long term. The BuCy regimen probably has less effects on growth than TBI.[43] In terms of disease control Cy-TBI has equal or better control of AML, especially for advanced disease. In general, older trials have used TBI and more recent ones have used Bu. Four days of Bu at 4 mg/kg/day followed by 4 days of Cy at 50 mg/kg/day is the only regimen in which therapeutic drug monitoring for Bu has been shown to reduce the rate of subsequent VOD and is still widely used for pediatric AML.[44] A recent review of registry data showed comparable outcome results with this approach and TBI-based regimens (S. Davies, personal communication).

Myelodysplasia and Juvenile Myelomonocytic Leukemia

Myelodysplasia syndrome and juvenile myelomonocytic leukemia (JMML) are rare pediatric diagnoses. Both represent hematopoietic stem cell disorders that are curable only by allogeneic BMT. The natural history of MDS in childhood is poor, with an estimated survival of 36% at 10 years, with 32% of patients developing acute leukemia, usually within 2 years of diagnosis.[45]

Upfront allogeneic transplant as an approach to treat JMML was best described by Locatelli,[46] who reported a cohort of 100 JMML patients transplanted using a combination of busulfan, melphalan, and cyclophosphamide (Bu/MLP/Cy). Donors were related (48) or unrelated (52), with 5-year EFS being the same (55% and 49%). Prior splenectomy and the receipt of intensive chemotherapy had no effect on EFS. Relapse remained the major cause of treatment failure.

A recent European Group for Blood and Marrow Transplant review recommended matched related or unrelated

BMT as a standard for pediatric patients with MDS.[47] The JMML series quoted above has been part of the broader use of Bu/MLP/Cy in Europe, and 89 pediatric patients with MDS were reported using this combination.[48] Prior AML-type therapy and blast percentage in the marrow at BMT had no impact on outcome. Transplant-related mortality was higher with unrelated donors (36%) than with family donors (14%). These outcomes are comparable to those of a single-institution Seattle report.[49] Both studies confirmed that allogeneic HCT is more likely to be successful early in the course of MDS.

Chronic Myelogenous Leukemia

Therapy for adults with this rare disease, characterized by a t(9;22) translocation between the BCR and ABL genes, has been dramatically altered by the introduction of imatinib mesylate (gleevec) and second-generation tyrosine kinase inhibitors (dasatinib, nilotinib). The fact that more than 80% of patients treated with imatinib remain progression-free at 5 years has overshadowed the well-established practice of allogeneic transplantation in chronic myelogenous leukemia (CML), which results in cure rates exceeding 80% when performed in early-phase disease.[50,51] Because cure with imatinib has yet to be established and transplant outcomes are excellent, the parents of some younger patients continue to choose upfront transplant therapy.[52] Others wait until resistance to imatinib and/or a second-generation agent has been noted. A key challenge in approaching this group is that transplant outcomes after the disease advances to accelerated or blast phases are dramatically worse, so close monitoring and detection of resistance early is essential. Because CML is highly sensitive to immunologic therapy and GvL, it is an ideal disease for which to consider reduced-intensity transplant approaches. Such approaches have demonstrated outcomes equivalent to myeloablative approaches in patients with early chronic phase,[53] but the role of these approaches in advanced-phase disease has not been fully established.

Hodgkin Disease (HD) and Non-Hodgkin Lymphoma (NHL)

The majority of pediatric patients with Hodgkin disease (HD) and non-Hodgkin lymphoma (NHL) have chemosensitive tumors that respond well to frontline chemotherapy; hence HCT is rarely necessary. For patients who relapse or have shown inadequate response to frontline therapy, however, a percentage can be salvaged with dose escalation and autologous HCT.

In the past, most groups would agree that a patient with HD who has residual disease or relapse after MOPP or ABVD is a good candidate for autologous HCT. However, the use of less-intensive chemotherapy regimens up front makes it more difficult to assess if a patient has truly failed conventional therapy.

Patients with HD who have chemosensitive disease have a good response to autologous HCT; in a cohort of 41 pediatric patients with mainly relapsed HD, the 5-year EFS was 53%.[54] As opposed to other types of lymphoma, a subset of patients with resistant HD may also be cured with autologous HCT. Although some studies have suggested a role for chemotherapy alone for a subset of patients with responsive disease after relapse,[55] most patients will benefit from autologous HCT at first relapse. An HD patient who has residual disease after multiagent chemotherapy including anthracyclines and has received mediastinal or cardiac irradiation is at high risk of TRM with an allograft, and autografts are generally preferred. However, an allograft does protect against relapse, as well as against myelodysplasia/secondary AML that is sometimes seen after autografts in HD.[56] Some centers are using reduced-intensity-regimen allogeneic approaches after failed autografts.

Most NHLs in pediatrics can be cured with standard chemotherapy. Early relapses are often chemoresistant, and the benefits of HCT with refractory or resistant disease are limited.[57] If a response to salvage chemotherapy can be achieved, autologous HCT will cure a proportion of patients.[58] Because of the overlap between categories of pediatric NHL and leukemia, the argument for a meaningful GvL effect is compelling. From a pediatric perspective, a patient with a high-grade T-cell lymphoma that relapses as leukemia is easily identified as a candidate for an allograft if a suitable donor is available. However, a retrospective comparison of allogeneic and autologous BMT in lymphoblastic lymphoma showed that the increased TRM associated with an allograft offset the reduced relapse rate, and disease-free survival was superimposable.[59] This study must be put into perspective, however, because transplant physicians generally reserve allogeneic approaches for their highest-risk patients.

When patients with lymphoma undergo HCT, there are no studies that have demonstrated superiority of one regimen over another, and there have been no randomized studies looking at the role of TBI-containing regimens.[57] Most centers use a chemotherapy combination such as BEAM (carmustine; etoposide, ara-C, melphalan) or BVC (carmustine, etoposide, cytoxan) for autografts, and more standard TBI-based regimens for allografts.

Hematopoietic Cell Transplantation for Solid Tumors

As described above, high-dose myeloablative therapy followed by HPC rescue allows dose escalation, to take advantage of the dose response curve and kill several more logs of disease than is possible with a lower dose. The general principles are:

- The drugs should be active for the disease in question.
- The limiting toxicity has to be myelosuppression.
- The higher dose that can be used with HPC support achieves a significantly higher cell kill of the disease.

Neuroblastoma

High-risk neuroblastoma is the most common indication for autologous HCT in a pediatric solid tumor. Even with cisplatin-based therapy, the historical survival has been poor with chemotherapy alone.[60] Neuroblastoma was one of the first diseases for which autologous HCT was performed.[61] The first study of the European Neuroblastoma Study Group randomized patients between chemotherapy and melphalan and showed an advantage for the autograft.[62] Later protocols intensified the conditioning, leading to a 25% to 50% EFS compared with the historical 6%.

A large CCG randomized study demonstrated improved survival with a TBI-containing HCT regimen and cis-retinoic acid added post HCT, given as a differentiating agent.[63] Antibody therapies are also now being used by some groups and tested in a randomized fashion for patients with minimal residual disease. Attempts are currently being made to reduce treatment toxicity by removing TBI from the regimen and including local irradiation post BMT.

Ongoing studies in the United States will assess whether 2 courses of myeloablative therapy are better than 1. A recently completed effort through the COG looked at whether purging of neuroblastoma cells from a collected stem cell product affects outcome, and an updated analysis shows no benefit to purging.

Central Nervous System Tumors

Surgical resection and radiation have been the mainstay of therapy for CNS tumors for many years, but recently these approaches have been augmented by a number of effective chemotherapy regimens. High-dose therapy followed by autologous HCT fits into this approach, increasing the amount of drug able to cross the blood-brain barrier. Several groups have developed high-dose regimens; generally they involve thiotepa or melphalan in combination with other agents such as cyclophosphamide, busulfan, or etoposide. Remission rates vary with tumor and are better when (1) patients have chemotherapy responsive disease pretransplant, (2) patients undergo a gross total resection of residual tumor or the tumor shrinks to a very small size with chemotherapy, and/or (3) patients can receive further posttransplant radiation.

As opposed to the excellent cure rates for upfront medulloblastoma with current therapy (60% to 80%),[64] relapsed medulloblastoma outcomes are poor. Small studies of autologous HCT have shown long-term survival between 25% and 50%.[65,66] Metastatic disease at recurrence was noted to be a poor risk factor. Primitive neuroectodermal tumors have similarly been salvaged at rates of 29% to 40% in very small studies.[67,68]

Recurrent astrocytomas have occasionally benefited from transplant approaches, with a study of 36 patients showing a 4-year progression-free survival of 22%.[69] The strongest predictive factor was < 3cm of residual disease at the time of transplant. High-dose HCT outcomes for recurrent ependymomas have been poor, with long-term survival less than 10% to 20%.[68] Similarly, brain stem gliomas fare poorly with any therapeutic modality, including HCT. Although oligodendrogliomas seem to be chemosensitive tumors, insufficient data have been published to understand the role of HCT in treating these tumors.

Another rare set of tumors with promising early data utilizing transplant approaches is recurrent CNS germ cell tumors (GCT). A recent series demonstrated 4-year event-free survival of 78% of patients with germinoma and 33% of patients with nongerminomatous-GCT.[70] Patients with complete responses to the transplant fared much better than those with stable or partially responsive disease.

Finally, high-dose autologous HCT has been used to avoid early radiotherapy in infants with a variety of CNS tumors. A triple high-dose therapy approach was performed by the CCG, and results of this study are forthcoming. The use of high-dose therapy is currently being explored by a number of single-center and cooperative group studies, and the next few years should bring a better understanding of the role of HCT approaches in high-risk pediatric CNS tumors.

Retinoblastoma

Although the prognosis for the majority of patients with retinoblastoma is good, some patients have widespread aggressive disease at diagnosis or relapse. It has been suggested that consolidation with high-dose therapy and HPC rescue may be appropriate for patients with extraocular disease and who are chemosensitive.[71] This strategy has been used in a number of patients, particularly in Europe, using conditioning regimens similar to those used for CNS tumors or neuroblastoma.[72]

Germ Cell Tumors

Cisplatin-based chemotherapy approaches have led to cure in the large majority of patients with germ cell tumors; even metastatic disease can be cured 70% to 80% of the time. Poor-risk, recurrent, or refractory tumors have long-term survival as low as 20%, prompting investigation of autologous HCT in this clinical scenario. Responsive disease is associated with better outcome, and the presence of tumor markers such as α-fetoprotein or human chorionic gonadotropin (HCG) has made it easier to follow response very sensitively. In treating patients with relapsed disease, long-term survival has been achieved in 15% to 40% of patients, with patients going to transplant after multiple recurrences falling on the lower end of that spectrum.[73,74] Patients with primary mediastinal disease do not seem to benefit from high-dose approaches. Some studies have suggested a role for upfront transplant in patients with high-risk features such as progressive disease, primary mediastinal tumor, cisplatin-refractory, and HCG > 1000 IU/L prior to transplant,[75] but further study is needed to clarify the best approach, and very little pediatric literature addresses this topic directly.

Autologous HCT Approaches to Other Solid Tumors

High-dose chemotherapy followed by HCT has been attempted in several other relapsed, poor-risk metastatic, or refractory solid tumors. Patients with metastatic or relapsed Ewing sarcoma have been reported in small series to have long-term survival outcomes in the 20% to 40% range,[76] but a prospective CCG study of transplant used as consolidation for patients with metastatic disease to bone or marrow did not demonstrate a benefit over historical controls.[77] The role of HCT in first-remission Ewing disease is unclear; currently, a large study randomizing continued chemotherapy with transplant in patients with isolated lung metastases is under way. For patients with isolated, nonmetastatic relapse, there is some evidence to suggest a benefit to high-dose therapy, but convincing studies are difficult to carry out in this rare situation.

Wilms tumor is a chemo/radiotherapy-responsive solid tumor with a high cure rate in spite of metastatic disease at presentation. Early-stage relapses can often be salvaged with chemotherapy alone, but the role of transplant in high-risk relapse is unclear. As with other solid tumors, studies have clearly shown that chemotherapy-resistant progressive relapse does not benefit from autologous HCT, but there may be a role for HCT in patients with high-risk relapse that is responsive to chemotherapy.[78]

Studies of autologous HCT in patients with high-risk osteosarcoma, rhabdomyosarcoma, desmoplastic small round cell tumor, and other solid tumors have shown mixed results. Osteosarcoma outcomes have been universally poor, but newer approaches using radioisotopes requiring HPC rescue may hold some promise. Rhabdomyosarcoma outcomes have been mixed, with some series showing very poor outcomes and others a degree of salvage.[79] Desmoplastic small round cell tumor patients have had prolongation of life with aggressive surgical resection, chemotherapy, and HCT; however, long-term outcomes have been poor.[80] The role of autologous HCT in most tumors that are refractory to standard-dose chemotherapy is limited. Newer approaches using radioconjugates (MIBG, Samarium, etc), biologic modifiers such as cis-retinoic acid, or immunologic approaches (reduced-intensity allogeneic transplants) performed in the context of minimal residual disease after HCT may improve outcomes of these difficult tumors in the future.

Summary and Emerging Transplant Approaches to Cancer Care

As chemotherapeutic approaches intensify and referral for HCT is delayed, patients in this era presenting for transplant consultation are more therapy resistant and have high rates of infection and organ damage. Methods of decreasing toxicity and preventing relapse are currently being developed and will be key to the success of future HCT approaches. Current research is focusing on immune therapy posttransplant, graft manipulation to enhance GvL, choosing graft sources with increased GvL effect, and nonimmunologic posttransplant therapies aimed at prolonging remission.

Although a number of these approaches will require years of development to determine whether they improve outcomes, reduced-intensity conditioning (RIC, also called nonmyeloablative or mini-transplantation) approaches are now firmly established in adult transplantation. Reduced-intensity conditioning regimens use new, potent immune suppressive agents to promote engraftment of donor cells without traditional intensive myeloablative therapies. The approach depends upon a GvL effect for cancer control and generally results in successful engraftment with low morbidity. Patients at high risk for TRM using standard myeloablative approaches (those who are older, have organ damage, had a previous transplant, etc) have been shown to benefit from these approaches. Because of a concern that relapse occurs more often after RIC regimens, use of these regimens in pediatrics has been limited.[81] Data are emerging, however, that indicate the approach is safe and offers a potentially curative alternative to patients not otherwise eligible for myeloablative HCT. Whether cancers susceptible to GvL will have better outcomes with RIC regimens will require further study.

As new therapeutic approaches improve transplant practice, and as nontransplant chemotherapeutic approaches also improve, indications for transplantation for a given disease will change. But with the introduction of novel cellular therapeutics and improvements in our understanding of the immunology of transplant, HCT-based treatments will continue to be a core part of comprehensive cancer care.

References

1. Bortin MM. A compendium of reported human bone marrow transplants. *Transplantation.* 1970;9:571–587.
2. Thomas ED, Lochte HL, Jr, Cannon JH, Sahler OD, Ferrebee JW. Supralethal whole body irradiation and isologous marrow transplantation in man. *J Clin Invest.* 1959;38:1709–1716.
3. Flomenberg N, Baxter-Lowe LA, Confer D, et al. Impact of HLA class I and class II high-resolution matching on outcomes of unrelated donor bone marrow transplantation: HLA-C mismatching is associated with a strong adverse effect on transplantation outcome. *Blood.* 2004;104:1923–1930.
4. Petersdorf EW, Kollman C, Hurley CK, et al. Effect of HLA class II gene disparity on clinical outcome in unrelated donor hematopoietic cell transplantation for chronic myeloid leukemia: the US National Marrow Donor Program Experience. *Blood.* 2001;98:2922–2929.
5. Petersdorf EW, Longton GM, Anasetti C, et al. Definition of HLA-DQ as a transplantation antigen. *Proc Natl Acad Sci USA.* 1996;93:15358–15363.
6. Varney MD, Lester S, McCluskey J, Gao X, Tait BD. Matching for HLA DPA1 and DPB1 alleles in unrelated bone marrow transplantation. *Hum Immunol.* 1999;60:532–538.
7. Gluckman E, Rocha V, Boyer-Chammard A, et al. Outcome of cord-blood transplantation from related and unrelated donors. Eurocord Transplant Group and the European Blood and Marrow Transplantation Group. *N Engl J Med.* 1997;337:373–381.
8. Rubinstein P, Carrier C, Scaradavou A, et al. Outcomes among 562 recipients of placental-blood transplants from unrelated donors. *N Engl J Med.* 1998; 339:1565–1577.
9. Ferrara JL, Reddy P. Pathophysiology of graft-versus-host disease. *Semin Hematol.* 2006;43:3–10.
10. Filipovich AH, Weisdorf D, Pavletic S, et al. National Institutes of Health consensus development project on criteria for clinical trials in chronic graft-versus-host disease: I. Diagnosis and staging working group report. *Biol Blood Marrow Transplant.* 2005;11:945–956.
11. Pavletic SZ, Martin P, Lee SJ, et al. Measuring therapeutic response in chronic graft-versus-host disease: National Institutes of Health Consensus Development Project on Criteria for Clinical Trials in Chronic Graft-versus-Host Disease: IV. Response Criteria Working Group report. *Biol Blood Marrow Transplant.* 2006;12:252–266.
12. Couriel D, Carpenter PA, Cutler C, et al. Ancillary therapy and supportive care of chronic graft-versus-host disease: National Institutes of Health consensus development project on criteria for clinical trials in chronic graft-versus-host disease: V. Ancillary Therapy and Supportive Care Working Group Report. *Biol Blood Marrow Transplant.* 2006;12:375–396.
13. Sanders JE, Im HJ, Hoffmeister PA, et al. Allogeneic hematopoietic cell transplantation for infants with acute lymphoblastic leukemia. *Blood.* 2005;105: 3749–3756.

14. Sanders J. Growth and development after hematopoietic cell transplantation. In: Blume KG, Forman S, Appelbaum F, eds. *Thomas' Hematopoietic Cell Transplantation*. 3rd ed. London: Blackwell Publishing Ltd; 2003:929–943.

15. Sanders JE, Hawley J, Levy W, et al. Pregnancies following high-dose cyclophosphamide with or without high-dose busulfan or total-body irradiation and bone marrow transplantation. *Blood*. 1996;87:3045–3052.

16. Bhatia S, Bhatia R. *Secondary Malignancies after Hematopoietic Cell Transplantation*. 3rd ed. London: Blackwell Publishing Ltd; 2003.

17. Gaynon PS, Trigg ME, Heerema NA, et al. Children's Cancer Group trials in childhood acute lymphoblastic leukemia: 1983–1995. *Leukemia*. 2000;14:2223–2233.

18. Pui CH, Evans WE. Acute lymphoblastic leukemia. *N Engl J Med*. 1998;339:605–615.

19. Schrappe M, Reiter A, Zimmermann M, et al. Long-term results of four consecutive trials in childhood ALL performed by the ALL-BFM study group from 1981 to 1995. Berlin-Frankfurt-Munster. *Leukemia*. 2000;14:2205–2222.

20. Hahn T, Wall D, Camitta B, et al. The role of cytotoxic therapy with hematopoietic stem cell transplantation in the therapy of acute lymphoblastic leukemia in children: an evidence-based review. *Biol Blood Marrow Transplant*. 2005;11:823–861.

21. Davies SM, Ramsay NK, Klein JP, et al. Comparison of preparative regimens in transplants for children with acute lymphoblastic leukemia. *J Clin Oncol*. 2000;18:340–347.

22. Eapen M, Raetz E, Zhang MJ, et al. Outcomes after HLA-matched sibling transplantation or chemotherapy in children with B-precursor acute lymphoblastic leukemia in a second remission: a collaborative study of the Children's Oncology Group and the Center for International Blood and Marrow Transplant Research. *Blood*. 2006;107:4961–4967.

23. Arico M, Valsecchi MG, Camitta B, et al. Outcome of treatment in children with Philadelphia chromosome-positive acute lymphoblastic leukemia. *N Engl J Med*. 2000;342:998–1006.

24. Singhal S, Powles R, Henslee-Downey PJ, et al. Allogeneic transplantation from HLA-matched sibling or partially HLA-mismatched related donors for primary refractory acute leukemia. *Bone Marrow Transplant*. 2002;29:291–295.

25. Hilden JM, Dinndorf PA, Meerbaum SO, et al. Analysis of prognostic factors of acute lymphoblastic leukemia in infants: report on CCG 1953 from the Children's Oncology Group. *Blood*. 2006;108:441–451.

26. Eapen M, Rubinstein P, Zhang MJ, et al. Comparable long-term survival after unrelated and HLA-matched sibling donor hematopoietic stem cell transplantations for acute leukemia in children younger than 18 months. *J Clin Oncol*. 2006;24:145–151.

27. Gaynon PS, Qu RP, Chappell RJ, et al. Survival after relapse in childhood acute lymphoblastic leukemia: impact of site and time to first relapse—the Children's Cancer Group Experience. *Cancer*. 1998;82:1387–1395.

28. Rivera GK, Hudson MM, Liu Q, et al. Effectiveness of intensified rotational combination chemotherapy for late hematologic relapse of childhood acute lymphoblastic leukemia. *Blood*. 1996;88:831–837.

29. Sadowitz PD, Smith SD, Shuster J, Wharam MD, Buchanan GR, Rivera GK. Treatment of late bone marrow relapse in children with acute lymphoblastic leukemia: a Pediatric Oncology Group study. *Blood*. 1993;81:602–609.

30. Barrett AJ, Horowitz MM, Pollock BH, et al. Bone marrow transplants from HLA-identical siblings as compared with chemotherapy for children with acute lymphoblastic leukemia in a second remission. *N Engl J Med*. 1994;331:1253–1258.

31. Bleakley M, Shaw PJ, Nielsen JM. Allogeneic bone marrow transplantation for childhood relapsed acute lymphoblastic leukemia: comparison of outcome in patients with and without a matched family donor. *Bone Marrow Transplant*. 2002;30:1–7.

32. Borgmann A, von Stackelberg A, Hartmann R, et al. Unrelated donor stem cell transplantation compared with chemotherapy for children with acute lymphoblastic leukemia in a second remission: a matched-pair analysis. *Blood*. 2003;101:3835–3839.

33. Boulad F, Steinherz P, Reyes B, et al. Allogeneic bone marrow transplantation versus chemotherapy for the treatment of childhood acute lymphoblastic leukemia in second remission: a single-institution study. *J Clin Oncol*. 1999;17:197–207.

34. Chessells JM, Veys P, Kempski H, et al. Long-term follow-up of relapsed childhood acute lymphoblastic leukaemia. *Br J Haematol*. 2003;123:396–405.

35. Feig SA, Harris RE, Sather HN. Bone marrow transplantation versus chemotherapy for maintenance of second remission of childhood acute lymphoblastic leukemia: a study of the Children's Cancer Group (CCG-1884). *Med Pediatr Oncol*. 1997;29:534–540.

36. Henze G, Fengler R, Hartmann R, et al. Six-year experience with a comprehensive approach to the treatment of recurrent childhood acute lymphoblastic leukemia (ALL-REZ BFM 85). A relapse study of the BFM group. *Blood*. 1991;78:1166–1172.

37. Locatelli F, Zecca M, Messina C, et al. Improvement over time in outcome for children with acute lymphoblastic leukemia in second remission given hematopoietic stem cell transplantation from unrelated donors. *Leukemia*. 2002;16:2228–2237.

38. Torres A, Alvarez MA, Sanchez J, et al. Allogeneic bone marrow transplantation vs chemotherapy for the treatment of childhood acute lymphoblastic leukaemia in second complete remission (revisited 10 years on). *Bone Marrow Transplant*. 1999;23:1257–1260.

39. Dahlke J, Kroger N, Zabelina T, et al. Comparable results in patients with acute lymphoblastic leukemia after related and unrelated stem cell transplantation. *Bone Marrow Transplant*. 2006;37:155–163.

40. Stevens RF, Hann IM, Wheatley K, Gray RG. Marked improvements in outcome with chemotherapy alone in paediatric acute myeloid leukemia: results of the United Kingdom Medical Research Council's 10th AML trial. MRC Childhood Leukaemia Working Party. *Br J Haematol*. 1998;101:130–140.

41. Woods WG, Neudorf S, Gold S, et al. A comparison of allogeneic bone marrow transplantation, autologous bone marrow transplantation, and aggressive chemotherapy in children with acute myeloid leukemia in remission. *Blood*. 2001;97:56–62.

42. Bleakley M, Lau L, Shaw PJ, Kaufman A. Bone marrow transplantation for paediatric AML in first remission: a systematic review and meta-analysis. *Bone Marrow Transplant*. 2002;29:843–852.

43. Afify Z, Shaw PJ, Clavano-Harding A, Cowell CT. Growth and endocrine function in children with acute myeloid leukaemia after bone marrow transplantation using busulfan/cyclophosphamide. *Bone Marrow Transplant*. 2000;25:1087–1092.

44. Grochow LB. Busulfan disposition: the role of therapeutic monitoring in bone marrow transplantation induction regimens. *Semin Oncol*. 1993;20:18–25; quiz 26.

45. Luna-Fineman S, Shannon KM, Atwater SK, et al. Myelodysplastic and myeloproliferative disorders of childhood: a study of 167 patients. *Blood*. 1999;93:459–466.

46. Locatelli F, Nollke P, Zecca M, et al. Hematopoietic stem cell transplantation (HSCT) in children with juvenile myelomonocytic leukemia (JMML): results of the EWOG-MDS/EBMT trial. *Blood*. 2005;105:410–419.

47. Ljungman P, Urbano-Ispizua A, Cavazzana-Calvo M, et al. Allogeneic and autologous transplantation for haematological diseases, solid tumours and immune disorders: definitions and current practice in Europe. *Bone Marrow Transplant*. 2006;37:439–449.

48. Stary J, Locatelli F, Niemeyer CM. Stem cell transplantation for aplastic anemia and myelodysplastic syndrome. *Bone Marrow Transplant*. 2005;35(suppl 1):S13–S16.

49. Yusuf U, Frangoul HA, Gooley TA, et al. Allogeneic bone marrow transplantation in children with myelodysplastic syndrome or juvenile myelomonocytic leukemia: the Seattle experience. *Bone Marrow Transplant*. 2004;33:805–814.

50. Hansen JA, Gooley TA, Martin PJ, et al. Bone marrow transplants from unrelated donors for patients with chronic myeloid leukemia. *N Engl J Med*. 1998;338:962–968.

51. Radich JP, Gooley T, Bensinger W, et al. HLA-matched related hematopoietic cell transplantation for chronic-phase CML using a targeted busulfan and cyclophosphamide preparative regimen. *Blood*. 2003;102:31–35.

52. Pulsipher MA. Treatment of CML in pediatric patients: should imatinib mesylate (STI-571, Gleevec) or allogeneic hematopoietic cell transplant be front-line therapy? *Pediatr Blood Cancer*. 2004;43:523–533.

53. Or R, Shapira MY, Resnick I, et al. Nonmyeloablative allogeneic stem cell transplantation for the treatment of chronic myeloid leukemia in first chronic phase. *Blood*. 2003;101:441–445.

54. Lieskovsky YE, Donaldson SS, Torres MA, et al. High-dose therapy and autologous hematopoietic stem-cell transplantation for recurrent or refractory pediatric Hodgkin's disease: results and prognostic indices. *J Clin Oncol*. 2004;22:4532–4540.

55. Stoneham S, Ashley S, Pinkerton CR, Wallace WH, Shankar AG. Outcome after autologous hemopoietic stem cell transplantation in relapsed or refractory childhood Hodgkin disease. *J Pediatr Hematol Oncol*. 2004;26:740–745.

56. Akpek G, Ambinder RF, Piantadosi S, et al. Long-term results of blood and marrow transplantation for Hodgkin's lymphoma. *J Clin Oncol*. 2001;19:4314–4321.

57. Shipp MA, Abeloff MD, Antman KH, et al. International Consensus Conference on High-Dose Therapy with Hematopoietic Stem Cell Transplantation in Aggressive Non-Hodgkin's Lymphomas: report of the jury. *J Clin Oncol*. 1999;17:423–429.

58. Ladenstein R, Pearce R, Hartmann O, Patte C, Goldstone T, Philip T. High-dose chemotherapy with autologous bone marrow rescue in children with poor-risk Burkitt's lymphoma: a report from the European Lymphoma Bone Marrow Transplantation Registry. *Blood*. 1997;90:2921–2930.

59. Armitage JO, Carbone PP, Connors JM, Levine A, Bennett JM, Kroll S. Treatment-related myelodysplasia and acute leukemia in non-Hodgkin's lymphoma patients. *J Clin Oncol*. 2003;21:897–906.

60. McWilliams NB, Hayes FA, Green AA, et al. Cyclophosphamide/doxorubicin vs. cisplatin/teniposide in the treatment of children older than 12 months of age with disseminated neuroblastoma: a Pediatric Oncology Group Randomized Phase II study. *Med Pediatr Oncol*. 1995;24:176–180.

61. McElwain TJ, Hedley DW, Gordon MY, Jarman M, Millar JL, Pritchard J. High dose melphalan and non-cryopreserved autologous bone marrow treatment of malignant melanoma and neuroblastoma. *Exp Hematol*. 1979;7(suppl 5):360–371.

62. Pritchard J, Cotterill SJ, Germond SM, Imeson J, de Kraker J, Jones DR. High dose melphalan in the treatment of advanced neuroblastoma: results of a

randomised trial (ENSG-1) by the European Neuroblastoma Study Group. *Pediatr Blood Cancer.* 2005;44:348–357.

63. Matthay KK, Villablanca JG, Seeger RC, et al. Treatment of high-risk neuroblastoma with intensive chemotherapy, radiotherapy, autologous bone marrow transplantation, and 13-cis-retinoic acid. Children's Cancer Group. *N Engl J Med.* 1999;341:1165–1173.

64. Packer RJ, Goldwein J, Nicholson HS, et al. Treatment of children with medulloblastomas with reduced-dose craniospinal radiation therapy and adjuvant chemotherapy: A Children's Cancer Group Study. *J Clin Oncol.* 1999;17:2127–2136.

65. Dunkel IJ, Boyett JM, Yates A, et al. High-dose carboplatin, thiotepa, and etoposide with autologous stem-cell rescue for patients with recurrent medulloblastoma. Children's Cancer Group. *J Clin Oncol.* 1998;16:222–228.

66. Dupuis-Girod S, Hartmann O, Benhamou E, et al. Will high dose chemotherapy followed by autologous bone marrow transplantation supplant craniospinal irradiation in young children treated for medulloblastoma? *J Neurooncol.* 1996;27:87–98.

67. Broniscer A, Nicolaides TP, Dunkel IJ, et al. High-dose chemotherapy with autologous stem-cell rescue in the treatment of patients with recurrent non-cerebellar primitive neuroectodermal tumors. *Pediatr Blood Cancer.* 2004;42:261–267.

68. Graham ML, Herndon JE, 2nd, Casey JR, et al. High-dose chemotherapy with autologous stem-cell rescue in patients with recurrent and high-risk pediatric brain tumors. *J Clin Oncol.* 1997;15:1814–1823.

69. Dunkel IJ, Finlay JL. High-dose chemotherapy with autologous bone marrow rescue for high-grade astrocytomas. *Bone Marrow Transplant.* 1994;14:64s.

70. Modak S, Gardner S, Dunkel IJ, et al. Thiotepa-based high-dose chemotherapy with autologous stem-cell rescue in patients with recurrent or progressive CNS germ cell tumors. *J Clin Oncol.* 2004;22:1934–1943.

71. Jubran RF, Erdreich-Epstein A, Butturini A, Murphree AL, Villablanca JG. Approaches to treatment for extraocular retinoblastoma: Children's Hospital Los Angeles experience. *J Pediatr Hematol Oncol.* 2004;26:31–34.

72. Namouni F, Doz F, Tanguy ML, et al. High-dose chemotherapy with carboplatin, etoposide and cyclophosphamide followed by a haematopoietic stem cell rescue in patients with high-risk retinoblastoma: a SFOP and SFGM study. *Eur J Cancer.* 1997;33:2368–2375.

73. Broun ER, Nichols CR, Mandanas R, et al. Dose escalation study of high-dose carboplatin and etoposide with autologous bone marrow support in patients with recurrent and refractory germ cell tumors. *Bone Marrow Transplant.* 1995;16:353–358.

74. Margolin K, Doroshow JH, Ahn C, et al. Treatment of germ cell cancer with two cycles of high-dose ifosfamide, carboplatin, and etoposide with autologous stem-cell support. *J Clin Oncol.* 1996;14:2631–2637.

75. Bhatia S, Abonour R, Porcu P, et al. High-dose chemotherapy as initial salvage chemotherapy in patients with relapsed testicular cancer. *J Clin Oncol.* 2000;18:3346–3351.

76. Paulussen M, Ahrens S, Burdach S, et al. Primary metastatic (stage IV) Ewing tumor: survival analysis of 171 patients from the EICESS studies. European Intergroup Cooperative Ewing Sarcoma Studies. *Ann Oncol.* 1998;9:275–281.

77. Meyers PA, Krailo MD, Ladanyi M, et al. High-dose melphalan, etoposide, total-body irradiation, and autologous stem-cell reconstitution as consolidation therapy for high-risk Ewing's sarcoma does not improve prognosis. *J Clin Oncol.* 2001;19:2812–2820.

78. Campbell AD, Cohn SL, Reynolds M, et al. Treatment of relapsed Wilms' tumor with high-dose therapy and autologous hematopoietic stem-cell rescue: the experience at Children's Memorial Hospital. *J Clin Oncol.* 2004;22:2885–2890.

79. Pinkerton CR. Megatherapy for soft tissue sarcomas. EBMT experience. *Bone Marrow Transplant.* 1991;7(suppl 3):120–122.

80. Kushner BH, LaQuaglia MP, Wollner N, et al. Desmoplastic small round-cell tumor: prolonged progression-free survival with aggressive multimodality therapy. *J Clin Oncol.* 1996;14:1526–1531.

81. Pulsipher MA, Woolfrey A. Nonmyeloablative transplantation in children. Current status and future prospects. *Hematol Oncol Clin North Am.* 2001;15:809–834, vii–viii.

Clinical Trials in Pediatric Oncology: Design and Conduct

CHAPTER 11

Mark Krailo and Gregory H. Reaman

Introduction

In this chapter we will review the important contributions to evidence-based standards of care for children with cancer made possible by therapeutic research as well as the state of the art in clinical trials, with particular reference to pediatric cancer research. We broadly define a clinical trial as any form of planned therapeutic experiment that involves patients and is designed to elucidate the most appropriate treatment of future patients with a given medical condition.[1] Important in the pediatric oncology setting is the principle that appropriate treatment encompasses that which not only achieves improvements in outcome (survival, event-free survival, cure) but does so with the least likelihood of resulting in severe short-term and late toxicity impacting quality of life and survivorship. The rationale for conducting clinical trials in pediatric cancer extends beyond the demonstration of clinical utility of a therapeutic approach to reach accurate conclusions from investigational observations about the benefit of highly toxic and expensive therapies. Anything other than controlled clinical trials risks reaching conclusions about a therapy that may actually be harmful or useless and potentially jeopardize progress in curing childhood cancer.

In oncology, clinical trials are usually divided into 3 broad classifications. A Phase I study is the primary means to establish a safe and feasible way to deliver a novel therapy; a Phase II study is employed to screen new therapies for evidence of efficacy; and a Phase III study provides the primary means of determining whether a new therapeutic approach is preferred to the current standard.

This paradigm of development of new therapies through well-defined stages has been used with profound success in treatment of some childhood cancers, as demonstrated by the steady increase in ultimate cure of children with acute lymphoblastic leukemia[2] (see Figure 11-1).

Conducting clinical trials in childhood cancer presents unique challenges. Cancer in individuals under 20 years old is a relatively low-incidence disease. Data from the Surveillance, Epidemiology, and End Results program of the US National Cancer Institute (NCI) indicate that approximately 15 000 new cases of cancer are diagnosed

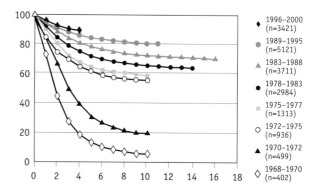

Figure 11-1 Survival comparison COG ALL study series.

in individuals under the age of 20 in the United States each year.[3] Robust, protocol-based research in this setting can be conducted only by multidisciplinary teams in a cooperative group setting.[4] The organization and execution of cooperative group trials have been a hallmark of pediatric cancer research and the primary reason for the advancement of cure of these diseases.[5]

Phase I, II, and III studies in pediatric cancer research each have their own special considerations for both study design and conduct as well as ethical consideration. In the sections that follow, we will review these concerns for each type of study.

Phase I Clinical Trials

Phase I clinical trials are the first step in human exposure to potential new treatments. In these situations, the safe and feasible approach to delivery of a new treatment must be established and the biological effects of the therapy on the patient have yet to be characterized. In the discussions that ensue, we describe the Phase I process for drug development, but the principles are similar for other types of investigational therapeutic interventions.

In the pediatric setting, new agents usually become available for investigation after safe and tolerable doses and schedules have been established in adults. Experience

151

has demonstrated that doses and schedules in adults are not directly applicable to children,[6] and thus Phase I studies of children are necessary. The therapeutic effects of such a new agent in childhood cancer, however, generally are not known. Because of this, enrollment in Phase I studies is restricted generally to patients for whom no known curative therapy exists. Most often, this restricts enrollment to patients with recurrent or refractory disease, but newly diagnosed patients with a low likelihood of cure, such as those with brain stem glioma, can be considered candidates for Phase I studies. Adequate hepatic and renal function are required, both for the protection of the patient and in order to accurately assess the agent's effects on the patient. Adequate organ function of other systems, including hematological and cardiac, are required depending on the disease studied (solid tumor vs leukemia) and the known or putative mechanism of toxicity of the new agent.

Because new agents are of unknown benefit, Phase I studies are designed to minimize the number of patients exposed to large doses or prolonged schedules, since these are associated with an increased chance of toxicity. Conventionally, Phase I studies are designed to start with the administration of 80% of the adult recommended dose, and subsequent dose levels to be investigated are determined according to a modified Fibonacci scheme. The starting dose is initially given to a small cohort of children. Each patient is assessed for the occurrence of a dose-limiting toxicity (DLT) over a fixed time frame, often 1 month, after treatment is started. Dose-limiting toxicity is defined to be a toxicity that prevents further administration of the agent at that level. Grade 3 or 4 adverse events as defined by the NCI common toxicity criteria (http://ctep.cancer.gov), with the specific exception of complications such as nausea and vomiting that can be controlled with appropriate supportive care measures, usually constitute DLTs, although prolonged grade 2 toxicities can be considered DLTs depending on the schedule of drug administration. The decision to escalate the drug is based on the results in the current cohort. A typical example of such a decision rule at a particular dose level is shown in Table 11-1.

The study proceeds until dose escalation or reduction is no longer possible. There are other design options for Phase I studies. Accelerated titration designs[7] provide for 1 or 2 patients to be enrolled to each dose level at the start of the escalation process and require larger cohorts only after toxicities are observed. Such methods are more appropriate when the adult recommended dose is not established so that the first dose levels may be low compared with the eventual maximum tolerated dose (MTD). Other methods, such as the continual reassessment method[8] and Escalation with Overdose Control,[9] model the relationship between dose and toxicity and use this relationship to determine the dose escalation to be used. All methods have in common the approach of escalating to higher doses only after low doses have proven to be tolerable. The designs have similar statistical properties,[10] so the choice of methods can be made

on considerations such as the number of patients available for enrollment.

Phase I studies provide a unique opportunity to assess the biologic effects of a new agent. Generally, patients are treated at several dose levels so that the relationship between dose and biologic effects can be explored. Such analyses can be key to the rational development of a new drug.[11,12] Detailed study of pharmacokinetics and pharmacodynamics are often performed; many studies also include other measures of biologic effects, such as immune modulation, depending on the putative method of action of the agent. Because the primary aim of Phase I studies is to establish the MTD or schedule, the target enrollment for a Phase I trial is established for those criteria and not planned to identify target differences in biologic measurements across dose levels. By implication, patients must be specifically consented for participation in biologic investigations; requiring participation in these studies as a condition of enrollment is defensible only when the results will be used to modify the treatment for that patient or other patients enrolled on the study.[13]

Children and adolescents represent a vulnerable population according to the US Code of Federal Regulations, part 46, subpart D. The consent process for enrollment on a Phase I trial, as in all clinical trials, including Phase II and III trials, must avoid coercion of the legal guardians as well as the child when the child is old enough to provide consent. By their nature, therapies considered in Phase I trials have not demonstrated efficacy in either controlling disease or prolonging life. Unlike the consent process for later-phase trials, the consent process for a Phase I study may not imply that there will be direct therapeutic benefit for the participant. A small survey[14] demonstrated that physician-investigators believed that the parents of children entering Phase I studies understood that the chance of cure was small and had realistic expectations regarding toxicity. Although there is limited empirical evidence on the informed consent process, personal interaction between health care professionals and patients and guardians is critical to achieve informed consent.[15]

Phase II Clinical Trials

Once the safe and tolerable dose and schedule of a therapy have been established, its effectiveness must be tested to determine whether the agent(s) have potential to become part of standard therapy. Few data regarding efficacy are available from Phase I studies, because usually fewer than 10 patients are enrolled at the recommended dose. The primary purpose of a Phase II study is to screen efficiently for potentially effective therapies that could be incorporated into, or become, standard treatment.

Because the efficacy of the new therapy generally is not known, enrollment in Phase II studies is restricted to patients for whom conventional curative therapy approaches have been exhausted. Adequate hepatic and renal function are required, both for the protection of the patient and to assess the agent's effects on the patient accurately. Adequate organ function of other

Table 11-1

Dose level escalation decision.

Number of Patients Previously Enrolled at the Dose Level	Number of Patients Evaluable for DLT	Total Number of Patients with DLT at the Dose Level	Escalation Decision
0	3	0	Escalate to the next dose level in the next cohort.
0	3	2 or more	The dose level is not tolerable. Reduce the dose in the next cohort enrolled unless 6 patients have been evaluated at the reduced dose.
0	3	1	Enroll 3 more patients at the current dose level.
3	3	0 or 1	Escalate to the next dose level unless that dose level is considered not tolerable.
3	3	2 or more	The dose level is not tolerable. Reduce the dose in the next cohort enrolled unless 6 patients have been evaluated at the reduced dose.

systems, including hematological and cardiac, are required depending on the disease studied (solid tumor vs leukemia) or the putative mechanism of action of toxicity. In addition, a patient must have a disease that can be objectively evaluated. This is generally referred to as "measurable disease." The definition and measurement is different for solid-tumor patients when compared with those with leukemia.

The efficacy of a therapy considered in a Phase II study is usually evaluated using a putative marker of disease sensitivity that can be determined within a short time frame. The reduction in tumor burden, as quantified by the Response Evaluation Criteria In Solid Tumors criteria,[16] is often employed for patients with solid tumors. Quantitative changes in bone marrow morphology[17] have been used for patients with leukemia. For certain diseases, such as neuroblastoma and brain tumors, alternative criteria involving multidimensional lesion measurements and semiquantitative imaging are employed to measure disease burden.

The agent(s) are screened by comparing the observed percentage of patients who demonstrate sufficient reduction in tumor burden ("response") with a target rate derived either from historical data or from a contemporaneous control. The agent is considered for further development if observed efficacy rate is consistent with the target.

Generally, reduction in tumor burden is chosen rather than other characteristics such as alleviation of symptoms, because the measurement of drug effect must be objective and reproducible by different investigators. Further, reduction in tumor burden may be a surrogate for prolonged survival, although this has not been confirmed for all disease types.

Results of Phase II studies must be reported within the context of a specific disease. Phase II trials in children generally enroll 20 to 30 patients with a particular disease. Most designs entail enrolling patients in 2 or more stages,[18,19] although 2-stage designs are used predominantly in studies of children.[17] In this way, agents can be screened rapidly while minimizing the number of patients enrolled on studies of therapies that do not reduce tumor burden. An example of a 2-stage rule developed using the methodology proposed by Simon[18] follows:

1. Enroll 9 patients. If no patient demonstrates response, terminate the trial with the conclusion that agent is not associated with a sufficiently high response rate; otherwise

2. Enroll an additional 19 patients. If 4 or more of 28 patients demonstrate response, the agent is considered for further development. Otherwise, the agent is considered inactive.

The probability of accepting an agent with a response rate of 10% in relapsed patients is only 0.15 whereas the probability of accepting an agent with a response rate of 30% is 0.85.

Many authors have described Phase II designs that incorporate prior information on the response probability.[20,21] When there are 2 or more candidate therapies, randomization among those regimens can be employed.[22,23] Because of the heterogeneity of the patients enrolled, particularly with respect to prior therapy, the outcome measures used, and the sample size requirements, randomized Phase II studies are intended to screen treatments for efficacy only. The results of such studies are not definitive and are a prelude to a definitive Phase III trial.

Phase II studies present a unique opportunity for refining early observations made in Phase I studies, because the new therapy is often combined with standard treatment in

Phase III studies. Limiting sampling pharmacokinetic techniques have been used successfully to obtain estimates of the pharmacology parameters of a drug administered at a dose considered tolerable and for which estimates of efficacy will be obtained.[24,25] Assessment of therapeutic modulation of a putative biologic target has also been incorporated into Phase II studies.[26,27] The primary aim of most Phase II studies, however, is to screen for new, potentially effective agents. By implication, patients must be specifically consented for participation in correlative biologic investigations and biological specimen acquisition.

Phase III Clinical Trials

Once a therapy has shown promise in the context of high-risk patients, investigation of its role in the treatment of newly diagnosed patients is warranted. This is best accomplished in the setting of a Phase III study. The primary objective of a Phase III trial is to provide definitive evidence on the safety and relative efficacy of interventions that can be delivered in real-world practice. In order to accomplish this, such trials are comparative;[1] that is, they involve assigning patients who are homogeneous with respect to disease type and prognosis to 2 or more different treatments and following these individuals until an event of interest, such as disease progression or death, is observed. Randomization is the most scientifically sound method of treatment assignment[28] and is a hallmark of most Phase III studies.

Successful treatments for childhood cancer are multidisciplinary. Primary therapy for patients generally requires close collaboration among oncologists, surgeons, pathologists, radiation therapists, nurses, and psychosocial providers. Protocol-based research must take this collaboration into account if the therapies studied are to meet the test of being applicable to real-world practice. In order to describe study treatments adequately and thus provide sound study conclusions, protocols must include guidelines for all modalities that are relevant to the treatment of the disease. Indeed, most Phase III studies have aims that address modality-specific questions. These aims are reflected in data collection and analysis plans that specifically address how such questions will be evaluated.

The particular design used varies according to the disease and hypothesis being tested. We list below some common components.

Eligibility: Eligibility criteria describe the patient population for whom the therapies under study is appropriate. Phase III studies should have broad-ranging and simple eligibility criteria, since the results of these trials will dictate subsequent clinical practice. These criteria usually describe the diagnostic criteria to be met to ensure that a patient has the disease of interest and the organ function criteria required and thus all the treatments that could be assigned to the patient can be given safely.

Eligibility should be determined by data that are available at the time the patient is to be enrolled in a study. If a patient's eligibility cannot be fully confirmed, enrollment in the particular clinical trial may jeopardize safety, since

the patient may not be appropriate for 1 or more of the therapies to be used in the study. Eligibility criteria should be precisely stated and not subject to interpretation.

Endpoints: The endpoints chosen to evaluate relative efficacy quantify clinical benefit to the patient. The endpoints most often chosen are: (1) time from study enrollment to death; or (2) time from study enrollment to first adverse disease event, where an adverse disease event is considered disease progression, diagnosis of a second malignant neoplasm, or death from causes other than disease (usually treatment toxicity).

Clinically Relevant Differences: Protocols for comparative Phase III studies designate the difference in outcome between regimens that are of interest and can be detected with high probability. Phase III studies in childhood cancer are generally designed to detect differences in long-term outcome of 15% or less between regimens. This figure represents a reduction in rate of failure of 50% or less for most types of malignancy.

Number of Patients Required to Evaluate Primary Study Questions: Phase III studies are designed to identify, with high probability, the best regimen with respect to the study endpoints when the candidate regimes differ by at least the stated clinically relevant difference. Sample size requirements for Phase III studies are dependent on rate at which the event of interest occurs in the study population rather than just the total number of patients enrolled.[29] The statistical methodology for such calculations is well developed and is available in statistical software packages such as EaST[30] and PASS.[31]

Interim Monitoring Strategy: Most Phase III studies of childhood cancer require at least 3 years of patient enrollment with 1 or more additional years of follow-up. A well-designed study incorporates a plan to terminate patient enrollment if the study regimens prove to be different with respect to the primary outcome early in the course of patient enrollment. Such a plan takes into account that the proportion of the expected information on the event rate will be available each time an interim comparison is performed.[32] This form of monitoring protects patients' interests by ensuring that patients are not treated with a regimen associated with significantly inferior outcome.

Increasingly, randomized studies include a futility monitoring rule.[33] In contrast to stopping a trial because of apparent treatment differences, this strategy entails stopping a randomized trial when, at an interim analysis, the study regimens have similar outcome and there is a small probability that further data will lead to the identification of a superior regimen according to study criteria.

Independent Data Monitoring Committee: An independent data and safety monitoring committee (DSMC) is essential to the conduct of Phase III studies.[34,35] A DSMC must be appointed, and the DSMC roles established, before a study is opened.[35] The primary role of the DSMC is to protect the interests of currently enrolled patients and patients who may be enrolled in the future.[35] The DSMC members discharge their duties by overseeing the execution of the interim monitoring strategy and reviewing the results of other investigations as they affect the relevance of the study.[35] The elements of the DSMC charter for cancer clinical trials sponsored by the NCI are described elsewhere.[34] Although the specific details of a DSMC charter may vary between studies, common to all practices is that unmasked analyses describing outcome are presented only to the DSMC during the time that data are being accumulated to answer the primary study questions.

Clinical Trial Planning and Conduct

All clinical trials have common requirements for design, implementation, and ethical conduct, as discussed below.

The process of planning a clinical trial includes the generation of a protocol that is essentially a written guide to the therapeutic experiment to be conducted. As a written guide, the protocol document should ensure that the experiment is conducted uniformly such that the clinical trial results in a definitive answer to the question(s) being asked or definitive proof of the hypothesis being tested. The critical elements of the protocol are listed in Table 11-2. Documentation of compliance with study requirements (regulatory, eligibility criteria, investigational intervention, response and/or toxicity assessment, data acquisition and reporting, biologic specimen procurement, handling, and testing) should encompass the obligation of the investigators and sponsor(s) to also ensure that the conduct of the study falls within legal and ethical guidelines set forth by regulatory agencies, eg, the Good Clinical Practice (GCP) Guidance document adopted by the US Food and Drug Administration and equivalent regulatory agencies in other countries.

The investigators at each institution must obtain appropriate review of the protocol by the Institutional Review Board with assurance of the Office of Human Research Protections, US Department of Health and Human Services, as required by federal law, to ensure that human subjects participating in clinical research are adequately protected from research risks. Central to the concept of human subjects protection is the concept of informed consent in which there is full disclosure of potential risks and benefits shared with the general population (justice). The risks to the individual must be minimized and the benefits maximized (beneficence) and the rights of the individual to decide whether to assume research risks must be observed (respect for persons). In most cases, particularly for children who have not reached the age of majority, informed consent actually constitutes parental (or legal guardian) permission. Because children are considered a highly vulnerable population, they are afforded the additional protection including the general requirement that they stand to benefit from participating in the research that exposes them to anything more than minimal risks. Excellent and meritorious scientific design of the clinical trial is an absolute requirement for protection of human subjects, not only because potential benefits will be maximized and risks minimized, but because less than a scientifically sound study will be unable to answer the research question fully and neither study participant nor society will derive benefit to offset the risks of the study.

The required critical elements of the informed consent process are listed in Table 11-3. A clear statement of study objective(s) limited to the actual research question is essential and clearly distinguishes a protocol document describing a clinical trial from a patient management guideline and is key to the development of a research plan. A well-prepared presentation of supporting background data/experiences leading to a rationale for the planned therapeutic experiment is essential for evaluating the significance of the impact of a study critical to determining scientific merit.

The protocol document should precisely define the patient population to be studied, regardless of the degree of homogeneity the investigator deems necessary. Careful selection and clearly stated eligibility criteria, including diagnosis, extent of disease (stage), age, prior therapy and performance status, and organ function will ensure the integrity of the investigation and the applicability of results to a specific patient population. To ensure compliance, eligibility criteria should be so clearly stated that nothing is left to interpretation. Generally, homogeneity of the patient population is more important in Phase I and II studies in which accurate toxicity assessment or biologic activity is being determined.

Concern for generalizability of study results is more important for Phase III studies in which treatment effect on an entire patient population is being assessed. Critical eligibility criteria for Phase II studies that seek to evaluate specific treatment response or other biologic effect are the existence of measurable disease and a definition of the methods of disease assessment at study entry.

The treatment plan should be clear, succinct, and precise to provide uniformity of that portion of the clinical experiment. Care should be taken to clarify that the protocol document dictates protocol-mandated therapy and not flexible treatment guidelines. Recommendations and guidelines (eg, supportive care) should be clearly distinguished from protocol requirements. If schematics are

Table 11-2
Critical sections of the protocol.
Objectives (specific aims to address hypothesis)
Background and rationale
Eligibility criteria
Study design (methods)
Treatment plan
Drug information
Response assessment: Methods; criteria
Clinical and laboratory data requirements
Statistical considerations
Informed consent document
References
Appendixes

Table 11-3

Essential elements of the informed consent document.

1. Clear statement of the research question as distinct from clinical care
   - Study purpose
   - Duration of participation
   - Experimental aspect of new drug, technique, route of drug delivery
   - Procedures, studies required
2. Clear statement of risks attributable to specific drugs or interventions
3. Statement of expected benefits (if any) to participation
4. Statement of alternative treatment approach to clinical trial participation
5. Assurance of confidentiality of research records with disclosure that they may be made available to NCI, FDA, other regulatory agencies, pharmacy company sponsor (if appropriate).
6. Statement of institutional policy for compensation for study-related injury and emergency injury management.
7. Identification of institutional officials (with contact information), staff, study personnel to answer questions.
8. Clear statement of voluntary nature of participation.
   - Refusal or discontinuation of study participation and impact on patient benefits and continuation of care.

used, they should be unambiguous and accurately reflect written text.

The criteria for response and/or toxicity assessment (clinical, laboratory investigations, imaging studies, histopathology, etc) should be clearly stated, individual specific parameters well defined, and the methodology for their measurement clearly described. In addition, the specific time points at which assessment is required should be stated. The importance with which clarity, specificity, and accuracy relate to eligibility criteria, uniformity of treatment intervention, and response assessment cannot be overstated when quality assurance of study conduct and data integrity are assessed.

Clinical and laboratory data required for the conduct of the study mandate judicious consideration of the study endpoints as well as the specific aims and are clearly different in Phase I, II, and III studies wherein the objective of assessment of toxicity vs response varies considerably. Requests for superfluous data (not required to address a study-specific aim) result in the potential for missed critical evaluations and threaten the quality of study data and subsequent analysis and results.

Clinical Trial Conduct and Management

Data required to address the goals of a study are often not recorded directly in a patient's medical record. Further, most clinical trials in pediatric oncology require the cooperation of, and enrollment from, 2 or more institutions. Because of this, clinical trials data, encompassing information to address the primary study questions and patient safety data, must be recorded on data-capture instruments distinct from a patient's medical record. The design of the data-capture instrument, whether paper or electronic, is an extremely important undertaking in the planning and conduct of a clinical trial. Consideration should be given to involve those clinical research staff

ultimately responsible for the capture and reporting of data elements in the design and execution of the instruments to maximize compliance and efficiency. Errors and ambiguities can be frequently avoided by "piloting" the use of such instruments. Significant attention should be given to "user-friendly" features to ensure accuracy, quality, and timeliness of data submitted. Submission schedules should be established in advance. Again, only data that are critical to answering study questions/objectives, as clearly stated in the protocol, should be requested.

Enrollment and treatment assignment should be done at a central facility. As much as is possible, a patient should be enrolled in a study prior to the start of any study-specified intervention. Prior to enrollment, the investigator who is requesting study entry should be asked to verify that the patient is eligible. Similarly, treatment assignment should be made by a central authority. All requirements for treatment assignment should be verified before the assignment is made, particularly if the assignment is randomly generated. Random treatment assignment should be made as closely as possible to the time when the assigned treatment will start. Pediatric cooperative group studies use a Web-based enrollment and treatment allocation system to meet these requirements.

Significant attention should also focus on methods to ensure quality control of study conduct and data obtained for analysis. Complex studies may require focused educational sessions for investigators, particularly when multidisciplinary treatment interventions are involved. A system should be developed to alert investigators and research staff of required observations and interventions as well as errors in data submitted to a central data management and analysis center. These generally are in place for pediatric cancer clinical trials. On-site auditing to evaluate compliance with protocol-specified treatment and observations as well as verification of accuracy of data submitted through validation of primary source documents (medical records, etc) are requisites for GCP compliance.

All research data used for analysis of a study should be maintained in a computer system. Documentation of the data structures, variables, and codes should be sufficiently complete to allow data analytic staff not associated with the study to retrieve data from the computer files and replicate key analyses performed for the study. In addition to the quality assurance systems noted above, rigorous computerized data validation checks should be part of the quality control system for a clinical trial. Data as originally submitted by institutional investigators should be retrievable from the computerized data system along with any other information obtained through review of data-capture instruments and laboratory investigations performed on patient samples.

All studies should have a system for data monitoring for untoward events and interim analysis. As mentioned previously, there are special considerations for Phase III clinical trials that entail, as part of writing the protocol, a plan for stopping a study early because of interim results and a process involving a data-monitoring committee to have these results reviewed by a body independent of the trial's organizers. In addition to monitoring for differences in the primary outcome measures, standardized toxicity displays, including a summary of all deaths attributable to treatment complications, should be reviewed by the trial organizers on a regular basis to ensure that the trial therapies are safe and tolerable for the patient population under study.

Reporting the outcomes of clinical trials in a timely fashion in peer-reviewed communications is a critical aspect of clinical trials execution.[36] The trial planning process should include designation of the primary manuscripts that will arise from the study. In this way, data collection and analysis needs can be targeted toward these needs. Once a manuscript is published, the data set and documentation used to produce the results should be archived so the analysis can be reproduced at a later time, if necessary. As the improvement in treatment outcomes for any childhood cancers are directly attributable to properly conducted, well-designed, multicenter, multidisciplinary clinical trials, the unequivocal responsibility of investigators to communicate the results of a clinical trial, whether positive or negative, to benefit society, cannot be overstated.

References

1. Pocock SJ. *Clinical Trials: A Practical Approach*. New York: John Wiley and Sons; 1983.
2. Gaynon PS, Trigg ME, Heerema NA, et al. Children's Cancer Group trials in childhood acute lymphoblastic leukemia: 1983–1995. *Leukemia*. 1997;14:2223–2233.
3. Surveillance, Epidemiology, and End Results (SEER) Program (www.seer.cancer.gov) SEER*Stat Database: Populations—Total U.S. (1969–2002), National Cancer Institute, DCCPS, Surveillance Research Program, Cancer Statistics Branch, released April 2005.
4. Reaman GH. Pediatric cancer research from past successes through collaboration to future transdisciplinary research. *J Pediatr Oncol Nurs*. 2004;21:123–127.
5. Bleyer WA. The U.S. pediatric cancer clinical trials programmes: international implications and the way forward. *Eur J Cancer*. 1997;33:1439–1447.
6. Lee DP, Skolnik JM, Adamson PC. Pediatric phase I trials in oncology: an analysis of study conduct efficiency. *J Clin Oncol*. 2005;23:8431–8441.
7. Simon RM, Freidlin B, Rubin LV, Arbuck S, Collins J, Christian M. Accelerated titration designs for phase I clinical trials in oncology. *J Natl Cancer Inst*. 1997;89:1138–1147.
8. O'Quigley J, Pepe M, Fisher M. Continual reassessment method: a practical design for phase I clinical trials in cancer. *Biometrics*. 1990;46:33–38.
9. Babb J, Rogatako A, Zacks SA. Cancer phase I clinical trials: efficient dose escalation with overdose control. *Stat Med*. 1998;7:1103–1120.
10. Ahn C. An evaluation of phase I cancer trials designs. *Stat Med*. 1998;17:1537–1549.
11. Panetta JC, Iacono LC, Adamson PC, Stewart CF. The importance of pharmacokinetic limited sampling models for childhood cancer drug development. *Clin Cancer Res*. 2003;9:5068–5077.
12. Smith M, Bernstein M, Bleyer WA, et al. Conduct of phase I trials in children with cancer. *J Clin Oncol*. 1998;16:966–978.
13. Anderson BD, Adamson PC, Weiner SL, McCabe MS, Smith MA. Tissue collection for correlative studies in childhood cancer clinical trials: ethical considerations and special imperatives. *J Clin Oncol*. 2004;22:4846–4850.
14. Estlin EJ, Cotterill S, Pratt CB, Pearson AD, Bernstein M. Phase I trials in pediatric oncology: perceptions of pediatricians from the United Kingdom Children's Cancer Study Group and the Pediatric Oncology Group. *J Clin Oncol*. 2000;18:1900–1905.
15. Albrecht TL, Franks MM, Ruckdeschel JC. Communication and informed consent. *Curr Opin Oncol*. 2005;17:336–339.
16. Therasse P, Arbuck SG, Eisenhauer A, et al. New guideline to evaluate response to treatment in solid tumors. *J Natl Cancer Inst*. 92:205–216.
17. Angiolillo AL, Whitlock J, Chen Z, Krailo M, Reaman G. Phase II study of gemcitabine in children with relapsed acute lymphoblastic leukemia or acute myelogenous leukemia (ADVL0022): A Children's Oncology Group Report. *Pediatr Blood Cancer*. 2006;46:193–197.
18. Simon R. Optimal two stage designs for phase II clinical trials. *Controlled Clin Trials*. 1989;10:1–10.
19. Chen T. Optimal three-stage designs for phase II clinical trials. *Stat Med*. 1997;16:2701–2711.
20. Thall PF, Simon RM, Estey EH. Bayesian sequential monitoring designs for single-arm clinical trials with multiple outcomes. *Stat Med*. 1995;14:357–379.
21. Tan S-B, Machin D. Bayesian two-stage designs for phase II clinical trials. *Stat Med*. 2002;21:1991–2012.
22. Simon R, Wittes RE, Ellenberg SS. Randomized phase II clinical trials. *Cancer Treat Rep*. 1985;69:1375–1381.
23. Rubenstein LV, Korn EL, Freidlin B, Hunsberger S, Ivy SP, Smith MA. Design issues of randomized phase II trials and a proposal for phase II screening trials. *J Clin Oncol*. 2005;23:7199–7206.
24. Vaughan WP, Carey D, Perry S, Westfall AO, Salzman DE. A limited sampling strategy for pharmacokinetic directed therapy with intravenous busulfan. *Biol Blood Marrow Transplant*. 2002;8:619–624.
25. Van Kesteren C, Mathjt RA, Lopez-Lazaro L, et al. A comparison of limited sampling strategies for the prediction of Ecteinascidin 743 clearance when administered as a 24-hour infusion. *Cancer Chemo Pharmacol*. 2001;48:459–466.
26. Kindler HL, Friberg G, Singh DA, et al. Phase II trial of bevacizumab plus gemcitabine in patients with advanced pancreatic cancer. *J Clin Oncol*. 2005;23:8033–8040.
27. Olson JJ, James CD, Lawson D, Hunter S, Tang G, Billingsley J. Correlation of the response of recurrent malignant gliomas treated with interferon alpha with tumor interferon alpha gene content. *Int J Oncol*. 2004;25:419–427.
28. Sprott DA, Farewell VT. Some thoughts on randomization and causation. *SSC Liaison*. 1992;6:6–10.
29. Curran D, Sylvester RJ, Hoctin Boes G. Sample size estimation in phase III cancer clinical trials. *Eur J Surg Oncol*. 1999;25:244–250.
30. *EaST (Early Stopping in Clinical Trials)*. Cambridge, MA: Cytel Software Corp; 1992.
31. PASS. Kaysville, UT: Number Cruncher Statistical Systems; 2004.
32. Lan KKG, DeMets DL. Group sequential procedures: calendar versus information time. *Stat Med*. 1989;8:1191–1198.
33. Whitehead J, Matsushita T. Stopping clinical trials because of treatment ineffectiveness: a comparison of a *futility design* with a method of stochastic curtailment. *Stat Med*. 2003;22:677–687.
34. Smith MA, Ungerleider RS, Korn EL, Rubinstein L, Simon R. Role of independent data-monitoring committees in randomized clinical trials sponsored by the National Cancer Institute. *J Clin Oncol*. 1997;15:2736–2743.
35. Wilhelmsen L. Role of the Data and Safety Monitoring Committee (DSMC). *Stat Med*. 2002;21:2823–2829.
36. Girling DJ. Important issues in planning and conducting multi centre randomised trials in cancer and publishing their results. *Crit Rev Oncol Hematol*. 2000;36:13–25.

Tumors in Children

Acute Lymphoblastic Leukemia

CHAPTER

12

Naomi J. Winick, Elizabeth A. Raetz, Joerg Ritter, and William L. Carroll

Introduction

The dramatic improvement in outcome for children with acute lymphoblastic leukemia (ALL) ranks as one of the most successful advances in the war against cancer. Many factors led to the remarkable cure rates, now approaching 80%. These include: (1) the identification of effective drug combinations through empiric, highly disciplined clinical trials; (2) the recognition of sanctuary sites and the routine use of presymptomatic central nervous system (CNS) directed therapy; (3) the intensification of therapy using existing agents; and (4) the identification of clinical and biologic variables predictive of outcome and their use in stratifying treatment. In spite of these advances, numerous challenges remain, including the development of better treatment for the significant minority of patients who relapse and the development of less-toxic therapy. Breakthroughs in basic science now provide an opportunity to target therapy to the abnormal biologic pathways that drive tumor growth and to minimize host toxicity.

Incidence and Epidemiology

Acute lymphoblastic leukemia is the most common childhood cancer, accounting for close to 25% of newly diagnosed cancers in children less than 15 years of age. Leukemia incidence rates are reasonably constant at 5 per 100 000 person-years, with 80% of the cases being ALL. A variety of hypotheses regarding the etiology and potential pathogenic mechanisms of childhood ALL have been described.[1,2] As with other cancers, multiple steps lead to clinically detectable leukemia from a preleukemic precursor cell. Consistent with Knudson's two-hit hypothesis,[3] neonatal events can play a role in the development of childhood ALL because evidence of the leukemic clone can be detected at birth in many cases.[1,4,5] Molecular techniques using the polymerase chain reaction (PCR) have documented the presence of the same leukemia-specific fusion-gene sequences in neonatal blood spots as are present in diagnostic samples from children with leukemia.[6] There is a higher concordance rate in mono-

chorionic twins than in dichorionic twins or in siblings.[1] Leukemias with the (4,11) translocation and the MLL-AF4 fusion product have a very high concordance rate and a brief latency, while others, such as those with the TEL-AML1 fusion gene, may present with disease after a long, several-year latency period.[7] Children with Down syndrome are at significantly increased risk for developing leukemia, while polymorphisms of the gene coding for methylenetetrahydrofolate reductase may protect individuals from developing leukemia by decreasing the incidence of uracil incorporation into DNA, thereby decreasing the likelihood of DNA strand breaks and chromosomal damage.[8–10]

Environmental factors may also play a role. Maternal exposures to the DNA-damaging agents dipyrone (a nonsteroidal anti-inflammatory agent) and baygon (a carbamate pesticide) have been linked to the diagnosis of ALL,[11] as has maternal exposure to indoor insecticides and pesticides in the garden.[11,12] The risk associated with these exposures appears to be enhanced by the presence of CYP-1A1m1 and CYP-1A1m2 polymorphisms.[13]

Infection may also be linked to childhood leukemia,[14,15] with the ubiquitous John Cunningham virus demonstrating specificity for B-lymphocytes and interacting with p53.[15] The largest epidemiologic study of childhood ALL published to date,[14] however, did not find a correlation between day care attendance or time in day care and the risk of developing ALL, despite the increase in common childhood infections associated with early day care. Breastfeeding was associated with a decreased risk of ALL, with the risk declining further for those infants breastfed for six months or longer.[16] Whether the protective effect stems from the transmission of maternal antibodies, macrophages, and lymphocytes; the transmission of cytokines and growth factors; or another immunomodulatory effect has yet to be defined.[16]

Although inciting events for the development of leukemia in the overwhelming majority of children remain unclear, future studies will define complex relationships between host genetic polymorphisms, environmental exposures, and infections in the development of childhood ALL.

Molecular Pathogenesis

The development of techniques to analyze chromosome structure in human cancers led to the recognition that many tumors contained structural alterations including gains and/or losses of chromosomes, as well as rearrangements between chromosomes (eg, translocations). In some cases these rearrangements were quite specific for tumor subtypes, indicating a direct role in tumor pathogenesis. Further refinement of classic cytogenetic techniques and the development of additional approaches including PCR and fluorescence in situ hybridization (FISH) now show that more than 85% of childhood ALL cases contain recurring chromosomal abnormalities.[17] Recombinant DNA technology has identified many of the genes that are altered by the observed gross chromosomal changes, and subsequently a variety of in vitro and in vivo experiments established a direct role for these genetic abnormalities in the transformation to leukemia.[18, 19] No single lesion is solely responsible for transforming a benign lymphoid precursor to leukemia but, as mentioned, multiple defects appear to cooperate in this process.

Approximately one-third of newly diagnosed B-precursor ALL samples contain excess chromosomes with two-thirds of these cases having modal chromosome numbers >50 (Table 12-1). An additional 25% of B-precursor cases contain a t(12;21)(p13;q22) that results in a chimeric mRNA linking the TEL (or ETV6) and AML1 (or RUNX1) genes. It is important to note that this translocation is rarely detected using conventional cytogenetics but can be seen using FISH.[20] The presence of hyperdiploidy[21,22] or TEL-AML1 correlates with a good prognosis,[23] so the detection of these and other prognostically important genetic abnormalities is an essential part of the initial evaluation of a child with ALL. Exactly how TEL-AML1 contributes to leukemogenesis is uncertain, but both genes are transcription factors required for normal hematopoiesis. The t(1;19)(q23;p130), seen in many B-precursor ALL cases, likewise juxtaposes two other genes encoding transcription factors resulting in the E2A-PBX fusion gene.[24,25] Translocations involving the MLL gene are uncommon in childhood ALL but are seen in approximately 70% of infant ALL cases.[26] The rearrangements at the MLL locus (11q23) involve more than 30 different reciprocal partners, with t(4;11)(q21;q23)(MLL-AF4) being the most common subtype.[26] The "downstream" consequences of these cytogenetic changes are now being elucidated to discover tumor-specific targets for the future development of molecularly targeted therapy. For example, the FMS-like tyrosine kinase-3 (FLT-3) receptor is a member of the class III receptor tyrosine kinase family that includes c-Kit and platelet-derived growth factor receptor (PDGFR). FLT-3 is aberrantly expressed in up to one-third of hyperdiploid ALL samples, and 18% of MLL-rearranged ALLs contain mutations in the kinase or juxtamembrane regions that result in activation of the receptor.[27,28] A number of pharmacological inhibitors of FLT-3 have now been developed, and preclinical data confirm that FLT-3 inhibition results in leukemia cell death.[29] These agents are now in clinical trials in adults and children with ALL and acute myeloid leukemia (AML).[30]

The Philadelphia (Ph) chromosome deserves special emphasis because it was the first chromosome abnormality observed in cancer cells. Initially described as an abnormally short chromosome 22, it was subsequently discovered that the Ph chromosome was actually the result of a reciprocal translocation between c-ABL oncogene sequences on chromosome 9 and the "breakpoint cluster region" (BCR) gene on chromosome 22, t(9;22)(q34;q11).[21] Although the Ph chromosome was initially associated with chronic myelogenous leukemia (CML), it was also identified in 2% to 3% of childhood ALL and is the most common genetic abnormality in adult ALL, occurring in approximately one-third of cases.[21] Subtle differences exist in the chromosomal breakpoints in BCR-ABL between CML and ALL with most ALLs

---

Table 12-1

Common chromosomal abnormalities in ALL.

Abnormality	ALL Subtype	Genes/Chromosomes	Approximate Frequency	Prognostic Significance
Hyperdiploidy	Early B-lineage	4, 10, and 17	30%	Favorable
Hypodiploidy	Early B-lineage	<44	3%	Unfavorable
t(4;11)(q21;q23)	Pro-B, Infants	MLL-AF4	2%	Unfavorable
t(1;19)(q23;p13)	Pre-B ALL	E2A-PBX1	5%	Neutral
t(9;22)(q34;q11)	Early B-lineage	BCR-ABL	2%	Unfavorable
t(12;21)(p13;q22)	Early B-lineage	TEL-AML1	25%	Favorable
t(1;14)(p33;q11)[a]	T-ALL	TAL1	25% T-ALL	Neutral
t(10;14)(q24;q11)	T-ALL	HOX11-TCR δ	10% T-ALL	Favorable (?)
t(8;14)(q24;q11)	B-Lymphoblasts	MYC-IgH	1% to 3%	Burkitt Tx.

[a]Most patients have submicroscopic deletions in TAL1 locus (1p33) rather than translocation.

containing a smaller BCR-ABL protein (185kDa, p185).[31] BCR-ABL encodes a constitutively active tyrosine kinase that is capable of transforming cells in culture and leading to tumors in animal models. The search for inhibitors of the tyrosine kinase activity of BCR-ABL led to the identification of the first truly molecularly targeted drug, imatinib mesylate (formally known as STI571, Gleevec), which is a potent inhibitor of ABL tyrosine kinases, platelet-derived growth factor, and KIT.[32, 33] The drug has had striking success in the treatment of CML, and early results indicate significant activity when used at diagnosis in patients with Ph+ ALL in conjunction with chemotherapy.[34–36] Although imatinib resistance due to mutations in BCR-ABL and/or gene amplification has been observed, new-generation TK inhibitors have been shown to inhibit such clones.[37]

Hyperdiploidy is uncommon in T-ALL, but approximately 25% of cases harbor translocations involving the T-cell receptor genes.[38] One of the most common examples is the t(10;14)(q24;q11), which fuses the TCR-δ locus to the HOX11 gene.[39] In contrast to translocations seen in B-precursor ALL that result in chimeric fusion mRNAs, this translocation results in up-regulation of an intact HOX11 gene because of its close proximity to strong enhancers within the TCR locus.[40] Another common abnormality in T-ALL is up-regulation of the TAL1 (aka TCL5 or SCL) gene either through translocation with the TCR α/δ locus or more commonly through a submicroscopic deletion that juxtaposes TAL1 next to SIL (SCL-interrupting locus).[41–43]

A rare t(7;9)(q34;q34) that juxtaposes the TCR-γ locus to the NOTCH1 gene provided important clues to the pathogenesis of T-cell ALL.[44,45] NOTCH1 encodes a transmembrane receptor that upon ligand binding undergoes proteolytic cleavage into an active form that regulates genes critical in T-cell development.[46] The translocation results in the formation of truncated constitutively activated forms of NOTCH1. Subsequently it has been shown that approximately 55% of pediatric T-cell ALL samples contain at least one mutation in the NOTCH1 gene that results in activation of the pathway.[46,47] It is noteworthy that activation of the NOTCH1 receptor requires final cleavage mediated by the γ-secretase complex.[44] Inhibitors of γ-secretase result in cell cycle arrest in T-cell lines in vitro, and these agents are in early-phase clinical trials.[48]

The genetic abnormalities described above are cancer specific and are not shared by normal cells. Translocations in particular can be attractive targets to detect small numbers of tumor cells in a large background of normal cells. As mentioned previously, investigators have been able to "back track" leukemia, showing that the translocation can be detected many years before a clinical diagnosis of ALL. This long latency suggests that the translocation by itself is incapable of transforming cells completely and that additional steps are required to convert a preleukemic cell to ALL. In addition, when neonatal blood spots were assayed for the presence of the TEL-AML1 fusion it was detected at a frequency 100 times greater[7] than the incidence of childhood ALL, indicating that in the great majority of cases, these additional steps in transformation do not occur. Recent analysis of DNA from ALL samples using single

nucleotide polymorphism arrays ("SNP chips") also shows that the genome of ALL cells contain specific gene copy number abnormalities that correlate with biologic subtypes. Overall deletions were more common than amplifications, and commonly these aberrations were detected in genes such as PAX5 and IKZF1 that control B-cell development.[49] Thus it appears that an essential step in leukemogenesis is arrested differentiation due to mutations that then collaborate with genetic lesions, such as the translocations mentioned above.

Evidence also suggests that many cancers actually arise from rare "cancer stem cells" that are responsible for colonizing the more-differentiated, clinically detectable bulk tumor population that leads to the initial diagnosis. Leukemic stem cells (LSCs) were first described in CML but now have been isolated in ALL, AML, myelodysplastic syndrome (MDS), and many solid tumors.[50–52] They share many properties with normal hematopoietic stem cells (HSCs), including the capacity for self-renewal. Acute lymphoblastic leukemia LSCs have an antigenic profile that is similar to HSCs in that they reside in a CD34+CD38– subpopulation and they often lack antigens that characterize the more differentiated B-precursor blasts that they give rise to.[53] However, recent evidence suggests that ALL LSCs display a more committed immunophenotype compared with HSCs with expression of CD19 in at least a subset of ALL LSCs. The cancer stem cell model has many ramifications for successful therapy because drugs that target the more differentiated pool of blasts may fail to eradicate the LSCs, creating a potential reservoir for the emergence of relapsed clones.

Clinical Presentation

Children with ALL commonly present with signs and symptoms of marrow failure with clinically detectable extramedullary disease being rare. It is a common misperception that significant lymphadenopathy and hepatosplenomegaly are frequent findings at presentation in the majority of children with B-lineage leukemia. Instead, nonspecific symptoms including fatigue, irritability, and anorexia are common, as is low-grade fever without a clear etiology. Bone pain is common (one-third of patients) and severe bone pain, especially involving the long bones, may lead to a limp or refusal to walk. The pain is most often out of proportion to the physical findings, with joint effusions rarely seen. Pallor, bruising, and petechiae are also common, leading parents to seek medical attention for their children.

The differential diagnosis includes other disorders that compromise marrow function. Nonmalignant conditions may include aplastic anemia and idiopathic thrombocytopenic purpura. Infections including mononucleosis with associated adenopathy and atypical lymphocytes may lead to a suspicion of leukemia; pertussis and parapertussis may also be in the differential as they may present with marked leukocytosis and lymphocytosis. Lastly, other malignancies including lymphomas, neuroblastoma, medulloblastoma, retinoblastoma, and rhabdomyosarcoma may involve the marrow, but these malignancies usually have distinct physical findings. Clearly, in the case of lymphomas there may be marked overlap in clinical presentation, and some consider subtypes of non-Hodgkin lymphoma (NHL) and ALL as part of a spectrum of the same disease. When staging NHL, by convention, the disease is labeled leukemia when the child has greater than 25% blasts in the marrow whereas a child with 5% to 25% blasts is classified as having stage IV NHL.

Laboratory Findings

The initial complete blood count (CBC), with very rare exception, is abnormal. Half of the children will have a white blood cell (WBC) count $>10\,000/\mu l$; with 20% showing a WBC $>50\,000/\mu l$. Anemia (hemoglobin $<10\,g/dL$) is present in approximately 80% of patients at diagnosis. It is most often normochromic, normocytic anemia with marrow failure evident by the absence of an appropriate reticulocyte response. A platelet count $<100\,000/\mu l$ is present in 75% of children at diagnosis. Note, however, that the platelet count may be in the low normal range. Should a child present with a mild leukocytosis, neutropenia, and mild thrombocytopenia, a short follow-up CBC or bone marrow aspirate should be considered. Other abnormal laboratory findings may include elevated liver enzymes and lactate dehydrogenase. An elevated uric acid may reflect a large tumor burden, while hypercalcemia may result from leukemic infiltration of bone or from the production of an abnormal parathormone-like substance.[54] Hypocalcemia may be secondary to hyperphosphatemia, as seen in the tumor lysis syndrome. Abnormal renal function from uric acid nephropathy or renal infiltration by leukemia may be present and calls for a rapid assessment for possible mechanical obstruction. Barring this, hydration, careful monitoring of electrolytes and other chemistries, and rapid correction of the hyperuricemia may preclude the need for emergency dialysis.

An anterior mediastinal mass, often associated with T-cell leukemias and lymphomas, may cause airway or pulmonary compromise. It is critical to observe the child, noting his or her preferred posture and position. Kneeling or leaning forward, especially with a history of cough or dyspnea and/or a change in sleeping habits, indicates significant airway compromise from the mass. Since the child may be using gravitational forces to alleviate lower airway obstruction, laying the child supine for a diagnostic procedure or administering sedative medications may result in severe respiratory distress or arrest, not readily alleviated by intubation because the obstruction may be below the tip of the endotracheal tube.

Plain films of the long bones may demonstrate radiolucent metaphyseal bands, often called "growth arrest" lines, periosteal elevation, diffuse osteoporosis, and, rarely, osteolytic lesions. Children with severe bone pain often have hemoglobin, neutrophil, and platelet counts that are closer to normal than those of children with less-significant bone pain.

Involvement of the CNS occurs in fewer than 5% of children with ALL at the time of diagnosis.[55] When present, CNS involvement is usually detected in an asymptomatic child with analysis of the cerebrospinal fluid (CSF) revealing a leukocytosis and the presence of lymphoblasts. CNS1 status describes a patient without detectable blasts in the diagnostic CSF; CNS2 indicates the presence of blasts with <5 WBC/μl, and CNS 3 includes patients with cranial nerve involvement or >5 WBC/μl with blasts. Traumatic lumbar punctures are defined as a CSF with >10 red blood cells (RBC)/μl, with or without blasts (TLP+ or TLP–). Symptoms of CNS disease, if present, reflect increased intracranial pressure with vomiting, headache, papilledema, lethargy, irritability, and possible seizures. Visual disturbances may result from the increased pressure or involvement of the cranial nerve nuclei. Testicular leukemia, presenting as painless testicular swelling, occurs rarely but is commonly associated with additional high-risk features.

Morphological and Immunological Classification of Acute Lymphoblastic Leukemia

It has long been recognized that ALL is a biologically and clinically heterogeneous disease. A number of classification systems have been proposed to classify ALL into subgroups to optimize therapy. One of the earliest international classification systems for both ALL and AML was proposed by the French-American-British Cooperative group in 1976.[56] Their original proposal, as well as subsequent revisions, divided ALL into three subtypes; L1, L2, and L3, on the basis of morphological characteristics (Figure 12-1). L1 lymphoblasts are typically smaller with scant cytoplasm and less-prominent nucleoli. L2 lymphoblasts are larger with more abundant cytoplasm, more heterogeneity in size, and prominent nucleoli. L3 blasts are characterized by deeply basophilic cytoplasm and cytoplasmic vacuolization. With the exception of the L3 subtype, which corresponds in almost all cases to mature B-ALL containing *myc* translocations (8q24), these distinctions hold little to no practical value.

The development of monoclonal antibodies targeted to distinct lineage-restricted cell surface antigens greatly aided the development of a biologically based classification system for ALL, based on cell lineage and differentiation stage rather than morphology alone. It has been recognized that ALL subtypes correspond to distinct stages of lymphocyte maturation,[57] and depending on where differentiation is blocked, leukemias can be classified into early and later stages of cellular maturation. However, leukemia cells may also often demonstrate aberrant antigen expression that is not reflective of normal lymphocyte ontogeny.[58] Whether this asynchronous antigen expression is related to disordered gene expression due to leukemia-specific genetic rearrangements, or whether such profiles exist in a very small population of cells under normal circumstances, is uncertain. However, leukemia-specific patterns of antigen expression allow for a convenient method to detect minimal residual disease (MRD) using flow cytometry.

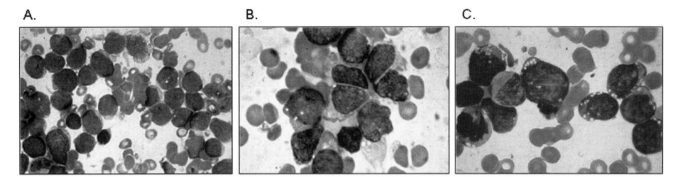

Figure 12-1 Morphological classification of ALL. French American and British (FAB) morphological classification of lymphoblasts. (A) L1 blasts. (B) L2 blasts. (C) L3 blasts. **See Plate 36 for color image.**

In the past, specific criteria for "positive" antigen expression were established—namely, 20% cell surface expression, or 10% cytoplasmic expression, depending on the antigen being expressed. However, with the development of multiparameter flow cytometry, many antigens can now be analyzed simultaneously on the surface and in the cytoplasm of leukemic blasts. Currently, diagnosis is established by recognizing multivariate patterns of antigen expression. The great majority (>98%) of leukemia subtypes can be easily classified into well-established subgroups. Previously, cytochemical stains were used routinely in the diagnostic evaluation of leukemia, but flow cytometry has obviated the need for these studies in ALL, especially since myeloperoxidase (a strong myeloid antigen) expression can be determined using flow cytometry.

The expression of a number of lineage-specific antigens can be used to classify leukemia, and those used routinely are listed in Table 12-2. Typical patterns are: CD19/CD22/CD79a (B-lineage), CD7/cytoplasmicCD3 (T-lineage), and CD13/CD33/CD65/MPO (myeloid).[59] Cases can be further classified according to discrete stages that mirror normal lymphocyte development (Table 12-3). Although immunophenotyping is essential for distinguishing ALL from AML and B-lineage from T-lineage disease, its prognostic importance in B-lineage ALL subclasses has been neutralized by the identification of blast cytogenetic features and early disease response characteristics that strongly correlate with outcome. Nonetheless, patients with T-cell immunophenotypes require more aggressive therapy than their B-lineage counterparts when matched for age and WBC count at diagnosis.[60–62]

Although antigen expression is used to assign lineage, significant promiscuity of certain antigens is observed frequently. For example, CD13 and CD33 are myeloid (My) antigens, expressed on almost all AML cases, but they can also be expressed in up to one-third of ALL blasts (My+ ALL). Likewise, terminal deoxynucleotidyl transferase (TdT) expression is characteristic of ALL but

Table 12-2

Common cell-surface antigens used to classify acute leukemia.

Antigen	Cell Type	B-lineage	T-lineage	Myeloid
CD45	Hematopoietic	+/−	+	+
CD19	Pan B-lineage	+	−	+/−
CD22	Precursor and mature B	+	−	−
CD79a	Precursor and mature B including plasma cells	+	−	+/−
CD7	T, NK, and stem cells	−	+	+/−
CD3	Thymic and mature T	−	+	−
MPO	Myeloid	−	−	+/−
CD13	Myeloid/monocytic progenitors	+/−	+/−	+/−
CD33	Myeloid/monocytic progenitor cells, early erythro- and megakaryoblasts	+/−	+/−	+/−
CD117	Hematopoietic stem cells	−	−/+	+/−
CD10 (CALLA)	Lymphoid precursors	+/−	+/−	−
TdT	Early lymphoid	+/−	+/−	+/−

Table 12-3

Immunological classification of ALL[70]

Subtype	Immunophenotype
B-lineage	CD19 and/or CD79a and/or CD22+ (at least 2)
Pro-B	Absent expression of other B-cell differentiation antigens
Common	CD10+
Pre-B	cyIgμ+
Mature B	cyIg or sIgκ+ or sIgλ+
T lineage	cy/m CD3+
Pro-T	CD7+
Pre-T	CD2 and/or CD5 and/or CD8+
Cortical T	CD1a+
Mature T	mCD3+, CD1a−
My+ALL	ALL with the presence of myeloid antigens

Abbreviations: cy, cytoplasmic; m, membrane

intensity is tailored according to the predicted likelihood of relapse. The recent merger of the Pediatric Oncology Group (POG) and Children's Cancer Group (CCG) allowed a large-scale analysis of many clinical and biologic variables used for risk classification.[71] Those markers, proven to be significant in both groups, irrespective of differences in therapy, are now used in the current COG classification system for patients with newly diagnosed B-precursor ALL. Age, initial WBC count, the presence of extramedullary disease, blast cytogenetics, and early treatment response are used to stratify patients with newly diagnosed B-precursor into one of four risk groups: low, standard, high, and very high risk, and other pediatric groups use similar classification systems (Table 12-4). Patients with T-ALL and infant ALL are classified and treated separately.

Although risk stratification has been an essential factor in improving outcomes for childhood ALL, current classification systems have limitations. Namely, it is difficult to accurately identify those children who are likely to be cured with less-intensive therapy, sparing toxicity. Furthermore, it is difficult to identify the 20% of patients who ultimately relapse as evidenced by the fact that the majority of the patients who relapse have favorable or neutral prog-

can be seen in approximately 10% of AML cases (Ly+ AML). Although early studies suggested that patients with My+ ALL had an adverse prognosis compared with more typical ALL,[63-66] subsequent studies[67,68] did not support this conclusion, leading to the treatment of My+ ALL in accordance with the same set of variables used to risk-stratify other patients. The coexpression of My antigens on ALL cells (My+ ALL), or the reverse (Ly+ AML) should be distinguished from those cases that cannot be assigned to either the My or lymphoid lineage. Such cases include both undifferentiated leukemias as well as cases referred to as bilineal or biphenotypic leukemia. The term *biphenotypic leukemia* is used to describe a leukemia in which a single dominant population of blasts simultaneously coexpresses both My and lymphoid antigens. Leukemias in which two distinct populations of blasts exist, each constituting a single lineage, are referred to as acute bilineal leukemia, although there is growing evidence that these are not distinct entities, because some leukemias have features of both biphenotypic and bilineal leukemia, and some patients may evolve from one leukemia to another over time. The distinction between biphenotypic and bilineal leukemia historically has not been well established, and acceptance of common nomenclature for these rare leukemias will help to establish a better understanding of underlying biology and optimal treatment strategies.[69]

Risk Classification

Children with ALL are routinely classified into one of several risk groups at diagnosis. A number of clinical and biologic variables are used for classification, and treatment

Table 12-4

B-precursor ALL risk groups.

	COG Risk Group Definitions for B-precursor ALL
Low	• NCI standard risk
	• No extramedullary disease
	• Rapid early response[a]
	• *TEL-AML1* or favorable trisomies
Standard	• NCI standard risk without favorable genetic features
	• Rapid early response[a]
	• Neutral cytogenetics
High	• NCI high risk
	• Rapid early response
	• No adverse cytogenetics
Very High	• Any NCI risk group
	• Slow response[b], induction failure, or
	• t(9;22), or
	• Extreme hypodiploidy (44 chromosomes), or
	• *MLL* translocation with slow early response

[a]Rapid early response: M1 marrow by day 15 and end-induction MRD<0.1%

[b]Slow early response: not M1 marrow by day 15 and/or end-induction MRD≥0.1% (the cutoff based on the best available data at the time this system was implemented).

nostic features at diagnosis. Recent advances in genomics and pharmacogenetics offer promise for future refinements in existing risk classification schemes.

Clinical Features

A number of clinical features are used for risk assessment. Among these, age at diagnosis and initial WBC count have consistently emerged as the most useful prognostic markers.[72] Both age and WBC are continuous variables and any cutoff is somewhat arbitrary. The commonly accepted National Cancer Institute (NCI) criteria classify NCI standard-risk (SR) ALL as children 1 to 10 years of age with a WBC $< 50\,000/\mu l$, whereas NCI high-risk ALL is defined as age ≥ 10 years or WBC $\geq 50\,000/\mu l$. Using these definitions, approximately two-thirds of the cases of B-cell precursor ALL are defined as SR while one-third of T-ALL cases fall into this category. The better outcomes observed in younger children are in part due to the fact that they have blasts with more favorable cytogenetic features. Gender is also prognostic, with girls faring better than boys and requiring a shorter treatment duration on some protocols.[73,74] It should be emphasized that more recent efforts to intensify therapy have neutralized the significance of some prognostic markers, such as the presence of organomegaly.

Blast Cytogenetics

Genetic features of blasts have emerged as some of the most important prognostic variables currently used for risk stratification.[19,21,75,76] Patients with high hyperdiploid blasts (> 50 chromosomes) and trisomies of chromosomes 4, 10, and 17 ("triple trisomies") have a very favorable prognosis with a 5-year event-free survival (EFS) rate of 90%.[22,77,78] Similarly, the presence of the TEL-AML1 fusion gene, resulting from t(12;12) translocations, is also associated with a superior EFS rate.[20,23,79,80] The triple trisomy and TEL-AML1 positive cases account for up to 50% of standard-risk B-cell precursor ALL cases,[19] and when associated with a favorable early response to treatment (see below), they constitute the "low-risk" group of patients on COG protocols.

In contrast, patients with hypodiploid blasts containing < 44 chromosomes and those individuals with Ph chromosome–positive (Ph+) ALL do poorly, with overall EFS rates generally $< 50\%$. These patients may be candidates for bone marrow transplantation,[81,82] though as described below, the addition of imatinib to aggressive chemotherapy for the treatment of Ph+ ALL may alter treatment outcome and the need for transplant. Hypodiploidy (≤ 45 chromosomes) occurs in 6% to 9% of cases of childhood ALL, with the vast majority having 45 chromosomes, and approximately 1% of individuals having < 44 chromosomes. While the outcomes for children with a modal chromosome number of 44 to 45 is intermediate, and similar to that observed with pseudodiploid and low-hyperdiploid ALL (47-50 chromosomes), outcomes for children with < 44 chromosomes are particularly poor, and this group now is classified as very high risk.[71,81,83–86] The worst outcomes are observed in patients with near-

haploid ALL (24-28 chromosomes), with reported EFS rates of 25% or less.[81,86–89] As a part of clonal evolution, doubling of the hypodiploid clone can occur, and caution should be taken not to mistake these cases for hyperdiploid ALL.

The Philadelphia chromosome is formed by a reciprocal translocation of the long arms of chromosomes 9 and 22, and it is present in 3% to 5% of childhood leukemias.[21] Although a complete remission is initially obtained in more than 80% of the pediatric patients, the prognosis has been poor, with 4- to 5-year EFS rates of 20% to 38%.[82, 90–97] Children treated on early POG or CCG protocols had overall 5-year EFS rates of 27.4% and 33.3%, respectively.[71] While applying traditional prognostic criteria such as age, initial WBC, and early treatment response to those with Ph+ disease did identify a subgroup with a better prognosis, the best group, treated prior to the addition of imatinib, still had a 5-year EFS rate of approximately 50%.[90] Early response as determined by peripheral blood blast clearance on day 8 after treatment with 1 week of prednisone and a single dose of intrathecal methotrexate was prognostic, although significantly fewer children with Ph+ disease have a prednisone good response, defined as < 1000 blasts/μl at day 8,[97] than their non-Ph+ B-precursor counterparts. Even the Ph+ prednisone good responders, however, still had a 4-year EFS of only 55% with intensive chemotherapy, with or without marrow transplant. Matched sibling donor transplant currently offers a lower risk of treatment failure in Ph+ ALL, with a relative risk of death from any cause of 0.4 (95% confidence interval 0.2 to 0.7, $p \pm 0.002$).[90] Although Wheeler et al[98] did not find an advantage to bone marrow transplant overall for patients with high-risk disease transplanted in first remission, among the 26 children with Ph+ ALL, 2 of 14 treated with chemotherapy, without a tyrosine kinase inhibitor, survived versus 8 of the 14 treated with transplantation. Current and future trials, using both a comprehensive risk classification system that incorporates clinical features and quantitative measurements of MRD in concert with aggressive therapies that include a tyrosine kinase inhibitor, seek to identify a group of patients with Ph+ disease with a good prognosis with a non-transplant-based regimen.

MLL rearrangements (eg, t(4;11), MLL-AF4; t(11;19), MLL-ENL; and t(9;11), MLL-AF9), which are seen in up to 70% of infants with ALL, are another unfavorable cytogenetic subgroup.[99] Infants, especially those under 6 months of age, commonly present with poor risk features: WBC $> 50\,000/\mu l$, CNS involvement, bulky extramedullary disease, and common ALL antigen (CALLA or CD10) negativity by flow cytometry.[100] The extremely poor prognosis associated with these leukemias often results from prenatal translocation of the mixed lineage leukemia (MLL) gene at chromosome band 11q23, a gene critical to the differentiation of hematopoietic cells.[100] Because MLL gene rearrangements are also common to epipodophyllotoxin or topoisomerase II-inhibitor induced leukemias,[101–103] it follows that a polymorphism in the system that detoxifies dietary topoisomerase II inhibitors could enhance the risk of developing infant leukemia.[104] Modest successes in therapy have allowed for the identification of risk groups among even the infant population, with the most critical feature being the presence of an abnormality of the *MLL* gene at 11q23. Age greater than 6 months and a good response to a prednisone window are also better prognostic features.[105,106] In non-infant patients, *MLL* translocations are also associated with inferior responses, particularly when associated with slow early responses to chemotherapy.[71,99,107,108] On the recently completed CCG-1961 study, non-infant patients with t(4;11) and an M3 marrow at day 7 had an extremely poor prognosis, with only 1 of 9 remaining in remission.[71]

The biologic basis for the association of certain genetic abnormalities and outcome is not known, but *in vitro* drug sensitivity studies do show that some cytogenetic subtypes of ALL blasts show preferential sensitivity to certain agents. *TEL-AML1+* blasts, for example, have unusual sensitivity to L-asparaginase, which may explain the very good outcome of these patients using regimens employing intensive asparaginase therapy.[79,109] Similarly, hyperdiploid blasts have been shown to accumulate very high levels of methotrexate polyglutamates, making them particularly sensitive to methotrexate cytotoxicity. This may explain in part the excellent outcomes for these patients when using regimens in which methotrexate is a primary component of continuation therapy.[110]

Early Response/Minimal Residual Disease

The rapidity of response to initial treatment is one of the most important prognostic indicators. Historically, failure to achieve a complete clinical remission at the end of induction has been associated with an extremely poor prognosis,[111] but more recently, physicians have tracked disease response at earlier points in induction. Early response has been studied extensively using conventional morphology to assess the regression of tumor burden. Gaynon et al[112] reviewed 15 large trials that included more than 10 000 children and found that early response, as determined by a quantitative assessment of marrow blast content on day 7 or day 14 or the persistence of peripheral blasts beyond day 7, correlated with outcome and was a consistent, independent prognostic feature. Those with slow early responses defined by either persistence of marrow disease in a day 7 or 14 marrow or persistence of blasts in peripheral blood at the end of the first week of induction were 1.5 to 6.1 (median 2.7) times as likely to have an adverse event.

In CCG studies conducted from 1989 to 1995, day 7 marrow status was routinely determined by conventional morphology. Among non-infant patients who achieved remission at end-induction, 52%, 23%, and 25% were M1 (5% blasts), M2 (5% to 25% blasts), or M3 (>25% blasts) on day 7 of induction, and their EFS was $80 \pm 1\%$, $74 \pm 2\%$, and $68 \pm 2\%$, respectively.[113] Similarly, the combined impact of the day 7 and 14 marrow response on outcome was investigated in CCG studies CCG-1952 for NCI standard-risk ALL (1996–2000) and CCG-1961 for NCI high-risk ALL (1996–2002). The outcomes for both SR

and high-risk patients who achieved an M1 marrow by day 14 were superior to those who did not, with a 5-year EFS of 84.4% vs 66.6% for NCI SR patients and 77% vs 59% for NCI high-risk patients, despite augmentation in therapy for those with slow early responses.[71] Other investigators have examined the fall in peripheral blood blast count after the first week of induction or following the administration of a single dose of intrathecal methotrexate and 7 days of oral prednisone. These studies have similarly shown that the persistence of disease early in therapy is associated with a poor long-term outcome.[114,115]

Technological advances have allowed for the detection of disease below the threshold detected by conventional morphology, and MRD can now be identified with lower limits of sensitivity of 1 in 10^4 to 1 in 10^6 cells.[116–125] Flow cytometric methods are generally cost effective, reproducible, and applicable to greater than 90% of children diagnosed with ALL.[118] "Real-time" PCR can be used to detect clone-specific rearrangements of antigen receptor genes and fusion genes characteristic of ALL. These assays may allow for greater sensitivity ($1/10^6$ vs $1/10^4$) but are expensive and labor intensive.[126]

Three large, prospective studies[117,118,125] provide strong evidence that quantitative measures of MRD represent the most accurate way of predicting patients at higher risk for relapse. Children without any evidence of MRD at the end of induction have a superior outcome (3-year EFS >90%) compared with those with high levels > 10^{-2} (3-year EFS 25%). Approximately 25% of children with B-lineage ALL have detectable MRD at the end of induction compared with 70% of children with T-ALL and 80% of children with Ph+ ALL.[117,118,123–125,127] Patients with intermediate levels of MRD can be further distinguished by MRD at a later time point. Recent data gathered as part of the POG protocol 9900 from 2000 to 2005 again document the powerful prognostic impact of end-induction MRD (Figure 12-2). These results were kept blinded and were not provided to treating physicians or used to alter therapy. Day 28 MRD specimens were sent to the reference lab for 97% (2100/2157) of patients enrolled on the clinical trials linked to COG P9900. Informative flow cytometry MRD results with a sensitivity of at least 1 of 10 000 (0.01%) were available for 1975/2100 patients (94%) within 24 to 48 hours of specimen receipt, with the remainder being informative at a level of 0.1% (96) or yielding indeterminate results (29). Day 28 MRD was a strong predictor of outcome (p 0.0001; Figure 12-2). While end-induction MRD was highly prognostic, approximately half of treatment failures occurred in the end-induction marrow MRD negative group. Day 8 peripheral blood MRD was used to identify a very favorable risk group; the 4-year EFS of day 8 blood MRD-negative patients in COG 9900 was $92 \pm 2\%$, with only 16% of treatment failures derived from this group.[128]

Currently, risk algorithms are used initially to assign children with newly diagnosed ALL to a standard-risk (3-drug) or high-risk (4-drug) induction based on the presence of testicular disease, age, and initial WBC count. At

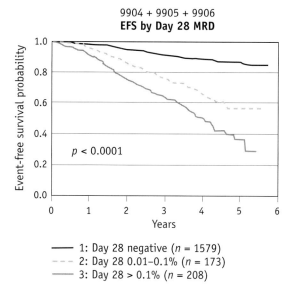

9904 + 9905 + 9906
EFS by Day 28 MRD

$p < 0.0001$

— 1: Day 28 negative ($n = 1579$)
- - - 2: Day 28 0.01–0.1% ($n = 173$)
—— 3: Day 28 > 0.1% ($n = 208$)

Figure 12-2 Outcomes of children based on end-induction MRD status: Event-free survival of children treated on frontline Pediatric Oncology Group studies 9904 (low risk), 9905 (standard and intermediate risk), and 906 (high risk) based on day 28 MRD response.

the end of induction, further data on CNS status, lymphoblast cytogenetics, and ploidy, as well as early morphological response and end-induction MRD, are used to refine assignments into 1 of 4 risk groups: low, standard, high, and very high risk (see Table 12-4). This risk algorithm, applied to children on recently completed CCG and POG studies, predicted these outcomes (Figure 12-3).

Acute Lymphoblastic Leukemia in the "Genomic Era"

The recent sequencing of the human genome offers enormous potential to better understand the underlying defects that drive leukemogenesis as well as genetic differ-

ences in the host that may be associated with susceptibility to leukemia, response to therapy, and side effects of treatment. The genomic era began in 2003 when the complete sequence of the genome was published, almost 50 years after James Watson and Francis Crick discovered the basic structure of the DNA molecule. The human genome contains approximately 30 000 genes, and 40% of these genes display alternative splice forms that account for the increased complexity of the human genome. Although remarkable similarity of gene sequence exists between individuals, subtle variation is always present, most commonly in the form of single nucleotide differences or polymorphisms (SNPs).

Single nucleotide polymorphisms may effect the expression, splicing, and/or amino acid sequence of genes, and there is an ever-increasing number of examples in which SNPs have been implicated in disease pathogenesis and outcome. One of the best-known examples is observed in children with ALL who are intolerant of maintenance chemotherapy. The enzyme thiopurine methyltransferase (TPMT) inactivates thiopurines like 6-mercaptopurine, and three relatively common polymorphisms influence the stability of the enzyme such that activity is low in individuals who inherit a variant allele.[129,130] Ten percent of Caucasians are heterozygotes, and 0.6% of patients are homozygous for 2 variant TPMT alleles. Low activity is associated with higher thioguanine nucleotide concentrations, more frequent episodes of myelosuppression, and an EFS rate at least comparable to that seen in patients with wild type enzyme, despite the administration of only 10% of the usual dose of 6-MP.[131,132] The glutathione S-transferase (GST) family of enzymes detoxifies many antileukemia drugs. The "non-null" *GSTM1* genotype, which is associated with higher GSTM1 expression, is associated with an increased risk of relapse. Within these patients prognosis was further impacted by a 3-base pair repeat in the *thymidylate synthetase* enhancer (*TYMS 3/3* genotype), which results

A.

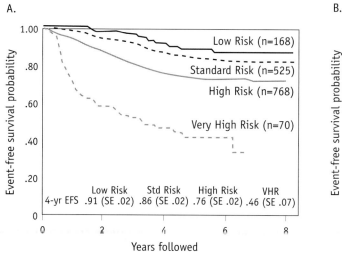

B.

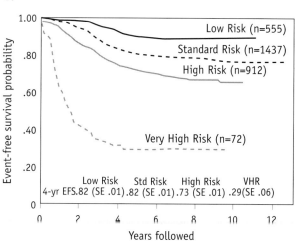

Figure 12-3 Predicted outcomes of children with newly diagnosed B-precursor ALL according to end-induction risk group: Predicted EFS using current COG risk algorithm for children with newly diagnosed B-precursor low-, standard-, high-, and very high risk ALL treated on recently completed CCG-1950s/60s (A) and POG ALinC 16 (A) trials.

in increased expression.[133] Because TYMS is a target for methotrexate, higher expression would be expected to blunt drug activity. The field of pharmacogenetics is rapidly advancing and in the near future will be used routinely to optimize treatment in individual patients.

Technical advances have now led to the ability to assess the expression of all genes within a cancer sample simultaneously, and comparisons across cancer subtypes and/or with normal cells have led to the identification of pathways responsible for biological behavior. DNA microarrays or "chips" have been used to define previously unrecognized leukemia and have been shown to classify conventional subtypes accurately. Gene expression "signatures" that correlate with outcome might provide a more accurate system to stratify patients into different treatment protocols. Finally, there are now numerous examples in which microarray analysis has led to the identification of targets for novel therapeutic intervention, such as the identification of *FLT3* in MLL-rearranged ALLs.[134] A number of recent reviews summarize these advances and future applications.[135–140]

Therapy

Marrow remissions were first described in 1953 when children with ALL were treated with an anti-fol, aminopterin.[141] Curative therapy did not become a reality, however, until the initiation of St Jude Total Study V (1967–1971), wherein investigators incorporated 2400 centigray (cGy) cranial radiation and 5 doses of intrathecal methotrexate (MTX) and demonstrated that CNS disease could be prevented.[142] Prior to this, therapies were associated with CNS relapse rates as high as 75%, with death from subsequent marrow failure the rule. Since then, the marriage of biologic science and disciplined clinical trials has led to a dramatic improvement in outcome for children with ALL (Figure 12-4).

The recognition of clinical and, more recently, biologic variables that correlate with prognosis has led to the implementation of risk-adapted therapies. Variations in the content and intensity of the basic phases of combina-tion therapy, in combination with new agents, will continue to improve the cure rate while minimizing side effects for children with ALL.

Induction Therapy

The Goldie-Coldman hypothesis addresses the issue of tumor cell heterogeneity and the inevitable development of drug resistance.[143] Based on this hypothesis, the goal of an induction regimen is to eliminate, rapidly, as great a proportion as possible of the malignant cell load. Should the frequency of mutation to resistance of a lymphoblast to Drug A be 1×10^6, and to Drug B 1×10^5, only 1 in 10^{11} would be doubly resistant. The delivery of multiple effective agents, each with a different mechanism of action, to an untreated leukemic cell population will not only result in maximal cell kill but may also prevent the emergence of resistant disease.

Vincristine (VCR) and prednisone (PDN) alone will induce remissions in approximately 85% of children with ALL. The addition of L-asparaginase (ASP) or an anthracycline or both induce a remission by day 28 in approximately 95% of patients. Importantly, the addition of a third agent to VCR/PDN induction not only improved the remission induction rate but significantly prolonged the duration of remission. It is unclear as to whether or not the addition of the fourth agent also has an impact on the duration of subsequent remission. Nevertheless, current high-risk therapies that include a 4-drug induction, intensive consolidation, and postconsolidation therapies have improved EFS for high-risk patients.

Most controversial in induction regimens is the choice of glucocorticoid. Dexamethasone (DEX) has better CNS penetration,[144] affords better CNS protection than prednisone,[145] and has also been associated with better *in vitro* leukemia cell kill.[146] Early studies using DEX reported an excellent EFS with tolerable induction toxicity.[145,147] In a large, randomized trial, for children with standard risk features (CCG-1992), DEX was associated with a superior EFS at 4 years (88% vs 81%).[148] In addition, the Medical Research Council (MRC) UKALLR1 trial for children with recurrent ALL included DEX during reinduction at a dose of 10 mg/m² per day for two weeks, in combination with VCR, ASP, and epirubicin.[149] This regimen was highly effective and well tolerated, with 95% of patients entering a second remission. Though epirubicin is less potent than adriamycin, this trial supported the belief that DEX could be safely administered as part of a 4-drug induction. In contrast, a Dana-Farber Cancer Institute study,[150] a POG/CCG infant trial, 2 POG trials for standard and high-risk patients, and a recent COG trial for children in first relapse were closed secondary to excessive morbidity and mortality associated with the use of DEX as part of a 4-drug induction most often in conjunction with an anthracycline. Ongoing trials in the United States and Europe are attempting to define a safe and efficacious DEX-based therapy for high-risk patients that includes the administration of an anthracycline.

Asparaginase is commonly used during induction therapy, though the specific product, dose, route, and sched-

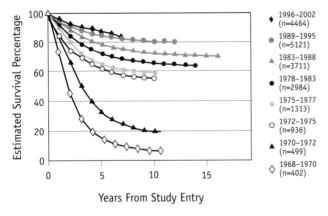

Figure 12-4 Improvements in outcome for childhood ALL. Estimated survival percentage for consecutive CCG ALL study eras from 1968 to 2002. The number of patients enrolled in trials per era is indicated at right.

ule of administration vary. Current and future COG leukemia trials largely incorporate polyethylene glycol (PEG) asparaginase, based on a CCG trial[151] suggesting that children receiving PEG as opposed to native ASP during induction therapy were more likely to achieve a rapid early response and less likely to develop neutralizing antibodies to ASP during later phases of therapy. The relatively long half-life of PEG asparaginase allows for dosing at 2- to 4-week intervals.[152] Controversy remains, however, with 2 studies suggesting that PEG does not deplete CSF asparagine to the same extent as native ASP.[153] Current and future studies in North America as well as established studies in Europe and Scandinavia have or will use intravenous preparations,[154–156] decreasing the pain associated with intramuscular injections and potentially diminishing immunogenicity.[157,158] Vincristine is given universally during induction therapy, though one can still debate whether or not the dose of this important agent should be capped to avoid prohibitive neurotoxicity. Lastly, intrathecal chemoprophylaxis is always initiated during the induction phase, although the doses and patterns vary.

Central Nervous System Prophylaxis/Consolidation

Central nervous system leukemia developed in up to 75% of children who survived in marrow remission beyond 2 years between 1958 and 1970. The St Jude Total Study V (1967–1971) was the first to affect cure with the administration of 2400 cGy cranial radiation and 5 concurrent doses of intrathecal methotrexate[142] during a consolidation phase after the achievement of marrow remission. The occurrence of long-term neurologic and neuroendocrine sequelae, as well as the risk of secondary CNS malignancies, ultimately prompted investigators to provide adequate CNS prophylaxis through the use of systemic and intrathecal chemotherapy, avoiding the use of cranial radiation for the majority of patients. A metaanalysis of 43 trials[159] that included more than 2800 patients concluded that radiotherapy and long-term intrathecal therapy were associated with similar outcomes, with no difference in EFS. Intravenous methotrexate reduced the number of non-CNS as opposed to CNS relapses and was associated with a 17% reduction in event rate.[159] Current CNS preventive regimens have reduced the incidence of isolated CNS relapse to less than 5%. Cranial radiation is reserved for those with CNS disease at diagnosis and those with high-risk features, although continued improvements in systemic chemotherapy may further limit the use of radiotherapy. For example, a small retrospective cohort study of 26 young children with T-cell ALL, treated on the same high-risk leukemia protocol, demonstrated that high-dose methotrexate was associated with an equivalent, excellent, EFS at 5 years when compared with the same systemic chemotherapy administered with 1800 cGy cranial radiation.[160]

The appropriate therapy and prognostic significance of the presence of blasts in a diagnostic CSF with fewer than 5 white cells per microliter (CNS2) remains controversial.

Therapies wherein CNS2 status has a greater impact include those that utilize prednisone, not dexamethasone, as a systemic glucocorticoid, perform a diagnostic lumbar puncture without the concomitant installation of intrathecal chemotherapy, delay the second dose of intrathecal chemotherapy until the third or later week of initial induction, and/or make no provision for the administration of additional intrathecal therapy for those with CSF blasts.[161] In addition, there are data suggesting that a traumatic lumbar puncture (≥ 10 RBC/μl CSF) with blasts present is also associated with a decrease in EFS.[114,162] Possible explanations include the iatrogenic introduction of lymphoblasts, the failure to recognize CNS3 cases because of the confounding peripheral blood contamination, and/or the impact of blood in the epidural or subarachnoid space on the distribution of subsequent doses of intrathecal therapy. To minimize the risk of traumatic lumbar punctures, all diagnostic punctures should be done by an experienced clinician under optimal conditions, with a child properly sedated. The use of prophylactic platelet transfusions prior to the diagnostic lumbar puncture may also minimize the risk of bleeding at the time of initial lumbar puncture.[163] Future DEX-based trials, designed to enroll large numbers of children classified by age, WBC count, blast cytogenetics, rapidity of response, and the presence of minimal residual disease at the end of induction, will allow for a broad-based assessment of the impact of CNS2 status on outcome. Thus, the consolidation phase is largely designed to expose leukemia cells to non–cross-resistant drug combinations following induction and to provide CNS prophylaxis. There is significant variation in the intensity of the systemic therapy delivered during this phase, and the impact of various schedules remains unclear. A recent COG trial for NCI standard-risk patients will determine the value of more intensive systemic therapy during this phase for this set of patients.

Postinduction Intensification or "Delayed" Intensification Therapy

Intensification of therapy, after remission has been achieved, is now universal, though the drugs, doses, and schedules vary. The best approach to postinduction intensification is inexorably linked to the population treated—ie, low, intermediate, high, or very high risk patients—as well as the makeup of the other components of a given therapy. Treating patients with both T- and B-precursor ALL of all risk groups, the UKALL trials supported the use of postremission intensification. Patients randomized to receive two 5-day blocks of intensified therapy fared better, with a 71% 5-year EFS vs 61% and 62% for patients randomized to receive a single block at week 5 or 20, versus 57% for those who did not receive any intensification. Subsequently, a third block, given at week 35, was also proven to be of benefit.[73,161] A 7-week delayed intensification (DI) phase was introduced with the BFM-76 protocol, beginning at week 16.[165] Hoping to prevent the emergence of resistance, drugs were altered, slightly. Prednisone given during induction was replaced with DEX, daunomycin was replaced with adriamycin, and thioguanine was substituted for mercaptopurine. This DI phase was tested in CCG-105 with those patients randomized to receive the DI having a significantly better EFS at 5 years than those in the control arm (73% vs 61%, $p = 0.006$).[166]

Subsequent trials have focused on augmenting DI where the dose intensity of VCR, ASP, and MTX are significantly enhanced. This approach includes 2-week courses of VCR and ASP during the periods of neutropenia that follow the consolidation and intensification blocks, and escalating doses of intravenous (IV) MTX without leucovorin rescue, combined with VCR and ASP, in a Capizzi pattern, instead of oral MTX and 6-MP during the interim maintenance phase (IM). This augmented therapy significantly improved outcome for NCI high-risk patients with an M3 marrow on day 7 (Slow Early Responders)[167] and was tested in CCG-1961 in NCI high-risk patients who had had a rapid early response to induction therapy. In that trial, a 2×2 factorial design was used to compare standard to augmented IM/DI phases and to compare 1 IM/DI phase to the administration of 2 of each of these phases. The results of this trial have defined ABFM (augmented BFM) therapy with a single IM/DI as standard of care for children with high-risk ALL enrolled on frontline ALL trials with an overall EFS of 80% for NCI high-risk patients and the elimination of older age as a prognostic factor.[168] The augmented DI and IM phases are now being tested in NCI standard-risk patients so as to determine if these components will enhance efficacy. Note that NCI standard-risk patients, treated in CCG-1922, with a DEX-based induction have a comparable EFS to those treated in CCG-1952 with 2 DI phases but a PDN-based induction.[148,169] Pediatric Oncology Group 9905 will determine the impact of a single DI in the context of a DEX-based induction. Both CCG-1961 for NCI high-risk patients and 1991 for SR patients included discontinuous DEX during the DI phase, with DEX given during only the first and third, not second, weeks of the DI phase. This approach to steroid administration has significantly lowered the incidence of osteonecrosis without appearing to compromising outcome.

The ASP preparation has also been modified. Augmented BFM therapy originally included *E coli* ASP, but the 9 doses of native product given during induction and the subsequent doses given during the DI phases were replaced with PEG asparaginase. A concomitant pharmacokinetic trial compared asparagine depletion, the formation of ASP antibodies, and the impact of *E coli* versus PEG asparaginase on early morphologic marrow response, demonstrating a lower incidence of neutralizing antibody formation and a greater likelihood of achieving an early morphologic remission with the PEG product.[151] Close attention will be paid to CNS relapse rates, however, with the pegylated product associated with less depletion of CSF asparagines.[170] Intensive ASP, another form of postremission intensification, has also been associated with a good overall EFS. The Dana Farber Cancer Institute trial 91-01 documented a superior outcome for patients receiving at least 26 weeks of continuous ASP therapy versus those who received less ASP (5-year EFS 90% vs 73%,

p 0.01),[171] and the International Berlin-Frankfurt-Muenster Study Group found a statistically significant improvement in disease-free survival, favoring the use of intensive ASP, when children with intermediate-risk disease were randomized to receive or not receive 20 weekly doses of L-ASP.[172]

Intensification of antimetabolite therapy has also been associated with an improvement in EFS, most clearly for patients with T-ALL. Pediatric Oncology Group study 9404 demonstrated an improvement in outcome for T-lineage NCI standard- and high-risk patients thru the addition of HDMTX,[173] and BFM-90 produced a superior EFS as compared with BFM-86 with an increase in the MTX dose[155] from 0.5 to 5.0 gm/m^2. This outcome was not surprising perhaps, because *in vitro* and *ex vivo* studies of T-lymphoblasts demonstrate a decrease in accumulation and polyglutamation of MTX when compared with B-lineage blasts.[174–178] Investigators at St Jude improved EFS for patients through the use of targeted MTX dose adjustments,[179] and many older trials have demonstrated an improvement in outcome with the addition of parenteral MTX infusions at doses ranging from 500 mg to 5 gms/m^2, to regimens for patients with both T- and B-lineage disease.[180–182] Other trials have not described an improvement in outcome with IV MTX.[183–185] This result may reflect a variety of confounding variables that include the dose and schedule of MTX administration, the timing and dose of leucovorin, the population treated (T- vs B-lineage), and the other components of the regimen.

As risk-adapted therapy is refined, the various approaches to intensification will be linked to tumor biology and response, possibly with antimetabolite-based therapy used for low-risk patients, low-dose anthracycline, and alkylating agent therapy for intermediate-risk patients, and more intensive cytotoxic therapy reserved for those with high-risk disease. The use of new, targeted therapies, linked to an understanding of important interactions with host polymorphisms, will provide a less-toxic, disease- and risk-specific approach to ALL therapy.

Maintenance Therapy

Unique among therapies for malignancies is the prolonged maintenance phase of ALL treatment regimens. Commonly incorporating oral 6-mercaptopurine (MP) and MTX, with variable use of vincristine/steroid pulses and intrathecal therapy, the maintenance phase extends to cover a minimum of 2 years from the achievement of a morphologic complete remission. Early on, no statistically significant difference in outcome was seen among patients randomized to 5 versus 3 years[186] of maintenance therapy, but a dramatically shorter, 6-month maintenance phase was associated with an inferior outcome.[187] Vincristine/steroid pulses were associated with a small reduction in the risk of relapse or death in a large metaanalysis,[188] although more recent data suggest that in the face of more intensive regimens, these pulses may not contribute to EFS.[189] Similarly, although prolonged intrathecal therapy is needed to provide adequate CNS protection, in the absence of radiation therapy the number of doses of IT therapy needed has yet to be firmly established, with the number likely impacted by other treatment and disease variables, including the steroid delivered (dexamethasone vs prednisone) and the immunophenotype of the leukemia treated (B-precursor vs T-ALL).

Potential reasons for the failure of maintenance therapy may reflect *de novo* or acquired resistance in the leukemia or unintentionally diminished therapy secondary to poor compliance, diminished bioavailability, variations in drug distribution, metabolism and transport, clearance and elimination, and/or host tolerance. Clearest among these variables is the relationship between 6-MP metabolism and thiopurine methyltransferase (TPMT) activity, described above.[129,190] Patients with TPMT deficiency have very high concentrations of thioguanine nucleotides (TGN) and an EFS at least comparable to those with wild type activity, despite receiving 10% of the standard MP dose.[132] Also suggesting that TGN are important to outcome, 17 of the 19 patients who relapsed on UKALL trials VII-X had RBC TGN concentrations below the group median.[191]

The Nordic Society of Paediatric Haematology and Oncology (NOPHO) ALL-88 protocol linked EFS to the product of the RBC concentrations of MTX and TGN.[192] Based on this, the NOPHO ALL-92 trial randomized patients to a regimen wherein doses of MP and MTX were adjusted using traditional blood count criteria versus therapy with dose adjustments designed to achieve the targeted product of the red cell concentration of TGN and MTX.[193] The failure of this rationally targeted therapy to enhance outcome may reflect, as the authors suggested, an increase in the frequency of neutropenia and the resultant decrease in therapy delivered and/or the use of the red cell TGN concentrations. Though these endpoints may represent the only pragmatic choice, the RBC TGN may be a poor surrogate for lymphoblast TGN.[194] Most important, an increasing understanding of pharmacokinetics, pharmacodynamics, pharmacogenomics, and the complex genetics of lymphoblast sensitivity and resistance as well as host biology and its relationship to drug response and sensitivity will ultimately allow for the rational administration of individualized therapy.[195-201]

Resistant Disease/Relapse

Despite dramatic improvements in the treatment of children with ALL over the past several decades, 20% to 30% of children will relapse, and their prognosis is generally poor, with approximately only one-third of all relapse patients surviving long-term.[202] One of the greatest challenges is that relapse often occurs unpredictably in patients with favorable or neutral prognostic features at diagnosis. Furthermore, response to salvage therapy is less predictable, as evidenced by lower remission reinduction rates, higher levels of end-induction MRD, and less-durable remissions with early second failures in up to one-third of patients after an initial remission is achieved.[203]

Although there are fewer prognostic markers at relapse compared with those at initial diagnosis, 3 factors have consistently emerged, regardless of initial therapy: timing of relapse, site of relapse, and blast immunophenotype.[204-207] These variables frequently form the basis for treatment decisions made at the time of relapse, and allocation to allogeneic stem cell transplantation (allo-SCT). The earlier the relapse occurs, the more difficult it is to treat. While the definition of early vs late marrow relapse varies, many groups define "early" as an initial marrow recurrence within 36 months from initial diagnosis, and "late" as marrow recurrence ≥ 36 months from diagnosis. In contrast to newly diagnosed ALL, in which >95% of children achieve remission, remission rates after first marrow relapse range from 66% to 82% for B-lineage ALL after an early relapse and around 90% to 95% for late B-lineage marrow relapse.[149,203,204,207-216] Although many reinduction regimens utilize the established 4-drug platform of vincristine, corticosteroid, asparaginase, and anthracycline,[217] others use alternate approaches such as the use of idarubicin and cytarabine.[216] Differences in the intensity and the composition of the reinduction regimens generally have not resulted in improvement in salvage rates, however, and reinduction regimens have reached the limit of tolerability with toxic death rates of 3% to 8% on average, but with reports of up to 19%.[210] Even if a second remission is achieved, however, many patients may relapse again before reaching the average time to SCT. Longer-term overall EFS rates for early relapse are approximately 10% to 20%, compared with EFS rates of approximately 40% to 50% for late marrow relapse, even when intensive salvage strategies including allo-SCT are employed.[203,204] In a recent analysis of patients with first marrow relapses occurring within 12 months of completion of initial therapy, 3-year EFS rates from relapse occurring < 18 months, 18 to 30 months, and >30 months from initial diagnosis were, $4 \pm 2\%$, $10 \pm 4\%$ and $41 \pm 6\%$, respectively.[203] It is striking that these outcomes have been remarkably consistent internationally over recent decades, irrespective of differences in the components of salvage regimens. Outcomes for second or greater relapse are even worse.[202,205] Although third remissions (CR3) can be achieved in approximately 40% of patients,[205] responses are not sustained, and there are few long-term survivors. Among 235 patients who achieved a third complete remission (CR) after a second marrow relapse following frontline therapy in UK Medical Research Council (MRC) studies, only 8% survived.[218]

Site of relapse is also an important prognostic variable. Isolated marrow relapses are the most challenging to treat, whereas isolated extramedullary relapses have more favorable outcomes and combined relapses have an intermediate prognosis. The distinction between early and late extramedullary relapse is generally 18 months from initial diagnosis (compared with 36 months for marrow relapse) and those children with a late isolated CNS relapse (≥ 18 months from diagnosis) still appear to have a very good prognosis with EFS rates of 83.3% and 76.4% on the two most recently completed POG studies.[219,220] However, children with early isolated CNS relapse (18 months diagnosis) have inferior outcomes with EFS rates of 41% to 46.2% on recently completed POG studies.[219, 220] Early isolated extramedullary relapses also fared poorly with a 5-year EFS of 20% on the UKALL R2 regimen[214] and 29% overall survival rates in Nordic studies.[202]

Another important prognostic determinant at the time of relapse is blast immunophenotype. T-cell relapses at any time are more difficult to salvage than B-precursor ones, with a T-cell phenotype portending a risk ratio of 2.1 in a multivariate Cox regression analysis.[204] In a recent analysis of children relapsing after treatment on frontline St Jude ALL studies, remission reinduction rates for T-ALL were 60%, and 5-year EFS rates were only $5 \pm 3.4\%$.[207] Similarly, on the recently complete COG AALL01P2 study, there were no survivors among 7 T-cell patients. [221]

Given the prognostic importance of end-induction MRD burden in children with newly diagnosed ALL, the role of MRD is also being explored in relapse. Prior studies in relapse have suggested that patients with a disease burden of $< 10^{-3}$ at the end of reinduction have better outcomes.[222] Furthermore, patients with no detectable MRD prior to allo-SCT have been shown to fare significantly better than those with persistent MRD.[223,224] Minimal residual disease was measured by flow cytometry at the completion of each of 3 individual blocks of reinduction therapy on the recently completed COG AALL01P2 study. Minimal residual disease was detected at the end of the first month of reinduction in 79% and 50% of patients with early and late marrow relapse, respectively.[221] These values are much higher than the 25% incidence of MRD at the end of induction in children with newly diagnosed ALL. Important to note is that the majority of those patients who responded favorably to the initial month of reinduction therapy continued to have further regression of MRD burden with subsequent blocks of reinduction therapy. Minimal residual disease in conjunction with morphological remission rates may prove to be a useful measure for determining the merit of reinduction strategies.

Even though some of the most heated debates within pediatric leukemia circles focus on the relative benefit of allo-SCT versus intensive chemotherapy for second-line treatment, neither strategy enjoys an optimal therapeutic ratio. Furthermore, transplant is a limited option due to donor availability and failures prior to the initiation of the transplant.[202] An analysis from the CCG-1941 study reported that greater than 50% of patients died, failed reinduction, or relapsed again before the median time to BMT,[203] highlighting the need for the early integration of new agents into salvage regimens to improve remission rates and spare toxicity.

Although a benefit for allo-SCT has been established for early marrow relapse, case-control analyses have shown the outcomes for transplant versus chemotherapy to be similar for late marrow relapse, with perhaps a slight advantage for transplant from an HLA-identical sibling donor.[225–232] In the absence of a randomized study comparing transplant and chemotherapy outcomes in relapse, transplant from any donor source is commonly recommended for early B-lineage and T-cell relapse occurring at any time due to the dismal outcomes with chemotherapy alone. In late B-lineage marrow relapse, transplantation is generally reserved for cases in which a matched identical sibling donor is available. The role of transplant for early extramedullary disease has not yet been defined, and the majority of late extramedullary relapses can be salvaged with intensive chemotherapy and radiation therapy. Although further improvements will come from an enhanced understanding of classic pharmacology and pharmacogenetics of standard drugs,[233–236] there is an urgent need for new agents and new strategies.

New Agents in ALL

One of the top priorities in pediatric ALL is the identification of new agents to improve outcomes for high-risk patient populations such as those with relapse, T-ALL, infant ALL, and Ph+ disease. For several high-risk populations, new agents of promise with unique and selective mechanisms of action are now being combined with established chemotherapeutic regimens. Nelarabine is a pro-drug of the deoxyguanosine analogue 9-β-D-arabino-furanosylguanine (ara-G) with selective cytotoxicity for T-cells, secondary to greater accumulation and prolonged retention of the cytotoxic triphosphate, ara-GTP in T-lymphoblasts versus B-lymphoblasts.[237,238] Ara-GTP substitutes for GTP in many essential biological processes, including DNA replication, and this substitution causes inhibition of DNA synthesis and resultant cell death.[239] Nelarabine produced response rates (complete plus partial responses) of 55% and 27% following first or second or greater T-cell marrow relapse, respectively, in a recently completed Phase II study.[240] Given these promising single-agent response rates, nelarabine has now been incorporated into a frontline treatment study for children with newly diagnosed high-risk T-ALL. Dose-limiting neurological toxicity was seen in the Phase I and II trials of nelarabine. Should nelarabine prove tolerable in combination with intensive chemotherapy for patients with high-risk T-cell ALL, a larger, randomized trial of patients with T-ALL will address the efficacy of the addition of nelarabine.

Imatinib, one of the most celebrated molecularly targeted compounds, inhibits the abnormal ABL protein tyrosine kinase common to Ph+ leukemias.[32,33] Complete hematologic responses, with minimal systemic toxicities, were documented in 53 of 54 patients with Ph+ CML and 4 of 20 with lymphoid blasts crisis or Ph+ ALL in early trials.[32] Second- and third-generation kinase inhibitors (such as dasatinib), which have broader and more potent kinase inhibition and which are effective in cases of imatinib resistance, are producing promising results in adult Phase I and II trials.[37] The Children's Oncology Group recently completed trials using imatinib in combination with chemotherapy for both newly diagnosed (AALL0031) and relapsed (AALL01P2) Ph+ ALL. Recent analysis shows that the integration of imatinib improves early outcome for children with Ph+ ALL in first remission.[36,221] A future COG study is being planned that will evaluate dasatinib in combination with chemotherapy for Ph+ ALL.

Infant ALL presents another challenge, with poor outcomes, particularly in the 70% to 80% of children with *MLL* rearrangements. Aberrant expression of the tyrosine kinase FLT3 has been shown to play an important role in the pathogenesis of *MLL*-rearranged leukemias.[241] *MLL*-rearranged leukemias are characterized by high levels of FLT3 expression, and FLT3 inhibition is now actively being explored as a therapeutic strategy in *MLL*-rearranged ALL and AML.[242,243] Lestaurtinib (CEP-701) is a selective small-molecule FLT3 tyrosine kinase inhibitor that has been shown to have promising preclinical activity in primary ALL cells in combination with chemotherapy.[29] Promising results have also been observed with lestaurtinib monotherapy in a Phase II study in adults with AML.[30] In the near future, lestaurtinib will be studied in combination with chemotherapy in infants with *MLL*-rearranged ALL.

There is also an urgent need for novel agents for relapsed ALL, particularly early marrow and T-cell recurrences. Given the baseline toxicity with current reinduction regimens, identifying promising agents, with favorable toxicity profiles, presents a challenge. However, given the poor response rates to single-agent therapy in this patient population, combination therapy is optimal. One class of drugs that is being investigated for marrow relapse is monoclonal antibodies targeting leukemia-specific antigens. As reviewed by Multani and Grossbard,[244] multiple steps, evolving since 1953, have led to the synthesis of multiple monoclonal antibodies that target specific antigens. These drugs have unique mechanisms of action and generally have limited and nonoverlapping toxicities when compared with cytotoxic agents, making them attractive candidates for combined therapy. The success of rituximab, an anti-CD20 monoclonal antibody, in the treatment of adult patients with non-Hodgkin lymphoma[245,246] suggests that monoclonal antibodies will play an important role in the therapy of hematopoietic malignancies.

A COG study using Campath-1H, a monoclonal antibody directed against CD52, with chemotherapy was recently completed, and a study using epratuzumab, an anti-CD22 IgG1 monoclonal antibody,[247] is presently under way. Epratuzumab has been shown to be tolerable and effective in the treatment of adult non-Hodgkin lymphoma, as a single agent, and also in combination with rituximab and chemotherapy.[248–252] After the successful completion of a safety phase, children with CD22-positive marrow relapse are now receiving epratuzumab in combination with a standard 3-block reinduction platform.[253] Clinical evaluation of these promising agents will require a creative approach to the traditional Phase I and Phase II designs, as monoclonal antibodies may prove valuable even if their use as single agents does not produce complete or partial responses in patients with bulk disease. Measures of early morphological response, end-induction MRD, and 4-month EFS are presently being used to measure the activity of these combinations and to define regimens of promise for further study in the future.

Clofarabine is another new agent, which is being studied in relapse. Clofarabine is a new-generation nucleoside analog, which combines the most favorable properties of fludarabine and cladribine and inhibits DNA synthesis through inhibition of DNA polymerases and ribonucleotide reductase. After promising 30% overall response rates were observed in heavily pretreated pediatric patients with refractory or relapsed ALL, this agent was granted accelerated approval by the US Federal Drug Administration in 2004 for the treatment of children with relapsed or refractory ALL after at least 2 prior regimens.[254,255] Trials using clofarabine in combination with cytarabine, and also etoposide and cyclophosphamide, are currently under way.[256]

Bortezomib, a selective inhibitor of the 26S proteasome, stabilizes many cell cycle–regulatory proteins and appears to sensitize malignant cells to apoptosis.[257–259] The antitumor effects of bortezomib in lymphoid tumors have been attributed to NF-κB inhibition,[260] and evidence suggests that bortezomib also sensitizes leukemic cells to chemotherapy.[258] Single-agent Phase I studies of bortezomib in relapsed/refractory pediatric leukemia[261] and solid tumors[262] have been completed, establishing a recommended Phase II dose in children. Bortezomib has also been safely combined with several chemotherapy platforms in adults with hematologic malignancies, and plans are currently under way to study this agent in combination with standard 4-drug reinduction therapy for children with marrow relapse.

Another class of agents of promise for advanced B- and T-lineage hematopoietic malignancies is mammalian target of rapamycin (mTOR) inhibitors. The mammalian target of rapamycin is a protein kinase that is a crucial regulator of cell metabolism, growth, and proliferation.[263,264] Mammalian target of rapamycin is a downstream effector of the phosphatidylinositol 3-kinase (PI3K)/AKT signaling pathway, and activation of the mTOR pathway has been observed in several human cancers, including leukemias.[265,266] Preclinical studies have demonstrated the activity of the mTOR inhibitors, sirolimus, and the rapamycin analog, CCI-779, *in vitro* in leukemia cell lines as well as in animal models of advanced hematopoietic tumors.[267–269] Synergy between mTOR inhibitors and other chemotherapeutic agents has also been observed in B- and T-lineage ALL cell lines and preclinical models.[270,271] These findings have fostered enthusiasm for investigating this class of agents in children with recurrent ALL.

Because the majority of failures occur early in the high-risk populations, it is hoped that regimens combining new agents with conventional chemotherapy will improve early outcomes, such as remission induction rates, and that some of the agents, if proven effective in these groups, may be suitable candidates for incorporation into frontline therapies in the future.

Long-Term Toxicities

Intensification of therapy has dramatically improved cure rates for children with ALL over the past 50 years. Two landmark studies[272,273] that included more than 33 000 individuals, alive >5 years from the diagnosis of ALL, found that 90% of these patients were alive 5 to 35 years later. Nevertheless, there was a standardized mortality ratio (observed: expected) of 10.8. The excess mortality was largely due to recurrence of the primary cancer, but approximately 20% of the deaths were due to a second malignant neoplasm or a therapy-related complication. Long-term toxicities associated with significant morbidity may include neurologic, cardiac, and orthopedic complications.

The Children's Oncology Group *Long-Term Follow-Up Guidelines for Survivors of Childhood, Adolescent, and Young Adult Cancers* were developed for health care providers and survivors, through the Nursing Discipline and Late Effects Committees. The guidelines provide recommendations for screening and management of late effects, based on a review of the literature as well as the collective clinical experience of the task force members, panel of experts, and a multidisciplinary review panel composed of nurses, physicians, behavioral specialists, and patient/parent advocates. Accessible at www.survivorguidelines.org, these guidelines will be updated periodically.

Neurotoxicity

Current predictions state that by 2010, 1 in 540 adults aged 20 to 34 years will be a childhood cancer survivor. An important finding is that for those children alive a minimum of 10 years from the diagnosis, not radiated during therapy, rates of death, marriage, employment, and having health insurance coverage were the same as age- and sex-adjusted national averages.[274] This picture is dramatically different, however, from that portrayed by Armstrong wherein 40% of children treated with intravenous methotrexate, without radiation, had full-scale IQs below 85.[275] The majority of published studies describe better neurocognitive outcomes for children treated with chemotherapy alone versus cranial radiation plus chemotherapy, although the extent to which chemotherapy alone causes neurocognitive dysfunction is unclear.[276–279] Overall, approximately two-thirds of published reports find a significant decrement in one or more aspects of cognitive function.[278] Impairment in nonverbal function and academic achievement has been described with specific deficits usually in 4 primary areas of function: short-term memory, processing speed, visuomotor coordination, and sequencing ability.[280] Defining the true incidence of neurotoxicity is difficult, however, as the child's baseline level of neurocognitive function, the timing of the testing, and the outcome measures used impact study conclusions. Perhaps most important, neuropsychological outcome measures are determined after completion of therapy, wherein study participants often represent a small proportion of the total population originally entered on the therapeutic trial. This introduces significant selection bias wherein participation is skewed toward those who are experiencing significant problems in school, for whom the participation and testing is of value.

The pathogenesis of leukoencephalopathy is multifactorial, difficult to predict, and dependent on a variety of treatment and host-related factors. In addition to radiotherapy, intravenous and intrathecal methotrexate have most commonly been implicated in causing leukoencephalopathy, although there is no simple dose response relationship. For example, neither 30 infants who received IV MTX[281] at 33.6 gm/m^2 nor children given weekly doses of IV MTX[282] at 2 gm/m^2 as part of multiagent therapy experienced acute neurotoxicity while on therapy, or neurocognitive abnormalities or school problems following the completion of therapy. In contrast, approximately 8% of children receiving 12 courses of IV MTX[283] at 1.0 gm/m^2 developed significant neurotoxicity despite the administration of leucovorin rescue, and patients receiving only intensive oral MTX[284] experienced unexpected acute neurotoxicity, before the addition of leucovorin. Acute neurotoxicities such as seizures do not necessarily predict chronic encephalopathy, and learning disabilities may appear without a history of acute neurologic toxicity; objective measures such as plasma MTX concentrations, the presence of other MTX-related toxicities, and magnetic resonance imaging have failed to correlate with clinical outcome.[282,283,285–290] Methotrexate-induced disturbances in folate homeostasis may play a role,[291,292] although a prospective trial failed to establish a correlation between neurologic toxicity and measures of CSF and/or plasma homocysteine.[293] Steroids have also been linked to brain atrophy and neurotoxicity, with concern raised as to whether or not dexamethasone, with its increased potency and better CNS penetration,[146,294,295] will be associated with more toxicity than prednisone.[296] Current and future COG trials seek to correlate host polymorphisms, corticosteroid use, and MTX administration with neurocognitive outcome, with trials designed to assess the relative toxicity of high-dose methotrexate with leucovorin rescue versus lower-dose IV MTX without leucovorin.

Cardiac Toxicity

Anthracyclines have become an integral part of the treatment of children with ALL, despite the risk of long-term cardiac toxicity. An extensive review[297] (30 studies; 12 507 patients) designed to determine the frequency of and risk factors for anthracycline-induced heart failure in children describes a frequency of clinical congestive heart failure (CHF) of 0% to 16% overall, with the one study, restricted to survivors of ALL who had received a cumulative dose of ≤ 270 mg/m^2, reporting CHF in 1 out of 120 (0.8%) survivors. Similarly, neither Hudson et al[298] nor Lipshultz et al[299] report clinical CHF among long-term survivors of ALL, a median of 9 and 11.5 years from the completion of therapy. However, assuming an age at diagnosis of < 20 years, few if any of these survivors would have yet reached the age of 40. Although Hudson et al[298] did not find significant echocardiographic abnormalities among 39 survivors who received less than 100 mg/m^2, Lipshultz et al[299] described decreased left ventricular mass and dimension among 18 survivors of ALL treated with total doses of adriamycin 45 mg/m^2.

Proposals to limit long-term cardiac toxicities[300,301] have included: decreasing the total dose, using a less-cardiotoxic anthracycline; adjusting doses for patients who appear to be at higher risk (female and younger patients); and perhaps altering doses in response to changes in parameters, such as echocardiographic changes and/or a rise in cardiac troponin T levels. The use of dexrazoxane, a potent iron-chelating agent,[302,303] has been associated with a statistically significant decrease in the decline of the left ventricular ejection fraction per 100 mg/m^2 of doxorubicin.[304] Recently closed, a large, prospective randomized trial for children with T-cell malignancies was designed to address the potential impact of dexrazoxane on efficacy, leukopenia, the incidence of secondary AML, and whether its use would protect children from chronic cardiac toxicity as well.[305] Preliminary data suggest that dexrazoxane does not impact the efficacy of leukemia therapy, but longer follow-up is needed to determine the impact of dexrazoxane on long-term cardiac dysfunction and the risk of second malignancies.[306,307]

Current COG frontline trials limit the total anthracycline dose to 75 mg/m^2 for standard-risk patients and 175 mg/m^2 for high-risk patients with a rapid early response. A low-risk group, identified by age, initial white cell count, blast cell cytogenetics, measures of early response, and minimal residual disease may be candidates for therapy with no anthracycline; emphasizing the importance of risk classification in balancing the risk of long-term toxicity with the need to cure leukemia. Detailed guidelines with respect to cardiac surveillance among long-term survivors are available at www.survivorguidelines.org.

Bone Toxicity

The use of higher doses and more potent glucocorticoids provide a survival advantage for children with ALL[308–312] but also increase the incidence of osteonecrosis (ON). Glucocorticoid-induced ON may arise from increased expression of specific genes and decreased expression of type I collagen and osteocalcin mRNA as well as from an increase in osteocyte apoptosis leading to a cumulative irreversible defect that ultimately causes avascular necrosis and femoral head collapse.[313–315] The "statins" are lipid-lowering agents that prevent the fatty change that precedes glucocorticoid-induced osteonecrosis.[316] These drugs, however, are substrates for the cytochrome P450 system, raising concerns about the potential for complex interactions between these agents and the drugs used to treat leukemia.[317] Advances in the identification of those patients at greatest risk[318] may identify a population for whom the risk:benefit ratio falls in favor of introducing prophylactic therapy with statins, a change in steroid dose, or other intervention designed to prevent ON while preserving antileukemic efficacy.

The two largest pediatric trials[319,320] describing bone disease found that teenagers were more likely to develop ON than younger children, but the Boston study[320] found that males were at greater risk and the CCG trial[319] found that females developed more ON. Although steroid dose is an important determinant in the development of ON, the relationship is complex. High-risk patients received 3 times the steroid dose of the standard-risk patients but did not have a higher incidence of ON in the Boston trial, and girls were more likely affected in CCG-1882, despite receiving a lesser total dose. Approximately 75% of those affected have multiple bones involved. The absence of a simple dose response, the incidence of 7.9%, and the severity of disease in those affected imply variable host susceptibility. Relling et al,[318] in work designed to identify those at greatest risk of bone morbidity, found that in addition to age and race, the vitamin D receptor *FokI* start site CC genotype and the *thymidylate synthase* low-activity 2/2 enhancer repeat genotype were associated with the development of ON. Work on ON-related polymorphisms is ongoing with hopes of a therapeutic intervention for those at highest risk in the near future.

Summary: Optimal Therapy

The development of ALL is linked to the acquisition of specific chromosomal abnormalities, possibly in a preleukemic stem cell. Defined genetic alterations can be used in diagnosis and treatment refinement along with other important variables including age and WBC at diagnosis, and early response to therapy. Currently, optimal therapy includes a 3- to 4-drug induction followed by a consolidation phase using non–cross-resistant chemotherapy. Coincident with consolidation, CNS prophylaxis with intrathecal methotrexate should be applied and CNS-directed therapy should be continued at least through the first year of therapy. Few patients require CNS radiotherapy, which should be reserved for patients with CNS disease and possibly high-risk T-cell patients. All treatment regimens benefit from some form of intensification, which might be antimetabolite-based for low-risk patients, but strong evidence supports the need for a reinduction/reconsolidation strategy (delayed intensification) to optimize outcome for patients with standard- and high-risk disease. The optimal duration of maintenance has not been defined, but most regimens currently rely on 2 years, with a longer duration for males in some cases.

Twenty years ago, Dr Howard Skipper wrote, "Cancer chemotherapy is many things. It is not just 'screening,' as some seem to think, nor is it just organic chemistry, biochemistry, cell population kinetics, pharmacology, or sophisticated experimental therapeutics in model systems and in man. It is all of these things and many more, but most of all it is discovery, development, collaboration across disciplines, and application to man with (for good reasons) a prevailing sense of urgency. We want and need and seek better guidance and are gaining it, but we cannot afford to sit and wait for the promise of tomorrow so long as stepwise progress can be made with the tools at hand today."[321] The progress made to date in the treatment of childhood ALL represents the unprecedented, worldwide cooperation of families, physicians, basic scientists, pharmacologists, nurses, psychologists, social workers, and others. Future success depends on a better understanding of leukemia and host biology and their interactions.

References

1. Biondi A, Masera G. Molecular pathogenesis of childhood acute lymphoblastic leukemia. *Haematologica*. 1998;83(7):651–659.
2. Pui CH, Relling MV, Downing JR. Acute lymphoblastic leukemia. *N Engl J Med*. 2004;350(15):1535–1548.
3. Knudson AG, Jr. Mutation and cancer: statistical study of retinoblastoma. *Proc Natl Acad Sci USA*. 1971;68(4):820–823.
4. Ross JA, Davies SM, Potter JD, Robison LL. Epidemiology of childhood leukemia, with a focus on infants. *Epidemiol Rev*. 1994;16(2):243–272.
5. Shu XO, Ross JA, Pendergrass TW, Reaman GH, Lampkin B, Robison LL. Parental alcohol consumption, cigarette smoking, and risk of infant leukemia: a Children's Cancer Group study. *J Natl Cancer Inst*. 1996;88(1):24–31.
6. Gale KB, Ford AM, Repp R, et al. Backtracking leukemia to birth: identification of clonotypic gene fusion sequences in neonatal blood spots. *Proc Natl Acad Sci USA*. 1997;94(25):13950–13954.
7. Greaves M. Childhood leukaemia. *BMJ*. 2002;324(7332):283–287.
8. Franco RF, Simoes BP, Tone LG, Gabellini SM, Zago MA, Falcao RP. The methylenetetrahydrofolate reductase C677T gene polymorphism decreases the risk of childhood acute lymphocytic leukaemia. *Br J Haematol*. 2001;115(3):616–618.
9. Skibola CF, Smith MT, Kane E, et al. Polymorphisms in the methylenetetrahydrofolate reductase gene are associated with susceptibility to acute leukemia in adults. *Proc Natl Acad Sci USA*. 1999;96(22):12810–12815.
10. Wiemels JL, Smith RN, Taylor GM, Eden OB, Alexander FE, Greaves MF. Methylenetetrahydrofolate reductase (MTHFR) polymorphisms and risk of molecularly defined subtypes of childhood acute leukemia. *Proc Natl Acad Sci USA*. 2001;98(7):4004–4009.
11. Alexander FE, Patheal SL, Biondi A, et al. Transplacental chemical exposure and risk of infant leukemia with *MLL* gene fusion. *Cancer Res*. 2001;61(6):2542–2546.
12. Zahm SH, Ward MH. Pesticides and childhood cancer. *Environ Health Perspect*. 1998;106(suppl 3):893–908.
13. Infante-Rivard C, Labuda D, Krajinovic M, Sinnett D. Risk of childhood leukemia associated with exposure to pesticides and with gene polymorphisms. *Epidemiology*. 1999;10(5):481–487.
14. Neglia JP, Linet MS, Shu XO, et al. Patterns of infection and day care utilization and risk of childhood acute lymphoblastic leukaemia. *Br J Cancer*. 2000;82(1):234–240.
15. Smith M. Considerations on a possible viral etiology for B-precursor acute lymphoblastic leukemia of childhood. *J Immunother*. 1997;20(2):89–100.
16. Shu XO, Linet MS, Steinbuch M, et al. Breast-feeding and risk of childhood acute leukemia. *J Natl Cancer Inst*. 1999;91(20):1765–1772.
17. Kearney L, Horsley SW. Molecular cytogenetics in haematological malignancy: current technology and future prospects. *Chromosoma*. 2005;114(4):286–294.
18. Rubnitz JE, Look AT. Molecular basis of leukemogenesis. *Curr Opin Hematol*. 1998;5(4):264–270.
19. Armstrong SA, Look AT. Molecular genetics of acute lymphoblastic leukemia. *J Clin Oncol*. 2005;23(26):6306–6315.
20. Shurtleff SA, Buijs A, Behm FG, et al. TEL/AML1 fusion resulting from a cryptic t(12;21) is the most common genetic lesion in pediatric ALL and defines a subgroup of patients with an excellent prognosis. *Leukemia*. 1995;9(12):1985–1989.
21. Mrozek K, Heerema NA, Bloomfield CD. Cytogenetics in acute leukemia. *Blood Rev*. 2004;18(2):115–136.
22. Trueworthy R, Shuster J, Look T, et al. Ploidy of lymphoblasts is the strongest predictor of treatment outcome in B-progenitor cell acute lymphoblastic leukemia of childhood: a Pediatric Oncology Group study. *J Clin Oncol*. 1992;10(4):606–613.
23. Rubnitz JE, Downing JR, Pui CH, et al. TEL gene rearrangement in acute lymphoblastic leukemia: a new genetic marker with prognostic significance. *J Clin Oncol*. 1997;15(3):1150–1157.
24. Hunger SP, Galili N, Carroll AJ, Crist WM, Link MP, Cleary ML. The t(1;19)(q23;p13) results in consistent fusion of E2A and PBX1 coding sequences in acute lymphoblastic leukemias. *Blood*. 1991;77(4):687–693.
25. Nourse J, Mellentin JD, Galili N, et al. Chromosomal translocation t(1;19) results in synthesis of a homeobox fusion mRNA that codes for a potential chimeric transcription factor. *Cell*. 1990;60(4):535–545.
26. Pui CH, Kane JR, Crist WM. Biology and treatment of infant leukemias. *Leukemia*. 1995;9(5):762–769.
27. Armstrong SA, Mabon ME, Silverman LB, et al. FLT3 mutations in childhood acute lymphoblastic leukemia. *Blood*. 2004;103(9):3544–3546.
28. Brown P, Levis M, Shurtleff S, Campana D, Downing J, Small D. FLT3 inhibition selectively kills childhood acute lymphoblastic leukemia cells with high levels of FLT3 expression. *Blood*. 2005;105(2):812–820.
29. Brown P, Levis M, McIntyre E, Griesemer M, Small D. Combinations of the FLT3 inhibitor CEP-701 and chemotherapy synergistically kill infant and childhood *MLL*-rearranged ALL cells in a sequence-dependent manner. *Leukemia*. 2006;20(8):1368–1376.
30. Smith BD, Levis M, Beran M, et al. Single-agent CEP-701, a novel FLT3 inhibitor, shows biologic and clinical activity in patients with relapsed or refractory acute myeloid leukemia. *Blood*. 2004;103(10):3669–3676.
31. Kurzrock R, Kantarjian HM, Druker BJ, Talpaz M. Philadelphia chromosome-positive leukemias: from basic mechanisms to molecular therapeutics. *Ann Intern Med*. 2003;138(10):819–830.
32. Druker BJ, Sawyers CL, Kantarjian H, et al. Activity of a specific inhibitor of the BCR-ABL tyrosine kinase in the blast crisis of chronic myeloid leukemia and acute lymphoblastic leukemia with the Philadelphia chromosome. *N Engl J Med*. 2001;344:1038–1042.
33. Druker BJ, Talpaz M, Resta DJ, Peng B, Buchdunger E, Ford JM. Efficacy and safety of a specific inhibitor of the BCR-ABL tyrosine kinase in chronic myeloid leukemia. *N Engl J Med*. 2001;344:1031–1037.
34. Lee KH, Lee JH, Choi SJ, et al. Clinical effect of imatinib added to intensive combination chemotherapy for newly diagnosed Philadelphia chromosome-positive acute lymphoblastic leukemia. *Leukemia*. 2005;19(9):1509–1516.
35. Wassmann B, Pfeifer H, Goekbuget N, et al. Alternating versus concurrent schedules of imatinib and chemotherapy as front-line therapy for Philadelphia-positive acute lymphoblastic leukemia (Ph+ ALL). *Blood*. 2006;108(5):1469–1477.
36. Schultz KR, Bowman WP, Slayton WB, et al. Improved early event-free survival (EFS) in children with Philadelphia chromosome-positive (Ph+) acute lymphoblastic leukemia (ALL) with intensive imatinib in combination with high dose chemotherapy: Children's Oncology Group (COG) Study AALL0031. *Blood*. 2007;110(11):Abstract #4.
37. Hochhaus A, Kantarjian HM, Baccarani M, et al. Dasatinib induces notable hematologic and cytogenetic responses in chronic-phase chronic myeloid leukemia after failure of imatinib therapy. *Blood*. 2007;109(6):2303–2309.
38. Graux C, Cools J, Michaux L, Vandenberghe P, Hagemeijer A. Cytogenetics and molecular genetics of T-cell acute lymphoblastic leukemia: from thymocyte to lymphoblast. *Leukemia*. 2006;20(9):1496–1510.
39. Schneider NR, Carroll AJ, Shuster JJ, et al. New recurring cytogenetic abnormalities and association of blast cell karyotypes with prognosis in childhood T-cell acute lymphoblastic leukemia: a Pediatric Oncology Group report of 343 cases. *Blood*. 2000;96(7):2543–2549.
40. Hatano M, Roberts CW, Minden M, Crist WM, Korsmeyer SJ. Deregulation of a homeobox gene, HOX11, by the t(10;14) in T-cell leukemia. *Science*. 1991;253(5015):79–82.
41. Aplan PD, Lombardi DP, Reaman GH, Sather HN, Hammond GD, Kirsch IR. Involvement of the putative hematopoietic transcription factor SCL in T-cell acute lymphoblastic leukemia. *Blood*. 1992;79(5):1327–1333.
42. Janssen JW, Ludwig WD, Sterry W, Bartram CR. SIL-TAL1 deletion in T-cell acute lymphoblastic leukemia. *Leukemia*. 1993;7(8):1204–1210.
43. Brown L, Cheng JT, Chen Q, et al. Site-specific recombination of the tal-1 gene is a common occurrence in human T cell leukemia. *Embo J*. 1990;9(10):3343–3351.
44. Grabher C, von Boehmer H, Look AT. Notch 1 activation in the molecular pathogenesis of T-cell acute lymphoblastic leukaemia. *Nat Rev Cancer*. 2006;6(5):347–359.
45. Ellisen LW, Bird J, West DC, et al. TAN-1, the human homolog of the Drosophila notch gene, is broken by chromosomal translocations in T lymphoblastic neoplasms. *Cell*. 1991;66(4):649–661.
46. Weng AP, Ferrando AA, Lee W, et al. Activating mutations of NOTCH1 in human T cell acute lymphoblastic leukemia. *Science*. 2004;306(5694):269–271.
47. Breit S, Stanulla M, Flohr T, et al. Activating NOTCH1 mutations predict favorable early treatment response and long-term outcome in childhood precursor T-cell lymphoblastic leukemia. *Blood*. 2006;108(4):1151–1157.
48. Aster JC. Deregulated NOTCH signaling in acute T-cell lymphoblastic leukemia/lymphoma: new insights, questions, and opportunities. *Int J Hematol*. 2005;82(4):295–301.
49. Mulligan CG, Goorha S, Radtke I, et al. Genome-wide analysis of genetic alterations in acute lymphoblastic leukaemia. *Nature*. 2007;446(7137):758–764.
50. Huntly BJ, Gilliland DG. Cancer biology: summing up cancer stem cells. *Nature*. 2005;435(7046):1169–1170.
51. Reya T, Morrison SJ, Clarke MF, Weissman IL. Stem cells, cancer, and cancer stem cells. *Nature*. 2001;414(6859):105–111.
52. Polyak K, Hahn WC. Roots and stems: stem cells in cancer. *Nat Med*. 2006;12(3):296–300.
53. Huntly BJ, Gilliland DG. Leukaemia stem cells and the evolution of cancer-stem-cell research. *Nat Rev Cancer*. 2005;5(4):311–321.
54. Inukai T, Hirose K, Inaba T, et al. Hypercalcemia in childhood acute lymphoblastic leukemia: frequent implication of parathyroid hormone-related peptide and E2A-HLF from translocation 17;19. *Leukemia*. 2007;21(2):288–296.
55. Bleyer WA. Central nervous system leukemia. *Pediatr Clin North Am*. 1988;35(4):789–814.
56. Bennett JM, Catovsky D, Daniel MT, et al. Proposals for the classification of the acute leukaemias. French-American-British (FAB) co-operative group. *Br J Haematol*. 1976;33(4):451–458.
57. Korsmeyer SJ, Hieter PA, Ravetch JV, Poplack DG, Waldmann TA, Leder P. Developmental hierarchy of immunoglobulin gene rearrangements in human leukemic pre-B-cells. *Proc Natl Acad Sci USA*. 1981;78(11):7096–7100.
58. Greaves MF, Chan LC, Furley AJ, Watt SM, Molgaard HV. Lineage promiscuity in hemopoietic differentiation and leukemia. *Blood*. 1986;67(1):1–11.
59. Campana D, Behm FG. Immunophenotyping of leukemia. *J Immunol Methods*. 2000;243(1–2):59–75.
60. Hammond GD, Sather H, Bleyer WA, Coccia P. Stratification by prognostic factors in the design and analysis of clinical trials for acute lymphoblastic leukemia. *Haematol Blood Transfus*. 1987;30:161–166.
61. Kalwinsky DK, Roberson P, Dahl G, et al. Clinical relevance of lymphoblast biological features in children with acute lymphoblastic leukemia. *J Clin Oncol*. 1985;3(4):477–484.

62. Buchner T, Schellong G, Hiddemann Wea. *Acute Leukemias: Prognostic Factors and Treatment Strategies*. Berlin, New York: Springer-Verlag; 1987.
63. Cantu-Rajnoldi A, Putti C, Saitta M, et al. Co-expression of myeloid antigens in childhood acute lymphoblastic leukaemia: relationship with the stage of differentiation and clinical significance. *Br J Haematol.* 1991;79(1):40–43.
64. Fink FM, Koller U, Mayer H, et al. Prognostic significance of myeloid-associated antigen expression on blast cells in children with acute lymphoblastic leukemia. The Austrian Pediatric Oncology Group. *Med Pediatr Oncol.* 1993;21(5):340–346.
65. Kurec AS, Belair P, Stefanu C, Barrett DM, Dubowy RL, Davey FR. Significance of aberrant immunophenotypes in childhood acute lymphoid leukemia. *Cancer.* 1991;67(12):3081–3086.
66. Wiersma SR, Ortega J, Sobel E, Weinberg KI. Clinical importance of myeloid-antigen expression in acute lymphoblastic leukemia of childhood. *N Engl J Med.* 1991;324(12):800–808.
67. Putti MC, Rondelli R, Cocito MG, et al. Expression of myeloid markers lacks prognostic impact in children treated for acute lymphoblastic leukemia: Italian experience in AIEOP-ALL 88–91 studies. *Blood.* 1998;92(3):795–801.
68. Uckun FM, Sather HN, Gaynon PS, et al. Clinical features and treatment outcome of children with myeloid antigen positive acute lymphoblastic leukemia: a report from the Children's Cancer Group. *Blood.* 1997;90(1):28–35.
69. Weir EG, Ali Ansari-Lari M, Batista DA, et al. Acute bilineal leukemia: a rare disease with poor outcome. *Leukemia.* 2007;21(11):2264–2270.
70. Bene MC, Castoldi G, Knapp W, et al. Proposals for the immunological classification of acute leukemias. European Group for the Immunological Characterization of Leukemias (EGIL). *Leukemia.* 1995;9(10):1783–1786.
71. Schultz KR, Pullen DJ, Sather HN, et al. Risk and response-based classification of childhood B-precursor acute lymphoblastic leukemia: a combined analysis of prognostic markers from the Pediatric Oncology Group (POG) and Children's Cancer Group (CCG). *Blood.* 2006;109(3):926–935.
72. Smith M, Arthur D, Camitta B, et al. Uniform approach to risk classification and treatment assignment for children with acute lymphoblastic leukemia. *J Clin Oncol.* 1996;14(1):18–24.
73. Chessells JM, Bailey C, Richards SM. Intensification of treatment and survival in all children with lymphoblastic leukaemia: results of UK Medical Research Council trial UKALL X. Medical Research Council Working Party on Childhood Leukaemia. *Lancet.* 1995;345(8943):143–148.
74. Shuster JJ, Wacker P, Pullen J, et al. Prognostic significance of sex in childhood B-precursor acute lymphoblastic leukemia: a Pediatric Oncology Group Study. *J Clin Oncol.* 1998;16(8):2854–2863.
75. Forestier E, Johansson B, Gustafsson G, et al. Prognostic impact of karyotypic findings in childhood acute lymphoblastic leukaemia: a Nordic series comparing two treatment periods. For the Nordic Society of Paediatric Haematology and Oncology (NOPHO) Leukaemia Cytogenetic Study Group. *Br J Haematol.* 2000;110(1):147–153.
76. Secker-Walker LM, Swansbury GJ, Hardisty RM, et al. Cytogenetics of acute lymphoblastic leukaemia in children as a factor in the prediction of long-term survival. *Br J Haematol.* 1982;52(3):389–399.
77. Look AT, Roberson PK, Williams DL, et al. Prognostic importance of blast cell DNA content in childhood acute lymphoblastic leukemia. *Blood.* 1985;65(5):1079–1086.
78. Sutcliffe MJ, Shuster JJ, Sather HN, et al. High concordance from independent studies by the Children's Cancer Group (CCG) and Pediatric Oncology Group (POG) associating favorable prognosis with combined trisomies 4, 10, and 17 in children with NCI Standard-Risk B-precursor Acute Lymphoblastic Leukemia: a Children's Oncology Group (COG) initiative. *Leukemia.* 2005;19(5):734–740.
79. Loh ML, Goldwasser MA, Silverman LB, et al. Prospective analysis of TEL/AML1–positive patients treated on Dana-Farber Cancer Institute Consortium Protocol 95–01. *Blood.* 2006;107(11):4508–4513.
80. McLean TW, Ringold S, Neuberg D. TEL/AML1 dimerizes and is associated with a favorable outcome in childhood acute lymphoblastic leukemia. *Blood.* 1996;88:4252–4258.
81. Heerema NA, Nachman JB, Sather HN, et al. Hypodiploidy with less than 45 chromosomes confers adverse risk in childhood acute lymphoblastic leukemia: a report from the children's cancer group. *Blood.* 1999;94(12):4036–4045.
82. Uckun FM, Nachman JB, Sather HN, et al. Clinical significance of Philadelphia chromosome positive pediatric acute lymphoblastic leukemia in the context of contemporary intensive therapies: a report from the Children's Cancer Group. *Cancer.* 1998;83(9):2030–2039.
83. Nachman JB, Heerema NA, Sather H, et al. Outcome of treatment in children with hypodiploid acute lymphoblastic leukemia. *Blood.* 2007;110(4):1112–1115.
84. Gadner H, Masera G, Schrappe M, et al. The Eighth International Childhood Acute Lymphoblastic Leukemia Workshop ('Ponte di legno meeting') report: Vienna, Austria, April 27–28, 2005. *Leukemia.* 2006;20(1):9–17.
85. Pui CH, Williams DL, Raimondi SC, et al. Hypodiploidy is associated with a poor prognosis in childhood acute lymphoblastic leukemia. *Blood.* 1987;70(1):247–253.
86. Raimondi SC, Zhou Y, Mathew S, et al. Reassessment of the prognostic significance of hypodiploidy in pediatric patients with acute lymphoblastic leukemia. *Cancer.* 2003;98(12):2715–2722.
87. Brodeur GM, Williams DL, Look AT, Bowman WP, Kalwinsky DK. Near-haploid acute lymphoblastic leukemia: a unique subgroup with a poor prognosis? *Blood.* 1981;58(1):14–19.

88. Chessels JM, Swansbury GJ, Reeves B, Bailey CC, Richards SM. Cytogenetics and prognosis in childhood lymphoblastic leukaemia: results of MRC UKALL X. Medical Research Council Working Party in Childhood Leukaemia. *Br J Haematol.* 1997;99(1):93–100.
89. Pui CH, Carroll AJ, Raimondi SC, et al. Clinical presentation, karyotypic characterization, and treatment outcome of childhood acute lymphoblastic leukemia with a near-haploid or hypodiploid less than 45 line. *Blood.* 1990;75(5):1170–1177.
90. Arico M, Valsecchi MG, Camitta B, et al. Outcome of treatment in children with Philadelphia chromosome-positive acute lymphoblastic leukemia. *N Engl J Med.* 2000;342(14):998–1006.
91. Crist W, Carroll A, Shuster J, et al. Philadelphia chromosome positive childhood acute lymphoblastic leukemia: clinical and cytogenetic characteristics and treatment outcome. A Pediatric Oncology Group study. *Blood.* 1990;76(3):489–494.
92. Radich JP. Philadelphia chromosome-positive acute lymphocytic leukemia. *Hematol Oncol Clin North Am.* 2001;15(1):21–36.
93. Ribeiro RC, Abromowitch M, Raimondi SC, Murphy SB, Behm F, Williams DL. Clinical and biologic hallmarks of the Philadelphia chromosome in childhood acute lymphoblastic leukemia. *Blood.* 1987;70(4):948–953.
94. Ribeiro RC, Broniscer A, Rivera GK, et al. Philadelphia chromosome-positive acute lymphoblastic leukemia in children: durable responses to chemotherapy associated with low initial white blood cell counts. *Leukemia.* 1997;11(9):1493–1496.
95. Roberts WM, Rivera GK, Raimondi SC, et al. Intensive chemotherapy for Philadelphia-chromosome-positive acute lymphoblastic leukaemia. *Lancet.* 1994;343(8893):331–332.
96. Russo C, Carroll A, Kohler S, et al. Philadelphia chromosome and monosomy 7 in childhood acute lymphoblastic leukemia: a Pediatric Oncology Group study. *Blood.* 1991;77(5):1050–1056.
97. Schrappe M, Arico M, Harbott J, et al. Philadelphia chromosome-positive (Ph+) childhood acute lymphoblastic leukemia: good initial steroid response allows early prediction of a favorable treatment outcome. *Blood.* 1998;92(8):2730–2741.
98. Wheeler KA, Richards SM, Bailey CC, et al. Bone marrow transplantation versus chemotherapy in the treatment of very high-risk childhood acute lymphoblastic leukemia in first remission: results from Medical Research Council UKALL X and XI. *Blood.* 2000;96(7):2412–2418.
99. Behm FG, Raimondi SC, Frestedt JL, et al. Rearrangement of the *MLL* gene confers a poor prognosis in childhood acute lymphoblastic leukemia, regardless of presenting age. *Blood.* 1996;87(7):2870–2877.
100. Felix CA, Lange BJ. Leukemia in infants. *Oncologist.* 1999;4(3):225–240.
101. Albain KS, Le Beau MM, Ullirsch R, Schumacher H. Implication of prior treatment with drug combinations including inhibitors of topoisomerase II in therapy-related monocytic leukemia with a 9;11 translocation. *Genes Chromosomes Cancer.* 1990;2(1):53–58.
102. Pui CH, Behm FG, Raimondi SC, et al. Secondary acute myeloid leukemia in children treated for acute lymphoid leukemia. *N Engl J Med.* 1989;321(3):136–142.
103. Whitlock JA, Greer JP, Lukens JN. Epipodophyllotoxin-related leukemia. Identification of a new subset of secondary leukemia. *Cancer.* 1991;68(3):600–604.
104. Wiemels JL, Cazzaniga G, Daniotti M, et al. Prenatal origin of acute lymphoblastic leukaemia in children. *Lancet.* 1999;354(9189):1499–1503.
105. Dordelmann M, Reiter A, Borkhardt A, et al. Prednisone response is the strongest predictor of treatment outcome in infant acute lymphoblastic leukemia. *Blood.* 1999;94(4):1209–1217.
106. Ferster A, Benoit Y, Francotte N, et al. Treatment outcome in infant acute lymphoblastic leukemia. Children Leukemia Cooperative Group—EORTC. European Organization for Research and Treatment of Cancer. *Blood.* 2000;95(8):2729–2731.
107. Pui CH, Chessells JM, Camitta B, et al. Clinical heterogeneity in childhood acute lymphoblastic leukemia with 11q23 rearrangements. *Leukemia.* 2003;17(4):700–706.
108. Pui CH, Gaynon PS, Boyett JM, et al. Outcome of treatment in childhood acute lymphoblastic leukaemia with rearrangements of the 11q23 chromosomal region. *Lancet.* 2002;359(9321):1909–1915.
109. Ramakers-van Woerden NL, Pieters R, Loonen AH, et al. TEL/AML1 gene fusion is related to *in vitro* drug sensitivity for L-asparaginase in childhood acute lymphoblastic leukemia. *Blood.* 2000;96(3):1094–1099.
110. Whitehead VM, Vuchich MJ, Lauer SJ, et al. Accumulation of high levels of methotrexate polyglutamates in lymphoblasts from children with hyperdiploid (greater than 50 chromosomes) B-lineage acute lymphoblastic leukemia: a Pediatric Oncology Group study. *Blood.* 1992;80(5):1316–1323.
111. Silverman LB, Gelber RD, Young ML, Dalton VK, Barr RD, Sallan SE. Induction failure in acute lymphoblastic leukemia of childhood. *Cancer.* 1999;85(6):1395–1404.
112. Gaynon PS, Desai AA, Bostrom BC, et al. Early response to therapy and outcome in childhood acute lymphoblastic leukemia: a review. *Cancer.* 1997;80(9):1717–1726.
113. Gaynon PS, Trigg ME, Heerema NA, et al. Children's Cancer Group trials in childhood acute lymphoblastic leukemia: 1983–1995. *Leukemia.* 2000;14(12):2223–2233.
114. Gajjar A, Ribeiro R, Hancock ML, et al. Persistence of circulating blasts after 1 week of multiagent chemotherapy confers a poor prognosis in childhood acute lymphoblastic leukemia. *Blood.* 1995;86(4):1292–1295.

115. Schrappe M, Reiter A, Riehm H. Cytoreduction and prognosis in childhood acute lymphoblastic leukemia. *J Clin Oncol.* 1996;14(8):2403–2406.

116. Biondi A, Valsecchi MG, Seriu T, et al. Molecular detection of minimal residual disease is a strong predictive factor of relapse in childhood B-lineage acute lymphoblastic leukemia with medium risk features. A case control study of the International BFM study group. *Leukemia.* 2000;14(11):1939–1943.

117. Cave H, van der Werff ten Bosch J, Suciu S, et al. Clinical significance of minimal residual disease in childhood acute lymphoblastic leukemia. European Organization for Research and Treatment of Cancer—Childhood Leukemia Cooperative Group. *N Engl J Med.* 1998;339(9):591–598.

118. Coustan-Smith E, Sancho J, Hancock ML, et al. Clinical importance of minimal residual disease in childhood acute lymphoblastic leukemia. *Blood.* 2000;96(8):2691–2696.

119. Evans PA, Short MA, Owen RG, et al. Residual disease detection using fluorescent polymerase chain reaction at 20 weeks of therapy predicts clinical outcome in childhood acute lymphoblastic leukemia. *J Clin Oncol.* 1998;16(11):3616–3627.

120. Goulden NJ, Knechtli CJ, Garland RJ, et al. Minimal residual disease analysis for the prediction of relapse in children with standard-risk acute lymphoblastic leukaemia. *Br J Haematol.* 1998;100(1):235–244.

121. Panzer-Grumayer ER, Schneider M, Panzer S, Fasching K, Gadner H. Rapid molecular response during early induction chemotherapy predicts a good outcome in childhood acute lymphoblastic leukemia. *Blood.* 2000;95(3):790–794.

122. Roberts WM, Estrov Z, Ouspenskaia MV, Johnston DA, McClain KL, Zipf TF. Measurement of residual leukemia during remission in childhood acute lymphoblastic leukemia. *N Engl J Med.* 1997;336(5):317–323.

123. Schmiegelow K, Nyvold C, Seyfarth J, et al. Post-induction residual leukemia in childhood acute lymphoblastic leukemia quantified by PCR correlates with in vitro prednisolone resistance. *Leukemia.* 2001;15(7):1066–1071.

124. Uckun FM, Stork L, Seibel N, et al. Residual bone marrow leukemic progenitor cell burden after induction chemotherapy in pediatric patients with acute lymphoblastic leukemia. *Clin Cancer Res.* 2000;6(8):3123–3130.

125. van Dongen JJ, Seriu T, Panzer-Grumayer ER, et al. Prognostic value of minimal residual disease in acute lymphoblastic leukaemia in childhood. *Lancet.* 1998;352(9142):1731–1738.

126. Pongers-Willemse MJ, Verhagen OJ, Tibbe GJ, et al. Real-time quantitative PCR for the detection of minimal residual disease in acute lymphoblastic leukemia using junctional region specific TaqMan probes. *Leukemia.* 1998;12(12):2006–2014.

127. Pui CH, Campana D. New definition of remission in childhood acute lymphoblastic leukemia. *Leukemia.* 2000;14(5):783–785.

128. Borowitz MJ, Devidas M, Bowman WP, et al. Prognostic significance of minimal residual disease (MRD) in childhood B-precursor ALL and its relation to other risk factors. A Children's Oncology Group (COG) Study. *Blood.* 2006;108(11):Abstract #219.

129. Weinshilboum R. Thiopurine pharmacogenetics: clinical and molecular studies of thiopurine methyltransferase. *Drug Metab Dispos.* 2001;29(4 Pt 2):601–605.

130. Weinshilboum RM, Sladek SL. Mercaptopurine pharmacogenetics: monogenic inheritance of erythrocyte thiopurine methyltransferase activity. *Am J Hum Genet.* 1980;32(5):651–662.

131. Lennard L, Lilleyman JS, Van Loon J, Weinshilboum RM. Genetic variation in response to 6-mercaptopurine for childhood acute lymphoblastic leukaemia. *Lancet.* 1990;336(8709):225–229.

132. Relling MV, Hancock ML, Boyett JM, Pui CH, Evans WE. Prognostic importance of 6-mercaptopurine dose intensity in acute lymphoblastic leukemia. *Blood.* 1999;93(9):2817–2823.

133. Cheok MH, Evans WE. Acute lymphoblastic leukaemia: a model for the pharmacogenomics of cancer therapy. *Nat Rev Cancer.* 2006;6(2):117–129.

134. Armstrong SA, Kung AL, Mabon ME, et al. Inhibition of FLT3 in MLL. Validation of a therapeutic target identified by gene expression based classification. *Cancer Cell.* 2003;3(2):173–183.

135. Armstrong SA, Hsieh JJ, Korsmeyer SJ. Genomic approaches to the pathogenesis and treatment of acute lymphoblastic leukemias. *Curr Opin Hematol.* 2002;9(4):339–344.

136. Bhojwani D, Moskowitz N, Raetz EA, Carroll WL. Potential of gene expression profiling in the management of childhood acute lymphoblastic leukemia. *Paediatr Drugs.* 2007;9(3):149–156.

137. Carroll WL, Bhojwani D, Min DJ, Moskowitz N, Raetz EA. Childhood acute lymphoblastic leukemia in the age of genomics. *Pediatr Blood Cancer.* 2006;46(5):570–578.

138. Golub TR. Genomic approaches to the pathogenesis of hematologic malignancy. *Curr Opin Hematol.* 2001;8(4):252–261.

139. Ferrando AA, Look AT. DNA microarrays in the diagnosis and management of acute lymphoblastic leukemia. *Int J Hematol.* 2004;80(5):395–400.

140. Mullighan CG, Flotho C, Downing JR. Genomic assessment of pediatric acute leukemia. *Cancer J.* 2005;11(4):268–282.

141. Farber S, Diamond LK, Mercer RD, Sylvester RF, Wolff JA. Temporary remissions in acute leukemia in children produced by folic acid antagonist, 4-aminopteroyl-glutamic acid (aminopterin). *N Engl J Med.* 1948;238:787–793.

142. Simone J, Aur RJ, Hustu HO, Pinkel D. "Total therapy" studies of acute lymphocytic leukemia in children: current results and prospects for cure. *Cancer.* 1972;30(6):1488–1494.

143. Goldie JH, Coldman AJ. The genetic origin of drug resistance in neoplasms: implications for systemic therapy. *Cancer Res.* 1984;44(9):3643–3653.

144. Balis FM, Lester CM, Chrousos GP, Heideman RL, Poplack DG. Differences in cerebrospinal fluid penetration of corticosteroids: possible relationship to the prevention of meningeal leukemia. *J Clin Oncol.* 1987;5(2):202–207.

145. Jones B, Freeman AI, Shuster JJ, et al. Lower incidence of meningeal leukemia when prednisone is replaced by dexamethasone in the treatment of acute lymphocytic leukemia. *Med Pediatr Oncol.* 1991;19(4):269–275.

146. Ito C, Evans WE, McNinch L, et al. Comparative cytotoxicity of dexamethasone and prednisolone in childhood acute lymphoblastic leukemia. *J Clin Oncol.* 1996;14(8):2370–2376.

147. Veerman AJ, Hahlen K, Kamps WA, et al. High cure rate with a moderately intensive treatment regimen in non-high-risk childhood acute lymphoblastic leukemia. Results of protocol ALL VI from the Dutch Childhood Leukemia Study Group. *J Clin Oncol.* 1996;14(3):911–918.

148. Bostrom BC, Sensel MR, Sather HN, et al. Dexamethasone versus prednisone and daily oral versus weekly intravenous mercaptopurine for patients with standard-risk acute lymphoblastic leukemia: a report from the Children's Cancer Group. *Blood.* 2003;101(10):3809–3817.

149. Lawson SE, Harrison G, Richards S, et al. The UK experience in treating relapsed childhood acute lymphoblastic leukaemia: a report on the medical research council UKALLR1 study. *Br J Haematol.* 2000;108(3):531–543.

150. Hurwitz CA, Silverman LB, Schorin MA, et al. Substituting dexamethasone for prednisone complicates remission induction in children with acute lymphoblastic leukemia. *Cancer.* 2000;88(8):1964–1969.

151. Avramis VI, Sencer S, Periclou AP, et al. A randomized comparison of native Escherichia coli asparaginase and polyethylene glycol conjugated asparaginase for treatment of children with newly diagnosed standard-risk acute lymphoblastic leukemia: a Children's Cancer Group study. *Blood.* 2002;99(6):1986–1994.

152. Graham ML. Pegaspargase: a review of clinical studies. *Adv Drug Deliv Rev.* 2003;55(10):1293–1302.

153. Vieira Pinheiro JP, Lanvers C, Wurthwein G, et al. Drug monitoring of PEG asparaginase treatment in childhood acute lymphoblastic leukemia and non-Hodgkin's lymphoma. *Leuk Lymphoma.* 2002;43(10):1911–1920.

154. Gustafsson G, Schmiegelow K, Forestier E, et al. Improving outcome through two decades in childhood ALL in the Nordic countries: the impact of high-dose methotrexate in the reduction of CNS irradiation. Nordic Society of Pediatric Haematology and Oncology (NOPHO). *Leukemia.* 2000;14(12):2267–2275.

155. Schrappe M, Reiter A, Ludwig WD, et al. Improved outcome in childhood acute lymphoblastic leukemia despite reduced use of anthracyclines and cranial radiotherapy: results of trial ALL-BFM 90. German-Austrian-Swiss ALL-BFM Study Group. *Blood.* 2000;95(11):3310–3322.

156. Silverman LB, Stevenson K, Neuberg D, O'Brien J, Supko J, Sallan S. Intravenous PEG asparaginase during remission induction for childhood ALL. *Blood* 2006;108:Abstract #1854.

157. Albertsen BK, Schroder H, Jakobsen P, et al. Antibody formation during intravenous and intramuscular therapy with Erwinia asparaginase. *Med Pediatr Oncol.* 2002;38(5):310–316.

158. Douer D, Yampolsky H, Cohen LJ, et al. Pharmacodynamics and safety of intravenous pegaspargase during remission induction in adults aged 55 years or younger with newly diagnosed acute lymphoblastic leukemia. *Blood.* 2007;109(7):2744–2750.

159. Clarke M, Gaynon P, Hann I, et al. CNS-directed therapy for childhood acute lymphoblastic leukemia: Childhood ALL Collaborative Group overview of 43 randomized trials. *J Clin Oncol.* 2003;21(9):1798–1809.

160. Nathan PC, Maze R, Spiegler B, Greenberg ML, Weitzman S, Hitzler JK. CNS-directed therapy in young children with T-lineage acute lymphoblastic leukemia: High-dose methotrexate versus cranial irradiation. *Pediatr Blood Cancer.* 2004;42(1):24–29.

161. Pui CH. Central nervous system disease in acute lymphoblastic leukemia: prophylaxis and treatment. *Hematology Am Soc Hematol Educ Program.* 2006:142–146.

162. Burger B, Zimmermann M, Mann G, et al. Diagnostic cerebrospinal fluid examination in children with acute lymphoblastic leukemia: significance of low leukocyte counts with blasts or traumatic lumbar puncture. *J Clin Oncol.* 2003;21(2):184–188.

163. Howard SC, Gajjar AJ, Cheng C, et al. Risk factors for traumatic and bloody lumbar puncture in children with acute lymphoblastic leukemia. *JAMA.* 2002;288(16):2001–2007.

164. Hann I, Vora A, Richards S, et al. Benefit of intensified treatment for all children with acute lymphoblastic leukaemia: results from MRC UKALL XI and MRC ALL97 randomised trials. UK Medical Research Council's Working Party on Childhood Leukaemia. *Leukemia.* 2000;14(3):356–363.

165. Henze G, Langermann HJ, Bramswig J, et al. [The BFM 76/79 acute lymphoblastic leukemia therapy study (author's transl)]. *Klin Padiatr.* 1981;193(3):145–154.

166. Tubergen DG, Gilchrist GS, O'Brien RT, et al. Improved outcome with delayed intensification for children with acute lymphoblastic leukemia and intermediate presenting features: a Children's Cancer Group Phase III trial. *J Clin Oncol.* 1993;11(3):527–537.

167. Nachman JB, Sather HN, Sensel MG, et al. Augmented post-induction therapy for children with high-risk acute lymphoblastic leukemia and a slow response to initial therapy. *N Engl J Med.* 1998;338(23):1663–1671.

168. Seibel NL, Steinherz PG, Sather HN, et al. Early post-induction intensification therapy improves survival for children and adolescents with high-risk acute lymphoblastic leukemia and a rapid early response to induction therapy: a report from the Children's Oncology Group. *Blood.* 2008;111(5):2548–2555.

169. Matloub Y, Lindemulder S, Gaynon PS, et al. Intrathecal triple therapy decreases central nervous system relapse but fails to improve event-free survival when compared with intrathecal methotrexate: results of the Children's Cancer Group (CCG) 1952 study for standard-risk acute lymphoblastic leukemia, reported by the Children's Oncology Group. *Blood.* 2006;108(4):1165–1173.

170. Rizzari C, Citterio M, Zucchetti M, et al. A pharmacological study on pegylated asparaginase used in front-line treatment of children with acute lymphoblastic leukemia. *Haematologica.* 2006;91(1):24–31.

171. Silverman LB, Gelber RD, Dalton VK, et al. Improved outcome for children with acute lymphoblastic leukemia: results of Dana-Farber Consortium Protocol 91–01. *Blood.* 2001;97(5):1211–1218.

172. Pession A, Valsecchi MG, Masera G, et al. Long-term results of a randomized trial on extended use of high dose L-asparaginase for standard risk childhood acute lymphoblastic leukemia. *J Clin Oncol.* 2005;23(28):7161–7167.

173. Asselin B, Shuster J, Amylon M, et al. Improved event free survival (EFS) with high dose methotrexate (HDM) in T-cell lymphoblastic leukemia (T-ALL) and advanced lymphoblastic lymphoma (T-NHL): a Pediatric Oncology Group (POG) study. *ASCO.* 2001;20:367a.

174. Barredo JC, Synold TW, Laver J, et al. Differences in constitutive and post-methotrexate folylpolyglutamate synthetase activity in B-lineage and T-lineage leukemia. *Blood.* 1994;84(2):564–569.

175. Galpin AJ, Schuetz JD, Masson E, et al. Differences in folylpolyglutamate synthetase and dihydrofolate reductase expression in human B-lineage versus T-lineage leukemic lymphoblasts: mechanisms for lineage differences in methotrexate polyglutamylation and cytotoxicity. *Mol Pharmacol.* 1997;52(1):155–163.

176. Goker E, Lin JT, Trippett T, et al. Decreased polyglutamylation of methotrexate in acute lymphoblastic leukemia blasts in adults compared to children with this disease. *Leukemia.* 1993;7(7):1000–1004.

177. Rots MG, Pieters R, Peters GJ, et al. Role of folylpolyglutamate synthetase and folylpolyglutamate hydrolase in methotrexate accumulation and polyglutamylation in childhood leukemia. *Blood.* 1999;93(5):1677–1683.

178. Synold TW, Relling MV, Boyett JM, et al. Blast cell methotrexate-polyglutamate accumulation in vivo differs by lineage, ploidy, and methotrexate dose in acute lymphoblastic leukemia. *J Clin Invest.* 1994;94(5):1996–2001.

179. Evans WE, Relling MV, Rodman JH, Crom WR, Boyett JM, Pui CH. Conventional compared with individualized chemotherapy for childhood acute lymphoblastic leukemia. *N Engl J Med.* 1998;338(8):499–505.

180. Abromowitch M, Ochs J, Pui CH, et al. High-dose methotrexate improves clinical outcome in children with acute lymphoblastic leukemia: St Jude Total Therapy Study X. *Med Pediatr Oncol.* 1988;16(5):297–303.

181. Freeman AI, Boyett JM, Glicksman AS, et al. Intermediate-dose methotrexate versus cranial irradiation in childhood acute lymphoblastic leukemia: a ten-year follow-up. *Med Pediatr Oncol.* 1997;28(2):98–107.

182. Reiter A, Schrappe M, Ludwig WD, et al. Chemotherapy in 998 unselected childhood acute lymphoblastic leukemia patients. Results and conclusions of the multicenter trial ALL-BFM 86. *Blood.* 1994;84(9):3122–3133.

183. Hill FG, Richards S, Gibson B, et al. Successful treatment without cranial radiotherapy of children receiving intensified chemotherapy for acute lymphoblastic leukaemia: results of the risk-stratified randomized central nervous system treatment trial MRC UKALL XI (ISRC TN 16757172). *Br J Haematol.* 2004;124(1):33–46.

184. Lange BJ, Blatt J, Sather HN, Meadows AT. Randomized comparison of moderate-dose methotrexate infusions to oral methotrexate in children with intermediate risk acute lymphoblastic leukemia: a Children's Cancer Group study. *Med Pediatr Oncol.* 1996;27(1):15–20.

185. Schaison G, Leblanc T, Perel Y, et al. Randomized trial comparing low dose methotrexate (LDMTX) versus high dose methotrexate (HDMTX) in low and intermediate risk pre B acute lymphoblastic leukemia (ALL) in children. Results of French protocol FRALLE 93. *Proc Am Soc Clin Oncol.* 1998;17: 2026a.

186. Miller DR, Leikin SL, Albo VC, Sather H, Hammond GD. Three versus five years of maintenance therapy are equivalent in childhood acute lymphoblastic leukemia: a report from the Children's Cancer Study Group. *J Clin Oncol.* 1989;7(3):316–325.

187. Toyoda Y, Manabe A, Tsuchida M, et al. Six months of maintenance chemotherapy after intensified treatment for acute lymphoblastic leukemia of childhood. *J Clin Oncol.* 2000;18(7):1508–1516.

188. Group CAC. Duration and intensity of maintenance chemotherapy in acute lymphoblastic leukaemia: overview of 42 trials involving 12 000 randomised children. *Lancet.* 1996;29;347(9018):1783–1788.

189. Conter V, Valsecchi MG, Silvestri D, et al. Pulses of vincristine and dexamethasone in addition to intensive chemotherapy for children with intermediate-risk acute lymphoblastic leukaemia: a multicentre randomised trial. *Lancet.* 2007;369(9556):123–131.

190. Coulthard SA, Matheson EC, Hall AG, Hogarth LA. The clinical impact of thiopurine methyltransferase polymorphisms on thiopurine treatment. *Nucleosides Nucleotides Nucleic Acids.* 2004;23(8–9):1385–1391.

191. Lilleyman JS, Lennard L. Mercaptopurine metabolism and risk of relapse in childhood lymphoblastic leukaemia. *Lancet.* 1994;343(8907):1188–1190.

192. Schmiegelow K, Schroder H, Gustafsson G, et al. Risk of relapse in childhood acute lymphoblastic leukemia is related to RBC methotrexate and mercaptopurine metabolites during maintenance chemotherapy. Nordic Society for Pediatric Hematology and Oncology. *J Clin Oncol.* 1995;13(2):345–351.

193. Schmiegelow K, Bjork O, Glomstein A, et al. Intensification of mercaptopurine/methotrexate maintenance chemotherapy may increase the risk of relapse for some children with acute lymphoblastic leukemia. *J Clin Oncol.* 2003;21(7):1332–1339.

194. Duley JA, Florin TH. Thiopurine therapies: problems, complexities, and progress with monitoring thioguanine nucleotides. *Ther Drug Monit.* 2005;27(5):647–654.

195. Evans WE, Relling MV. Moving towards individualized medicine with pharmacogenomics. *Nature.* 2004;429(6990):464–468.

196. Lugthart S, Cheok MH, den Boer ML, et al. Identification of genes associated with chemotherapy crossresistance and treatment response in childhood acute lymphoblastic leukemia. *Cancer Cell.* 2005;7(4):375–386.

197. Pui CH, Relling MV. Can the genotoxicity of chemotherapy be predicted? *Lancet.* 2004;364(9438):917–918.

198. Rocha JC, Cheng C, Liu W, et al. Pharmacogenetics of outcome in children with acute lymphoblastic leukemia. *Blood.* 2005;105(12):4752–4758.

199. Stanulla M, Cario G, Meissner B, et al. Integrating molecular information into treatment of childhood acute lymphoblastic leukemia: a perspective from the BFM Study Group. *Blood Cells Mol Dis.* 2007;39(2):160–163.

200. Zaza G, Cheok M, Yang W, et al. Gene expression and thioguanine nucleotide disposition in acute lymphoblastic leukemia after in vivo mercaptopurine treatment. *Blood.* 2005;106(5):1778–1785.

201. Carroll WL, Raetz EA. Building better therapy for children with acute lymphoblastic leukemia. *Cancer Cell.* 2005;7(4):289–291.

202. Saarinen-Pihkala UM, Heilmann C, Winiarski J, et al. Pathways through relapses and deaths of children with acute lymphoblastic leukemia: role of allogeneic stem-cell transplantation in Nordic data. *J Clin Oncol.* 2006;24(36):5750–5762.

203. Gaynon PS, Harris RE, Altman AJ, et al. Bone marrow transplantation versus prolonged intensive chemotherapy for children with acute lymphoblastic leukemia and an initial bone marrow relapse within 12 months of the completion of primary therapy: Children's Oncology Group study CCG-1941. *J Clin Oncol.* 2006;24(19):3150–3156.

204. Einsiedel HG, von Stackelberg A, Hartmann R, et al. Long-term outcome in children with relapsed ALL by risk-stratified salvage therapy: results of trial acute lymphoblastic leukemia-relapse study of the Berlin-Frankfurt-Munster Group 87. *J Clin Oncol.* 2005;23(31):7942–7950.

205. Gaynon PS. Childhood acute lymphoblastic leukaemia and relapse. *Br J Haematol.* 2005;131(5):579–587.

206. Gaynon PS, Qu RP, Chappell RJ, et al. Survival after relapse in childhood acute lymphoblastic leukemia: impact of site and time to first relapse—the Children's Cancer Group Experience. *Cancer.* 1998;82(7):1387–1395.

207. Rivera GK, Zhou Y, Hancock ML, et al. Bone marrow recurrence after initial intensive treatment for childhood acute lymphoblastic leukemia. *Cancer.* 2005;103(2):368–376.

208. Abshire TC, Pollock BH, Billett AL, Bradley P, Buchanan GR. Weekly polyethylene glycol conjugated L-asparaginase compared with biweekly dosing produces superior induction remission rates in childhood relapsed acute lymphoblastic leukemia: a Pediatric Oncology Group Study. *Blood.* 2000;96(5):1709–1715.

209. Buchanan GR, Rivera GK, Boyett JM, Chauvenet AR, Crist WM, Vietti TJ. Reinduction therapy in 297 children with acute lymphoblastic leukemia in first bone marrow relapse: a Pediatric Oncology Group study. *Blood.* 1988;72(4):1286–1292.

210. Feig SA, Ames MM, Sather HN, et al. Comparison of idarubicin to daunomycin in a randomized multidrug treatment of childhood acute lymphoblastic leukemia at first bone marrow relapse: a report from the Children's Cancer Group. *Med Pediatr Oncol.* 1996;27(6):505–514.

211. Giona F, Testi AM, Rondelli R, et al. ALL R-87 protocol in the treatment of children with acute lymphoblastic leukaemia in early bone marrow relapse. *Br J Haematol.* 1997;99(3):671–677.

212. Henze G, Fengler R, Hartmann R, et al. Six-year experience with a comprehensive approach to the treatment of recurrent childhood acute lymphoblastic leukemia (ALL-REZ BFM 85). A relapse study of the BFM group. *Blood.* 1991;78(5):1166–1172.

213. Rivera GK, Hudson MM, Liu Q, et al. Effectiveness of intensified rotational combination chemotherapy for late hematologic relapse of childhood acute lymphoblastic leukemia. *Blood.* 1996;88(3):831–837.

214. Roy A, Cargill A, Love S, et al. Outcome after first relapse in childhood acute lymphoblastic leukaemia: lessons from the United Kingdom R2 trial. *Br J Haematol.* 2005;130(1):67–75.

215. Sadowitz PD, Smith SD, Shuster J, Wharam MD, Buchanan GR, Rivera GK. Treatment of late bone marrow relapse in children with acute lymphoblastic leukemia: a Pediatric Oncology Group study. *Blood.* 1993;81(3):602–609.

216. Testi AM, Del Giudice I, Arcese W, et al. A single high dose of idarubicin combined with high-dose ARA-C for treatment of first relapse in childhood "high-risk" acute lymphoblastic leukaemia: a study of the AIEOP group. *Br J Haematol.* 2002;118(3):741–747.

217. Reaman GH, Ladisch S, Echelberger C, Poplack DG. Improved treatment results in the management of single and multiple relapses of acute lymphoblastic leukemia. *Cancer.* 1980;45(12):3090–3094.

218. Chessells JM, Veys P, Kempski H, et al. Long-term follow-up of relapsed childhood acute lymphoblastic leukaemia. *Br J Haematol.* 2003;123(3): 396–405.

219. Ritchey AK, Pollock BH, Lauer SJ, Andejeski Y, Barredo J, Buchanan GR. Improved survival of children with isolated CNS relapse of acute lymphoblastic leukemia: a Pediatric Oncology Group study. *J Clin Oncol.* 1999;17(12): 3745–3752.

220. Barredo JC, Devidas M, Lauer SJ, et al. Isolated CNS relapse of acute lymphoblastic leukemia treated with intensive systemic chemotherapy and delayed CNS radiation: a Pediatric Oncology Group study. *J Clin Oncol.* 2006;24(19):3142–3149.

221. Raetz EA, Borowitz MJ, Devidas M, et al. Outcomes of children with first marrow relapse: Results from Children's Oncology Group (COG) Study AALL01P2. *Blood.* 2006;108:abstract #1871.

222. Eckert C, Biondi A, Seeger K, et al. Prognostic value of minimal residual disease in relapsed childhood acute lymphoblastic leukaemia. *Lancet.* 2001; 358(9289):1239–1241.

223. Bader P, Hancock J, Kreyenberg H, et al. Minimal residual disease (MRD) status prior to allogeneic stem cell transplantation is a powerful predictor for post-transplant outcome in children with ALL. *Leukemia.* 2002;16(9): 1668–1672.

224. Knechtli CJ, Goulden NJ, Hancock JP, et al. Minimal residual disease status before allogeneic bone marrow transplantation is an important determinant of successful outcome for children and adolescents with acute lymphoblastic leukemia. *Blood.* 1998;92(11):4072–4079.

225. Barrett AJ, Horowitz MM, Pollock BH, et al. Bone marrow transplants from HLA-identical siblings as compared with chemotherapy for children with acute lymphoblastic leukemia in a second remission. *N Engl J Med.* 1994;331(19):1253–1258.

226. Borgmann A, von Stackelberg A, Hartmann R, et al. Unrelated donor stem cell transplantation compared with chemotherapy for children with acute lymphoblastic leukemia in a second remission: a matched-pair analysis. *Blood.* 2003;101(10):3835–3839.

227. Boulad F, Steinherz P, Reyes B, et al. Allogeneic bone marrow transplantation versus chemotherapy for the treatment of childhood acute lymphoblastic leukemia in second remission: a single-institution study. *J Clin Oncol.* 1999;17(1):197–207.

228. Dopfer R, Henze G, Bender-Gotze C, et al. Allogeneic bone marrow transplantation for childhood acute lymphoblastic leukemia in second remission after intensive primary and relapse therapy according to the BFM- and CoALL-protocols: results of the German Cooperative Study. *Blood.* 1991; 78(10):2780–2784.

229. Eapen M, Raetz E, Zhang MJ, et al. Outcomes after HLA-matched sibling transplantation or chemotherapy in children with B-precursor acute lymphoblastic leukemia in a second remission: a collaborative study of the Children's Oncology Group and the Center for International Blood and Marrow Transplant Research. *Blood.* 2006;107(12):4961–4967.

230. Harrison G, Richards S, Lawson S, et al. Comparison of allogeneic transplant versus chemotherapy for relapsed childhood acute lymphoblastic leukaemia in the MRC UKALL R1 trial. MRC Childhood Leukaemia Working Party. *Ann Oncol.* 2000;11(8):999–1006.

231. Uderzo C, Dini G, Locatelli F, Miniero R, Tamaro P. Treatment of childhood acute lymphoblastic leukaemia after the first relapse: curative strategies. *Haematologica.* 2000;85(suppl 11):47–53.

232. Wheeler K, Richards S, Bailey C, Chessells J. Comparison of bone marrow transplant and chemotherapy for relapsed childhood acute lymphoblastic leukaemia: the MRC UKALL X experience. Medical Research Council Working Party on Childhood Leukaemia. *Br J Haematol.* 1998;101(1):94–103.

233. Evans WE, Johnson JA. Pharmacogenomics: the inherited basis for interindividual differences in drug response. *Annu Rev Genomics Hum Genet.* 2001; 2:9–39.

234. Kaspers GJ, Veerman AJ, Pieters R, et al. In vitro cellular drug resistance and prognosis in newly diagnosed childhood acute lymphoblastic leukemia. *Blood.* 1997;90(7):2723–2729.

235. Relling MV, Dervieux T. Pharmacogenetics and cancer therapy. *Nat Rev Cancer.* 2001;1(2):99–108.

236. Yates CR, Pui CH, Evans WE. Pharmacodynamic monitoring of cancer chemotherapy: childhood acute lymphoblastic leukemia as a model. *Ther Drug Monit.* 1998;20(5):453–458.

237. Aguayo A, Cortes JE, Kantarjian HM, et al. Complete hematologic and cytogenetic response to 2-amino-9-beta-D-arabinosyl-6-methoxy-9H-guanine in a patient with chronic myelogenous leukemia in T-cell blastic phase: A case report and review of the literature. *Cancer.* 1999;85:58–64.

238. Kisor DF, Plunkett W, Kurtzberg J, et al. Pharmacokinetics of nelarabine and 9-beta-D-arabinofuranosyl guanine in pediatric and adult patients during a Phase I study of nelarabine for the treatment of refractory hematologic malignancies. *Journal of Clinical Oncology.* 2000;18:995–1003.

239. Cohen MH, Johnson JR, Massie T, et al. Approval summary: nelarabine for the treatment of T-cell lymphoblastic leukemia/lymphoma. *Clin Cancer Res.* 2006;12(18):5329–5335.

240. Berg SL, Blaney SM, Devidas M, et al. Phase II study of nelarabine (compound 506U78) in children and young adults with refractory T-cell malignancies: a report from the Children's Oncology Group. *J Clin Oncol.* 2005;23(15): 3376–3382.

241. Stam RW, den Boer ML, Schneider P, et al. Targeting FLT3 in primary *MLL*-gene-rearranged infant acute lymphoblastic leukemia. *Blood.* 2005;106(7): 2484–2490.

242. Armstrong SA, Staunton JE, Silverman LB, et al. *MLL* translocations specify a distinct gene expression profile that distinguishes a unique leukemia. *Nat Genet.* 2002;30(1):41–47.

243. Brown P, Small D. FLT3 inhibitors: a paradigm for the development of targeted therapeutics for paediatric cancer. *Eur J Cancer.* 2004;40(5):707–721, discussion 722–704.

244. Multani PS, Grossbard ML. Monoclonal antibody-based therapies for hematologic malignancies. *Journal of Clinical Oncology.* 1998;16:3691–3710.

245. Czuczman MS, Fallon A, Mohr A, Stewart C, Bernstein ZP. Rituximab in combination with CHOP or fludarabine in low-grade lymphoma. *Seminars in Oncology.* 2002;29:36–40.

246. Grillo-Lopez AJ, Hedrick E, Rashford M, Benyunes M. Rituximab: Ongoing and future clinical development. *Seminars in Oncology.* 2002;29:105–112.

247. Carnahan J, Stein R, Qu Z, et al. Epratuzumab, a CD22-targeting recombinant humanized antibody with a different mode of action from rituximab. *Mol Immunol.* 2007;44(6):1331–1341.

248. Goldenberg DM. Epratuzumab in the therapy of oncological and immunological diseases. *Expert Rev Anticancer Ther.* 2006;6(10):1341–1353.

249. Leonard JP, Coleman M, Ketas J, et al. Combination antibody therapy with epratuzumab and rituximab in relapsed or refractory non-Hodgkin's lymphoma. *J Clin Oncol.* 2005;23(22):5044–5051.

250. Leonard JP, Coleman M, Ketas JC, et al. Phase I/II trial of epratuzumab (humanized anti-CD22 antibody) in indolent non-Hodgkin's lymphoma. *J Clin Oncol.* 2003;21(16):3051–3059.

251. Micallef IN, Kahl BS, Maurer MJ, et al. A pilot study of epratuzumab and rituximab in combination with cyclophosphamide, doxorubicin, vincristine, and prednisone in patients with previously untreated, diffuse large B-cell lymphoma. *Cancer.* 2006;107(12):2826–2832.

252. Strauss SJ, Morschhauser F, Rech J, et al. Multicenter Phase II trial of immunotherapy with the humanized anti-CD22 antibody, epratuzumab, in combination with rituximab, in refractory or recurrent non-Hodgkin's lymphoma. *J Clin Oncol.* 2006;24(24):3880–3886.

253. Raetz EA, Cairo M, Borowitz MJ, et al. Chemoimmunotherapy reinduction with epratuzumab in children with ALL with marrow relapse: A Children's Oncology Group (COG) pilot study (ADVL04P2). *Proc Am Soc Clin Onc.* 2007:Abstract # 9513.

254. Jeha S, Gandhi V, Chan KW, et al. Clofarabine, a novel nucleoside analog, is active in pediatric patients with advanced leukemia. *Blood.* 2004;103(3): 784–789.

255. Pui CH, Jeha S. Clofarabine. *Nat Rev Drug Discov.* 2005;(suppl):S12–13.

256. Hijiya N, Franklin J, Rytting M, et al. A Phase I study of clofarabine in combination with cyclophosphamide and etoposide: a new regimen in pediatric patients with refractory or relapsed acute leukemia. *Proc ASCO.* 2007: Abstract # 9529.

257. Adams J, Palombella VJ, Elliott PJ. Proteasome inhibition: a new strategy in cancer treatment. *Invest New Drugs.* 2000;18(2):109–121.

258. Horton TM, Gannavarapu A, Blaney SM, D'Argenio DZ, Plon SE, Berg SL. Bortezomib interactions with chemotherapy agents in acute leukemia *in vitro. Cancer Chemother Pharmacol.* 2006;58(1):13–23.

259. Masdehors P, Merle-Beral H, Maloum K, Omura S, Magdelenat H, Delic J. Deregulation of the ubiquitin system and p53 proteolysis modify the apoptotic response in B-CLL lymphocytes. *Blood.* 2000;96(1):269–274.

260. Hideshima T, Chauhan D, Richardson P, et al. NF-kappa B as a therapeutic target in multiple myeloma. *J Biol Chem.* 2002;277(19):16639–16647.

261. Horton TM, Pati D, Plon SE, et al. A Phase 1 study of the proteasome inhibitor bortezomib in pediatric patients with refractory leukemia: a Children's Oncology Group study. *Clin Cancer Res.* 2007;13(5):1516–1522.

262. Blaney SM, Bernstein M, Neville K, et al. Phase I study of the proteasome inhibitor bortezomib in pediatric patients with refractory solid tumors: a Children's Oncology Group study (ADVL0015). *J Clin Oncol.* 2004;22(23): 4804–4809.

263. Chiang GG, Abraham RT. Targeting the mTOR signaling network in cancer. *Trends Mol Med.* 2007;13(10):433–442.

264. Guertin DA, Sabatini DM. Defining the role of mTOR in cancer. *Cancer Cell.* 2007;12(1):9–22.

265. Giles FJ, Albitar M. Mammalian target of rapamycin as a therapeutic target in leukemia. *Curr Mol Med.* 2005;5(7):653–661.

266. Smolewski P. Recent developments in targeting the mammalian target of rapamycin (mTOR) kinase pathway. *Anticancer Drugs.* 2006;17(5):487–494.

267. Brown VI, Fang J, Alcorn K, et al. Rapamycin is active against B-precursor leukemia *in vitro* and in vivo, an effect that is modulated by IL-7-mediated signaling. *Proc Natl Acad Sci USA.* 2003;100(25):15113–15118.

268. Teachey DT, Obzut DA, Axsom K, et al. Rapamycin improves lymphoproliferative disease in murine autoimmune lymphoproliferative syndrome (ALPS). *Blood.* 2006;108(6):1965–1971.

269. Teachey DT, Obzut DA, Cooperman J, et al. The mTOR inhibitor CCI-779 induces apoptosis and inhibits growth in preclinical models of primary adult human ALL. *Blood.* 2006;107(3):1149–1155.

270. Chan SM, Weng AP, Tibshirani R, Aster JC, Utz PJ. Notch signals positively regulate activity of the mTOR pathway in T-cell acute lymphoblastic leukemia. *Blood.* 2007;110(1):278–286.

271. Teachey DT, Reid G, Fish J, et al. mTOR inhibitors are synergistic with methotrexate: an effective combination to treat acute lymphoblastic leukemia (ALL). *Pediatric Blood and Cancer.* 2007;48(6):abstract # 5725.5724.

272. Mertens AC, Yasui Y, Neglia JP, et al. Late mortality experience in five-year survivors of childhood and adolescent cancer: the Childhood Cancer Survivor Study. *J Clin Oncol.* 2001;19(13):3163–3172.

273. Moller TR, Garwicz S, Barlow L, et al. Decreasing late mortality among five-year survivors of cancer in childhood and adolescence: a population-based study in the Nordic countries. *J Clin Oncol.* 2001;19(13):3173–3181.

274. Pui CH, Cheng C, Leung W, et al. Extended follow-up of long-term survivors of childhood acute lymphoblastic leukemia. *N Engl J Med.* 2003;349(7):640–649.

275. Armstrong FD, Reaman GH. Psychological research in childhood cancer: the Children's Oncology Group perspective. *J Pediatr Psychol.* 2005;30(1):89–97.

276. Butler RW, Haser JK. Neurocognitive effects of treatment for childhood cancer. *Ment Retard Dev Disabil Res Rev.* 2006;12(3):184–191.

277. Moore BD, 3rd. Neurocognitive outcomes in survivors of childhood cancer. *J Pediatr Psychol.* 2005;30(1):51–63.

278. Moleski M. Neuropsychological, neuroanatomical, and neurophysiological consequences of CNS chemotherapy for acute lymphoblastic leukemia. *Arch Clin Neuropsychol.* 2000;15(7):603–630.

279. Spiegler BJ, Kennedy K, Maze R, et al. Comparison of long-term neurocognitive outcomes in young children with acute lymphoblastic leukemia treated with cranial radiation or high-dose or very high-dose intravenous methotrexate. *J Clin Oncol.* 2006;24(24):3858–3864.

280. Cousens P, Ungerer JA, Crawford JA, Stevens MM. Cognitive effects of childhood leukemia therapy: a case for four specific deficits. *J Pediatr Psychol.* 1991;16(4):475–488.

281. Kaleita TA, Reaman GH, MacLean WE, Sather HN, Whitt JK. Neurodevelopmental outcome of infants with acute lymphoblastic leukemia. *Cancer.* 1999;85:1859–1865.

282. Kingma A, van Dommelen RI, Mooyaart EL, Wilmink JT, Deelman BG, Kamps WA. Slight cognitive impairment and magnetic resonance imaging abnormalities but normal school levels in children treated for acute lymphoblastic leukemia with chemotherapy only. *J Pediatr.* 2001;139:413–420.

283. Mahoney DH, Jr., Shuster JJ, Nitschke R, et al. Acute neurotoxicity in children with B-precursor acute lymphoid leukemia: an association with intermediate-dose intravenous methotrexate and intrathecal triple therapy: a Pediatric Oncology Group study. *J Clin Oncol.* 1998;16(5):1712–1722.

284. Winick NJ, Bowman WP, Kamen BA, et al. Unexpected acute neurologic toxicity in the treatment of children with acute lymphoblastic leukemia. *J Natl Cancer Inst.* 1992;84(4):252–256.

285. Asato R, Akiyama Y, Ito M, et al. Nuclear magnetic resonance abnormalities of the cerebral white matter in children with acute lymphoblastic leukemia and malignant lymphoma during and after central nervous system prophylactic treatment with intrathecal methotrexate. *Cancer.* 1997;70:1997–2004.

286. Bleyer WA. Neurologic sequelae of methotrexate and ionizing radiation: a new classification. *Cancer Treat Rep.* 1981;65(suppl 1):89–98.

287. Harila-Saari AH, Paakko EL, Vainionpaa LK, Pyhtinen J, Lanning BM. A longitudinal magnetic resonance imaging study of the brain in survivors in childhood acute lymphoblastic leukemia. *Cancer.* 1998;83(12):2608–2617.

288. Kay HE, Knapton PJ, O'Sullivan JP, et al. Encephalopathy in acute leukaemia associated with methotrexate therapy. *Arch Dis Child.* 1972;47(253):344–354.

289. Paakko E, Vainionpaa I., Pyhtinen J, Lanning M. Minor changes on cranial MRI during treatment in children with acute lymphoblastic leukaemia. *Neuroradiology.* 1996;38(3):264–268.

290. Wilson DA, Nitschke R, Bowman ME, Chaffin MJ, Sexauer CL, Prince JR. Transient white matter changes on MR Images in children undergoing chemotherapy for acute lymphocytic leukemia: correlation with neuropsychologic deficiencies. *Radiology.* 1991;180:205–209.

291. Millot F, Dhondt JL, Mazingue F, Mechinaud F, Ingrand P, Guilhot F. Changes of cerebral biopterin and biogenic amine metabolism in leukemic children receiving 5 g/m2 intravenous methotrexate. *Pediatr Res.* 1995;37(2):151–154.

292. Quinn CT, Griener JC, Bottiglieri T. Elevation of homocysteine and excitatory amino acid neurotransmitters in the CSF of children who receive methotrexate for the treatment of cancer. *J Clin Oncol.* 1997;15:2800–2806.

293. Kishi S, Griener J, Cheng C, et al. Homocysteine, pharmacogenetics, and neurotoxicity in children with leukemia. *J Clin Oncol.* 2003;21(16):3084–3091.

294. Balis FM, Lester CM, Chrousos GP. Differences in cerebrospinal fluid penetration of corticosteroids: possible relationship to the preventing of meningeal leukemia. *J Clin Oncol.* 1987;5:202–207.

295. Kaspers GJL, Pieters R, Van Zantwijk V, Van Wering ER, Van Der Does-Van Den Berg A, Veerman AJP. Prednisolone resistance in childhood acute lymphoblastic leukemia: vitro-vivo correlations and cross-resistance to other drugs. *Blood.* 1998;92:259–266.

296. Waber DP, Carpentieri SC, Klar N, et al. Cognitive sequelae in children treated for acute lymphoblastic leukemia with dexamethasone or prednisone. *J Pediatr Hematol Oncol.* 2000;22(3):206–213.

297. Kremer LC, van Dalen EC, Offringa M, Voute PA. Frequency and risk factors of anthracycline-induced clinical heart failure in children: a systematic review. *Ann Oncol.* 2002;13(4):503–512.

298. Hudson MM, Rai SN, Nunez C, et al. Noninvasive evaluation of late anthracycline cardiac toxicity in childhood cancer survivors. *J Clin Oncol.* 2007;25(24):3635–3643.

299. Lipshultz SE, Lipsitz SR, Sallan SE, et al. Chronic progressive cardiac dysfunction years after doxorubicin therapy for childhood acute lymphoblastic leukemia. *J Clin Oncol.* 2005;23(12):2629–2636.

300. Kremer LCM, van Dalen EC, Offringa M, Ottenkamp J, Voûte PA. Anthracycline-induced clinical heart failure in a cohort of 607 children: long-term follow-up study. *J Clin Oncol.* 2001;19:191–196.

301. Singal PK, Iliskovic N. Doxorubicin-induced cardiomyopathy. *N Engl J Med.* 1998;339:900–905.

302. Hasinoff BB. The interaction of the cardioprotective agent ICRF-187 ((+)-1,2-bis(3,5–dioxopiperazinyl-1-yl)propane); its hydrolysis product (ICRF-198); and other chelating agents with the Fe(III)(and Cu(II) complexes of adriamycin. *Agents Actions.* 1989;26:378–385.

303. Sobol MM, Amiet RG, Green MD. *In vitro* evidence for direct complexation of ADR-529/ICRF-187 [(+)-1,2bis-(3,5–dioxo-piperazin-1-yl)propane] onto an existing ferric-anthracycline complex. *Mol Pharmacol.* 1991;41:8–16.

304. Wexler I H, Andrich MP, Venzon D, et al. Randomized trial of the cardioprotective agent ICRF-187 in pediatric sarcoma patients treated with doxorubicin. *J Clin Oncol.* 1996;14:362–372.

305. Lipshultz SE. Dexrazoxane for protection against cardiotoxic effects of anthracyclines in children. *J Clin Oncol.* 1996;14(2):328–331.

306. Lipshultz SE, Rifai N, Dalton VM, et al. The effect of dexrazoxane on myocardial injury in doxorubicin-treated children with acute lymphoblastic leukemia. *N Engl J Med.* 2004;351(2):145–153.

307. Tebbi CK, London WB, Friedman D, et al. Dexrazoxane-associated risk for acute myeloid leukemia/myelodysplastic syndrome and other secondary malignancies in pediatric Hodgkin's disease. *J Clin Oncol.* 2007;25(5):493–500.

308. Bostrom B, Gaynon PS, Sather H, et al. Dexamethasone (DEX) decreases central nervous system (CNS) relapse and improves event-free survival (EFS) in lower risk acute lymphoblastic leukemia (ALL). *Proceedings of the American Society of Clinical Oncology.* 1998;17:2024.

309. Gaynon PS, Carrel AL. Glucocorticosteroid therapy in childhood acute lymphoblastic leukemia. *Advances in Experimental Medicine and Biology.* 1999;457:593–605.

310. Niemeyer CM, Gelber RD, Tarbell NJ. Low-dose versus high-dose methotrexate during remission induction in childhood acute lymphoblastic leukemia. *Blood.* 1991;78:2514–2519.

311. Riehm H, Gadner H, Henze G, et al. Results and significance of six randomized trials in four consecutive ALL-BFM studies. *Haematol Blood Transfus.* 1990;33:439–450.

312. Schwartz CL, Thompson EB, Gelber RD, et al. Improved response with higher corticosteroid dose in children with acute lymphoblastic leukemia. *J Clin Oncol.* 2001;19:1040–1046.

313. Chang JK, Ho ML, Yeh CH, Chen CH, Wang GJ. Osteogenic gene expression decreases in stromal cells of patients with osteonecrosis. *Clin Orthop Relat Res.* 2006;453:286–292.

314. Wang GJ, Cui Q, Balian G. The Nicolas Andry award. The pathogenesis and prevention of steroid-induced osteonecrosis. *Clin Orthop Relat Res.* 2000 (370):295–310.

315. Weinstein RS, Nicholas RW, Manolagas SC. Apoptosis of osteocytes in glucocorticoid-induced osteonecrosis of the hip. *J Clin Endocrinol Metab.* 2000; 85(8):2907–2912.

316. Pritchett JW. Statin therapy decreases the risk of osteonecrosis in patients receiving steroids. *Clin Orthop Relat Res.* 2001(386):173–178.

317. Schmitz G, Schmitz-Madry A, Ugocsai P. Pharmacogenetics and pharmacogenomics of cholesterol-lowering therapy. *Curr Opin Lipidol.* 2007;18(2):164–173.

318. Relling MV, Yang W, Das S, et al. Pharmacogenetic risk factors for osteonecrosis of the hip among children with leukemia. *J Clin Oncol.* 2004;22(19):3930–3936.

319. Mattano LA, Sather HN, Trigg ME, Nachman JB. Osteonecrosis as a complication of treating acute lymphoblastic leukemia in children: a report from the Children's Cancer Group. *J Clin Oncol.* 2000;18:3262–3272.

320. Strauss AJ, Su JT, Kimball Dalton VM, Gelber RD, Sallan SE, Silverman LB. Bony morbidity in children treated for acute lymphoblastic leukemia. *J Clin Oncol.* 2001;19:3066–3072.

321. Skipper HE. Foreword. In: Bruchovsky N, Goldie JH, eds. *Drug and Hormone Resistance in Neoplasia.* Vol 1. Boca Raton: CRC Press; 1982.

Myeloid Leukemias and Myelodysplastic Syndromes

Robert J. Arceci and Patrick A. Brown

Introduction

Acute myeloid leukemia (AML) is a malignancy characterized by clonal proliferation of variably differentiated myeloid precursors in the bone marrow. Although AML is significantly less common than acute lymphoblastic leukemia (ALL) in childhood, it has considerably greater mortality, with only half as many children likely to be cured with standard therapy. In addition, the typical treatment for AML is among the most toxic of treatments for any pediatric cancer, including intensive multiagent chemotherapy and often hematopoietic stem cell transplantation (HSCT). Given the poor prognosis and toxicity of therapy for AML, novel molecularly targeted therapies are being aggressively pursued to improve the outcome for children with AML.

Epidemiology

In the United States, the incidence of AML in children younger than 20 years old is approximately 7 per million per year, or approximately 600 new cases per year.[1] This accounts for 19% of leukemia in childhood, with the remainder being ALL (76%) and the rare chronic leukemias of childhood (5%). The incidence of AML in children aged 0 to 19 years in the United States increased at a rate of 1.3% per year from 1975 to 2004.

Unlike with ALL, the incidence of AML in children does not have an obvious age peak, although there are subtle increases in incidence in the neonatal and the adolescent age periods. After age 20, the incidence of AML increases steadily with age so that in adults, AML is approximately 4 times as common as ALL. The incidence of AML is not significantly different in boys and girls.

There is evidence of variation in childhood AML incidence with race, ethnicity, and geography. In the United States, Hispanic children have a significantly higher incidence of AML (9 per million), which is primarily due to an increased incidence of the acute promyelocytic leukemia (APML) subtype.[2,3] The most recent US Surveillance, Epidemiology, and End Results data indicate no significant difference in the incidence of AML between Caucasian and African American children.[1]

Internationally, the highest incidences of AML are seen in Japan (8 per million), Australia (8 per million), and Zimbabwe (11 per million).[4]

The incidence of secondary AML after treatment for other malignancies is increasing in pediatrics, likely as a result of increased survivorship and increased use of epipodophyllotoxins (such as etoposide) for the treatment of many solid tumors of childhood.[5] Risk of secondary AML has been linked to use not only of epipodophyllotoxins but also of anthracyclines (which, like epipodophyllotoxins, inhibit topoisomerase II), alkylating chemotherapy agents, and irradiation.[6]

Predisposition

Although the vast majority of cases of AML in children occur in patients with no known predisposition and can be considered sporadic, several inherited and acquired risk factors have been shown to be associated with increased risk of AML in childhood.

Inherited

Trisomy 21 and Down Syndrome

The most common inherited predisposition to develop leukemia is Down syndrome (DS). Children with DS have an approximately 10- to 20–fold increased risk of leukemia compared with other children. During the first 3 years of life, children with DS have a particularly high risk of the megakaryoblastic subtype of AML (French-American-British subtype FAB M7).[7] Overall, patients with DS constitute approximately 10% of pediatric patients with AML. In addition, approximately 10% of neonates with DS manifest a transient myeloproliferative disorder (TMD). This disorder mimics congenital AML but usually improves spontaneously within 4 to 6 weeks. Retrospective surveys indicate that 20% to 30% of infants with DS and TMD will develop M7 AML before 3 years of age.[8] Children who lack the phenotypic features of DS but exhibit mosaicism for trisomy 21 in the bone marrow and peripheral blood demonstrate a similar increased risk of TMD and leukemia.

The biologic basis of the increased risk of AML and TMD in children with trisomy 21 is not completely clear. The possibility that there is a gene on chromosome 21 (such as the *RUNX1/AML1* gene, which is known to be involved in some forms of AML and ALL) that predisposes to leukemia when present in 3 copies has been investigated but not conclusively demonstrated. The important discovery of acquired somatic mutations of the GATA1 transcription factor in the vast majority of cases of DS–associated M7 AML and TMD implicates these mutations as an early event in development of these diseases.[9] It is likely that the development of M7 AML results from the acquisition of additional mutations by myeloid progenitor clones that harbor 3 copies of chromosome 21 and mutant GATA1.

Bone Marrow Failure Syndromes and Other Rare Inherited Syndromes Predisposing to Acute Myeloid Leukemia

Inherited bone marrow failure syndromes represent distinctive disorders that affect cellular pathways involving DNA damage responses and repair, chromosomal stability, telomere maintenance, ribosome biogenesis, and hematopoietic growth factor signaling. They are also commonly associated with congenital anomalies and a predisposition to various cancers, including AML. Some of these syndromes result in trilineage failure (eg, Fanconi anemia, dyskeratosis congenital) while others primarily affect one or two hematopoietic lineages (eg, Kostmann syndrome, Diamond-Blackfan anemia, Schwachman-Diamond syndrome, congenital amegakaryoctyic thrombocytopenia). Other inherited disorders associated with an increased incidence of developing AML but not typically characterized by bone marrow failure include Li-Fraumeni syndrome, Bloom syndrome, familial platelet disorder (FPD) with a propensity to develop AML (FPD/AML), neurofibromatosis type 1 (NF1), and Noonan syndrome. Table 13-1 summarizes the major clinical, genetic, and molecular features of these conditions, which are quite rare and account for only a small fraction of all cases of childhood AML. Nonetheless, important clues to the genetic and molecular pathogenesis of AML, and cancer generally, have come from the discovery of the specific mutation(s) responsible for many of these disorders.

Twins and Siblings

Being a twin or sibling of a patient with acute leukemia (AML or ALL) confers an increased risk of developing leukemia.[10] For monozygotic twins, when the index case is diagnosed prior to the age of 1 year, the risk of the second twin developing leukemia is exceedingly high (the concordance is nearly 100%) and the latency is typically short. If the index case is between 1 and 6 years at diagnosis, the concordance is lower (approximately 20%), and the latency is typically longer. Finally, if the index case is older than 6 years at diagnosis, the risk to the second twin is only slightly increased from the general population, suggesting that a common prenatal preleukemic event does not occur in these cases or that the event leads to a

change with limited consequences for cell longevity. Dizygotic twins and siblings of children with acute leukemia also appear to have a slightly (less than 2-fold) increased risk of developing leukemia.[11] The implications of these epidemiologic observations on the biology of leukemogenesis are discussed in the section on genetic and molecular pathogenesis later in this chapter.

Familial Acute Myeloid Leukemia

There have been rare reports of kindreds with several cases of AML occurring over multiple generations where no known predisposing syndrome or other condition has been identified, but where a common constitutional chromosomal abnormality has been detected.[12–15] Monosomy 7 has been the most common abnormality noted. The parental origin of the deleted segment of chromosome 7 differs between affected members of the same family, suggesting a "mutator gene" as the underlying inherited genetic defect.[16] A family with 3 affected members over 2 generations has been described where all affected members (and no unaffected members) had an identical heterozygous mutation in the gene encoding the transcription factor CEBPA, which is known to regulate myeloid differentiation.[17]

Acquired Predispositions

Several acquired conditions have been associated with an increased risk of AML. Patients with severe aplastic anemia (SAA) treated with immunosuppressive regimens and recombinant human granulocyte colony-stimulating factor (G-CSF) have been noted to have a significant risk (up to 20%) of developing myelodysplastic syndrome (MDS) or AML.[18–20] The relative contribution of each potential leukemogenic factor (SAA, immunosuppression, and G-CSF administration) is not clear from these studies. The related disorder, paroxysmal nocturnal hemoglobinuria, is also associated with an increased risk of developing MDS and AML[21] but occurs less frequently than SAA in the pediatric age group.[22] Myelodysplastic syndrome is considered a predisposing condition for developing AML in any age group, but AML arising from MDS is far more common in adults than children.[23] Myelodysplastic syndrome in children differs in many respects from MDS in adults, and several groups have proposed classification schemes taking these unique features into account (see below).[24,25] Some examples of the differences include higher incidence of cases of MDS arising from an inherited predisposing condition (such as one of the congenital bone marrow failure syndromes) and the relative rarity of 5q- syndrome and refractory anemia with ringed sideroblasts (RARS).

Environmental Exposures

Several lines of evidence implicate various environmental exposures as etiologic agents of AML. High doses of ionizing radiation clearly played a significant role in the observed 20-fold increase in incidence of AML that peaked 6 to 8 years after the atomic bomb detonations in Hiroshima and Nagasaki during World War II.[26] Interestingly, no increased incidence in AML was documented in

Table 13-1

Inherited pediatric disorders with an acute myeloid leukemia predisposition.

Disorder	Inheritance	Associated Myeloid Malignancy	Clinical Features	Molecular Genetic Features
			Bone Marrow Failure Syndromes	
Fanconi anemia	AR	MDS, AML (cumulative risk up to 50%)	characteristic congenital abnormalities (skeletal, renal, mental retardation), progressive bone marrow failure	Mutations in one of several components of FA/BRCA multiprotein complex involved in homology-directed DNA repair, resulting in chromosomal instability, increased sensitivity to genotoxic agents (mitomycin C, diepoxybutane), cancer risk
Dyskeratosis congenita	XR, AD, AR	MDS, AML	abnormal skin pigmentation, nail dystrophy, leukoplakia, progressive bone marrow failure	DKC1 (XR) or TERC (AD) (components of telomerase complex) mutations, resulting in defective telomere maintenance
Diamond-Blackfan anemia	AD	AML	pure red cell aplasia, characteristic congenital abnormalities (facial, skeletal, genitourinary)	RPS19 and RPS24 mutations, affecting rRNA processing and 40S subunit biogenesis
Kostmann syndrome	AR	MDS, AML	severe congenital neutropenia	ELA2 (elastase) mutations, resulting in agranulocytosis; secondary activating mutations of G-CSF receptor often responsible for progression to AML
Schwachman-Diamond syndrome	AR	MDS, AML	Neutropenia, exocrine pancreatic insufficiency, skeletal abnormalities	SBDS mutations, affecting rRNA processing and 40S subunit biogenesis
Congenital amegakaryocytic thrombocytopenia	AR	MDS, AML	congenital thrombocytopenia, progressive bone marrow failure	MPL (thrombopoietin receptor) mutations
			Other	
Bloom syndrome	AR	AML	characteristic congenital abnormalities (dwarfism, facies), sun sensitivity	BLM (a RecQ helicase family member) mutations, resulting in chromosomal instability, sister chromatid exchanges, cancer risk (many types)
Li-Fraumeni syndrome	AD	AML	cancer predisposition (mostly solid tumors, leukemia less common)	P53 mutations
Neurofibromatosis type 1	AD	JMML, MDS, AML	characteristic neurocutaneous syndrome	NF1 mutations, resulting in enhanced SHP2/RAS signaling
Noonan syndrome	AD	JMML, MDS, AML	characteristic congenital abnormalities (cardiac, short stature, facies, webbed neck)	PTPN11 mutations, resulting in enhanced SHP2/RAS signaling
Familial platelet disorder with predisposition to AML	AD	AML	qualitative and quantitative platelet defects	AML1 (myeloid transcription factor) mutations

children born after in utero exposure to radiation from the atomic bombs.[27] Although prenatal exposure to diagnostic x-rays has been fairly convincingly implicated in increased risk of childhood ALL, this association has not been demonstrated for AML.[28,29] There is no convincing evidence that electromagnetic field exposure due to proximity to power lines increases the risk of children developing leukemia of any kind.[30]

Maternal consumption of various genotoxic agents (eg, alcohol, tobacco, and marijuana) during pregnancy has been associated with increased risk of AML in offspring by some studies, but none of these have been conclusive.[31–33] A very interesting theory proposes an association between infant leukemia and maternal consumption of various substances (eg, flavonoids, catechins as in green tea, caffeine, and quinolones as certain classes of antibiotics) that contain chemicals known to be inhibitors of topoisomerase II.[34–36] Support for this theory is provided by the fact that the most common molecular abnormality in infant leukemia is rearrangement of the *MLL* gene at chromosome 11q23, which is the same abnormality most commonly seen in AML arising secondary to exposure to the epipodophyllotoxin class of chemotherapeutic agents, such as etoposide and teniposide, whose major mechanism of action is topoisomerase II inhibition. There is also in vitro evidence that dietary bioflavonoids can induce *MLL* rearrangements in primary human CD34+ hematopoietic stem/progenitor cells.[37]

One potent etiologic risk factor for AML that has become increasingly problematic as childhood cancer survivorship has increased is prior exposure to chemotherapeutics. Agents that cause direct DNA damage (alkylating agents, radiation, anthracyclines) and agents that inhibit topoisomerase II (epipodophyllotoxins, anthracyclines) are most frequently implicated in the etiology of treatment-related MDS and AML (t-MDS/t-AML). There are differences in the presentation of t-MDS/t-AML based on the suspected etiologic agent. Alkylating agents and radiation are associated with long (5–7 year) latency from exposure to onset of t-MDS/t-AML, with a preceding MDS phase, and monosomy or long-arm deletions in chromosomes 5 and 7. Topoisomerase II inhibitors are associated with shorter latency (median 2 years), lack of a preceding MDS phase, and "classic" translocations (most commonly involving 11q23, but also t(8;21), t(15;17), t(9;22), and inv(16)).[38] Regardless of age at presentation or etiology, t-MDS/t-AML tends to be more refractory to therapy than de novo MDS or AML.[39,40]

Clinical Presentation

Most symptoms and signs of childhood AML are the result of the propensity of leukemia cells to replace the bone marrow and infiltrate multiple other organs throughout the body. It is estimated that approximately 10^{12} leukemia cells are commonly present in a patient's body at diagnosis. It is important to recognize that newly diagnosed AML is a medical emergency, because there are several potentially life-threatening complications that may be present at diagnosis or may develop within a short period of time after diagnosis.

The replacement of normal bone marrow with leukemic blasts is responsible for the characteristic abnormal blood counts, which in most cases include the triad of neutropenia, anemia, and thrombocytopenia. Depending on the number of circulating leukemic blasts in the peripheral blood, the total white blood cell (WBC) count may be low, normal, or high. The neutropenia is often profound (absolute neutrophil count less than 500/μL) and is associated with an increased risk of serious, life-threatening infection. Blood cultures and broad spectrum intravenous antibiotic coverage are indicated in any newly diagnosed leukemia patient with fever.[41,42] Anemia is often manifested by fatigue, lethargy, headache, and pallor. Congestive heart failure (CHF) is less common at presentation, but care should be taken to transfuse packed red blood cells slowly to avoid precipitating CHF. Thrombocytopenia often leads to bruising and petechiae, and more rarely frank bleeding. Platelet transfusion is indicated for bleeding or for very low platelet counts (less than 10,000/μL). Infiltration of organs other than the bone marrow with leukemia cells is responsible for additional presenting clinical features. Table 13-2 summarizes the organ systems most frequently involved in AML and the typical clinical manifestations.

Life-threatening bleeding is another potential complication of leukemia. Although all patients with thrombocy-

Table 13-2	
Organ system involvement in pediatric AML.	
Organ System	**Clinical Manifestation(s)**
Bone marrow	Pancytopenia, bone pain
Reticuloendothelial system	Lymphadenopathy, hepatosplenomegaly (particularly prominent in M4 and M5)
Bones	Bone pain common, fractures and chloromas rare
Gums	Gingival hypertrophy (M4 and M5)
Skin	Leukemia cutis/chloromas (M2, M4, and M5 AML, infant leukemia)
Central nervous system	Meningitis, cranial nerve palsies, rarely intracranial, epidural, or orbital chloromas (M4 and M5 AML)
Kidneys	Often infiltrated/enlarged, rarely acute renal failure (except in tumor lysis syndrome)

topenia are at risk, patients with concomitant coagulopathy due to disseminated intravascular coagulation (DIC) are at particularly high risk.[43] The leukemia subtype most commonly complicated by DIC and serious bleeding is acute promyelocytic leukemia (M3 AML).[44] This association is due to the release of thromboplastin from the cytoplasmic granules in promyelocytic blasts. Aggressive blood product support and early treatment with the differentiation-inducing agent all-trans retinoic acid (ATRA) has been shown to decrease the risk of bleeding in APL.[45] Despite these measures, up to 10% of patients will die of bleeding complications during the initial weeks of therapy, and additional patients will suffer lasting morbidity from retinal hemorrhages and nonfatal central nervous system (CNS) hemorrhages.

Hyperleukocytosis becomes a potential clinical problem when the WBC count rises above 100,000/μL.[46] Circulating blood can become hyperviscous with markedly elevated WBCs, leading to sludging of blood in brain, lungs, kidneys, and other organs. Clinical features of hyperleukocytosis are summarized in Table 13-3. The risk of hyperviscosity is higher with AML than ALL, because myeloblasts are generally larger and more adherent than lymphoblasts. Management consists of treating the leukemia as soon as possible, and exchange transfusion or leukopheresis should be done in cases where initial symptoms are prominent.[47]

A rare but important presentation of AML is spinal cord compression, which results from a chloroma (a solid tumor resulting from the localized proliferation of myeloblasts) in the paraspinal/epidural region.[48] Chloromas are present most commonly in skin or bones, but they can occur anywhere in the body. They are most frequently seen in FAB M2 AML, and, in particular, cases with the t(8;21) translocation that results in the *AML1-ETO* fusion gene.[49] Chloromas are also commonly observed in patients with FAB M4 and M5 subtypes. Chloromas may occur in approximately 10% of patients with AML. Rarely, patients can present with a chloroma in the absence of detectable bone marrow or other systemic involvement.[50,51] The term *granulocytic sarcoma* is often used to refer to these aleukemic myeloid neoplasms. In nearly all such cases, the AML will become systemic if the patient is not treated with conventional AML therapy. The management of chloromas has been addressed in a report from the Children's Cancer Group (CCG) in which the event-free survival (EFS) and local recurrence rates were not found to be different for patients who received local irradiation to a chloroma along with systemic therapy compared with those who received only systemic therapy.[52] Thus, irradiation is reserved for situations in which a chloroma is not responding to intensive, combination therapy or when the chloroma runs the risk of causing significant morbidity, such as loss of vision or spinal cord compression.[52]

Tumor lysis syndrome (TLS) is a complication resulting from the rapid lysis of large numbers of tumor cells, releasing intracellular contents. Although TLS is seen most often after initial treatment with chemotherapy, it may also be present prior to the initiation of therapy due to spontaneous lysis. Risk factors include high WBC count, lymphadenopathy, hepatosplenomegaly, high mitotic index, and a diagnosis of ALL (especially Burkitt leukemia/lymphoma and T-cell ALL), although both spontaneous and treatment-associated TLS is a significant problem in AML as well. Tumor lysis syndrome is characterized by hyperuricemia, hyperkalemia, and hyperphosphatemia (with secondary hypocalcemia). Renal insufficiency may develop due to the nephrotoxic effects of precipitated urate crystals in the renal tubules; in severe cases, dialysis may be necessary. Management consists of aggressive hydration to reduce tubular uric acid concentration and alkalinization of urine to promote solubility of urate crystals. Frequent electrolyte monitoring with standard management of abnormal levels is essential. Allopurinol is a xanthine oxidase inhibitor routinely used at the outset of leukemia management to decrease the production of uric acid. Rasburicase (recombinant urate oxidase) is a new agent used in severe cases of TLS to rapidly convert uric acid to the more soluble allantoin.[53]

Differential Diagnosis

Although leukemia should be at least considered in cases of isolated neutropenia, anemia, or thrombocytopenia, the vast majority of leukemia patients present with depressions in more than 1 cell line. In suspected cases of immune thrombocytopenic purpura (ITP), for example, a careful review of the peripheral blood smear should be performed to rule out the presence of circulating leukemic blasts. Bone marrow aspiration should be reserved for cases with features atypical for ITP, such as concomitant anemia or neutropenia, hepatosplenomegaly, bone pain, or significant weight loss.

Pancytopenia or multiple cytopenias can be caused by diseases other than leukemia. Some viral infections have a propensity to suppress bone marrow function and cause low counts, including Epstein-Barr virus (EBV), herpes simplex virus, human herpes virus 6, influenza, hepatitis viruses, and human immunodeficiency virus.[54-56] Infectious mononucleosis from EBV infection can be particularly difficult to differentiate from leukemia, because patients will often have hepatosplenomegaly and circulating atypical lymphocytes (which can appear very similar to leukemic blasts). Pancytopenia on the basis of bone

Table 13-3	
Clinical features of hyperleukocytosis in AML.	
Organ System	**Clinical Manifestation(s)**
CNS	Decreased level of consciousness, stroke, intracranial bleeding
Respiratory	Hypoxia, respiratory distress, diffuse infiltrates
Renal	Renal insufficiency (multifactorial, exacerbated by renal infiltration, tumor lysis syndrome)

marrow failure (from acquired aplastic anemia or rare inherited bone marrow failure syndromes) can be distinguished from leukemia by bone marrow biopsy for assessment of overall marrow cellularity. Certain solid tumors have a tendency to metastasize to the bone marrow and cause cytopenias, including neuroblastoma, rhabdomyosarcoma, and retinoblastoma, but it is rare for the pancytopenia to be the presenting feature in these cases.[57] Joint pain, fever, hepatosplenomegaly, and pallor are common presenting features in both systemic onset juvenile rheumatoid arthritis (JRA) and leukemia. A bone marrow aspirate should be performed to rule out leukemia prior to treatment with steroids in suspected cases of systemic-onset JRA.[58]

Diagnosis and Classification

The diagnosis of AML is typically made by examination of the bone marrow. Morphologic evaluation is performed by standard light microscopy of bone marrow aspirate smears stained with Wright-Giemsa or similar stains. In addition, several histochemical stains (such as myeloperoxidase, PAS, Sudan Black B, and esterase) may be used to help distinguish myeloid versus lymphoid lineage and, within the myeloid lineage, whether there is any evidence of specific myeloid lineage differentiation. This histochemical evaluation has largely been replaced by flow cytometric assessment of surface antigen expression, which has proven a more definitive approach to classifying leukemia. Acute myeloid leukemia was initially defined by evidence for the replacement of at least 30% of the cellularity of the bone marrow with myeloblasts. Increasingly important adjuncts to the diagnosis of AML include various assays to detect cytogenetic and molecular abnormalities with diagnostic, prognostic, or therapeutic significance.

The first comprehensive classification system for AML was developed by the French-American-British (FAB) Cooperative Group and was first published in 1976 and revised in 1985.[59,60] This system classifies AML into 10 major subtypes based primarily on morphology and immunohistochemical and/or immunophenotypic detection of lineage markers (Table 13-4).

Table 13-4

French-American-British (FAB) classification of AML.

	AML Subtype	Comments
M0	AML without differentiation	Difficult to distinguish from ALL; diagnosis requires expression of surface markers such as CD13, CD33, and CD117 (c-kit) in the absence of lymphoid differentiation
M1	AML with minimal differentiation	Myeloperoxidase detectable by special stains/flow cytometry
M2	AML with differentiation	Auer rods; common t(8;21) -> *AML1–ETO* fusion, good prognosis, chloromas
M3	Acute promyelocytic leukemia (APL), hypergranular type	Auer rods; DIC/bleeding; t(15;17) -> *PML-RARα* fusion, good prognosis with ATRA therapy
M3v	APL, microgranular variant	Cytoplasm of promyelocytes demonstrates a fine granularity, and nuclei are often folded. Same clinical, cytogenetic, and therapeutic implications as FAB M3.
M4	Acute myelomonocytic leukemia (AMML)	Mixture of myeloblasts (at least 20%) and monocytic blasts; often with peripheral monocytosis
M4Eo	AMML with eosinophilia	AMML with >5% abnormal eosinophil precursors in marrow (with basophilic granules), common inv(16), good prognosis
M5	Acute monocytic leukemia	>80% of bone marrow nonerythroid cells are monocytic; M5a: monoblastic; M5b: monocytic (more differentiated); for both M4 and M5: infant age, *MLL* 11q23 rearrangements, CNS involvement, chloromas, gingival hyperplasia
M6	Acute erythroblastic leukemia	Rare in children
M7	Acute megakaryoblastic leukemia	Seen mostly in children with Down syndrome (good prognosis if ≤2 years old; *GATA1* mutations) or mosaicism for trisomy 21; rare in normal children (poor prognosis, t(1;22) -> *OTT-MAL* fusion, often infants); myelofibrosis common

In 2000, the European Association of Pathologists and the Society for Hematopathology published the first report describing the World Health Organization (WHO) classification of hematologic malignancies.[61] The WHO classification, summarized in Table 13-5, differs from the FAB classification in that it incorporates clinical, morphologic, immunophenotypic, cytogenetic, and molecular data. Another difference is that the threshold for the diagnosis of AML is reduced from 30% to 20% blasts in the blood or marrow. In addition, patients with the clonal, recurring cytogenetic abnormalities t(8;21)(q22;q22), inv(16)(p13q22) or t(16;16) (p13;q22), and t(15;17)(q22;q12) are considered to have AML regardless of the blast percentage.

The use of monoclonal antibodies to determine cell surface antigen expression of AML cells serves in virtually all cases to reinforce the histologic diagnosis and in some cases is absolutely essential to making the correct diagnosis (eg, in cases of minimally differentiated AML and certain cases of megakaryoblastic leukemia).[62] Various monoclonal antibodies that detect lineage-related antigens on AML cells should be used at the time of initial diagnostic workup, along with a battery of lineage-specific T-lymphocyte and B-lymphocyte markers to help distinguish AML from ALL and bilineal or biphenotypic leukemias. The expression of various proteins, termed cluster designations (CD), that are relatively lineage specific for AML include CD33, CD13, CD14, CDw41 (or platelet antiglycoprotein IIb/IIIa), CD15, CD11B, CD36, and CD235a (glycophorin A). Lineage-associated B-lymphocytic antigens CD10, CD19, CD20, CD22, and CD24 may be present in 10% to 20% of AML, but monoclonal surface immunoglobulin and cytoplasmic immunoglobulin heavy chains are usually absent; similarly, the T-lymphocyte associated antigens CD2, CD3, CD5, and CD7 are present in 20% to 40% of AML. Although the aberrant expression of lymphoid-associated antigens by AML cells is relatively common, it has not been shown to have prognostic significance.[63,64]

Table 13-5

World Health Organization (WHO) classification of AML.

I. Acute myeloid leukemia with recurrent genetic abnormalities
- Acute myeloid leukemia with t(8;21)(q22;q22), (*AML1-ETO*)
- Acute myeloid leukemia with abnormal bone marrow eosinophils and inv(16)(p13q22) or t(16;16)(p13;q22), (*CBFβ-MYH11*)
- Acute promyelocytic leukemia with t(15;17)(q22;q12), (*PML-RARα*), and variants
- Acute myeloid leukemia with 11q23 (*MLL*) abnormalities

II. Acute myeloid leukemia with multilineage dysplasia
- Following MDS or MDS/MPD
- Without antecedent MDS or MDS/MPD, but with dysplasia in at least 50% of cells in 2 or more myeloid lineages

III. Acute myeloid leukemia and myelodysplastic syndromes, therapy related
- Alkylating agent/radiation-related type
- Topoisomerase II inhibitor-related type (some may be lymphoid)
- Others

IV. Acute myeloid leukemia of ambiguous lineage
- Acute undifferentiated leukemia
- Acute biphenotypic leukemia (one population of leukemic blasts that co-expresses myeloid and lymphoid antigens)
- Acute bilineal leukemia (two distinct populations of leukemic blasts of different lineages)

V. Acute myeloid leukemia, not otherwise categorized
- Acute myeloid leukemia, minimally differentiated (FAB M0)
- Acute myeloid leukemia without maturation (FAB M1)
- Acute myeloid leukemia with maturation (FAB M2)
- Acute myelomonocytic leukemia (FAB M4)
- Acute monoblastic/acute monocytic leukemia (FAB M5)
- Acute erythroid leukemia (erythroid/myeloid and pure erythroleukemia) (FAB M6)
- Acute megakaryoblastic leukemia (FAB M7)
- Acute basophilic leukemia
- Acute panmyelosis with myelofibrosis
- Myeloid sarcoma

Immunophenotyping can also be helpful in distinguishing some FAB subtypes of AML. Testing for the presence of HLA-DR can be helpful in identifying APL. Overall, HLA-DR is expressed on 75% to 80% of AML but rarely expressed or expressed very low levels in APL or sometimes at low levels. In addition, APL cases with *PML-RARα* were noted to express CD33/CD15 and demonstrate a heterogeneous pattern of CD13 expression.[65] Testing for the presence of glycoprotein Ib, glycoprotein IIb/IIIa, or factor VIII antigen expression is helpful in making the diagnosis of M7 (megakaryocytic leukemia). Glycophorin expression is helpful in making the diagnosis of M6 AML (erythroleukemia).

Chromosomal analyses should be performed on children with AML because they are important diagnostic and prognostic markers.[66,67] Clonal chromosomal abnormalities have been identified in the leukemic blasts of about 75% of children with AML and are useful in defining subtypes with particular characteristics (eg, t(8;21) with M2, t(15;17) with M3, inv(16) with M4Eo, 11q23 abnormalities with M4 and M5, t(1;22) with M7). Leukemias with the chromosomal abnormalities t(8;21) and inv(16) are called core-binding factor leukemias; core-binding factor (a transcription factor involved in hematopoietic stem cell [HSC] differentiation) is disrupted by each of these chromosomal abnormalities. Molecular probes and cytogenetic techniques such as fluorescence in situ hybridization can detect cryptic abnormalities that were not evident by standard cytogenetic banding studies.[68] This is clinically important when optimal therapy differs, as in APL. Use of these techniques can identify cases of APL when the diagnosis is suspected, but the t(15;17) is not identified by routine cytogenetic evaluation.[69]

Cellular Pathogenesis

Perturbations in 4 fundamental cellular processes constitute the functional hallmarks of leukemia cells (and cancer cells, generally): enhanced proliferative capacity, impaired differentiation, impaired apoptosis, and enhanced metastatic/infiltrative potential.

The clonal nature of leukemia has been well established. Traditional descriptions of leukemogenesis have involved transformation of an immature hematopoietic precursor (at a stage of maturation that correlated with the morphology of the disease at diagnosis) followed by uncontrolled proliferation of a clone of leukemia cells that are identical to each other functionally. In this model, the goal of antileukemic therapy is simply to eradicate every leukemia cell in a patient's body by exposing the patient to an effective therapeutic regimen at a sufficient dose and over a sufficient duration to achieve this goal. More recent research has called this traditional understanding of leukemogenesis into question, and it has become clear that there is a remarkable similarity between leukemogenesis and normal hematopoiesis. Normal hematopoiesis is characterized by a hierarchical progression of a single HSC with unlimited self-renewal capacity and minimal differentiation to a tremendous number of mature blood cells with no self-renewal capacity and full functional differentiation. It is now clear that myeloid leukemogenesis is similarly hierarchical, with a "leukemic stem cell" (LSC) with unlimited self-renewal and minimal differentiation giving rise, through various stages of precursors, to the bulk leukemia cells, which do not have self-renewal capacity and a variable degree of myeloid differentiation.[70] This model has clear implications for antileukemic therapy, because according to the model, eradication of the LSC would seem to be the most relevant goal of therapy. Because antileukemic therapies have traditionally been selected for development based on response criteria reflective of an agent's effect on bulk leukemia cells, there has been little correlation between this initial assessment of "activity" and the ability to cure a patient of his or her disease. This suggests a differential between an antileukemic agent's efficacy against bulk leukemia cells and the LSC. Better understanding of the molecular bases of this differential, and of the differential features of the LSC and the normal HSC, is an area of intense research that has the potential to lead to improved outcomes for patients.

Genetic and Molecular Pathogenesis

Several lines of evidence suggest that childhood AML is a disease that results from an accumulation of 2 or more perturbations in the function of certain oncogenes. The most common recurrent cytogenetic abnormality in children and adults with AML is the t(8;21) translocation, which results in expression of the AML1–ETO fusion protein. Greaves et al examined DNA isolated from the archived neonatal screening blood spot cards (Guthrie cards) of children who developed t(8;21)/AML1–ETO AML up to 10 years later and found that the t(8;21)/AML1–ETO was detectable at birth in most of these children.[71] This study provided evidence that a significant proportion of childhood AML cases originate in utero, with the appearance of a myeloid precursor that becomes "preleukemic" as the result of a first, "permissive" mutation. Only later, sometimes years later, does one of these preleukemic precursors acquire the second, "promotional" mutation that results in a full-blown case of leukemia. A similar phenomenon has been demonstrated in children with ALL with the t(12;21)/TEL-AML1 and the t(4;11)/MLL-AF4 cytogenetic abnormalities, as well.[72,73]

A question naturally arose from these studies: Is every newborn with a detectable preleukemic genetic abnormality, such as t(8;21)/AML1–ETO, destined to develop leukemia? This question was answered in another study by Greaves, which examined an unselected group of cord blood samples and found evidence of a preleukemic fusion gene (t(12;21)/TEL-AML1 or t(8;21)/AML1–ETO) in approximately 1% of the samples.[74] Because the incidence of the corresponding leukemias in children is approximately 100-fold less than 1%, this established that the vast majority of newborns with detectable preleukemic abnormalities do not, in fact, go on to acquire the second mutation required for the development of overt leukemia.

Studies of leukemia concordance in identical (monozygotic) twins have provided further evidence in support of the prenatal origin of some types of childhood leukemia.[75]

Approximately 70 pairs of monozygotic twins with concordant leukemia have been recorded in the medical literature. Analysis of these cases reveals a striking relationship between the age that the first of the twin pair develops leukemia, and the nature of the risk of leukemia in the second twin. When the first twin is diagnosed with leukemia in infancy, the concordance rate approaches 100%, and the latency is typically very short (on the order of days or weeks). Nearly all of these cases have involved rearrangements in the *MLL* gene at 11q23, which is present in the majority of infant leukemia cases. In cases where detailed molecular testing was available, the common, clonal origin of the leukemia was confirmed by the presence of clonotypic breakpoints in the *MLL* gene in both cases. These data in infants suggest that the *MLL* rearrangement first arises in a hematopoietic precursor in one twin, which then expands and transfers to the co-twin via shared placental circulation; second, *MLL* rearrangements appear to be remarkably potent oncogenes and may not require an additional, promotional mutation or may be associated with the rapid development of additional mutations as mentioned earlier. When the first twin is diagnosed between the ages of 1 and 6 years, the concordance rate decreases to approximately 20%, and the latency is substantially longer (up to 8 years in one case). In several of these cases, the leukemic cells in both twins have been demonstrated to have arisen from a common clone (by sharing clonotypic breakpoints in the *TEL-AML1* fusion, for example). These data suggest that concordant leukemia in older twins is also the result of intrauterine transfer of cells arising from a common preleukemic precursor, but that at least one additional mutation, which in most cases does not occur in both twins, is needed for overt leukemia to develop. Finally, if the first twin develops leukemia after the age of 6, the risk of leukemia in the second twin is no greater than it is for a sibling or dizygotic twin, which is about double the risk of leukemia in a child with no leukemic relatives and which suggests that these cases of leukemia do not originate prenatally.

Various murine models are also supportive of the concept of multi-hit leukemogenesis for AML. Conditional knock-in[76] or targeted transgenic expression[77] of the *AML1–ETO* fusion gene in hematopoietic cells of mice does not, by itself, cause leukemia. When additional mutations are either randomly induced with mutagens[76] or specifically engineered as with retroviral infection of normal murine bone marrow with both *FLT3* internal tandem duplication (ITD) and *AML1–ETO* constructs, followed by marrow transplantation,[78] acute leukemia results. A model of myeloid leukemogenesis has emerged in which mutations that primarily cause impaired differentiation, such as *AML1–ETO* and *PML-RARα*, cooperate with mutations that confer a proliferative/survival advantage, such as *FLT3* or *RAS* mutations, to cause AML.[79]

The specific recurring cytogenetic and molecular abnormalities that have been associated with AML can be broadly classified as chimeric transcription factors, mutationally activated oncogenes, or other miscellaneous abnormalities. Because many of these abnormalities have been shown to impact on prognosis and risk stratification,

a detailed description of each abnormality is presented in the section on prognostic factors and risk stratification.

Prognostic Factors and Risk Stratification in Childhood Acute Myeloid Leukemia

The concept of "risk stratification" in the treatment of leukemia has gained widespread acceptance driven largely by the success of this approach in improving the overall outlook for children with ALL. The basic strategy in risk stratification is to treat patients who have a comparatively higher risk of relapse with more intensive, and potentially more toxic, therapies, and, conversely, to treat patients that have a lower risk of relapse with lower-intensity regimens that ideally will maintain the low risk of relapse while reducing the risk of toxicity. The classification of patients into higher or lower relapse risk groups is generally based on prognostic factors that were identified initially by retrospective analysis and then verified by prospective analysis, in the context of prior clinical trials. Because many of these factors are interdependent, it is important for each to be evaluated in multivariate analyses, which allow adjustment for other established prognostic factors in determining the independent contribution of the novel putative prognostic factor. The specific prognostic factors that have proven more or less useful in defining risk groups vary among leukemia subtypes, among age groups within a given subtype, and among different treatment regimens given to similar groups of patients. Therefore, it is important to evaluate each prognostic factor in a specific and well-defined context. Prognostic factors can be broadly categorized into host characteristics and disease characteristics.

Host Characteristics

Host factors, such as gender, age, race, and constitutional abnormalities have been associated with outcome in pediatric patients with AML. Females may do slightly better than males, although this association has not been strong enough to include in therapeutic stratification. Although some reports have described inferior outcomes for infants with AML, most current studies treat infants in a fashion similar to older children with equal or slightly better outcomes.[80,81] Racial variation may have a stronger influence on clinical outcome. Nonwhite patients appear to have a significantly worse outcome than Caucasians treated with identical chemotherapy regimens. In a recent study of nearly 1600 children treated on CCG-2891 and -2961, African American and Hispanic patients had an overall survival of approximately 35% compared with survival of 48% for the Caucasian patients.[82]

Constitutional trisomy 21 has been shown to impact the outcome of children with AML. Acute myeloid leukemia patients with DS, particularly those under age 4 years, appear to be extremely sensitive to the cytotoxic therapy, because they show increased toxicity as well as an improved outcome with less-intensive therapy with a remission rate of 90% and an overall survival of 80%. These patients are now treated with reduced intensity, alternative approaches.[83–85]

Variance from ideal body weight of AML patients at the time of diagnosis has recently been shown to impact clinical outcome. In CCG-2961, children with AML who were either underweight (≤10th percentile) or overweight (>95th percentile) at diagnosis had a nearly 2-fold higher risk of mortality. The increased mortality was due to excess treatment-related mortality (as opposed to excess relapse risk) in both underweight and overweight patients.[86]

Additional host factors are being studied that might influence response to therapy and/or toxicity in terms of pharmacologic metabolism of drugs. For example, inherited alterations in the detoxification enzyme, GST θ, that result in a null phenotype are associated with a significantly decreased survival due to excess toxicity.[87] This association of toxicity with GST genotype is likely associated with the specific drug combinations used in different AML therapy platforms.

Disease Characteristics

Characteristics of an individual case of AML that have been investigated as prognostic factors have included diagnostic WBC count, morphologic classification (FAB subtype), and biologic characteristics such as cytogenetics. With advances in molecular diagnostics and genomic and proteomic profiling, there has been a rapid increase in the number of disease markers that could potentially improve classification and prognostication, provide a deeper understanding of leukemogenesis, and lead to the development of novel therapies able to target aberrant molecular pathways selectively.

White Blood Cell Count and Morphology

Diagnostic WBC count has been demonstrated to be a prognostic factor in AML. A WBC count of less than 20,000 cells/μL has been associated with improved prognosis, and a WBC count of greater than 100,000 cells/μL has been linked to an unfavorable outcome.[88] Diagnostic WBC count has been shown to be a continuous variable for outcome because increasing the WBC count is associated with incremental decline in outcome. Such a continuous variable has thus far been difficult to incorporate into risk stratification strategies in AML, as many molecular events that mediate myeloid leukemogenesis lead to leukocytosis (ie, FLT3/ITD). Thus, identification of the underlying biologic mechanisms responsible for leukemic proliferation and survival characteristics leading to a leukocytosis should provide more definitive means for assessing risk of treatment failure.

Historically, AML has been classified based on morphologic appearance using the FAB classification. Due to the subjective nature of such classification and lack of uniformity or correlation with underlying biology, WHO recently developed a system for comprehensive AML classification based on cytogenetics, disease biology, and clinical history (Table 13-5). Scrutiny of the FAB subtypes (eg, FAB M6 and M7) that have traditionally been associated with poor outcome has revealed that high-risk cytogenetics are significantly over-represented in those with FAB M6/M7, and that

prognostic significance of these subtypes may be due to the predominance of cytogenetics groups associated with poor outcomes. The WHO classification schema for AML relies mainly on recurrent cytogenetic alterations and clinical history.[61]

Cytogenetic and Molecular Abnormalities

The specific recurring cytogenetic and molecular abnormalities that have been associated with AML can be broadly classified as chimeric transcription factors, mutationally activated oncogenes, or other miscellaneous abnormalities. Many have proven important in prognosis and risk stratification.

Chimeric Transcription Factors The chimeric transcription factors are generally produced as a result of chromosomal translocations that fuse a DNA-binding domain of a transcriptional activator to a transcriptional repressor. The transcriptional repressor is thereby redirected to target genes of the transcriptional activator, many of which have been shown to play important roles in myeloid differentiation. Functionally, this is thought to produce the block in differentiation that characterizes acute leukemia. The presence of one of these translocations in an individual case of AML may have significant prognostic and therapeutic implications.

Acute Myeloid Leukemia with t(8;21) and AML1–ETO Fusion In leukemic cells with t(8;21), the DNA-binding domain of the transcriptional activator AML1 (RUNX1, CBFA2) on chromosome 21q22 is fused with the transcriptional repressor ETO on chromosome 8q22. The t(8;21) translocation is associated with characteristic clinical, morphologic, and immunophenotypic features. Chloromas (extramedullary collections of leukemia cells, also known as granulocytic sarcoma) occur in approximately 20% of cases.[49,89] More than 80% of t(8;21) cases are classified as FAB type M2; conversely, of all cases classified as FAB M2, approximately 40% will be found to harbor t(8;21).[89] The immunophenotype of cases with t(8;21) often includes expression of the B-cell antigen CD19 and the natural killer cell antigen CD56.[90] In both adults and children, t(8;21) is associated with a favorable prognosis.[66,67,91,92] In adults, improved outcome for patients with t(8;21) was reported to be associated with dose intensity of cytarabine treatment.[93]

Acute Myeloid Leukemia with inv(16) or t(16;16) and CBFB-MYH11 Fusion In leukemic cells with inv(16) or t(16;16), the CBFB gene at chromosome band 16q22 is fused with the MYH11 gene at chromosome band 16p13. CBFB encodes the beta subunit of the core binding factor (CBF) transcriptional complex, which normally heterodimerizes with AML1 (or CBFA2, which encodes the alpha subunit of CBF). The fusion of CBFB with the multimerization domain of the myosin-heavy chain gene MYH11 results in decreased CBF transcriptional activity. The inv(16) and t(16;16) abnormalities are essentially pathognomonic for the FAB M4Eo subtype, and both confer a favorable prognosis for both adults and children with AML.[66,67,88,94]

Acute Myeloid Leukemia with (15;17) and PML-RARα fusion (and Variants)

Acute myeloid leukemia with t(15;17) is invariably associated with APML, a distinct subtype of AML that is treated differently than other types of AML because of its marked sensitivity to the differentiating effects of ATRA. The t(15;17) translocation leads to the production of a fusion protein involving the retinoid acid receptor alpha and PML. Other much less common translocations involving the retinoic acid receptor alpha (RARα) can also result in APML (eg, t(11;17) involving the PLZF gene).[95] Identification of cases with the t(11;17) translocation is important because of their decreased sensitivity to ATRA.

Acute Myeloid Leukemia with MLL Gene Rearrangements

Translocations of chromosomal band 11q23 involving the MLL gene, including most AML secondary to epipodophyllotoxin,[96] are associated with monocytic differentiation (FAB M4 and M5) and generally have an unfavorable prognosis. One exception to the poor prognostic significance of translocations at chromosome band 11q23 may be for children with t(9;11) in which the MLL gene is fused with the AF9 gene. In some reports, outcome has been relatively favorable for children whose leukemia cells have t(9;11),[94,97,98] although favorable outcome has not been observed in other series.[66] The t(10;11) translocation has been reported to define a group at particularly high risk of relapse in bone marrow and the CNS.[99] Some cases with the t(10;11) translocation have fusion of the MLL gene with the AF10 (MLLT10) gene on chromosome 10, with most of these cases having the FAB M5 subtype.[100] Acute myeloid leukemia with t(10;11) may also have fusion of the CALM gene on chromosome 11 with the AF10 gene.[101] Based on the limited number of cases reported, prognosis appears poor for cases with t(10;11) regardless of the type of gene fusion present.[102]

Acute Myeloid Leukemia with t(1;22) and OTT-MAL Fusion

The t(1;22)(p13;q13) translocation is restricted to acute megakaryoblastic leukemia (AMKL) and occurs in as many as one-third of AMKL cases in children. In leukemias with t(1;22), the OTT (RBM15) gene on chromosome 1 is fused to the MAL (MLK1) gene on chromosome 22.[103,104] Cases with detectable OTT/MAL fusion transcripts in the absence of t(1;22) have been reported as well. In the small number of children reported, the presence of the t(1;22) translocation appears to be associated with poor prognosis, although long-term survivors have been noted following intensive therapy.[105,106]

Mutationally Activated Oncogenes

Acute Myeloid Leukemia with FLT3 mutations

Internal tandem duplication mutations of FLT3 occur in approximately 25% of adults with AML and are associated with poor prognosis, particularly when both alleles are mutated or there is a high ratio of the mutant allele to the normal allele.[91,107,108] FLT3/ITD mutations occur with lower frequency (10%-15%) in childhood AML but have a similar negative prognostic impact.[109–113] Mutations in the kinase domain (KD) of FLT3 have also been identified in about 7% of adults and children with AML.[114–116] FLT3/KD mutations do not have the same negative prognostic significance as FLT3/ITD mutations.[109,117] FLT3 mutations occur in 30% to 40% of children and adults with APML, and FLT3/ITD mutations are strongly associated with the microgranular variant (M3v) and with hyperleukocytosis. It remains unclear whether FLT3 mutations are associated with poorer prognosis in patients with APL who are treated with modern therapy that includes ATRA.[111,118,119]

Acute Myeloid Leukemia with RAS or c-KIT mutations

RAS (N-RAS or K-RAS) mutations occur in approximately 20% and c-KIT mutations in approximately 5% of pediatric AML.[114,120] However, activating c-KIT mutations occur in 20% to 40% cases of AML with t(8;21) and inv(16), and patients with these mutations are associated with a relatively poor prognosis when compared with similar patients without c-KIT mutations.[121,122]

Acute Myeloid Leukemia with t(9;22) and BCR-ABL Fusion

The presence of the Philadelphia chromosome and/or BCR-ABL fusion in children with AML most likely represents chronic myelogenous leukemia (CML) that has transformed to AML rather than de novo AML.

Miscellaneous Abnormalities

Chromosomal abnormalities associated with poorer prognosis in adults with AML include those involving chromosome 7 (monosomy 7 and del(7q)), chromosome 5 (monosomy 5 and del(5q)), and the long arm of chromosome 3 (inv(3)(q21;q26) or t(3;3)(q21;q26)).[67] These cytogenetic subgroups are also associated with poor prognosis in children with AML, although abnormalities of the long arm of chromosome 3q and 5q are extremely rare in children with AML.[123]

GATA1

GATA1 mutations are present in most, if not all, DS children with either TMD or AMKL.[124–126] GATA1 mutations are not observed in non–DS children with AMKL nor in DS children with other types of leukemia.[9,125] GATA1 is a transcription factor that is required for normal development of erythroid cells, megakaryocytes, eosinophils, and mast cells. GATA1 mutations confer increased sensitivity to cytarabine, possibly by decreasing cytidine deaminase expression and thus providing an explanation for the superior outcome of children with DS and M7 AML when treated with cytarabine-containing regimens.[127]

CEBPA and NPM

Novel mutations in CEBPA and NPM genes that may have clinical implications have been identified in AML. The presence of CEBPA mutations, which modulate granulocytic differentiation and lead to maturational arrest, have been identified in nearly 10% of adult AML, and their expression has been associated with favorable outcome.[128] Prevalence of

CEBPA mutations in pediatric AML is somewhat lower, and their clinical significance in children has not been clearly defined.[129] Nucleophosmin (NPM), a nucleocytoplasmic shuttling protein with prominent nucleolar localization, regulates the ARF-p53 tumor-suppressor pathway.[130] Mutations in *NPM* that lead to the abnormal cytoplasmic localization of the affected protein have been reported in 30% to 50% of adult AML[131] and correlate with favorable outcome in patients with normal karyotype without *FLT3/ITD*.[132–134] Brown et al examined *NPM* mutations in 295 children with newly diagnosed AML treated on a large cooperative group clinical trial (Pediatric Oncology Group study POG-9421), finding that *NPM* mutations are relatively rare in childhood AML (incidence of 8%), particularly in younger children (no mutations in 71 children under 3 years old).[135] There was a trend toward a favorable impact of *NPM* mutations on survival in children lacking *FLT3/ITD*, which was similar in magnitude to the favorable impact of t(8;21) and inv(16). Thus, *NPM* mutations do not appear to completely abrogate the negative prognostic influence of *FLT3/ITD* mutations but may contribute to risk stratification in children who lack *FLT3/ITD* mutations by identifying a group with superior prognosis.

Gene Expression

In addition to function-altering mutations, regulation of expression level of various transcription factors may have biologic and prognostic significance. Expression level of the Wilms tumor gene (*WT1*) has been implicated in pathogenesis and prognosis in AML. Although *WT1* expression level at the time of diagnosis has been correlated with clinical outcome,[136] such findings have not been uniformly observed. However, it has been demonstrated that patients with high *WT1* expression level at the end of induction have a worse clinical outcome, suggesting the use of *WT1* expression as a useful marker of minimal residual disease (MRD) at the time of clinical remission.[137] Telomerase activity has been implicated in leukemogenesis, and there are data to suggest that telomerase activity may have prognostic significance in pediatric AML.[138] *BAALC* (brain and acute leukemia, cytoplasmic) is a gene whose elevated expression has been recently associated with adverse outcome in adults with AML.[139] *AF1q*, an *MLL* fusion partner whose expression regulates hematopoietic differentiation, is differentially expressed in AML; high expression of *AF1q* has been shown to be associated with undifferentiated phenotype and worse outcome.[140] Vasoactive endothelial growth factor (VEGF) ligand expression has been shown to be elevated in leukemias, and early data suggest that high VEGF ligand expression (and subsequent autocrine/paracrine stimulation) may be associated with poor outcome.[141] Substantiation of all novel prognostic markers should be done in multicenter trials with sufficient numbers of patients to achieve proper statistically powered endpoints, preferably analyzed prospectively prior to their use in therapeutic planning and stratification. In addition, there is a growing need for evaluation of all putative prognostic markers in the same patient population in order to delineate overlap and possible interaction among prognostic factors as well as with the type of treatment used.

New technologies allowing determination of gene and protein expression profiles have opened up an important era in refining diagnostic subtyping of AML, identification of new prognostic factors, and drug development. DNA microarray analysis has allowed disease classification based on gene expression profiling. Genomic classification of relapse risk is being applied to pediatric AML, and early data are encouraging. Lacayo et al used DNA microarray technology to evaluate relapse risk in a cohort of patients with pediatric AML with *FLT3* mutations.[142] They determined an expression profile that identified patients with *FLT3* mutations and were further able to separate into high-risk and low-risk subpopulations among the patients with *FLT3* mutations. Furthermore, they were able to validate their microarray findings using quantitative reverse transcriptase–polymerase chain reaction (RT-PCR), where they assigned relapse risk using the expression level of 2 genes previously identified by microarray profiling. Yagi et al used gene expression profiling to evaluate diagnostic marrow specimens from 54 pediatric patients with AML.[143] They identified 35 genes whose expression pattern correlated with clinical outcome. More recent studies in adult AML used microarrays to identify specific expression profiles that correlated with disease response and clinical outcome.[144,145] Such studies have demonstrated that the clustering was primarily driven by the presence of chromosomal alterations. This finding highlights the significant impact of the underlying cytogenetic characteristics of the leukemia and its profound prognostic significance. Larger studies using gene expression profiling for prognostic determination from pediatric cooperative group studies are required to establish the role of genomic profiling in risk identification in pediatric AML as well as in the identification of therapeutic targets. Similarly, genomic and epigenomic analyses along with proteomic profiling may play increasingly important roles in prognostication and therapeutic target identification.

Multidrug Resistance Superfamily Expression

Therapeutic resistance is a major obstacle in the treatment of AML. Such resistance has been associated with rapid drug efflux mediated by the multidrug resistance gene 1 (*MDR1*) encoding P-glycoprotein (PgP) as well as expression of other proteins conferring multidrug resistance such as *MRP1* (multidrug resistance–associated protein 1) and lung resistance protein. It would be expected that expression level of genes that mediate drug resistance may correlate with response to chemotherapy and clinical outcome. Evaluation of *MDR* gene expression in pediatric patients has failed to demonstrate prognostic significance. Sievers et al demonstrated a prevalence of 13% for the expression of PgP in a group of 130 pediatric AML patients treated on CCG-2891.[146] However, the clinical outcome of those with or without PgP expression was not different. Additional pediatric studies have demonstrated that *MDR1* expression is not higher overall in patients with relapsed AML.[147] Although MDR expression may not be an independent prognostic factor, it may be a useful therapeutic target in the management of AML. Several agents have been shown to impair the function of proteins encoded by *MDR* genes, which may potentially sensitize cells to the therapeutic effects of the specific chemotherapy agents.[148]

Response to Therapy

Response to therapy has been an important predictor of clinical outcome in leukemias. Historically, response to therapy has been measured by morphologic presence of disease at defined periods after start of induction therapy. In addition, the presence of disease below the level of morphologic detection has been evaluated.

Primary Induction Failure

Studies evaluating the morphologic presence of disease at end induction has shown that such patients have a dismal outcome even if they are reinduced into remission. The Medical Research Council (MRC) studies methodically evaluated the role of response to therapy as a part of the MRC 10 AML trials, where they demonstrated that patients with >15% marrow blast prior to the start of a second induction course had a significantly worse outcome than those with <15% disease.[81,149] They established this clinical cutoff by demonstrating that patients with partial remission (5%-15% blast) at the end of induction had a survival rather similar to those with <5% blast, whereas the survival for those with greater than 15% to 20% blast was poor and mirrored the outcome for those with >20% marrow blast. Based on these findings, the MRC used the threshold of 15% morphologically evident disease to define refractory disease. Many clinical trials, including Children's Oncology Group (COG) pediatric AML trials, are now using the threshold of 15% to define primary induction failure (PIF). Patients with AML and PIF have an extraordinarily poor prognosis, and current COG approaches are studying unrelated donor stem cell transplantation in this very high risk group.

Minimal Residual Disease

Because morphologic disease response has been shown to be such a powerful prognostic factor, the role of disease persistence below the detection at the morphologic level (MRD) has also been evaluated as a prognostic factor in AML. More than 80% of pediatric patients with AML who undergo induction therapy achieve a complete remission as assessed by morphologic evaluation of the marrow at the end of induction therapy. However, nearly half of these patients are destined for relapse and poor outcome. Identification of occult disease in patients in morphologic remission may identify patients at high risk of impending relapse. Appropriate intervention in this group of patients could potentially prevent morphologic relapse and be more effective. Despite its potential in risk management in AML, the clinical utility of MRD, which represents an in vivo measure of response to therapy, is related to several factors. First, MRD should have general applicability and be able to identify a significant proportion of patients at

risk of relapse. Second, there should be adequate time from detection of MRD to morphologic relapse to allow for intervention. And most important, therapy of MRD should lead to improved outcome; otherwise, detection of MRD would be clinically meaningless.

The majority of data on detection of MRD in AML has been generated using PCR-based methods where detection of unique fusion genes has been correlated with morphologic relapse.[150,151] The only AML subtype where MRD has been conclusively demonstrated to be of clinical utility is APML characterized by the t(15;17) fusion product *PML-RARα*. In APML, detection of persistent t(15;17) fusion product is significantly associated with a high risk of relapse, and early therapeutic intervention, prior to morphologic relapse, has been shown to improve outcome.[152,153] In contrast, the t(8;21) translocation-generated fusion product not only may be present in the general population but can remain positive by PCR for many years in patients with AML in morphologic remission.[154,155] However, Weisser et al have reported that an increasing, quantitative RT-PCR detection of t(8;21) transcripts can effectively predict relapse.[156] Thus, mere detection of an abnormal transcript at a single time point may not always be clinically meaningful. The question of whether therapeutic intervention in the context of molecular MRD in CBF leukemias improves clinical outcome needs to be addressed.

Leukemic blasts usually express aberrant surface antigen patterns that differ from the pattern observed in normal progenitors. This difference has been exploited to develop flow cytometric–based MRD assays where the presence of one cell with leukemic immunophenotype can be detected in 1000 to 10 000 normal nucleated cells. The advantage of flow cytometry over PCR-based technology is that it is applicable to most patients with AML. Recent studies have evaluated the utility of multidimensional flow cytometry to detect disease presence in patients in morphologic remission and correlated the presence of MRD to clinical outcome. In evaluation of 126 adult AML patients in clinical remission, San Miguel et al used flow cytometry to determine the presence of MRD.[157] They demonstrated that patients with occult disease detected by flow cytometry had a significantly greater risk of relapse than patients without measurable MRD. In a CCG study of 252 pediatric patients with AML in morphologic remission, Sievers et al established flow cytometric detection of MRD as a viable means of identifying patients at high risk of relapse.[158] Approximately 16% of the patients in complete remission were identified as having occult disease by flow cytometry. These patients had a 5-fold higher risk of relapse than the MRD-negative patients with relapse-free survival from remission of 35% compared with 65% for the MRD-negative patients. In a multivariate analysis, flow cytometric detection of MRD showed the strongest correlation with relapse-free survival. This study thus demonstrated that flow cytometry can be utilized to screen for clinically relevant, occult disease in pediatric AML. This study also showed that the median time to relapse for the MRD-positive population was 173 days, more than adequate for intervention. In contrast, a Berlin-Frankfurt-Munster (BFM) cooperative group report has shown that MRD detection did not provide additional, prognostic information than that of more traditional risk factors, although there were relatively small numbers of patients analyzed, a significant percentage of patients who did not have samples analyzed, and the inclusion of morphologically evident disease in the analysis.[159] The question of how to manage such MRD-positive patients optimally, however, has not been resolved. There are currently no data to suggest whether intervention in MRD-positive patients would alter their overall clinical outcome.

Therapy

Newly Diagnosed Acute Myeloid Leukemia

Remission Induction

Initial success inducing remission in patients with AML involved the use of a combination of cytarabine arabinoside (ARAC; 100 mg/m^2 by continuous infusion over 7 days) and an anthracycline (eg, daunomycin at 45 mg/m^2/day for 3 days). The continuous infusion approach with ARAC was based on its mechanism of action and incorporation into DNA during the S phase of the cell cycle. This "7 and 3" regimen achieved remission rates of approximately 60% to 70% and became a standard backbone for induction of remission.[160,161] Several important studies have tested different strategies for altering the standard induction chemotherapy backbone in an attempt to improve remission induction rates. These strategies can be broadly categorized as changes in ARAC dosing, duration, or schedule; use of alternative anthracyclines; timed sequential therapy; and use of other agents in addition to ARAC and anthracycline. Individual trials have frequently tested more than one of these strategies simultaneously. Improvements in supportive care, such as preemptive use of broad-spectrum antibiotics and the use of hematopoietic growth factors, have also been investigated as a strategy for improving induction outcomes.

Cytarabine Arabinoside Duration, Dosing, and/or Schedule
Several groups have studied increase duration and/or dose of ARAC in a nonrandomized fashion and noted improved complete remission (CR) rates compared with historical controls. The Cancer and Leukemia Group B 7921 study used a "10 and 3" schedule and noted improved CR rates compared with its experience with the "7 and 3" regimen.[162] The MRC AML 9 trial demonstrated that a "10 and 3" schedule of ARAC and daunorubicin with thioguanine resulted in improved remission rates of 91% compared with MRC AML 8, which used a "5 and 1" schedule.[163] The French studies, Leucemie Aigue Myeloblastique Enfant (LAME) 89 and 91, used 7 days of ARAC at 200 mg/m^2 per day by continuous infusion along with 5 days of mitoxantrone at 12 mg/m^2 per day with CR rates of 85% and 90%, respectively.[164] The Nordic Society for Pediatric Hematology and Oncology (NOPHO) AML 88 and 93 used ARAC at 200 mg/m^2 per day plus mitoxantrone and achieved CR rates of 83% and 92%, respectively.[94] However, in direct ran-

domized comparisons of different ARAC dosing regimens (ranging from 100 mg/m^2 per day as a continuous infusion for 7 days to 3000 mg/m^2 per day divided every 12 hours usually for 5 days), no significant differences have been observed in remission rates.[165–167] For example, POG 9421 compared remission rates for patients randomly assigned to receive ARAC at 100 mg/m^2 per day by continuous infusion or ARAC at 1 gm/m^2 per dose every 12 hours for 7 consecutive days along with the same schedule of daunorubicin and thioguanine.[168] The results showed no significant difference in remission rates (88% and 91%, respectively).

Use of Alternative Anthracyclines
The use of alternative anthracyclines or anthracenediones has not resulted in clear-cut improvements in outcome. The BFM AML 93 study randomized patients to idarubicin (IDA) versus daunorubicin in combination with ARAC and etoposide during induction. Although a more rapid clearing of leukemic blasts at day 15 of induction was noted in the IDA group, the 5-year EFS and disease-free survival (DFS) were similar in the two groups.[169] The CCG-2941 pilot trial attempted to deliver 2 consecutive cycles of IDA as part of the CCG-2891 DCTER/DCTER regimen (dexamethasone, cytarabine, thioguanine, etopside, and rubidomycin) but observed the combination with idarubicin to be too toxic; this led to the use of IDA/DCTER followed by DCTER/DCTER in the CCG-2961 study.[170,171] A metaanalysis of several randomized trials comparing IDA, mitoxantrone, and daunorubicin suggested that remission rates were highest with IDA, intermediate with mitoxantrone, and lowest with daunorubicin; however, no significant differences were observed in DFS.[172]

Timed Sequential Therapy
The LAME SP study attempted to improve remission induction rates further by using timed sequential therapy including ARAC 200 mg/m^2 per day on days 1 to 4 by continuous infusion along with mitoxantrone at 12 mg/m^2 per day on days 1 to 3, followed 8 to 14 days later with 3 days of the ARAC infusion and 2 days of mitoxantrone. The CR rate for 32 patients was 84% with 3% induction deaths, but with unacceptable delays in consolidation therapy, with neutrophil and platelet recovery times of 51 and 47 days, respectively, compared with previous studies with approximately 30-day recovery periods.[164] The CCG-2891 trial attempted to directly test the hypothesis that intensively timed or timed sequential chemotherapy would lead to improved remission rates and overall outcomes. This trial randomized standard timing (ie, the second cycle of chemotherapy given upon marrow recovery, which usually was at about day 30 after the first cycle) versus an intensively timed approach (ie, the second cycle given on days 10 to 13 following the first course of treatment regardless of the status of the bone marrow). In each arm, the 5-drug DCTER regimen was used for each cycle of treatment.[173,174] The CR rates for the intensive and standard timing arm were 78% and 74%, respectively (not significantly different).[173,174] Although this result seemed disappointing in terms of the lack of improvement in the

CR rates, the overall survival and EFS were significantly better for patients who received the intensively timed induction therapy.[173,174] This was true regardless of whether postremission therapy was chemotherapy, autologous HSCT, or allogeneic HSCT.[174,175] This result remains intriguing and strongly suggests that the quality of remission has an important impact on subsequent outcomes. Of interest, however, is that the more rapid response and lower level of leukemic burden observed with IDA compared with daunorubicin during induction on the BFM AML 93 trial did not translate into improved EFS.[169] Thus, the elements of remission induction therapy that are critical to achieving improved long-term outcome remain unclear.

Use of Other Agents in Addition to Cytarabine Arabinoside and Anthracyclines
The issue of adding additional agents to the basic "7 and 3" combination has not always been addressed in a systematic and randomized fashion. An exception was the MRC AML 10 trial, which randomized patients during induction to receive either thioguanine or etoposide along with daunorubicin and ARAC (DAT vs ADE regimens, respectively). The results showed no difference in remission rate (81% for DAT and 83% for ADE), although the toxicities were different, with ADE showing slightly higher deaths during induction and more nonhematologic toxicities, such as mucositis.[176] Postremission outcomes also did not differ, with survival at 6 years being 40% for both induction regimens. [176]

Supportive Care
In order to reduce treatment-related deaths during remission, supportive care interventions have also been tested. Several groups have examined whether hematopoietic cytokines, such as G-CSF, can reduce the length of neutropenia during induction and thereby decrease serious infections and improve overall outcomes.[177–179] The addition of G-CSF to the intensively timed arm of the CCG-2891 was reported to reduce fatal infections, leading to an improved CR rate of 82% compared with the 78% without the cytokine, but the lack of a prospective, randomized methodology prevented definitive conclusions.[180] The BFM AML 98 trial randomized newly diagnosed pediatric patients with AML to receive or to not receive G-CSF during the first two courses of therapy.[181,182] The duration of neutropenia after both courses of therapy was significantly reduced in the G-CSF group from 23 to 18 days after the first course of therapy and from 16 to 11 days after the second course of therapy, but there were no differences in relapse rates, EFS, incidence of secondary malignancies, or the incidence of episodes of febrile neutropenia, microbiologically documented infections, or infection-associated mortality.[182]

Summary and Future Directions
The past several decades have led to significant advances in the ability to achieve remission in patients with newly diagnosed AML. The approaches have involved primarily intensively dosed or timed multiagent chemotherapeutic agents along with aggressive, preemptive supportive care measures. Despite these advances, 10% to 20% of patients are still not able to achieve remission. Improved remission induction regimens are needed, and improvements are likely to come from novel agents that provide increased antileukemic effects without adding significant toxicity to current regimens. Furthermore, the fact that higher induction remission rates do not necessarily translate into improved cure rates emphasizes that postremission treatment is essential to cure patients effectively.

Postremission Therapy

Is there a role for extended-duration, low-intensity maintenance therapy?
In part based on treatment approaches in ALL, many early AML trials employed the use of relatively low-dose maintenance therapy. The CCG-213 trial randomized patients after a 4-month postremission intensification to receive either 2 years of maintenance therapy with the PATCO regimen (prednisolone, ARAC, 6-thioguanine, cyclophosphamide, and vincristine) or no further therapy.[183] An improved 5-year survival of 68% was observed in the intensification-only arm versus 44% in the maintenance arm, demonstrating that in the setting of postremission intensification, there is no benefit of maintenance therapy.[175,183] In a similar study design, the LAME 91 trial randomized patients after postremission intensification to receive either an 18-month maintenance regimen (daily 6-mercaptopurine and monthly 4-day pulses of subcutaneous ARAC) or no maintenance. Again, the DFS was superior in patients who did not receive maintenance therapy (62% vs 51%). Most groups now omit maintenance therapy.[164,184] An exception is the BFM group. Based on the results of the BFM-87 trial, in which a maintenance phase was beneficial to a low-risk group of patients not receiving HSCT, BFM studies continue to use maintenance chemotherapy.[185] Thus, most studies support the conclusion that maintenance therapy does not lead to improved outcomes in patients with AML if dose and/or timing intensification of induction and several courses of postremission treatment are given. In addition, there is some evidence that relapsing after maintenance phase therapy may result in more resistant disease and therefore less chance of cure. However, as more targeted approaches to treatment become available, the role of maintenance therapy may need to be readdressed. How many postremission courses of therapy are needed also remains an important question.

What is the optimal number of postremission treatment courses?
There is little information to definitively answer this question, which, in light of the significant morbidity and mortality associated with each course of intensive therapy, is more than just an academic query. The CCG-2961 study gave patients a total of 3 courses of intensive chemotherapy with comparable results to other trials, suggesting that more courses may not be necessary. For example, out of 901 enrolled patients under the age of 21 years, the 5-year EFS was

$42 \pm 3\%$ and overall survival $52 \pm 4\%$.[170] The MRC AML 12 study directly asked whether a total of 4 compared with 5 total courses of therapy is preferable. Preliminary results from this study suggest no difference between 4 and 5 courses, with an overall survival of 81% for 4 courses compared with 78% for 5 courses ($p = 0.5$).[163] Of note, there was also no difference in the percentage of deaths in CR for the 4 versus 5 courses. Although these results might suggest that 4 courses of MRC 12 therapy is better than 3 courses of CCG-2961 therapy, it is impossible to definitively compare the two studies and study populations at this time, although with similar follow-up, this comparison would potentially be informative. The current COG trial for patients with newly diagnosed AML uses 5 courses of MRC AML 12–like therapy and should help to determine whether similar results are obtained in the United States population. Unfortunately, no trial has directly compared 3 courses versus 4 courses of therapy in a prospective fashion in children and adolescents. However, with survival rates being 50% or less overall and worse in the very high risk groups of patients, testing whether 3 courses versus 4 courses of therapy is better might need to be done only for patients with favorable-risk AML, in which survival rates are above 70% and the ability to salvage patients following relapse is excellent.

Which patients should receive a hematopoietic stem cell transplant in first remission?
As chemotherapy regimens have improved the outcome for pediatric patients with AML, the role for HSCT has become more restricted. A key to the evolution of the role of HSCT has been subgroup analysis of patients in different risk groups.[186]

Autologous Hematopoietic Stem Cell Transplantation
Several randomized studies have compared autologous HSCT with chemotherapy and have not shown an overall survival advantage for transplantation.[174,187] Such results have been used to suggest that chemotherapy is preferable to autologous HSCT. However, the MRC AML 10 study showed a significantly improved DFS and lower relapse rate in patients who received an autologous HSCT compared with those receiving no further treatment.[176] The overall survival rates were not significantly different, however, due to the increased ability to salvage with second-line treatment patients who had not received autologous HSCT. With equivalency of overall outcome between autologous HSCT and chemotherapy, one might also conclude that either approach would be a reasonable, evidence-based recommendation.[186] For example, receiving an autologous HSCT after induction and consolidation may be preferable to receiving 4 or more courses of severely myelosuppressive therapy with chemotherapy. A cost-benefit analysis, including quality-of-life issues, has not been done comparing these two modalities. In addition, there has not been a detailed subgroup analysis of outcome for patients receiving autologous HSCT versus chemotherapy.

Allogeneic Hematopoietic Stem Cell Transplantation
The majority of randomized clinical trials have shown a consistent advantage in terms of DFS for allogeneic HSCT compared with chemotherapy or autologous HSCT.[174,187–189] These data have strongly suggested that the ablative preparative regimen along with an allogeneic antileukemic effect play important roles in preventing leukemic relapse. However, in light of the potential for improved disease control as well as balancing treatment-related toxicities, the role of allogeneic HSCT in specific subgroups of patients needs to be carefully considered.[188–190]

The MRC AML trials have been particularly helpful in defining which subgroups of patients have or do not have an outcome advantage with allogeneic HSCT. In the MRC AML 10 trial, outcome was analyzed based on whether or not a donor was available. Of the 85 children with donors, 61 received HSCT, including 12 of 21 classified as good risk.[163] Although the relapse rate was significantly lower for those with a donor (30% versus 45%), there was no statistically significant difference in overall survival between those children with (68%) or without (59%) a donor ($p = 0.3$) at 10 years. Of note, survival at 5 years from the time of relapse was 57%, 14%, and 8% for good-, standard-, and poor-risk groups, respectively ($p = 0.0003$), leading the MRC and other groups to recommend that good-risk patients receive allogeneic HSCT only in the case of relapse. For patients in the standard- and poor-risk groups, these data suggest that receiving allogeneic HSCT in first remission may be advantageous. However, when data from MRC AML 10 and 12 studies were combined, allogeneic HSCT was not shown to provide a statistically significant survival advantage for any risk group.[163] These conclusions are similar to those obtained from recent BFM studies.[169]

Studies from cooperative groups in the United States have reported somewhat different data and conclusions. In both the POG 8821 and 9421 studies, allogeneic transplantation resulted in the best chance for cure, although detailed subgroup analyses have not been reported.[168,187,191] Analysis of postremission treatment of 1464 children less than age 21 years on five consecutive CCG trials from 1979 to 1996 has shown an advantage to those patients assigned an HSCT in terms of overall survival (OS) ($p = 0.026$), DFS ($p = 0.005$), and relapse rate ($p < 0.001$).[175,192] Analysis of subgroups demonstrated that HSCT was associated with improved survival for patients with WBC count greater than $50,000/\mu L$ and for those with normal karyotype but was not beneficial for patients with inv(16) or t(8;21). Data from the CCG-2961 trial showed no statistically significant advantage of HSCT donor availability in terms of OS or DFS in either the study group as a whole or in the subgroup of patients with inv(16) or t(8;21) chromosomal translocations.[170] A detailed analysis of the effect of donor availability on patients with standard- and poor-risk features has not been reported. Overall, these results appear to be consistent with those reported from the MRC AML trials.[163]

Information regarding outcomes with HSCT compared with chemotherapy alone in molecular subgroups of AML is emerging but remains inconclusive. For example, *FLT3/ITD* mutations, especially when present in a high ratio of mutant to normal alleles, have been associated with a very poor prognosis in adult and pediatric patients.[108–110] Data from BFM AML studies have shown that those with an *FLT3/ITD* to normal allelic ratio of >0.69 was associated with an extremely poor prognosis compared with those with a lower ratio, which in turn was not different from that in patients without an *FLT3/ITD* mutation.[110] A subsequent report from CCG AML trials 2941 and 2961 demonstrated that an *FLT3/ITD* to normal allelic ratio of ≥0.4 was associated with a significantly worse progression-free survival than those with a lower ratio.[109] There are some data that suggest that increased intensity of treatment, including allogeneic HSCT, may partially abrogate the poor prognosis of patients with AML characterized by a high *FLT3/ITD* to normal allelic ratio.[109,193–195] For instance, the data from the CCG-2941 and 2961 studies showed a borderline significant difference for the relapse rate for patients with *FLT3/ITD*-positive AML who received an allogeneic matched sibling donor HSCT (27% ± 27%) compared with those treated with only chemotherapy (65% ± 15%, $p = 0.05$). Overall survival at 4 years from the end of the second course of treatment was 64% ± 29% for those with *FLT3/ITD* AML who received an allogeneic HSCT compared with 48% ± 17% for those treated only with chemotherapy, but this was not significantly different ($p = 0.4$).[109] An analysis of 1135 young adult patients from the MRC AML 10 and 12 trials concluded that there was no strong evidence to consider *FLT3* status in deciding whether patients should receive an HCST.[196] This conclusion was based in part on the lack of statistically significant differences for DFS or OS in patients with *FLT3/ITD* AML who did or did not receive a transplant. Based on a donor versus no donor analysis, OS was not found to be significantly improved by having a donor in patients with *FLT3/ITD*-positive or -negative AML: thus, this report concluded that an allogeneic HSCT may not overcome the chemoresistance or radiation resistance inherent in *FLT3/ITD*-positive AML.

Most pediatric cooperative groups now recommend that patients with favorable-risk cytogenetics and good early responses to induction therapy receive allogeneic HSCT only in the case of relapse and after a second remission has been achieved. In MRC and BFM trials, HLA-matched or one antigen-mismatched family donor allogeneic HSCT is offered in first remission only for patients with high-risk cytogenetics or those patients not achieving remission after two courses of induction therapy. The current COG strategy, which uses an MRC-like backbone of chemotherapy, offers matched family donor HSCT to patients with standard- or high-risk features. The COG is also piloting the use of any form of donor (eg, HLA-matched or partially matched family donors, cord blood, matched unrelated, mismatched unrelated, or haploidentical) for patients with high-risk cytogenetic/molecular features (monosomy 7, 5q-, *FLT3/ITD* with high mutant-to-wild type allelic ratio) or with primary refractory disease. It remains unclear what the role of allogeneic HSCT is in this setting of highly refractory disease. Hematopoietic stem cell transplant is not recommended in first remission for patients with APL or patients

younger than 4 years with DS and megakaryoblastic leukemia because of the distinctive biology of these leukemias and their excellent outcomes with chemotherapy.

Is cranial prophylaxis necessary for patients with acute myeloid leukemia?
Morphologic subtypes of AML with the highest incidence of CNS involvement are FAB M4 and M5, especially in cases with very high peripheral leukemic blast counts.[197,198] The frequency of CNS involvement by AML at the time of diagnosis in children has been reported to be between 3% and 20%.[94,163,164,169,175,191] Contemporary studies have reported CNS relapse rates of approximately 2% to 8%, most of them combined with concomitant bone marrow relapse.[94,163,164,169,175,191] Trials in most cooperative groups have empirically included 3 to 10 lumbar punctures with intrathecal ARAC or methotrexate. The introduction of high-dose systemic ARAC, which has significant ability to penetrate the CNS and CSF, is also thought to contribute to the treatment and prophylaxis of CNS AML. The BFM group has taken a somewhat different approach to CNS prophylaxis. The BFM AML 87 study randomized children at diagnosis without CNS disease to receive either CNS radiation (1800 centigray) or no radiation. All patients with evidence of CNS disease at diagnosis and/or a presenting WBC count of >70,000/μl received radiation. For the CNS-negative patients, a significant decrease in the 5-year cumulative incidence of systemic relapse was seen in patients who received radiation (29% compared with 50% for those not irradiated, $p = 0.001$). However, the randomization was stopped before the conclusion of the trial, and when only randomized patients were included in the analysis, the difference in relapse risk was no longer significant.[169,199] These results suggest that the delivery of cranial radiation decreases the chance of later systemic relapse, but lack of a significant difference when only randomized patients were included as well as the similar systemic and/or CNS relapse rates to other contemporary studies indicates that cranial irradiation is not necessary in the context of modern therapy.

Treatment of Special Subtypes
Down Syndrome   Several reports from the 1980s and 1990s convincingly demonstrated that patients with DS and AML had a better outcome than patients without DS.[85,123,200–205] The intensity of treatment has also shown to be a factor in outcome. For example, the CCG-2891 trial randomized patients, including those with DS, to receive intensively timed or standard-timing induction treatment.[206] A 90% CR rate was observed for the standard-timing arm and an approximately 60% CR rate for the intensively timed induction. Quite significantly, the primary reason for this difference was treatment-related mortality of 32% for the intensively timed arm and only 3% for the standard timing. Of note, treatment-related mortality did not differ significantly between patients with DS and those without DS in subsequent courses of therapy, suggesting that children with DS did not have increased sensitivity to high-dose ARAC containing postinduction regimens. In addition, the postremission

DFS for children with DS who received an allogeneic HSCT was 33% compared with 89% for those treated with chemotherapy alone. Thus, the best outcome for patients with DS was achieved with standard-timing induction therapy and postinduction chemotherapy, which resulted in an 86% relapse-free survival. In contrast, children without DS who received standard timing had only a 38% relapse-free survival.[206] Age at diagnosis has emerged as a clear prognostic indicator for DS AML patients. Children older than 4 years (who account for less than 10% of DS AML patients) have a significantly worse prognosis, with 4-year EFS of only 28% being reported.[83,206] There is currently no optimized therapeutic strategy for these older children with DS, although recommendations are to include them on more dose-intensive clinical trials designed for children without DS. In the COG, children with DS and AML who are younger than 4 years are treated on a separate protocol that intensifies ARAC and decreases exposure to anthracycline.

As noted above, TMD is a self-limited condition that will usually resolve within weeks to months. However, infants with TMD can experience significant morbidity, and a significant number die from complications of the disorder, which can include hydrops fetalis, massive hepatomegaly, and hepatic fibrosis resulting in respiratory distress, hepatic failure or hepatorenal syndrome, and DIC. Hepatic fibrosis in TMD may be related to the expression of platelet-derived growth factor (PDGF) and TGF-β by infiltrating megakaryoblasts.[207] Initial therapy for these infants with TMD involves aggressive support care. However, with progression of the disease and associated signs and symptoms, interventions such as exchange transfusion or low-dose ARAC have proven to be effective.[206–208] The optimal treatment for patients who develop hepatic failure due to fibrosis is unclear, but the use of PDGF inhibitors is being considered for testing in clinical trials. Approximately 25% to 30% of infants who survive TMD will develop AML, so these patients need to be closely followed through their early childhood years, particularly up to age 3 years.

Acute Promyelocytic Leukemia

Acute promyelocytic leukemia is a distinct subtype of AML that is treated differently than other types of AML because of its marked sensitivity to "differentiating agents" such as ATRA and arsenic trioxide (ATO).[209] The t(15;17) translocation is present in the vast majority of APML cases and leads to the production of a fusion protein involving the RARα and PML. The PML/RARα fusion protein is believed to result in the repression of genes involved in promyelocytic differentiation. Upon binding PML/RARα, ATRA is thought to alter its ability to interact with chromatin remodeling complexes, inducing the expression of genes leading to both terminal differentiation and apoptosis of the leukemic promyelocytes. Other much less common translocations involving the retinoic acid receptor alpha can also result in APML (eg, t(11;17) involving the PLZF gene).[95] Identification of cases with the t(11;17) translocation is important because of their decreased sensitivity to ATRA.[95] An important prognostic factor in APML is WBC count at diagnosis. In most studies, a presenting WBC count of 10,000/μL or greater has been associated with high risk and significantly poorer outcome.[210] Of note, higher count in APML is closely associated with the microgranular morphologic variant, the presence of FLT3/ITD mutation, and bcr3 PML breakpoints.[211–213]

When administered as a single agent, ATRA results in a greater than 90% remission rate in patients with the t(15;17) translocation.[214] However, if no additional therapy is given, leukemic relapse usually occurs within approximately 3 months. Optimal treatment using combination ATRA and chemotherapy during induction followed by maintenance with ATRA and low-dose antimetabolite therapy with 6-mercaptopurine and methotrexate results in leukemia-free survival of between 70% and 80%.[214–217] The use of ATRA in combination with chemotherapy during induction therapy has the important advantage of preventing progressive leukocytosis, a complication that can predispose to induction deaths from hemorrhage. However, approximately 3% of patients, i.e., around half of induction failures, still die from hemorrhagic complications.[218] The use of ATRA in maintenance has also proven to result in superior outcomes, including improving overall survival and reducing relapses.[219,220] It is also important to consider the toxicities associated with ATRA. These significant toxicities include pseudotumor cerebri and the development of acute pulmonary edema. The latter toxicity is termed ATRA syndrome or "differentiation" syndrome, because it can also occur with other differentiating agents such as arsenic.[221] Early diagnosis of the ATRA syndrome should allow temporary cessation of ATRA and treatment with dexamethasone.[221]

Arsenic trioxide has produced excellent remission rates of approximately 80% to 85% when used in patients with relapsed APML.[222–225] Alternative approaches have included chemotherapy, usually including IDA plus ATRA, ATRA alone or in combination with arsenic or combinations of ATRA, and/or arsenic with anti-CD33/calicheamicin (Mylotarg) conjugated antibody.[226–229] The high percentage of responses in patients with relapsed APML to ATO has led to its introduction into treatment regimens for newly diagnosed patients. Preliminary results from the North American Intergroup Protocol C9710 showed that the addition of two courses of ATO significantly improved EFS and OS in adults with APML.[230] Event-free survival/overall survival at 3 years was 77%/86% for the arsenic group compared with 59%/77% for the no arsenic groups ($p = 0.0013/0.029$). In order to build on the excellent activity of ATO and to try to reduce the anthracycline exposure of young patients, the COG has proposed in its next planned trial to replace an anthracycline-based consolidation with an ATRA/ATO combination.

Hematopoietic stem cell transplantation for patients with APML is typically reserved for patients who relapse and achieve a second complete remission.[231] Furthermore, for patients with relapsed APML who achieve a second molecular remission, autologous HSCT has proven efficacious, with one study reporting 80% relapse-free survival,

60% OS, and 6% treatment-related mortality for autologous HSCT in adults.[232] In the same study, patients treated with allogeneic HSCT had similar survival, but with a 39% treatment-related mortality. In comparison, patients not receiving some type of HSCT had a relapse-free survival of 38% and an overall survival of 40%. Thus, if a patient achieves a second molecular remission and lacks a matched related donor, autologous HSCT appears to be a reasonable option. When a matched related donor is available, the choice is more difficult, with no definitive prospective data available to guide decision making. If a molecular remission cannot be obtained, then matched family or unrelated donor HSCT is a reasonable approach.

Congenital and Infant Acute Myeloid Leukemia

Congenital leukemia is defined by presentation within the first month of life; the presence of abnormally high numbers of immature myeloid, lymphoid, or erythroid cells; infiltration of clonal, immature hematopoietic cells into nonhematopoietic tissues; and the absence of other etiologies.[233] Approximately two-thirds of these patients will show signs of leukemia cutis, often mimicking the appearance of a "blueberry muffin," also seen in this age group with other metastatic small, blue, round malignancies, particularly neuroblastoma.[234] Central nervous system involvement is also more commonly observed in this age group, with an incidence of approximately 50%.[234] Marked hepatosplenomegaly and lymphadenopathy are common, WBC count is usually higher than observed in older children with AML, and there is a predominance of monocytic features.[233,234] A significant proportion of these patients have 11q23 chromosomal abnormalities.[163,233,234] Although spontaneous remissions and responses to exchange transfusion have been reported,[235] systemic AML-directed chemotherapy is nearly always required, but with OS rates that appear significantly worse than for older children.[96,233,236] For infants (patients older than 1 month and less than 1 year), comparable results to older children have been reported when treatment includes intensive, contemporary regimens.[163] The role of HSCT in this group of patients is controversial, underscoring the need for novel therapeutic approaches.

Treatment of Relapsed Acute Myeloid Leukemia

The expected outcome for patients with relapsed AML depends upon several factors, including the biology (particularly the cytogenetics) of the leukemia, previous therapy, time to relapse from first remission, host comorbidities, and the site of relapse.[237,238] For patients with inv(16) or t(8;21) on the MRC AML10 trial who relapsed, treatment with reinduction chemotherapy followed by allogeneic HSCT resulted in 5-year survival from relapse of 57%. By comparison, for patients in the standard- and poor-risk groups that relapsed, survival was only 14% and 8%, respectively.[163,239] Patients who relapse on therapy or within 6 months from diagnosis after obtaining an initial remission have been reported to have less than 20% survival at 5 years.[238,240,241] An analysis of NOPHO results from 1988 to 2003 showed that 2 critical prognostic factors were the duration of the first remission and whether a patient had a relapse after receiving HSCT.[242] For example, for patients having a less than 1-year remission, survival at 5 years was 21% compared with 48% for those with later relapses. Patients who relapsed after having received either an autologous or allogeneic HSCT had a less than 20% survival at 5 years compared with 41% for those who relapsed after having received only chemotherapy.[242]

Reinduction of a second remission provides an optimal pretransplant condition. A variety of reinduction regimens have been used successfully, including combination chemotherapy with some of the agents used during the patient's initial therapy. Such combinations include mitoxantrone and high-dose ARAC, fludarabine and high-dose ARAC plus G-CSF (FLAG), and IDA with FLAG (IDA-FLAG).[243–247] In addition, several trials have used immunotargeted agents, such as anti-CD33/calicheamicin (gemtuzumab ozogamicin), either alone or in combination with chemotherapy, with reasonable safety profiles and activity.[248] Newer agents, such as clofarabine in combination with high-dose ARAC or other agents, are also being tested to reduce the exposure of patients to further anthracycline exposure as well as introducing a novel agent.[249–251] Clinical trials using other novel agents are also under way, as discussed below.

The overall strategy for approaching the patient with relapsed AML is to evaluate the above characteristics, ideally enter the patient on a clinical trial for relapsed AML, and proceed to allogeneic HSCT with an ablative preparative regimen and the best donor available. A definitive role for nonablative, allogeneic HSCT for relapsed AML in pediatrics has not been established but may provide an approach to deliver an allogeneic antileukemic effect while reducing toxicity.[252] Patients who relapse again after HSCT have a nearly 100% mortality, although survival after a second HSCT has been occasionally reported.[253]

Therapeutics in Development

With current therapy, only about half of children with AML are expected to be long-term survivors despite receiving intensive postremission therapies that have been pushed to the limits of tolerable toxicity and are associated with significant rates of treatment-related morbidity and mortality. There are two interdependent and complementary areas of research that are most likely to lead to the development of more-effective and less-toxic therapies for AML. The first is the discovery and characterization of molecular alterations that are important in the pathogenesis of AML and that can be potentially targeted by novel therapeutics. The second is an improved understanding of the biology of the LSC, since eradication of the LSC (as opposed to mere reduction in the numbers of bulk leukemia cells) is emerging as a potentially relevant goal of AML therapy. In AML, the prototype of molecularly targeted therapy is APML characterized by t(15;17), in which a differentiation block induced by the PML-RARα fusion protein has been successfully targeted with ATRA. The addition of ATRA to chemotherapy has turned what was previously a poor-prognosis disease into one in which most cases are cured. In this case, the APML stem cell appears to be effectively eradicated by this approach. Interestingly, the APML stem cell appears to have distinct characteristics compared with the stem cell for other subtypes of AML in that it has the more differentiated phenotype of a committed myeloid precursor (as opposed to the primitive phenotype reminiscent of the normal HSC, which is characteristic of the other subtypes of AML).[254] This may in part explain the relative ease with which APML can be treated successfully in children and adults. The ability to move beyond standard cytogenetic approaches for the discovery and characterization of molecular alterations in AML, and the relationship of these alterations with the LSC, will hopefully pave the way for development of additional novel, targeted therapies that will improve the outcome for children with AML. This section will review recent efforts in this regard.

Targeted Immunotherapy

More than 3 decades have passed since the discovery of how to generate monoclonal antibodies. Several of these highly specific antibodies have been shown to be effective antileukemic agents. In AML, one of the primary targets has been CD33, a sialic acid–dependent cell adhesion molecule that is differentially expressed during myeloid differentiation.[255] Gemtuzumab ozogamicin (GO; Mylotarg™) is a humanized, IgG4 subtype, monoclonal antibody conjugated to calicheamicin and directed against CD33 that has demonstrated significant activity in AML.[256] Clinical trials in adults and children with AML have shown response rates to be approximately 30% to 35% when GO is used as a single agent for patients with relapsed or primary refractory disease.[248,256] In a pediatric Phase I/II trial, the response in children with primary refractory disease was the same as that for patients with relapsed disease who had achieved a prior remission, suggesting that some conventional resistance mechanisms can be circumvented with this agent.[248] The maximal tolerated dose for children was determined to be 6 mg/m², although two patients tolerated 7.5 mg/m² on the pediatric Phase I study. The main toxicity was myelosuppression. There was a 24% (7 of 29 patients) overall incidence of veno-occlusive disease (VOD) with 6 of 13 (40%) developing VOD during a subsequent HSCT. Veno-occlusive disease was most frequently observed in patients undergoing allogeneic SCT in less than 3.5 months from receiving GO. The COG recently completed 2 clinical trials that included GO. The first was a pilot study evaluating the safety and efficacy of adding GO to high-dose cytarabine–based reinduction chemotherapy in children with relapsed, refractory, or secondary AML. The second was a pilot study evaluating the safety of adding GO to intensive MRC-based chemotherapy, with GO added to the first induction course (cytarabine, daunomycin, and etoposide) and the second intensification course (mitoxantrone and cytarabine). The current COG randomized Phase III study for de novo AML will test the hypothesis

that GO added to a standard chemotherapy backbone (MRC-based chemotherapy) will improve overall survival by reducing primary refractory disease and by reducing later relapses without increasing treatment-related mortality. Because it is unclear that CD33 is consistently expressed on the LSC in CD33+ AML, there is some concern that despite its proven cytoreductive activity, the addition of GO to standard therapy may not reduce the risk of relapse.

Kinase Inhibitors/Farnesyltransferase Inhibitors

Laboratory investigations on the importance of expression and function of cytokine receptors and downstream signaling pathways in normal hematopoiesis led to the documentation that these same pathways contributed significantly to the development and clinical behavior of AML. Several of these cytokine receptors, such as FLT3 and c-KIT, have been shown to have activating mutations in patients with AML leading to altered proliferative, survival, and drug-resistant patterns.[112,114,116,257,258] In addition, as discussed, patients with FLT3/ITD mutations have a poor outcome in both pediatric and adult AML. Such observations have provided the rationale to target these mutant receptors and their downstream signaling pathways. Several inhibitors of FLT3/ITD have been developed, and preclinical models suggest that they may prove to be promising to test in clinical trials.[259–262] One of these inhibitors, lestaurtinib (CEP-701), is being tested in COG AAML06P1 in combination with chemotherapy for pediatric patients with relapsed AML that is characterized by FLT3 mutation. The decision to use cytarabine as one of the chemotherapeutic agents is based on preclinical information showing synergy for this combination and schedule.[261] Another important observation regarding FLT3/ITD is that at least some cases of AML appear to have the mutation in a leukemia-repopulating subset of cells as well as their progeny, thus in part addressing the issues raised above concerning the targeting of the right cell as well as the right molecular target.[263] In addition, recognition of the increased expression of wild type FLT3 in AML, and in particular infant leukemia, may lead to an expanded therapeutic role for FLT3 inhibitors in AML.[259,264]

RAS signaling is an important downstream component of cytokine receptor signaling. Activating mutations of N-RAS have been observed in approximately 25% of AML and/or MDSs.[120] In addition, signaling through the RAS pathway has been shown to play a significant role in leukemogenesis in AML as well as in juvenile myelomonocytic leukemia (JMML).[265] Farnesyltransferase inhibitors (FTI) were initially tested in patients with AML[266–268] as a means of inhibiting RAS activity, which is dependent on post-translational farnesylation.[269] Phase I/II studies have been completed in pediatric patients with leukemia and neurofibromatosis with results that have been sufficiently encouraging to develop additional, randomized trials. Tipifarnib (R115777, Zarnestra™), a potent FTI, is planned for testing in pediatric patients with relapsed AML as a randomized question in the postallogeneic SCT setting (ADVL0522).

This study is built upon Phase I and II studies in adults demonstrating response rates of 14% to 33% in relapsed/refractory AML and in poor-risk de novo AML.[266] In addition, COG has recently completed a Phase I study of tipifarnib in refractory leukemia, which subsequently led to a Phase II window study in JMML (AAML0122). Tipifarnib is being considered for use in a randomized study in patients with newly diagnosed AML following CR as well as in a trial of patients with relapsed AML following HSCT.

Proteosome Inhibitors

Nuclear factor kB (NF-kB) is an important regulator of transcription and mediator of tumor cell survival. NF-kB has also been shown to be differentially expressed in the hematopoietic system during differentiation but also in myeloid malignancies. For example, NF-kB expression has been shown to be highly expressed and activated in AML samples but, possibly most important, also in the quiescent leukemia stem cell population.[270] These observations led Guzman et al to test whether inhibition of NF-kB would differentially induce killing in the leukemia stem cell population compared with normal, hematopoietic stem cells.[271] The class of drugs that inhibits proteosome function has also been shown to augment NF-kB degradation through their inhibition of degradation of IkB alpha, a negative regulator of NF-kB. Guzman et al therefore treated normal bone marrow progenitors and leukemia samples with the proteosome inhibitor MG-132 in combination with IDA. They observed a significant augmentation of selective killing of the LSCs compared with normal progenitors.[271] Such observations have now led to the development of clinical trials using the proteosome inhibitor bortezomib alone and in combination with IDA-containing chemotherapy regimens.

Demethylating Agents/HDAC Inhibitors

Epigenetic modifications, such as histone deacetylation and promoter CpG island methylation, are important regulators of gene expression and have been shown to result in the transcriptional silencing of tumor suppressor genes in myeloid malignancies. Of central importance to AML are the observations that link the presence of fusion proteins resulting from chromosomal translocations to the repression of genes regulating hematopoietic cell maturation. Some of these fusion conjugates, such as the t(15;17)/PML-*RAR*α in APL, those involving core binding factors such as AML1-ETO resulting from t(8;21) or those involving the *MLL* gene product, have been demonstrated to recruit repression-associated chromatin remodeling protein complexes.[272,273] These molecular events, as well as those that are not completely understood, usually result in AML blasts that show a degree of global genomic hypomethylation and hypermethylation of selected promoters.[274,275] Novel agents that may alter these epigenetic modifications in order to favor leukemic cell maturation and death have thus become an important avenue of therapeutic targeting. Small-molecule inhibitors of histone deacetylases (such as valproic

acid and MS275) and DNA methyltransferases (such as decitabine and azacytidine) are currently being tested in pediatric patients with AML. The relatively favorable toxicity profile of these agents may provide an advantageous therapeutic ratio. In addition, by affecting at least one of the primary genetic characteristics of AML blasts, these transcriptional or epigenetic therapeutic strategies may prove more important in eradicating more primitive, self-repopulating leukemic stem cells.

Myelodysplastic and Myeloproliferative Disorders

The myelodysplastic (MDS) and myeloproliferative (MPS) syndromes are a heterogeneous group of disorders with the former usually presenting with cytopenias and the latter with increased peripheral WBC, erythrocyte, or platelet counts. Myelodysplastic syndrome is characterized by ineffective hematopoiesis and increased cell death, while MPS is associated with increased progenitor proliferation and survival. Because they both represent disorders of very primitive, multipotential HSCs, curative therapeutic approaches nearly always require allogeneic stem cell transplantation. These disorders combined represent less than 10% of myeloid malignancies in children.[24] The FAB and WHO classification systems of MDS and MPS have been difficult to apply to pediatric patients. Alternative classification systems for children have been proposed, but none have been uniformly adopted.[24,276]

Myelodysplastic Syndrome

In MDSs the bone marrow is characterized by hypercellularity, dysplastic changes in myeloid precursors, and clonal evolution with eventual development of AML. The percentage of abnormal blasts is less than 20%. The rarer, hypocellular MDS can be distinguished from aplastic anemia in part by its marked dysplasia, clonal nature, and higher percentage of CD34+ precursors.[277,278] Thus MDS is a HSC disorder that in time usually will develop into AML. For patients with clinically significant cytopenias, supportive care with transfusions and prophylactic antibiotics is indicated. In addition, the use of hematopoietic growth factors can improve the hematopoietic status, but there is some concern that such treatment could accelerate conversion to AML.[279–283] Hormonal therapy has also been used, including glucocorticoids and androgens, with mixed results.[284] Other treatment approaches, such as scavenging free oxygen radicals with amifostine, or the use of differentiation-promoting agents, such as retinoids, DNA methylation inhibitors, and histone deacetylase inhibitors, have all shown some positive responses.[285] Azacytidine has been approved by the Food and Drug Administration (FDA) for the treatment of MDS in adults based on randomized studies.[286] Based on the observations of increased angiogenic activity in the bone marrow of patients with MDS, anti-angiogenic agents such as lenalidomide, an analog of thalidomide, have been tested.[287] While the mechanism is unclear, lenalidomide has shown the best responses in patients with 5q- syndrome and is now FDA approved for use in this group. Some patients with MDS have responded to immunosuppression with antithymocyte globulin and/or cyclosporine.[288,289]

In spite of the hematopoietic responses from several different types of approaches, none of them have proven to be curative, although the possibility exists that some form of differentiation or selectively targeted therapy could eliminate over time the abnormal MDS clonal cell. Currently, allogeneic HSCT is the only known curative therapy for these disorders. A major question that arises, however, is what the optimal timing of HSCT should be. Some patients may have prolonged periods where they require minimal supportive care. Such patients can be closely followed and HSCT planned for signs of progression, as assessed by increased need for transfusions, repeated infections due to neutropenia, karyotypic/clonal evolution, or rising blast percentages. Another potentially useful guide, termed the International Prognostic Scoring System, can help to determine which patients should proceed to HSCT.[290-292] This system is particularly useful when considered in the context of the subtype of MDS according to the WHO classification or modifications of it. In practice, close follow-up will usually allow for HSCT before conversion of MDS to AML.

The optimal preparative regimen for HSCT has not been established in randomized, clinical trials. Most regimens, however, use either a conventional total body irradiation with cyclophosphamide or busulfan plus cyclophosphamide. Disease-free survival rates of approximately 50% to 70% have been reported with allogeneic HSCT.[293,294] Furthermore, outcomes for unrelated donors compare favorably with HLA-matched or partially mismatched family donors.[295-297] The use of nonablative approaches in order to reduce long-term adverse sequelae but retaining potential graft-versus-leukemia effects is of interest but has not been established as equivalent to ablative HSCT regimens.

Progression of MDS is characterized by increased blast counts and transformation to AML. The question of whether to attempt remission induction with chemotherapy prior to HSCT in this setting remains controversial. Several reports have demonstrated that AML arising from MDS or what used to be called refractory anemia with excess blasts in transission to AML (RAEB-T) responds to conventional AML induction therapy, albeit with a lower response rate and increased treatment-related mortality.[293,298] An analysis based on CCG-2891 has confirmed the overall lower survival for patients with MDS (along with FAB subtypes M6 and M7, which resemble MDS) compared with those with FAB subtypes M0 to M5.[39] Of particular interest, however, was that DFS and OS as measured from the successful completion of induction therapy did not show significant differences.[39] These findings suggest that if patients with RAEB and RAEB-T enter remission with chemotherapy induction, they have about 50% 5-year OS.[39] Similar conclusions were obtained in a study from Great Britain.[298] Thus, many centers currently recommend chemotherapy induction for patients with AML that has transformed from MDS prior to HSCT, although this approach cannot be considered uniformly accepted. For patients with MDS with a low percentage of blasts, patients should go directly to HSCT.

Myelodysplastic Syndrome/ Myeloproliferative Syndrome

The MDS/MPS category includes several rare conditions, with juvenile myelomonocytic leukemia (JMML) being the most relevant for pediatric patients. The diagnostic criteria for JMML have evolved with the introduction of new information.[24,299] Of note, none of the criteria are by themselves diagnostic, but a combination of several of the criteria in the context of a young child is critical in helping to define this disorder. The median age of diagnosis is 2 years, with diagnosis beyond 5 years being very rare. Males with JMML outnumber females by a 2 to 1 ratio. Common clinical features include massive hepatosplenomegaly and lymphadenopathy and rashes caused by myelomonocytic infiltration. Monosomy 7, the most common acquired abnormality in children with MDS, is also observed in JMML, where it does not correlate with any significant clinical differences.[300-302] Juvenile myelomonocytic leukemia is considered to be derived from a very early hematopoietic precursor or stem cell. Juvenile myelomonocytic leukemia myeloid progenitor cells have been characterized in the laboratory by marked hypersensitivity to granulocyte-macrophage-colony stimulating factor.

Although treatments designed to cytoreduce the leukemic burden prior to HSCT have been utilized, there are no definitive data that demonstrate a benefit in outcome compared with going directly to allogeneic HSCT.[24,303] A European Working Group of MDS in Childhood study that used a busulfan, cyclophosphamide, and melphalan preparative regimen for both HLA-matched family and unrelated donors reported EFS and OS to be 52% and 64%, respectively.[294,304] The primary cause of failure was relapse, which usually occurred within the first 2 to 4 months post-HSCT. Although early relapse has been successfully treated with the withdrawal of immunosuppressive therapy and/or infusion of donor lymphocytes, this approach is mostly unsuccessful.[289,305,306] The early detection of increasing host chimerism post-HSCT is a useful way to pick up disease recurrence; more specific molecular methods for detecting MRD in JMML are being developed based on *PTPN11* or *RAS* mutations. There is also precedent for disease eradication with a second or third HSCT.[307]

Based on the known activation of the *RAS* oncogene pathway in JMML, as well as the dependence of *RAS* activation on the posttranslational addition of a farnesyl tether to the inner cell membrane, a clinical trial using a farnesyl transferase inhibitor has been conducted by the North American JMML Study Group and COG.[308] In addition, this trial utilized pre-HSCT chemotherapy with the FLAG regimen and recommended splenectomy at the treating clinician's discretion in order to reduce the risk of graft failure and accelerate hematopoietic recovery. Finally, a TBI/cyclophosphamide HSCT preparative regimen was used as well as post-HSCT cis-retinoic acid. Although initial results appeared encouraging in terms of clinical and hematologic response to this approach, the definitive results from this study have not yet been reported.

Myeloproliferative Syndromes

The traditional myeloproliferative syndromes represent primarily include BCR-ABL-positive chronic myelogenous leukemia (CML) in addition to the much rarer polycythemia vera (PV) and other polycythemia disorders, essential thrombocythemia (ET), and idiopathic myelofibrosis. Chronic myelogenous leukemia is characterized by chronic, accelerated, and blast crisis phases. The chronic phase, which usually lasts about 3 to 5 years, presents with marked leukocytosis with a "left shift" and with all stages of differentiation present; thrombocytosis is common. The bone marrow is hypercellular and primarily granulocytic with relatively normal maturation. The accelerated phase of CML is characterized by ≥ 10% but < 30% blasts in peripheral blood or bone marrow. In addition, the percentage of blasts plus promyelocytes may be elevated to ≥ 20% as well as a basophilia in peripheral blood or bone marrow. Thrombocytopenia unrelated to any treatment is common. Progressive splenomegaly and additional chromosomal abnormalities along with the Philadelphia chromosome are observed. Blast crisis mimics acute leukemia, with two-thirds of cases being myeloid and the remaining mostly early B cell. The bone marrow usually shows greater than 30% blasts, and increased chromosomal abnormalities are frequent.

Polycythemia in children may in rare cases be due to PV but may also be due to primary (familial/congenital) polycythemia as well as a variety of secondary causes such as those related to hemoglobinopathies or excess erythropoietin. Congenital PV has been reported with mutations of the erythropoietin receptor.[309,310] In addition, a familial form of secondary PV, known as Chuvash polycythemia, has been described and is due to mutations in the von Hippel-Lindau gene.[309,310] Polycythemia vera is characterized by an increased red blood cell mass, manifested by an increased hematocrit/hemoglobin along with increased WBC count and platelets. Patients also may show a ruddy complexion as well as suffer from headaches, night sweats, pruritis, and thrombotic problems secondary to hyperviscosity. Although bone marrow examination is not essential for the diagnosis of PV, characteristics include hypercellularity in most but not all cases along with relatively normal percentages of trilineage hematopoiesis. In some cases, increased numbers of megakaryocytes and pronormoblasts, often in clusters, can be seen. The PV Study Group has established diagnostic criteria for adults with PV,[311] although it has been argued that separate criteria should be developed for children who appear to have some distinguishing features, particularly in terms of JAK2 mutations and their frequency.[312,313]

Similarly, diagnostic criteria have been developed for ET, which presents with a persistently increased platelet count, the presence of large or giant platelets on peripheral blood smear, the absence of cytogenetic abnormalities, normal serum erythropoietin levels, and the absence of underlying alternative causes that would lead to a reactive thrombocytosis. The bone marrow shows normal granulopoiesis and erythropoiesis but with increased numbers of often clustered, enlarged, mature megakaryocytes.[311] Mutations in the signaling molecule JAK2 are commonly observed in PV and ET.[311] It has also been reported that pediatric patients with ET have a milder course and a lower percentage of JAK2 mutations.[314,315] In contrast, gain of function mutations of TPO or cMPL are found in congenital ET.[311]

Idiopathic myelofibrosis is extremely rare in children. It often presents with cytopenias, particularly anemia characterized by anisocytosis and poikilocytosis with variable WBC and platelet counts accompanied by a leukoerythroblastic peripheral blood smear. Splenomegaly, often caused by extramedullary hematopoiesis, is common. The bone marrow has increased reticulum on biopsy and aspirations are typically "dry taps." Of note, megakaryoblastic (FAB M7) AML can also present with similar findings. In addition, PV can evolve into MDS and myelofibrosis as well.

Each of the MPS disorders arises from pluripotential, hematopoietic stem cells, and thus the use of allogeneic HSCT has been considered the only curative therapy. Although such an approach has been reasonable in the past, new developments in agents that target critical signal transduction pathways are now challenging this approach in some situations. Hematopoietic stem cell transplantation is usually recommended for patients with PV who develop significant thrombotic complications or who develop MDS, myelofibrosis, or AML. For patients with essential thrombocytosis, platelet cytoreductive therapy with agents such as hydroxyurea, anagrelide, or interferon alpha is preferred to HSCT; however, HSCT is used for patients who suffer adverse consequences of the high platelet counts such as thrombotic events or to myelofibrosis and AML. The choice between HSCT and drug therapy for patients with CML is more complex.

Chronic myelogenous leukemia is the most common MPS in children, although it still represents less than 5% of pediatric leukemia. Chronic myelogenous leukemia presents most commonly in chronic phase. When the presenting WBC count is very high and signs/symptoms of hyperviscosity are observed, then cytoreduction with imatinib (Gleevec) and/or hydroxyurea is indicated. Since the introduction of imatinib, intensive multiagent chemotherapy is no longer recommended as frontline treatment, even in patients who present in accelerated or blastic phases. Similarly, the role of interferon alpha has decreased because imatinib has shown significantly higher responses.

Prognosis is in part dependent on whether a patient is in chronic, accelerated, or blast crisis phase of the disease, with estimated relative risks for mortality being about 1.5 and 2.5 for accelerated and blast crisis compared to chronic phase.[316,317] An interim of greater than 1 year from diagnosis to HSCT has been associated with a decreased survival rate, with a relative risk estimated to be about 1.5.[316,318] Ablative HSCT has been the only accepted curative therapy for patients with CML. Results in children and adolescents show that outcomes for HLA-matched related and unrelated donors are comparable with long-term survival in the 60% to 75% range.[318,319] T-cell depletion of the graft without at least a partial T cell "add back" is not recommended for patients with CML because of an increased risk of relapse, suggesting that a graft-versus-leukemia effect is important in eradicating CML.[320–322] Cord blood donors have been successfully used, but this modality does not allow the use of donor lymphocytes post-HSCT to treat early relapse, which has been reported to be successful in up to 60% of patients with early recurrent disease.[321,323,324]

The introduction of imatinib for the treatment of CML has changed the decision algorithm considerably in terms of when and whether to do an HSCT.[325] Imatinib, as well as several other subsequently developed agents, selectively targets the proliferative and survival pathways resulting from the action of the BCR-ABL fusion protein that characterizes CML.[325] The International Randomized Study of Interferon and STI571 0106 study initially showed that at 18 months 87% and 76% of patients on 400 mg per day of imatinib obtained major and complete cytogenetic responses, respectively.[326] This report also showed a 97% estimated rate of being free from progression to accelerated or blast crisis phase.[326] An update of these data at 2.5 years' follow-up showed a 90% and 82% major and complete cytogenetic responses, respectively, in the imatinib-treated group. Although the pediatric experience with imatinib is limited in terms of published reports, a COG Phase I trial has established that 260 to 340 mg/m^2 daily in children achieves systemic exposures similar to those observed in adults.[327,328] There is also evidence that increasing the daily dose and exposure to imatinib results in a statistically significant increase in complete cytogenetic and molecular remissions.[329]

As with most chemotherapeutic agents, the development of resistance to imatinib has been observed at the time of diagnosis, or more commonly while on therapy. The resistance can be due to mutations or amplification of the BCR-ABL fusion gene as well as up-regulation of alternative pathways.[330] The use of non-cross-resistant, alternative signal transduction inhibitors, such as nilotinib or dasatinib, are often effective in obtaining a second hematologic and cytogenetic response. For instance, dasatinib has been reported to produce major cytogenetic responses after first-line imatinib failure in 52% of patients and 40% complete cytogenetic responses.[331] Combinations of such signal transduction inhibitors are currently being studied in clinical trials. Nevertheless, the progression to a sudden blast crisis while on imatinib therapy remains low (about 0.7%).[332] Close cytogenetic and molecular monitoring are therefore quite useful in the clinical assessment of patients with newly diagnosed CML treated with imatinib. The early detection of BCR-ABL mutations that lead to imatinib resistance appears to identify a high-risk group of patients who may then be considered for alternative treatments with other signal transduction inhibitors or allogeneic HSCT.

Questions have been raised as to whether targeted therapeutics such as imatinib are able to eradicate the LSC effectively. It is possible that CML stem cells may escape killing from agents such as imatinib through inherent resistant mechanisms, and thus persist following cytogenetic remission.[333,334] If so, one would predict that CML patients treated with imatinib are destined to recur after stopping treatment. This prediction has been tested in a limited number of adult patients with CML, as in a report of 3 patients who achieved molecular remissions lasting 1 to 2 years who discontinued use of imatinib; all of them subsequently recurred in 6 to 8 months.[335] Another patient who was initially treated with interferon alpha and obtained a complete cytogenetic remission and then a molecular remission on imatinib for 17 months recurred within 2 months after stopping therapy.[336] Rousselot et al reported on 12 patients with a median period of being in a molecular remission on imatinib of 32 months, and the median time on treatment with imatinib was 45 months.[337] Six of these 12 patients had a recurrence of detectable BCR-ABL transcripts within 5 months of stopping imatinib, while the other 6 patients remained in molecular remission with a median follow-up of 18 months.[337] Although longer follow-up with a larger number of patients is needed, such results suggest that imatinib therapy, if given for a sufficiently long period, may eradicate CML stem cells. Of interest, such observations have been observed with interferon alpha as well; the mechanism of killing the BCR-ABL-positive cells appears to be different for interferon alpha and imatinib, providing the possibility of developing possible combination treatment schedules.[336]

Thus, there remain significant differences of opinion as to the optimal treatment for patients with CML, even among pediatric oncologists. A survey based on several clinical scenarios led to the conclusion that most pediatric transplant physicians favor HSCT as an early treatment while hematologist/oncologists favor the use of imatinib.[338] Most pediatric patients will be started on imatinib following their initial diagnosis. Then, depending on the patient and family choices in conjunction with the recommendations of their treating physicians, some patients will be brought to allogeneic HSCT, especially if an HLA-matched family donor is available. However, a reasonable argument can now be made to continue patients on imatinib with close molecular monitoring with the hope of obtaining a molecular remission that is sustainable. If emergence of BCR-ABL positivity occurs or mutations in BCR-ABL are identified, then HSCT can be rapidly pursued. For patients without an HLA-matched family donor, a similar approach is also reasonable. As new drugs become available that can treat imatinib-resistant disease or even more selectively target the CML stem cell, the use of HSCT in these patients may decrease.

Late Effects and Monitoring of Survivors of Childhood Acute Myeloid Leukemia

Approximately 50% of children with AML will be cured of their disease, in that they will be in a state of complete continuous remission following treatment. However, many of these children will continue to be challenged by treatment-related late effects. Although several investigators have reported on late effects in childhood AML,[339–343] population-based studies following recent intensive therapies are not yet available.

Leung et al reported on 77 patients surviving more than 10 years from diagnosis, with a median follow-up of 17 years.[339,344] Of the 77 patients, 44 had been treated with chemotherapy only, 18 with chemotherapy and cranial irradiation, and 15 with chemotherapy, total body irradiation, and allogeneic bone marrow transplantation. Common late effects included growth delay (30%), endocrine abnormalities (16%), cataracts (12%), and cardiac abnormalities (8%). Increasing radiation dose and younger age at diagnosis and initiation of radiation therapy were risk factors for growth delay, infertility, academic difficulties, cataracts, and hypothyroidism. Patients receiving total body irradiation had lower cumulative anthracycline doses (204 mg/m^2 vs 335 mg/m2) but did not have a lower rate of cardiomyopathy. Another study by the same group estimated that 15 years from diagnosis of childhood AML, the cumulative incidence of second malignancy is 1.3% (approximately 10-fold higher than expected in the general population).[344] However, this risk is small compared with the risk of death due to the primary AML and early complication of its treatment.

Pediatric oncology centers nearly always have late-effects programs to conduct surveillance for the development of these problems and provide follow-up care to patients who develop late complications of therapy. In addition, excellent resources have been developed to assist medical providers in caring for long-term survivors of childhood AML and other malignancies, such as the COG's *Long-Term Follow-Up Guidelines for Survivors of Childhood, Adolescent, and Young Adult Cancers* (available at www.survivorshipguidelines.org). An important element in the success of survivorship care is the completion by the treating oncologist of a "comprehensive treatment summary" that the patient can share with subsequent medical providers. Excellent templates have been created to assist oncologists in preparing these summaries (examples include the Cancer Survivor's Treatment Record available at www.patientcenters.com, and the Cancer Survivor's Medical Treatment Summary available at www.livestrong.org).

References

1. Ries L, Melbert D, Krapcho M, et al. *SEER Cancer Statistics Review, 1975–2004.* Bethesda, MD: National Cancer Institute; 2007.
2. Douer D, Preston-Martin S, Chang E, Nichols PW, Watkins KJ, Levine AM. High frequency of acute promyelocytic leukemia among Latinos with acute myeloid leukemia. *Blood.* 1996;87:308–313.
3. Glazer ER, Perkins CI, Young JL, Jr, Schlag RD, Campleman SL, Wright WE. Cancer among Hispanic children in California, 1988–1994: comparison with non-Hispanic white children. *Cancer.* 1999;86:1070–1079.
4. Stiller CA. Epidemiology and genetics of childhood cancer. *Oncogene.* 2004;23:6429–6444.
5. Le Deley MC, Leblanc T, Shamsaldin A, et al. Risk of secondary leukemia after a solid tumor in childhood according to the dose of epipodophyllotoxins and anthracyclines: a case-control study by the Société Francaise d'Oncologie Pédiatrique. *J Clin Oncol.* 2003;21:1074–1081.
6. Sandoval C, Pui CH, Bowman LC, et al. Secondary acute myeloid leukemia in children previously treated with alkylating agents, intercalating topoisomerase II inhibitors, and irradiation. *J Clin Oncol.* 1993;11:1039–1045.
7. Ross JA, Spector LG, Robison LL, Olshan AF. Epidemiology of leukemia in children with Down syndrome. *Pediatr Blood Cancer.* 2005;44:8–12.
8. Homans AC, Verissimo AM, Vlacha V. Transient abnormal myelopoiesis of infancy associated with trisomy 21. *Am J Pediatr Hematol Oncol.* 1993;15:392–399.
9. Wechsler J, Greene M, McDevitt MA, et al. Acquired mutations in GATA1 in the megakaryoblastic leukemia of Down syndrome. *Nat Genet.* 2002;32:148–152.
10. Greaves MF, Maia AT, Wiemels JL, Ford AM. Leukemia in twins: lessons in natural history. *Blood.* 2003;102:2321–2333.
11. Kadan-Lottick NS, Kawashima T, Tomlinson G, et al. The risk of cancer in twins: a report from the childhood cancer survivor study. *Pediatr Blood Cancer.* 2006;46:476–481.
12. Escher R, Jones A, Hagos F, et al. Chromosome band 16q22–linked familial AML: exclusion of candidate genes, and possible disease risk modification by NQO1 polymorphisms. *Genes Chromosomes Cancer.* 2004;41:278–282.
13. Gao Q, Horwitz M, Roulston D, et al. Susceptibility gene for familial acute myeloid leukemia associated with loss of 5q and/or 7q is not localized on the commonly deleted portion of 5q. *Genes Chromosomes Cancer.* 2000;28:164–172.
14. Olopade OI, Roulston D, Baker T, et al. Familial myeloid leukemia associated with loss of the long arm of chromosome 5. *Leukemia.* 1996;10:669–674.
15. Siebert R, Jhanwar S, Brown K, Berman E, Offit K. Familial acute myeloid leukemia and DiGuglielmo syndrome. *Leukemia.* 1995;9:1091–1094.
16. Minelli A, Maserati E, Giudici G, et al. Familial partial monosomy 7 and myelodysplasia: different parental origin of the monosomy 7 suggests action of a mutator gene. *Cancer Genet Cytogenet.* 2001;124:147–151.
17. Smith ML, Cavenagh JD, Lister TA, Fitzgibbon J. Mutation of CEBPA in familial acute myeloid leukemia. *N Engl J Med.* 2004;351:2403–2407.
18. Imashuku S, Hibi S, Nakajima F, et al. A review of 125 cases to determine the risk of myelodysplasia and leukemia in pediatric neutropenic patients after treatment with recombinant human granulocyte colony-stimulating factor. *Blood.* 1994;84:2380–2381.
19. Ohara A, Kojima S, Hamajima N, et al. Myelodysplastic syndrome and acute myelogenous leukemia as a late clonal complication in children with acquired aplastic anemia. *Blood.* 1997;90:1009–1013.
20. Shannon KM, Turhan AG, Chang SS, et al. Familial bone marrow monosomy 7. Evidence that the predisposing locus is not on the long arm of chromosome 7. *J Clin Invest.* 1989;84:984–989.
21. Devine DV, Gluck WL, Rosse WF, Weinberg JB. Acute myeloblastic leukemia in paroxysmal nocturnal hemoglobinuria: evidence of evolution from the abnormal paroxysmal nocturnal hemoglobinuria clone. *J Clin Invest.* 1987;79:314–317.
22. van den Heuvel-Eibrink MM, Bredius RG, te Winkel ML, et al. Childhood paroxysmal nocturnal haemoglobinuria (PNH), a report of 11 cases in the Netherlands. *Br J Haematol.* 2005;128:571–577.
23. Luna-Fineman S, Shannon KM, Atwater SK, et al. Myelodysplastic and myeloproliferative disorders of childhood: a study of 167 patients. *Blood.* 1999;93:459–466.
24. Hasle H, Niemeyer CM, Chessells JM, et al. A pediatric approach to the WHO classification of myelodysplastic and myeloproliferative diseases. *Leukemia.* 2003;17:277–282.
25. Mandel K, Dror Y, Poon A, Freedman MH. A practical, comprehensive classification for pediatric myelodysplastic syndromes: the CCC system. *J Pediatr Hematol Oncol.* 2002;24:596–605.
26. Shimizu Y, Schull WJ, Kato H. Cancer risk among atomic bomb survivors. The RERF Life Span Study. Radiation Effects Research Foundation. *JAMA.* 1990;264:601–604.
27. Jablon S, Kato H. Childhood cancer in relation to prenatal exposure to atomic-bomb radiation. *Lancet.* 1970;2:1000–1003.
28. Doll R, Wakeford R. Risk of childhood cancer from fetal irradiation. *Br J Radiol.* 1997;70:130–139.
29. Mole RH. Childhood cancer after prenatal exposure to diagnostic X-ray examinations in Britain. *Br J Cancer.* 1990;62:152–168.
30. Linet MS, Hatch EE, Kleinerman RA, et al. Residential exposure to magnetic fields and acute lymphoblastic leukemia in children. *N Engl J Med.* 1997;337:1–7.
31. Chang JS, Selvin S, Metayer C, Crouse V, Golembesky A, Buffler PA. Parental smoking and the risk of childhood leukemia. *Am J Epidemiol.* 2006;163:1091–1100.
32. Menegaux F, Ripert M, Hemon D, Clavel J. Maternal alcohol and coffee drinking, parental smoking and childhood leukaemia: a French population-based case-control study. *Paediatr Perinat Epidemiol.* 2007;21:293–299.
33. McNally RJ, Parker L. Environmental factors and childhood acute leukemias and lymphomas. *Leuk Lymphoma.* 2006;47:583–598.
34. Strick R, Strissel PL, Borgers S, Smith SL, Rowley JD. Dietary bioflavonoids induce cleavage in the *MLL* gene and may contribute to infant leukemia. *Proc Natl Acad Sci USA.* 2000;97:4790–4795.
35. Abe T. Infantile leukemia and soybeans: a hypothesis. *Leukemia.* 1999;13:317–320.
36. Spector LG, Xie Y, Robison LL, et al. Maternal diet and infant leukemia: the DNA topoisomerase II inhibitor hypothesis: a report from the Children's Oncology Group. *Cancer Epidemiol Biomarkers Prev.* 2005;14:651–655.
37. van Waalwijk van Doorn-Khosrovani SB, Janssen J, Maas LM, Godschalk RW, Nijhuis JG, van Schooten FJ. Dietary flavonoids induce *MLL* translocations in primary human CD34+ cells. *Carcinogenesis.* 2007;28:1703–1709.
38. Barnard DR, Woods WG. Treatment-related myelodysplastic syndrome/acute myeloid leukemia in survivors of childhood cancer: an update. *Leuk Lymphoma.* 2005;46:651–663.

39. Barnard DR, Alonzo TA, Gerbing RB, Lange B, Woods WG. Comparison of childhood myelodysplastic syndrome, AML FAB M6 or M7, CCG 2891: report from the Children's Oncology Group. *Pediatr Blood Cancer.* 2007;49: 17–22.

40. Barnard DR, Lange B, Alonzo TA, et al. Acute myeloid leukemia and myelodysplastic syndrome in children treated for cancer: comparison with primary presentation. *Blood.* 2002;100:427–434.

41. Jagarlamudi R, Kumar L, Kochupillai V, Kapil A, Banerjee U, Thulkar S. Infections in acute leukemia: an analysis of 240 febrile episodes. *Med Oncol.* 2000; 17:111–116.

42. Miranda-Novales MG, Belmont-Martinez L, Villasis-Keever MA, Penagos-Paniagua M, Bernaldez-Rios R, Solorzano-Santos F. Empirical antimicrobial therapy in pediatric patients with neutropenia and fever: risk factors for treatment failure. *Arch Med Res.* 1998;29:331–335.

43. Barbui T, Falanga A. Disseminated intravascular coagulation in acute leukemia. *Semin Thromb Hemost.* 2001;27:593–604.

44. Ventura GJ, Hester JP, Dixon DO, Khorana S, Keating MJ. Analysis of risk factors for fatal hemorrhage during induction therapy of patients with acute promyelocytic leukemia. *Hematol Pathol.* 1989;3:23–28.

45. Kawai Y, Watanabe K, Kizaki M, et al. Rapid improvement of coagulopathy by all-trans retinoic acid in acute promyelocytic leukemia. *Am J Hematol.* 1994; 46:184–188.

46. Creutzig U, Ritter J, Budde M, Sutor A, Schellong G. Early deaths due to hemorrhage and leukostasis in childhood acute myelogenous leukemia: associations with hyperleukocytosis and acute monocytic leukemia. *Cancer.* 1987; 60:3071–3079.

47. Zarkovic M, Kwaan HC. Correction of hyperviscosity by apheresis. *Semin Thromb Hemost.* 2003;29:535–542.

48. Brown LM, Daeschner CD, Timms J, Crow W. Granulocytic sarcoma in childhood acute myelogenous leukemia. *Pediatr Neurol.* 1989;5:173–178.

49. Tallman MS, Hakimian D, Shaw JM, Lissner GS, Russell EJ, Variakojis D. Granulocytic sarcoma is associated with the 8;21 translocation in acute myeloid leukemia. *J Clin Oncol.* 1993;11:690–697.

50. Reinhardt D, Creutzig U. Isolated myelosarcoma in children: update and review. *Leuk Lymphoma.* 2002;43:565–574.

51. Landis DM, Aboulafia DM. Granulocytic sarcoma: an unusual complication of aleukemic myeloid leukemia causing spinal cord compression. A case report and literature review. *Leuk Lymphoma.* 2003;44:1753–1760.

52. Dusenbery K, Arthur D, Howells W, et al. Granulocytic sarcomas (chloromas) in pediatric patients with newly diagnosed acute myeloid leukemia. *Proc Am Soc Clin Oncol.* 1996;15:369A.

53. Goldman SC, Holcenberg JS, Finklestein JZ, et al. A randomized comparison between rasburicase and allopurinol in children with lymphoma or leukemia at high risk for tumor lysis. *Blood.* 2001;97:2998–3003.

54. Rice J, Resar LM. Hematologic abnormalities associated with influenza A infection: a report of 3 cases. *Am J Med Sci.* 1998;316:401–403.

55. Iishi Y, Kosaka M, Mizuguchi T, et al. Suppression of hematopoiesis by activated T-cells in infectious mononucleosis associated with pancytopenia. *Int J Hematol.* 1991;54:65–73.

56. Kagialis-Girard S, Durand B, Mialou V, et al. Human herpes virus 6 infection and transient acquired myelodysplasia in children. *Pediatr Blood Cancer.* 2006;47:543–548.

57. Sandberg AA, Stone JF, Czarnecki L, Cohen JD. Hematologic masquerade of rhabdomyosarcoma. *Am J Hematol.* 2001;68:51–57.

58. Ostrov BE, Goldsmith DP, Athreya BH. Differentiation of systemic juvenile rheumatoid arthritis from acute leukemia near the onset of disease. *J Pediatr.* 1993;122:595–598.

59. Bennett JM, Catovsky D, Daniel MT, et al. Proposals for the classification of the acute leukaemias. French-American-British (FAB) co-operative group. *Br J Haematol.* 1976;33:451–458.

60. Bennett JM, Catovsky D, Daniel MT, et al. Proposed revised criteria for the classification of acute myeloid leukemia: a report of the French-American-British Cooperative Group. *Ann Intern Med.* 1985;103:626–629.

61. Jaffe ES, Harris NL, Diebold J, Muller-Hermelink HK. World Health Organization classification of neoplastic diseases of the hematopoietic and lymphoid tissues: a progress report. *Am J Clin Pathol.* 1999;111:S8–S12.

62. Hanson CA, Gajl-Peczalska KJ, Parkin JL, Brunning RD. Immunophenotyping of acute myeloid leukemia using monoclonal antibodies and the alkaline phosphatase-antialkaline phosphatase technique. *Blood.* 1987;70:83–89.

63. Kuerbitz SJ, Civin CI, Krischer JP, et al. Expression of myeloid-associated and lymphoid-associated cell-surface antigens in acute myeloid leukemia of childhood: a Pediatric Oncology Group study. *J Clin Oncol.* 1992;10:1419–1429.

64. Smith FO, Lampkin BC, Versteeg C, et al. Expression of lymphoid-associated cell surface antigens by childhood acute myeloid leukemia cells lacks prognostic significance. *Blood.* 1992;79:2415–2422.

65. Orfao A, Chillon MC, Bortoluci AM, et al. The flow cytometric pattern of CD34, CD15 and CD13 expression in acute myeloblastic leukemia is highly characteristic of the presence of PML-RARalpha gene rearrangements. *Haematologica.* 1999;84:405–412.

66. Raimondi SC, Chang MN, Ravindranath Y, et al. Chromosomal abnormalities in 478 children with acute myeloid leukemia: clinical characteristics and treatment outcome in a cooperative pediatric oncology group study-POG 8821. *Blood.* 1999;94:3707–3716.

67. Grimwade D, Walker H, Oliver F, et al. The importance of diagnostic cytogenetics on outcome in AML: analysis of 1,612 patients entered into the MRC AML 10 trial. The Medical Research Council Adult and Children's Leukaemia Working Parties. *Blood.* 1998;92:2322–2333.

68. Haferlach T, Bacher U, Kern W, Schnittger S, Haferlach C. Diagnostic pathways in acute leukemias: a proposal for a multimodal approach. *Ann Hematol.* 2007;86:311–327.

69. Grimwade D, Howe K, Langabeer S, et al. Establishing the presence of the t(15;17) in suspected acute promyelocytic leukaemia: cytogenetic, molecular and PML immunofluorescence assessment of patients entered into the MRC ATRA trial. MRC Adult Leukaemia Working Party. *Br J Haematol.* 1996;94: 557–573.

70. Bonnet D, Dick JE. Human acute myeloid leukemia is organized as a hierarchy that originates from a primitive hematopoietic cell. *Nature Med.* 1997;3: 730–737.

71. Wiemels JL, Xiao Z, Buffler PA, et al. In utero origin of t(8;21) *AML1–ETO* translocations in childhood acute myeloid leukemia. *Blood.* 2002;99:3801–3805.

72. Wiemels JL, Cazzaniga G, Daniotti M, et al. Prenatal origin of acute lymphoblastic leukaemia in children. *Lancet.* 1999;354:1499–1503.

73. Ford AM, Bennett CA, Price CM, Bruin MC, Van Wering ER, Greaves M. Fetal origins of the *TEL-AML1* fusion gene in identical twins with leukemia. *Proc Natl Acad Sci USA.* 1998;95:4584–4588.

74. Mori H, Colman SM, Xiao Z, et al. Chromosome translocations and covert leukemic clones are generated during normal fetal development. *Proc Natl Acad Sci USA.* 2002;99:8242–8247.

75. Greaves M. Pre-natal origins of childhood leukemia. *Rev Clin Exp Hematol.* 2003;7:233–245.

76. Higuchi M, O'Brien D, Kumaravelu P, Lenny N, Yeoh EJ, Downing JR. Expression of a conditional *AML1–ETO* oncogene bypasses embryonic lethality and establishes a murine model of human t(8;21) acute myeloid leukemia. *Cancer Cell.* 2002;1:63–74.

77. Fenske TS, Pengue G, Mathews V, et al. Stem cell expression of the AML1/ETO fusion protein induces a myeloproliferative disorder in mice. *Proc Natl Acad Sci USA.* 2004;101:15184–15189.

78. Schessl C, Rawat VP, Cusan M, et al. The *AML1–ETO* fusion gene and the FLT3 length mutation collaborate in inducing acute leukemia in mice. *J Clin Invest.* 2005;115:2159–2168.

79. Gilliland DG, Griffin JD. The roles of FLT3 in hematopoiesis and leukemia. *Blood.* 2002;100:1532–1542.

80. Webb DK, Wheatley K, Harrison G, Stevens RF, Hann IM. Outcome for children with relapsed acute myeloid leukaemia following initial therapy in the Medical Research Council (MRC) AML 10 trial. MRC Childhood Leukaemia Working Party. *Leukemia.* 1999;13:25–31.

81. Wheatley K, Burnett AK, Goldstone AH, et al. A simple, robust, validated and highly predictive index for the determination of risk-directed therapy in acute myeloid leukaemia derived from the MRC AML 10 trial. United Kingdom Medical Research Council's Adult and Childhood Leukaemia Working Parties. *Br J Haematol.* 1999;107:69–79.

82. Aplenc R, Alonzo TA, Gerbing RB, et al. Ethnicity and survival in childhood acute myeloid leukemia: a report from the Children's Oncology Group. *Blood.* 2006;108:74–80.

83. Gamis AS. Acute myeloid leukemia and Down syndrome evolution of modern therapy: state of the art review. *Pediatr Blood Cancer.* 2005;44:13–20.

84. Creutzig U, Ritter J, Ludwig WD, et al. Acute myeloid leukemia in children with Down syndrome. *Klin Padiatr.* 1995;207:136–144.

85. Ravindranath Y, Abella E, Krischer JP, et al. Acute myeloid leukemia (AML) in Down's syndrome is highly responsive to chemotherapy: experience on Pediatric Oncology Group AML Study 8498. *Blood.* 1992;80:2210–2214.

86. Lange BJ, Gerbing RB, Feusner J, et al. Mortality in overweight and underweight children with acute myeloid leukemia. *JAMA.* 2005;293:203–211.

87. Davies SM, Robison LL, Buckley JD, Radloff GA, Ross JA, Perentesis JP. Glutathione S-transferase polymorphisms in children with myeloid leukemia: a Children's Cancer Group study. *Cancer Epidemiol Biomarkers Prev.* 2000;9: 563–566.

88. Creutzig U, Zimmermann M, Ritter J, et al. Definition of a standard-risk group in children with AML. *Br J Haematol.* 1999;104:630–639.

89. Rubnitz JE, Raimondi SC, Halbert AR, et al. Characteristics and outcome of t(8;21)-positive childhood acute myeloid leukemia: a single institution's experience. *Leukemia.* 2002;16:2072–2077.

90. Hurwitz CA, Raimondi SC, Head D, et al. Distinctive immunophenotypic features of t(8;21)(q22;q22) acute myeloblastic leukemia in children. *Blood.* 1992;80:3182–3188.

91. Whitman SP, Archer KJ, Feng L, et al. Absence of the wild-type allele predicts poor prognosis in adult de novo acute myeloid leukemia with normal cytogenetics and the internal tandem duplication of FLT3: a cancer and leukemia group B study. *Cancer Res.* 2001;61:7233–7239.

92. Felice MS, Zubizarreta PA, Alfaro EM, et al. Good outcome of children with acute myeloid leukemia and t(8;21)(q22;q22), even when associated with granulocytic sarcoma: a report from a single institution in Argentina. *Cancer.* 2000;88:1939–1944.

93. Byrd JC, Dodge RK, Carroll A, et al. Patients with t(8;21)(q22;q22) and acute myeloid leukemia have superior failure-free and overall survival when repetitive cycles of high-dose cytarabine are administered. *J Clin Oncol.* 1999;17: 3767–3775.

94. Lie SO, Abrahamsson J, Clausen N, et al. Long-term results in children with AML: NOPHO-AML Study Group: report of three consecutive trials. *Leukemia.* 2005;19:2090–2100.

95. Licht JD, Chomienne C, Goy A, et al. Clinical and molecular characterization of a rare syndrome of acute promyelocytic leukemia associated with translocation (11;17). *Blood.* 1995;85:1083–1094.

96. Pui CH, Kane JR, Crist WM. Biology and treatment of infant leukemias. *Leukemia.* 1995;9:762–769.

97. Rubnitz JE, Raimondi SC, Tong X, et al. Favorable impact of the t(9;11) in childhood acute myeloid leukemia. *J Clin Oncol.* 2002;20:2302–2309.

98. Swansbury GJ, Slater R, Bain BJ, Moorman AV, Secker-Walker LM. Hematological malignancies with t(9;11)(p21–22;q23): a laboratory and clinical study of 125 cases. European 11q23 Workshop participants. *Leukemia.* 1998; 12:792–800.

99. Casillas JN, Woods WG, Hunger SP, McGavran L, Alonzo TA, Feig SA. Prognostic implications of t(10;11) translocations in childhood acute myelogenous leukemia: a report from the Children's Cancer Group. *J Pediatr Hematol Oncol.* 2003;25:594–600.

100. Van Limbergen H, Poppe B, Janssens A, et al. Molecular cytogenetic analysis of 10;11 rearrangements in acute myeloid leukemia. *Leukemia.* 2002;16:344–351.

101. Carlson KM, Vignon C, Bohlander S, Martinez-Climent JA, Le Beau MM, Rowley JD. Identification and molecular characterization of CALM/AF10 fusion products in T cell acute lymphoblastic leukemia and acute myeloid leukemia. *Leukemia.* 2000;14:100–104.

102. Dreyling MH, Schrader K, Fonatsch C, et al. MLL and CALM are fused to AF10 in morphologically distinct subsets of acute leukemia with translocation t(10;11): both rearrangements are associated with a poor prognosis. *Blood.* 1998;91:4662–4667.

103. Ma Z, Morris SW, Valentine V, et al. Fusion of two novel genes, *RBM15* and *MKL1*, in the t(1;22)(p13;q13) of acute megakaryoblastic leukemia. *Nature Genet.* 2001;28:220–221.

104. Mercher T, Coniat MB, Monni R, et al. Involvement of a human gene related to the Drosophila spen gene in the recurrent t(1;22) translocation of acute megakaryocytic leukemia. *Proc Natl Acad Sci USA.* 2001;98:5776–5779.

105. Duchayne E, Fenneteau O, Pages MP, et al. Acute megakaryoblastic leukaemia: a national clinical and biological study of 53 adult and childhood cases by the Groupe Francais d'Hematologie Cellulaire (GFHC). *Leuk Lymphoma.* 2003;44:49–58.

106. Bernstein J, Dastugue N, Haas OA, et al. Nineteen cases of the t(1;22)(p13; q13) acute megakaryblastic leukaemia of infants/children and a review of 39 cases: report from a t(1;22) study group. *Leukemia.* 2000;14:216–218.

107. Schnittger S, Schoch C, Dugas M, et al. Analysis of FLT3 length mutations in 1003 patients with acute myeloid leukemia: correlation to cytogenetics, FAB subtype, and prognosis in the AMLCG study and usefulness as a marker for the detection of minimal residual disease. *Blood.* 2002;100:59–66.

108. Thiede C, Steudel C, Mohr B, et al. Analysis of FLT3–activating mutations in 979 patients with acute myelogenous leukemia: association with FAB subtypes and identification of subgroups with poor prognosis. *Blood.* 2002;99: 4326–4335.

109. Meshinchi S, Alonzo TA, Stirewalt DL, et al. Clinical implications of FLT3 mutations in pediatric AML. *Blood.* 2006;108:3654–3661.

110. Zwaan CM, Meshinchi S, Radich JP, et al. FLT3 internal tandem duplication in 234 children with acute myeloid leukemia: prognostic significance and relation to cellular drug resistance. *Blood.* 2003;102:2387–2394.

111. Arrigoni P, Beretta C, Silvestri D, et al. FLT3 internal tandem duplication in childhood acute myeloid leukaemia: association with hyperleucocytosis in acute promyelocytic leukaemia. *Br J Haematol.* 2003;120:89–92.

112. Meshinchi S, Woods WG, Stirewalt DL, et al. Prevalence and prognostic significance of Flt3 internal tandem duplication in pediatric acute myeloid leukemia. *Blood.* 2001;97:89–94.

113. Iwai T, Yokota S, Nakao M, et al. Internal tandem duplication of the FLT3 gene and clinical evaluation in childhood acute myeloid leukemia. The Children's Cancer and Leukemia Study Group, Japan. *Leukemia.* 1999;13: 38–43.

114. Meshinchi S, Stirewalt DL, Alonzo TA, et al. Activating mutations of RTK/ras signal transduction pathway in pediatric acute myeloid leukemia. *Blood.* 2003;102:1474–1479.

115. Abu-Duhier FM, Goodeve AC, Wilson GA, Care RS, Peake IR, Reilly JT. Identification of novel FLT-3 Asp835 mutations in adult acute myeloid leukaemia. *Br J Haematol.* 2001;113:983–988.

116. Yamamoto Y, Kiyoi H, Nakano Y, et al. Activating mutation of D835 within the activation loop of FLT3 in human hematologic malignancies. *Blood.* 2001;97:2434–2439.

117. Mead AJ, Linch DC, Hills RK, Wheatley K, Burnett AK, Gale RE. FLT3 tyrosine kinase domain mutations are biologically distinct from and have a significantly more favorable prognosis than FLT3 internal tandem duplications in patients with acute myeloid leukemia. *Blood.* 2007;110:1262–1270.

118. Shih LY, Kuo MC, Liang DC, et al. Internal tandem duplication and Asp835 mutations of the FMS-like tyrosine kinase 3 (FLT3) gene in acute promyelocytic leukemia. *Cancer.* 2003;98:1206–1216.

119. Noguera NI, Breccia M, Divona M, et al. Alterations of the FLT3 gene in acute promyelocytic leukemia: association with diagnostic characteristics and analysis of clinical outcome in patients treated with the Italian AIDA protocol. *Leukemia.* 2002;16:2185–2189.

120. Farr C, Gill R, Katz F, Gibbons B, Marshall CJ. Analysis of ras gene mutations in childhood myeloid leukaemia. *Br J Haematol.* 1991;77:323–327.

121. Shimada A, Taki T, Tabuchi K, et al. KIT mutations, and not FLT3 internal tandem duplication, are strongly associated with a poor prognosis in pediatric acute myeloid leukemia with t(8;21): a study of the Japanese Childhood AML Cooperative Study Group. *Blood.* 2006;107:1806–1809.

122. Schnittger S, Kohl TM, Haferlach T, et al. KIT-D816 mutations in AML1–ETO-positive AML are associated with impaired event-free and overall survival. *Blood.* 2006;107:1791–1799.

123. Stevens RF, Hann IM, Wheatley K, Gray RG. Marked improvements in outcome with chemotherapy alone in paediatric acute myeloid leukemia: results of the United Kingdom Medical Research Council's 10th AML trial. MRC Childhood Leukaemia Working Party. *Br J Haematol.* 1998;101:130–140.

124. Groet J, McElwaine S, Spinelli M, et al. Acquired mutations in GATA1 in neonates with Down's syndrome with transient myeloid disorder. *Lancet.* 2003;361:1617–1620.

125. Rainis L, Bercovich D, Strehl S, et al. Mutations in exon 2 of GATA1 are early events in megakaryocytic malignancies associated with trisomy 21. *Blood.* 2003;102:981–986.

126. Hitzler JK, Cheung J, Li Y, Scherer SW, Zipursky A. GATA1 mutations in transient leukemia and acute megakaryoblastic leukemia of Down syndrome. *Blood.* 2003;101:4301–4304.

127. Ge Y, Stout ML, Tatman DA, et al. GATA1, cytidine deaminase, and the high cure rate of Down syndrome children with acute megakaryocytic leukemia. *J Natl Cancer Inst.* 2005;97:226–231.

128. Preudhomme C, Sagot C, Boissel N, et al. Favorable prognostic significance of CEBPA mutations in patients with de novo acute myeloid leukemia: a study from the Acute Leukemia French Association (ALFA). *Blood.* 2002;100: 2717–2723.

129. Liang DC, Shih LY, Huang CF, et al. CEBPα mutations in childhood acute myeloid leukemia. *Leukemia.* 2005;19:410–414.

130. Colombo E, Marine JC, Danovi D, Falini B, Pelicci PG. Nucleophosmin regulates the stability and transcriptional activity of p53. *Nature Cell Biol.* 2002;4: 529–533.

131. Falini B, Mecucci C, Tiacci E, et al. Cytoplasmic nucleophosmin in acute myelogenous leukemia with a normal karyotype. *N Engl J Med.* 2005;352: 254–266.

132. Verhaak RG, Goudswaard CS, van Putten W, et al. Mutations in nucleophosmin (NPM1) in acute myeloid leukemia (AML): association with other gene abnormalities and previously established gene expression signatures and their prognostic significance. *Blood.* 2005;106:3747–3754.

133. Schnittger S, Schoch C, Kern W, et al. Nucleophosmin gene mutations are predictors of favorable prognosis in acute myelogenous leukemia with a normal karyotype. *Blood.* 2005;106:3733–3739.

134. Boissel N, Renneville A, Biggio V, et al. Prevalence, clinical profile, and prognosis of NPM mutations in AML with normal karyotype. *Blood.* 2005;106: 3618–3620.

135. Brown P, McIntyre E, Rau R, et al. The incidence and clinical significance of nucleophosmin mutations in childhood AML. *Blood.* 2007;110:979–985.

136. Bergmann L, Maurer U, Weidmann E. Wilms tumor gene expression in acute myeloid leukemias. *Leuk Lymphoma.* 1997;25:435–443.

137. Lapillonne H, Renneville A, Auvrignon A, et al. High WT1 expression after induction therapy predicts high risk of relapse and death in pediatric acute myeloid leukemia. *J Clin Oncol.* 2006;24:1507–1515.

138. Verstovsek S, Manshouri T, Smith FO, et al. Telomerase activity is prognostic in pediatric patients with acute myeloid leukemia: comparison with adult acute myeloid leukemia. *Cancer.* 2003;97:2212–2217.

139. Baldus CD, Thiede C, Soucek S, Bloomfield CD, Thiel E, Ehninger G. BAALC expression and FLT3 internal tandem duplication mutations in acute myeloid leukemia patients with normal cytogenetics: prognostic implications. *J Clin Oncol.* 2006;24:790–797.

140. Tse W, Meshinchi S, Alonzo TA, et al. Elevated expression of the *AF1q* gene, an *MLL* fusion partner, is an independent adverse prognostic factor in pediatric acute myeloid leukemia. *Blood.* 2004;104:3058–3063.

141. de Bont ES, Fidler V, Meeuwsen T, Scherpen F, Hahlen K, Kamps WA. Vascular endothelial growth factor secretion is an independent prognostic factor for relapse-free survival in pediatric acute myeloid leukemia patients. *Clin Cancer Res.* 2002;8:2856–2861.

142. Lacayo NJ, Meshinchi S, Kinnunen P, et al. Gene expression profiles at diagnosis in de novo childhood AML patients identify FLT3 mutations with good clinical outcomes. *Blood.* 2004;104:2646–2654.

143. Yagi T, Morimoto A, Eguchi M, et al. Identification of a gene expression signature associated with pediatric AML prognosis. *Blood.* 2003;102:1849–1856.

144. Valk PJ, Verhaak RG, Beijen MA, et al. Prognostically useful gene-expression profiles in acute myeloid leukemia. *N Engl J Med.* 2004;350:1617–1628.

145. Wilson CS, Davidson GS, Martin SB, et al. Gene expression profiling of adult acute myeloid leukemia identifies novel biologic clusters for risk classification and outcome prediction. *Blood.* 2006;108:685–696.

146. Sievers EL, Smith FO, Woods WG, et al. Cell surface expression of the multidrug resistance P-glycoprotein (P-170) as detected by monoclonal antibody MRK-16 in pediatric acute myeloid leukemia fails to define a poor prognostic group: a report from the Children's Cancer Group. *Leukemia.* 1995;9:2042–2048.

147. den Boer ML, Pieters R, Kazemier KM, et al. Relationship between major vault protein/lung resistance protein, multidrug resistance-associated protein, P-glycoprotein expression, and drug resistance in childhood leukemia. *Blood.* 1998;91:2092–2098.

148. Arceci RJ. Can multidrug resistance mechanisms be modified? *Br J Haematol.* 2000;110:285–291.

149. Riley LC, Hann IM, Wheatley K, Stevens RF. Treatment-related deaths during induction and first remission of acute myeloid leukaemia in children treated on the Tenth Medical Research Council acute leukaemia trial (MRC AML10). The MCR Childhood Leukaemia Working Party. *Br J Haematol.* 1999;106:436–444.

150. Viehmann S, Teigler-Schlegel A, Bruch J, Langebrake C, Reinhardt D, Harbott J. Monitoring of minimal residual disease (MRD) by real-time quantitative reverse transcription PCR (RQ-RT-PCR) in childhood acute myeloid leukemia with AML1/ETO rearrangement. *Leukemia.* 2003;17:1130–1136.

151. Buonamici S, Ottaviani E, Testoni N, et al. Real-time quantitation of minimal residual disease in inv(16)-positive acute myeloid leukemia may indicate risk for clinical relapse and may identify patients in a curable state. *Blood.* 2002; 99:443–449.

152. Diverio D, Rossi V, Avvisati G, et al. Early detection of relapse by prospective reverse transcriptase–polymerase chain reaction analysis of the PML/ RARalpha fusion gene in patients with acute promyelocytic leukemia enrolled in the GIMEMA-AIEOP multicenter "AIDA" trial. GIMEMA-AIEOP Multicenter "AIDA" Trial. *Blood.* 1998;92:784–789.

153. Martinelli G, Ottaviani E, Testoni N, et al. Disappearance of PML/RAR alpha acute promyelocytic leukemia-associated transcript during consolidation chemotherapy. *Haematologica.* 1998;83:985–988.

154. Basecke J, Cepek L, Mannhalter C, et al. Transcription of AML1/ETO in bone marrow and cord blood of individuals without acute myelogenous leukemia. *Blood.* 2002;100:2267–2268.

155. Nucifora G, Larson RA, Rowley JD. Persistence of the 8;21 translocation in patients with acute myeloid leukemia type M2 in long-term remission. *Blood.* 1993;82:712–715.

156. Weisser M, Haferlach C, Hiddemann W, Schnittger S. The quality of molecular response to chemotherapy is predictive for the outcome of AML1–ETO-positive AML and is independent of pretreatment risk factors. *Leukemia.* 2007;21:1177–1182.

157. San Miguel J, Martinez A, Macedo A, et al. Immunophenotyping investigation of minimal residual disease is a useful approach for predicting relapse in acute myeloid leukemia patients. *Blood.* 1997;90:2465.

158. Sievers EL, Lange BJ, Alonzo TA, et al. Immunophenotypic evidence of leukemia after induction therapy predicts relapse: results from a prospective Children's Cancer Group study of 252 patients with acute myeloid leukemia. *Blood.* 2003;101:3398–3406.

159. Langebrake C, Creutzig U, Dworzak M, et al. Residual disease monitoring in childhood acute myeloid leukemia by multiparameter flow cytometry: the MRD-AML-BFM Study Group. *J Clin Oncol.* 2006;24:3686–3692.

160. Buckley JD, Lampkin BC, Nesbit ME, et al. Remission induction in children with acute non-lymphocytic leukemia using cytosine arabinoside and doxorubicin or daunorubicin: a report from the Children's Cancer Study Group. *Med Pediatr Oncol.* 1989;17:382–390.

161. Yates J, Glidewell O, Wiernik P, et al. Cytosine arabinoside with daunorubicin or Adriamycin for therapy of acute myelocytic leukemia: a CALGB study. *Blood.* 1982;60:454–462.

162. Preisler H, Bjornsson S, Henderson ES, et al. Remission induction in acute nonlymphocytic leukemia: comparison of a seven-day and ten-day infusion of cytosine arabinoside in combination with adriamycin. *Med Pediatr Oncol.* 1979;7:269–275.

163. Gibson BE, Wheatley K, Hann IM, et al. Treatment strategy and long-term results in paediatric patients treated in consecutive UK AML trials. *Leukemia.* 2005;19:2130–2138.

164. Perel Y, Auvrignon A, Leblanc T, et al. Treatment of childhood acute myeloblastic leukemia: dose intensification improves outcome and maintenance therapy is of no benefit: multicenter studies of the French LAME (Leucemie Aigue Myeloblastique Enfant) Cooperative Group. *Leukemia.* 2005;19:2082–2089.

165. Dillman RO, Davis RB, Green MR, et al. A comparative study of two different doses of cytarabine for acute myeloid leukemia: a Phase III trial of Cancer and Leukemia Group B. *Blood.* 1991;78:2520–2526.

166. Bishop JF, Matthews JP, Young GA, et al. A randomized study of high-dose cytarabine in induction in acute myeloid leukemia. *Blood.* 1996;87:1710–1717.

167. Weick JK, Kopecky KJ, Appelbaum FR, et al. A randomized investigation of high-dose versus standard-dose cytosine arabinoside with daunorubicin in patients with previously untreated acute myeloid leukemia: a Southwest Oncology Group study. *Blood.* 1996;88:2841–2851.

168. Becton D, Dahl GV, Ravindranath Y, et al. Randomized use of cyclosporin A (CsA) to modulate P-glycoprotein in children with AML in remission: Pediatric Oncology Group Study 9421. *Blood.* 2006;107:1315–1324.

169. Creutzig U, Zimmermann M, Ritter J, et al. Treatment strategies and long-term results in paediatric patients treated in four consecutive AML-BFM trials. *Leukemia.* 2005;19:2030–2042.

170. Lange BJ, Smith FO, Feusner J, et al. Outcomes in CCG-2961, a Children's Oncology Group Phase 3 trial for untreated pediatric acute myeloid leukemia (AML): a report from the Children's Oncology Group. *Blood.* 2007.

171. Lange BJ, Dinndorf P, Smith FO, et al. Pilot study of idarubicin-based intensive-timing induction therapy for children with previously untreated acute myeloid leukemia: Children's Cancer Group Study 2941. *J Clin Oncol.* 2004; 22:150–156.

172. Wheatley K. Meta-analysis of randomized trials of idarubicin (IDAR) or metozantrone (Mito) versus daunorubicin (DNR) as induction therapy for acute myeloid leukaemia (AML). *Blood.* 1995;86:43A.

173. Woods WG, Kobrinsky N, Buckley JD, et al. Timed-sequential induction therapy improves postremission outcome in acute myeloid leukemia: a report from the Children's Cancer Group. *Blood.* 1996;87:4979–4989.

174. Woods WG, Neudorf S, Gold S, et al. A comparison of allogeneic bone marrow transplantation, autologous bone marrow transplantation, and aggressive chemotherapy in children with acute myeloid leukemia in remission. *Blood.* 2001;97:56–62.

175. Smith FO, Alonzo TA, Gerbing RB, Woods WG, Arceci RJ. Long-term results of children with acute myeloid leukemia: a report of three consecutive Phase III trials by the Children's Cancer Group: CCG 251, CCG 213 and CCG 2891. *Leukemia.* 2005;19:2054–2062.

176. Hann IM, Stevens RF, Goldstone AH, et al. Randomized comparison of DAT versus ADE as induction chemotherapy in children and younger adults with acute myeloid leukemia. Results of the Medical Research Council's 10th AML trial (MRC AML10). Adult and Childhood Leukaemia Working Parties of the Medical Research Council. *Blood.* 1997;89:2311–2318.

177. Heil G, Hoelzer D, Sanz MA, et al. A randomized, double-blind, placebo-controlled, Phase III study of filgrastim in remission induction and consolidation therapy for adults with de novo acute myeloid leukemia. The International Acute Myeloid Leukemia Study Group. *Blood.* 1997;90:4710–4718.

178. Schiffer CA. Hematopoietic growth factors and the future of therapeutic research on acute myeloid leukemia. *N Engl J Med.* 2003;349:727–729.

179. Witz F, Sadoun A, Perrin MC, et al. A placebo-controlled study of recombinant human granulocyte-macrophage colony-stimulating factor administered during and after induction treatment for de novo acute myelogenous leukemia in elderly patients. Groupe Ouest Est Leucemies Aigues Myeloblastiques (GOELAM). *Blood.* 1998;91:2722–2730.

180. Alonzo TA, Kobrinsky NL, Aledo A, Lange BJ, Buxton AB, Woods WG. Impact of granulocyte colony-stimulating factor use during induction for acute myelogenous leukemia in children: a report from the Children's Cancer Group. *J Pediatr Hematol Oncol.* 2002;24:627–635.

181. Creutzig U, Zimmermann M, Lehrnbecher T, et al. Less toxicity by optimizing chemotherapy, but not by addition of granulocyte colony-stimulating factor in children and adolescents with acute myeloid leukemia: results of AML-BFM 98. *J Clin Oncol.* 2006;24:4499–4506.

182. Lehrnbecher T, Zimmermann M, Reinhardt D, Dworzak M, Stary J, Creutzig U. Prophylactic human granulocyte colony-stimulating factor after induction therapy in pediatric acute myeloid leukemia. *Blood.* 2007;109:936–943.

183. Wells RJ, Woods WG, Lampkin BC, et al. Impact of high-dose cytarabine and asparaginase intensification on childhood acute myeloid leukemia: a report from the Children's Cancer Group. *J Clin Oncol.* 1993;11:538–545.

184. Perel Y, Auvrignon A, Leblanc T, et al. Impact of addition of maintenance therapy to intensive induction and consolidation chemotherapy for childhood acute myeloblastic leukemia: results of a prospective randomized trial, LAME 89/91. Leucamie Aique Myeloide Enfant. *J Clin Oncol.* 2002;20:2774–2782.

185. Creutzig U, Ritter J, Zimmermann M, Schellong G. Does cranial irradiation reduce the risk for bone marrow relapse in acute myelogenous leukemia? Unexpected results of the Childhood Acute Myelogenous Leukemia Study BFM-87. *J Clin Oncol.* 1993;11:279–286.

186. Oliansky DM, Rizzo JD, Aplan PD, et al. The role of cytotoxic therapy with hematopoietic stem cell transplantation in the therapy of acute myeloid leukemia in children: an evidence-based review. *Biol Blood Marrow Transplant.* 2007;13:1–25.

187. Ravindranath Y, Yeager AM, Chang MN, et al. Autologous bone marrow transplantation versus intensive consolidation chemotherapy for acute myeloid leukemia in childhood. Pediatric Oncology Group. *N Engl J Med.* 1996;334:1428–1434.

188. Burnett AK, Wheatley K, Goldstone AH, et al. The value of allogeneic bone marrow transplant in patients with acute myeloid leukaemia at differing risk of relapse: results of the UK MRC AML 10 trial. *Br J Haematol.* 2002;118:385–400.

189. Chen AR, Alonzo TA, Woods WG, Arceci RJ. Current controversies: which patients with acute myeloid leukaemia should receive a bone marrow transplantation?—an American view. *Br J Haematol.* 2002;118:378–384.

190. Creutzig U, Reinhardt D. Current controversies: which patients with acute myeloid leukaemia should receive a bone marrow transplantation?—a European view. *Br J Haematol.* 2002;118:365–377.

191. Ravindranath Y, Chang M, Steuber CP, et al. Pediatric Oncology Group (POG) studies of acute myeloid leukemia (AML): a review of four consecutive childhood AML trials conducted between 1981 and 2000. *Leukemia.* 2005;19:2101–2116.

192. Alonzo TA, Wells RJ, Woods WG, et al. Postremission therapy for children with acute myeloid leukemia: the Children's Cancer Group experience in the transplant era. *Leukemia.* 2005;19:965–970.

193. Bornhauser M, Illmer T, Schaich M, Soucek S, Ehninger G, Thiede C. Improved outcome after stem-cell transplantation in FLT3/ITD-positive AML. *Blood.* 2007;109:2264–2265; author reply 2265.

194. Doubek M, Muzik J, Szotkowski T, et al. Is FLT3 internal tandem duplication significant indicator for allogeneic transplantation in acute myeloid leukemia? An analysis of patients from the Czech Acute Leukemia Clinical Register (ALERT). *Neoplasma.* 2007;54:89–94.

195. Yoshimoto G, Nagafuji K, Miyamoto T, et al. FLT3 mutations in normal karyotype acute myeloid leukemia in first complete remission treated with autologous peripheral blood stem cell transplantation. *Bone Marrow Transplant.* 2005;36:977–983.

196. Gale RE, Hills R, Kottaridis PD, et al. No evidence that FLT3 status should be considered as an indicator for transplantation in acute myeloid leukemia (AML): an analysis of 1135 patients, excluding acute promyelocytic leukemia, from the UK MRC AML10 and 12 trials. *Blood.* 2005;106:3658–3665.
197. Grier HE, Gelber RD, Camitta BM, et al. Prognostic factors in childhood acute myelogenous leukemia. *J Clin Oncol.* 1987;5:1026–1032.
198. Pui C-H, Dahl G, Kalwinsky DK. Central nervous system leukemia in children with acute nonlymphoblstic leukemia. *Blood.* 1985;66:1062.
199. Creutzig U, Ritter J, Heyen P, et al. Effect of cranial irradiation on rate of recurrence in children with acute myeloid leukemia: initial results of the AML-BFM-87 study. The AML-BFM Study Group. *Klin Padiatr.* 1992;204:236–245.
200. Craze JL, Harrison G, Wheatley K, Hann IM, Chessells JM. Improved outcome of acute myeloid leukaemia in Down's syndrome. *Arch Dis Child.* 1999;81:32–37.
201. Creutzig U, Ritter J, Vormoor J, et al. Myelodysplasia and acute myelogenous leukemia in Down's syndrome: a report of 40 children of the AML-BFM Study Group. *Leukemia.* 1996;10:1677–1686.
202. Kojima S, Sako M, Kato K, et al. An effective chemotherapeutic regimen for acute myeloid leukemia and myelodysplastic syndrome in children with Down's syndrome. *Leukemia.* 2000;14:786–791.
203. Lie SO, Jonmundsson G, Mellander L, Siimes MA, Yssing M, Gustafsson G. A population-based study of 272 children with acute myeloid leukaemia treated on two consecutive protocols with different intensity: best outcome in girls, infants, and children with Down's syndrome. Nordic Society of Paediatric Haematology and Oncology (NOPHO). *Br J Haematol.* 1996;94:82–88.
204. Ravindranath Y, Steuber CP, Krischer J, et al. High-dose cytarabine for intensification of early therapy of childhood acute myeloid leukemia: a Pediatric Oncology Group study. *J Clin Oncol.* 1991;9:572–580.
205. Robison LL, Nesbit ME, Sather HN, et al. Down syndrome and acute leukemia in children: a 10-year retrospective survey from Children's Cancer Study Group. *J Pediatr.* 1984;105:235–242.
206. Gamis AS, Woods WG, Alonzo TA, et al. Increased age at diagnosis has a significantly negative effect on outcome in children with Down syndrome and acute myeloid leukemia: a report from the Children's Cancer Group Study 2891. *J Clin Oncol.* 2003;21:3415–3422.
207. Hattori H, Matsuzaki A, Suminoe A, Ihara K, Nakayama H, Hara T. High expression of platelet-derived growth factor and transforming growth factor-beta 1 in blast cells from patients with Down syndrome suffering from transient myeloproliferative disorder and organ fibrosis. *Br J Haematol.* 2001;115:472–475.
208. Zipursky A, Thorner P, De Harven E, Christensen H, Doyle J. Myelodysplasia and acute megakaryoblastic leukemia in Down's syndrome. *Leuk Res.* 1994;18:163–171.
209. Grignani F, Fagioli M, Alcalay M, et al. Acute promyelocytic leukemia: from genetics to treatment. *Blood.* 1994;83:10–25.
210. Sanz MA, Martin G, Gonzalez M, et al. Risk-adapted treatment of acute promyelocytic leukemia with all-trans-retinoic acid and anthracycline monochemotherapy: a multicenter study by the PETHEMA group. *Blood.* 2004;103:1237–1243.
211. Au WY, Fung A, Chim CS, et al. FLT-3 aberrations in acute promyelocytic leukaemia: clinicopathological associations and prognostic impact. *Br J Haematol.* 2004;125:463–469.
212. Reiter A, Lengfelder E, Grimwade D. Pathogenesis, diagnosis and monitoring of residual disease in acute promyelocytic leukaemia. *Acta Haematol.* 2004;112:55–67.
213. Lo-Coco F, Breccia M, Diverio D. The importance of molecular monitoring in acute promyelocytic leukaemia. *Best Pract Res Clin Haematol.* 2003;16:503–520.
214. Tallman MS. All-trans-retinoic acid in acute promyelocytic leukemia and its potential in other hematologic malignancies. *Semin Hematol.* 1994;31:38–48.
215. Asou N, Adachi K, Tamura J, et al. All-trans retinoic acid therapy for newly diagnosed acute promyelocytic leukemia: comparison with intensive chemotherapy. The Japan Adult Leukemia Study Group (JALSG). *Cancer Chemother Pharmacol.* 1997;40:S30–35.
216. Fenaux P, Chevret S, Guerci A, et al. Long-term follow-up confirms the benefit of all-trans retinoic acid in acute promyelocytic leukemia. European APL group. *Leukemia.* 2000;14:1371–1377.
217. Tallman MS, Andersen JW, Schiffer CA, et al. All-trans-retinoic acid in acute promyelocytic leukemia. *N Engl J Med.* 1997;337:1021–1028.
218. Falanga A, Rickles FR. Pathogenesis and management of the bleeding diathesis in acute promyelocytic leukaemia. *Best Pract Res Clin Haematol.* 2003;16:463–482.
219. Fenaux P, Chastang C, Chevret S, et al. A randomized comparison of all trans-retinoic acid (ATRA) followed by chemotherapy and ATRA plus chemotherapy and the role of maintenance therapy in newly diagnosed acute promyelocytic leukaemia: the European APL Group. *Blood.* 1999;94:1192–1200.
220. Sanz M, Martinez JA, Barragan E, Martin G, Lo Coco F. All-trans retinoic acid and low-dose chemotherapy for acute promyelocytic leukaemia. *Br J Haematol.* 2000;109:896–897.
221. Fenaux P, De Botton S. Retinoic acid syndrome. Recognition, prevention and management. *Drug Saf.* 1998;18:273–279.
222. Dombret H, Castaigne S, Fenaux P, Chomienne C, Degos L. Induction treatment of acute promyelocytic leukemia using all-trans retinoic acid: controver-

223. Niu C, Yan H, Yu T, et al. Studies on treatment of acute promyelocytic leukemia with arsenic trioxide: remission induction, follow-up, and molecular monitoring in 11 newly diagnosed and 47 relapsed acute promyelocytic leukemia patients. *Blood.* 1999;94:3315–3324.
224. Shen ZX, Chen GQ, Ni JH, et al. Use of arsenic trioxide (As2O3) in the treatment of acute promyelocytic leukemia (APL): II. Clinical efficacy and pharmacokinetics in relapsed patients. *Blood.* 1997;89:3354–3360.
225. Soignet SL, Maslak P, Wang ZG, et al. Complete remission after treatment of acute promyelocytic leukemia with arsenic trioxide. *N Engl J Med.* 1998;339:1341–1348.
226. Wang G, Li W, Cui J, et al. An efficient therapeutic approach to patients with acute promyelocytic leukemia using a combination of arsenic trioxide with low-dose all-trans retinoic acid. *Hematol Oncol.* 2004;22:63–71.
227. Sanz MA. Treatment of acute promyelocytic leukemia. *Hematol Am Soc Hematol Educ Program.* 2006:147–155.
228. Lo-Coco F, Cimino G, Breccia M, et al. Gemtuzumab ozogamicin (Mylotarg) as a single agent for molecularly relapsed acute promyelocytic leukemia. *Blood.* 2004;104:1995–1999.
229. Giles F, Estey E, O'Brien S. Gemtuzumab ozogamicin in the treatment of acute myeloid leukemia. *Cancer.* 2003;98:2095–2104.
230. Powell BL. Effect of consolidation with arsenic trioxide (As$_2$O$_3$) on event-free survival (EFS) and overall survival (OS) among patients with newly diagnosed acute promyelocytic leukemia (APL): North American Intergroup Protocol C9710. ASCO Annual Meeting Proceedings. *J Clin Oncol.* 2007;25 (theme issue):1S.
231. Sanz MA, Labopin M, Gorin NC, et al. Hematopoietic stem cell transplantation for adults with acute promyelocytic leukemia in the ATRA era: a survey of the European Cooperative Group for Blood and Marrow Transplantation. *Bone Marrow Transplant.* 2007;39:461–469.
232. de Botton S, Fawaz A, Chevret S, et al. Autologous and allogeneic stem-cell transplantation as salvage treatment of acute promyelocytic leukemia initially treated with all-trans-retinoic acid: a retrospective analysis of the European acute promyelocytic leukemia group. *J Clin Oncol.* 2005;23:120–126.
233. Ishii E, Oda M, Kinugawa N, et al. Features and outcome of neonatal leukemia in Japan: experience of the Japan infant leukemia study group. *Pediatr Blood Cancer.* 2006;47:268–272.
234. Bresters D, Reus AC, Veerman AJ, van Wering ER, van der Does-van den Berg A, Kaspers GJ. Congenital leukaemia: the Dutch experience and review of the literature. *Br J Haematol.* 2002;117:513–524.
235. Grundy RG, Martinez A, Kempski H, Malone M, Atherton D. Spontaneous remission of congenital leukemia: a case for conservative treatment. *J Pediatr Hematol Oncol.* 2000;22:252–255.
236. Sande JE, Arceci RJ, Lampkin BC. Congenital and neonatal leukemia. *Semin Perinatol.* 1999;23:274–285.
237. Tavernier E, Le QH, Elhamri M, Thomas X. Salvage therapy in refractory acute myeloid leukemia: prediction of outcome based on analysis of prognostic factors. *Leuk Res.* 2003;27:205–214.
238. Estey EH. Treatment of relapsed and refractory acute myelogenous leukemia. *Leukemia.* 2000;14:476–479.
239. Gibson BE, Webb D, Wheatley K. Does transplant in first CR have a role in pediatric AML? A review of the MRC10 and 12 trials. *Blood.* 2000;96:522a.
240. Casper J, Camitta B, Truitt R, et al. Unrelated bone marrow donor transplants for children with leukemia or myelodysplasia. *Blood.* 1995;85:2354–2363.
241. Davies SM, Wagner JE, Shu XO, et al. Unrelated donor bone marrow transplantation for children with acute leukemia. *J Clin Oncol.* 1997;15:557–565.
242. Abrahamsson J, Clausen N, Gustafsson G, et al. Improved outcome after relapse in children with acute myeloid leukaemia. *Br J Haematol.* 2007;136:229–236.
243. Dahl GV, Lacayo NJ, Brophy N, et al. Mitoxantrone, etoposide, and cyclosporine therapy in pediatric patients with recurrent or refractory acute myeloid leukemia. *J Clin Oncol.* 2000;18:1867–1875.
244. Ferrara F, Melillo L, Montillo M, et al. Fludarabine, cytarabine, and G-CSF (FLAG) for the treatment of acute myeloid leukemia relapsing after autologous stem cell transplantation. *Ann Hematol.* 1999;78:380–384.
245. Fleischhack G, Graf N, Hasan C, et al. IDA-FLAG (idarubicin, fludarabine, high dosage cytarabine and G-CSF): an effective therapy regimen in treatment of recurrent acute myeloid leukemia in children and adolescents. Initial results of a pilot study. *Klin Padiatr.* 1996;208:229–235.
246. Steinmetz HT, Schulz A, Staib P, et al. Phase II trial of idarubicin, fludarabine, cytosine arabinoside, and filgrastim (Ida-FLAG) for treatment of refractory, relapsed, and secondary AML. *Ann Hematol.* 1999;78:418–425.
247. Wells RJ, Adams MT, Alonzo TA, et al. Mitoxantrone and cytarabine induction, high-dose cytarabine, and etoposide intensification for pediatric patients with relapsed or refractory acute myeloid leukemia: Children's Cancer Group Study 2951. *J Clin Oncol.* 2003;21:2940–2947.
248. Arceci RJ, Sande J, Lange B, et al. Safety and efficacy of gemtuzumab ozogamicin in pediatric patients with advanced CD33+ acute myeloid leukemia. *Blood.* 2005;106:1183–1188.
249. Karp JE, Ricklis RM, Balakrishnan K, et al. A Phase I clinical-laboratory study of clofarabine followed by cyclophosphamide for adults with refractory acute leukemias. *Blood.* 2007.

250. Faderl S, Verstovsek S, Cortes J, et al. Clofarabine and cytarabine combination as induction therapy for acute myeloid leukemia (AML) in patients 50 years of age or older. *Blood.* 2006;108:45–51.

251. Jeha S, Gandhi V, Chan KW, et al. Clofarabine, a novel nucleoside analog, is active in pediatric patients with advanced leukemia. *Blood.* 2004;103:784–789.

252. Valcarcel D, Martino R, Sureda A, et al. Conventional versus reduced-intensity conditioning regimen for allogeneic stem cell transplantation in patients with hematological malignancies. *Eur J Haematol.* 2005;74:144–151.

253. Meshinchi S, Leisenring WM, Carpenter PA, et al. Survival after second hematopoietic stem cell transplantation for recurrent pediatric acute myeloid leukemia. *Biol Blood Marrow Transplant.* 2003;9:706–713.

254. Grimwade D, Enver T. Acute promyelocytic leukemia: where does it stem from? *Leukemia.* 2004;18:375–384.

255. Brashem-Stein C, Flowers DA, Smith FO, Staats SJ, Andrews RG, Bernstein ID. Ontogeny of hematopoietic stem cell development: reciprocal expression of CD33 and a novel molecule by maturing myeloid and erythroid progenitors. *Blood.* 1993;82:792–799.

256. Larson RA, Sievers EL, Stadtmauer EA, et al. Final report of the efficacy and safety of gemtuzumab ozogamicin (Mylotarg) in patients with CD33–positive acute myeloid leukemia in first recurrence. *Cancer.* 2005;104:1442–1452.

257. Kiyoi H, Naoe T, Nakano Y, et al. Prognostic implication of FLT3 and N-RAS gene mutations in acute myeloid leukemia. *Blood.* 1999;93:3074–3080.

258. Kiyoi H, Towatari M, Yokota S, et al. Internal tandem duplication of the FLT3 gene is a novel modality of elongation mutation which causes constitutive activation of the product. *Leukemia.* 1998;12:1333–1337.

259. Brown P, Levis M, McIntyre E, Griesemer M, Small D. Combinations of the FLT3 inhibitor CEP-701 and chemotherapy synergistically kill infant and childhood *MLL*-rearranged ALL cells in a sequence-dependent manner. *Leukemia.* 2006;20:1368–1376.

260. Levis M, Allebach J, Tse KF, et al. A FLT3–targeted tyrosine kinase inhibitor is cytotoxic to leukemia cells in vitro and in vivo. *Blood.* 2002;99:3885–3891.

261. Levis M, Pham R, Smith BD, Small D. In vitro studies of a FLT3 inhibitor combined with chemotherapy: sequence of administration is important to achieve synergistic cytotoxic effects. *Blood.* 2004;104:1145–1150.

262. Smith BD, Levis M, Beran M, et al. Single-agent CEP-701, a novel FLT3 inhibitor, shows biologic and clinical activity in patients with relapsed or refractory acute myeloid leukemia. *Blood.* 2004;103:3669–3676.

263. Levis M, Murphy KM, Pham R, et al. Internal tandem duplications of the FLT3 gene are present in leukemia stem cells. *Blood.* 2005;106:673–680.

264. Brown P, Levis M, Shurtleff S, Campana D, Downing J, Small D. FLT3 inhibition selectively kills childhood acute lymphoblastic leukemia cells with high levels of FLT3 expression. *Blood.* 2005;105:812–820.

265. Loh ML, Vattikuti S, Schubbert S, et al. Mutations in PTPN11 implicate the SHP-2 phosphatase in leukemogenesis. *Blood.* 2004;103:2325–2331.

266. Karp JE. Farnesyl protein transferase inhibitors as targeted therapies for hematologic malignancies. *Semin Hematol.* 2001;38:16–23.

267. Karp JE. Farnesyl transferase inhibition in hematologic malignancies. *J Natl Compr Cancer Netw.* 2005;3(suppl 1):S37–S40.

268. Gotlib J. Farnesyltransferase inhibitor therapy in acute myelogenous leukemia. *Curr Hematol Rep.* 2005;4:77–84.

269. Emanuel PD, Snyder RC, Wiley T, Gopurala B, Castleberry RP. Inhibition of juvenile myelomonocytic leukemia cell growth in vitro by farnesyltransferase inhibitors. *Blood.* 2000;95:639–645.

270. Guzman ML, Neering SJ, Upchurch D, et al. Nuclear factor-κB is constitutively activated in primitive human acute myelogenous leukemia cells. *Blood.* 2001;98:2301–2307.

271. Guzman ML, Swiderski CF, Howard DS, et al. Preferential induction of apoptosis for primary human leukemic stem cells. *Proc Natl Acad Sci USA.* 2002; 99:16220–16225.

272. Nie Z, Yan Z, Chen EH, et al. Novel SWI/SNF chromatin-remodeling complexes contain a mixed-lineage leukemia chromosomal translocation partner. *Mol Cell Biol.* 2003;23:2942–2952.

273. Wood A, Schneider J, Shilatifard A. Cross-talking histones: implications for the regulation of gene expression and DNA repair. *Biochem Cell Biol.* 2005; 83:460–467.

274. Galm O, Herman JG, Baylin SB. The fundamental role of epigenetics in hematopoietic malignancies. *Blood Rev.* 2006;20:1–13.

275. Baylin SB. Mechanisms underlying epigenetically mediated gene silencing in cancer. *Semin Cancer Biol.* 2002;12:331–337.

276. Occhipinti E, Correa H, Yu L, Craver R. Comparison of two new classifications for pediatric myelodysplastic and myeloproliferative disorders. *Pediatr Blood Cancer.* 2005;44:240–244.

277. Kasahara S, Hara T, Itoh H, et al. Hypoplastic myelodysplastic syndromes can be distinguished from acquired aplastic anaemia by bone marrow stem cell expression of the tumour necrosis factor receptor. *Br J Haematol.* 2002;118: 181–188.

278. Orazi A. Histopathology in the diagnosis and classification of acute myeloid leukemia, myelodysplastic syndromes, and myelodysplastic/myeloproliferative diseases. *Pathobiology.* 2007;74:97–114.

279. Hershman D, Neugut AI, Jacobson JS, et al. Acute myeloid leukemia or myelodysplastic syndrome following use of granulocyte colony-stimulating factors during breast cancer adjuvant chemotherapy. *J Natl Cancer Inst.* 2007; 99:196–205.

280. Montero AJ, Estrov Z, Freireich EJ, Khouri IF, Koller CA, Kurzrock R. Phase II study of low-dose interleukin-11 in patients with myelodysplastic syndrome. *Leuk Lymphoma.* 2006;47:2049–2054.

281. Mannone L, Gardin C, Quarre MC, et al. High-dose darbepoetin alpha in the treatment of anaemia of lower risk myelodysplastic syndrome results of a Phase II study. *Br J Haematol.* 2006;133:513–519.

282. Balleari E, Rossi E, Clavio M, et al. Erythropoietin plus granulocyte colony-stimulating factor is better than erythropoietin alone to treat anemia in low-risk myelodysplastic syndromes: results from a randomized single-centre study. *Ann Hematol.* 2006;85:174–180.

283. Zwierzina H, Suciu S, Loeffler-Ragg J, et al. Low-dose cytosine arabinoside (LD-AraC) vs LD-AraC plus granulocyte/macrophage colony stimulating factor vs LD-AraC plus Interleukin-3 for myelodysplastic syndrome patients with a high risk of developing acute leukemia: final results of a randomized phase III study (06903) of the EORTC Leukemia Cooperative Group. *Leukemia.* 2005;19:1929–1933.

284. Chan G, DiVenuti G, Miller K. Danazol for the treatment of thrombocytopenia in patients with myelodysplastic syndrome. *Am J Hematol.* 2002;71:166–171.

285. Sadek I, Zayed E, Hayne O, Fernandez L. Prolonged complete remission of myelodysplastic syndrome treated with danazol, retinoic acid and low-dose prednisone. *Am J Hematol.* 2000;64:306–310.

286. Silverman LR, Demakos EP, Peterson BL, et al. Randomized controlled trial of azacitidine in patients with the myelodysplastic syndrome: a study of the cancer and leukemia group B. *J Clin Oncol.* 2002;20:2429–2440.

287. List A, Dewald G, Bennett J, et al. Lenalidomide in the myelodysplastic syndrome with chromosome 5q deletion. *N Engl J Med.* 2006;355:1456–1465.

288. Yazji S, Giles FJ, Tsimberidou AM, et al. Antithymocyte globulin (ATG)-based therapy in patients with myelodysplastic syndromes. *Leukemia.* 2003; 17:2101–2106.

289. Yoshimi A, Baumann I, Fuhrer M, et al. Immunosuppressive therapy with anti-thymocyte globulin and cyclosporine A in selected children with hypoplastic refractory cytopenia. *Haematologica.* 2007;92:397–400.

290. Nosslinger T, Reisner R, Koller E, et al. Myelodysplastic syndromes, from French-American-British to World Health Organization: comparison of classifications on 431 unselected patients from a single institution. *Blood.* 2001; 98:2935–2941.

291. Cutler CS, Lee SJ, Greenberg P, et al. A decision analysis of allogeneic bone marrow transplantation for the myelodysplastic syndromes: delayed transplantation for low-risk myelodysplasia is associated with improved outcome. *Blood.* 2004;104:579–585.

292. Hasle H, Baumann I, Bergstrasser E, et al. The International Prognostic Scoring System (IPSS) for childhood myelodysplastic syndrome (MDS) and juvenile myelomonocytic leukemia (JMML). *Leukemia.* 2004;18:2008–2014.

293. Woods WG, Barnard DR, Alonzo TA, et al. Prospective study of 90 children requiring treatment for juvenile myelomonocytic leukemia or myelodysplastic syndrome: a report from the Children's Cancer Group. *J Clin Oncol.* 2002; 20:434–440.

294. Locatelli F, Niemeyer C, Angelucci E, et al. Allogeneic bone marrow transplantation for chronic myelomonocytic leukemia in childhood: a report from the European Working Group on Myelodysplastic Syndrome in Childhood. *J Clin Oncol.* 1997;15:566–573.

295. Davies SM, Wagner JE, Defor T, et al. Unrelated donor bone marrow transplantation for children and adolescents with aplastic anaemia or myelodysplasia. *Br J Haematol.* 1997;96:749–756.

296. Anderson JE, Anasetti C, Appelbaum FR, et al. Unrelated donor marrow transplantation for myelodysplasia (MDS) and MDS-related acute myeloid leukaemia. *Br J Haematol.* 1996;93:59–67.

297. Jurado M, Deeg HJ, Storer B, et al. Hematopoietic stem cell transplantation for advanced myelodysplastic syndrome after conditioning with busulfan and fractionated total body irradiation is associated with low relapse rate but considerable nonrelapse mortality. *Biol Blood Marrow Transplant.* 2002;8:161–169.

298. Webb DK, Passmore SJ, Hann IM, Harrison G, Wheatley K, Chessells JM. Results of treatment of children with refractory anaemia with excess blasts (RAEB) and RAEB in transformation (RAEBt) in Great Britain 1990–99. *Br J Haematol.* 2002;117:33–39.

299. Niemeyer CM, Kratz C. Juvenile myelomonocytic leukemia. *Curr Oncol Rep.* 2003;5:510–515.

300. Hasle H, Arico M, Basso G, et al. Myelodysplastic syndrome, juvenile myelomonocytic leukemia, and acute myeloid leukemia associated with complete or partial monosomy 7. European Working Group on MDS in Childhood (EWOG-MDS). *Leukemia.* 1999;13:376–385.

301. Hasle H, Alonzo TA, Auvrignon A, et al. Monosomy 7 and deletion /q in children and adolescents with acute myeloid leukemia: an international retrospective study. *Blood.* 2007;109:4641–4647.

302. Niemeyer CM, Arico M, Basso G, et al. Chronic myelomonocytic leukemia in childhood: a retrospective analysis of 110 cases. European Working Group on Myelodysplastic Syndromes in Childhood (EWOG-MDS). *Blood.* 1997;89: 3534–3543.

303. Hasle H. Myelodysplastic and myeloproliferative disorders in children. *Curr Opin Pediatr.* 2007;19:1–8.

304. Locatelli F, Nollke P, Zecca M, et al. Hematopoietic stem cell transplantation (HSCT) in children with juvenile myelomonocytic leukemia (JMML): results of the EWOG-MDS/EBMT trial. *Blood.* 2005;105:410–419.

305. Yoshimi A, Niemeyer CM, Bohmer V, et al. Chimaerism analyses and subsequent immunological intervention after stem cell transplantation in patients with juvenile myelomonocytic leukemia. *Br J Haematol.* 2005;129:542–549.

306. Yoshimi A, Bader P, Matthes-Martin S, et al. Donor leukocyte infusion after hematopoietic stem cell transplantation in patients with juvenile myelomonocytic leukemia. *Leukemia.* 2005;19:971–977.

307. Faraci M, Micalizzi C, Lanino E, et al. Three consecutive related bone marrow transplants for juvenile myelomonocytic leukaemia. *Pediatr Transplant.* 2005;9:797–800.

308. Castleberry RP, Emanuel PD, Zuckerman KS, et al. A pilot study of isotretinoin in the treatment of juvenile chronic myelogenous leukemia. *N Engl J Med.* 1994;331:1680–1684.

309. Cario H. Childhood polycythemias/erythrocytoses: classification, diagnosis, clinical presentation, and treatment. *Ann Hematol.* 2005;84:137–145.

310. Cario H, Schwarz K, Debatin KM, Kohne E. Congenital erythrocytosis and polycythemia vera in childhood and adolescence. *Klin Padiatr.* 2004;216: 157–162.

311. Michiels JJ, De Raeve H, Berneman Z, et al. The 2001 World Health Organization and updated European clinical and pathological criteria for the diagnosis, classification, and staging of the Philadelphia chromosome-negative chronic myeloproliferative disorders. *Semin Thromb Hemost.* 2006;32:307–340.

312. Van Maerken T, Hunninck K, Callewaert L, Benoit Y, Laureys G, Verlooy J. Familial and congenital polycythemias: a diagnostic approach. *J Pediatr Hematol Oncol.* 2004;26:407–416.

313. Teofili L, Giona F, Martini M, et al. The revised WHO diagnostic criteria for Ph-negative myeloproliferative diseases are not appropriate for the diagnostic screening of childhood polycythemia vera and essential thrombocythemia. *Blood.* 2007.

314. Randi ML, Putti MC, Scapin M, et al. Pediatric patients with essential thrombocythemia are mostly polyclonal and V617FJAK2 negative. *Blood.* 2006;108: 3600–3602.

315. Papageorgiou T, Theodoridou A, Kourti M, Nikolaidou S, Athanassiadou F, Kaloutsi V. Childhood essential thrombocytosis. *Pediatr Blood Cancer.* 2006; 47:970–971.

316. Weisdorf DJ, Anasetti C, Antin JH, et al. Allogeneic bone marrow transplantation for chronic myelogenous leukemia: comparative analysis of unrelated versus matched sibling donor transplantation. *Blood.* 2002;99:1971–1977.

317. Pocock C, Szydlo R, Davis J, et al. Stem cell transplantation for chronic myeloid leukaemia: the role of infused marrow cell dose. *Hematol J.* 2001;2: 265–272.

318. Pulsipher MA. Treatment of CML in pediatric patients: should imatinib mesylate (STI-571, Gleevec) or allogeneic hematopoietic cell transplant be front-line therapy? *Pediatr Blood Cancer.* 2004;43:523–533.

319. Millot F, Esperou H, Bordigoni P, et al. Allogeneic bone marrow transplantation for chronic myeloid leukemia in childhood: a report from the Société Francaise de Greffe de Moelle et de Therapie Cellulaire (SFGM-TC). *Bone Marrow Transplant.* 2003;32:993–999.

320. Chalandon Y, Roosnek E, Mermillod B, Waelchli L, Helg C, Chapuis B. Can only partial T-cell depletion of the graft before hematopoietic stem cell transplantation mitigate graft-versus-host disease while preserving a graft-versus-leukemia reaction? A prospective Phase II study. *Biol Blood Marrow Transplant.* 2006;12:102–110.

321. Novitzky N, Rubinstein R, Hallett JM, du Toit CE, Thomas VL. Bone marrow transplantation depleted of T cells followed by repletion with incremental doses of donor lymphocytes for relapsing patients with chronic myeloid leukemia: a therapeutic strategy. *Transplantation.* 2000;69:1358–1363.

322. Drobyski WR, Hessner MJ, Klein JP, et al. T-cell depletion plus salvage immunotherapy with donor leukocyte infusions as a strategy to treat chronic-phase chronic myelogenous leukemia patients undergoing HLA-identical sibling marrow transplantation. *Blood.* 1999;94:434–441.

323. Simula MP, Marktel S, Fozza C, et al. Response to donor lymphocyte infusions for chronic myeloid leukemia is dose-dependent: the importance of escalating the cell dose to maximize therapeutic efficacy. *Leukemia.* 2007;21: 943–948.

324. Cummins M, Cwynarski K, Marktel S, et al. Management of chronic myeloid leukaemia in relapse following donor lymphocyte infusion induced remission: a retrospective study of the Clinical Trials Committee of the British Society of Blood & Marrow Transplantation (BSBMT). *Bone Marrow Transplant.* 2005;36:1065–1069.

325. Deininger M, Buchdunger E, Druker BJ. The development of imatinib as a therapeutic agent for chronic myeloid leukemia. *Blood.* 2005;105:2640–2653.

326. O'Brien SG, Guilhot F, Larson RA, et al. Imatinib compared with interferon and low-dose cytarabine for newly diagnosed chronic-phase chronic myeloid leukemia. *N Engl J Med.* 2003;348:994–1004.

327. Champagne MA, Capdeville R, Krailo M, et al. Imatinib mesylate (STI571) for treatment of children with Philadelphia chromosome-positive leukemia: results from a Children's Oncology Group Phase 1 study. *Blood.* 2004;104: 2655–2660.

328. Millot F, Guilhot J, Nelken B, et al. Imatinib mesylate is effective in children with chronic myelogenous leukemia in late chronic and advanced phase and in relapse after stem cell transplantation. *Leukemia.* 2006;20:187–192.

329. Kantarjian H, Talpaz M, O'Brien S, et al. High-dose imatinib mesylate therapy in newly diagnosed Philadelphia chromosome-positive chronic phase chronic myeloid leukemia. *Blood.* 2004;103:2873–2878.

330. Gorre ME, Sawyers CL. Molecular mechanisms of resistance to STI571 in chronic myeloid leukemia. *Curr Opin Hematol.* 2002;9:303–307.

331. Kantarjian H, Pasquini R, Hamerschlak N, et al. Dasatinib or high-dose imatinib for chronic-phase chronic myeloid leukemia after failure of first-line imatinib: a randomized Phase 2 trial. *Blood.* 2007;109:5143–5150.

332. Jabbour E, Kantarjian H, O'Brien S, et al. Sudden blastic transformation in patients with chronic myeloid leukemia treated with imatinib mesylate. *Blood.* 2006;107:480–482.

333. Bhatia R, Holtz M, Niu N, et al. Persistence of malignant hematopoietic progenitors in chronic myelogenous leukemia patients in complete cytogenetic remission following imatinib mesylate treatment. *Blood.* 2003;101:4701–4707.

334. Holtz MS, Forman SJ, Bhatia R. Nonproliferating CML CD34+ progenitors are resistant to apoptosis induced by a wide range of proapoptotic stimuli. *Leukemia.* 2005;19:1034–1041.

335. Cortes J, O'Brien S, Kantarjian H. Discontinuation of imatinib therapy after achieving a molecular response. *Blood.* 2004;104:2204–2205.

336. Breccia M, Diverio D, Pane F, et al. Discontinuation of imatinib therapy after achievement of complete molecular response in a Ph(+) CML patient treated while in long lasting complete cytogenetic remission (CCR) induced by interferon. *Leuk Res.* 2006;30:1577–1579.

337. Rousselot P, Huguet F, Rea D, et al. Imatinib mesylate discontinuation in patients with chronic myelogenous leukemia in complete molecular remission for more than 2 years. *Blood.* 2007;109:58–60.

338. Thornley I, Perentesis JP, Davies SM, Smith FO, Champagne M, Lipton JM. Treating children with chronic myeloid leukemia in the imatinib era: a therapeutic dilemma? *Med Pediatr Oncol.* 2003;41:115–117.

339. Leung W, Hudson M, Zhu Y, et al. Late effects in survivors of infant leukemia. *Leukemia.* 2000;14:1185–1190.

340. Liesner RJ, Leiper AD, Hann IM, Chessells JM. Late effects of intensive treatment for acute myeloid leukemia and myelodysplasia in childhood. *J Clin Oncol.* 1994;12:916–924.

341. Huma Z, Boulad F, Black P, Heller G, Sklar C. Growth in children after bone marrow transplantation for acute leukemia. *Blood.* 1995;86:819–824.

342. Leahey AM, Teunissen H, Friedman DL, Moshang T, Lange BJ, Meadows AT. Late effects of chemotherapy compared to bone marrow transplantation in the treatment of pediatric acute myeloid leukemia and myelodysplasia. *Med Pediatr Oncol.* 1999;32:163–169.

343. Michel G, Socie G, Gebhard F, et al. Late effects of allogeneic bone marrow transplantation for children with acute myeloblastic leukemia in first complete remission: the impact of conditioning regimen without total-body irradiation: a report from the Société Francaise de Greffe de Moelle. *J Clin Oncol.* 1997;15:2238–2246.

344. Leung W, Hudson MM, Strickland DK, et al. Late effects of treatment in survivors of childhood acute myeloid leukemia. *J Clin Oncol.* 2000;18:3273–3279.

Non-Hodgkin Lymphoma and Lymphoproliferative Disorders in Children

Mitchell S. Cairo

Introduction

Approximately 9% of all childhood cancers diagnosed in the United States each year are of the non-Hodgkin lymphoma (NHL) subtype.[1,2] The vast majority of childhood NHLs are high-grade tumors with aggressive clinical behavior. In comparison, the majority of adult NHLs are low- to intermediate-grade tumors with indolent clinical behavior.[1-3] Currently, four major histologic subtypes of childhood NHL are recognized: Burkitt and Burkitt-like (BL and BLL), lymphoblastic lymphoma (LL), diffuse large B-cell lymphoma (DLBCL), and anaplastic large-cell lymphoma (ALCL). The distribution of these four main histologic subtypes is approximately 40% BL/BLL, 30% LL, 20% DLBCL, and 10% ALCL (Table 14-1).[1,4] Another increasingly large group of NHL in children includes those with posttransplant lymphoproliferative disorders (PTLD). The largest group of children with PTLD includes those on immunosuppressive medications following solid organ transplantation.[5,6]

Clinical Presentation and Staging

The majority (70%) of children who present with NHL have advanced disease (ie, Murphy stage III or IV) and/or have metastatic involvement including bone marrow, central nervous system [CNS], and/or bone.[1,7] Children in equatorial Africa with BL (endemic) will commonly present with head and neck involvement, especially jaw involvement, and, less commonly, orbital and paraspinal disease. The sporadic form of BL more common in North America and Europe presents with abdominal involvement and much less commonly with head and neck or paraspinal disease.[1,3,8] The sporadic forms of BL and BLL often are associated with metastatic spread to the bone marrow and/or the CNS. Patients with bone marrow involvement will present with cytopenias and have evidence of L3 lymphoblasts within the bone marrow (Figure 14-1A). Children with greater than 25% involvement with L3 lymphoblasts in the bone marrow are often referred to as B-ALL (acute lymphoblastic leukemia). Children with CNS involvement often present with meningeal involvement (Figure 14-1B), spinal cord compression, cranial and/or peripheral nerve palsies, and/or seizures.[1,3,9]

Childhood lymphoblastic lymphoma commonly presents with a supradiaphragmatic mass, usually either intrathoracic and/or mediastinal. The clinical presentation often includes various forms of respiratory distress and/or signs and symptoms associated with a superior vena caval syndrome.[1,3,8] Besides involving an intrathoracic mass, lymphoblastic lymphoma in children often includes bilateral pleural effusions and splenomegaly and may also involve spread to the bone marrow and/or the CNS. Children presenting with more than 25% of lymphoblastic lymphoma cells in the bone marrow are often diagnosed and treated as having acute T-lymphoblastic leukemia (T-ALL) and treated on ALL treatment protocols.[1,3,8]

Diffuse large B-cell lymphoma in children presents similarly to other forms of B-cell small noncleaved-cell lymphoma (ie, BL and BLL). Approximately 75% of children with DLBCL have advanced disease—ie, stage III (70%)

Table 14-1

Distribution of non-Hodgkin lymphoma in children.

Histology	%	Organs Involved
Burkitt (BL) & Burkitt-like (BLL)	40	Abdomen, head, neck, BM, CNS
Lymphoblastic lymphoma (LL)	30	Mediastinum, lymph nodes, CNS, BM, bone
Diffuse large B-cell lymphoma (DLBCL)	20	Mediastinum, abdomen
Anaplastic large cell lymphoma (ALCL)	10	Skin, mediastinum, liver, spleen, abdomen

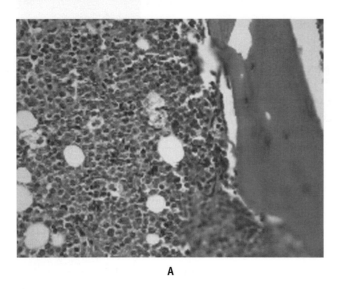
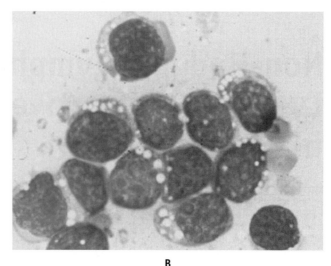

| A | B |

Figure 14-1 (A) Burkitt leukemia involving the bone marrow with complete effacement of normal bone marrow architecture (H&E section, 400X magnification). (B) Cytologic preparation demonstrating Burkitt cells in a cerebral spinal fluid preparation (Wrights stain, 1000X magnification). **See Plates 37 and 38 for color images.**

or, rarely, stage IV (5%).[4] The majority of children with advanced DLBCL present with an abdominal primary lesion and, to a lesser extent, a primary lesion in the mediastinum. Diffuse large B-cell lymphoma in children, however, rarely involves either the CNS and/or bone marrow (fewer than 3% of cases).[10]

Anaplastic large-cell lymphoma has a somewhat different clinical presentation resulting in two categories, systemic and primary cutaneous ALCL.[11] The majority of children with ALCL have advanced stage III/IV disease at diagnosis.[12] In systemic ALCL, 40% to 60% of patients have extranodal disease, most commonly involving the skin, bone, and soft tissue. In contrast, primary cutaneous ALCL is limited to the skin and tends to occur in older patients.[13-15]

Correct staging is critically important at the time of diagnosis in children with NHL because the vast majority present with advanced disease. Historically, the staging system for childhood NHL entailed a modification of the Ann Arbor staging system for Hodgkin disease.[3] The St Jude Children's Research Hospital NHL staging classification, modified from the Ann Arbor system, took into consideration the common presentations of childhood NHL including extranodal involvement, metastatic spread to the bone marrow and CNS, and noncutaneous spread of disease (Table 14-2).[16,17] However, St Jude NHL staging classification is unclear on the definition of extensive primary disease and considers all primary abdominal and thoracic tumors as extensive stage III disease, despite original surgical debulking.[16] Recently, a new French, American, and British (FAB) childhood NHL staging classification was developed (Table 14-3)[18] that better defines the staging of childhood DLBCL, BL, and BLL. This staging classification was utilized in the DLBCL, BL, and BLL international study (FAB/LMB 96) by the Children's Cancer Group (CCG), United Kingdom Children's Cancer

Group (UKCCSG), and the Société Française d'Oncologie Pédiatrique (SFOP) study groups.[19]

Emergent Treatment Principles

Newly diagnosed childhood NHL is associated with several acute emergent conditions that require specific methods of immediate treatment. Because of the high tumor burden and short doubling time in several forms of childhood NHL, especially in BL and LL, children are susceptible to several complications including uric acid (UA) nephropathy and acute tumor lysis syndrome (TLS).[1,20] In addition to the high risk of acute TLS, children are susceptible to other emergencies including superior vena caval syndrome, respiratory distress, acute abdominal emergencies, cardiac tamponade, and/or cranial and peripheral nerve compression and/or palsies.[1] Acute superior vena caval syndrome due to tumor mass compression of the superior vena cava requires emergent use of either local radiotherapy and/or systemic steroids. Tumor lysis syndrome requires rapid treatment with vigorous hydration, diuresis, and hypouricemic therapy with either allopurinol or recombinant urate oxidase enzyme (rasburicase) therapy.[21] A nonrecombinant form of urate oxidase purified from cultures of *Aspergillis flavus* was previously demonstrated by Pui et al[22] to significantly reduce UA levels (median maximal level) (2.3 vs 3.9 mg/dl) ($p < .001$) compared with historical controls in children with hematologic malignancies at risk of TLS. However, there was a 5% incidence of significant allergic complications. We recently demonstrated in a randomized prospective trial comparing rasburicase, the new recombinant form of urate oxidase, and allopurinol in children with hematologic malignancies and a high risk of TLS that rasburicase versus allopurinol significantly lowered mean uric acid $AUC_{0->96}$ (128 ± 70 vs 329 ± 129 mg/dL/h)

Table 14-2

St Jude staging classification for childhood non-Hodgkin lymphoma.

Stage I

A single tumor (extranodal) or single anatomic area (nodal) with the exclusion of mediastinum or abdomen

Stage II

A single tumor (extranodal) with regional node involvement

Two or more nodal areas on the same side of the diaphragm

Two single (extranodal) tumors with or without regional node on the same side of the diaphragm

A primary gastrointestinal tract tumor with or without mesenteric nodes, grossly and completely excised

Stage III

Two single tumors (extranodal) on opposite sides of the diaphragm

Two or more nodal areas above and below the diaphragm

All of the primary intrathoracic tumors (mediastinal, pleural, thymic)

All extensive primary intra-abdominal disease

All paraspinal or epidural tumors, regardless of the other tumor site(s)

Stage IV

Any of the above with initial CNS and/or bone marrow involvement ($<$ 25% malignant cells)

Source: Reproduced from Murphy SB. *N Engl J Med*. 1978; 299:1446.

Table 14-3

FAB staging system for childhood DLBCL, BL, and BLL.

Group A

Completely resected stage I (Murphy)

Completely resected abdominal stage II (Murphy)

Group B

All patients not eligible for Group A or Group C

Group C

Any CNS involvement and/or bone marrow involvement ($\geq$ 25% blasts)

Abbreviations: FAB, French, American, British; CNS, any L3 blast, cranial nerve palsy or compression, intracerebral mass, and/or para-meningeal compression.

Source: Cairo et al. *Med Pediatr Oncol*. 1997; 29:320a.

($p<0.0001$) and 4-hours-post UA by 86% versus 12%, respectively ($p<0.0001$).[21] Furthermore, in the hyperuricemic group, the baseline creatinine level decreased from 144% to 102% by 96 hours following rasburicase.[21] In contrast, the hyperuricemic allopurinol treatment group had a baseline of 132%, which increased over 4 days to 147% of the mean.[21]

Burkitt and Burkitt-like Lymphoma
Pathology of Burkitt and Burkitt-like Lymphoma

Burkitt and Burkitt-like lymphomas are both considered under the combination of small noncleaved-cell lymphomas. Whereas BL is a well-defined clinical, morphologic, and cytogenetic entity, BLL is poorly defined. Due to difficulties among pathologists in diagnostic reproducibility[23] and heterogeneous molecular, cytogenetic, and morphologic features, BLL is considered only as a provisional diagnostic category in the Revised European American Lymphoma (REAL) classification.[24] Burkitt-like lymphoma is not a recognized specific category in the World Health Organization (WHO) classification, where it is included under Burkitt lymphoma as "atypical Burkitt's or Burkitt-like" lymphoma.[11]

The morphologic features of BL include a diffuse, homogeneous proliferation of intermediately sized cells that are larger in size than a lymphocyte but smaller than a centrocyte or large cell (Table 14-4). The cells have smooth round to ovoid nuclear contours and usually 3 to 5 inconspicuous nucleoli. The cytoplasm is moderate to large in size, is intensely basophilic due to a high content of polyribosomes, and contains numerous cytoplasmic vacuoles that are filled with lipid that may be demonstrated with neutral fat stains. These cells are analogous to those seen in ALL-L3 leukemias. Burkitt lymphoma has an extremely high proliferative rate (doubling time of 24 hours),[24] and a starry-sky pattern of reactive macrophages

Table 14-4

Morphologic and immunologic features in childhood NHL.

	DLBCL	Burkitt	Lymphoblastic	ALCL
Morphology				
Cell size	Large	Intermediate	Small to intermediate	Small to large
Nuclear chromatin	Clumped, vesicular	Coarse	Fine, blastic	Clumped, vesicular
Nucleoli	Variable	Variable	Absent	Variable
Cytoplasm	Moderate to abundant	Moderate to scanty with prominent vacuoles	Scanty	Moderate to abundant
Nodal pattern	Diffuse	Diffuse, starry-sky pattern	Diffuse, starry-sky pattern	Sinusoidal or diffuse
Immunophenotype	CD20+, CD22+	CD20+, CD22+	CD2 (80%), CD19 (20%)	T-cell, null cell, CD30+, ALK+

DLBCL, diffuse large B-cell lymphoma; ALCL, anaplastic large-cell lymphoma.

is present. Burkitt-like lymphomas share many morphologic features with BL but tend to display more cellular pleomorphism, variable nuclear irregularities, and variable numbers of nucleoli (Figure 14-2A).

Immunophenotypic features of both BL and BLL are identical. Both are mature B cells, expressing CD19, CD20, CD22, CD10, and cell surface immunoglobulin (usually IgM) that is light chain restricted.[25] We recently demonstrated 100% of children with BL to express CD20 and CD22 in the international FAB study.[26] More variability in cell-surface antigen expression (CD10) and mitotic rate is seen in the BLL or atypical BL.[27] Some studies also suggest that BLL has a higher immunophenotypic expression of BCL-6, similar to that of B-LCL, than does BL.[28]

Genetic Features of Burkitt and Burkitt-like Lymphomas

Cytogenetic analysis of BL has demonstrated characteristic translocations involving the c-myc oncogene locus on chromosome 8, including t(8;14)(q24;q32) in about 80% of cases, with the remaining 20% of cases demonstrating t(2;8)(p11;q24) or t(8;22)(q24;q11) translocations. These translocations will juxtapose c-myc to immunoglobulin genes (heavy chain, kappa, or lambda light chain loci) leading to inappropriate overexpression of the oncogene.[29,30] The translocations seen in BLL are much more heterogeneous and include translocations involving one or more components of the c-myc locus, the BCL-2 locus, or other sporadic translocations that are not associated with c-myc.

We recently analyzed the cytogenetics in 182 cases of BL and 18 cases of BLL in children with advanced B-NHL treated on the FAB/LMB96 study. This study represents the largest series (200 cases) of cytogenetic cases of childhood BL and BLL analyzed to date.[31,32] C-myc rearrangements were identical in 92% of BL and 83% of BLL. The next

most common abnormality identified was dup (1q) in 27% of the c-myc rearrangement cases. Additionally, cytogenetic abnormalities with the c-myc rearrangement included 13q deletion or rearrangement (17%), del (6q) (11%), del (17p) (5%), and 11q abnormalities (2.5%). In only approximately one-third of cases was c-myc rearrangement the only clonal abnormality (Table 14-5).[31,32]

Treatment of Limited-Disease Burkitt Lymphoma and Burkitt-like Lymphoma

Similar to the case with limited-disease DLBCL, children with limited-disease BL and BLL, either Murphy stage I/stage II, CCG limited stage, or FAB Group A, have a superb prognosis with an estimated 5-year event-free survival (EFS) equal to or exceeding 95% (Table 14-6). As with limited-disease childhood DLBCL, any radiotherapy has been eliminated in the treatment regimen. Surgery is critically important for diagnosis and accurate staging. With minimal chemotherapy (from 6 weeks to 6 months), the prognosis is superb (exceeding 95% 5-year EFS).[33–38] There are several multiagent chemotherapy regimens that have been utilized by a variety of pediatric cooperative groups that have resulted in this excellent outcome, including cyclophosphamide, vincristine, prednis(ol)one, and doxorubicin (COPAD) (6 weeks' duration) (SFOP) (FAB), cyclophosphamide, vincristine, methotrexate, and prednisone (COMP) (3 to 6 months' duration) (CCG and Pediatric Oncology Group [POG]), or cyclophosphamide and prednisone (CP) followed by dexamethasone/ifosfamide/Ara-C/VP-16/methotrexate and dexamethasone/cyclophosphamide/methotrexate/doxorubicin Berlin-Frankfurt-Münster (BFM) (12 weeks' duration) (Table 14-6).[33–38] In the FAB study of children with Group A or limited-stage disease, 83 patients had either BL or BLL and received 2 cycles (6 weeks' duration) of COPAD and had a 3-year EFS of 99%.[38]

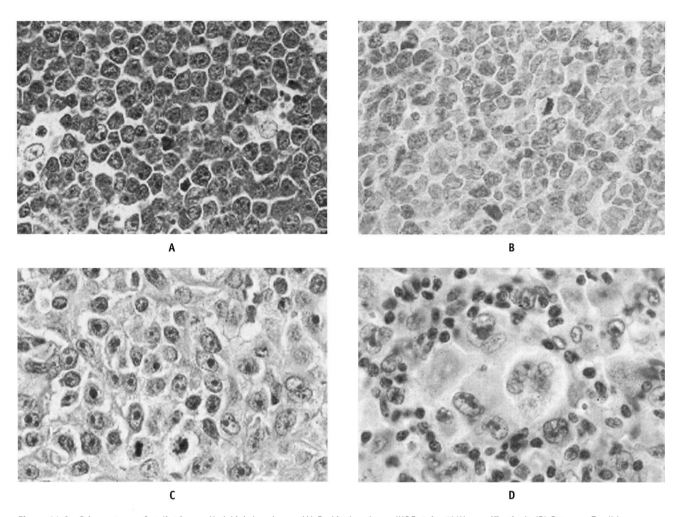

Figure 14-2 Primary types of pediatric non-Hodgkin's lymphoma. (A) Burkitt lymphoma (H&E stain, 400X magnification). (B) Precursor T-cell lymphoblastic lymphoma/leukemia (H&E stain of lymph node, 400X magnification). (C) Diffuse large B-cell lymphoma (H&E stain, 400X magnification). (D) Anaplastic large-cell lymphoma, *CD30* positive and *ALK-1* positive (H&E stain, 400 X magnification). **See Plates 39–42 for color images.**

Table 14-5

Genetic features of childhood non-Hodgkin lymphoma.

DLBCL	Burkitt	Lymphoblastic	Anaplastic Large Cell
t(8;14)(q24;q32)	t(8;14)(q24;q32)	T-cell receptor rearrangements (Tα, Tβ, Tδ, Tγ)	t(2;5)(p23;q25)
12 gain	t(8;22)(q24;q11)	*TCL-1* t(7;14)(q35;q32) t(14;14) (q11;q32)	*ALK* translocation with chromosome 1, 2, 3, 17
21 gain	t(2;8)(q11;q24)	*TCL-2* t(11;13)(p13;q11)	
15 loss	1q duplication	*TCL-3* t(10;14)(q24;q11)	
3q27 rearrangements	13q abnormality	*TAL-1* t(1;14)(q32;q11)	
6q deletion	6q deletion		
7q gain	17p abnormality		
11q gain	11q abnormality		

Table 14-6

Limited disease DLBCL, BL, and BLL in children.

	CCG Meadows et al[35]	POG Link et al[36]	SFOP Patte et al[34]	BFM Reiter et al[37]	FAB/LMB 96 Gerrard et al[38]
Patients (N)	52	27	52	71	137
Protocol	COMP	COMP	COPAD	CP, DX, IFOS, MTX, Ara-C, VP-16 DX, MTX, CTX, DOX COPAD	
Duration (mo)	6	8	1.5	3	1.5
5-yr EFS (Est)	95%	88%	99%	100%	99%

Abbreviations: DLBCL, diffuse large B-cell lymphoma; BL, Burkitt lymphoma; BLL, Burkitt-like lymphoma; EFS, event-free survival; COMP, cyclophosphamide, vincristine, methotrexate, prednisone; COPAD, cyclophosphamide, vincristine, prednisone, doxorubicin; CP, cyclophosphamide, prednisone; DX, dexamethasone; IFOS, ifosfamide; MTX, methotrexate; Ara-C, cytosine arabinoside; VP-16, etoposide; CTX, cyclophosphamide; DOX, doxorubicin; Est, estimate; mo, months; yr, year.

Treatment of Advanced-Disease Burkitt Lymphoma and Burkitt-like Lymphoma

Four consecutive CCG studies from 1977 through 1995 showed a steady improvement in the 3-year disease-free survival (DFS) in children with advanced BL and BLL.[39] In the original CCG-551 study conducted from 1977 through 1983 utilizing COMP or LSA$_2$L$_2$, the 3-year DFS for advanced-disease BL and BLL was approximately 45%.[39] In the most recent CCG study, CCG-5911, conducted from 1993 through 1995 and utilizing short but intensive chemotherapy consisting of cyclophosphamide, doxorubicin, vincristine, and prednisone (CHOP), ifosfamide + etoposide, and dexamethasone, etoposide, cisplatin, cytosine arabinoside [Ara-C], and L-asparaginase (DECAL) or LMB-89 type therapy, the 3-year DFS improved significantly to 82%.[39,40] Similarly, Patte et al, utilizing an LMB-type regimen of cyclophosphamide, vincristine, prednisone (COP) reduction, cyclophosphamide, vincristine, prednis(ol)one, doxorubicin, and high-dose methotrexate (COPADM) intensification, and cytabarine and etoposide consolidation in children with advanced BL and BLL, demonstrated a 90% 3-year DFS (Table 14-7).[34] Reiter et al, utilizing a BFM approach (BFM95) (R2 and R3) regimens in children with advanced BL and BLL, reported an estimated 4-year EFS of 89% and 74% for bulky-disease B-BL and B-ALL, respectively.[37] Additionally, building on the original success of Total-B therapy, the POG has intensified Total-B therapy with the addition of VP-16 and Ara-C and has recently reported a 83% 3-year DFS in children with advanced BL and BLL (Table 14-7).[41]

We recently reported the results of the international FAB study in children with advanced BL and BLL.[42,43] In patients with BL and BLL with intermediate-risk Group B disease, patients randomized to 13 weeks of therapy with a deletion of maintenance COPADM3 and a 50% reduction in the cyclophosphamide dose in COPADM2 had a greater than 90% 3-year EFS.[42,43] Patients with more advanced disease (BM with or without CNS involvement) receiving standard FAB therapy (Group C) also had an estimated 3-year EFS of 90% (Table 14-7).[43] There were two major subgroups of patients with Group C disease who had a significantly poorer outcome with standard

Table 14-7

Advanced-disease BL and BLL in children.

	CCG Cairo et al[40]	POG Schwenn et al[41]	SFOP Patte et al[34]	BFM Reiter et al[37]	FAB Patte et al[42] Cairo et al[43]
Patients (N)	46	327	368	322	864
Protocol	"ORANGE"	"TOTAL B" + ARA-C/VP-16	"LMB" Group B & C	"BFM" R2 & R3	"FAB/LMB 96" Group B & C
Duration	6 mo	4–5 mo	6 mo	5 mo	31–60 mo
EFS	82%	83%	92%	89%	90%

EFS, event-free survival; mo, months; ORANGE, CHOP + (IFOS + VP-16) + DECAL.

FAB therapy: patients either with a poor response to COP reduction (less than 20% tumor reduction) or with both BM and CNS disease.[44] Furthermore, patients with CNS disease had cranial irradiation omitted in the FAB/LMB 96 study and had a similar outcome to that of patients receiving cranial irradiation treated with similar therapy in LMB89 (80%-85% 3-year EFS).[34,44] These data along with the BFM-NHL 90 and BFM 95 studies suggest that cranial irradiation is not required for patients with CNS involvement at presentation.

Lymphoblastic Lymphoma

Pathology of Lymphoblastic Lymphoma

The term "lymphoblastic lymphoma" embraces a wide spectrum of disease well delineated in both the REAL[24] and WHO[11] classifications, including both precursor T (or B) lymphoblastic leukemia/lymphomas. The designation "lymphoblastic lymphoma" is commonly given when the primary presentation is as a mass lesion with minimal blood and bone marrow involvement, whereas acute lymphoblastic leukemia is commonly used for patients whose primary presentation is in the blood and who have greater than 25% blasts present in the marrow.[11,24] When the primary presentation pattern is not clear, the designation of "leukemia/lymphoma" may be appropriate. Whereas precursor B-cell disease predominates in ALL, most of the lymphomatous presentations are of precursor T-cell derivation (80%-90% T-cell vs 10%-20% B-cell). Precursor T-cell LLs tend to present as mediastinal or upper torso nodal masses, whereas precursor B-cell LLs are more likely to present in the skin, soft tissues, bone, tonsils, or peripheral lymph nodes.[25,45–47]

Morphologic features of LL include diffuse or partial effacement of lymph nodes that may infiltrate interfollicular zones with sparing of benign, reactive follicles. Due to rapid proliferation, a starry-sky pattern derived from the presence of macrophages ingesting apoptotic debris may be present. Cytologically, the neoplastic cells are indistinguishable from those seen in precursor B- or T-ALL. The cells have an immature, blastlike appearance with fine chromatin, inconspicuous or absent nucleoli, and scanty cytoplasm that ranges from pale to slightly basophilic in color with high proliferative rates (Table 14-4).[11,24,25] Some "large-cell" variants may have more abundant cytoplasm and visible nucleoli as well as significant nuclear pleomorphism, corresponding to the L2 morphologic variant seen in precursor B-ALL (Table 14-4, Figure 14-2B).[48,49]

Most immature B- or T-lymphoid blasts express terminal deoxynucleotidyl transferase (TdT).[25] T-cell LL commonly expresses CD1, CD2, CD5, and CD7 along with coexpression of CD4 and/or CD8. Occasionally, both CD4 and CD8 may be absent. CD10 is expressed in 15% to 40% of cases, and occasionally natural killer antigens such as CD57 or CD16 may be seen.[25,49] Precursor B-lymphoblastic lymphomas most often display the immunophenotype of early pre-B or pre B-phenotypes (CD19, CD10, and TdT

with variable CD20, CD22, HLA-Dr, and cytoplasmic immunoglobulin).[25,47]

Genetics of Lymphoblastic Lymphoma in Children

Molecular and cytogenetic features of LL are similar to those commonly found in ALL.[49–51] Precursor T-lymphoblastic lymphomas will commonly display early T-cell gene rearrangements (TCRδ, TCRγ, TCRα, and/or TCRβ).[51] Precursor B-lymphoblastic lymphomas commonly demonstrate clonal immunoglobulin gene rearrangements and lack evidence of somatic hypermutation.[52] Cytogenetic abnormalities are common (50 to 80%) in both B- and T-lymphoblastic lymphomas.[49] T-lymphoblastic lymphoma chromosomal breakpoints have included T-cell receptor (TCR) genes or specific oncogenes TCRαδ (14q11), TRCβ (7q32–36), and TCRγ (7p15). Often the TCR enhancer or promoter elements are translocated and juxtaposed to putative transcription factors.[49,51] Specific oncogenes associated with T-lymphoblastic lymphomas include TCL-1 (14q32) involved in t(7;14)(q35;q32) or t(14;14)(q11;q32), TCL-2 oncogene (11p13) involved in t(11;13)(p13;q11), TCL-3 oncogene (10q24) seen in t(10;14)(q24;q11), and TAL-1 (1p32) involved in t(1;14)(q32;q11) (Table 14-5). Approximately 30% of precursor T-cell neoplasms will demonstrate cytogenetic abnormalities involving these specific loci.[30] Cytogenetic abnormalities in B-lymphoblastic lymphoma include hyperdiploidy and additional material from the 21q locus (near the locus involved in the t(12;21) translocation that gives rise to the TEL/AML1 fusion gene).[47]

Treatment of Limited-Disease Lymphoblastic Lymphoma

Children with limited-disease LL, Murphy stages I and II, have a favorable prognosis with long-term overall survival (OS) of 85% to 90%,[1] but with DFS rates of only 63% to 73%, however (Table 14-8).[35,53,54] The excellent OS rates have been attributed to effective salvage strategies for children who have relapsed after initial less-intensive therapies. In general, children with limited-stage LL have achieved better DFS with ALL-based treatment protocols (Table 14-8).[54–57]

Over the past 20 years, the need for local radiotherapy, especially to the mediastinum, has been virtually eliminated.[33] Although surgery plays a major role in the diagnosis and/or complete resection of limited disease, combination chemotherapy is the mainstay of treatment. Therapeutic approaches have varied and have included CHOP with mercaptopurine and methotrexate (POG),[36] LSA$_2$L$_2$ and COMP (CCG),[35,57] and modified LSA$_2$L$_2$ with the addition of high-dose methotrexate[54] (Table 14-8). Due to the reports of treatment failures after less-intensive B-NHL limited-disease chemotherapy,[35,36,55,57] many pediatric cooperative groups have now adopted histology-specific treatment strategies for limited disease that are similar or identical to the treatment approaches used for advanced-stage (III or IV) LL.[54,56,58,59]

Table 14-8

Limited disease lymphoblastic lymphoma in children.

	CCG Meadows et al[35]	POG Link et al[53]	SFOP Patte et al[54]
Patients (N)	15	50	8
Protocol	COMP	CHOP, MP, MTX	LMT81
Duration (mo)	6–18	2–8	24
5-yr EFS (Est)	67%	63%	73%
5-yr OS (Est)	95%	90–95%	90%

Abbreviations: EFS, event-free survival; OS, overall survival; COMP, cyclophosphamide, vincristine, methotrexate, prednisone; CHOP, cyclophosphamide, doxorubicin, vincristine, prednisone; MP, 6-mercaptopurine; MTX, methotrexate; LMT8, modified LSA$_2$L$_2$ with high-dose methotrexate; Est, estimate; mo, months.

Treatment of Advanced-Disease Lymphoblastic Lymphoma

The prognosis for children with advanced LL improved significantly after the introduction of the 10-drug LSA$_2$L$_2$ regimen by Wollner and colleagues.[60] The selective advantage of this regimen in the treatment of lymphoblastic compared with nonlymphoblastic lymphoma also helped to identify the importance of histology-based treatment strategies in childhood NHL. For example, the 5-year EFS for children with advanced-disease LL treated with LSA$_2$L$_2$ in comparison with COMP were significantly better (64% vs 34%, $p = 0.001$).[55] Recent excellent results have also been demonstrated without the addition of local radiotherapy.[59] Treatment approaches for advanced LL have varied, with many groups adopting ALL-based therapeutic regimens.[59,61,62] Sixty percent to 80% OS has been demonstrated using a variety of multiagent chemotherapy regimens ranging from 12 to 32

months of therapy (Table 14-9).[56,62–67] More recently, superb results have been demonstrated with the BFM NHL-90 protocol. The BFM NHL-90 regimen, which utilizes high-dose methotrexate, dexamethasone, moderate doses of anthracyclines and cyclophosphamide, as well as prophylactic cranial irradiation, with a treatment stratification based upon tumor response to induction therapy, resulted in a 90% EFS.[59] Similarly, the POG has reported improved outcomes for patients with advanced LL with the addition of high-dose methotrexate (HD-MTX) to a Dana-Farber Leukemia Consortium regimen including vincristine, prednisone, doxorubicin, asparaginase, mercaptopurine, and prophylactic cranial radiation therapy. The 3-year EFS in children receiving HD-MTX was 86%, compared with 72% in those who received the same regimen without HD-MTX.[61]

Relapsed Lymphoblastic Lymphoma

The prognosis for children who develop recurrent disease is poor, with less than 10% 5-year OS.[55] In an effort to improve outcome for patients with relapsed disease, intensive reinduction chemotherapy followed by stem cell transplantation (SCT) improved DFS to between 23% and 58%.[68–73] Retrieval chemotherapy is similar to that employed in relapsed childhood ALL. Intensive NHL regimens such as DECAL (dexamethasone, etoposide, cisplatin, high-dose cytarabine, and L-asparaginase)[73] or ICE (ifosfamide, carboplatin, etoposide)[74] have been utilized. The response to salvage chemotherapy is an important predictor of outcome following SCT with improved survival after SCT seen in those patients with chemosensitive disease.[69,71,75] Outcomes following autologous versus allogeneic SCT for recurrent LL from the International Bone Marrow Transplant Registry and Autologous Blood and Marrow Transplant Registry were recently compared.[76] Significantly lower relapse rates were observed following allogeneic SCT; however, higher treatment-related mortality offset any survival benefit. Potential benefits of an allogeneic stem cell source include a graft-versus-lymphoma effect,[75] as well as elimination of the risk of infusing tumor cells, or stem cells damaged by prior therapy.

Table 14-9

Advanced-disease lymphoblastic lymphoma in children.

	BFM Reiter et al[56]	St Jude Dahl et al[62]	EORTC-CLCG Millot et al[63]	DFCI Weinstein et al[65]	UKCCSG Eden et al[67]	CCG Abromowitch et al[68]
Patients (N)	101	24	60	21	95	102
Protocol	NHL-BFM-90	Total Therapy-X	EORTC 58881	APO	UKCCSG 8503	CCG 5941
Duration (mo)	24	32	24	24	24	12
EFS (Est) 3–6 yrs	90%	73%	76%	58%	65%	79%

Abbreviations: EFS, event-free survival; Est, estimate; mo, months; yrs, years.

Diffuse Large B-Cell Lymphoma

Pathologic Features of Childhood Diffuse Large B-Cell Lymphoma

Diffuse large B-cell lymphoma is characterized by a mature B-cell phenotype and B-cell gene rearrangements. Unlike DLBCL in adults, where follicular architecture is more common, childhood DLBCLs are predominantly diffuse neoplasms occurring in lymph nodes or the mediastinum.[25] A small proportion (less than 1% of B-LCL) may be predominantly follicular, with a high proportion occurring in extranodal sites such as the testis.[77] Similar to the case with adult DLBCL, specific subtypes such as primary mediastinal large B-cell lymphoma[78] or T-cell rich large B-cell lymphoma[79] have been described in childhood and adolescent populations. Diffuse large B-cell lymphoma may arise in both nodal and extranodal sites and commonly occur in underlying immunodeficiency states.[25]

Diffuse large B-cell lymphoma displays a large number of morphologic features including large noncleaved cells, large cleaved cells, polylobated cells, and immunoblastic cells (exhibiting a single prominent eosinophilic nucleolus). Although in earlier classifications these morphologic subtypes were separated out, in the REAL and WHO classifications they are all considered together as DLBCL.[11,24] The neoplastic cells demonstrate a nucleus that is larger than the size of a tissue histiocyte or twice the size of a small lymphocyte. The cytoplasm varies from pale to plasmacytoid on some occasions. There may be a significant accompanying infiltrate of reactive T cells accompanying the malignant cells that in some cases may obscure the malignant large B cells (Table 14-4; Figure 14-2C).[79]

All DLBCLs demonstrate a mature B-cell immunophenotype including expression of CD20, CD22, and CD79a in paraffin sections[80] and CD19, CD20, and CD22 by flow cytometry.[25] Most will demonstrate monoclonal cell surface expression of immunoglobulin light chains but will lack CD10, CD5, or TdT.[24] We recently analyzed 94 cases of DLBCL registered and treated on FAB/LMB 96.[26] CD20 was expressed in 98% of cases of DLBCL, CD22 was expressed in 100% of cases, and CD3 was absent in all cases.[26]

Genetics of Childhood Diffuse Large B-Cell Lymphoma

About 30% of adult cases with DLBCL will have a t(14;18)(q32;q21), the translocation seen in follicular center-cell lymphomas involving the BCL-2 oncogene and associated with BCL-2 protein expression that is detectable by immunohistochemistry.[81] However, this translocation has not been well described in childhood DLBCL.[30] We analyzed 29 DLBCL cases by cytogenetics in children treated on the FAB/LMB 96 study.[82] Two children (6.5%) had a 3q27 rearrangement (BCL-6), which occurs in approximately 35% of adults with DLBCL. Translocations associated with the c-myc oncogene, such as t(8;14), may also be seen in childhood DLBCL, suggesting a possible relationship with BLs.[83] Eleven of 29 cases (38%) had evidence of a c-myc rearrangement (8q24) in the international FAB

childhood DLBCL study.[81] Furthermore, gains of chromosomes 12 and/or 21 and loss of chromosome 15 were also frequently observed in children with DLBCL treated on the international FAB study (Table 14-5).[82] These findings suggest a genetic difference between childhood and adult DLBCL.

Treatment of Limited-Disease Diffuse Large B-Cell Lymphoma

Children with limited-disease DLBCL, either Murphy stage I and II, CCG limited stage, or FAB Group A, have a superb prognosis, with an estimated 5-year EFS equal to or exceeding 95% (Table 14-6). Over the past 20 years, there has been significant progress in reducing the amount of therapy required for limited-disease DLBCL and eliminating any need for local radiotherapy. Surgery plays an important role in the diagnosis and/or complete resection of limited-disease DLBCL, and multiagent chemotherapy accounts for the excellent survival recently reported.[34–38] The length of treatment for childhood limited-disease DLBCL ranges from as little as 6 weeks to 6 months of multiagent chemotherapy. Current chemotherapy regimens that have been successfully utilized in this clinical setting include COMP (cyclophosphamide, vincristine, methotrexate, prednisone) (CCG and POG) (3 to 6 months), COPAD (cyclophosphamide, vincristine, prednisone, doxorubicin) (6 weeks' duration) (SFOP), or cyclophosphamide and prednisone (CP) followed by dexamethasone/ifosfamide/Ara-C/VP-16/methotrexate and dexamethasone/cyclophosphamide/methotrexate/doxorubicin (12 weeks' duration) (BFM) (Table 14-6).[33–38] The largest and most recent series to date was reported by the FAB/LMB 96 International Study consisting of the SFOP, the CCG, and the UKCCSG. This international study group reported a 99% 3-year EFS in 44 children and adolescents with DLBCL who received 2 cycles of COPAD, completed their therapy within 6 weeks, and did not require local radiotherapy.[38]

Treatment of Advanced-Disease DLBCL

The prognosis of advanced childhood DLBCL has improved significantly over the past decade.[34,37,40,42,43,84–88] The chemotherapy combinations that have been used for advanced large B-cell (non-anaplastic) childhood lymphoma include "APO" (doxorubicin, prednisone, vincristine) + Ara-C/V-16 (POG), "Orange" (CCG), LMB (SFOP), BFM-NHL (BFM) and FAB/LMB (FAB).[34,37,40,43,85,87,88] The recent use, however, of short but intense chemotherapy such as LMB-89 (SFOP), CCG ("Orange"), BFM-NHL, and FAB/LMB 96 has now resulted in a greater than 90% 3-year survival rate in children with advanced DLBCL.[34,37,40,42,43] The CCG hybrid regimen "Orange," which consists of CHOP-based induction, VP-16/ifosfamide intensification and DECAL intensification, and a similar maintenance phase with a slight decrease in intensity, results in a 90% overall survival rate in children with advanced DLBCL.[40,73] Similarly, Patte et al, utilizing an LMB-type regimen of COP reduction, COPADM (cyclophosphamide, vincristine, prednisone, doxorubicin, methotrexate) intensification, and CYM

(Ara-C and methotrexate) consolidation in children and adolescents with advanced DLBCL, demonstrated a 90% 5-year EFS.[84] Reiter et al, utilizing a BFM approach of cyclophosphamide/prednisone, ifosfamide, methotrexate, dexamethasone, Ara-C, VP-16 and cytarabine/methotrexate/cyclophosphamide/dexamethasone/doxorubicin, demonstrated a 95% 3-year EFS.[37] All three of the above advanced DLBCL approaches have utilized a chemotherapy regimen designed to treat Burkitt and Burkitt-like B-cell NHL. Laver et al, however, utilizing an approach more designed for DLBCL (APO + MTX/Ara-C), demonstrated only a 56% to 70% EFS with this approach.[87] Most recently, the FAB International Study Committee investigated the possibility of reducing therapy in the LMB protocol design in children with advanced DLBCL. Children were randomized to standard LMB Group B (B1) therapy or deletion of the maintenance course (COPADM3) (B2), reduced cyclophosphamide by 50% in COPADM2 (B3), or both (B4). Three-year EFS was equal to or greater than 90% in all arms, demonstrating that COPADM3 could be eliminated from maintenance therapy and cyclophosphamide reduced by 50% in the COPADM2 arm. This new FAB therapy now requires only 13 weeks of therapy (Table 14-10).[42,89]

We recently analyzed the results of both DLBCL and ALCL in children and adolescents registered on NHL protocols in CCG from 1977 through 1995.[90] There were 67 with localized and 212 with advanced disease. The 5-year EFS for localized LCL was 92 ± 3.3%.[90] Patients with advanced disease with an increased lactate dehydrogenase or age less than 5 years had a significantly poorer outcome.[90] The results of the FAB study mentioned above, however, suggest that the prognosis for advanced DLBCL with FAB therapy results in greater than or equal to 80% EFS.[42,89]

Anaplastic Large-Cell Lymphoma

Pathology of Anaplastic Large-Cell Lymphoma

Anaplastic large-cell lymphoma is considered predominantly a peripheral T-cell lymphoma, occasionally null cell or rarely B cell, characterized by expression of CD30 (Ki-1) and two major histological subtypes, systemic (S-ALCL) and primary cutaneous ALCL (C-ALCL).[11] Anaplastic large-cell lymphoma histology is usually characterized by large, pleomorphic, multinucleated cells or cells with eccentric horseshoe-shaped nuclei and abundant clear to basophilic cytoplasm with an area of eosinophilia near the nucleus (termed "hallmark cells").[91] These "hallmark cells" may resemble Reed-Sternberg cells found in Hodgkin disease, although they tend to have less-conspicuous nucleoli compared with Reed-Sternberg cells (Figure 14-2D).

There is morphologic diversity in ALCL, and several morphologic variants have been identified in the REAL and WHO classifications.[11,24] These include the common variant (75%) composed primarily of hallmark cells, the lymphohistiocytic variant (10%) that has a large number of benign histiocytes admixed with neoplastic cells, and the small-cell variant (10%) in which small neoplastic cells predominate and only scattered hallmark cells are visualized. Other (<5%) less well described variants include a sarcomatoid variant, signet ring variant, neutrophil rich variant, and giant cell variant (Table 14-4).[14,92] In the lymph nodes, the neoplastic cells tend to infiltrate in a sinusoidal pattern, mimicking metastatic disease, although diffuse effacement of nodes may also be demonstrated. There is a high propensity of S-ALCL to spread to extranodal tissues (skin, bone, soft tissues) either as the only sites of disease or, more commonly, in association with nodal disease.[92]

Cutaneous ALCL is part of a spectrum of CD30+ T-cell lymphoproliferative disorders that includes the benign entity of lymphomatoid papulosis.[14,93,94] Because CD30-cutaneous lymphoproliferative disorders share overlapping pathologic and clinical features, diagnosis requires careful assessment of clinical, histologic, immunophenotypic, and genetic features. Cutaneous ALCL is a T-cell lymphoma of large, anaplastic cells that are CD30 positive and is limited to the skin. Cutaneous ALCL usually presents as a solitary tumor, nodule, or papule that is composed of larger, pleomorphic cells that infiltrate the upper and deep dermis and extend into the subcutaneous tissues. Epidermal invasion is uncommon, and surrounding inflammation is usually present (Figure 14-3).[94]

Both S-ALCL and C-ALCL express CD30 on the surface by immunohistochemistry.[95] CD30 can also be expressed in DLBCL as well as on the surface of benign cells. The majority of ALCLs have been shown to be of T-cell phenotype (CD2, CD3, CD5, CD7, CD45RO, CD43) or may fail

Table 14-10

Advanced-disease DLBCL in children.

	CCG Cairo et al[40]	POG Laver et al[87]	SFOP Patte et al[34]	BFM Reiter et al[37]	FAB Patte et al[42]
Patients (N)	18	33	62	56	155
Protocol	ORANGE	APO + MTX/ARA-C	LMB-89	BFM	FAB/LMB 96
Duration (mo)	6	12	6	5	3.5
3-yr EFS (Est)	90%	56–70%	90%	95%	90%

Abbreviations: DLBCL, diffuse large B-cell lymphoma; EFS, event-free survival; ORANGE, CHOP + (IFOS + VP-16) + DECAL; APO+, doxorubicin, prednisone, vincristine + VP-16, Ara-C; FAB/LMB, French American British/Lymphoma Mature B-cell; Est, estimate; mo, months; yr, year.

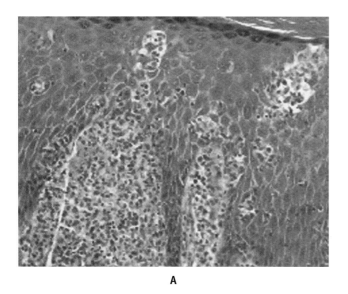
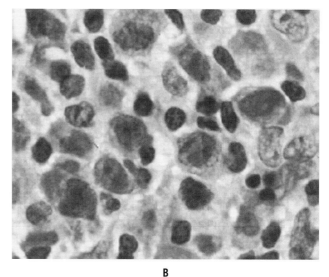

A   B

Figure 14-3 Anaplastic large-cell lymphoma, primary to skin. (A) Section of the skin (H&E stain, 1000X magnification). (B) Malignant infiltrates from primary cutaneous anaplastic large-cell lymphoma demonstrating large anaplastic cells (H&E stain, 1000X magnification). **See Plates 43 and 44 for color images.**

to demonstrate staining with either T- or B-cell markers (null cell). Antigen deletion, especially of CD3, CD5, and/or CD7, is common. Most tumors will express CD4. Expression of cytotoxic antigens, such as TIA-1 or granzyme, and epithelial membrane antigen is commonly observed. *ALK* expression (P80) detects the fusion protein generated by translocations associated with S-ALCL. *ALK* staining is very specific for S-ALCL and is otherwise noted only in brain cells, some rhabdomyosarcomas, and inflammatory myofibroblastic tumors. *ALK* staining is absent in C-ALCL, and if observed, indicates the likelihood that systemic disease is present.[96]

Genetics of Anaplastic Large-Cell Lymphoma

Most S-ALCLs and C-ALCLs demonstrate T-cell receptor gene rearrangements, even when immunophenotypic analysis fails to demonstrate expression of T-cell antigens.[16] Cytogenetic and molecular analyses often demonstrate a characteristic genetic alteration involving the ALK locus on chromosome 2. Classically, this is manifested as the t(2;5)(p23;q35) translocation that places a nucleolar phosphoprotein gene (*NPM1*) adjacent to the *ALK* (anaplastic lymphoma kinase) tyrosine kinase gene.[97] Less common translocations include translocation of *ALK* to partner genes on chromosomes 1, 2, 3, and 17 that also result in up-regulation of *ALK* expression (Table 14-5).[98,99] *ALK* translocations may be detected by conventional cytogenetics, polymerase chain reaction, or fluorescent in situ hybridization using *ALK*-specific probes. The pattern of *ALK* staining is usually nuclear with or without cytoplasmic staining for the t(2;5) and is in the cytoplasm only for many of the alternative translocations.[14] There are greater than 90% *ALK* translocations present in advanced childhood S-ALCL. *ALK* translocations are absent in C-ALCL

and seen with lower frequency in adults.[14,98,99] The presence of an *ALK* translocation or *ALK* protein expression, however, appears to be associated with a better prognosis in adults.[14,81]

Treatment of Limited-Disease Anaplastic Large-Cell Lymphoma

The treatment for limited-disease ALCL has included both intensive B-NHL therapy[100–103] and precursor T-ALL-type protocols based upon the T-cell immunophenotypes that are commonly present in these tumors.[57,104–106] However, optimal therapeutic approaches for limited disease have not been well defined.[12] In a recent report, children with localized (stage I/stage II resected) ALCL achieved 100% EFS with 2 months of chemotherapy including dexamethasone, ifosfamide, methotrexate, cytarabine, etoposide, and prophylactic intrathecal therapy.[100] A 75% EFS has been reported in a small number of children with localized CD30+ large-cell lymphoma, presumably ALCL, treated at St Jude Children's Research Hospital with 3 courses of CHOP, either with or without maintenance with 6–mercaptopurine and methotrexate.[102]

Treatment of Advanced-Disease Anaplastic Large-Cell Lymphoma

The use of CHOP-based therapies over a 6-month period has resulted in greater than 75% 3-year OS.[102,107] Cooperative European studies, using either BFM-NHL or HM 89–91, and the POG study, using an APO regimen (doxorubicin, prednisone, vincristine) in children with advanced-disease ALCL, have demonstrated 65% to 75% 3- to 5-year EFS (Table 14-11).[40,100,101,103,104,108] Children with advanced-disease ALCL treated on NHL-BFM 90 have achieved EFS rates of 76% after receiving short courses of intensive B-NHL therapy, stratified according to disease

Table 14-11

Advanced anaplastic large-cell lymphoma in children.

	BFM Seidemann et al[100]	POG Laver et al[87]	SFOP Brugieres et al[101]	St Jude Sandlund et al[102]	MSKCC Mora et al[104]	CCG Abromowitch et al[108]
Patients (N)	89	67	82	18	19	80
Protocol	NHL-BFM 90	POG 9315	HM89–91	CHOP-based	LSA$_2$L$_2$, LSA$_4$	CCG-5941
Duration (mo)	2–5	12	7–8	6–18	14–36	12
EFS (Est) 2–5 yrs	76%	73%	66%	57%	56%	73%
OS 2–5 yrs	NR	93%	83%	84%	84%	83%

Abbreviations: EFS, event-free survival; Est, estimate; mo, months; OS, overall survival; yrs, years

stage, without local radiotherapy. The maximal duration of treatment was 5 months. Features of this regimen that may have contributed to its success were the use of dexamethasone versus prednisone, the incorporation of ifosfamide, and 24-hour methotrexate infusions with delayed leucovorin rescue.

We recently reported the results of a pilot study (CCG-5941) in children with stage III/IV ALCL (Table 14-11).[108] This study utilized a T-lymphoblastic protocol as a pilot to treat advanced ALCL. Induction therapy consisted of vincristine, prednisone, daunomycin, cyclophosphamide, and L-asparaginase. The intensification phase followed with vincristine, cytosine arabinoside (Ara-C), etoposide (VP-16), high-dose methotrexate, 6–Thioguanine (6 TG), and L-asparaginase. Maintenance therapy consisted of alternating pulses of (1) cyclophosphamide and 6TG; (2) vincristine, prednisone, and doxorubicin; (3) vincristine and high-dose methotrexate; and (4) Ara-C and VP-16. The 3-year EFS and OS rates were 73 ± 6% and 83 ± 5%, respectively.[108]

Several prognostic parameters have been identified in children with advanced-disease ALCL. With small numbers of patients enrolled on current studies and heterogeneous treatment approaches, however, the findings have been inconsistent. Poor-risk prognostic factors that have been identified include organ involvement (liver, lung, spleen), mediastinal involvement, an elevated LDH, and/or disseminated skin disease.[101,109] In the NHL-BFM 90, only the presence of B symptoms was significantly associated with a poor outcome in multivariate analysis.[100] *ALK* expression has not been associated with outcome in children with advanced ALCL, in contrast to adults with ALCL, in whom it has been associated with a favorable outcome.[13]

Relapsed Anaplastic Large-Cell Lymphoma

Chemosensitivity at the time of relapse is a hallmark feature of childhood ALCL and has made salvage strategies for ALCL generally very effective.[100,104,106,107] Relapses in ALCL also tend to occur later than in other histologic subtypes of childhood NHL.[104] The clinical behavior after relapse has been variable, with some patients developing rapidly progressive disease and others having an indolent waxing and waning course.[103] These differences have made uniform treatment approaches difficult.

The outcomes for 41 patients treated for consecutive relapses of ALCL following initial treatment on a series of three clinical trials in France over two decades were recently reported.[110] Three-year OS and DFS rates were 69% and 44%, respectively. Fifteen patients underwent myeloablative therapy with autologous or allogeneic SCT in second remission (CR2). Twenty-one patients received chemotherapy alone, commonly with CBVA (CCNU, bleomycin, vinblastine, Ara-C) or, alternatively, with weekly vinblastine alone. Higher risk for treatment failure included earlier relapse and more intensive initial treatment. Three-year DFS was not significantly different in patients who underwent ablative SCT in CR2 versus those treated with chemotherapy alone (45% vs 52% 3-year DFS).[110] Furthermore, the chemosensitivity of relapsed disease was highlighted by the unexpectedly favorable outcome of 12 children treated with weekly vinblastine alone. Ten of these 12 children achieved a complete remission, and the overall CR2 rate with chemotherapy alone was 85%.

Posttransplant Lymphoproliferative Disorders

Pathology of Posttransplant Lymphoproliferative Disorders

The Society of Hematopathology has developed a classification that recognizes three major morphologic categories of PTLDs: (1) lymphoid hyperplasia, (2) polymorphic PTLD, and (3) lymphomatous or monomorphic PTLD.[110] This classification also recognizes another category that includes other unusual presentations of PTLD such as plasmacytoma, myeloma, Hodgkin disease, and T-cell PTLD.[111,112] The majority of cases express B-cell markers such as CD20 or CD79a.[113] Furthermore, 90% of PTLDs demonstrate intratumoral Epstein-Barr virus (EBV) by either in situ hybridization, EBV early RNA (EBER), or

LMP-1 by immunohistochemistry.[111,114,121] Posttransplant lymphoproliferative disorders following solid organ transplantation in children occurs most commonly in the following highest-risk groups: lung, bowel, combined organ solid organ transplantation, use of OKT3 antibody or tacrolimus, EBV seronegativity at time of transplant, and age less than 5 years.[5,115–118] In contrast, the risk of PTLD following allogeneic SCT in children occurs most commonly in the following high-risk groups: unrelated adult stem cell donors, mismatched donors, T-cell depletion, and recipients who develop grade II-IV acute graft-versus-host disease.[119,120] The most prominent immune defect in both groups of children who develop PTLD following either a solid organ graft or allogeneic stem cell graft is delayed T-cell reconstitution or suppression of specific T-cell EBV cytotoxic T-lymphocytes (EBV-CTL).[118,120]

Genetics in Posttransplant Lymphoproliferative Disorders

Because of the variety of histologic variants, there are not well-described genetic features of PTLD following solid organ transplantation. Polymorphic and monomorphic PTLDs are more likely to show monoclonal gene rearrangements, but they also may be oligoclonal or polyclonal.[111–113] T-cell PTLDs will commonly exhibit clonal T-cell receptor gene rearrangements.[112,122] In patients with monomorphic or lymphomatous PTLD, molecular abnormalities of p53, n-RAS, and/or c-myc have been previously described.[123] Recently, up to 40% of polymorphic PTLDs have been described to have BCL-6 mutations, which have been associated with refractoriness to therapy.[124]

Treatment of Posttransplant Lymphoproliferative Disorders in Children

The mainstay of treatment of PTLD following solid organ transplantation has been a reduction in the intensity of immunosuppressive medications.[125,126] Although this approach has a reasonable success rate in patients with polymorphic histology, less than one-third of children with monomorphic histology respond to simple reduction of immunosuppressive medications.[126] Furthermore, reducing immunosuppressive medications following solid organ transplantation for the treatment of PTLD significantly increases the risk of organ allograft rejection. Successful treatment of PTLD requires controlling EBV-induced B-cell proliferation and transformation and enhancing the development of specific EBV cytotoxic T lymphocytes (EBV-CTLs).[127] Antiviral therapy including acyclovir and, recently, ganciclovir has been suggested as a potential therapeutic approach for EBV-associated PTLD but has not been demonstrated to be effective.[128–130]

Immunomodulation with interferon and/or intravenous gamma globulin has been studied in patients with PTLD following solid organ transplantation but has been associated with mixed results.[131,132] The most successful therapy for EBV-associated PTLD following allogeneic SCT has been the infusion of donor leuko-

cytes from the original donor.[133] Recently, patients with PTLD post solid organ transplantation have also received partially HLA-matched allogeneic EBV-specific CTLs from a frozen bank of CTLs derived from healthy blood donors.[134]

Patients that do not respond to reduction/withdrawal of immunosuppression or develop allograft rejection (refractory PTLD) have had a poor prognosis due to increased risk of treatment-related toxicity. Chemotherapy has been utilized for refractory PTLD because it provides cytotoxic therapy for B-cell lymphoproliferation and immunosuppression to prevent/treat allograft rejection. Results in the treatment of PTLD come mainly from single center, small series—ie, fewer than 20 patients, with nonuniformly treated patients.[132,135–137] Due to the concerns of toxicity and the theoretical risk of conventional dose chemotherapy inhibiting EBV T-cell immunity development, Gross et al conducted an institutional pilot study using a low-dose chemotherapy regimen of cyclophosphamide and prednisone (Cy/Pred) for 36 children with refractory PTLD and demonstrated Cy/Pred to be safe and effective, with a 69% 2-year EFS, but the relapse rate was higher than expected (22%), and there was a 10% allograft failure rate.[138,139]

Early studies with anti-B-cell monoclonal antibodies (anti-CD21 and anti-CD24) suggested a high response rate, but only a 50% long-term DFS in a small number of solid organ transplant recipients who developed PTLD.[140] In further studies with monoclonal anti-B-cell antibodies in patients with PTLD following solid organ transplantation, the long-term DFS is still only around 50% to 55%.[141] A recently developed chimeric antibody that consists of variable regions from the heavy and light chains of the murine anti-CD20 antibody and human IgG1 and kappa constant regions (rituximab) was demonstrated to induce significant responses with and without chemotherapy in adults with low and intermediate non-PTLD-associated B-NHL.[142,143] Most recently, Coiffier et al demonstrated that chemoimmunotherapy (utilizing rituximab and CHOP chemotherapy) compared with chemotherapy alone with CHOP in elderly patients with DLBCL resulted in a significant improvement in DFS and OS.[144] In vitro studies with rituximab and glucocorticoids have demonstrated supra-additive cytotoxicity (apoptosis, complement-dependent cytotoxicity, antibody-dependent cellular cytotoxicity) against nine B-NHL cell lines.[145] Furthermore, rituximab-induced tumor cytotoxicity may be significantly enhanced by antigen-presenting cell (APC)/dendritic cell activation.[146]

Initial studies utilizing monoimmunotherapy (rituximab) in patients with PTLD reported a 65% response rate, with an 18% relapse rate and a 16% mortality rate following rituximab alone.[147] However, in a much larger cohort and with longer follow-up in a multicenter open-label Phase II trial of rituximab therapy in patients with PTLD, the overall response rate was only 46%, with the remainder of patients either progressing or dying on study.[148] These results suggest that while single-agent rituximab therapy may be of some benefit in controlling

EBV-transformed B-cell proliferation, single-agent immunotherapy is not likely to result in a high percentage of long-term sustained complete remissions.

We recently conducted a pilot study combining Cy/Pred with rituximab (CPR).[149] Six children, 2 with fulminant PTLD, were treated with cyclophosphamide (600 mg/m² day 1), prednisone (2 mg/kg/day for 5 days), and rituximab (375 mg/m²/dose intravenous weekly for 3 weeks) for 2 to 4 courses of therapy. Two patients each had a cardiac, liver, and renal transplant with a median onset of PTLD of 39 (10 to 144) months post solid organ allograft. The overall response rate was 100% (5 complete and 1 partial response). All 5 complete responders are currently without disease, and the one partial responder with fulminant PTLD eventually developed progressive disease and died.[149] These data have suggested the potential benefit of combined chemoimmunotherapy and have led to a Children's Oncology Group (COG) trial of CPR in children who develop PTLD following solid organ transplantation following reduced immunosuppression (COG study ANHL0221).

Summary

The prognosis for children with both limited- and advanced-disease NHL has improved significantly over the past 30 years. The 5-year OS rates for limited and advanced disease are approximately 95% and 80%, respectively. The improved survival for childhood NHL, however, is associated with significant morbidity and sometimes prolonged hospitalization. The use of short but intense chemotherapy has resulted in severe hematopoietic and nonhematopoietic toxicity. Furthermore, long-term complications or late effects such as sterility, cardiomyopathy, and secondary malignancies may still develop following multiagent chemotherapy in children with advanced NHL.

The introduction of targeted immunotherapy may not only enhance the prognosis but also provide a synergistic strategy of using combination chemotherapy and immunotherapy in hopes of decreasing the acute and chronic long-term morbidity associated with current multiagent chemotherapy regimens. The COG is currently piloting a new protocol combining rituximab with FAB-type therapy (COMRAP) in their current advanced DLBCL and BL trial (COG ANHL01P1). Furthermore, COG is also investigating the safety and efficacy of targeted radioimmunotherapy (ibritumomab-tiuxetin-Y90) (anti-CD20–Yttrium-90) (Zevalin®) in children with recurrent/refractory DLBCL, BL, BLL, and precursor BLL.

Future considerations should include investigating the genomics of childhood NHL. Recent advances in genomic scale gene expression profiling of adult DLBCL have identified subgroups of adults with DLBCL with genetic signatures.[150] Staudt et al, utilizing a "Lymphochip" developed at the National Cancer Institute, performed microarray analyses in a large cohort of adults with DLBCL.[151,152] They demonstrated the clustering of 5 genetic signatures that predicted for prognoses ranging between 15% and 75% with similar CHOP-based chemotherapy.[152,153] Within the current COG ANHL01P1 study, gene expression profiling in childhood and adolescent DLBCL, BL,

and BLL is being performed to determine if similar diagnostic and prognostic subgroups can be identified by this molecular genetic approach.

Future therapeutic strategies for childhood NHL will likely incorporate the development of therapies directed toward surface targets and/or cytogenetic and genetic features. Surface, intracellular, and molecular targets will likely be identified that will alter our treatment approach over the next decade. New approaches for treatment of CNS B-NHL are also required. Furthermore, prevention of the initial transformation to childhood NHL and/or the reduction of acute and long-term complications will be two major themes to investigate in years to come.

Acknowledgments

This research and education was supported in part from grants from the Pediatric Cancer Research Foundation, the Andrew J. Gargiso Foundation, and the National Cancer Institute (P30–CA13696).

The authors would like to thank Linda Rahl for her editorial assistance in the preparation of this manuscript, and Erin Morris, RN, for her assistance in the development of this manuscript. The authors would also like to thank Sherrie Perkins, MD, PhD, and Elizabeth Raetz, MD, for their contributions to this subject matter.

References

1. Sandlund JT, Downing JR, Crist WM. Non-Hodgkin's lymphoma in childhood. *N Engl J Med.* 1996;334:1238–1248.
2. Young JL Jr, Ries LG, Silverberg E, Horm JW, Miller RW. Cancer incidence, survival, and mortality for children younger than age 15 years. *Cancer.* 1986;58:598–602.
3. Perkins SL, Segal GH, Kjeldsberg CR. Classification of non-Hodgkin's lymphomas in children. *Semin Diagn Pathol.* 1995;12:303–313.
4. Cairo MS. Current advances and future strategies in B-large cell lymphoma in children and adolescents. In: Perry MC, ed. *American Society of Clinical Oncology Educational Book.* Alexandria VA: American Society of Clinical Oncology; 2002:512–519.
5. Ho M, Jaffe R, Miller G, et al. The frequency of Epstein-Barr virus infection and associated lymphoproliferative syndrome after transplantation and its manifestations in children. *Transplantation.* 1988;45:719–727.
6. Dror Y, Greenberg M, Taylor G, et al. Lymphoproliferative disorders after organ transplantation in children. *Transplantation.* 1999;67:990–998.
7. Murphy SB, Fairclough DL, Hutchison RE, Berard CW. Non-Hodgkin's lymphomas of childhood: an analysis of the histology, staging, and response to treatment of 338 cases at a single institution. *J Clin Oncol.* 1989;7:186–193.
8. Rappaport H. Tumors of the hematopoietic system. In: *Atlas of Tumor Pathology.* Washington, DC: Armed Forces Institute of Pathology; 1966:241–243.
9. Cairo MS, Sposto R, Perkins SL, et al. Burkitt's and Burkitt-like lymphoma in children and adolescents: a review of the Children's Cancer Group experience. *Br J Haematol.* 2003:120:660–670.
10. Hoover-Regan M, Meadows AT, Sposto R, et al. Treatment and outcome of pediatric large cell lymphoma over 18 years (*n* = 279): The Children's Cancer Group (CCG) experience. *Proc Am Soc Clin Oncol.* 1997(abstract);16:517a.
11. Jaffe E, Harris N, Stein H, Vardiman J, eds. *World Health Organization Classification of Tumors: Tumours of Haematopoietic and Lymphoid Tissues.* Washington, DC: IARC Press; 2000.
12. Murphy SB. Pediatric lymphomas: recent advances and commentary on Ki-1–positive anaplastic large-cell lymphomas of childhood. *Ann Oncol.* 1994;5:31–33.
13. Falini B, Pileri S, Zinzani PL, et al. ALK+ lymphoma: clinico-pathological findings and outcome. *Blood.* 1999;93:2697–2706.
14. Stein H, Foss HD, Durkop H, et al. CD30(+) anaplastic large cell lymphoma: a review of its histopathologic, genetic, and clinical features. *Blood.* 2000;96:3681–3695.
15. Kinney MC, Kadin ME. The pathologic and clinical spectrum of anaplastic large cell lymphoma and correlation with ALK gene dysregulation. *Am J Clin Pathol.* 1999;111:S56–S67.
16. Murphy SB. Classification, staging and end results of treatment of childhood non-Hodgkin's lymphoma: dissimilarities from lymphomas in adults. *Semin Oncol.* 1980;7:332–339.
17. Murphy SB. Childhood non-Hodgkin's lymphoma. *N Engl J Med.* 1978;299:1446.

18. Cairo et al. Matched related allogeneic BMT (ALBMT) in first remission (CR) of acute lymphoblastic leukemia (ALL) with ultra high risk features. *Med Pediatr Oncol.* 1997;29:320a.

19. Cairo MS, Gerrard M, Patte C. A new protocol for treatment of mature B-cell lymphoma/leukaemia (BCLL): FAB LMB 96, a SFOP LMB 96/CCG-5961/UKCCSG NHL 9600 international cooperative study. *Med Pediatr Oncol.* 1997(abstract);29:320a.

20. Shad A, Magrath I. Malignant non-Hodgkin's lymphomas in children. In: Pizzo PA, Poplack DG, eds. *Principles and Practice of Pediatric Oncology.* 3rd ed. Philadelphia: Lippincott-Raven; 1997:545–587.

21. Goldman SC, Holcenberg JS, Finklestein JZ, et al. A randomized comparison between rasburicase and allopurinol in children with lymphoma or leukemia at high risk for tumor lysis. *Blood.* 2001;97:2998–3003.

22. Pui CH, Relling MV, Lascombes F, et al. Urate oxidase in prevention and treatment of hyperuricemia associated with lymphoid malignancies. *Leukemia.* 1997;11:1813–1816.

23. Lones MA, Auperin A, Raphael M, et al. Mature B-cell lymphoma/leukemia in children and adolescents: intergroup pathologist consensus with the revised European-American Lymphoma Classification. *Ann Oncol.* 2000;11:47–51.

24. Harris N, Jaffe E, Stein H, et al. A revised European-American classification of lymphoid neoplasms: a proposal from the International Lymphoma Study Group. *Blood.* 1994;84:1361–1392.

25. Perkins SL. Work-up and diagnosis of pediatric non-Hodgkin's lymphomas. *Pediatr Dev Pathol.* 2000;3:374–390.

26. Perkins SL, Lones MA, Davenport V, Cairo MS. B-cell non-Hodgkin's lymphoma in children and adolescents: surface antigen expression and clinical implications for future targeted bioimmune therapy. A Children's Cancer Group report. *Clin Adv Hematol Oncol.* 2003;1:314–317.

27. Braziel RM, Arber DA, Slovak ML, et al. The Burkitt-like lymphomas: a Southwest Oncology Group study delineating phenotypic, genotypic, and clinical features. *Blood.* 2001;97:3713–3720.

28. Hutchison RE, Finch C, Kepner J, et al. Burkitt lymphoma is immunophenotypically different from Burkitt-like lymphoma in young persons. *Ann Oncol.* 2000;11:35–38.

29. Macpherson N, Lesack D, Klasa R, et al. Small noncleaved, non-Burkitt's (Burkitt-like) lymphoma: cytogenetics predict outcome and reflect clinical presentation. *J Clin Oncol.* 1999;17:1558–1567.

30. Goldsby RE, Carroll WL. The molecular biology of pediatric lymphomas. *J Pediatr Hematol Oncol.* 1998;20:282–296.

31. Sanger WG, Swansbury J, Poirel H, et al. Primary (8q24) and secondary chromosome abnormalities (1q, 6q, 13q, & 17p) are similar in pediatric Burkitt lymphoma/Burkitt leukemia and Burkitt-like lymphoma: a report of the international pediatric B-cell non-Hodgkin lymphoma study (FAB/LMB 96). *Blood.* 2003 (abstract);102:1355.

32. Poirel H, Heerema N, Swansbury J, et al. Prognostic value of recurrent chromosomal alterations in pediatric B-cell non Hodgkin lymphoma (NHL): report of 238 cases from the international FAB/LMB96 study. *Blood.* 2003 (abstract);102:1420.

33. Link MP, Donaldson SS, Berard CW, Shuster JJ, Murphy SB. Results of treatment of childhood localized non-Hodgkin's lymphoma with combination chemotherapy with or without radiotherapy. *N Engl J Med.* 1990;322:1169–1174.

34. Patte C, Auperin A, Michon J, et al. The Societe Francaise d'Oncologie Pediatrique LMB89 protocol: highly effective multiagent chemotherapy tailored to the tumor burden and initial response in 561 unselected children with B-cell lymphomas and L3 leukemia. *Blood.* 2001;97:3370–3379.

35. Meadows AT, Sposto R, Jenkin RD, et al. Similar efficacy of 6 and 18 months of therapy with four drugs (COMP) for localized non-Hodgkin's lymphoma of children: a report from the Children's Cancer Study Group. *J Clin Oncol.* 1989;7:92–99.

36. Link MP, Shuster JJ, Donaldson SS, Berard CW, Murphy SB. Treatment of children and young adults with early-stage non-Hodgkin's lymphoma. *N Engl J Med.* Oct 30 1997;337(18):1259–1266.

37. Reiter A, Schrappe M, Tiemann M, et al. Improved treatment results in childhood B-cell neoplasms with tailored intensification of therapy: A report of the Berlin-Frankfurt-Munster Group Trial NHL-BFM 90. *Blood.* 1999;94:3294–3306.

38. Gerrard M, Cairo MS, Weston C, et al. Excellent survival following two courses of COPAD chemotherapy in children and adolescents with resected localized B-cell non-Hodgkin's lymphoma: results of the FAB/LMB 96 international study. *Br J Haematol.* 2008;doi:10.111/j.1365–2141.2008.07144.x

39. Cairo MS, Sposto R, Perkins SL, et al. Burkitt's and Burkitt-like lymphoma in children and adolescents: a review of the Children's Cancer Group experience. *Br J Haematol.* 2003;120:660–670.

40. Cairo MS, Krailo MD, Morse M, et al. Long-term follow-up of short intensive multiagent chemotherapy without high-dose methotrexate ("Orange") in children with advanced non-lymphoblastic non-Hodgkin's lymphoma. A Children's Cancer Group report. *Leukemia.* 2002;16:594–600.

41. Schwenn MR, Mahmoud HH, Bowman WP, Hutchison RE, Kepner J, Murphy SM. Successful treatment of small noncleaved cell (SNCC) lymphoma and B cell acute lymphoblastic leukemia (B-ALL) with central nervous system (CNS) involvement: a Pediatric Oncology Group (POG) study. *Proc Am Soc Clin Oncol.* 2000 (abstract);19:580a.

42. Patte C, Gerrard M, Auperin A, et al. Results of the randomised international trial FAB LMB 96 for the "intermediate risk" childhood and adolescent B-cell lymphoma: reduced therapy is efficacious. *Proc Am Soc Clin Oncol.* 2003 (abstract);22:796.

43. Cairo MS, Gerrard M, Sposto R, et al. Results of a randomized FAB LMB96 international study in children and adolescents (C+A) with advanced (bone marrow [BM] [B-ALL] and/or CNS) B-NHL (large cell [LCL], Burkitt's [BL] and Burkitt-like [BLL]): Pts with L3 leukemia/CNS– have an excellent prognosis. *Proc Am Soc Clin Oncol.* 2003 (abstract);22:796.

44. Cairo MS, Gerrard M, Sposto R, et al. Results of a randomized international study of high-risk central nervous system B non-Hodgkin lymphoma and B acute lymphoblastic leukemia in children and adolescents. *Blood.* 2007;109:2736–2743.

45. Soslow RA, Baergen RN, Warnke RA. B-lineage lymphoblastic lymphoma is a clinicopathologic entity distinct from other histologically similar aggressive lymphomas with blastic morphology. *Cancer.* 1999;85:2648–2654.

46. Lin P, Jones D, Dorfman DM, Medeiros LJ. Precursor B-cell lymphoblastic lymphoma: a predominantly extranodal tumor with low propensity for leukemic involvement. *Am J Surg Pathol.* 2000;24:1480–1490.

47. Maitra A, McKenna RW, Weinberg AG, Schneider NR, Kroft SH. Precursor B-cell lymphoblastic lymphoma: a study of nine cases lacking blood and bone marrow involvement and review of the literature. *Am J Clin Pathol.* 2001;115:868–875.

48. Picozzi VJ, Jr., Coleman CN. Lymphoblastic lymphoma. *Semin Oncol.* 1990;17:96–103.

49. Thomas DA, Kantarjian HM. Lymphoblastic lymphoma. *Hematol Oncol Clin North Am.* 2001;15:51–95.

50. Raimondi SC. Current status of cytogenetic research in childhood acute lymphoblastic leukemia. *Blood.* 1993;81:2237–2251.

51. Pilozzi E, Muller-Hermelink HK, Falini B, et al. Gene rearrangements in T-cell lymphoblastic lymphoma. *J Pathol.* 1999;188:267–270.

52. Hojo H, Sasaki Y, Nakamura N, Abe M. Absence of somatic hypermutation of immunoglobulin heavy chain variable region genes in precursor B-lymphoblastic lymphoma: a study of four cases in childhood and adolescence. *Am J Clin Pathol.* 2001;116:673–682.

53. Link MP, Shuster JJ, Donaldson SS, Berard CW, Murphy SB. Treatment of children and young adults with early-stage non-Hodgkin's lymphoma. *N Engl J Med.* 1997;337:1259–1266.

54. Patte C, Kalifa C, Flamant F, et al. Results of the LMT81 protocol, a modified LSA2L2 protocol with high dose methotrexate, on 84 children with non-B-cell (lymphoblastic) lymphoma. *Med Pediatr Oncol.* 1992;20:105–113.

55. Anderson J, Jenkin R, Wilson J, et al. Long-term follow-up of patients treated with COMP or LSA₂L₂ therapy for childhood non-Hodgkin's lymphoma: a report of CCG-551 from the Children's Cancer Group. *J Clin Oncol.* 1993;11:1024–1032.

56. Reiter A, Schrappe M, Parwaresch R, et al. Non-Hodgkin's lymphomas of childhood and adolescence: results of a treatment stratified for biologic subtypes and stage—a report of the Berlin-Frankfurt-Munster group. *J Clin Oncol.* 1995;13:359–372.

57. Anderson J, Wilson J, Jenkin D, et al. Childhood non-Hodgkin's lymphoma: the results of a randomized therapeutic trial comparing a 4-drug regimen (COMP) with a 10-drug regimen (LSA₂-L₂). *N Engl J Med.* 1983;308:559–565.

58. Neth O, Seidemann K, Jansen P, et al. Precursor B-cell lymphoblastic lymphoma in childhood and adolescence: clinical features, treatment, and results in trials NHL-BFM 86 and 90. *Med Pediatr Oncol.* 2000;35:20–27.

59. Reiter A, Schrappe M, Ludwig WD, et al. Intensive ALL-type therapy without local radiotherapy provides a 90% event-free survival for children with T-cell lymphoblastic lymphoma: a BFM group report. *Blood.* 2000;95:416–421.

60. Wollner N, Burchenal JH, Lieberman PH, Exelby P, D'Angio G, Murphy ML. Non-Hodgkin's lymphoma in children: a comparative study of two modalities of therapy. *Cancer.* 1976;37:123–134.

61. Asselin B, Shuster JJ, Amylon M, et al. Improved event-free survival (EFS) with high dose methotrexate (HDM) in T-cell lymphoblastic leukemia (T-ALL) and advanced lymphoblastic lymphoma (T-NHL): a Pediatric Oncology Group (POG) study. *Proc Am Soc Clin Oncol.* 2001 (abstract 1464);20:1464.

62. Dahl GV, Rivera G, Pui CH, et al. A novel treatment of childhood lymphoblastic non-Hodgkin's lymphoma: early and intermittent use of teniposide plus cytarabine. *Blood.* 1985;66:1110–1114.

63. Millot F, Suciu S, Philippe N, et al. Value of high-dose cytarabine during interval therapy of a Berlin-Frankfurt-Munster-based protocol in increased-risk children with acute lymphoblastic leukemia and lymphoblastic lymphoma: results of the European Organization for Research and Treatment of Cancer 58881 randomized Phase III trial. *J Clin Oncol.* 2001;19:1935–1942.

64. Sullivan MP, Boyett J, Pullen J, et al. Pediatric Oncology Group experience with modified LSA2–L2 therapy in 107 children with non-Hodgkin's lymphoma (Burkitt's lymphoma excluded). *Cancer.* 1985;55:323–336.

65. Weinstein HJ, Cassady JR, Levey R. Long-term results of the APO protocol (vincristine, doxorubicin [adriamycin], and prednisone) for treatment of mediastinal lymphoblastic lymphoma. *J Clin Oncol.* 1983;1:537–541.

66. Hvizdala EV, Berard C, Callihan T, et al. Lymphoblastic lymphoma in children: a randomized trial comparing LSA2– L2 with the A-COP+ therapeutic regimen. A Pediatric Oncology Group study. *J Clin Oncol.* 1988;6:26–33.

67. Eden OB, Hann I, Imeson J, Cotterill S, Gerrard M, Pinkerton CR. Treatment of advanced stage T cell lymphoblastic lymphoma: results of the United Kingdom Children's Cancer Study Group (UKCCSG) protocol 8503. *Br J Haematol.* 1992;82:310–316.

68. Abromowitch M, Sposto R, Perkins S, Finlay J, Cairo MS. Results of CCG-5941: intensified multiagent chemotherapy and non-cross resistant maintenance therapy for advanced lymphoblastic lymphoma in children and adolescents.

Presented at the American Society of Hematology Annual Meeting, 2006. *Blood.* 2006;108(11):#533.

69. Bureo E, Ortega JJ, Munoz A, et al. Bone marrow transplantation in 46 pediatric patients with non-Hodgkin's lymphoma. Spanish Working Party for Bone Marrow Transplantation in Children. *Bone Marrow Transplant.* 1995;15: 353–359.

70. Hartmann O, Pein F, Beaujean F, et al. High-dose polychemotherapy with autologous bone marrow transplantation in children with relapsed lymphomas. *J Clin Oncol.* 1984;2:979–985.

71. Mills W, Chopra R, McMillan A, Pearce R, Linch DC, Goldstone AH. BEAM chemotherapy and autologous bone marrow transplantation for patients with relapsed or refractory non-Hodgkin's lymphoma. *J Clin Oncol.* 1995;13:588–595.

72. Sweetenham JW, Liberti G, Pearce R, Taghipour G, Santini G, Goldstone AH. High-dose therapy and autologous bone marrow transplantation for adult patients with lymphoblastic lymphoma: results of the European Group for Bone Marrow Transplantation. *J Clin Oncol.* 1994;12:1358–1365.

73. Kobrinsky NL, Sposto R, Shah NR, et al. Outcomes of treatment of children and adolescents with recurrent non-Hodgkin's lymphoma and Hodgkin's disease with dexamethasone, etoposide, cisplatin, cytarabine, and l-asparaginase, maintenance chemotherapy, and transplantation: Children's Cancer Group Study CCG-5912. *J Clin Oncol.* 2001;19:2390–2396.

74. Kleiner S, Kirsch A, Schwaner I, et al. High-dose chemotherapy with carboplatin, etoposide and ifosfamide followed by autologous stem cell rescue in patients with relapsed or refractory malignant lymphomas: a Phase I/II study. *Bone Marrow Transplant.* 1997;20:953–959.

75. Jones RJ, Ambinder RF, Piantadosi S, Santos GW. Evidence of a graft-versus-lymphoma effect associated with allogeneic bone marrow transplantation. *Blood.* 1991;77:649–653.

76. Levine JE, Harris RE, Loberiza FR Jr, et al. A comparison of allogeneic and autologous bone marrow transplantation for lymphoblastic lymphoma. *Blood.* 2003;101(7):2476–2482.

77. Finn LS, Viswanatha DS, Belasco JB, et al. Primary follicular lymphoma of the testis in childhood. *Cancer.* 1999;85:1626–1635.

78. Lones MA, Perkins SL, Sposto R, et al. Large-cell lymphoma arising in the mediastinum in children and adolescents is associated with an excellent outcome: a Children's Cancer Group report. *J Clin Oncol.* 2000;18:3845–3853.

79. Lones MA, Cairo MS, Perkins SL. T-cell-rich large B-cell lymphoma in children and adolescents: a clinicopathologic report of six cases from the Children's Cancer Group Study CCG-5961. *Cancer.* 2000;88:2378–2386.

80. Chu PG, Chang KL, Arber DA, Weiss LM. Practical applications of immunohistochemistry in hematolymphoid neoplasms. *Ann Diagn Pathol.* 1999;3: 104–133.

81. Gascoyne RD, Adomat SA, Krajewski S, et al. Prognostic significance of Bcl-2 protein expression and Bcl-2 gene rearrangement in diffuse aggressive non-Hodgkin's lymphoma. *Blood.* 1997;90:244–251.

82. Heerema N, Poirel H, Swansbury J, et al. Chromosomal abnormalities of pediatric (ped) and adult diffuse large B-cell lymphoma (DLBCL) differ and may reflect potential differences in oncogenesis: an international pediatric mature B-cell non-Hodgkin lymphoma study (FAB/LMB96). *Blood.* 2003 (abstract 3139);102:3139.

83. Le Beau MM, Rowley JD. Chromosomal abnormalities in leukemia and lymphoma: clinical and biological significance. *Adv Hum Genet.* 1986;15:1–54.

84. Patte C, Philip T, Rodary C, et al. High survival rate in advanced-stage B-cell lymphomas and leukemias without CNS involvement with a short intensive polychemotherapy: results from the French Pediatric Oncology Society of a randomized trial of 216 children. *J Clin Oncol.* 1991;9:123–132.

85. Weinstein H, Lack E, Cassady J. APO therapy for malignant lymphoma on large cell "histiocytic" type of childhood: analysis of treatment for 29 patients. *Blood.* 1984;64:422–426.

86. Hvizdala EV, Berard C, Callihan T, et al. Nonlymphoblastic lymphoma in children: histology and stage-related response to therapy. A Pediatric Oncology Group study. *J Clin Oncol.* 1991;9:1189–1195.

87. Laver JH, Kraveka JM, Hutchison RE, et al. Advanced-stage large-cell lymphoma in children and adolescents: results of a randomized trial incorporating intermediate-dose methotrexate and high-dose cytarabine in the maintenance phase of the APO regimen: a Pediatric Oncology Group phase III trial. *J Clin Oncol.* 2005;23(3):541–547.

88. Sposto R, Meadows AT, Chilcote RR, et al. Comparison of long-term outcome of children and adolescents with disseminated non-lymphoblastic non-Hodgkin lymphoma treated with COMP or daunomycin-COMP: a report from the Children's Cancer Group. *Med Pediatr Oncol.* 2001;37:432–441.

89. Patte C, Auperin A, Gerrard M, et al. Results of the randomized international FAB/LMB96 trial for intermediate risk B-cell non-Hodgkin lymphoma in children and adolescents: it is possible to reduce treatment for the early responding patients. *Blood.* 2007;109:2773–2780.

90. Cairo MS, Sposto R, Hoover-Regan M, et al. Childhood and adolescent large-cell lymphoma (LCL): a review of the Children's Cancer Group experience. *Am J Hematol.* 2003;72:53–63.

91. Benharroch D, Meguerian-Bedoyan Z, Lamant L, et al. ALK-positive lymphoma: a single disease with a broad spectrum of morphology. *Blood.* 1998; 91:2076–2084.

92. Jaffe ES. Anaplastic large cell lymphoma: the shifting sands of diagnostic hematopathology. *Mod Pathol.* 2001;14:219–228.

93. Willemze R, Beljaards RC. Spectrum of primary cutaneous CD30 (Ki-1)-positive lymphoproliferative disorders: a proposal for classification and guidelines for management and treatment. *J Am Acad Dermatol.* 1993;28:973–980.

94. Vergier B, Beylot-Barry M, Pulford K, et al. Statistical evaluation of diagnostic and prognostic features of CD30+ cutaneous lymphoproliferative disorders: a clinicopathologic study of 65 cases. *Am J Surg Pathol.* 1998;22:1192–1202.

95. Falini B, Pileri S, Pizzolo G, et al. CD30 (Ki-1) molecule: a new cytokine receptor of the tumor necrosis factor receptor superfamily as a tool for diagnosis and immunotherapy. *Blood.* 1995;85:1–14.

96. DeCoteau JF, Butmarc JR, Kinney MC, Kadin ME. The t(2;5) chromosomal translocation is not a common feature of primary cutaneous CD30+ lymphoproliferative disorders: comparison with anaplastic large-cell lymphoma of nodal origin. *Blood.* 1996;87:3437–3441.

97. Morris SW, Kirstein MN, Valentine MB, et al. Fusion of a kinase gene, *ALK*, to a nucleolar protein gene, *NPM*, in non-Hodgkin's lymphoma. *Science.* 1994; 263:1281–1284.

98. Drexler HG, Gignac SM, von Wasielewski R, Werner M, Dirks WG. Pathobiology of *NPM-ALK* and variant fusion genes in anaplastic large cell lymphoma and other lymphomas. *Leukemia.* 2000;14:1533–1559.

99. Duyster J, Bai RY, Morris SW. Translocations involving anaplastic lymphoma kinase (ALK). *Oncogene.* 2001;20:5623–5637.

100. Seidemann K, Tiemann M, Schrappe M, et al. Short-pulse B-non-Hodgkin lymphoma-type chemotherapy is efficacious treatment for pediatric anaplastic large cell lymphoma: a report of the Berlin-Frankfurt-Munster Group Trial NHL-BFM 90. *Blood.* 2001;97:3699–3706.

101. Brugieres L, Deley MC, Pacquement H, et al. CD30(+) anaplastic large-cell lymphoma in children: analysis of 82 patients enrolled in two consecutive studies of the French Society of Pediatric Oncology. *Blood.* 1998;92:3591–3598.

102. Sandlund JT, Pui CH, Santana VM, et al. Clinical features and treatment outcome for children with CD30+ large-cell non-Hodgkin's lymphoma. *J Clin Oncol.* 1994;12:895–898.

103. Reiter A, Schrappe M, Tiemann M, et al. Successful treatment strategy for Ki-1 anaplastic large-cell lymphoma of childhood: a prospective analysis of 62 patients enrolled in three consecutive Berlin-Frankfurt-Munster group studies. *J Clin Oncol.* 1994;12:899–908.

104. Mora J, Filippa DA, Thaler HT, Polyak T, Cranor ML, Wollner N. Large cell non-Hodgkin lymphoma of childhood: analysis of 78 consecutive patients enrolled in 2 consecutive protocols at the Memorial Sloan-Kettering Cancer Center. *Cancer.* 2000;88:186–197.

105. Massimino M, Gasparini M, Giardini R. Ki-1 (CD30) anaplastic large-cell lymphoma in childhood. *Ann Oncol.* 1995;6:915–920.

106. Vecchi V, Burnelli R, Pileri S, et al. Anaplastic large cell lymphoma (Ki-1+/ CD30+) in childhood. *Med Pediatr Oncol.* 1993;21:402–410.

107. Sandlund JT, Pui CH, Roberts WM, et al. Clinicopathologic features and treatment outcome of children with large-cell lymphoma and the t(2;5)(p23; q35). *Blood.* 1994;84:2467–2471.

108. Abromowitch M, Sposto R, Perkins SL, Zwick D, Finlay J. Preliminary results of CCG-5941 a pilot study in children and adolescents with anaplastic large cell lymphoma. *Ann Oncol.* 2002(abstract 96);13.

109. Massimino M, Spreafico F, Luksch R, Giardini R. Prognostic significance of p80 and visceral involvement in childhood CD30 anaplastic large cell lymphoma (ALCL). *Med Pediatr Oncol.* 2001;37:97–102.

110. Brugieres L, Quartier P, Le Deley MC, et al. Relapses of childhood anaplastic large-cell lymphoma: treatment results in a series of 41 children. A report from the French Society of Pediatric Oncology. *Ann Oncol.* 2000;11:53–58.

111. Harris NL, Ferry JA, Swerdlow SH. Posttransplant lymphoproliferative disorders: summary of Society for Hematopathology Workshop. *Semin Diagn Pathol.* 1997;14:8–14.

112. Nalesnik MA. The diverse pathology of post-transplant lymphoproliferative disorders: the importance of a standardized approach. *Transpl Infect Dis.* 2001;3:88–96.

113. Pickhardt PJ, Siegel MJ, Hayashi RJ, Kelly M. Posttransplantation lymphoproliferative disorder in children: clinical, histopathologic, and imaging features. *Radiology.* 2000;217:16–25.

114. Ifthikharuddin JJ, Mieles LA, Rosenblatt JD, Ryan CK, Sahasrabudhe DM. CD-20 expression in post-transplant lymphoproliferative disorders: treatment with rituximab. *Am J Hematol.* 2000;65:171–173.

115. Opelz G, Henderson R. Incidence of non-Hodgkin lymphoma in kidney and heart transplant recipients. *Lancet.* 1993;342:1514–1516.

116. Morgan G, Superina RA. Lymphoproliferative disease after pediatric liver transplantation. *J Pediatr Surg.* 1994;29:1192–1196.

117. Cox KL, Lawrence-Miyasaki LS, Garcia-Kennedy R, et al. An increased incidence of Epstein-Barr virus infection and lymphoproliferative disorder in young children on FK506 after liver transplantation. *Transplantation.* 1995; 59:524–529.

118. Haque T, Thomas JA, Parratt R, Hunt BJ, Yacoub MH, Crawford DH. A prospective study in heart and lung transplant recipients correlating persistent Epstein-Barr virus infection with clinical events. *Transplantation.* 1997; 64:1028–1034.

119. Gross TG, Steinbuch M, DeFor T, et al. B cell lymphoproliferative disorders following hematopoietic stem cell transplantation: risk factors, treatment and outcome. *Bone Marrow Transplant.* 1999;23:251–258.

120. Curtis RE, Travis LB, Rowlings PA, et al. Risk of lymphoproliferative disorders after bone marrow transplantation: a multi-institutional study. *Blood.* 1999;94:2208–2216.

121. Lucas KG, Small TN, Heller G, Dupont B, O'Reilly RJ. The development of cellular immunity to Epstein-Barr virus after allogeneic bone marrow transplantation. *Blood.* 1996;87:2594–2603.

122. Sivaraman P, Lye WC. Epstein-Barr virus-associated T-cell lymphoma in solid organ transplant recipients. *Biomed Pharmacother.* 2001;55:366–368.

123. Knowles DM, Cesarman E, Chadburn A, et al. Correlative morphologic and molecular genetic analysis demonstrates three distinct categories of post-transplantation lymphoproliferative disorders. *Blood.* 1995;85:552–565.

124. Cesarman E, Chadburn A, Liu YF, Migliazza A, Dalla-Favera R, Knowles DM. BCL-6 gene mutations in posttransplantation lymphoproliferative disorders predict response to therapy and clinical outcome. *Blood.* 1998;92:2294–2302.

125. Starzl TE, Nalesnik MA, Porter KA, et al. Reversibility of lymphomas and lymphoproliferative lesions developing under cyclosporin-steroid therapy. *Lancet.* 1984;1:583–587.

126. Hayashi RJ, Kraus MD, Patel AL, et al. Posttransplant lymphoproliferative disease in children: correlation of histology to clinical behavior. *J Pediatr Hematol Oncol.* 2001;23:14–18.

127. Gross TG. Treatment of Epstein-Barr virus-associated posttransplant lymphoproliferative disorders. *J Pediatr Hematol Oncol.* 2001;23:7–9.

128. Cohen JI. Epstein-Barr virus lymphoproliferative disease associated with acquired immunodeficiency. *Medicine (Baltimore).* 1991;70:137–160.

129. Katz BZ, Raab-Traub N, Miller G. Latent and replicating forms of Epstein-Barr virus DNA in lymphomas and lymphoproliferative diseases. *J Infect Dis.* 1989;160:589–598.

130. Sixbey JW, Pagano JS. Epstein-Barr virus transformation of human B lymphocytes despite inhibition of viral polymerase. *J Virol.* 1985;53:299–301.

131. Shapiro RS, Chauvenet A, McGuire W, et al. Treatment of B-cell lymphoproliferative disorders with interferon alfa and intravenous gamma globulin. *N Engl J Med.* 1988;318:1334.

132. Davis CL, Wood BL, Sabath DE, Joseph JS, Stehman-Breen C, Broudy VC. Interferon-alpha treatment of posttransplant lymphoproliferative disorder in recipients of solid organ transplants. *Transplantation.* 1998;66:1770–1779.

133. Papadopoulos EB, Ladanyi M, Emanuel D, et al. Infusions of donor leukocytes to treat Epstein-Barr virus-associated lymphoproliferative disorders after allogeneic bone marrow transplantation. *N Engl J Med.* 1994;330:1185–1191.

134. Haque T, Wilkie GM, Taylor C, et al. Treatment of Epstein-Barr-virus-positive post-transplantation lymphoproliferative disease with partly HLA-matched allogeneic cytotoxic T cells. *Lancet.* 2002;360:436–442.

135. Swinnen LJ, Mullen GM, Carr TJ, Costanzo MR, Fisher RI. Aggressive treatment for postcardiac transplant lymphoproliferation. *Blood.* 1995;86:3333–3340.

136. Mamzer-Bruneel MF, Lome C, Morelon E, et al. Durable remission after aggressive chemotherapy for very late post-kidney transplant lymphoproliferation: a report of 16 cases observed in a single center. *J Clin Oncol.* 2000;18:3622–3632.

137. Morrison VA, Dunn DL, Manivel JC, Gajl-Peczalska KJ, Peterson BA. Clinical characteristics of post-transplant lymphoproliferative disorders. *Am J Med.* 1994;97:14–24.

138. Gross TG. Low-dose chemotherapy for treatment of children with PT-LPD. In: Oertel SH, Riess HB, eds. *Recent Results in Cancer Research, Immunosurveillance, Immunodeficiencies and Lymphoproliferations.* Berlin: Springer-Verlag; 2002.

139. Gross TG, Park J, Bucuvalas J, et al. Low-dose chemotherapy for refractory EBV associated post-transplant lymphoproliferative disease (PTLD) following solid organ transplant (SLT) in children. *Blood.* 2002(abstract);100:159a.

140. Fischer A, Blanche S, Le Bidois J, et al. Anti-B-cell monoclonal antibodies in the treatment of severe B-cell lymphoproliferative syndrome following bone marrow and organ transplantation. *N Engl J Med.* 1991;324:1451–1456.

141. Benkerrou M, Jais JP, Leblond V, et al. Anti-B-cell monoclonal antibody treatment of severe posttransplant B-lymphoproliferative disorder: prognostic factors and long-term outcome. *Blood.* 1998;92:3137–3147.

142. Maloney DG, Grillo-Lopez AJ, Bodkin DJ, et al. IDEC-C2B8: results of a Phase I multiple-dose trial in patients with relapsed non-Hodgkin's lymphoma. *J Clin Oncol.* 1997;15:3266–3274.

143. Czuczman MS, Grillo-Lopez AJ, White CA, et al. Treatment of patients with low-grade B-cell lymphoma with the combination of chimeric anti-CD20 monoclonal antibody and CHOP chemotherapy. *J Clin Oncol.* 1999;17:268–276.

144. Coiffier B, Lepage E, Briere J, et al. CHOP chemotherapy plus rituximab compared with CHOP alone in elderly patients with diffuse large-B-cell lymphoma. *N Engl J Med.* 2002;346:235–242.

145. Rose AL, Smith BE, Maloney DG. Glucocorticoids and rituximab in vitro: synergistic direct antiproliferative and apoptotic effects. *Blood.* 2002;100:1765–1773.

146. Selenko N, Maidic O, Draxier S, et al. CD20 antibody (C2B8)-induced apoptosis of lymphoma cells promotes phagocytosis by dendritic cells and cross-priming of CD8+ cytotoxic T cells. *Leukemia.* 2001;15:1619–1626.

147. Milpied N, Vasseur B, Parquet N, et al. Humanized anti-CD20 monoclonal antibody (Rituximab) in post transplant B-lymphoproliferative disorder: a retrospective analysis on 32 patients. *Ann Oncol.* 2000;11:113–116.

148. Choquet S, Leblond V, Herbrecht R, et al. Efficacy and safety of rituximab in B-cell post-transplantation lymphoproliferative disorders: results of a prospective multicenter phase 2 study. *Blood.* 2006;107(8):3053–3057.

149. Orjuela M, Gross TG, Cheung YK, Alobeid B, Morris E, Cairo MS. A pilot study of chemoimmunotherapy (cyclophosphamide, prednisone, and rituximab) in patients with post-transplant lymphoproliferative disorder following solid organ transplantation. *Clin Cancer Res.* 2003;9:3945S-3952S.

150. Alizadeh AA, Eisen MB, Davis RE, et al. Distinct types of diffuse large B-cell lymphoma identified by gene expression profiling. *Nature.* 2000;403:503–511.

151. Klein U, Tu Y, Stolovitzky GA, et al. Gene expression profiling of B cell chronic lymphocytic leukemia reveals a homogeneous phenotype related to memory B cells. *J Exp Med.* 2001;194:1625–1638.

152. Staudt LM. Genomic-scale gene expression profiling of lymphoid malignancies reveals new cancer types. *Proc Am Soc Clin Oncol.* 2001;19:252–255.

153. Rosenwald A, Wright G, Chan WC, et al. The use of molecular profiling to predict survival after chemotherapy for diffuse large-B-cell lymphoma. *N Engl J Med.* 2002;346:1937–1947.

Hodgkin Lymphoma

James Nachman

Introduction

Hodgkin lymphoma is a unique malignant neoplasm. It is the only malignant neoplasm in which the malignant cell, the so-called Reed-Sternberg (RS) cell or lymphocytic and histiocytic (L&H) cell, represents only a small proportion of the cells making up the tumor; the majority of cells are small lymphocytes, histiocytes, neutrophils, plasma cells, and fibroblasts in different proportions dependent on the histologic subtype. In the most common subtype of classical Hodgkin lymphoma, nodular sclerosis (NS), thick collagen bands separate individual tumor nodules. It is thought that cytokines and other chemicals produced by RS cells and L&H cells elicit the background inflammatory infiltrate and fibrosis. It was only recently that the clonal nature of the RS cell population in a given tumor was confirmed.[1]

Hodgkin lymphoma commonly presents as a single area or multiple areas of lymphadenopathy, most commonly in the upper torso. Approximately 25% of patients present with one or more systemic symptoms including high, spiking fever, weight loss, night sweats, and pruritus. Hodgkin lymphoma is highly sensitive to both chemotherapy and irradiation; event-free survival (EFS) for pediatric Hodgkin lymphoma patients is approximately 80% to 85%, and overall survival is approximately 90% to 95%.[2,3] For adult patients, most early trials focused on the use of high-dose extended-field radiotherapy with curative intent in patients with disease limited to nodal sites; chemotherapy was reserved for patients who had disseminated extranodal disease (stage IV) or those who recurred following irradiation. However, high-dose radiation therapy, when used in skeletally immature pediatric patients, produced unacceptable stunting of skeletal growth, particularly in the neck and upper chest regions.[4,5] Therefore, the primary treatment for pediatric Hodgkin lymphoma has been chemotherapy with or without additional low-dose limited-field radiotherapy. Because of the significant long-term side effects of high-dose extended-field radiotherapy that have now been observed in long-term adult Hodgkin lymphoma survivors (breast cancer and coronary artery disease, for example), many adult oncologists are now adapting the pediatric treatment strategy of chemotherapy with or without low-dose involved-field irradiation. Because cure rates for pediatric Hodgkin lymphoma are high, treatment-related late effects such as second malignant neoplasms and cardiovascular damage take on paramount importance.

Pathology

Hodgkin lymphoma can be divided into two broad classes, classical Hodgkin lymphoma and nodular lymphocyte-predominant Hodgkin lymphoma.[6,7]

The defining feature of classical Hodgkin lymphoma is the RS cell.[8] The RS cell is generally a binucleate or multinucleated giant cell. The typical RS cell has a bilobed nucleus with two large nucleoli that produces the characteristic "owl's eye" appearance. Reed-Sternberg cells are usually widely scattered in a nonmalignant reactive cell population of T lymphocytes, macrophages, granulocytes, and eosinophils. Reed-Sternberg cells do not express typical B-lymphocytic antigens such as CD45, CD19, or CD79A. Almost all RS cells express CD30, and greater than 80% express CD15. CD20, another B-lymphocytic antigen, is expressed on approximately 20% of RS cells.[9] Classical Hodgkin lymphoma is divided into four subgroups. Lymphocyte-rich classic Hodgkin lymphoma is a recently recognized subtype, which may have a nodular appearance and lack the classic RS cell. This form of classical Hodgkin lymphoma can be differentiated from nodular lymphocyte-predominant Hodgkin lymphoma by the immune phenotype that is characteristic of the classic RS cell. It accounts for only a small percentage of cases of pediatric Hodgkin lymphoma. In mixed-cellularity Hodgkin lymphoma, RS cells are frequently seen in an abundant background of benign reactive elements including T lymphocytes, plasma cells, histiocytes, and eosinophils. Mixed-cellularity Hodgkin lymphoma is more common in young patients than in adolescents. Nodular sclerosis Hodgkin lymphoma is characterized by broad bands of collagen that separate the lymph node into visible nodules. An RS cell variant referred to as a "lacunar cell" is often found in lymph nodes showing NS histology. There is controversy as to whether or not the presence of greater or fewer RS cells in an involved lymph node (NS-1 and NS-2) has any prognostic significance. Lymphocyte-depleted Hodgkin lymphoma is characterized by large numbers of RS cells and a scant reactive background infiltrate. This subtype is extremely rare in children and young adults and when it occurs is frequently associated with a variety of congenital or acquired immunodeficiency states.

Nodular lymphocytic-predominant Hodgkin lymphoma is characterized by the L&H cell or "popcorn" cell.[10,11] Lymphocytic and histiocytic cells have a very different phenotype than that of the RS cell, expressing B-lymphocytic surface antigens such as CD19, CD20, CD22, and CD79A and not expressing CD15. Nodular lymphocyte-predominant Hodgkin lymphoma may be confused with progressive transformation of germinal centers, a benign condition, or T lymphocyte–rich B-cell lymphoma. Nodular lymphocyte-predominant Hodgkin lymphoma is most common in younger children, usually presenting as an asymptomatic nonbulky localized mass (Table 15-1).

Biology

Research on the biology of the malignant cell in Hodgkin lymphoma, the RS cell or the L&H cell, has been extremely difficult due to the rarity of these cells within the tumor tissue. Microdissection techniques have now allowed the isolation of individual RS and L&H cells. It appears that the malignant cell in the vast majority of Hodgkin lymphoma cases originates from a germinal-center B lymphocyte. The biology of the malignant cells differs between the lymphocyte-predominant and the classical forms of Hodgkin lymphoma.

Classical Hodgkin *Lymphoma*

The RS cell, characteristic of classic Hodgkin lymphoma, expresses CD15 and CD30 but rarely expresses CD20 or other surface antigens characteristic of B lymphocytes. Expression of CD20 on RS cells may confer an adverse prognosis.[9] A recent study found that RS cells lack several intracellular signaling molecules found in normal B cells including protein tyrosine kinase, B cell linker protein, and phospholipase gamma 2.[12]

In classical Hodgkin lymphoma, clonality of the RS cell can be demonstrated through unique rearrangements in the variable region of immunoglobulin genes. B lymphocytes in the germinal center generally undergo one of two processes. B lymphocytes with productive immunoglobulin gene rearrangements (resulting in the expression of functional surface immunoglobulin) persist and undergo somatic hypermutation to generate high-affinity immunoglobulin receptor–positive B lymphocytes. Cells with nonproductive immunoglobulin gene rearrangements undergo apoptosis and are eliminated. Reed-Sternberg cells appear to derive from germinal-center B lymphocytes that do not produce functional immunoglobulin but escape apoptosis and continue to proliferate. In about 25% of cases, mutations are found that render functional gene rearrangements nonfunctional (nonsense, deletion mutations).[13] In the majority of cases, however, it is likely that defects in the transcriptional machinery result in the lack of production of functional immunoglobulin. Transcription factors such as OCT2, BOB1, and PU1 may be down-regulated in cells of classical Hodgkin lymphoma.[14]

Because germinal-center B lymphocytes that do not produce functional immunoglobulin normally undergo apoptosis, investigators have sought out the mechanisms by which RS cells are able to avoid apoptosis. Much of the research has focused on the NF-kB pathway.[15] NFkB is a transcription factor that is up-regulated in most patients with classical Hodgkin lymphoma. Under normal conditions, NFkB is found in the cytoplasm attached to an inhibitor IkB. Certain stimuli such as CD40 ligand and LMP-1 activate an Ik kinase that phosphorylates IkB, leading to ubiquitination and degradation of IkB by the 26S proteasome, thus liberating NFkB. NFkB then translocates to the nucleus, where it can activate multiple genes that promote resistance to apoptosis. In certain cases, mutations in the IkB molecule have been demonstrated.

One of the unique features of Hodgkin lymphoma is the reactive cellular infiltrate and/or fibrosis that make up most of the tumor. It is thought that the cellular infiltrate and fibrosis are due to the large number of cytokines produced by the RS cell, including interleukin-1 (IL-1), IL-6, and tumor necrosis factor-α.[16,17] IL-5, a cytokine-producing eosinophilia, is secreted by RS cells. Transforming growth factor-β may be responsible for the fibrosis seen in cases of NS histology. High levels of IL-6 are associated with "B" symptoms.

Table 15-1

Distinction between Reed-Sternberg cell and lymphocyte and histiocytic cell.

Feature	Reed-Sternberg Cell	L&H Cell
CD30	+	−
CD15	+	−
CD20	20%	+
CD79a	−	+
Oct-2; BOB-1 Expression	Down-regulated	Up-regulated

Lymphocyte-Predominant Hodgkin Lymphoma

In contradistinction to the RS cell in classical Hodgkin lymphoma, the L&H cell of nodular lymphocyte-predominant Hodgkin lymphoma expresses a B-lymphocytic phenotype (CD20 positive) and generally does not express CD15 or CD30. OCT2 is significantly overexpressed in nodular lymphocyte-predominant Hodgkin lymphoma, while OCT2 is generally down-regulated in the RS cell.[18]

Somatic hypermutation of immunoglobulin genes occurs in nodular lymphocyte-predominant Hodgkin lymphoma. Lyn-kinase, a B-lymphocyte signaling molecule, appears to be absent in a large majority of L&H cells.[19] Presence or absence of Lyn-kinase may allow distinction between nodular lymphocyte-predominant Hodgkin lymphoma and the benign disorder referred to as progressive transformation of germinal centers.

Epidemiology

Hodgkin lymphoma accounts for 6% of childhood cancer. The incidence is 14 cases per 100 000 for patients younger than 15 years. In a recent large clinical trial, only 16% of cases occurred in patients younger than 10 years.[2] Table 15-2 shows the demographic features for pediatric Hodgkin lymphoma. For patients younger than 10 years, there is a striking male predominance. Younger patients have a higher incidence of lymphocyte-predominant and mixed-cellularity histology compared with older patients. Younger patients have a higher incidence of early-stage disease and a lower incidence of symptoms at diagnosis. Nodular-sclerosis histology accounts for the vast majority of cases in adolescents. Siblings have a 2- to 5-fold increased risk of developing Hodgkin lymphoma; the risk is 9-fold in same-sex siblings.[20–22] One study reported a 99-fold increased risk in monozygotic twins of patients but no higher risk in dizygotic twins.[23] A deficiency in cellular immunity characterized by a decrease in naive T lymphocytes and an increased sensitivity of effector T lymphocytes to suppressor monocytes and suppressor T lymphocytes is seen in newly diagnosed adolescent patients with Hodgkin lymphoma.[24] Hodgkin lymphoma occurs in patients infected with the human immunodeficiency virus and is characterized by advanced stage, "B" symptoms, extranodal involvement, and a poor response to therapy. For children and adolescents in the United States, there is a direct relationship between parental income, parental education level, and Hodgkin lymphoma incidence and an inverse relationship between sibling number and Hodgkin lymphoma incidence.[25]

Epstein-Barr Virus and Pediatric Hodgkin Lymphoma

Epstein-Barr virus (EBV) DNA can be detected in the genome of RS cells of classic Hodgkin lymphoma in approximately 40% to 60% of cases.[26] Epstein-Barr virus DNA is rarely present in the L&H cells of nodular lymphocyte-predominant patients. Epstein-Barr virus–positive Hodgkin lymphoma is most commonly seen in younger patients (less than 10 years) with mixed-cellularity histology. Among cases of classical Hodgkin lymphoma, EBV expression is lowest in adolescents with nodular sclerosis histology. Patients with serologically confirmed infectious mononucleosis (either clinical or subclinical) had a 3- to 4.5-fold increased risk for developing EBV-positive Hodgkin lymphoma; there was no increased risk for EBV-negative Hodgkin lymphoma.[27] LMP1, a protein expressed by EBV,

Table 15-2. Comparison of presenting features and outcome for children and adolescents with Hodgkin lymphoma.

Feature	Overall	< 10 Yrs	≥ 10 Yrs
Stage I, II A	57.4%	68%	55.1%
"B" symptoms	25.4%	16%	27.7%
Bulk disease	29%	17.5%	32.5%
Nodular sclerosis	78.5%	82.9%	83.1%
5-year EFS	85.1%	90.4%	83.4%

Abbreviations: EFS, event-free survival; yrs, years.

activates NFkB. Increased expression of NFkB is seen in a large percentage of RS cells. LMP1 also activates IL-10, which may lead to down-regulation of cytotoxic T lymphocyte function. The literature concerning the prognostic significance of EBV positivity in pediatric Hodgkin lymphoma is contradictory.[28] Recently, a study has suggested that within the subset of pediatric Hodgkin lymphoma cases associated with EBV, measurement of EBV DNA in plasma may be a sensitive indicator for response and/or relapse.[29]

Presentation, Staging, and Workup

The majority of pediatric and adolescent patients with Hodgkin lymphoma present with painless adenopathy, most commonly in the neck or supraclavicular region. Approximately 20% to 25% of patients will have one or more systemic manifestations including high, spiking fever, drenching night sweats, and weight loss of greater than 10% (collectively referred to as "B" symptoms). Some patients may have significant pruritus at the time of presentation. Patients with large anterior mediastinal masses may present with cough or shortness of breath and may show superior vena cava compression syndrome. The diagnosis of Hodgkin lymphoma is usually made by means of an incisional or excisional biopsy of a suspicious lymph node. Before giving general anesthesia to a patient with Hodgkin lymphoma, a careful assessment of the patient's airway must be undertaken. A chest radiograph must be performed prior to any lymph node biopsy. Needle aspiration for cytology is often nondiagnostic in Hodgkin lymphoma. Once the diagnosis of Hodgkin lymphoma is made, a computerized tomographic scan of the neck, chest, abdomen, and pelvis should be performed. Bone marrow aspiration and biopsy should be performed for patients with disease on both sides of the diaphragm and/or "B" symptoms at diagnosis. Bone scans should be undertaken only in patients with pain in bony sites. All patients should have some type of functional as well as anatomic imaging. Until recently, the standard functional imaging procedure was gallium scanning,[30] but this imaging modality is being replaced by positron emission tomographic (PET) scanning utilizing radiolabeled glucose.[31–35] Functional imaging is particularly important in cases of NS histology, because residual masses are often seen at the end of treatment, and the anatomical distinction of scar from active tumor is not possible. In patients with a suspicious pulmonary nodule or nodules, biopsy should be performed to confirm the presence of Hodgkin lymphoma. At the conclusion of the staging workup, a clinical stage is assigned based on the Ann Arbor staging system (see Table 15-3).[36] The type of initial treatment is usually determined by the Ann Arbor stage, the presence or absence of "B" symptoms, and the presence or absence of bulk disease. The erythrocyte sedimentation rate (ESR) should be performed in all patients, because a low ESR is a favorable prognostic factor. Recently, a radiographically documented rapid early anatomic response to chemotherapy has been identified as a potentially important prognostic factor in patients with Hodgkin lymphoma. Many modern protocols are evaluating early PET response as a possible prognostic factor.

Treatment of Pediatric Hodgkin Lymphoma

Since the recognition that standard-dose radiotherapy provided unacceptable consequences for skeletal growth, the primary therapeutic modality for children and adolescents with Hodgkin lymphoma has been combination chemotherapy. The initial chemotherapy treatment for Hodgkin lymphoma consisted of nitrogen mustargen, oncovin/vincristine, procarbazine, and prednisone (MOPP).[37] Because of a disturbingly high incidence of therapy-related myeloid leukemia and male infertility, a non–cross-resistant regimen, adriamycin, bleomycin, vinblastine, dacarbazine (ABVD), was developed.[38] In clinical trials comparing the efficacy of these two regimens, ABVD generally provided better results. The primary long-term late effects of ABVD include cardiac and pulmonary dysfunction. In an effort to reduce toxicity and improve efficacy, investigators used combinations of MOPP and ABVD, either alternating monthly courses or combining half cycles of MOPP and ABVD in a single course.[39] These hybrid regimens or other such hybrids form the basis for many current Hodgkin lymphoma protocols. By limiting the amount of alkylating agents (cytoxan and procarbazine) and the amount of anthracycline and bleomycin, investigators hoped to lessen the frequency of significant late effects. VP-16 was added by some investigators, while others chose to eliminate alkylating agents altogether. Regimens such as vinblastine, adriamycin, methotrexate, prednisone and vincristine, epirubicin, etoposide, and prednisone were developed.[40,41]

These non–alkylator-containing regimens worked reasonably well for patients with early-stage disease, but they were generally less effective in patients with advanced-stage disease.

Most early pediatric oncology trials utilized low-dose (15 to 25 gy) involved-field radiation following completion of chemotherapy. In some studies, higher doses of radiation were used in patients showing only partial responses to initial therapy.

Because all pediatric patients with Hodgkin lymphoma receive chemotherapy, a logical question was whether or not pediatric patients with Hodgkin lymphoma could be successfully treated with chemotherapy alone. In a Children's Cancer Group (CCG) trial for patients with advanced-stage disease, patients were randomized between 12 cycles of MOPP/ABVD and 6 cycles of MOPP/ABVD plus low-dose involved-field radiation therapy (IFRT).[42] In a Pediatric Oncology Group trial for patients with advanced-stage disease, patients were randomized to 8 cycles of MOPP/ABVD versus 6 cycles of MOPP/ABVD and IFRT.[43] In each trial the results for the chemotherapy alone and chemotherapy plus radiation arms were equivalent. Because of the additional radiation given to patients who received lower-intensity chemotherapy, these trials did not answer the question as to whether low-dose IFRT given following a complete response to initial chemotherapy would improve EFS, overall survival, or both.

Two recent trials, one performed by the CCG and the other by the German pediatric oncology group, were designed to answer this question.[2,3] In both trials, the intensity of initial chemotherapy was determined by a combination of prognostic features such as stage, presence or absence of symptoms, presence or absence of bulk disease, number of nodal regions involved, and presence or absence of hilar adenopathy. In the CCG trial, patients who attained a complete response were randomized to receive or not receive radiation therapy, while in the German pediatric trial, patients achieving a complete response were nonrandomly assigned to no further treatment.

Before describing the results of the trials, a brief comment on the rationale and evaluation techniques used for the studies is in order. The goal of each of the two studies was to determine whether or not elimination of radiation therapy for patients achieving a complete response would adversely effect outcome. In most pediatric malignancies, EFS is a good measure of outcome because the salvage rates following relapse are low. Thus, EFS generally predicts ultimate survival. This is not the case for pediatric Hodgkin lymphoma. Most patients with pediatric Hodgkin lymphoma who experience a relapse attain a second remission, and 30% to 50% of patients who relapse may be cured. There are suggestions from a number of adult studies that survival following relapse when the initial treatment is chemotherapy alone may be significantly better than for patients who relapse after chemotherapy plus radiation therapy.

The goal of eliminating radiation therapy for patients achieving a complete response to chemotherapy stems from the premise that eliminating radiation therapy will lead to a decrease in late effects. Evaluating late effects in patients with Hodgkin lymphoma has been a frustrating experience. Because late effects take long periods of time to appear, the therapies that led to an identified late effect have often been abandoned by the time the late effect is noted. For example, the majority of late-effects papers published to date concern patients who received high-dose extended-field radiation therapy. These studies are not particularly helpful in predicting what long-term toxicities to expect for patients who receive low-dose IFRT. Because the late effects of low-dose IFRT are not known, it is difficult to determine what decrement in EFS or survival would outweigh the presumed lesser long-term

Table 15-3

Ann Arbor staging system with Cotswold modifications for Hodgkin lymphoma.

Stage	Description
I	Involvement of a single lymph node region or lymphoid structure, eg, spleen, thymus, Waldeyer's ring, or single extralymphatic site (IE).
II	Involvement of 2 or more lymph node regions on the same side of the diaphragm, or localized contiguous involvement of only 1 extranodal organ/site and lymph node region on the same side of the diaphragm (IIE). The number of anatomic sites are indicated by the subscript (eg, II_3).
III	Involvement of lymph node regions on both sides of the diaphragm (III), which may be accompanied by involvement of the spleen (III_S) or by localized contiguous involvement of only 1 extranodal organ site (III_E) or both (III_{SE}).
III_1	With or without involvement of splenic hilar, celiac, or mesenteric nodes.
III_2	With involvement of paraaortic, iliac, or mesenteric nodes.
IV	Diffuse or disseminated involvement of one or more extranodal organs or tissues, with or without associated lymph node involvement.

Designations applicable to any stage

A	No symptoms.
B	Fever (temperature $> 38°C$), drenching night sweats, unexplained loss of $> 10\%$ of body weight within the preceding 6 months.
X	Bulky disease (a widening of the mediastinum by more than one-third or the presence of a nodal mass with a maximal dimension > 10 cm).
E	Involvement of a single extranodal site that is contiguous or proximal to the known nodal site.
CS	Clinical stage.
PS	Pathologic stage (as determined by laparotomy).

effects associated with chemotherapy alone, recognizing that patients requiring salvage therapy have a higher treatment burden and thus a greater potential incidence of late effects. In both studies, investigators chose EFS as the primary end point.

The CCG 5942 entered 829 eligible patients between January 1995 and December 1998. The study design is shown in Figure 15-1. Patients were assigned to initial chemotherapy groups, based on clinical stage, presence or absence of "B" symptoms, bulk disease, hilar adenopathy, and number of nodal regions involved (see Table 15-4). Patients who achieved a complete response were randomized to receive low-dose IFRT or no further therapy, while patients achieving a partial response were assigned to receive radiation. Complete response was defined as greater than 70% reduction in all tumor masses and a change from gallium positive to gallium negative if masses were initially gallium positive. No lower limit of residual mass size was used in determining complete response. The study was closed to accrual in December 1998 when a statistically significant difference in EFS favoring the treatment arm including low-dose IFRT was observed on a routine interim data monitoring review. Five hundred and one patients achieved a complete response to risk-adapted chemotherapy and were randomized to receive low-dose IFRT ($N = 251$) or to receive no further therapy ($N = 250$). Three-year EFS for

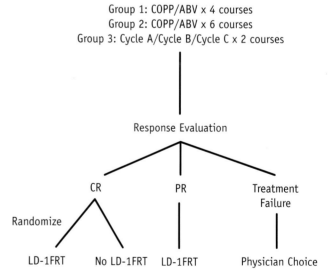

Group 1: COPP/ABV x 4 courses
Group 2: COPP/ABV x 6 courses
Group 3: Cycle A/Cycle B/Cycle C x 2 courses

Response Evaluation

CR PR Treatment Failure

Randomize

LD-1FRT No LD-1FRT LD-1FRT Physician Choice

Figure 15-1 Clinical group-specific chemotherapy.

patients randomized to low-dose IFRT was $92\% \pm 1.9\%$ versus $87 \pm 2.2\%$ for patients randomized to receive no further treatment ($P = 0.57$). However, 23 patients initially randomized to low-dose IFRT chose no further therapy, while 7 patients randomized to receive no further therapy actually received low-dose IFRT. In an "as

Table 15-4

Clinical group definitions.

Group 1

Stage I patients without adverse disease features

Stage II patients without adverse disease features and without clinical "B" symptoms

Group 2

Stage I patients with adverse disease features

Stage II patients with adverse disease features and/or with clinical "B" symptoms

Stage III patients

Group 3

Stage IV patients

Adverse disease features comprise 1 or more of the following: hilar adenopathy, involvement of more than 4 nodal regions; mediastinal tumor with diameter greater than or equal to one-third of the chest diameter, and node or nodal aggregate with a diameter greater than 10 cm.

Clinical B symptoms comprise 1 or more of the following: unexplained loss of more than 10% of body weight, unexplained recurrent fever greater than 38°C, and drenching night sweats.

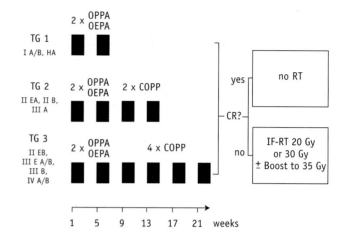

Protocol schedule GPOH-HD 95.

Figure 15-2 German pediatric oncology Hodgkin 95 study.

treated" analysis, 3-year EFS was $92 \pm 1.7\%$ for patients receiving low-dose IFRT and $85 \pm 2.3\%$ for patients receiving no further treatment ($P = .0024$). For patients who relapsed after chemotherapy alone, median time to relapse was 6 months, and 85% of relapses were confined to areas of initial involvement.

Three-year survival estimates for randomized patients receiving low-dose IFRT or no further therapy were 98% and 99%, respectively.

During a similar time frame, the German pediatric oncology group initiated the Hodgkin's Disease 95 study.[3] The study design is shown in Figure 15-2. All patients received risk-adapted chemotherapy; males received 2 initial cycles of oncovin, etoposide, prednisone, and adriamycin, while females received 2 initial cycles of oncovin, prednisone, procarbazine, and adriamycin. Patients in the most favorable group received only 2 cycles of chemotherapy: other patients received either 2 or 4 additional cycles of COPP chemotherapy. A reevaluation was performed at the end of chemotherapy. Patients achieving a complete response defined as no imageable disease or all residual tumor masses < 2 mL in volume received no further treatment, while other patients received IFRT with the radiation dose based on residual tumor volume, regardless of the intensity of initial chemotherapy. Of the 950 patients entered on the trial, 326 patients were assigned to group 1 (2 cycles of chemotherapy), 224 to group 2 (4 cycles), and 280 to group 3 (6 cycles). At the end of chemotherapy 23% of patients had a complete response and received no further therapy. Overall EFS was 90% at 3 years. The 3-year EFS for patients treated with and without radiation

was 93% and 89%, respectively ($P = NS$). However, when the analysis was restricted to patients in groups 2 and 3, EFS at 3 years was 92% for patients receiving IFRT versus 81% for those receiving no further treatment ($P = .01$). The overall survival for patients receiving and not receiving radiation was 97% in both groups.

The Children's Oncology Group has developed a new risk assignment strategy for children and adolescents with Hodgkin lymphoma. Patients with stage I, IIA, nonbulky (mediastinal mass < 1/3 maximal chest diameter: extramediastinal mass < 6 cm in maximal diameter) disease will be assigned to the favorable risk group. Patients with stage IIIB and IVB disease will be assigned to the unfavorable group. All other patients will be assigned to the intermediate-risk group.

Patients with favorable-risk lymphocyte-predominant Hodgkin lymphoma will be assigned to a separate clinical trial; all other patients with lymphocyte-predominant histology will be treated on the same protocol as patients with classical Hodgkin lymphoma.

For favorable-risk patients with lymphocyte-predominant histology, those patients who undergo complete excision of stage I disease will be observed without any therapy. For patients with nonresected stage I or stage II disease, 3 cycles of chemotherapy with adriamycin, vincristine, prednisone, and cytoxan (AVPC) will be given. Patients achieving a complete response (>80% reduction in all mass lesions and negative functional imaging) will receive no further therapy, while patients achieving a partial response will receive low-dose involved-field radiotherapy. Patients with favorable classical Hodgkin lymphoma will receive similar treatment, except all patients will receive 3 initial cycles of AVPC chemotherapy. Intermediate-risk patients with Hodgkin lymphoma will receive 2 initial cycles of chemotherapy with adriamycin, bleomycin, vincristine, etoposide, prednisone, and cytoxan (ABVE-PC). The protocol will evaluate a response-based paradigm of treatment assignment compared with a standard non–response-based regimen consisting of 4 cycles of chemotherapy and low-dose IFRT. Patients in the response-based arm who show a rapid response to the 2 initial cycles of chemotherapy will receive 3 additional cycles of ABVE-PC and no radiotherapy. Patients with slow response to initial chemotherapy will receive 2 cycles of ABVE-PC and 2 cycles of dexamethasone, etoposide, cisplatin, and Ara-C prior to the low-dose IFRT.

For patients with unfavorable-risk Hodgkin lymphoma, initial chemotherapy will consist of ABVE-PC with a higher dose of cytoxan. Patients who achieve a complete response to 5 cycles of chemotherapy will be randomized to standard involved-field radiotherapy or radiotherapy to initial sites of bulk disease only.

Late Effects

Hodgkin lymphoma appears to be a focal point for late-effects research. Cure rates are quite high, so large numbers of patients are long-term survivors. As late effects have been identified, changes to frontline therapy have been instituted in an effort to eliminate the late effects while maintaining high cure rates. Major late effects associated with chemotherapy for Hodgkin lymphoma include treatment-related second malignant neoplasms,[44,45] male infertility,[46] premature menopause[47] (alkylating agents), cardiac failure[48–50] (anthracycline), and pulmonary dysfunction[51] (bleomycin). In modern treatment programs, elements of the MOPP and ABVD chemotherapy program have been combined into hybrid regimens to reduce the overall exposure to alkylating agents, anthracycline, and bleomycin. There is a general consensus that limiting alkylating agent exposure decreases the risk for therapy-related myeloid leukemia. In protocols using cytoxan as the sole alkylating agent, limiting drug exposure to <9 gm/m^2 appears to markedly reduce the risk of male infertility.[52] Current pediatric Hodgkin lymphoma protocols generally limit anthracycline exposure to 140 to 210 mg/m^2, which is well below the dose usually associated with cardiac decompensation. Cytosine arabinoside containing combination chemotherapy may allow a reduction in alkylator and/or anthracycline exposure. A new combination, gemcitabine and vinorelbine, has shown promise in the relapse setting.[53] There are plans to incorporate this combination into frontline regimens that would also reduce alkylator and anthracycline exposure. However, the combined use of gemcitabine and bleomycin produced unacceptable pulmonary toxicity in a recent trial.[54]

High-dose radiation has been used extensively for adult patients with Hodgkin lymphoma. There is a significant incidence of second tumors in the radiation field. Breast cancer is of particular concern.[55] Other commonly noted late effects related to radiation include thyroid dysfunction, coronary artery disease, and pulmonary complications.

A number of recent publications have dealt with late effects of childhood Hodgkin lymphoma. In one study utilizing a self-reporting mechanism, hypothyroidism occurred in 7.6% of nonirradiated patients, 30% of patients receiving <35 Gy and 50% of those receiving >50 Gy. There was an 18-fold increased risk of thyroid cancer in

this population. All patients who developed thyroid cancer received >25 Gy.[56] In another large series, childhood Hodgkin lymphoma survivors were found to have an 18.5-fold increased risk of developing a second cancer compared with the general population.[57] The cumulative incidence of a second cancer was 10.6% at 20 years and 26.3% at 30 years. The risk for breast cancer in female survivors of Hodgkin lymphoma increases with increasing radiation dose.[58] Even low-dose radiation (4 Gy) may increase the risk for subsequent breast cancer (3.2-fold increase in 1 study). The use of alkylating agents in combination with radiation decreased the risk of breast cancer. The risk for developing therapy-related leukemia peaks at 5 years, while the incidence of second solid tumors gradually increases with time.

In the United States, current chemotherapy protocols for children and young adults with Hodgkin lymphoma utilize cytoxan as the sole alkylating agent, and cumulative dose is usually <6 gms/m^2, a dose usually associated with preserved fertility in males. Anthracycline dose is generally limited to <200 mg/m^2. Radiation, when given, is limited to 20 to 25 Gy. Low-dose IFRT has now been used in children for approximately 20 years, so reliable late-effects data should become available for this cohort in approximately 5 to 10 years.

Recurrent Disease

Treatment failure occurs in approximately 20% of children and young adults with Hodgkin lymphoma.[2,3] Patients who do not respond to initial therapy have the lowest salvage rate. Pretreatment prognostic factors for patients who relapse after an initial complete response include time to relapse, treatment modalities utilized prior to relapse, site of relapse (initially involved site: new site), "B" symptoms at relapse, and extranodal involvement at relapse. Almost all children and young adults receive chemotherapy as the initial therapy for treatment failure. Multiple combination chemotherapy regimens have been utilized including ifosfamide, carboplatin, and etoposide[59]; cisplatin, ARA-C, and etoposide; and more recently ifosfamide and vinorelbine.[60] The combination of emcitabine and vinorelbine is also effective.[61] Initial response to salvage chemotherapy is an extremely important prognostic factor. Patients with low-risk relapse—that is, who relapse after minimal chemotherapy and no radiation, whose disease recurs in a site or sites of initial involvement only, and who achieve a complete response to salvage chemotherapy—may be cured with low-dose IFRT. For all other patients who relapse, autologous peripheral blood stem cell transplant ± additional involved field radiotherapy is utilized following initial salvage chemotherapy. The most commonly used preparative regimen prior to stem cell transplant includes BCNU, etoposide, ARA-C, and melphalan.[62]

There is controversy whether relapse patients who have had recurrence in a previously irradiated region derive benefit from additional radiation.[63] The salvage rate for patients with Hodgkin lymphoma who experience a relapse is 30%

to 50%, with a higher salvage rate for patients who fail following chemotherapy alone.[64-65] A recent study has suggested that even patients with primary refractory Hodgkin lymphoma may be salvaged with chemotherapy, peripheral blood stem cell transplant, and radiation.[66]

References

1. Kanzler H, Kuppers R, Hansmann ML, et al. Hodgkin and Reed-Sternberg cells in Hodgkin's disease represent the outgrowth of a dominant tumor clone derived from (crippled) germinal center B cells. *J Exp Med.* 1996;184:1495–1505.
2. Nachman JB, Sposto R, Herzog P, et al. Randomized comparison of low-dose involved-field radiotherapy and no radiotherapy for children with Hodgkin's disease who achieve a complete response to chemotherapy. *J Clin Oncol.* 2002;20:3765–3771.
3. Ruhl U, Albrecht M, Dieckmann K, et al. Response-adapted radiotherapy in the treatment of pediatric Hodgkin's disease: an interim report at 5 years of the German GPOHHD 95 trial. *Int J Radiat Oncol Biol Phys.* 2001;51:1209–1218.
4. Mauch PM, Weinstein H, Botnick L, et al. An evaluation of long-term survival and treatment complications in children with Hodgkin's disease. *Cancer.* 1983;51:925–932.
5. Jenkin D, Doyle J, Berry M, et al. Hodgkin's disease in children: treatment with MOPP and low-dose, extended field irradiation without laparotomy. Late results and toxicity. *Med Pediatr Oncol.* 1990;18:265–272.
6. Pileri SA, Ascani S, Leoncini L, et al. Hodgkin's lymphoma: the pathologist's viewpoint. *J Clin Pathol.* 2002;55:162–176.
7. Harris NL. Hodgkin's lymphomas: classification, diagnosis, and grading. *Semin Hematol.* 1999;36:220–232.
8. Cossman J, Messineo C, and Bagg A. Reed-Sternberg cell: survival in a hostile sea. *Lab Invest.* 1998;78:229–235.
9. Tzankov. A, Krugman J, Fend F, et al. Prognostic significance of CD20 expression in classical Hodgkin lymphoma: a clinico-pathologic study of 119 cases. *Clin Cancer Res.* 2003;9:1381–1386.
10. Marafioti T, Hummel M, Anagnostopoulos I, et al. Origin of nodular lymphocyte-predominant Hodgkin's disease from a clonal expansion of highly mutated germinal-center B cells. *N Engl J Med.* 1997;337:453–458.
11. Ohno T, Stribley JA, Wu G, et al. Clonality in nodular lymphocyte-predominant Hodgkin's disease. *N Engl J Med.* 1997;337:459–465.
12. Kadin ME, Carpenter C. Hidden identity of Hodgkin/Reed-Sternberg cells. *Blood.* 2004;103:7.
13. Kuppers R, Schwering I, Brauniger A, et al. Biology of Hodgkin's lymphoma. *Ann Oncol.* 2002;13(suppl 1):11–18.
14. Laddenkemper C, Anagnostopoulos I, Hummel M, et al. Differential Eu enhancer activity and expression of BOB.1/OBF.1, Oct-2, PU.1, and immunoglobulin in reactive B-cell populations, B-cell non Hodgkin lymphomas and Hodgkin lymphoma. *J Pathol.* 2004;202:60–69.
15. Fiumara P, Snell V, Li Y, et al. Functional expression of receptor activator of nuclear factor kappa B in Hodgkin disease cell lines. *Blood.* 2001;98:2784–2790.
16. Gruss HJ, Pinto A, Duyster J, et al. Hodgkin's disease: a tumor with disturbed immunological pathways. *Immunol Today.* 1997;18:156–163.
17. Skinnider BF, Mak TW. The role of cytokines in classical Hodgkin lymphoma. *Blood.* 2002;99:4283–4297.
18. Stein H, Marafioti T, Foss HD, et al. Down-regulation of BOB.1/OBF.1 and Oct2 in classical Hodgkin disease but not in lymphocyte predominant Hodgkin disease correlates with immunoglobulin transcription. *Blood.* 2001;97:496–501.
19. Marafioti T, Pozzobon M, Hansmann ML, et al. Expression of intracellular signaling molecules in classical and lymphocyte predominance Hodgkin disease. *Blood.* 2004;103:188–193.
20. MacMahon B. Epidemiological evidence on the nature of Hodgkin's disease. *Cancer.* 1957;10:1045–1054.
21. Grufferman S, Delsell E. Epidemiology of Hodgkin's disease. *Epidemiol Rev.* 1984;6:76–106.
22. Robertson SJ, Lowman JT, Grufferman S, et al. Familial Hodgkin's disease. A clinical and laboratory investigation. *Cancer.* 1987;59:1314–1319.
23. Mack TM, Cozen W, Shibata DK, et al. Concordance for Hodgkin's disease in identical twins suggesting genetic susceptibility to the young-adult form of the disease. *N Engl J Med.* 1995;332:413–418.
24. Schneider BF, Mak TW. The role of cytokines in classical Hodgkin's disease. *Blood.* 2002;99:4283–4297.
25. Grufferman S, Gilchrist GS, Pollock H, et al. Socioeconomic status, the Epstein Barr virus, and risk of Hodgkin's disease in childhood. *Leuk Lymphoma.* 2001;42(suppl 1):40.
26. Razzouk BI, Gan YJ, Mendonca C, et al. Epstein-Barr virus in pediatric Hodgkin disease: age and histiotype are more predictive than geographic region. *Med Pediatr Oncol.* 1997;28:248–254.
27. Hjalerim H, Askung J, Rostgaard K, et al. Characteristics of Hodgkin's lymphoma after infectious mononucleosis. *N Engl J Med.* 2003;349:1324–1332.
28. Flavell K, Billingham LJ, Biddulph JP. et al. The effects of Epstein-Barr virus status on outcome in age and sex-defined subgroups of patients with advanced Hodgkin's disease. *Ann Oncol.* 2003;14:282–290.
29. Wagner HJ, Schlager F, Clavier A, et al. Detection of Epstein-Barr virus in peripheral blood of pediatric patients with Hodgkin's disease by real time polymerase chain reaction. *Eur J Cancer.* 2001;37:1853–1857.
30. Weiner M, Leventhal B, Cantor A, et al. Gallium-67 scans as an adjunct to computed tomography scans for the assessment of a residual mediastinal mass in pediatric patients with Hodgkin's disease. A Pediatric Oncology Group study. *Cancer.* 1981;68:2478–2480.
31. Bar-Shalom R, Yefremov N, Haim N, et al. Camera-based FDG PET and 67Ga SPECT in evaluation of lymphoma: comparative study. *Radiology.* 2003;227:353–360.
32. Heultenschmidt B, Sautter-Bihl ML, Lang O, et al. Whole-body positron emission tomography in the treatment of Hodgkin disease. *Cancer.* 2001;91:302–310.
33. Jadvar H, Connoly L, Shulkin B, et al. Positron-emission tomography in pediatrics. In: Freeman LM, ed. *Nuclear Medicine Annual.* Philadelphia, PA: Lippincott Williams & Wilkins; 2000.
34. Jerusalem G, Beguin Y, Fassotte MF, et al. Whole-body positron emission tomography using 18F-fluorodeoxyglucose for posttreatment evaluation in Hodgkin's disease and non-Hodgkin's lymphoma has higher diagnostic and prognostic value than classical computed tomography scan imaging. *Blood.* 1999;94:429–433.
35. Wirth A, Seymour JF, Hicks RJ, et al. Fluorine-18 fluorodeoxyglucose positron emission tomography, gallium-67 scintigraphy, and conventional staging for Hodgkin's disease and non-Hodgkin's lymphoma. *Am J Med.* 2002;112:262–268.
36. Lister TA, Crowther D, Sutcliffe SB, et al. Report of a committee convened to discuss the evaluation and staging of patients with Hodgkin's disease: Cotswolds meeting. *J Clin Oncol.* 1989;7:1630–1636.
37. Donaldson SS, Link MP. Combined modality treatment with low-dose radiation and MOPP chemotherapy for children with Hodgkin's disease. *J Clin Oncol.* 1987;5:742–749.
38. Behrendt H, Brinkhuis M, Van Leeuwen EF. Treatment of childhood Hodgkin's disease with ABVD without radiotherapy. *Med Pediatr Oncol.* 1996;26:244–248.
39. Hunger SP, Link MP, Donaldson SS. ABVD/MOPP and low-dose involved-field radiotherapy in pediatric Hodgkin's disease: the Stanford experience. *J Clin Oncol.* 1994;12:2160–2166.
40. Donaldson SS, Hudson MM, Lamborn KR, et al. VAMP and low-dose, involved-field radiation for children and adolescents with favorable, early-stage Hodgkin's disease: results of a prospective clinical trial. *J Clin Oncol.* 2002;20:3081–3087.
41. Shankar AG, Ashley S, Atra A, et al. A limited role for VEEP (vincristine, etoposide, epirubicin, prednisolone) chemotherapy in childhood Hodgkin's disease. *Eur J Cancer.* 1998;34:2058–2063.
42. Fryer CJ, Hutchinson RJ, Krailo M, et al. Efficacy and toxicity of 12 courses of ABVD chemotherapy followed by low-dose regional radiation in advanced Hodgkin's disease in children: a report from the Children's Cancer Study Group. *J Clin Oncol.* 1990;8:1971–1980.
43. Weiner MA, Leventhal B, Breecher ML, et al. Randomized study of intensive MOPP-ABVD with or without low-dose total-nodal radiation therapy in the treatment of stages III A-2, III-B, and IV Hodgkin's disease in pediatric patients: a Pediatric Oncology Group study. *J Clin Oncol.* 1997;15:2769–2779.
44. Sankila R, Garwicz S, Olsen JH, et al. Risk of subsequent malignant neoplasms among 1641 Hodgkin's disease patients diagnosed in childhood and adolescence: a population-based cohort study in the five Nordic countries. Association of the Nordic Cancer Registries and the Nordic Society of Pediatric Hematology and Oncology. *J Clin Oncol.* 1996;14:1442–1446.
45. Metayer C, Lynch CF, Clarke EA, et al. Second cancers among long-term survivors of Hodgkin's disease diagnosed in childhood and adolescence. *J Clin Oncol.* 2000;18:235–244.
46. Anselmo AP, Cartoni C, Bellantuono P, et al. Risk of infertility in patients with Hodgkin's disease treated with ABVD vs MOPP vs ABVD/MOPP. *Haematologica.* 1990;75:155–158.
47. Byrne J, Fears TR, Gail MH, et al. Early menopause in long-term survivors of cancer during adolescence. *Am J Obstet Gynecol.* 1992;166:788–793.
48. Green DM, Gingell RL. Regarding cardiac function and morbidity in long-term survivors of Hodgkin's disease. *Int J Radiat Oncol Biol Phys.* 1998;41:971.
49. Hancock SL, Donaldson SS, Hoppe RT. Cardiac disease following treatment of Hodgkin's disease in children and adolescents. *J Clin Oncol.* 1993;11:1208–1215.
50. Green DM, Hyland A, Chung CS, et al. Cancer and cardiac mortality among 15-year survivors of cancer diagnosed during childhood or adolescence. *J Clin Oncol.* 1999;17:3207–3215.
51. Mertens AC, Yasui Y, Liu Y, et al. Pulmonary complications in survivors of childhood and adolescent cancer. A report from the Childhood Cancer Survivor Study. *Cancer.* 2002;95:2431–2441.
52. Bramswig JH, Heimes U, Heiermann E, et al. The effects of different cumulative doses of chemotherapy on testicular function. Results in 75 patients treated for Hodgkin's disease during childhood or adolescence. *Cancer.* 1990;65:1298–1302.
53. Ozkaynak MF, Jayabose S. Gemcitabine and vinorelbine as a salvage regimen for relapse in Hodgkin lymphoma after autologous hematopoietic stem cell transplantation. *Pediatr Hematol Oncol.* 2004;21:107–113.

54. Bredenfeld H, Franklin J, Nogova C. et al. Severe pulmonary toxicity in patients with advanced stage Hodgkin's disease treated with a modified bleomycin, doxorubicin, cyclophosphamide, vincristine, procarbazine, prednisone, and gemcitabine (BEACOPP) regimen is probably related to the combination of gemcitabine and bleomycin: a report of the German Hodgkin's Lymphoma Study Group. *J Clin Oncol*. 2004;22:2424–2429.

55. Cutuli B, Borel C, Dhermain F, et al. Breast cancer occurred after the treatment for Hodgkin's disease: analysis of 133 cases. *Radiother Oncol*. 2001;59:247–255.

56. Sklar C, Whitton J, Mertens A, et al. Abnormalities of the thyroid in survivors of Hodgkin's disease: data from the Childhood Cancer Survivor Study. *J Clin Endocrinol Metab*. 2000;85:3227–3232.

57. Bhatia S, Yasui Y, Robison L, et al. High risk of subsequent neoplasms continuing with extended follow-up of childhood Hodgkin's disease: report from the late effects study group. *J Clin Oncol*. 2003;21:4386–4394.

58. Travis LB, Hill DA, Dores GM, et al. Breast cancer following radiotherapy and chemotherapy among young women with Hodgkin's disease. *JAMA*. 2003;290:465–475.

59. Kobrinsky NL, Sposto R, Shah NR, et al. Outcomes of treatment of children and adolescents with recurrent non-Hodgkin's lymphoma and Hodgkin's disease with dexamethasone, etoposide, cisplatin, cytarabine, and l-asparaginase, maintenance chemotherapy, and transplantation: Children's Cancer Group Study CCG-5912. *J Clin Oncol*. 2001;19:2390–2396.

60. Moskowitz CH, Nimer SD, Zelenetz AD, et al. A 2-step comprehensive high-dose chemoradiotherapy second-line program for relapsed and refractory Hodgkin disease: analysis by intent to treat and development of a prognostic model. *Blood*. 2001;97:616–623.

61. Cairo MS, Shen V, Krailo MD, et al. Prospective randomized trial between two doses of granulocyte colony-stimulating factor after ifosfamide, carboplatin, and etoposide in children with recurrent or refractory solid tumors: a Children's Cancer Group Report. *J Pediatr Hematol Oncol*. 2001;23:30–38.

62. Bonfante V, Viviani S, Santoro A, et al. Ifosfamide and vinorelbine: an active regimen for patients with relapsed or refractory Hodgkin's disease. *Br J Haematol*. 1998;103:533–535.

63. Baker KS, Gordon BG, Gross TG, et al. Autologous hematopoietic stem-cell transplantation for relapsed or refractory Hodgkin's disease in children and adolescents. *J Clin Oncol*. 1999;17:825–831.

64. Cooney JP, Stiff PJ, Toor AA, et al. BEAM allogeneic transplantation for patients with Hodgkin's disease who relapse after autologous transplantation is safe and effective. *Biol Blood Marrow Transplant*. 2003;9:177–182.

65. Wadhwa P, Shina DC, Schenkein D, et al. Should involved-field radiation therapy be used as an adjunct to lymphoma autotransplantation? *Bone Marrow Transplant*. 2002;29:183–189.

66. Moskowitz CH, Kewalramani T, Nimer SD, et al. Effectiveness of high dose chemotherapy and autologous stem cell transplantation for patients with biopsy proven primary refractory Hodgkin's disease. *Br J Haematol*. 2004;124:645–652.

Histiocytic Disorders

Sheila Weitzman and R. Maarten Egeler

CHAPTER

16

Introduction

The histiocytic disorders are classified into two major subtypes, disorders of variable biologic behavior and those that are clearly malignant.[1] The aptly named disorders of variable biologic behavior encompass conditions in which the natural history varies from mild spontaneously regressing disease to widespread disease that is potentially fatal. This category is further subdivided into disorders of the antigen-presenting dendritic cell and disorders of the macrophage/monocyte line of cells (Table 16-1). Langerhans cell histiocytosis (LCH) is the major disorder of the antigen-presenting cell, while hemophagocytic lymphohistiocytosis (HLH) is the commonest disorder associated with the macrophage/monocyte line. The finding of more than one disorder in the same patient[2,3] reflects the ability of one cell type to give rise to another under the influence of different growth factors. Nonetheless, the Histiocyte Society classification provides a means of standardization of the nomenclature, making possible international cooperative studies and comparison of results of different studies.

Langerhans Cell Histiocytosis

Langerhans cell histiocytosis, the commonest of the histiocytic disorders, is characterized by clonal proliferation and excess accumulation of pathologic Langerhans cells (LCs). The disease varies widely in clinical presentation from localized involvement of a single bone to a widely disseminated life-threatening disease.

Diagnosis of Langerhans Cell Histiocytosis

The diagnosis is clearly based on classical clinical findings in addition to the histologic and immunohistochemical criteria (Table 16-2), to avoid misdiagnosis of reactive normal LCs found within lymph nodes in response to a variety of diseases, including some neoplasms.[4,5]

Histopathology

The histopathology of LCH is that of a granulomatous lesion containing pathologic LCs as well as normal inflammatory cells such as T cells, eosinophils, and macrophages,

---

Table 16-1

Classification of histiocytic disorder.

1. *Disorders of varying biologic behavior*
   a. *Dendritic-cell related*
      Langerhans cell histiocytosis
      Juvenile xanthogranuloma and related disorders
      Solitary histiocytomas with JXG phenotype
      Secondary dendritic cell disorders
   b. *Macrophage-related*
      Hemophagocytic lymphohistiocytosis
      Familial and sporadic
      Secondary hemophagocytic syndromes
      Infection associated
      Malignancy associated
      Autoimmune associated
      Other
      Sinus histiocytosis with massive lymphadenopathy (Rosai-Dorfman disease)
      Solitary histiocytoma of macrophage phenotype
2. *Malignant disorders*
   a. *Monocyte/Macrophage-related*
      Monocytic leukemias M4, M5A and B, CMML
      Extramedullary monocytic tumors or sarcoma (monocytic counterpart of granulocytic sarcoma)
      Macrophage-related-histiocytic sarcoma (localized or disseminated)
   b. *Dendritic-cell related*
      Histiocytic sarcoma (localized or disseminated) (specify phenotype: follicular dendritic cell, interdigitating dendritic cell, etc)

Source: Adapted from Favara et al.[1]

Table 16-2

Characteristics of histiocytes in health and disease.

	LC	IDC	DD*	M/M
Immunohistochem				
HLA-DR	+	+	−	+
CD1a	++	−	−	−
CD14	−	−	±	+
CD68	±	−	+	++
CD163	±	−	+	++
Factor XIIIa	−	−	+	−
Histochemical				
NSE	±	±	±	+
S100	+	+	−	±
Lysozyme	−	−	−	++
Langerin (BG)	++	−	−	−
Clinical disease	LCH	Inter-digitating cell sarcoma	JXG family	HLH SHML

LC = Langerhans cell   IDC = interdigitating cell   DD = dermal dendrocyte (origin is questioned, possibly plasmacytic histiocyte)   M/M = monocyte/macrophage   JXG = juvenile xanthogranuloma   HLH = hemophagocytic lymphohistiocytosis   SHML = sinus histiocytosis with massive lymphadenopathy.

together with multinucleated giant cells. In contrast to normal LCs, LCH cells are actively proliferating, and they have a rounded shape without marked dendritic extensions, a folded nucleus, a moderate amount of homogeneous pink, granular cytoplasm, and distinct cell margins. Birbeck granules (BG), typically rod- or racket-shaped intracytoplasmic granules, are found only in LCs. Langerhans cells typically express high levels of CD1a and of langerin (CD207), and positivity of these two markers now defines the normal LC phenotype.[6,7] Langerin is a mannose-specific lectin whose intracellular component is found in association with the BG, with 100% concordance.[8] The presence of BG can thus now be proven immunohistochemically, without the necessity of electron microscopy. Birbeck granules (and by association langerin positivity) are usually absent from brain and liver LCH, even when they are clinically involved.[9]

Pathogenesis

The major developments in the clinical arena of LCH have been complemented by productive research concerning the basic biology. Normal LCs, the sentinels of the immune system for foreign antigens, are strategically located at host/environmental interfaces such as the epidermis and respiratory and genital epithelia. Langerhans cells and keratinocytes form a network throughout the epidermis, bound together by adhesion molecules such as E-cadherin. Langerhans cells capture antigens, process them, express the antigenic peptides on their cell surface bound to major histocompatibility complex HLA molecules, migrate through lymphatics, and present antigen to peptide-specific naive and to central memory T lymphocytes[10] in the T-lymphocyte-predominant areas of draining nodes and spleen. These processes appear to be controlled by cytokines and chemokines produced by the keratinocytes, LCs, endothelial cells, and T cells.[7,11] Necessary for LC mobilization is down-regulation of CCR6, a receptor on the cell surface, which responds to a ligand within the epidermis, and up-regulation of CCR7, which responds to a chemokine within the lymph node. At the same time, reduction of expression of adhesion molecules and up-regulation of matrix metalloproteinases that allow passage across basement membranes[12] allow migration of the LC cell to the T-lymphocyte-rich areas of the lymph nodes. There up-regulation of MHC-II complexes and of the membrane-bound costimulatory receptor-coreceptor pairs, such as CD40-CD40L and CD28/CTLA4-CD80/CD86, binds the LCs and T lymphocytes, resulting in further activation and cytokine secretion by both cell types. In LCH, the pathologic LCH cells appear to be in an arrested state of activation and/or differentiation.[13] The immature lesional CD1a-positive cells fail to up-regulate CCR7 and are prevented from leaving their peripheral tissue sites, where they accumulate and express other inflammatory chemokines, resulting in their own recruitment and retention as well as that of other inflammatory cells, including T lymphocytes.[7,13] Ligation of CD40-positive LCH-cells by the high number of lesional CD40L-positive T lymphocytes results in activation of both cells and erratic and uncontrolled production of various cytokines,[14,15] creating a "cytokine storm." High expression of cytokines within the LCH lesion include interleukin-2 (IL-2), IL-4, IL-5, tumor necrosis factor-alpha (TNFα), IL-1α, granulocyte/monocyte-colony stimulating factor and interferon-gamma, IL-3, and IL-7.[16] The pattern of cytokine expression favors recruitment of LC progenitors, as well as their maturation and rescue from apoptosis, thereby explaining the pathologic accumulation of LCH cells.[15–17] The cytokines produced contribute directly to the pathological sequelae, including fibrosis, bone resorption, and necrosis. Thus the unique clinicopathologic picture of LCH results from the accumulation of abnormal LC cells, an aberrant interaction with T lymphocytes, and the effects of the cytokines produced by both cells. However, the findings to date do not provide insight into what initiates the process.

Etiology of Langerhans Cell Histiocytosis

The discovery that all forms of LCH tested are monoclonal[18,19] suggests that this may be a neoplastic process with varying biologic behavior. Circumstances exist in which a monoclonal population may persist for years without development of malignancy; however, all those described involve monoclonal expansion of T lymphocytes, and whether this can be readily translated to a clonal expansion of LCs is unknown. Recent findings of loss of heterozygosity on chromosomes 1, 4, 6, 7, 9, 16, 17, and 22, as well as chromosomal instability and elevated expression of cell-cycle related proteins or oncogene products, such as p53, H-ras, and c-myc, suggesting disrupted cell-cycle regulation, are more persuasive evidence of neoplasia.[7,20–22]

Studies on telomerase expression in LCH cells have also been done to try to address this question. Maintenance of telomere length is a requirement for unlimited proliferation. A recent study showed that the lesional CD1a+ cells express telomerase in patients with multisystem (MS) disease as well as all single-system (SS) skin LCH lesions. This is in contrast to SS bone lesions in which about 25% of the lesions analyzed contained LCH cells that expressed telomerase, suggesting that the LCH cells in bone lesions may have a more limited proliferative capacity and life span. This could explain the fact that many unifocal SS bone lesions require minimal treatment or resolve spontaneously and hardly ever recur. In contrast, the maintenance of the telomere length in MS LCH may support this subtype of LCH being of neoplastic origin.[23] However, these findings need to be repeated and extended, and arguments in favor of and against malignancy continue.[7]

Genetic and Ethnic Factors

Evidence in favor of a genetic predisposition for LCH include familial clustering, with 1% of probands having another first- or second-degree relative with the disease,[24] indicating that there is a germline mutation in some patients that predisposes them to LCH and the associated malignancies.[7]

Twin studies demonstrate an 87% concordance rate for monozygotic twins compared with 10% for dizygotic twins. Monozygotic twins also present at a younger median age and have a higher prevalence of MS disease.[24] A recent Nordic study found no association between HLA subtypes and the occurrence of LCH but raised the possibility that HLA-DRB1*03 plays a protective role against developing MS disease.[25] In view of the heterogeneity of LCH, differences in genetic predisposition between the subtypes may be possible, as suggested by the differences in telomerase expression discussed above.

Risk Factors for Langerhans Cell Histiocytosis

Defective immune function has long been suggested as being central to the pathogenesis of LCH. Many immune defects have been described, with the commonest being a decrease in CD8-suppressor T lymphocytes. Associated with the immune defects are abnormal thymus histology and an increase in thymic calcification seen radiographically. Administration of thymic extract was said to result in clinical improvement in some patients[26]; however, these studies could not be repeated. An alternative hypothesis is that this is a reactive disease, resulting from environmental or other triggers that lead to the aberrant reaction between LCs and T lymphocytes.[27] The known association between LCH and malignancy may support this hypothesis. The consistent finding that there is no seasonal or geographic clustering of LCH argues against an infectious etiology,[28] and viral studies have produced varying results. An analysis of 9 different viruses by in situ hybridization and polymerase chain reaction techniques failed to demonstrate an association,[29] as did a study of a possible relationship with human herpes viruses (HHV-8).[30] An association with HHV-6 was suggested in 1993,[31] and more recently HHV-6 was found in a high percentage of LCH lesional tissues.[27] Further studies to clarify the role of these viruses are necessary.

A recent large epidemiologic study of childhood LCH showed an increase in thyroid disease in the probands as well as an increased family history of thyroid disease. In infants with MS disease, no association was found with risk factors during pregnancy; however, an increase in postnatal infections and use of antibiotics was found.[32] An increased incidence of autoimmune diseases (3%), cancer (16%), and thyroid disease (5%) was found in the grandparents' generation in the twin study.[24] In adults, cigarette smoking is a clear risk factor for pulmonary LCH. The exact relationship of this sometimes polyclonal lung disease to the monoclonal forms of the disease remains to be elucidated, particularly in view of a Swedish study that raised the possibility of an increased risk for the development of lung LCH in adult survivors of pediatric LCH who smoke.[33]

Race, Age, and Gender in Langerhans Cell Histiocytosis

Langerhans cell histiocytosis can occur at any age from the neonatal period until old age.[34–35] A recent population-based study showed an overall incidence of 2.6 per million child years for children younger than 15 years, with an incidence of 9.0 and 4.6 cases per million years at risk for those younger than 1 year and 1 to 4 years of age, respectively.[36] These figures probably still underestimate the problem, because many patients with localized LCH are likely to go undiagnosed. Studies report a slight male preponderance overall, with a male to female ratio as high as 2 to 1 in MS disease patients.[35] Recent figures from a national incidence survey in the United Kingdom suggest that there are as many cases in adults as in children with a similar spectrum of disease.[7]

Clinical Presentation of Langerhans Cell Histiocytosis

Langerhans cell histiocytosis in children is very diverse, ranging from a spontaneously regressing single lesion to a life-threatening MS disorder with rapid progression and death. Between the two extremes are patients with MS disease without organ failure whose disease runs a fluctuating course and eventually "burns out," often leaving serious residual disabilities.[7]

The severity of disease tends to be age related, with MS LCH seen mainly in children under 2 years of age, multifocal SS disease in children between 2 and 5 years, while 50% of unifocal bone (UFB) disease occurs in children over

5 years of age.[37] Some forms require little if any treatment, and others need aggressive therapy. The need for "risk-adjusted" therapy was recognized early, and the Histiocyte Society defined two categories for disease extent—namely, SS-LCH and MS-LCH.[38] Approximately two-thirds of children present with SS disease, usually in bone.[7] Single-system disease is further subdivided as unifocal or multifocal, while MS disease is divided into limited (low-risk) MS-LCH (previously known as Hand-Schuller-Christian disease) and disseminated MS disease (previously called Letterer-Siwe disease). Single-system disease may progress to become limited MS disease with involvement of the hypothalamic-pituitary axis and the central nervous system (CNS). However, only very young babies tend to progress from SS-LCH (usually skin-only disease) to the disseminated potentially fatal form of the disease.[39] Although the prognosis for survival in SS disease and for limited MS-LCH is excellent, repeated reactivations may be associated with significant long-term complications. Disseminated MS-LCH has an extremely variable course and an unpredictable prognosis,[40] with a high mortality.[41]

Bone Involvement in Langerhans Cell Histiocytosis

Bone is the commonest single organ involved in childhood LCH, with approximately 80% of patients having bone disease, of whom about 80% have SS disease, and 20% of whom have bone disease as part of MS-LCH.[42] Involvement of a single bone (UFB) is seen in 78%, and 2 or more bones (multifocal bone, MFB) in 22% of cases.[42,43] Spontaneous healing of bone lesions is well known, and healing at one site at the same time as, or followed by, progression in another is not uncommon. Survival of patients with SS bone LCH is almost universal; however, reactivations may occur at a rate of 3%[44] to 12%[42] for UFB, 11% to 25% for MFB, and 50% to 70% for bone involvement as part of MS disease.[42] The greater the reactivation rate, the higher the incidence of diabetes insipidus (DI) and other late complications. "Risk" bones are those that give the highest risk of DI and include the facial bones and skull base, particularly if associated with an intracranial soft tissue mass.[45] A large study comprising 300 patients from Argentina who achieved a remission after initial therapy showed that most reactivations (88%) occurred within the first 2 years and that permanent consequences occurred in 71% and 25%, respectively, of patients with and without reactivations, and sequelae were generally more severe in patients with reactivations.[46]

Clinical Presentation of Bone Langerhans Cell Histiocytosis

The bone most commonly involved is the skull, and the commonest presentation of LCH in childhood is with a single mass lesion on the head. All bones may be involved, however, except for the hands and feet. In the extremity, proximal long bones are more commonly involved than distal, and diaphysis and metaphysis are equally involved,

while the epiphysis is commonly spared.[47] The majority of patients present with swelling and/or pain that may be present during activity and/or rest, and rarely a pathologic fracture may be present. Pain may be present only at night, particularly in the early stages. Approximately half of the bone lesions are asymptomatic and detected only by radiographic investigations.[48] Depending on the area involved, other symptoms and signs may be present. Jaw pain, swelling, and/or loose teeth occur in jaw LCH. Temporal bone LCH should be considered whenever chronic ear drainage, with dermatitis of the auricular canal, mastoiditis, and cholesteatoma, occurs in children younger than 3 years.[49,50] The external canal involvement is usually due to extension of skin rash into the external ear canal, while middle and inner ear disease usually suggests involvement of temporal bone. Orbital involvement may result in proptosis, swelling and redness of the eyelid, diplopia, and/or ophthalmoplegia.[51] Lower-extremity lesions may cause a limp or fracture, while spine involvement causes back pain and/or kyphoscoliosis or neurologic dysfunction including paraplegia.[52,53] Langerhans cell histiocytosis is the commonest cause of vertebra plana in children.[54] Most patients with SS bone disease are afebrile, but fever should not exclude the diagnosis. Blood counts may show mild eosinophilia but are otherwise normal, and the erythrocyte sedimentation rate is often mildly elevated. Because bone lesions may be asymptomatic, every patient should have a complete radiographic workup at diagnosis, irrespective of presentation.

Radiographic Investigation of Bone Langerhans Cell Histiocytosis

The extent of bone disease is best assessed by plain radiographs that are more sensitive and specific than Technetium-99 nuclear medicine bone scans.[55,56] However, both modalities are suggested for best assessment of initial bone lesions and of healing. Radiographic characteristics vary from the classic osteolytic lesion with sharply demarcated margins and little or no periosteal reaction (Figure 16-1a) to radiologically aggressive lesions resembling a malignant tumor (Figure 16-1b). These may be seen particularly in the facial bones but also occur in the long bones.[55,57] Computerized tomography and magnetic resonance imaging (MRI) scans are useful in delineating the extent of soft tissue involvement; however, neither is useful in distinguishing LCH from malignancy in radiologically aggressive lesions,[58,59] and the diagnosis should be proven by biopsy in all cases. Only in patients with vertebra plana without a soft tissue mass does the risk of biopsy outweigh the benefit, and these patients can be observed without biopsy. They should, however, be closely followed to exclude infections such as tuberculosis and malignancies such as Ewing sarcoma and lymphoma. The classic radiographic description of healing is disappearance of the soft tissue mass with development of a well-defined sclerotic rim, but assessment of response in bone is notoriously difficult, as residual soft tissue masses may occur without active LCH being present, and the bone scan may remain positive due to healing.

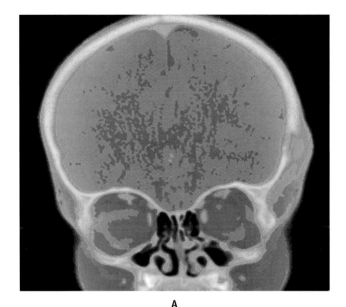

A

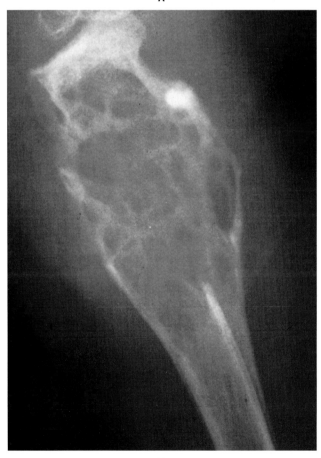

B

Figure 16-1 (A) Typical LCH lytic lesion in skull with overlying soft tissue mass. (B) Atypical LCH with periosteal elevation resembling a bone sarcoma.

18-fluorodeoxyglucose (18-FDG) positron emission tomography (PET) is a sensitive technique for identifying metabolically active LCH, but availability, expense, irradiation dose, and need for sedation in young children may limit its utility.[60]

Skin Involvement in Langerhans Cell Histiocytosis

Skin is the second most commonly involved organ in LCH, involved in about 50% of patients.[61] Isolated skin disease (skin-only LCH) is seen in 10% of cases, usually in very young children, but may occur in older patients and adults.[62] The commonest area involved is the scalp, followed by flexural creases, but any site may be involved, including the nails. The commonest presentation is with a "seborrhea-like" eruption, which may or may not be purpuric and is often initially misdiagnosed as "cradle cap." Many other skin manifestations are described such as papules, vesicles, crusted plaques, nodules, and purpuric nodules[61] (Figure 16-2). Involvement of skin of external auditory canal may lead to chronic discharge. *LCH should be considered whenever seborrheic dermatitis or diaper dermatitis fails to respond to therapy or keeps recurring.*

The natural history is variable; patients with skin-only LCH may have spontaneous regression, regression and reactivation in skin, or progression, particularly in the infant, to disseminated, sometimes fatal disease. Hashimoto and Pritzker described a particular form of skin LCH associated with spontaneous involution. Pathologically, the disease involves the dermis with epidermal sparing, and senescent mitochondria are seen as "myelin-dense" bodies on EM. Although a small percentage of babies with

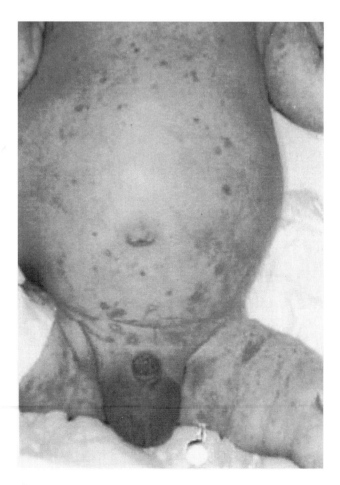

Figure 16-2 Skin LCH in a neonate with multisystem disease.

skin-only LCH fit this description, half of all babies with skin-only LCH will progress to MS disease.[39] It is safer to follow with close observation all young babies with skin-only LCH.[39,63,64]

Lymph Node Involvement in Langerhans Cell Histiocytosis

Lymph node enlargement may occur as the only organ system involved (SS-LCH) or more commonly as part of MS-LCH. On occasion, chronic involvement of a lymph node can lead to a chronically discharging sinus through the overlying skin.[65]

Multisystem Langerhans Cell Histiocytosis

The clinical presentation depends on the organs involved. Limited MS-LCH usually refers to involvement of bone and/or skin and/or the hypothalamic-pituitary axis. Disseminated MS-LCH usually occurs in children younger than 2 years and can involve any organ except the kidneys and gonads. The presentation is therefore with any or all of the following: fever, wasting, hepatosplenomegaly with abdominal distention, lymph node enlargement, pancytopenia, edema, tachypnea, and respiratory distress. Skin and bone involvement is common in MS disease, and the manifestations described above are also part of the clinical presentation of MS-LCH.

Liver and Spleen Involvement in Langerhans Cell Histiocytosis

Hepatosplenomegaly may indicate involvement by LCH, obstructive disease from enlarged nodes in the porta hepatis, or even secondary HLH (Figure 16-3). Liver dysfunction may be the most important prognosticator for poor outcome (Grois, personal communication) and is demonstrated by jaundice, hypoalbuminemia, and/or coagulopathy. Progression of cholestasis to sclerosing cholangitis, biliary cirrhosis, and liver failure may occur even after the disease becomes inactive. Hypersplenism may aggravate the pancytopenia.

Lung Involvement in Langerhans Cell Histiocytosis

Pulmonary LCH (P-LCH) occurs most commonly in adults who smoke cigarettes during the third decade[66] but may occur at any age, including in young children with MS-LCH. A dry cough or tachypnea with rib retraction is often the only clinical sign. In the early stages the diagnosis is suggested by a diffuse micronodular pattern on chest radiographs, which may progress to cyst formation and a "honeycomb lung" (Figure 16-4). In later stages large bullae may rupture, causing spontaneous pneumothoraces, although this finding is commoner in adults than in pediatric P-LCH. Emphysematous changes, along with increasing amounts of interstitial fibrosis, may occur in

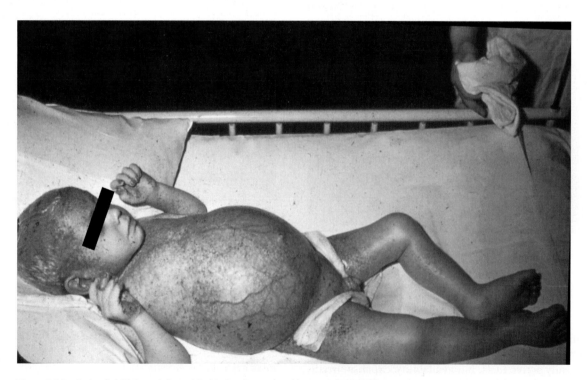

Figure 16-3 Systemic LCH in an infant with skin involvement and hepatosplenomegaly.

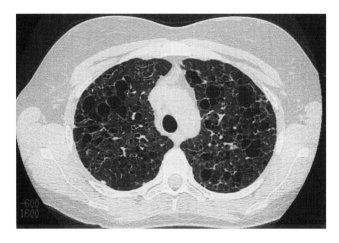

Figure 16-4 CT scan showing typical changes of lung LCH.

the final phase of P-LCH (discussed later). It has been suggested that more than 5% CD1a-positive cells in the broncho-alveolar fluid, where normally there should be fewer than 1% CD1a-positive cells, is diagnostic of P-LCH.[67] This appears to be true in children,[68] but lower levels are often seen in adult P-LCH.[69]

Hematopoietic System Involvement in Langerhans Cell Histiocytosis

Anemia, neutropenia, and/or thrombocytopenia are frequent findings in disseminated MS-LCH and are considered to be important risk factors. The absence of morphologic infiltration of bone marrow does not exclude hematopoietic involvement. In the LCH-I study, 18% of MS patients had documented marrow infiltration, and 36% had blood count abnormalities.[38,49] It may be associated with secondary hemophagocytosis, which may require specific therapy to prevent a fatal outcome. The pancytopenia may also be associated with marked hepatosplenomegaly and hypersplenism in particular, in the absence of marrow involvement.

Gastrointestinal Tract Involvement in Langerhans Cell Histiocytosis

Signs and symptoms of gastrointestinal involvement in LCH (GI-LCH) include "failure to thrive" due to malabsorption, vomiting, diarrhea with or without blood, and protein-losing enteropathy. Endoscopic biopsy is needed for diagnosis, and GI involvement, although not at present a criterion of "risk" disease, may suggest an inferior prognosis.[70]

Central Nervous System/Endocrine Involvement in Langerhans Cell Histiocytosis

Diabetes insipidus due to infiltration of the hypothalamic-pituitary axis is the commonest manifestation of endocrine LCH and occurs in about 13% of patients overall.[46] Dia-

betes insipidus may be the first presenting symptom of LCH or may occur subsequent to diagnosis, usually in patients with the chronically reactivating form of the disease.[71,72] The risk of DI is greatest in patients with lesions involving the facial bones and skull base[72] and is most common in patients with MS-LCH.[46,73] Gadolinium-enhanced MRI scans demonstrate loss of the posterior pituitary "bright spot," thickening of the pituitary stalk, a partial or completely empty sella, and sometimes a suprasellar mass.[74,75] Anterior pituitary deficits may follow the onset of DI by 0.1 to 6 years (median 3.5 years).[71] Growth hormone (GH) deficiency usually occurs first,[76] although growth failure in children with LCH is multi-factorial, with additional contributing factors being chronic illness, malabsorption, and prolonged cortico-steroid treatment.[49] Treatment with GH is safe and effective and does not appear to induce reactivations or second malignancies.[77] Other hypothalamic-pituitary axis abnormalities include precocious or delayed puberty, amenorrhea in adult females, hyperprolactinemia, morbid obesity,[78] sleeping disorders, and disorders of thermoregulation.[76] Thyroid deficiency may occur as a result of either hypothalamic-pituitary axis involvement or thyroid gland infiltration.[73,76,79]

Nonendocrine Central Nervous System Involvement in Langerhans Cell Histiocytosis

Involvement of the brain may also follow the onset of DI. Active CNS LCH is usually first seen as extraparenchymal lesions arising in areas where the blood-brain barrier (BBB) is deficient such as the leptomeninges, choroid plexus, or pineal gland. Active CNS disease may progress to a chronic neurodegenerative stage due either to demyelination and gliosis from cytokine- and chemokine-mediated neural damage[80] or to an autoimmune reaction to the preceding LCH.[72] This end-stage disease is observed in about 3% to 5% of patients with LCH but may occur in 10% or more of patients with DI. Central nervous system neurodegeneration can occasionally arise in the absence of other CNS involvement.[69] Clinical findings including ataxia, dysarthria, nystagmus, tremor, dysdiadochokinesia, dysphagia, psychomotor retardation, and neuropsychologic problems may develop years after the original diagnosis of LCH and may progress to produce severe disability and even death. It is unclear how many asymptomatic patients with radiographic neurodegeneration seen on MRI scans will progress to the debilitating symptomatic neurodegenerative phase. Brain 18-FDG PET scans may be helpful in defining active as well as burned-out lesions.[81] There is no known effective therapy for patients with late progressive CNS disease. At present, only DI heralds involvement of other parts of the brain resulting in global neurologic and neuropsychologic sequelae.[72,76] Prevention of the onset of DI is therefore likely to be very important. Attempts to detect partial DI before it becomes established have been largely unsuccessful. Urinary vasopressin (AVP) levels do not appear to be useful,[77] partly because of the wide range of AVP values in patients with partial DI.

Treatment of Langerhans Cell Histiocytosis

Therapeutic decisions are based on two major concerns, the probability of survival and the likelihood of development of late effects. Thus the recommendations vary for UFB compared with MFB, for those defined as having disease in "risk" bones, and within the setting of MS disease for those defined as having "risk" as compared to "low-risk" MS disease.

Treatment of Bone Langerhans Cell Histiocytosis

Effective therapies for bone LCH include observation, biopsy, curettage, intralesional injection of corticosteroids, nonsteroidal anti-inflammatory drugs (NSAIDs), bisphosphonates, antineoplastic chemotherapy, low-dose radiation therapy, and various forms of immunotherapy. Treatment decisions are based on the excellent survival rates for SS bone disease, the ability of bone lesions to undergo spontaneous regression, the fact that therapy does not appear to alter the rate of healing,[82–84] and the risk of long-term complications associated with multiple reactivations in bone. At first presentation, most UFB lesions undergo curettage to induce healing and provide tissue for diagnosis. Surgical resection is unnecessary, may lead to long-term deformity, and is contraindicated at any site. Observation is limited to lesions in "non-risk" bones in patients with a pathologic diagnosis. Patients with intense pain, restriction of motion, unacceptable deformity, involvement of a growth plate, and/or involvement of a bone likely to fracture usually require therapy.[85] Patients presenting with vertebra plana without a soft tissue mass or neurologic symptoms can be observed without a firm diagnosis but should be carefully followed. Where therapy is needed for a limited number of lesions, intralesional corticosteroid, best inserted under radiographic control, is effective and usually safe.[85,86] Around 10% of such patients require a repeat injection to achieve healing.[86] Low-dose radiation therapy (6 Gy to 10 Gy over 3 to 5 doses) remains an effective modality but is usually restricted to involvement of critical organs such as the spinal cord or optic nerve. At the suggested dose, long-term effects are unlikely, and it is preferable to mutilating surgery. For single or multiple lesions, indomethacin, a potent prostaglandin-E2 inhibitor, and other NSAIDs, have proven efficacious,[87,88] as has bisphosphonate therapy.[89–91] The use of bisphosphonates is supported by the report of da Costa et al, who demonstrated that the bony destruction is likely mediated by osteoclast-like giant cells that produce various matrix-degrading enzymes resulting in destructive lesions and the predominant symptom of bone pain.[92]

Toxicity has been tolerable in most patients treated. However, the role of NSAIDs and bisphosphonates in pre-venting reactivations and late complications is unclear, as is the long-term effect of bisphosphonates in young children. Patients with MFB or bone LCH in MS disease are usually treated with chemotherapy.

Treatment of Cutaneous Langerhans Cell Histiocytosis

A few case reports document progression of skin-only LCH to DI,[93–95] but in general skin-only LCH has a good prognosis and should not be overtreated. Careful observation for progression to advanced disease is necessary in the very young child. Surgical excision should be undertaken for small isolated lesions only, and no mutilating surgery is necessary. Local or systemic corticosteroids are the first-line therapy, but the effect is usually transient. Psoralen with ultraviolet therapy has been shown to be effective,[96,97] as has topical nitrogen mustard.[93,98] Despite the finding of no premalignant or malignant changes in the nitrogen mustard-treated skin of 20 children with median follow-up of 8.3 years,[93] concerns with regard to late skin cancer persist for both these therapies. There are anecdotal reports of successful use of topical tacrolimus even in very young babies. If a large surface area is treated, serum tacrolimus levels need to be followed. Numerous case reports attest to the efficacy of thalidomide in adult patients with cutaneous, mucosal, and vulvar LCH, but in most patients described, the disease recurred within variable periods after cessation of therapy. Retreatment with the same drugs, however, appears to be effective.[99–102] Dramatic responses of cutaneous and ano-genital lesions to the combination of thalidomide plus interferon have been reported.[103] Interferon-alpha (IFN-α) alone has been used in patients with progressive LCH,[88,104] and successes have been reported with prolonged IFN-α therapy, without apparent toxicity.[105,106] Finally, chemotherapy is usually effective in skin LCH but is usually limited to widespread symptomatic disease or skin as part of MS LCH. Successful prolonged use of oral etoposide without apparent adverse effects has been reported in adults.[107]

Treatment of Diabetes Insipidus in Langerhans Cell Histiocytosis

A few reports have been published of reversibility of DI by early therapy,[108] but in most cases DI is irreversible at the time of presentation. However, because of the significant neurologic consequences that may follow DI, the current recommendation is to treat recent-onset DI to try to prevent the uncommon but devastating late CNS disease. The optimal therapy, however, is unclear. Radiation therapy may be effective, but there is no evidence that "late" disease will respond to therapy,[109] and the potential for late effects means that irradiation should be restricted to nonresponsive growing masses. Because the pituitary is outside the BBB, standard LCH chemotherapy will likely treat the active disease. Theoretically, a drug such as 2-chlorodeoxyadenosine (2-CdA), which crosses the BBB and has successfully treated active CNS-LCH,[108,110,111] may be the best option both to treat active LCH in the hypothalamic-pituitary axis and to prevent late CNS disease. A recent study by Dhall et al found that 8 of 12 patients treated with 2-CdA for mass lesions in the CNS had a complete radiographic response, while the remaining 4 patients had a sustained partial response. Eleven of the 12 remained progression free at the time of reporting. There was, however, no reversal of neurocognitive dysfunction and/or DI that was already present at the time of therapy.[112]

Treatment of Multisystem Langerhans Cell Histiocytosis

Treatment of MS-LCH has dual aims: to improve survival and to prevent late sequelae of the disease or therapy. Patients with extensive disease but without involvement of the "risk" organs—namely, liver, spleen, and hematopoietic system—have an excellent survival rate with minimal therapy. For this group, therapy should be given to prevent DI and other late complications. Lung disease has conventionally been included as a "risk" organ, but recent work suggests that children with lung as the only "risk" organ do well and should be included with the low-risk patients. For patients with "risk"-organ MS-LCH, results of the large randomized cooperative group trials suggest that early therapy with relatively nontoxic chemotherapy improves survival and may reduce the incidence of late complications.[38,43,73,113,114] A different and conservative approach was suggested by McLelland, who reported that of 44 children with extensive disease, 36 required systemic therapy. Of the 36 patients, 17 responded to prednisolone alone, and 19 required the addition of vinblastine or etoposide. Overall survival was equivalent at 82%, but 60% of survivors had late effects, and 36% developed DI,[115] compared with 10% in the DAL-HX studies, supporting the use of early chemotherapy for MS-LCH. Comparison of the DAL-HX and LCH-I and -II studies of the Histiocyte Society demonstrated that around 80% of young children with MS-LCH survive long term.[40] All three studies, as well as a large French study,[73] showed that a lack of response to chemotherapy at 6 weeks was the single most important predictor of poor survival.[40,41,73] For patients who responded to initial therapy, survival was very good, and the ensuing problem was that of reactivation of disease in non-risk organs such as skin or bone, which was rarely fatal. However, permanent disease-related disabilities occurred in more than 40% of patients.[41] Recent data from the Japanese LCH study group, as well as a French pilot study, suggest that early switch of poor responders to intensive salvage regimens improves survival.[114,116]

These studies have allowed the development of risk-adapted therapy. Patients with extensive disease with "risk" organ involvement should be evaluated at the end of induction therapy, allowing allocation to a group of "responders" or "nonresponders."

The very high risk group of nonresponders (22% of "risk" patients on LCH-II) should be moved early to a salvage protocol. In this setting, toxicity and late effects become secondary considerations.

Salvage Therapies for Refractory/Recurrent Langerhans Cell Histiocytosis

The three groups of patients requiring salvage therapy are those with refractory MS disease, those with chronically relapsing disease associated with good survival but significant long-term complications, and patients with the late progressive involvement of liver, lung, and CNS. Many chemotherapy drugs have proved to be effective in the treatment of LCH, and a number of drug combinations have been tried in nonresponders to first-line protocols, including vinca alkaloids, alkylating agents, anthracyclines, and platinum drugs.[88] A combination of low-dose cytosine arabinoside (ara-C), vincristine, and prednisolone was shown to be effective in patients with organ dysfunction and those with relapsed or progressive disease.[117] However, these protocols did not improve the survival in refractory patients, nor have they been shown to prevent reactivations in the chronically relapsing patients. Early results of a prospective Histiocyte Society study utilizing 2-CdA suggest that 2-CdA is more effective in low-risk chronically relapsing patients, and that fewer than a third of refractory high-risk patients responded (Weitzman, personal communication). Similar results were seen with other promising agents such as cyclosporine-A,[118] thalidomide,[102,119] and IFN-α,[104] all drugs with significant activity in low-risk LCH such as skin, but results in refractory MS patients have been disappointing.[88] Results of a French pilot study of the combination of 2-CdA and ara-C in patients with progressive LCH show encouraging results,[116] and this combination is being tested in a Histiocyte Society salvage protocol. Tumor necrosis factor-alpha is an important cause of morbidity in LCH. Etanercept, a soluble TNF receptor/Fc fusion protein, was added to the therapy of a child with nonresponsive MS-LCH, with good effect and no toxicity. Prolonged therapy was necessary,[120] however, and this positive experience has not been repeated. A number of successful hematopoietic progenitor cell transplants have been reported in refractory LCH patients. A review of the literature found 35 patients transplanted for refractory LCH.[121] A summary of 27 well-documented cases shows that 15 of 27 (56%) patients were alive in continuous complete remission from 12+ to 144+ (median 25+) months. The major cause of failure was transplant-related mortality. Although there remains the likelihood of positive reporting bias, it nonetheless seems that allogeneic, but not autologous, transplant is potentially curative in poor-risk patients, particularly if the transplant-related mortality can be lowered by the use of reduced-intensity conditioning, as suggested by the survival of 9 of 11 patients in a recent study.[122] This concept is the subject of an open Histiocyte Society study designed for patients that fail the 2-CdA/ara-C salvage study.

Treatment of Late Chronic Langerhans Cell Histiocytosis

Late progressive chronic LCH is seen in liver, lung, and CNS as described above, and appears to be due to late fibrosis (or gliosis), possibly due to the effect of excess inflammatory cytokines such as transforming growth factor-beta (β).[123] Langerhans cell histiocytosis is unique in having exquisite tropism for the bile ducts,[4] and late chronic liver disease presents as sclerosing cholangitis and biliary cirrhosis progressing to liver failure. Patients may present with sclerosing cholangitis at diagnosis or following active liver involvement as part of MS-LCH.[124,125] In the lungs, fibrosis surrounds cystic spaces, giving the classic honeycomb lung. Progression to pulmonary fibrosis and respiratory failure may result in death.[69] Clinically and radiographically, it is difficult to discriminate active LCH from end-stage fibrosis.[66,126] Organ transplantation is the only proven effective therapy for end-stage lung and liver disease, and the results appear to be durable. A review of pediatric LCH patients transplanted for liver failure found that 78% of patients were alive,[127] with only 2 recurrences, and no cases of sclerosing cholangitis have been reported in the transplanted livers,[128] suggesting that posttransplant immunosuppression with drugs may prevent LCH recurrence. Similarly, 5 of 7 adult patients are alive and well from 15 to 90 months post-lung transplantation, with 2 recurrences of active LCH after resuming smoking.[129] An increased incidence in severity and frequency of rejection was found in several series.[130-132] A number of experimental antifibrotic drugs that ameliorate bleomycin-induced lung fibrosis in mice are being tested in humans and may prove useful in the future.[133,134]

Permanent Consequences of Langerhans Cell Histiocytosis

Results of the late effects study of the Histiocyte Society suggest that with a minimum of 3 years of follow-up, at least 71% of MS disease and 24% of SS disease patients have at least one permanent consequence, the most commonly reported being DI.[130]

In a large French study of 589 patients with pediatric-onset LCH, the estimated 10-year risk of pituitary involvement was $24.2 \pm 1.8\%$.[135] Growth hormone deficiency occurred in 61. The median age of onset of LCH was 2.8 years, of DI was 3.9 years, and of growth deficiency was 7.67 years. The most severe complication was neurodegenerative syndrome, affecting 4.3% and 10.8% of patients, respectively, at 5 and 15 years after diagnosis and appeared to be linked to pituitary involvement. Neurologic problems such as cerebellar ataxia, psychological problems, and learning difficulties may occur in as many as 40% of patients with MS disease if followed long enough.[136,137]

Other permanent consequences include orthopedic problems, facial asymmetry, residual proptosis, loss of teeth, and hearing loss, which may contribute to the learning problems. Second malignancies, particularly T acute lymphoblastic leukemia, occur in LCH patients with a much higher than expected frequency[138] and include solid tumors, lymphoma, as well as myeloid and lymphoid leukemias.

From the point of view of therapeutic decision making, most of the serious permanent consequences such as endocrine and CNS involvement occur in patients with MS disease and with lesions involving the facial bones and base of skull, especially for those whose disease has a chronically relapsing and remitting course, and particular attention needs to be paid to these patients. Extensive surgical resections should be avoided, and the use of carcinogenic drugs and radiation therapy should be limited to life-threatening situations.

Hemophagocytic Lymphohistiocytosis

In 1952, Farquhar and Claireaux[139] first reported 2 siblings with unexplained fevers, progressive pancytopenia, hepatosplenomegaly, and a proliferation of histiocytes showing erythrophagocytosis.[140] In 1979, Risdall et al described 19 patients with similar findings, most of whom proved to have a viral etiology.[141] Since that time, the underlying pathophysiology has been recognized and therapy much improved. Whatever the underlying etiology, an inappropriate immune reaction with excess proliferation of activated T lymphocytes and macrophages, associated with inadequate apoptosis of immunogenic agents, results in an excess of pro-inflammatory cytokines, which produce the clinical picture of HLH.[142,143] Hemophagocytic lymphohistiocytosis is subdivided into primary and secondary forms, with the majority of cases being due to secondary (acquired) disease and an important minority due to familial (hereditary) HLH (FHLH), an autosomal recessive disease that at a molecular level appears to be associated with a variety of abnormalities of the perforin/granzyme pathway. Assignment to FHLH is based on a family history of the disease and/or the finding of one of the newly described genetic mutations. Parental consanguinity should raise suspicion of FHLH.[140] Recent studies suggest that 20% to 40% of FHLH cases are due to perforin gene mutations,[144-147] but several other genetic mutations may underlie the HLH phenotype, including mutations in syntaxin-11, munc13.4, rab-27A (Griscelli-type 2), lyst (Chediak-Higashi), SAP/SH2-D1A (X-linked lymphoproliferative disease), and others.[148,149]

The estimated incidence of FHLH is 1 in 50 000 live births,[140] but this figure will almost certainly increase as more genetic defects are discovered. The male to female ratio is 1 to 1. There is an increased incidence of the disease in ethnic groups with higher rates of consanguinity.[150] The majority of patients present before the age of 1 year; however, with the description of the gene mutations, it has become obvious that some FHLH patients may present at a much older age than previously suspected.

Secondary HLH occurs as a result of macrophage activation by a known stimulus that can be infectious, malignant, and autoimmune, associated with metabolic diseases and the hyperlipidemia of total parenteral nutrition.[151] The commonest of the infection-associated hemophagocytic syndrome is viral-associated due to Epstein-Barr virus (EBV) and other herpes viruses, but bacterial[152] and other infections are also described. At least in children, EBV-HLH appears to occur at a young age with more than 50% of patients being younger than 3 years.[151] Epstein-Barr virus and other infections may also trigger the familial form of the disease, an important distinction when therapy is considered.[153] In adults, the commonest cause of HLH is malignant lymphoma.[154]

Clinical Presentation and Diagnosis

Hemophagocytic lymphohistiocytosis usually presents with fever, hepatosplenomegaly, and cytopenias. Lymphadenopathy, skin rash, jaundice, and edema may occur and neurologic symptoms are common. A retrospective study of 193 HLH patients treated on the HLH-94 study showed that 63% had either neurologic symptoms or abnormal cerebrospinal fluid (CSF) at diagnosis. The clinical abnormalities included seizures, meningismus, irritability, decreased level of consciousness, cranial nerve palsy, psychomotor retardation, ataxia, and hypotonia. Fifteen percent of survivors had significant neurologic sequelae, highest in the patients with both neurologic symptoms and abnormal CSF.[155]

Common laboratory findings at diagnosis include hypertriglyceridemia, hypercholesterolemia, hypofibrinogenemia, liver dysfunction, hyperferritinemia, which may reach extremely high levels, as well as the CSF pleocytosis.[154] Low natural killer (NK) cell activity is commonly found, and persistence of this finding may suggest FHLH, as may NK activity subtyping.[156–158] Activation of the coagulation and fibrinolytic pathways with resultant hemorrhagic diathesis occurs in severe cases. High soluble interleukin-2 receptor (IL-2r or SCD25) serum levels also appear to be of value in making this diagnosis.[159] Histopathologic findings show accumulation of lymphocytes and macrophages. Hemophagocytic lymphohistiocytosis can lead to severe liver damage. Although a portal lymphohistiocytic infiltrate is most characteristic, it is cytokine-mediated hepatocellular damage that can cause substantial functional impairment or even hepatic failure.[160] Hemophagocytosis may be seen, especially in the spleen, enlarged lymph nodes, bone marrow and liver, but absence of this finding, particularly early in the disease, does not exclude HLH.

Revised diagnostic criteria suggested by the Histiocyte Society HLH working group are shown in Table 16-3.

Treatment of Hemophagocytic Lymphohistiocytosis

Diagnosis of HLH is often delayed, and a high index of suspicion for the diagnosis among caregivers of ill young children is important.

Once the diagnosis is made, a search for an underlying disease as well as evaluation of risk factors are critical. Low-risk patients generally are older than 2 years with a negative family history, lack of severe neutropenia, no or mild disseminated intravascular coagulation, no CNS dis-

Table 16-3
Diagnostic guidelines for hemaphagocytic lymphohistiocytosis.

1 A molecular diagnosis consistent with HLH
2 Diagnostic criteria for HLH fulfilled (5 of 8 criteria below):

Clinical Criteria
- Fever
- Splenomegaly

Laboratory Criteria
- Cytopenias (affecting ≥ 2 of 3 lineages) Hemoglobin < 90 g/L. platelets $< 100 \times 10^9$/L Neutrophils $< 1.0 \times 10^9$/L Infants < 4 weeks: hemoglobin < 100 g/L
- Hypertriglyceridemia and/or hypofibrinogenemia
- low or absent NK cell activity
- ferritin ≥ 500 μg/L
- soluble CD25 ≥ 2400U/ml

Histopathologic criteria
- hemophagocytosis in bone marrow or spleen or nodes

Source: Adapted from Henter et al.[159]

ease, absence of EBV and underlying malignancy, and a good response to initial therapy. In this group, therapy of the underlying disease and prompt management of cytokine-induced symptoms by corticosteroids and intravenous immune gamma globulin may be all that is necessary, but failure of response should result in early addition of other drugs. For high-risk patients, which includes those with FHLH and severe secondary HLH, including most cases of EBV-HLH,[151,153] appropriate anti-HLH therapy and intensive supportive care should be started early while the etiology is sought. If an underlying condition is found, specific therapy should be started promptly. However, even when an underlying condition is obvious at onset, specific therapy of the hemophagocytic component may be necessary to prevent a fatal outcome. For high-risk patients, a combination of etoposide, high-dose corticosteroids, and cyclosporine-A (CSA) with intrathecal therapy form the basis of the Histiocyte Society frontline protocols (HLH-94/HLH-2004)[153,159] Cyclosporine-A has been shown to down-modulate the "cytokine storm" and appears to be an essential drug in high-risk HLH, with improved results if given early, particularly in neutropenic patients.[161] Despite concern about secondary leukemia, etoposide too has been shown to be an important drug in high-risk patients. Etoposide suppresses EBV nuclear antigen synthesis,[162] and therapy of EBV-HLH should include early use of etoposide in children[161] and adults.[153] Experience has shown that patients failing to respond to a standard combination of dexamethasone and etoposide may respond to higher doses of the two drugs, as well as earlier use of CSA. Therapy is given for 4 to 8 weeks, except for FHLH patients and those with refractory disease. Intrathecal methotrexate chemotherapy is added for patients with CNS disease that does not respond to dexamethasone therapy. Antithymocyte globulin, which replaces etoposide in a successful French protocol, may be particularly useful in patients with significant conjugated hyperbilirubinemia in whom etoposide use is problematic. It has not, however, been shown to be useful in patients who fail the HLH-94/2004 protocol therapy.[158] For patients refractory to frontline therapy, high-dose pulse methylprednisolone, the anti-CD52 antibody alemtuzumab, and the anti-TNF antibody infliximab have all been suggested as being potentially useful.[163]

Since 1986, when Fischer et al demonstrated that allogeneic bone marrow transplant could effect a cure in some patients,[164] it has become clear that despite initial response to therapy, all patients with FHLH will eventually relapse without an allogeneic stem cell transplant (alloSCT). Allogeneic stem cell transplant is therefore indicated for FHLH but may also be necessary in refractory secondary HLH.[153] Successful outcome after alloSCT is obtained in 64% of patients, 71% $\pm$ 18% for those with matched family donors, 70 $\pm$ 16% for matched unrelated donors, and 50 $\pm$ 24% for haploidentical donors.[159] Experience with the HLH-94 protocol has shown that alloSCT results are better in patients who respond to initial therapy, but failure to respond should not preclude an alloSCT.[159] Utilizing these principles, survival has improved from a 1-year survival close to 0% in 1983[165] to an estimated 3-year probability of survival of 55% ($\pm$9%) at present.[159]

Conclusion

Despite significant gains in knowledge with regard to the biology of histiocytes, as well as the dramatic improvement in survival in patients with HLH, much remains to be learned. The high incidence of significant late effects found in patients with MS-LCH has successfully demolished any tendency to complacency among treating physicians. Much work remains to be done, and only international cooperation in clinical trials is likely to lead to the improvements required for the successful treatment of these patients.

References

1. Favara BE, Feller AC, Pauli M, et al. Contemporary classification of histiocytic disorders. The WHO Committee on Histiocytic/Reticulum Cell Proliferations. Reclassification Working Group of the Histiocyte Society. *Med Pediatr Oncol.* 1997;29:157–166.
2. Gianotti R, Alessi E, Caputo R. Benign cephalic histiocytosis: a distinct entity or a part of a wide spectrum of histiocytic proliferative disorders of children? A histopathological study. *Am J Dermatopathol.* 1993;15:315–319.
3. Shani-Adir A, Chou P, Morgan E, et al. A child with both Langerhans and non-Langerhans cell histiocytosis. *Pediatr Dermatol.* 2002;19:419–422.
4. Jaffe R. The diagnostic histopathology of Langerhans cell histiocytosis. In: Weitzman S, Egeler RM, eds. Histiocytic disorders of children and adults. Cambridge: Cambridge University Press; 2005:4–39.
5. Christie LJ, Evans AT, Bray SE, et al. Lesions resembling Langerhans cell histiocytosis in association with other lymphoproliferative disorders: a reactive or neoplastic phenomenon? *Hum Pathol.* 2006;37:32–39.
6. Romani N, Holzmann S, Tripp CH, Koch F, Stoitzner P. Langerhans cells-dendritic cells of the epidermis. *APMIS.* 2003;111:725–740.
7. Beverley PC, Egeler RM, Arceci RJ, Pritchard J. The Nikolas Symposia and histiocytosis. *Nat Rev Cancer.* 2005;5:488–494.
8. Bechan GI, Egeler RM, Arceci RJ. Biology of Langerhans cells and Langerhans cell histiocytosis. *Int Rev Cytol.* 2006;254:1–43.
9. Ladisch S, Jaffe ES. Histiocytoses. In: Pizzo PA, Poplack DG, eds. *Principles and Practice of Pediatric Oncology.* Vol. 4. Philadelphia: Lippincott Williams and Wilkins; 2002:733–750.
10. Gunn MD, Tangemann K, Tam C, Cyster JG, Rosen SD, Williams LT. A chemokine expressed in lymphoid high endothelial venules promotes the adhesion and chemotaxis of naive T lymphocytes. *Proc Natl Acad Sci USA.* 1998;95:258–263.
11. Schroder JM, Reich K, Kabashima K, et al. Who is really in control of skin immunity under physiological circumstances—lymphocytes, dendritic cells or keratinocytes? *Exp Dermatol.* 2006;15:913–929.
12. Cumberbatch M, Dearman RJ, Griffiths CEM, Kimber I. Epidermal Langerhans cell migration and sensitisation to chemical allergens. *APMIS.* 2003;111:797–804.
13. Annels NE, da Costa CET, Prins FA, et al. Aberrant chemokine receptor expression and chemokine production by Langerhans cells underlies the pathogenesis of Langerhans cell histiocytosis. *J Exp Med.* 2003;197:1385–1390.
14. Egeler RM, Favara BE, Laman JD, Claassen E. Abundant expression of CD40 and CD40-ligand (CD154) in paediatric Langerhans cell histiocytosis lesions. *Eur J Cancer.* 2000;36:2105–2110.
15. Tazi A, Moreau J, Bergeron A, Dominique S, Hance AJ, Soler P. Evidence that Langerhans cells in adult pulmonary Langerhans cell histiocytosis are mature dendritic cells: importance of the cytokine microenvironment. *J Immunol.* 1999;163:3511–3515.
16. Egeler RM, Favara BE, van Meurs M, Laman JD, Claasen E. Differential in situ cytokine profiles of Langerhans-like cells and T cells in Langerhans cell histiocytosis: abundant expression of cytokines relevant to disease and treatment. *Blood.* 1999;94:4195–4201.
17. Geissmann F, Lepelletier Y, Fraitag S, et al. Differentiation of Langerhans cells in Langerhans cell histiocytosis. *Blood.* 2001;97:1241–1248.
18. Willman CL, Busque L, Griffiths BB, et al. Langerhans cell histiocytosis: a clonal proliferation of Langerhans cells. *New Engl J Med.* 1994;331:154–160.
19. Yu RC, Chu C, Buluwela L, Chu AC. Clonal proliferation of Langerhans cells in Langerhans cell histiocytosis. *Lancet.* 1994;343:767–768.
20. Murakami I, Gogusev J, Fournet JC, Glorion C, Jaubert F. Detection of molecular cytogenetic aberrations in Langerhans cell histiocytosis of bone. *Hum Pathol.* 2002;33:555–560.
21. Betts DR, Leibundgut KE, Feldges A, et al. Cytogenetic abnormalities in Langerhans cell histiocytosis. *Br J Cancer.* 1998;77:552–555.
22. Schouten B, Egeler RM, Leenen PJ, Taminiau AHM, van den Broek LJCM, Hogendoorn PCW. Expression of cell cycle-related gene products in Langerhans cell histiocytosis. *J Pediatr Hematol Oncol.* 2002;24:727–732.
23. da Costa CE, Egeler RM, Hoogeboom M, et al. Differences in telomerase expression by the CD1a+ cells in Langerhans cell histiocytosis reflect the diverse clinical presentation of the disease. *J Pathol.* 2007;212:188–197.
24. Aricò M, Scappaticci S, Danesino C. The genetics of Langerhans cell histiocytosis. In: Weitzman S, Egeler RM, eds. Histiocytic disorders of children and adults. Cambridge: Cambridge University Press; 2005:83–94.
25. Bernstrand C, Carstensen H, Jakobsen B, Svejgaard A, Henter J-I, Olerup O. Immunogenetic heterogeneity in single-system and multisystem Langerhans cell histiocytosis. *Pediatr Res.* 2003;54:30–36.
26. Osband ME, Lipton JM, Lavin O, et al. Histiocytosis X: demonstration of abnormal immunity, T-cell histamine H2 receptor deficiency, and successful treatment with thymic extract. *New Engl J Med.* 1981;304:146–153.
27. Glotzbecker MP, Carpentieri DF, Dormans JP. Langerhans cell histiocytosis: clinical presentation, pathogenesis and treatment from the LCH etiology research group at the Children's Hospital of Philadelphia. *UPOJ.* 2002;15:67–73.
28. Arceci RJ. The histiocytoses: the fall of the Tower of Babel. *Eur J Cancer.* 1999;35:747–767.
29. McClain K, Jin H, Gresik V, Favara B. Langerhans cell histiocytosis: lack of a viral etiology. *Am J Hematol.* 1994;47:16–20.
30. Slacmeulder M, Geissmann F, Lepelletier Y, et al. No association between Langerhans cell histiocytosis and human herpes virus 8. *Med Pediatr Oncol.* 2002;39:187–189.
31. Leahy MA, Krejci SM, Friednash M. Human Herpes virus 6 is present in lesions of Langerhans cell histiocytosis. *J Invest Dermatol.* 1993;101:642–645.
32. Bhatia S, Nesbit ME, Egeler RM, Buckley JD, Mertens A, Robison LL. Epidemiologic study of Langerhans cell histiocytosis in children. *J Pediatr.* 1997;130:774–784.
33. Bernstrand C, Cederlund K, Åhstrom L, Henter J-I. Smoking preceded pulmonary involvement in adults with Langerhans cell histiocytosis diagnosed in childhood. *Acta Paediatr.* 2000;89:1389–1392.
34. Karis J, Bernstrand C, Fadeel B, Henter J-I. The incidence of Langerhans Cell Histiocytosis in children in Stockholm County, Sweden 1992–2001. In: *Proceedings of the XIX Meeting of the Histiocyte Society.* Philadelphia; 2003:21
35. Carstensen H, Ornvold K. The epidemiology of Langerhans cell histiocytosis in children in Denmark, 1975–89. *Med Pediatr Oncol.* 1993;21:387–388.

36. Alston RD, Tatevossian RG, McNally RJQ, et al. Incidence and survival of childhood Langerhans Cell Histiocytosis in Northwest England from 1954 to 1998. *Pediatr Blood Cancer.* 2007;48:555–560.
37. Huang F, Arceci R. The histiocytoses of infancy. *Semin Perinatol.* 1999;23: 319–331.
38. Ladisch S, Gadner H, Aricó M, et al. A randomized trial of etoposide *versus* vinblastine in disseminated Langerhans cell histiocytosis. *Med Pediatr Oncol.* 1994;23:107–110.
39. Lau L, Krafchik B, Trebo M, Weitzman S. Cutaneous Langerhans Cell Histiocytosis in children under one year. *Pediatr Blood Cancer.* 2006;46:66–71.
40. Minkov M, Grois N, Heitger A, Potschger U, Westermeier T, Gadner H. Response to initial treatment of multisystem Langerhans cell histiocytosis: an important prognostic indicator. *Med Pediatr Oncol.* 2002;39:581–585.
41. Gadner H, Grois N, Arico M, et al. A randomized trial of treatment for multisystem Langerhans' cell histiocytosis. *J Pediatr.* 2001;138:728–734.
42. Stuurman KE, Lau L, Doda W, Weitzman S. Evaluation of the natural history and long term complications of patients with Langerhans cell histiocytosis of bone. In: *Proceedings of the XIX Meeting of the Histiocyte Society.* Philadelphia; 2003:13.
43. Titgemeyer C, Grois N, Minkov M, Flucher-Wolfram B, Gatterer-Menz, Gadner H. Pattern and course of single-system disease in Langerhans cell histiocytosis data from the DAL-HX 83- and 90 study. *Med Pediatr Oncol.* 2001;37: 108–114.
44. Howarth DM, Gilchrist GS, Mullan BP, Wiseman GA, Edmonson JH, Schomberg PJ. Langerhans cell histiocytosis: diagnosis, natural history, management and outcome. *Cancer.* 1999;85:2278–2290.
45. Nanduri V, Titgemeyer C, Brock P. Long term outcome of orbital involvement in Langerhans cell histiocytosis. In: *Proceedings of the XVII Meeting of the Histiocyte Society.* Stresa, Italy; 2001:176.
46. Pollono D, Rey G, Latella A, et al. Reactivation and risk of sequelae in Langerhans cell histiocytosis. *Pediatr Blood Cancer.* 2007;48:696–699.
47. Ghanem I, Tolo VT, D'Ambra P, Malogolowkin MH. Langerhans cell histiocytosis of bone in children and adolescents. *J Pediatr Orthop.* 2003;23:124–130.
48. Kilpatrick SE, Wenger DE, Gilchrist GS, et al. Langerhans cell histiocytosis (histiocytosis X) of bone. *Cancer.* 1995;76:2471–2484.
49. Aricò M, Egeler RM. Clinical aspects of Langerhans cell histiocytosis. *Hematol/Oncol Clin N America.* 1998;12:247–258.
50. Koch B. Langerhans cell histiocytosis of temporal bone: role of magnetic resonance imaging. *Top Magn Reson Imaging.* 2000;11:66–74.
51. Fernández-Latorre F, Menor-Serrano F, Alonso-Charterina S, Arenas-Jiménez J. Langerhans' cell histiocytosis of the temporal bone in pediatric patients. *Am J Roentgenol.* 2000;174:217–221.
52. Guzey FK, Bas NS, Emel E, Alatas I, Kebudi R. Polyostotic monosystemic calvarial and spinal Langerhans cell histiocytosis treated by surgery and chemotherapy. *Pediatr Neurosurg.* 2003;38:206–211.
53. Turgut M, Gurcay O. Multifocal histiocytosis X of bone in two adjacent vertebrae causing paraplegia. *Aust N Z J Surg.* 1992;62:241–244.
54. Kamimura M, Kinoshita T, Itoh H, Yuzawa Y, Takahashi J, Ohtsuka K. Eosinophilic granuloma of the spine: early spontaneous disappearance of tumor detected on magnetic resonance imaging. *J Neurosurg.* 2000;93(suppl 2):312–316.
55. Ruppert D, Oria RA, Kumar R, et al. Radiologic features of eosinophilic granuloma of bone. *Am J Radiol.* 153:1021–1026.
56. Meyer JS, Harty MP, Mabboubi S, et al. Langerhans cell histiocytosis: presentation and evolution of radiologic findings with clinical correlation. *Radiographics.* 1995;15:1135–1146.
57. Potepan P, Tesoro-Tess JD, Laffranchi A, et al. Langerhans cell histiocytosis mimicking malignancy: a radiologic appraisal. *Tumori.* 1996;82:603–609.
58. Hayes CW, Conway WF, Sundaram M. Misleading aggressive MR imaging appearance of some benign musculoskeletal lesions. *Radiographics.* 1992;12: 1119–1134.
59. Fisher AJ, Reinus WR, Friedland JA, Wilson AJ. Quantitative analysis of the plain radiographic appearance of eosinophilic granuloma. *Invest Radiol.* 1995;8:466–473.
60. Kaste SC, Rodriguez-Galindo C, McCarville ME, Shulkin BL. PET-CT in pediatric Langerhans cell histiocytosis. *Pediatr Radiol.* 2007;37:615–622.
61. Munn S, Chu AC. Langerhans cell histiocytosis of the skin. *Hematol/Oncol Clin N Am.* 1998;12:269–286.
62. Munn S, Murray S, Chu AC. Adult Langerhans cell histiocytosis: a review of 46 cases. In: *Proceedings of the XVII Meeting of the Histiocyte Society.* Stresa, Italy; 2001:222.
63. Longaker MA, Frieden IJ, Le Boit PT, Sherertz EF. Congenital "self-healing" Langerhans cell histiocytosis: the need for long term follow-up. *J Am Acad Dermatol.* 1994;31:910–916.
64. Esterly NB, Maurer HS, Gonzalez-Crussi F. Histiocytosis-X: a seven-year experience at a children's hospital. *J Am Acad Dermatol.* 1985;13:481–496.
65. Edelweiss M, Medeiros LJ, Suster S, Moran CA. Lymph node involvement by Langerhans cell histiocytosis: a clinicopathologic and immunohistochemical study of 20 cases. *Hum Pathol.* 2007;38:1463–1469.
66. Sundar KM, Gosselin MV, Chung HL, Cahill BC. Pulmonary Langerhans cell histiocytosis: emerging concepts in pathobiology, radiology, and clinical evolution of disease. *Chest.* 2003;123:1673–1683.
67. Auerswald U, Biwh J, Magnussen H. Value of CD–1-positive cells in bronchoalveolar lavage fluid for the diagnosis of pulmonary histiocytosis X. *Lungs.* 1991;169:305–309.
68. Réfabert L, Rambaud C, Mamou-Mani T, Scheinmann P, de Blic J. CD1a-positive cells in bronchoalveolar lavage samples from children with Langerhans cell histiocytosis. *J Pediatr.* 1996;129:913–915.
69. Tazi A, Hiltermann TJN, Vassallo R. Adult lung histiocytosis. In: Weitzman S, Egeler RM, eds. *Histiocytic Disorders of Children and Adults.* Cambridge: Cambridge University Press; 2005:187–207.
70. Choi SW, Bangaru BS, Wu CD, Finlay JL. Gastrointestinal involvement in disseminated Langerhans cell histiocytosis (LCH) with durable complete response to 2-chlorodeoxyadenosine and high-dose cytarabine. *J Pediatr Hematol Oncol.* 2003;25:503–506.
71. Maghnie M, Cosi G, Genovese E, et al. Central diabetes insipidus in children and young adults. *New Engl J Med.* 2000;343:998–1007.
72. Grois N, Prosch H, Lassmann H, et al. Central nervous system disease in Langerhans cell histiocytosis. In: Weitzman S, Egeler RM, eds. *Histiocytic Disorders of Children and Adults.* Cambridge: Cambridge University Press; 2005: 208–228.
73. The French LCH Study Group. A multicentre retrospective survey of LCH: 348 cases observed between 1983 and 1993. *Arch Dis Child.* 1996;75:17–24.
74. Maghnie M, Aricò M, Villa A, et al. MR of the hypothalamic-pituitary axis in Langerhans cell histiocytosis. *Am J Neuroradiol.* 1992;13:1365.
75. Prayer D, Grois N., Prosch H, et al. MR imaging presentation of intracranial disease associated with Langerhans cell histiocytosis. *Am J Neuroradiol.* 2004; 25:880–891.
76. Kaltsas GA, Powles TB, Evanson J, et al. Hypothalamo-pituitary abnormalities in adult patients with Langerhans cell histiocytosis: clinical, endocrinological and radiological features and response to treatment. *J Clin Endocrinol Metab.* 2000;85:1370–1376.
77. Maghnie M, Bossi G, Klersy C, Cosi G, Genovese E, Aricò M. Dynamic endocrine testing and Magnetic Resonance Imaging in the long term follow-up of childhood Langerhans cell histiocytosis. *J Clin Endocrinol Metab.* 1998; 83:3089–3094.
78. Municchi G, Marconcini S, D'Ambrosio A, Berardi R, Aquaviva A. Central precocious puberty in multisytem Langerhans cell histiocytosis: a case report. *Pediatr Hematol Oncol.* 2002;19:273–278.
79. Chong VF. Langerhans cell histiocytosis with thyroid involvement. *Eur J Radiol.* 1996;22:155.
80. Pritchard J. Acute ataxia complicating Langerhans cell histiocytosis. *Arch Dis Child.* 2003;88:178–179.
81. Calming U, Bernstrand C, Mosskin M, Elander SS, Ingvar M, Henter J-I. Brain 18-FDG PET scan in central nervous system Langerhans cell histiocytosis. *J Pediatr.* 2002;141:435–440.
82. Bollini G, Jouve JL, Gentet JC, Jacquemier M, Bouyals JM. Bone lesions in Histiocytosis X. *J Pediatr Orthop.* 1991;11:469–477.
83. Sartoris DJ, Parker BR. Histiocytosis X: rate and pattern of resolution of osseous lesions. *Radiology.* 1984;152:679–684.
84. Womer RB, Raney RB, D'Angio GJ. Healing rates of treated and untreated bone lesions in Histiocytosis X. *Pediatrics.* 1985;76:286–288.
85. Egeler RM, Thompson RC, Voûte PA, Nesbit ME. Intralesional infiltration of corticosteroids in localized Langerhans cell histiocytosis. *J Pediatr Orthop.* 1992;12:811–814.
86. Yasco AW, Fanning CV, Ayala AG, et al. Percutaneous techniques for the diagnosis and treatment of localized Langerhans cell histiocytosis (eosinophilic granuloma of bone). *J Bone Joint Surg.* 1998;80:219–228.
87. Munn SE, Olliver L, Broadbent V, Pritchard J. Use of indomethacin in Langerhans cell histiocytosis. *Med Pediatr Oncol.* 1999;32:247–249.
88. Arceci RJ, Brenner MK, Pritchard J. Controversies and new approaches to treatment of LCH. *Hematol/Oncol Clin N America.* 1998;12:339–357.
89. Brown RE. Bisphosphonates as anti-alveolar macrophage therapy in pulmonary Langerhans cell histiocytosis. *Med Pediatr Oncol.* 2001;36:641–664.
90. Farran RP, Zaretski E, Egeler RM. Treatment of Langerhans cell histiocytosis with pamidronate. *J Pediatr Hematol Oncol.* 2001;23:54–56.
91. Kamizono J, Okada Y, Shirahata A, Tanaka Y. Bisphosphonate induces remission of refractory osteolysis in Langerhans cell histiocytosis. *J Bone Joint Surg.* 2002;17:1926–1928.
92. da Costa CE, Annels NE, Faaij CM, Forsyth RG, Hogendoorn PC, Egeler RM. Presence of osteoclast-like multinucleated giant cells in the bone and nonostotic lesions of Langerhans cell histiocytosis. *J Exp Med.* 2005;201:687–693.
93. Hoeger PH, Nanduri VR, Harper JL, Atherton DA, Pritchard J. Long-term follow-up of topical mustine treatment for cutaneous Langerhans cell histiocytosis. *Arch Dis Child.* 2000;82:483–487.
94. Stein SL, Paller AS, Haut PR, Mancini AJ. Langerhans cell histiocytosis presenting in the neonatal period: a retrospective case series. *Arch Pediatr Adolesc Med.* 2001;155:778–783.
95. Minkov M, Prosch H, Steiner M, et al. Langerhans cell histiocytosis in neonates. *Pediatr Blood Cancer.* 2005;45:802–807.
96. Sakai H, Ibe M, Takahashi H, et al. Satisfactory remission achieved by PUVA therapy in Langerhans cell histiocytosis in an elderly patient. *J Dermatol.* 1996;23:42–46.

97. Kwon OS, Cho KH, Song KY. Primary cutaneous Langerhans cell histiocytosis treated with photochemotherapy. *J Dermatol.* 1997;24:54–56.

98. Gerlach B, Stein A, Fischer R, Wozel G, Dittert DD, Richter G. Langerhans cell histiocytosis in the elderly. *Hautarzt.* 1998;49:23–30.

99. Misery L, Larbre B, Lyonnet S, Faure M, Thivolet J. Remission of Langerhans cell histiocytosis with thalidomide treatment. *Clin Exp Dermatol.* 1993;18: 487.

100. Moraes M, Russo G. Thalidomide and its dermatologic uses. *Am J Med Sci.* 2001;321:321–326.

101. Lair G, Marie I, Cailleux N, et al. Langerhans cell histiocytosis in adults: cutaneous and mucous lesion regression after treatment with thalidomide. *Revue de Medicine Interne.* 1998;19:196–198.

102. Claudon A, Dietamann JL, Hamman De Compte A, Hassler P. Interest in thalidomide in cutaneo-mucous and hypothalamo-hypophyseal involvement of Langerhans cell histiocytosis. *Revue de Medicine Interne.* 2002;23:651–656.

103. Montero AJ, Diaz-Montero CM, Malpica A, Ramirez PT, Kavanagh JJ. Langerhans cell histiocytosis of the female genital tract: a literature review. *Int J Gynecol Cancer.* 2003;13:381–388.

104. Culic S, Jakobson À, Culik V, Kuzmic I, Scukanec-Spoljar M, Primorac D. Etoposide as the basic and interferon-alpha as the maintenance therapy for Langerhans cell histiocytosis. *Pediatr Hematol Oncol.* 2001;18:291–294.

105. Chang SE, Koh GJ, Choi JH, et al. Widespread skin-limited adult Langerhans cell histiocytosis: long term follow up with good response to interferon alpha. *Clin Exp Dermatol.* 2002;27:135–137.

106. Kwong YL, Chan ACL, Chan TK. Widespread skin-limited Langerhans cell histiocytosis: complete remission with interferon alpha. *J Am Acad Dermatol.* 1997;36:628–629.

107. Helmbold P, Hegemann B, Holzhausen H-J, Klapperstück T, Marsch WCh. Low dose oral etoposide monotherapy in adult Langerhans cell histiocytosis. *Arch Dermatol.* 1998;134:1275–1278.

108. Ottaviano F, Finlay JL. Diabetes insipidus and Langerhans cell histiocytosis: a case report of reversibility with 2-chlorodeoxyadenosine. *J Pediatr Hematol Oncol.* 2003;25:575–577.

109. Rosenzweig KE, Arceci R, Tarbell NJ. Diabetes insipidus secondary to Langerhans' cell histiocytosis: is radiation therapy indicated? *Med Pediatr Oncol.* 1997;29:36–40.

110. Watts J, Files B. Langerhans cell histiocytosis: central nervous system involvement treated successfully with 2-chlorodeoxyadenosine. *Pediatr Hematol Oncol.* 2001;18:199–204.

111. Giona F, Annino L, Bongarzoni V, et al. Unifocal Langerhans cell histiocytosis involving the central nervous system successfully treated with 2-chlorodeoxyadenosine. *Med Pediatr Oncol.* 2002;38:223.

112. Dhall G, Finlay JL, Dunkel IJ, et al. Analysis of outcome for patients with mass lesions of the central nervous system due to Langerhans cell histiocytosis treated with 2-chlorodeoxyadenosine. *Pediatr Blood Cancer.* 2008;50:72–79.

113. Gadner H, Heitger A, Grois N, Gaterer-Menz I, Ladisch S. Treatment strategy for disseminated Langerhans cell histiocytosis. *Med Pediatr Oncol.* 1994;23: 72–80.

114. Morimoto A, Ikushima S, Kinugawa N, et al. Improved outcome in the treatment of pediatric multifocal Langerhans cell histiocytosis. results from the Japan Langerhans cell histiocytosis study group–96 protocol. *Cancer.* 2006; 107:613–619.

115. McLelland J, Broadbent V, Yeomans E, Malone M, Pritchard J. Langerhans cell histiocytosis : the case for conservative therapy. *Arch Dis Child.* 1990;65:301–303.

116. Bernard F, Thomas C, Bertrand Y, et al. Multicentre pilot study of 2-chlorodeoxyadenosine and cytosine arabinoside combined chemotherapy in refractory Langerhans cell histiocytosis with haematological dysfunction. *Eur J Cancer.* 2005;41:2682–2689.

117. Egeler RM, de Kraker J, Voute PA. Cytosine arabinoside, vincristine and prednisolone in the treatment of children with disseminated Langerhans cell histiocytosis with organ dysfunction: experience at a single institution. *Med Pediatr Oncol.* 1993;21:265–270.

118. Minkov M, Grois N, Braier J, et al. Immunosuppressive therapy for chemotherapy-resistant multisystem Langerhans cell histiocytosis. *Med Pediatr Oncol.* 2003;40:253–256.

119. Mortazavi H, Ehsani A, Namazi MR, Hosseini M. Langerhans cell histiocytosis. *Dermatol Online J.* 2002;8:18.

120. Henter J-I, Karlén J, Calming U, Bernstrand C, Andersson U, Fadeel B. Successful treatment of Langerhans' cell histiocytosis with Etanercept. *New Engl J Med.* 2001;345:1577–1578.

121. Weitzman S, McClain K, Arceci R. Treatment of relapsed and/or refractory Langerhans cell histiocytosis. In: Weitzman S, Egeler RM, eds. *Histiocytic Disorders of Children and Adults.* Cambridge: Cambridge University Press; 2005: 254–271.

122. Steiner M, Matthes-Martin S, Attarbaschi A, et al. Improved outcome of treatment-resistant high-risk Langerhans cell histiocytosis after allogeneic stem cell transplantation with reduced-intensity conditioning. *Bone Marrow Transplant.* 2005;36:215–225.

123. Kelly M, Kolb M, Bonniaud P, Gauldie J. Re-evaluation of fibrogenic cytokines in lung fibrosis. *Curr Pharm Des.* 2003;9:39–49.

124. Marti L, Thomas C, Emilé JF, et al. Liver involvement in LCH: the French experience. *Proceedings of the XIX Meeting of the Histiocyte Society.* Philadelphia; 2003:20.

125. Braier J, Cioccca M, Latella A, de Davila MG, Drajer M, Imventarza O. Cholestasis, sclerosing cholangitis, and liver transplantation in Langerhans cell histiocytosis. *Med Pediatr Oncol.* 2002;38:178–182.

126. Soler P, Bergeron A, Kambouchner M, et al. Is high resolution computed tomography a reliable tool to predict the histopathological activity of pulmonary Langerhans cell histiocytosis? *Am J Resp Crit Care Med.* 2000;162: 264–270.

127. Rajwal SR, Stringer MD, Davison SM, et al. Use of basiliximab in pediatric liver transplantation for Langerhans cell histiocytosis. *Pediatr Transplant.* 2003;7:247–251.

128. Hadzic N, Pritchard J, Webb D, et al. Recurrence of Langerhans cell histiocytosis in the graft after pediatric liver transplantation. *Transplantation.* 2000; 15:815–819.

129. Etienne B, Bertocchi M, Gamondes J-P, et al. Relapsing pulmonary Langerhans cell histiocytosis after lung transplantation. *Am J Resp Crit Care Med.* 1998;157:288–291.

130. Newell KA, Alonso EM, Kelly SM, Rubin CM, Thistlethwaite JR, Whitington PF. Association between liver transplantation for Langerhans cell histiocytosis, rejection and development of post-transplantation lymphoproliferative disease in children. *J Pediatr.* 1997;131:98–104.

131. Stieber AC, Sever C, Starzl TE. Liver transplantation in patients with Langerhans' cell histiocytosis. *Transplantation.* 1990;50:338–340.

132. Woltman AM, de Fijter JW, Kamerling SWA, et al. Rapamycin induces apoptosis in monocyte-and CD34-derived dendritic cells but not in monocytes and macrophages. *Blood.* 2001;98:174–180.

133. Brewer GJ, Ullenbruch MR, Dick R, Olivarez L, Phan SH. Tetrathiomolybdate therapy protects against bleomycin-induced pulmonary fibrosis in mice. *J Lab Clin Med.* 2003;14:210–216.

134. Strieter RM. Mechanisms of pulmonary fibrosis: conference summary. *Chest.* 2003;120(suppl):77S–85S.

135. Donadieu J, Rolon MA, Pion I, et al. Incidence of growth hormone deficiency in pediatric-onset Langerhans cell histiocytosis: efficacy and safety of growth hormone treatment. *J Clin Endocrinol Metab.* 2004;89:604–609.

136. Nanduri VR, Barelle P, Pritchard J, Stanhope R. Growth and endocrine disorders in multisystem Langerhans cell histiocytosis. *Clin Endocrinol.* 2000;53: 509–515.

137. Willis B, Ablin A, Weinberg V, et al. Disease course and late sequelae of Langerhans' cell histiocytosis: a 25 year experience at the University of California, San Francisco. *J Clin Oncol.* 1996;14:2073–2082.

138. Haupt R, Nanduri V, Calevo MG, et al. Permanent consequences in Langerhans cell histiocytosis patients: a pilot study from the Histiocyte Society Late Effects Study Group. *Pediatr Blood Cancer.* 2004;42:438–444.

139. Farquhar J, Claireaux A. Familial haemophagocytic reticulosis. *Arch Dis Child.* 1952;27:519–525.

140. Filipovich AH. Hemophagocytic lymphohistiocytosis: a lethal disorder of immune regulation. *J Pediatr.* 1997;130:337–338.

141. Risdall RJ, McKenna RW, Nesbit ME, et al. Virus-associated hemophagocytic syndrome: a benign histiocytic proliferation distinct from malignant histiocytosis. *Cancer.* 1979;44:993–1002.

142. Henter J-I, Elinder G, Söder O, Hansson M, Andersson B, Andersson U. Hypercytokinemia in familial hemophagocytic lymphohistiocytosis. *Blood.* 1991;78:2918–2922.

143. Imashuku S, Teramura T, Morimoto A, Hibi S. Recent developments in the management of haemophagocytic lymphohistiocytosis. *Expert Opin Pharmacother.* 2001;2:1437–1448.

144. Goransdotter Ericson KG, Fadeel B, Nilsson-Ardnor S, et al. Spectrum of perforin gene mutations in familial hemophagocytic lymphohistiocytosis. *Am J Hum Genet.* 2001;68:590–597.

145. Ohadi M, Lalloz MRA, Sham P. Localization of a gene for familial hemophagocytic lymphohistiocytosis at chromosome 9q21.3–22 by homozygosity mapping. *Am J Hum Genet.* 1999;64:165–171.

146. Stepp SE, Dufourcq-Lagelouse R, Le Deist F, et al. Perforin gene defects in familial hemophagocytic lymphohistiocytosis. *Science.* 1999;286:1957–1959.

147. Dufourcq-Lagelouse R, Jabado N, Le Deist F, et al. Linkage of familial hemophagocytic lymphohistiocytosis to 10q21–22 and evidence for heterogeneity. *Am J Hum Genet.* 1999;64:172–179.

148. Feldmann J, Callebaut I, Raposo G, et al. Munc 13–4 is essential for cytolytic granules fusion and is mutated in a form of familial hemophagocytic lymphohistiocytosis (FHL3). *Cell.* 2003;115:461–473.

149. Zur Stadt U, Beutel K, Kolberg S, et al. Mutation spectrum in children with primary hemophagocytic lymphohistiocytosis: molecular and functional analyses of PRF1, UNC13D, STX11, and RAB27A. *Hum Mutation.* 2006;27: 62–68.

150. Henter J-I, Aricò M, Elinder G, Imashuku S, Janka G. Familial hemophagocytic lymphohisticytosis. *Hematol Oncol Clin N Am.* 1998;12:417–433.

151. Janka G, Imashuku S, Elinder G, Schneider M, Henter J-I. Infection- and malignancy-associated hemophagocytic syndromes: secondary hemophagocytic lymphohistiocytosis. *Hematol Oncol Clin N Am.* 1998;12: 435–444, 1998.

152. Risdall RJ, Brunning RD, Hernandez JI, Gordon DH. Bacteria-associated hemophagocytic syndrome. *Cancer.* 1984;54:2968–2972.

153. Imashuku S, Kuriyama K, Sakai R, et al. Treatment of Epstein-Barr virus–associated hemophagocytic lymphohistiocytosis (EBV-HLH) in young adults: a report from the HLH-Study Center. *Med Pediatr Oncol.* 2003;41:103–109.

154. Janka G, Henter J-I, Imashuku S. Clinical aspects and therapy of hemophagocytic lymphohistiocytosis. In: Weitzman S, Egeler RM, eds. *Histiocytic Disorders of Children and Adults*. Cambridge: Cambridge University Press; 2005: 353–379.

155. Horne AC, Trottestam H, Aricò M, et al. Frequency and spectrum of CNS involvement in 193 children with hemophagocytic lymphohistiocytosis. *Br J Haematol*. 2008;140(3):327–335.

156. Zheng C, Schneider EM, Samuelsson-Horne AC, et al. Natural killer cell activity subtypes provide therapeutic guidance in hemophagocytic lymphohistiocytosis. *Proceedings of the XIX Meeting of the Histiocyte Society*. Philadelphia; 2003.

157. Sullivan KE, Delaat CA, Douglas SD, Filipovich AH. Defective natural killer cell activity in patients with hemophagocytic lymphohistiocytosis and in first degree relatives. *Pediatr Res*. 1998;44:465–468.

158. Schneider EM, Lorenz I, Muller-Rosenberger M, et al. Hemophagocytic lymphohistiocytosis is associated with deficiencies of cellular cytolysis but normal expression of transcripts relevant to killer-cell-induced apoptosis. *Blood*. 2002;100:2891–2898.

159. Henter J-I, Horne AC, Aricó M, et al. HLH–2004: diagnostic and therapeutic guidelines for Hemophagocytic Lymphohistiocytosis. *Pediatr Blood Cancer*. 2007;48:124–131.

160. Jaffe R. The histopathology of hemophagocytic lymphohistiocytosis. In: Weitzman S, Egeler RM, eds. *Histiocytic Disorders of Children and Adults*. Cambridge: Cambridge University Press; 2005:321–336.

161. Imashuku S, Kuriyama K, Teramura T, et al. Requirement for etoposide in the treatment of Epstein-Barr virus-associated hemophagocytic lymphohistiocytosis. *J Clin Oncol*. 2001;19:2665–2673.

162. Kikuta H, Sakiyama Y. Etoposide (VP16) inhibits Epstein-Barr virus determined nuclear antigen (EBNA) synthesis. *Br J Haematol*. 1995;90:971–973.

163. Filipovich AH, Imashuku S, Henter JI, Sullivan KE. Healing hemophagocytosis. *Clin Immunol*. 2005;117:121–124.

164. Fischer A, Cerf-Bensussan N, Blanche S, et al. Allogeneic bone marrow transplantation for erythrophagocytic lymphohistiocytosis. *J Pediatr*. 1986;108: 267–270.

165. Janka GE. Familial Hemophagocytic Lymphohistiocytosis. *Eur J Pediatr*. 1983;140:221–230.

Gliomas

Ian F. Pollack and Regina I. Jakacki

Introduction

Approximately half of all central nervous system tumors of childhood are gliomas.[1,2] Low-grade gliomas account for almost 60% of supratentorial hemispheric tumors in children, 50% of supratentorial midline tumors, and 30% of infratentorial tumors. More than half of such lesions are grade I or II astrocytomas,[1,2] and the remainder are mixed gliomas, oligodendrogliomas, gangliogliomas, and a host of less common lesions, such as pleomorphic xanthoastrocytomas, dysembryoplastic neuroepithelial tumors (DNET), and desmoplastic infantile gangliogliomas (DIG), which are almost unique to the pediatric age group.[3–8] In contrast to the situation in adults, high-grade gliomas of the cerebral and cerebellar hemispheres account for a minority of gliomas in children but constitute the majority of intrinsic brainstem lesions.[1]

Epidemiology

Although a definite environmental or genetic "cause" for most gliomas is unknown, a subgroup of affected children does have an underlying genetic syndrome that predisposes the children to develop gliomas, such as type 1 neurofibromatosis (NF1), tuberous sclerosis, or Turcot syndrome. Type 1 neurofibromatosis is caused by a mutation in the neurofibromin gene on chromosome 17q11.2,[9] which encodes a protein with GTPase-activating properties that functions in signal transduction.[10] Although the most characteristic intracranial neoplasms in patients with NF1 are visual pathway gliomas, a small percentage of patients develop glial neoplasms, both low grade and high grade, in other locations.[11]

Patients with tuberous sclerosis typically have seizures, mental retardation, and adenoma sebaceum in addition to cortical and subependymal hamartomas (tubers), angioleiomyomas of the kidney, and rhabdomyomas of the heart. This syndrome has been linked to mutations in a gene on chromosome 9 and another on chromosome 16, the latter of which codes for a member of the ras-GTPase-activating protein signaling pathway that has been referred to as "tuberin."[12] Subependymal giant cell astrocytomas are the characteristic intracranial neoplasm in patients with tuberous sclerosis.

Pathology and Molecular Pathogenesis

Low-grade gliomas are subdivided into several groups, based on their histological appearance.[3] These are: (1) astrocytic tumors, including pilocytic and nonpilocytic astrocytomas, pleomorphic xanthoastrocytomas, and subependymal giant cell astrocytomas; (2) oligodendroglial tumors; (3) mixed gliomas; and (4) benign neuroepithelial tumors, such as gangliogliomas, DIGs and DNETs. High-grade or malignant gliomas are subdivided into anaplastic (grade III) astrocytomas, mixed gliomas, oligodendrogliomas, and glioblastoma multiforme.

Although tremendous energy has been directed at unraveling the steps in the development of adult astrocytomas, comparatively little work has been focused on pediatric tumors. However, recent reports have begun to shed light on this issue. For example, pilocytic astrocytomas often exhibit deletions of chromosome 17q,[13] the site of the neurofibromin gene that is commonly mutated in patients with NF1. However, an association with neurofibromin mutations has yet to be confirmed for sporadic gliomas. Studies of other pediatric low-grade gliomas have not demonstrated a consistent pattern of genetic abnormalities. Of interest, mutations of the *p53* gene are uncommon in low-grade pediatric astrocytomas.[14] This is in contrast to the situation in adult low-grade gliomas[15] and suggests that morphologically similar tumors in these two age groups may arise from different molecular events.

Pediatric high-grade gliomas have also been reported to differ from their adult counterparts in terms of their molecular abnormalities. Our own analysis of a cohort of gliomas that were classified as high grade using contemporary guidelines found *p53* mutations in approximately 40% of tumors, comparable to the frequency in adult gliomas.[15,16] In adult tumors, *p53* mutations represent an important milestone in the progression of so-called secondary malignant gliomas, which begin as low-grade nonpilocytic lesions, evolve into anaplastic astrocytomas, and ultimately become glioblastomas.[15,17,18] However, because this evolution is not as commonly observed in pediatric gliomas, it is uncertain whether such tumors are truly analogous to the secondary adult subgroup. Moreover, childhood malignant gliomas with *p53* mutations appear to have a worse prognosis than lesions that lack such changes, whereas no such association between *p53* status and outcome is apparent in adult malignant gliomas.[19] A second molecular pathway in gliomagenesis involves so-called de novo or primary development of a glioblastoma multiforme, which is characterized by loss of a portion of chromosome 10 in and around the region of the *PTEN* gene,[15,17,18] in association with amplification and/or rearrangement of the epidermal growth factor receptor (EGFR) gene but without mutation of the *p53* gene. Our studies indicate that *EGFR* amplification and *PTEN* deletion are observed in only about 10% of pediatric malignant gliomas, suggesting that this pathway is less commonly implicated than in adults.[20] A third group of malignant gliomas (in adults) arise by a distinct pathway, with characteristic deletions of chromosomes 1p and 19q.[21] Such tumors often have oligodendroglial morphology and tend to carry a better prognosis than other groups of malignant gliomas.[21] Although such changes are observed in about 20% of childhood gliomas, a favorable association between 1p/19q loss and outcome has not been observed.[22]

Notwithstanding the above differences between childhood and adult malignant gliomas, recent studies have identified an important similarity among these tumors in the prognostic significance of expression levels of the DNA repair protein methylguanine DNA methyltransferase (MGMT) in patients treated with alkylating agents, such as the nitrosoureas and temozolomide. Methylguanine DNA methyltransferase constitutes the proximal mechanism of resistance to such agents by removing drug-induced alkyl groups, and methylation of the MGMT promoter, a surrogate of MGMT silencing, has been noted to confer an improved prognosis in adults treated with temozolomide and irradiation.[23] Similarly, children treated with lomustine-based regimens whose tumors have low levels of MGMT expression have been noted to have a significantly better prognosis than those with MGMT overexpression,[24] and preliminary data suggest a similar association with outcome in children treated with temozolomide.[25]

Clinical Features

The mode of presentation of a brain tumor depends upon the age of the child and the location of the lesion. Brain tumors in infants often produce nonspecific symptoms, such as irritability, lethargy, failure to thrive, and macrocephaly. In older children, a larger percentage of tumors manifest with localizing symptoms and signs that, in conjunction with the clinical history, often suggest the site as well as the histologic identity of the tumor.[1] For example, cerebral hemispheric gliomas may produce headaches, seizures, and focal neurologic deficits, such as hemiparesis. Symptoms due to low-grade gliomas generally progress insidiously, while those due to malignant gliomas progress more rapidly. Chiasmatic-hypothalamic gliomas often present with visual loss, which can be difficult to assess in very young children, and are often accompanied by neuroendocrine dysfunction, behavioral and appetite disturbances, and failure to thrive.

Infratentorial tumors manifest in a variety of ways, depending on tumor type. Diffuse intrinsic brainstem gliomas typically produce rapidly progressive cranial neuropathies and long-tract signs, such as hemiparesis or quadriparesis. In contrast, cerebellar astrocytomas often exhibit a long history of ataxia and symptoms of increased intracranial pressure from obstruction of the fourth ventricle. With progressive tumor enlargement, neck pain may develop as a result of downward herniation of the cerebellar tonsils through the foramen magnum.

Diagnostic Evaluation

Either computed tomography or magnetic resonance imaging (MRI), performed with and without intravenous contrast, may be employed to establish the diagnosis of a brain tumor. Magnetic resonance imaging is preferred under most circumstances and, for some tumor types, such as diffuse intrinsic brainstem glioma[26] and chiasmatic gliomas in patients with NF1,[11] is often sufficient to establish the diagnosis without the need for surgical biopsy. Postoperative imaging provides an objective assessment of the extent of resection, which for several types of childhood glial tumors is of major prognostic significance. These studies should be performed within 48 hours of surgery, if possible, to minimize postsurgical enhancement around the operative bed, which complicates interpretation.

Treatment, Outcome, and Prognostic Factors for Specific Tumor Types

Cerebral Hemispheric Low-Grade Gliomas

Complete surgical resection, if feasible, is generally the initial management goal, but this may be difficult to achieve for nonpilocytic tumors, which rarely have distinct margins (Figure 17-1). Results from several series, including a large pediatric cooperative group natural history study, suggest that extent of resection is the most important predictor of outcome. After a gross total resection, 5-year survival rates exceed 90%.[27,28] Because of the low incidence of tumor progression in children undergoing complete resection, adjuvant therapy is usually not employed. Following incomplete resection, there is a growing trend, particularly for young children, either to treat the unresectable residual disease with chemotherapy[29,30] or to defer adjuvant therapy until there is tumor progression, because of the risks of radiation therapy to the developing nervous system[31–33] and the potential for irradiation-induced malignancies.[34] Attempts to define the role of radiotherapy for subtotally resected low-grade gliomas in the North American Children's Cancer Group/Pediatric Oncology Group CCG-9891/POG-8930 study were hampered by difficulties in accruing randomized patients. Because malignant degeneration of nonirradiated childhood low-grade gliomas is uncommon, lesions that progress after initial operation are often amenable to repeat resection.[27,35]

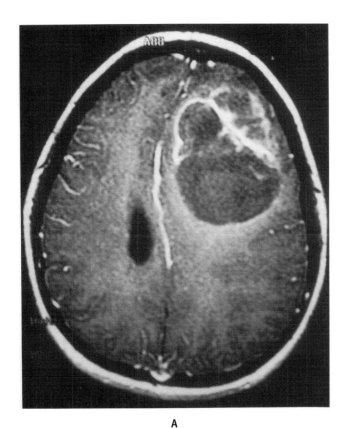

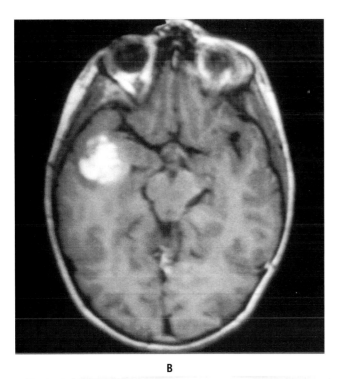

Figure 17-1 Cerebral hemispheric low-grade astrocytomas. (A) This large pilocytic astrocytoma has a plaque-like solid component with a large cystic component. (B) This non-pilocytic tumor shows indistinct borders with the surrounding brain. Both lesions were amenable to resection.

Supratentorial Malignant (High-Grade) Gliomas

In children older than 3 years, these lesions (Figure 17-2) are treated with maximal resection followed by irradiation to the tumor bed and a margin of surrounding brain. The use of adjuvant chemotherapy has been shown to enhance survival[36]; in the first CCG randomized controlled trial for malignant gliomas, CCG-943, children who received irradiation followed by lomustine, vincristine, and prednisone experienced a 5-year event-free survival of 46% versus only 18% for patients treated with radiotherapy alone. An attempt to improve on these results using the "8-in-1" regimen in the CCG-945 study showed no improvement in outcome compared to treatment with lomustine and vincristine alone.[37] This provided the impetus for a series of subsequent studies, which examined the efficacy of administering more-intensive chemotherapy regimens in a neoadjuvant (pre-irradiation) setting, as well as administering highly intensive regimens using myeloablative chemotherapy coupled with autologous bone marrow or peripheral blood stem cell rescue.[38,39] Although some studies suggested an improvement in outcome with these approaches,[40] the results were less convincing in others, and the potential for significant treatment-induced morbidity and mortality with some highly intensive regimens has also been a concern.[39] For example, the North American POG-9135 study examined the use of neoadjuvant cisplatin combined with carmustine versus cyclophosphamide combined with vincristine. The cisplatin-carmustine arm was associated with a 20% 5-year event-free survival, which was comparable to the results with adjuvant lomustine and vincristine, versus less than 5% for the cyclophosphamide-vincristine arm

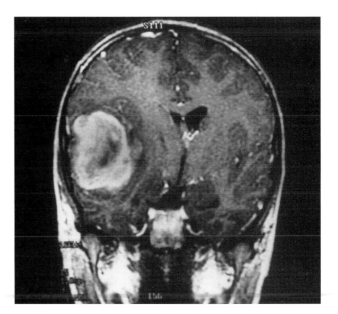

Figure 17-2 This large supratentorial glioblastoma multiforme had relatively well-defined margins, a situation rarely encountered in adult high-grade gliomas, and was amenable to gross total resection. This child remains disease-free 5 years after completing adjuvant therapy.

(p $0 < .05$). Subsequently, the CCG-9933 trial compared three alkylating agents (carboplatin, ifosfamide, and cyclophosphamide) combined with etoposide, before irradiation, for patients with postoperative residual disease. Although responses were observed with all three regimens, there was an unacceptably high rate of early disease progression, with a progression-free survival rate of only 15% at 2 years.[41] Similarly, the POG-9431 trial noted insufficient activity of neoadjuvant procarbazine and topotecan to warrant further study.[42] Although CCG-9922 noted an encouraging 2-year progression-free survival rate of 46% among 11 patients with newly diagnosed high-grade glioma who were treated with a highly intensive, myeloablative chemotherapy regimen that included carmustine, thiotepa, and etoposide, the 45% incidence of severe pulmonary and/or neurologic toxicity and the 18% toxic death rate dampened enthusiasm for further exploration of this regimen.[39]

In view of these disappointing results, more recent studies have focused on attempting to enhance the efficacy of adjuvant chemotherapy by administering active agents concurrently with, as well as following, irradiation.[43] The recently completed Children's Oncology Group (COG) ACNS0126 study evaluated the activity of administering temozolomide on a daily basis during irradiation and on a standard 5-day schedule after irradiation. This design was based upon the results of a recent study for adults with malignant gliomas that demonstrated that the addition of temozolomide to irradiation significantly improved outcome, particularly in patients whose tumors had MGMT silencing.[23,44] Unfortunately, preliminary results from the ACNS0126 cohort, although similar to those from the adult study, were no better than those achieved in the CCG-945 cohort using lomustine and vincristine.[45] A subsequent study (ACNS0423) attempted to build upon these results by combining temozolomide with lomustine, although outcome from this trial is currently pending.[46] In parallel with the latter study, recent protocols from both the COG and the Pediatric Brain Tumor Consortium (PBTC) have examined the activity of a series of agents targeted against growth-signaling pathways known to be abnormally activated in malignant gliomas, although the results to date have demonstrated objective tumor responses in only a small subset of patients.[47]

Despite the relatively limited advances that have been made in the adjuvant management of malignant gliomas, recent studies have provided prognostically useful informa-

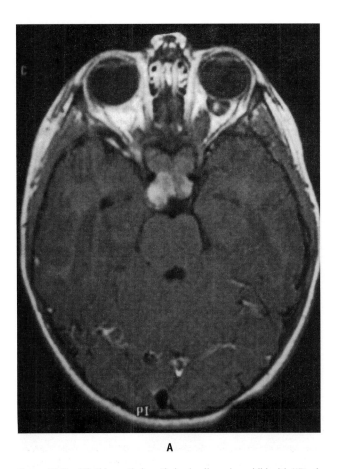
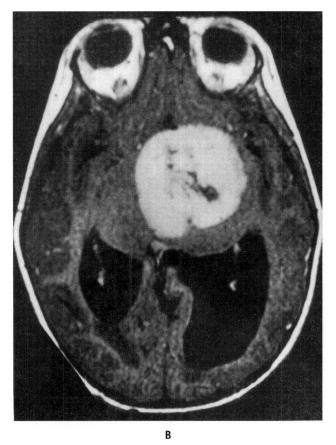

A   B

Figure 17-3 (A) Chiasmatic hypothalamic glioma in a child with NF1, demonstrating diffuse thickening of the chiasm. (B) This chiasmatic-hypothalamic glioma produced substantial local mass effect and biventricular hydrocephalus. A central tumor debulking was performed, which partially opened the cerebrospinal fluid pathways and relieved the patient's preoperative hemiparesis, but substantial residual tumor was apparent. After 6 months of chemotherapy with carboplatin and vincristine, the residual tumor had regressed dramatically. The patient is currently neurologically intact with normal vision and stable residual tumor, 6 years after diagnosis.

tion, calling attention to a striking association between extent of resection and outcome.[37,48] In the CCG-945 study, 3-year event-free survival was 54% for patients undergoing greater than 90% tumor resection versus only 17% for patients undergoing less than a 90% tumor resection.[37] However, it is impossible to exclude the possibility that certain tumors with more favorable biologic characteristics are inherently more amenable to radical resection.[48]

Histology is another factor that has been associated with outcome; children with glioblastoma multiforme fare worse than those with anaplastic astrocytomas, with 5-year progression-free survivals of 15% to 20% versus 30% to 40%, respectively.[36,37] High-grade gliomas with an oligodendroglial component seem to have a better prognosis than purely astrocytic malignant gliomas,[21,37] reflecting the greater sensitivity of oligodendroglial tumors to conventional chemotherapeutic agents.[21]

Optic-Hypothalamic Gliomas

Because optic-hypothalamic gliomas cannot be completely resected without unacceptable morbidity, and many lesions are either indolent or respond well to adjuvant chemotherapy, the operative indications remain controversial. In patients with NF1, the pathological identity of the radiographically evident tumor is rarely in question, and neither biopsy nor resection are usually pursued[49,50] (Figure 17-3a). In non-NF1 patients, resection is generally limited to tumors that are exophytic and causing mass effect or hydrocephalus[51] (Figure 17-3b). Although complete resection is not feasible because these lesions infiltrate the optic chiasm and hypothalamus, substantial cytoreduction can sometimes be achieved.[50,51] However, an alternative approach is to obtain a histologic diagnosis by stereotactic biopsy and then give chemotherapy initially, reserving resection for lesions that fail to respond and exhibit increasing mass effect. In some instances, a well-timed surgical debulking of tumor will stabilize the patient sufficiently so that additional chemotherapy or irradiation can be administered, leading to long-term tumor control.

Although optic-hypothalamic gliomas are generally low-grade tumors histologically, their biologic behavior varies widely.[52] Whereas some lesions exhibit decelerating growth over time, others enlarge rapidly despite treatment. In the review by Jenkin et al, survival was significantly better in the 38 patients with NF1 than in the 49 without this diagnosis ($p = .0007$).[53] Chiasmatic gliomas with extension into the hypothalamus carry a worse prognosis than lesions strictly localized to the chiasm.[52] In addition, tumors tend to behave more aggressively in infants than in older children.[50–52]

Radiation therapy had long been used in the treatment of these lesions, resulting in reported 5-year survival rates between 75% and 90%.[52,54] However, because this modality has significant long-term sequelae,[31–31] chemotherapy has become the preferred approach in recent years, particularly in patients younger than 10 years.[29,30] A variety of regimens have been employed (eg, carboplatin/vincristine and 6-thioguanine/procarbazine/lomustine/vincristine), with response or stabilization rates in excess of 75%.[29,30]

These two regimens were compared in terms of activity and tolerability in the CCG A9952 study,[55] the results of which are currently pending. Another agent that has demonstrated activity against low-grade gliomas is temozolomide,[56,57] and this agent was added to the carboplatin/vincristine "backbone" in the recently completed COG ACNS0223 study. Although some patients initially treated with chemotherapy later require radiotherapy for disease control, the deferral of irradiation for several years is beneficial in improving functional outcome. As an additional strategy to minimize late effects, the COG ACNS0221 study will examine the efficacy of conformal radiotherapy with 3-dimensional image-based treatment planning and delivery in children who require irradiation for these tumors.[58] It has also become clear that not all chiasmatic gliomas in patients with NF1 require treatment. Because tumors in children with NF1 often remain stable for years after diagnosis, adjuvant therapy for asymptomatic lesions is best deferred until progression is documented.[11] In contrast to these sometimes indolent tumors, a subset of hypothalamic gliomas with pilomyxoid features has been noted to have a more adverse prognosis, although distinctive management guidelines have yet to be formulated.[59]

Gangliogliomas and Low-Grade Neuroepithelial Tumors

Gangliogliomas are usually well-circumscribed lesions that are amenable to complete resection. In such cases, radiotherapy is not required, and the 10-year survival rate exceeds 90%.[60] The role of radiotherapy for incompletely resected low-grade gangliogliomas is uncertain.[60] Because hemispheric lesions tend to be indolent, irradiation is probably best reserved for tumors that progress after resection and remain incompletely resectable. Several other uncommon low-grade neuroepithelial tumors of childhood, such as DIGs,[7,8] DNETs,[6] and papillary glioneuronal tumors,[61] are also best managed surgically; adjuvant therapy is reserved for lesions that subsequently progress.

Cerebellar Astrocytomas

Posterior fossa juvenile pilocytic astrocytomas (Figure 17-4) have perhaps the best prognosis of any type of pediatric brain tumor, with 10-year survival rates exceeding 95%.[62,63] Nonpilocytic astrocytomas also have an excellent outcome if an extensive resection can be achieved.[63] The prognosis of these tumors is strongly affected by the extent of resection as assessed by postoperative imaging. Patients with no evidence of disease are followed with periodic MRI studies. If the postoperative scan shows resectable tumor, reoperation may be indicated to achieve complete resection. Patients with unresectable residual disease may be followed with observation until progression or treated, if symptomatic, with radiotherapy or chemotherapy. Although histologic features of malignancy in pilocytic astrocytomas do not necessarily indicate a poor prognosis,[64] the presence of malignant features in a nonpilocytic tumor is clearly an adverse prognostic factor. As with

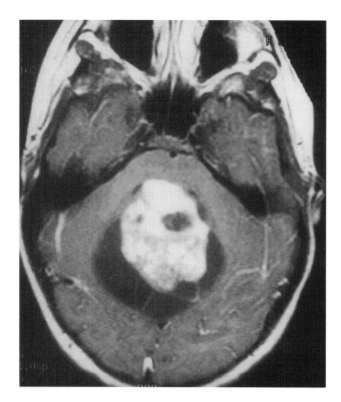

Figure 17-4 As is typical of pilocytic cerebellar astrocytomas, this partially cystic vermian lesion was well circumscribed from the surrounding brain, allowing a complete resection.

cerebral high-grade gliomas, such lesions are treated postoperatively with radiotherapy and chemotherapy.

Brainstem Gliomas

The prognosis of children with brainstem tumors can vary widely, depending on the growth characteristics of the tumor (ie, focal or diffuse), which is usually apparent on MRI.[26] The lowest-grade lesions are the intrinsic tectal tumors[65] (Figure 17-5a): in our series of more than 20 such lesions managed by cerebrospinal fluid diversion without specific treatment for the tumor, only about 25% have exhibited progression with a median follow-up in excess of 8 years. Focal midbrain, pontine and medullary tumors, and dorsally exophytic and cervicomedullary tumors are less indolent than the tectal tumors (Figure 17-5b) but nonetheless have an excellent prognosis with extensive resection.[66–68]

In contrast to the above groups, patients with diffuse intrinsic brainstem gliomas have a dismal prognosis, with a median survival of approximately 9 months.[69–73] The diagnosis is made based on the characteristic MRI features (Figure 17-5c) and clinical appearance. Treatment is nonoperative and has historically consisted of external beam irradiation (54 Gy to 60 Gy) to the tumor site. Although radiotherapy often induces temporary disease regression and symptomatic improvement, it is rarely curative. In addition, pre- and post-irradiation administration of a variety of conventional chemotherapeutic agents, either alone

or in combination, has failed to significantly improve prognosis. In the CCG-944 study of children with newly diagnosed brainstem glioma who were randomized to receive either irradiation alone or with the addition of lomustine, vincristine, and prednisone, there was no improvement in survival in the group who received chemotherapy.[70] More recent studies using intensive neoadjuvant chemotherapy and postirradiation myeloablative chemotherapy were similarly disappointing, with few responders and short survival times.[71–73]

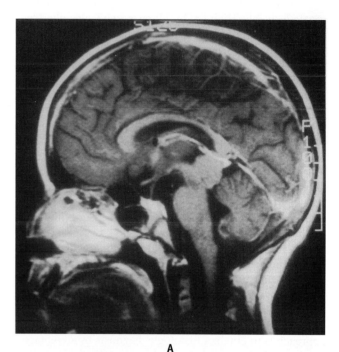

A

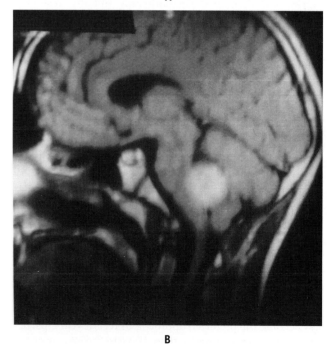

B

Figure 17-5 Various types of brainstem gliomas. (A) A low-grade intrinsic tectal tumor. (B) A dorsally exophytic brainstem glioma.

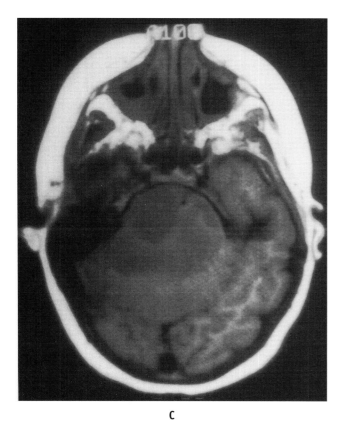

Figure 17-5 (continued)   (C) A diffuse intrinsic brainstem glioma.

Based on the efficacy of radiotherapy for achieving at least temporary disease regression in children with brainstem gliomas, and the realization that conventional chemotherapy has little activity against these tumors, differing radiation therapy administration strategies have been pursued to attempt to enhance tumor cytotoxicity and, potentially, survival. Unfortunately, studies from both CCG and POG demonstrated that escalation of the dose of irradiation to as high as 7800 cGy using hyperfractionated (twice daily) delivery failed to improve survival.[69,74] Accordingly, this approach has largely been abandoned.

An alternative strategy that is currently being pursued in a number of studies involves the administration of radiosensitizing agents concurrently with irradiation, with the goal of potentiating the efficacy of radiotherapy. A difference between this strategy and simple dose escalation of irradiation is that radiosensitization is theorized to synergistically potentiate the efficacy of irradiation within rapidly dividing tumor cells. A related approach, so-called chemoradiotherapy, combines radiotherapy with an agent that has demonstrated at least some activity against the tumor, in the hope of achieving additive tumor cell cytotoxicity. Ongoing Phase I studies of the COG and the PBTC are evaluating a series of such agents that have shown radiation-enhancing properties in preclinical and preliminary clinical studies. In addition, several studies of the PBTC are examining the efficacy of combining irradiation with molecularly targeted agents against growth-signaling pathways, although preliminary results have yet to demonstrate an improvement in outcome.[47]

Sequelae of Treatment

Many of the most troubling sequelae of treating childhood brain tumors manifest several years after diagnosis, which mandates long-term multidisciplinary follow-up. Sequential measurements of intelligence quotient in young children who received whole-brain irradiation have shown a gradual decline in intelligence during the first 2 years after treatment.[31,32] This appears to be less of a problem with focal irradiation, particularly if the medial temporal lobes and hypothalamus are outside the treatment volume.

Cranial irradiation has also been associated with carotid occlusive disease, particularly in patients irradiated for parasellar lesions, such as chiasmatic-hypothalamic gliomas. Endocrinopathies are also extremely common in children with such lesions.[33] Second neoplasms are an additional concern in children with a brain tumor, with an incidence that ranges from 1% to 5%.[34,75] The majority of such tumors are malignant gliomas, meningiomas, and sarcomas that occur within radiotherapy treatment fields 10 to 20 years after irradiation; an increased incidence of hematologic malignancies has been noted after chemotherapy.

Future Directions

Improvements in the outcome of children with hemispheric low-grade glial tumors will depend on continued evolution of surgical techniques, coupled with appropriate implementation of extraoperative and intraoperative imaging modalities, and physiologic monitoring, to enhance the percentage of tumors that are amenable to complete resection and reduce surgical morbidity. For patients with inherently unresectable low-grade gliomas, such as extensive chiasmatic-hypothalamic lesions, as well as those with malignant gliomas, improvements in outcome will depend on identifying and applying better multimodality treatment strategies that target the molecular pathways that are aberrantly activated in these tumors. These include pharmacologic agents designed to modulate such pathways and immunologic approaches directed at proteins that are selectively overexpressed in these tumors compared with normal brain tissue. In addition, the application of convection-enhanced delivery strategies has allowed the administration of high-molecular-weight immunotoxins targeting cell surface receptors overexpressed on tumor cells as well as active chemotherapeutic agents, thereby bypassing the delivery restrictions imposed by the blood-brain barrier. Pilot studies of each of the above approaches are currently in progress or under development.

Acknowledgment

This work was supported in part by NIH grant P01NS-40923 and R01NS37704.

References

1. Pollack IF. Brain tumors in children. *N Engl J Med.* 1994;331:1500–1507.
2. Young JL. Cancer incidence, survival, and mortality for children younger than 15 years. *Cancer.* 1986;58:561–568.
3. *Kleihues P, Burger PC, Scheithauer BW, et al. World Health Organization Histological Typing of Tumours of the Central Nervous System. New York: Springer-Verlag; 1993.*

4. Berger MS, Keles GE, Geyer JR. Cerebral hemispheric tumors of childhood. *Pediatr Neuro-Oncol.* 1992;3:839–852.

5. Giannini C, Scheithauer BW, Burger PC, et al. Pleomorphic xanthoastrocytoma: what do we really know about it? *Cancer.* 1995;85:2033–2045.

6. Daumas-Duport C, Scheithauer BW, Chodkiewicz J-P, et al. Dysembryoplastic neuroepithelial tumor (DNT): a surgically curable tumor of young subjects with intractable partial seizures. Report of 39 cases. *Neurosurgery.* 1988;23:545–556.

7. VandenBerg SR, May EE, Rubinstein LJ, et al. Desmoplastic supratentorial neuroepithelial tumors of infancy with divergent differentiation potential ("desmoplastic infantile gangliogliomas"): report on 11 cases of a distinctive embryonal tumor with a favorable prognosis. *J Neurosurg.* 1987;66:58–71.

8. Duffner PK, Burger PC, Cohen ME, et al. Desmoplastic infantile gangliogliomas: an approach to therapy. *Neurosurgery.* 1994;34:583–589.

9. Xu G, O'Connell P, Viskochil D, et al. The neurofibromatosis type 1 gene encodes a protein related to GAP. *Cell.* 1990;62:599–608.

10. Basu TN, Gutmann DH, Fletcher JA, et al. Aberrant regulation of ras proteins in malignant tumors cells from type 1 neurofibromatosis patients. *Nature.* 1992;356:713–715.

11. Pollack IF, Mulvihill JJ. Special issues in the management of gliomas in children with neurofibromatosis 1. *J Neuro-Oncol.* 1996;28:257–268.

12. The European chromosome 16 tuberous sclerosis consortium. Identification and characterization of the tuberous sclerosis gene on chromosome 16. *Cell.* 1993;75:1305–1315.

13. von Deimling A, Louis DN, Menon AG, et al. Deletions on the long arm of chromosome 17 in pilocytic astrocytoma. *Acta Neuropathol.* 1993;86:81–85.

14. Lang FF, Miller DC, Pisharody S, et al. High frequency of p53 protein accumulation without p53 gene mutation in human juvenile pilocytic, low grade and anaplastic astrocytomas. *Oncogene.* 1994;9:949–954.

15. Rasheed BKA, McLendon RE, Herndon RE, et al. Alterations of the *TP53* gene in human gliomas. *Cancer Res.* 1994;54:1324–1330.

16. Pollack IF, Finkelstein SD, Burnham J, et al. Age and *TP53* mutation frequency in childhood gliomas. Results in a multi-institutional cohort. *Cancer Res.* 2001;61:7404–7407.

17. Sidransky D, Mikkelsen T, Schwechheimer K, et al. Clonal expansion of p53 mutant cells is associated with brain tumor progression. *Nature.* 1992;355:846–847.

18. Collins VP. Progression as exemplified by human astrocytic tumors. *Cancer Biol.* 1999;9:267–276.

19. Pollack IF, Finkelstein SD, Woods J, et al. Expression of p53 and prognosis in malignant gliomas in children. *N Engl J Med.* 2002;346:420–427.

20. Pollack IF, Hamilton RL, James CD, et al. Rarity of PTEN deletions and EGFR amplification in malignant gliomas of childhood: results from the Children's Cancer Group 945 cohort. *J Neurosurg: Pediatr.* 2006;105:3431–3437.

21. Ino Y, Betensky RA, Zlatescu MC, et al. Molecular subtypes of anaplastic oligodendroglioma: implications for patient management at diagnosis. *Clin Cancer Res.* 2001;7:839–845.

22. Pollack IF, Finkelstein SD, Burnham J, et al. The association between chromosome 1p loss and outcome in pediatric malignant gliomas: Results from the CCG–945 cohort. *Pediatr Neurosurg.* 2003;39:114–121.

23. Hegi ME, Diserens AC, Gorlia T, et al. MGMT gene silencing and benefit from temozolomide in glioblastoma. *N Engl J Med.* 2005;352:997–1003.

24. Pollack IF, Hamilton RL, Sobol RW, et al. O⁶-methylguanine-DNA methyltransferase expression strongly correlates with outcome in childhood malignant gliomas: results from the CCG–945 cohort. *J Clin Oncol.* 2006;24:3431–3437.

25. Pollack IF, Hamilton RL, Burnham J, et al. Molecular predictors of outcome in childhood malignant gliomas: the Children's Oncology Group experience. *Neuro-Oncol.* 2007;9:188.

26. Albright AL, Packer RJ, Zimmerman R, et al. Magnetic resonance scans should replace biopsies for the diagnosis of diffuse brain stem gliomas: a report from the Children's Cancer Group. *Neurosurgery.* 1993;1026–1030.

27. Pollack IF, Claassen D, Al-Shboul Q, et al. Low-grade gliomas of the cerebral hemispheres in children: an analysis of 71 cases. *J Neurosurg.* 1995;82:536–547.

28. Sanford A, Kun L, Sposto R, et al. Low-grade gliomas of childhood: impact of surgical resection. A report from the Children's Oncology Group. *J Neurosurg.* 2002;96:427–428.

29. Packer RJ, Ater J, Allen J, et al. Carboplatin and vincristine chemotherapy for children with newly diagnosed progressive low-grade gliomas. *J Neurosurg.* 1997;86:747–754.

30. Petronio J, Edwards MSB, Prados M, et al. Management of chiasmal and hypothalamic gliomas of infancy and childhood with chemotherapy. *J Neurosurg.* 1991;74:701–708.

31. Ellenberg L, McComb JG, Siegel S, Stowe S. Factors affecting intellectual outcome in pediatric brain tumor patients. *Neurosurgery.* 1987;21:638–644.

32. Radcliffe J, Packer RJ, Atkins TE, et al. Three- and four-year cognitive outcome in children with noncortical brain tumors treated with whole-brain radiotherapy. *Ann Neurol.* 1992;32:551–554.

33. Livesey EA, Hindmarsh PC, Brook CGD, et al. Endocrine disorders following treatment of childhood brain tumours. *Br J Cancer.* 1990;61:622–625.

34. Dirks PB, Jay V, Becker LE, et al. Development of anaplastic changes in low-grade astrocytomas of childhood. *Neurosurgery.* 1994;34:68–78.

35. Bowers DC, Krause TP, Aronson LJ, et al. Second surgery for recurrent pilocytic astrocytoma. *Pediatr Neurosurg.* 2001;34:229–234.

36. Sposto R, Ertel IJ, Jenkin RDT, et al. The effectiveness of chemotherapy for treatment of high-grade astrocytoma in children: results of a randomized trial. *J Neuro-Oncol.* 1989;7:165–177.

37. Finlay J, Boyett J, Yates A, et al. Randomized Phase III trial in childhood high-grade astrocytoma comparing vincristine, lomustine, and prednisone with the eight-drugs-in-1-day regimen. *J Clin Oncol.* 1993;13:112–123.

38. Pollack IF, Boyett J, Finlay JL. Chemotherapy for high-grade gliomas of childhood. *Child's Nerv Syst.* 1999;15:529–544.

39. Grovas AC, Boyett JM, Lindsley K, et al. Regimen-related toxicity of myeloablastive chemotherapy with BCNU, thiotepa, and etoposide followed by autologous stem cell rescue for children with newly diagnosed glioblastoma multiforme: report from the Children's Cancer Group. *Med Pediatr Oncol.* 1999;33:83–87.

40. Wolff JE, Gnekow AK, Kortmann RD, et al. Preradiation chemotherapy for pediatric patients with high-grade glioma. *Cancer.* 2001;94:264–271.

41. Arenson E, Ater J, Bank J, et al. A randomized Phase II trial of high dose alkylating agents plus VP-16 in children with high grade astrocytoma. *J Pediatr Hematol Oncol.* 1999;21:325.

42. Chintagumpala M, Steward C, Burger P, et al. Response to topotecan in newly-diagnosed patients with high-grade gliomas: a Pediatric Oncology Group (POG) study. *Proceedings of the 9th International Symposium on Pediatric Neuro-Oncology.* San Francisco, CA; 2000:55.

43. Stupp R, Dietrich PY, Ostermann-Kraljevic S, et al. Promising survival with newly diagnosed glioblastoma multiforme treated with concomitant radiation plus temozolomide followed by adjuvant temozolomide. *J Clin Oncol.* 2002;20:1375–1382.

44. Stupp R, Mason WP, van den Bent MJ, et al; European Organisation for Research and Treatment of Cancer Brain Tumor and Radiotherapy Groups; National Cancer Institute of Canada Clinical Trials Group. Radiotherapy plus concomitant and adjuvant temozolomide for glioblastoma. *N Eng J Med.* 2005;352:987–996.

45. Cohen KJ, Heideman R, Zhou T, et al. Should temozolomide be the standard of care for children with newly diagnosed high-grade gliomas? results of the Children's Oncology Group ACNS0126 study. *Neuro Oncol.* 2007;9:188.

46. Jakacki R, Yates A, Zhou T, et al. Temozolomide as part of combination chemotherapy for pediatric brain tumors: the Children's Oncology Group experience. *Neuro Oncol.* 2007;9:188.

47. Pollack IF, Jakacki RI, Blaney SM, et al. Phase I trial of imatinib in children with newly diagnosed brainstem and recurrent malignant gliomas: a Pediatric Brain Tumor Consortium report. *Neuro Oncol.* 2007;9:145–160.

48. Campbell JW, Pollack IF, Martinez AJ, Shultz BL. High-grade astrocytomas in children: radiologically complete resection is associated with an excellent long-term prognosis. *Neurosurgery.* 1996;38:258–264.

49. Listernak R, Charrow J, Greenwald MJ, Esterly NB. Optic gliomas in children with neurofibromatosis type 1. *J Pediatr.* 1989;114:788–792.

50. Hoffman HJ, Humphreys RP, Drake JM, et al. Optic pathway/hypothalamic gliomas: a dilemma in management. *Pediatr Neurosurg.* 1993;19:186–195.

51. Wisoff JH, Abbott R, Epstein F. Surgical management of exophytic chiasmatic-hypothalamic tumors of childhood. *J Neurosurg.* 1990;73:661–667.

52. Alvord E Jr, Lofton S. Gliomas of the optic nene and chiasm. Outcome by patient's age, tumor site, and treatment. *J Neurosurg.* 1988;68:85–98.

53. Jenkin D, Angyalfi S, Becker L, et al. Optic glioma in children: surveillance, resection or irradiation? *Int J Radiat Oncol Biol Phys.* 1993;25:215–225.

54. Pierce SM, Barnes PD, Loeffler JS, et al. Definitive radiation therapy in the management of symptomatic patients with optic glioma: survival and long-term effects. *Cancer.* 1990;65:45–52.

55. Ater J, Mazewski C, Roberts W, et al. Phase 3 randomized study of two chemotherapy regimens for treatment of progressive low-grade glioma in young children: preliminary report from the Children's Oncology Group protocol A9952. *Neuro Oncol.* 2007;9:204.

56. Quinn JA, Reardon DA, Friedman AH, et al. Phase II trial of temozolomide in patients with progressive low-grade glioma. *J Clin Oncol.* 2003;21:646–651.

57. Kuo DJ, Weiner HL, Wisoff J, et al. Temozolomide is active in childhood, progressive, unresectable, low-grade gliomas. *J Pediatr Hematol Oncol.* 2003;25:372–378.

58. Nishihori T, Shirato H, Aoyama H, et al. Three-dimensional conformal radiotherapy for astrocytic tumors involving the eloquent area in children and young adults. *J Neuro Oncol.* 2002;60:177–183.

59. Komotar RJ, Burger PC, Carson BS, et al. Pilocytic and pilomyxoid hypothalamic/chiasmatic astrocytomas. *Neurosurgery.* 2004;54:72–79.

60. Lang FF, Epstein FJ, Ransohoff J, et al. Central nervous system gangliogliomas. Part 2: clinical outcome. *J Neurosurg.* 1993;79:867–873.

61. Rosenblum MK. The 2007 WHO Classification of Nervous System Tumors: newly recognized members of the mixed glioneuronal group. *Brain Pathol.* 2007;17:308–313.

62. Garcia DM, Latifi HR, Simpson JR, et al. Astrocytomas of the cerebellum in children. *J Neurosurg.* 1989;71:661–664.

63. Schneider JH, Raffel C, McComb JG. Benign cerebellar astrocytomas of childhood. *Neurosurgery.* 1992;30:58–63.

64. Tomlinson FH, Scheithauer BW, Hayostek CJ, et al. The significance of atypia and histologic malignancy in pilocytic astrocytoma of the cerebellum: a clinicopathologic and flow cytometric study. *J Child Neurol.* 1994;9:301–310.

65. Pollack IF, Pang D, Albright AL. The long-term outcome in children with late-onset aqueductal stenosis resulting from benign intrinsic tectal tumors. *J Neurosurg.* 1994;80:681–688.

66. Epstein F, McCleary EL. Intrinsic brain-stem tumors of childhood: surgical indications. *J Neurosurg*. 1988;64:11–15.
67. Epstein FJ, Wisoff JH. Intra-axial tumors of the cervicomedullary junction. *J Neurosurg*. 1987;67:483–487.
68. Pollack IF, Hoffman HJ, Humphreys RP, Becker L. The long-term outcome after surgical treatment of dorsally exophytic brain-stem gliomas. *J Neurosurg*. 1993;78:859–863.
69. Packer RJ, Boyett JM, Zimmerman RA, et al. Outcome of children with brain stem gliomas after treatment with 7800 cGy of hyperfractionated radiotherapy. *Cancer*. 1994;74:1827–1834.
70. Jenkin RDT, Boesel C, Ertel I, et al. Brain-stem tumors in childhood: a prospective randomized trial of irradiation with and without adjuvant CCNU, VCR, and prednisone. *J Neurosurg*. 1987;66:227–233.
71. Kretschmar CS, Tarbell NJ, Barnes PD, et al. Pre-irradiation chemotherapy and hyperfractionated radiation therapy 66Gy for children with brain stem tumors. *Cancer*. 1993;72:1404–1413.
72. Dunkel IJ, Garvin JH, Goldman S, et al. High dose chemotherapy with autologous bone marrow rescue for children with diffuse pontine brain stem tumors. *J Neuro Oncol*. 1998;37:67–73.
73. Jennings MT, Sposto R, Boyett JM, et al. Pre-radiation chemotherapy in primary high risk brain stem tumors: CCG-9941, a Phase II study of the Children's Cancer Group. *J Clin Oncol*. 2002;20:3431–3437.
74. Freeman CR, Krischer JP, Sanford RA, et al. Final results of a study of escalating doses of hyperfractionated radiotherapy in brain stem tumors in children: a Pediatric Oncology Group study. *Int J Radiat Oncol Biol Phys*. 1993;27:197–206.
75. Hawkins MM, Draper GJ, Kingston JE. Incidence of second primary tumors among childhood cancer survivors. *Br J Cancer*. 1987; 56:339–347.

Ependymoma

Richard Grundy and Thomas E. Merchant

Introduction

Pediatric ependymomas are intriguing tumors, and their clinical management remains one of the more difficult in pediatric neurooncology. Ependymomas constitute 6% to 12% of all childhood intracranial neoplasms and 30% of spinal tumors in childhood.[1,2] Interestingly, more than half of all intracranial ependymomas arise in children under 5 years, providing a significant management challenge.[1,2]

Clinical Presentation

Signs and Symptoms

Most childhood ependymomas arise in the posterior fossa, where they are intimately associated with the fourth ventricle. Ependymomas show a propensity to adhere to and invade the brain stem as well as to extend through the foramen of Luschka, often bilaterally, enveloping the lower cranial nerves.[3] The most common presentation is therefore nonspecific and related to raised intracranial pressure from obstructive hydrocephalus, but patients may also present with cerebellar or lower cranial nerve dysfunction. In young children, irritability and lethargy may be the only presenting symptoms. The duration of these symptoms prior to presentation varies greatly depending on site and may be prolonged, particularly in spinal tumors (Tables 18-1, 18-2, 18-3).

Table 18-1

Symptoms and signs of intracranial ependymoma.

Headache	Papilloedema
Nausea and vomiting	Cranial nerve palsies
Lethargy	Ataxia
Behavioral changes	Cerebellar signs
Slurred speech/visual disturbance	Torticollis

Table 18-2

Symptoms and signs of spinal ependymoma.

Pain: localized (backache) and radicular (sciatica)	Spastic paraparesis
	Hyper-reflexia
Gait disturbance	Suspended sensory level
Weakness	Bladder/bowel dysfunction
Sensory change	Scoliosis
Bladder/bowel dysfunction	

Table 18-3

Differential diagnosis of ependymoma.

Medulloblastoma/PNET	High-grade glioma
Exophytic brainstem gliomas	Pilocytic astrocytomas
	Choroid plexus tumors

Location

Ependymomas are thought to arise from the ependymal lining of the ventricles and of the central canal. In contradistinction to their clinical presentation in adults, approximately 90% of pediatric ependymomas are intracranial, and of these more than 70% arise in the posterior fossa[4,5] (Figures 18-1 and 18-2). Although ependymomas are most frequently associated with the ventricular cavities, they may occur anywhere in the neuraxis. Dissemination via cerebrospinal fluid (CSF) is reported in 7% to 22% of cases.[6] Spinal ependymomas may occur as intramedullary or as intradural extramedullary tumors (Figure 18-3), the latter arising predominantly in the caudal region—the filum terminale, where they are usually of the myxopapillary histologic subtype (see Table 18-1).[7]

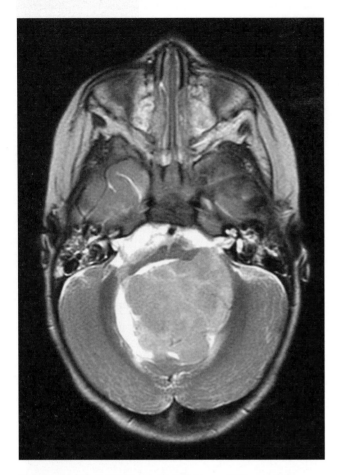

Figure 18-1 Transverse T2-weighted MR image of IVth ventricular ependymoma with extension into the foramen of Luschka on the left side.

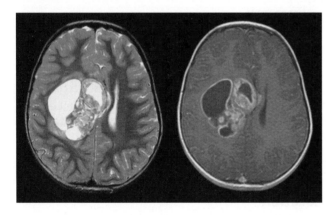

Figure 18-2 Transverse T2 and post-contrast T1-weighted MR images of left hemispheric ependymoma. The tumor has cystic and solid components with heterogeneous enhancement.

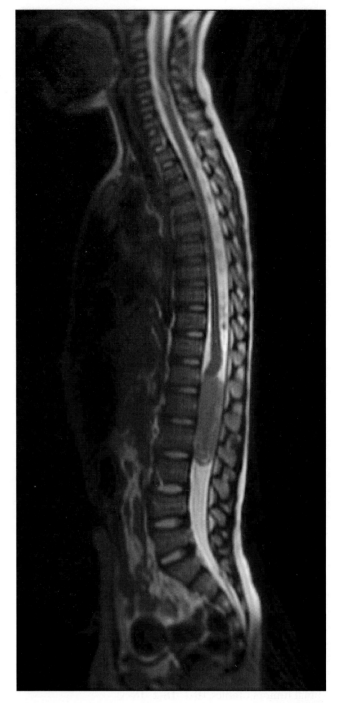

Figure 18-3 Sagittal T2-weighted MR image of the entire spine demonstrating a myxopapillary ependymoma arising from the terminal spinal cord.

Pathology

Consistent histologic grading of ependymomas has proven difficult, and several different classification systems have been proposed. The most frequently used system is the World Health Organization 2007.[8] The most common histologic subtypes occurring in children are classic ependymoma (grade II) and anaplastic ependymoma (grade III) (Table 18-4). However, a spectrum of pathologic features exists, and the distinction between classic and anaplastic is difficult. Indeed, in one recent study the pathologic diagnoses of the treating institution and the central review were discordant in 69% of cases,[9] and the relative proportion of grade III ependymoma in reported studies ranges from 10% to more than 80%.[4,5,10] A clear international consensus on this difficult issue is now required.

Table 18-4

World Health Organization Classification (2007) of ependymal tumors.

Grade I Ependymoma	Grade II Ependymoma	Grade III Ependymoma
Myxopapillary	Cellular	Anaplastic
Subependymoma	Papillary	
	Anycytic	

Source: Adapted from McLendon RE, Wiestler OD, Kros, JM, et al. Ependymoma; in DN Lewis, H Ohgaki, OD Wiestler, and WK Cavanle (eds): *Pathology & Genetics of Tumors of the Nervous System*. 3rd ed. Lyon, IARC, 2007; 72–80.

Diagnostic Evaluation

Imaging Studies

On computerized tomographic (CT) imaging, ependymomas are typically hyperdense and frequently contain cystic areas and calcifications.[11] On magnetic resonance imaging (MRI), ependymomas typically display iso- to hypo-intensity on T1-weighted images and hyperintensity on T2-weighted images, and they usually enhance heterogeneously with gadolinium contrast (Table 18-5). Areas of signal heterogeneity representing hemorrhage, necrosis, or calcification are common,[12] as are areas of nonenhancing tumor, which can confound pre- and postoperative assessments. Complete neuraxis imaging is essential to exclude leptomeningeal disease. Continued full neuraxis imaging is advised even in spinal tumors, including myxopapillary ependymomas which occasionally metastasize to the brain. An unresolved issue is exactly what surveillance protocol is optimal for children with ependymomas in order to maximize detection of recurrence without unduly wasting resources. The detection of asymptomatic recurrences through routine surveillance does appear to confer some benefit.[12] A widely accepted strategy is 3 to 4 monthly scans for up to 5 years, particularly in infants who have not been irradiated. Minimal residual visible spinal metastatic disease in the absence of intracranial metastases is uncommon.

Prognostic Factors

Although a number of prognostic factors have been identified, their veracity is uncertain. The literature abounds with single-institution retrospective series involving limited numbers of patients accrued over a time span covering many different attitudes to both the diagnosis and treatment of ependymoma. This situation is compounded by difficulties in standardizing the pathologic grading of ependymomas.

Surgery

The most widely accepted prognostic factor is the degree of surgical resection. Axiomatically, gross total resection is associated with a better prognosis.[6,8,13–17] However, a small number of studies have failed to demonstrate that a gross total resection confers a survival advantage.[18–20] Critically, the degree of postoperative resection needs to be confirmed by MRI within 48 hours of surgery. Surgical recollection is insufficiently reliable and does not correlate with outcome.[4,21] However, a recent United Kingdom study challenges this view, showing that surgical designation of completeness of surgery is more closely related to outcome than radiologic review.[5] Despite the importance of obtaining a gross total resection, a complete resection is obtained in only 50% to 85% of cases reported from a number of national trials.[4,5,8,21,22] Results in single-institution studies appear better: 84% of patients underwent a gross total resection in a recent series,[23] raising important questions about centralization of neurosurgical management.

Age

Older children (>greater than 3 years of age) appear to fare better, with a 5-year survival rate of 55% to 83% compared with 12% to 48% for children under 3 years.[6,8,13–17] In this regard a number of factors are likely to be important, such as surgical accessibility and a hitherto general reluctance to irradiate young children.

Location

Supratentorial location is considered relatively favorable, with 5-year survivals ranging from 12% to 68% for

Table 18-5

Magnetic resonance imaging features.

Intracranial MRI features	Spinal MRI features
T1—iso or hyperintense	Cord symmetrically expanded in intramedullary tumors
T2—hyperintense	T1
May enhance with contrast	• Intramedullary tumors—Isointense
	• Extramedullary tumors—hyperintense
	T2
	• Hyperintense
	• Occasional hemosiderin rim in myxopapillary tumors
	Cysts common

infratentorial tumors compared with 22% to 100% for supratentorial tumors.[4-6]

Tumor Grade

Despite a number of studies, the relationship between histologic grading and tumor outcome is unclear, making this the most controversial prognostic factor. Some studies have found that the presence of anaplasia carries a worse prognosis,[22,24] and others have found no difference.[5,8,16,25-28] The lack of uniformity in the grading system used across series makes it difficult to conclude which histological features are prognostic. The Ki-67 (or MIB-1) index, a surrogate immunohistochemical marker for tumor cell proliferation, has been shown to be a useful predictor of outcome in ependymoma.[29,30]

Genetics

The characterization of tumor-specific molecular abnormalities that predict biologically favorable or unfavorable disease is important. Not only may this characterization allow a more judicious use of current therapies such as radiotherapy, but it might also identify molecular targets against which new therapies can be directed.[31]

A number of biologic markers have now been identified and reported to be of prognostic significance, including Ki-67, survivin, the receptor tyrosine kinase I (RTK I) family, and hTERT, the catalytic subunit of telomerase. The proliferation marker Ki-67 has been widely reported as a predictor of outcome in ependymoma, although few studies on Ki-67 have been conducted exclusively in pediatric cases.[29-35] Survivin has been reported to function as a mitotic regulator.[36] Its prognostic significance in ependymoma has been reported with contrasting results,[37,38] confirming the need to further evaluate the prognostic value of survivin in ependymoma.[75] The RTK I family includes epidermal growth factor receptor, ERBB2 (HER2), ERBB3, and ERBB4, which are involved in many cellular processes including cell division, cell survival, and cell motility.[39,40] Coexpression of ERBB2 and ERBB4, high Ki-67 labeling index (LI) and degree of surgical resection are reported to be predictive of poor prognosis in ependymoma.[31] A recent study has reported that hTERT expression was the strongest predictor of outcome in pediatric ependymoma, independent of other clinical and pathologic prognostic markers.[41] However, more recent reports have reevaluated the target of the antibody NCL-hTERT (44F12), providing evidence to support specificity toward nucleolin.[42] Nucleolin is abundant in tumor cells.[43,44] A recent multivariate analysis of all the putative biologic markers listed above concluded that low nucleolin expression was the single most important biologic predictor of outcome in pediatric intracranial ependymoma. Moreover, Ki-67 and survivin correlated with histologic grade but not with outcome, and immunohistochemical analysis of the RTK family was not sufficiently robust to be used as a prognostic marker in clinical trial cohorts.[75]

A number of tumor-specific genetic abnormalities have now been identified in ependymoma; gain of 1q and loss of 6q and 22q are the most common chromosomal imbalances.[45-47] Emerging evidence suggests that genetic factors are important in predicting outcome in childhood ependymoma.[46] There is a clear need to better understand the underlying biology of this disease in order to improve the therapeutic options and outcomes.[5] However, prospective studies are now required to validate these factors, which will in turn require international collaboration.

Treatment

It is widely accepted that once a patient is stabilized, surgical resection should be the initial treatment with the aim of gross total resection. If such has not been accomplished at initial surgery, then a second surgical procedure is warranted with the goal of achieving this. Although surgery alone may cure patients with completely resected supratentorial disease,[48,49] it is widely accepted that adjuvant therapy is required in patients with incompletely resected or infratentorial disease. Concerns over the late effects of cranial irradiation in young children have led a number of national groups to use adjuvant chemotherapy in order to avoid or delay chemotherapy. The recently completed trial from the Children's Oncology Group will hopefully soon answer a number of important questions related to the role of observation after gross total resection for supratentorial ependymoma, the role of chemotherapy to facilitate gross total resection with second surgery, and disease control and functional outcome in a large cohort of children, including the very young, who received immediate postoperative radiation therapy. The trial accrued more than 350 patients between August 2003 and September 2007.

Chemotherapy

Chemotherapy undeniably has a role in the management of ependymoma, although it remains controversial.[5,54,60] There is increasing evidence that a proportion of ependymomas are chemo-responsive,[5,50,54] but debate exists over the degree of response,[50] and a convincing role for chemotherapy has still to be demonstrated.[51,52] This in part reflects the difficulties in interpretation of postchemotherapy imaging, and more sophisticated imaging studies are now needed.[53] Early studies reported a response rate of 48% in infants using a combination of vincristine and cyclophosphamide.[54] However, this finding was based on CT imaging. More recently, a complete response rate of 42%, based on MRI, was reported following preirradiation cisplatin, etoposide, cyclophosphamide, and vincristine.[50]

Furthermore, it is now clear that a proportion of infants can be cured following adjuvant chemotherapy without the use of radiotherapy[4,5,55] (Table 18-6). A recently reported United Kingdom study enrolled 89 children with intracranial ependymoma aged 3 years or younger at diagnosis who had not received prior drug or radiation treatment.[5] Following surgery, the children received alternating cycles of myelosuppressive and nonmyelosuppressive chemotherapy for 1 year. For the nonmetastatic patients, the 5-year cumulative incidence rate of freedom from radiotherapy was 42%. The 3-year and 5-year event-free survival rates for these patients were 47.6% and 41.8%, respectively. The overall survival rates for the nonmetastatic patients at 3 and at 5 years were 79.3% and 63.4%, respectively. Complete resection did not result in a better outcome, and overall and event-free survival rates were similar between groups with different age at diagnosis, site of disease, or histologic grade. The median time to progression for patients who progressed was 1.6 years, with a median age at radiotherapy of 3.6 years. Similar results were reported from the US Children's Cancer Group (CCG-9921): the 5-year overall survival of 59% was achieved with a radiotherapy-free survival of 40%.[55]

The United Kingdom study also provided further evidence that dose intensity may play a role in the treatment of ependymoma, in that the postchemotherapy 5-year overall survival for the patients with the highest relative dose intensity of chemotherapy was significantly better ($p = $. value $< .04$), at 76%, compared with those patients receiving the lowest dose intensity, at 52%. In another study, infants randomized to a dose-intense chemotherapy arm had a significantly better event-free survival than those receiving conventional dose therapy.[56] However, the overall survival was similar in both arms, despite the improved initial response.[56] The role of dose intensity in ependymoma deserves further study.

There is to date no evidence to support a role for high-dose, marrow ablative chemotherapy in childhood ependymoma.[57,58] Chemotherapy may improve outcome by enabling second-look surgery[59]; prospective studies to confirm or refute this finding are awaited.

In summary, there is increasing evidence that in a proportion of cases ependymomas are chemo-responsive and chemo-curable. The systematic laboratory analysis of ependymoma specimens may provide useful information as to which patients would benefit from chemotherapy, which from radiotherapy alone, and perhaps even those that can be observed.

Current recommendations for chemotherapy in ependymoma include (i) infants when the aim is to delay or avoid radiotherapy due to concerns over neurocognitive outcomes, particularly for those under 12 to 18 months, and (ii) patients with residual tumor after initial surgery. Importantly, we still need to define which drugs are active in ependymoma; this might be best achieved through Phase II window studies in patients with residual disease post surgery as proposed in a new European study (SIOP Ependymoma). Another important question to be addressed is whether the addition of chemotherapy to radiotherapy improves the cure rate, as we have seen in medulloblastoma. Defining which patients are likely to benefit from chemotherapy, which from radiation therapy, and which from both is clearly an important, albeit difficult, challenge.[60]

Radiation Therapy

Postoperative radiation therapy to the tumor bed is an important component in the treatment of localized ependymoma, and its role in the treatment of very young children is changing. Newer radiotherapy methods that incorporate 3-dimensional imaging have improved the treatment of ependymoma. Only two decades ago, ependymoma was treated with surgery and postoperative craniospinal irradiation with or without chemotherapy. The long-term event-free survival was less than 40%,[61] and most patients experienced tumor progression at the

Table 18-6

Comparative outcomes of major studies of ependymoma in young children.

Groups	Number of Patients	EFS (%) 3-Year	EFS (%) 5-Year	OS (%) 3-Year	OS (%) 5-Year	Relative Values of Freedom from RT
Pediatric Oncology[16,54] Group[2,21]	48	46*	27	58*	40.5	0
Children's Cancer Geyer et al[55]	15	26	18	Not available	Not available	Not available
SFOP[4]	73	40*	22	68*	52	22
CCG9921[55]	74	50*	32	65	59	20
St Jude[54]	48	69.5	55^^	Not available	Not available	0
UKCCSG[5]	89	42.7 (32.2 to 52.8)***	37.5 (27.3 to 47.7)	79.3 (68.5 to 86.8)***	63.4 (51.2 to 73.4)	42

primary site because a high proportion had residual tumor at the time of irradiation. Because of concern about neuraxis dissemination, especially in patients with high-grade tumors, 36 Gy craniospinal irradiation was administered to many patients, and 54 Gy was prescribed to the primary tumor site using conventional techniques that irradiated large volumes of normal tissue. Survivors treated with craniospinal irradiation experienced debilitating side effects. Craniospinal irradiation was abandoned when investigators learned that neuraxis dissemination at the time of diagnosis was uncommon, and tumor grade was no longer used to determine the treatment volume.[62,63] Further, the curability of patients with metastatic ependymoma using craniospinal irradiation has never been convincingly demonstrated.

The ability of newer treatment methods to limit the highest dose to the tumor bed and spare normal tissues has been objectively demonstrated in a recent prospective trial.[23] Eighty-eight children with ependymoma, including 48 children under the age of 3 years at the time of irradiation, were treated at St Jude Children's Research Hospital with conformal radiation therapy to 54 to 59.4 Gy using a 1-cm clinical target volume margin surrounding the postoperatively defined tumor bed. Preliminary results reveal a 3-year progression-free survival of 75% ± 6%. Patients were serially evaluated using objective measures of cognitive function that included testing of intelligence quotient (IQ), memory, academic achievement and adaptive behavior. No decline in cognitive function was observed among these patients. Historical comparison was made with the CCG-9942 study, which reported a 3-year event-free survival of 59% ± 6%. The differences in disease control may be attributed to the high rate of gross total resection in the St Jude series (84%) and improved targeting through the use of conformal treatment methods. The recently completed trial emanating from the US-based Children's Oncology Group included 3 treatment arms: observation for patients with differentiated supratentorial tumors after microscopically complete resection, conformal irradiation to 59.4 Gy for all other patients after gross total or near total resection, and chemotherapy followed by second surgery and postoperative conformal irradiation for patients after initial subtotal resection. Children as young as 12 months were irradiated.

Hyperfractionated radiation therapy (HFRT) has been proposed as an alternative means to increase disease control or reduce side effects in children with ependymoma. However, there is little objective evidence of benefit to further escalation of irradiation dose using HFRT.[22,64]

A spectrum of complications with various levels of severity has been observed for patients treated with radiation therapy, including cognitive decline, hearing loss, endocrine deficits, and abnormalities in growth and development. Rare but devastating complications such as symptomatic vasculopathy, brain and spinal cord necrosis, and secondary malignancies have been reported. Although functional outcomes after radiation therapy are directly related to the age of the patient at the time of irradiation and morbidity associated with the tumor and surgical intervention, there is a statistically significant relationship between cognitive function after radiation therapy and dosimetry to the supratentorial brain. Indeed, IQ after radiation therapy may be predicted on the basis of 3-dimensional radiation dosimetry.[65]

Craniospinal irradiation is reserved for the treatment of patients with obvious neuraxis dissemination from intracranial or spinal primary tumors. Although the curability of patients with metastatic ependymoma has never been convincingly demonstrated, long-term survivors have been reported. The effectiveness of craniospinal irradiation is likely to be related to the extent and bulk of neuraxis dissemination, ranging from cytologic involvement of CSF to isolated ventricular or spinal metastases to bulky tumor filling the subarachnoid spaces.

Spinal Cord Tumors

Spinal cord ependymomas in children are rare, and when completely resected do not require radiation therapy. In the setting of incomplete or piecemeal resection, radiation therapy is most often indicated. Treatment of spinal cord ependymoma is challenging and requires detailed neuraxis staging and delineation of the extent of disease. The known association of NF2 and ependymoma should prompt surgical evaluation of suspected metastatic disease.[66]

Experimental Therapy

Drug resistance in ependymoma appears to be multifactorial. Expression of the multiple resistance gene MDR-1 has been demonstrated at the protein level by two independent groups explaining resistance to some but not all active chemotherapy agents.[67,68] Overexpression of the DNA protein O6-methylguanine-DNA methyltransferase (MGMT) has also been demonstrated in ependymoma.[69] MGMT can be depleted by temozolomide, which may therefore have a role in the treatment of this disease.[70]

Recurrence and Patterns of Failure

The majority of tumor recurrences occur as a result of failure of local tumor control and are identified between 9 and 24 months after therapy.[71] The prognosis for relapse is relatively poor, and overall only 25% of children survive first or subsequent relapses.[72] Though children may be salvaged a number of times, the law of diminishing returns applies, and there are few long-term survivors of multiple relapses. Ependymomas may recur several years after seeming successful therapy, and long follow-up of the order of 10 to 15 years is essential.

Treatment options following relapse will depend on initial treatment. Surgery should always be considered in patients with local recurrence,[72] as should irradiation for infants in whom radiotherapy was not given as part of the primary treatment. The use of stereotactic radiotherapy in children who have already received radiotherapy should also be considered.[73] The role of chemotherapy in relapse remains uncertain, and international studies are now required.[71,74]

Table 18-7

Ongoing issues in ependymoma.

Improving duration of response and reducing local failure	Surgical issues
Defining prognostic factors	Role of chemotherapy—Which agents/dose intensity
Biologic factors	Role of radiotherapy
Pathologic factors	Neuropsychological outcome of infants
Assessing chemosensitivity—role of new imaging techniques	

In the absence of effective salvage therapy, reirradiation in various forms has been considered for patients who relapse after their initial course of radiation therapy. Single-dose radiosurgery and fractionated external beam reirradiation have both been employed successfully in patients with local recurrence after radiation therapy. The indications for reirradiation and the selection of the best modality are generally based on the feasibility of performing additional surgery at the time of relapse, the presence or absence of residual disease, and the perceived tolerance of the tissues to be encompassed within the reirradiated volume. More challenging is the use of reirradiation in patients who fail with disseminated disease after prior focal irradiation. The options for these patients range from single or multifocal radiosurgery to craniospinal irradiation. In patients with limited metastatic burden and for whom metastatectomy can be performed, craniospinal irradiation with overlap of the primary site is preferred. Shielding of the previously irradiated spinal cord may be indicated. Patients who remain controlled at the primary site appear to have a better outcome than those who have synchronous metastatic and primary recurrence.

Summary

A number of important issues remain to be addressed in childhood ependymoma. We need to arrive at an international consensus on tumor grade, identify biologic correlates of prognosis and outcome, investigate novel imaging methods for assessing chemosensitivity, investigate active chemotherapy or biologic agents, and assess the long-term outcomes and side effects of conformal radiotherapy from multicenter studies (Table 18-7). Clearly, the management of intracranial ependymoma in children and young adults will continue to present significant challenges in the years ahead.

References

1. Wiestler O, Schiffer D, Coons S, et al. Ependymoma. In: P Kleihues, WK Cavanee, eds. Pathology and Genetics of Tumours of the Nervous System. Lyon: IARC; 2000:71–81.
2. Kun LE, Kovnar EH, Sanford RA. Ependymomas in children. Pediatr Neurosci. 1988;14:57–63.
3. Ikezaki K, Matsushima T, Inoue T, et al. Correlation of microanatomical localization with postoperative survival in posterior fossa ependymomas. Neurosurgery. 1993;32:38–44.
4. Grill J, Le Deley MC, Gambarelli D, et al. Postoperative chemotherapy without irradiation for ependymoma in children under 5 years of age: a multicenter trial of the French Society of Pediatric Oncology. J Clin Oncol. 2001;19: 1288–1296.
5. Grundy R, Wilne S, Weston CL, et al. Primary postoperative chemotherapy without radiotherapy for intracranial ependymoma in children: the UKCCSG/SIOP prospective study. Lancet Oncol. 2007;8:696–705.
6. Pollack IF, Gerszten PC, Martinez AJ, et al. Intracranial ependymomas of childhood: long-term outcome and prognostic factors. Neurosurgery. 1995;37: 655–666; discussion 666–667.
7. DeSousa AL, Kalsbeck JE, Mealey J, Jr, et al. Intraspinal tumors in children. A review of 81 cases. J Neurosurg. 1979;51:437–445.
8. McLendon RE, Wiestler OD, Kros JM, et al. Ependymoma. In: Louis DN, Ohgaki H, Wiestler OD, Cavanee WK, eds. Pathology and Genetics of Tumours of the Nervous System. 3rd ed. Lyon: IARC; 2007:72–80.
9. Robertson PL, Zeltzer PM, Boyett JM, et al. Survival and prognostic factors following radiation therapy and chemotherapy for ependymomas in children: a report of the Children's Cancer Group. J Neurosurg. 1998;88:695–703.
10. Schiffer D, Chio A, Giordana MT, et al. Histologic prognostic factors in ependymoma. Child's Nerv Syst. 1991;7:177–182.
11. Comi AM, Backstrom JW, Burger PC, et al. Clinical and neuroradiologic findings in infants with intracranial ependymomas. Pediatric Oncology Group. Pediatr Neurol. 1998;18:23–29.
12. Good CD, Wade AM, Hayward RD, et al. Surveillance neuroimaging in childhood intracranial ependymoma: how effective, how often, and for how long? J Neurosurg. 2001;94:27–32.
13. Nazar GB, Hoffman HJ, Becker LE, et al. Infratentorial ependymomas in childhood: prognostic factors and treatment. J Neurosurg. 1990;72:408–417.
14. Rousseau P, Habrand JL, Sarrazin D, et al. Treatment of intracranial ependymomas of children: review of a 15-year experience. Int J Radiat Oncol Biol Phys. 1994;28:381–386.
15. Sutton LN, Goldwein J, Perilongo G, et al. Prognostic factors in childhood ependymomas. Pediatr Neurosurg. 1990;16:57–65.
16. Duffner PK, Krischer JP, Sanford RA, et al. Prognostic factors in infants and very young children with intracranial ependymomas. Pediatr Neurosurg. 1998;28:215–222.
17. Foreman NK, Love S, Thorne R. Intracranial ependymomas: analysis of prognostic factors in a population-based series. Pediatr Neurosurg. 1996:24:119–125.
18. Salazar OM, Castro-Vita H, VanHoutte P, et al. Improved survival in cases of intracranial ependymoma after radiation therapy: late report and recommendations. J Neurosurg. 1983;59:652–659.
19. Shaw EG, Evans RG, Scheithauer BW, et al. Postoperative radiotherapy of intracranial ependymoma in pediatric and adult patients. Int J Radiat Oncol Biol Phys. 1987;13:1457–1462.
20. Goldwein JW, Leahy JM, Packer RJ, et al. Intracranial ependymomas in children. Int J Radiat Oncol Biol Phys. 1990;19:1497–1502.
21. Healey EA, Barnes PD, Kupsky WJ, et al. The prognostic significance of postoperative residual tumor in ependymoma. Neurosurgery. 1991;28:666–671; discussion 671–672.
22. Massimino M, Gandola L, Giangaspero F, et al. Hyperfractionated radiotherapy and chemotherapy for childhood ependymoma: final results of the first prospective AIEOP (Associazione Italiana di Ematologia-Oncologia Pediatrica) study. Int J Radiat Oncol Biol Phys. 2004;58:1336–1345.
23. Merchant TE, Mulhern RK, Krasin MJ, et al. Preliminary results from a phase II trial of conformal radiation therapy and evaluation of radiation-related CNS effects for pediatric patients with localized ependymoma. J Clin Oncol. 2004;22: 3156–3162.
24. Merchant TE, Jenkins JJ, Burger PC, et al. Influence of tumor grade on time to progression after irradiation for localized ependymoma in children. Int J Radiat Oncol Biol Phys. 2002;53:52–57.
25. Horn B, Heideman R, Geyer R, et al. A multi-institutional retrospective study of intracranial ependymoma in children: identification of risk factors. J Pediatr Hematol Oncol. 1999;21:203–211.
26. Schiffer D, Chio A, Cravioto H, et al. Ependymoma: internal correlations among pathological signs: the anaplastic variant. Neurosurgery. 1991;29:206–210.
27. Heidermann RL, Packer RJ, Albright LA, et al. Tumours of the central nervous system. In: Pizzo PA, Poplack DG, eds. Principles and Practice of Paediatric Oncology. 3rd ed. Philadelphia: Lippincott; 1997:633–698.
28. Ross GW, Rubinstein LJ. Lack of histopathological correlation of malignant ependymomas with postoperative survival. J Neurosurg. 1989;70:31–36.

29. Wolfsberger S, Fischer I, Hoftberger R, et al. Ki-67 immunolabeling index is an accurate predictor of outcome in patients with intracranial ependymoma. *Am J Surg Pathol.* 2004;28:914–920.

30. Bennetto L, Foreman N, Harding B, et al. Ki-67 immunolabelling index is a prognostic indicator in childhood posterior fossa ependymomas. *Neuropathol Appl Neurobiol.* 1998;24:434–440.

31. Gilbertson RJ, Bentley L, Hernan R, et al. ERBB receptor signaling promotes ependymoma cell proliferation and represents a potential novel therapeutic target for this disease. *Clin Cancer Res.* 2002;8:3054–3064.

32. Figarella-Branger D, Civatte M, Bouvier-Labit C, et al. Prognostic factors in intracranial ependymomas in children. *J Neurosurg.* 2000;93:605–613.

33. Prayson RA. Clinicopathologic study of 61 patients with ependymoma including MIB-1 immunohistochemistry. *Ann Diagn Pathol.* 1999;3:11–18.

34. Ritter AM, Hess KR, McLendon RE, et al. Ependymomas: MIB-1 proliferation index and survival. *J Neuro-Oncol.* 1998;40:51–57.

35. Verstegen MJ, Leenstra DT, Ijlst-Keizers H, et al. Proliferation- and apoptosis-related proteins in intracranial ependymomas: an immunohistochemical analysis. *J Neuro-Oncol.* 2002;56:21–28.

36. Lens SM, Vader G, Medema RH. The case for Survivin as mitotic regulator. *Curr Opin Cell Biol.* 2006;18:616–622.

37. Altura RA, Olshefski RS, Jiang Y, et al. Nuclear expression of Survivin in paediatric ependymomas and choroid plexus tumours correlates with morphologic tumour grade. *Br J Cancer.* 2003;89:1743–1749.

38. Preusser M, Gelpi E, Matej R, et al. No prognostic impact of survivin expression in glioblastoma. *Acta Neuropathol.* 2005;109:534–538.

39. Herbst RS. Review of epidermal growth factor receptor biology. *Int J Radiat Oncol Biol Phys.* 2004;59:21–26.

40. Yarden Y, Sliwkowski MX. Untangling the ErbB signalling network. *Nat Rev Mol Cell Biol.* 2001;2:127–137.

41. Tabori U, Ma J, Carter M, et al. Human telomere reverse transcriptase expression predicts progression and survival in pediatric intracranial ependymoma. *J Clin Oncol.* 2006;24:1522–1528.

42. Wu YL, Dudognon C, Nguyen E, et al. Immunodetection of human telomerase reverse-transcriptase (hTERT) re-appraised: nucleolin and telomerase cross paths. *J Cell Sci.* 2006;119:2797–2806.

43. Grinstein E, Shan Y, Karawajew L, et al. Cell cycle-controlled interaction of nucleolin with the retinoblastoma protein and cancerous cell transformation. *J Biol Chem.* 2006;281:22223–22235.

44. Srivastava M, Pollard HB. Molecular dissection of nucleolin's role in growth and cell proliferation: new insights. *Faseb J.* 1999;13:1911–1922.

45. Carter M, Nicholson J, Ross F, et al. Genetic abnormalities detected in ependymomas by comparative genomic hybridisation. *Br J Cancer.* 2002;86:929–939.

46. Dyer S, Prebble E, Davison V, et al. Genomic imbalances in pediatric intracranial ependymomas define clinically relevant groups. *Am J Pathol.* 2002;161:2133–2141.

47. Hirose Y, Aldape K, Bollen A, et al. Chromosomal abnormalities subdivide ependymal tumors into clinically relevant groups. *Am J Pathol.* 2001;158:1137–1143.

48. Awaad YM, Allen JC, Miller DC, et al. Deferring adjuvant therapy for totally resected intracranial ependymoma. *Pediatr Neurol.* 1996;14:216–219.

49. Hukin J, Epstein F, Lefton D, et al. Treatment of intracranial ependymoma by surgery alone. *Pediatr Neurosurg.* 1998;29:40–45.

50. Garvin J, Sposto R, Stanley P, et al. Childhood ependymoma: improved survival for patients with incompletely resected tumors with the use of pre-irradiation chemotherapy. *Neuro Oncol.* 2004;6:456.

51. Bouffet E, Foreman N. Chemotherapy for intracranial ependymomas. *Child's Nerv Syst.* 1999;15:563–570.

52. Grill J, Pascal C, Chantal K. Childhood ependymoma: a systematic review of treatment options and strategies. *Paediatr Drugs.* 2003;5:533–543.

53. Peet A, Leach M, Pinkerton C, et al. The development of functional imaging in the diagnosis, management and understanding of childhood brain tumours. *Pediatr Blood Cancer.* 2006;44:103–113.

54. Duffner PK, Horowitz ME, Krischer JP, et al. Postoperative chemotherapy and delayed radiation in children less than three years of age with malignant brain tumors. *N Engl J Med.* 1993;328:1725–1731.

55. Geyer JR, Zeltzer PM, Boyett JM, et al. Survival of infants with primitive neuroectodermal tumors or malignant ependymomas of the CNS treated with eight drugs in 1 day: a report from the Children's Cancer Group. *J Clin Oncol.* 2008;12:1607–1615.

56. Strother D, Kepner J, Aronin P; International Society of Pediatric Oncology. Effects of the degree of surgical resection and intensity of chemotherapy on event free survival of children with ependymoma and medulloblastoma. *Med Pediatr Oncol.* 2000;35 (3).

57. Mason WP, Goldman S, Yates AJ, et al. Survival following intensive chemotherapy with bone marrow reconstitution for children with recurrent intracranial ependymoma: a report of the Children's Cancer Group. *J Neuro-Oncol.* 1998;37:135–143.

58. Grill J, Kalifa C, Doz F, et al. A high-dose busulfan-thiotepa combination followed by autologous bone marrow transplantation in childhood recurrent ependymoma. A Phase II study. *Pediatr Neurosurg.* 1996;25:7–12.

59. Foreman NK, Love S, Gill S, et al. Second-look surgery for incompletely resected fourth ventricle ependymomas: technical case report. *Neurosurgery.* 1997;40:856–860.

60. Grundy R. Intracranial ependymoma in children: reflection and reaction. *Lancet Oncol.* 2007;8:760–761.

61. Evans AE, Anderson JR, Lefkowitz-Boudreaux IB, Finlay JL. Adjuvant chemotherapy of childhood posterior fossa ependymoma: cranio-spinal irradiation with or without adjuvant CCNU, vincristine, and prednisone: a Children's Cancer Group study. *Med Pediatr Oncol.* 1996;27(1):8–14.

62. Vanuytsel L, Brada M. The role of prophylactic spinal irradiation in localized intracranial ependymoma. *Int J Radiat Oncol Biol Phys.* 1991;21:825–830.

63. Wallner KE, Wara WM, Sheline GE, Davis RL. Intracranial ependymomas: Results of treatment with partial or whole-brain irradiation without spinal irradiation. *Int J Radiat Oncol Biol Phys.* 1986;12:1937–1941.

64. Kovnar E, Curran W, Tomita T, et al. Hyperfractionated irradiation for childhood ependymoma: improved local control in subtotally resected tumors. *Child's Nerv Sys.* 1998;14:489.

65. Merchant TE, Kiehna EN, Li C, Xiong X, Mulhern RK. Radiation dosimetry predicts IQ after conformal radiation therapy in pediatric patients with localized ependymoma. *Int J Radiat Oncol Biol Phys.* 2005;63(5):1546–1554.

66. Wagner LM, Zhou H, Brockmeyer DL, Hedlund GL. Spinal cord schwannomas mimicking drop metastases in a patient with intramedullary ependymoma and neurofibromatosis 2. *J Pediatr Hematol Oncol.* 2004;26(1):56–59.

67. Geddes JF, Vowles GH, Ashmore SM, et al. Detection of multidrug resistance gene product (P-glycoprotein) expression in ependymomas. *Neuropathol Appl Neurobiol.* 1994;20:118–121.

68. Chou PM, Barquin N, Gonzalez-Crussi F, et al. Ependymomas in children express the multidrug resistance gene: immunohistochemical and molecular biologic study. *Pediatr Pathol Lab Med.* 1996;16:551–561.

69. Hongeng S, Brent TP, Sanford RA, et al. O6–Methylguanine-DNA methyltransferase protein levels in pediatric brain tumors. *Clin Cancer Res.* 1997;3:2459–2463.

70. Constanza A, Ducati A, Nobile M, et al. Does ependymoma respond to chemotherapy with temozolamide? *Neuro Oncol.* 2002;4:S21.

71. Goldwein JW, Glauser TA, Packer RJ, et al. Recurrent intracranial ependymomas in children: survival, patterns of failure, and prognostic factors. *Cancer.* 1990;66:557–563.

72. Messahel B, Robinson K, Weston C, et al. Relapsed ependymoma in children: a UKCCSG study, International Society of Paediatric Oncology. Oporto, 2002. *Med Pediatr Oncol.* 2002;39:342.

73. Stafford S, Pollock B, Foote R, et al. Stereotactic radiosurgery for recurrent ependymoma. *Cancer.* 2000;88:870–875.

74. Sexauer CL, Khan A, Burger PC, et al. Cisplatin in recurrent pediatric brain tumors: a POG Phase II study. A Pediatric Oncology Group Study. *Cancer.* 1985;56:1497–1501.

75. Ridley L, Rahman R, Bruhdler, MA, et al. Multifactorial analysis of predictors of outcome in pediatric intracranial ependymoma. *Neuro Oncol.* 2008.

Medulloblastoma and Other Central Nervous System Primitive Neuroectodermal Tumors

Barry L. Pizer, Steven C. Clifford, and Jeff M. Michalski

CHAPTER 19

Introduction

Primitive neuroectodermal tumors (PNETs) are highly cellular malignant embryonal tumors of unknown etiology, accounting for approximately 20% of central nervous system (CNS) cancers. This tumor type was first described in 1925 by Bailey and Cushing, who coined the term "medulloblastoma" as a tumor of primitive origin composed of small round blue cells that predominantly arose in the posterior fossa of young children. The concept of PNETs was originally proposed by Hart and Earle in 1973[1] in recognition of the similar histologic characteristics of cerebellar PNETs (medulloblastoma) and tumors occurring in the supratentorial region of the brain (supratentorial PNETs [ST-PNETs]) such as those arising from the cerebral hemispheres and pineal gland. Although the concept of PNETs has been generally accepted and is now included in the World Health Organization (WHO) classification of CNS tumors,[2] there remains doubt as to whether PNETs arise from a common cell of origin, with increasing evidence of differences between the molecular characterization of medulloblastoma and ST-PNETs, for example, on the basis of DNA microarray gene expres-

sion.[3] These tumors do, however, share common clinical features such as sensitivity to both radiotherapy and chemotherapy, and a propensity to leptomeningeal dissemination via the cerebrospinal fluid (CSF) pathways, such that whole CNS radiotherapy is a standard aspect of management. This chapter considers the features and treatment of PNETs and discusses specific management of these tumors in "older" children, aged at least 3 years. The treatment of PNETs in very young children is discussed elsewhere in this book.

Medulloblastoma

Medulloblastoma is the most common malignant brain tumor in childhood, accounting for between 15% and 20% of all childhood primary CNS cancers and around 80% of PNETs. The large majority occur within the first decade of life with a peak incidence at 5 years. There is a 2 to 1 male to female ratio. A report from the National Cancer Institute's Surveillance, Epidemiology, and End Results program found that in the United States the incidence of PNETs in persons under 20 years rose 23% from 4 per million person years in the period 1973 to 1977 to 4.9 per

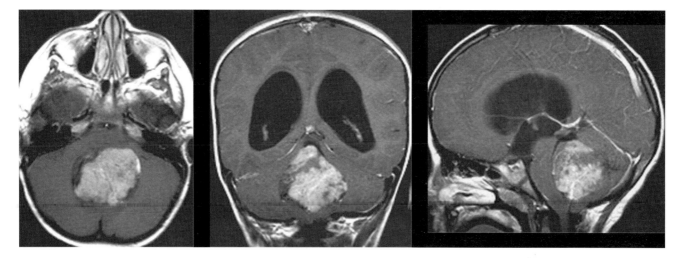

Figure 19-1 Axial, coronal, and sagittal gadolinium-enhanced T1-weighted MRI images of a child with medulloblastoma at diagnosis. Note the marked internal hydrocephalus due to the obstruction of the aqueduct of Sylvius.

million in the period 1993 to 1998.[4] Rates were 42% higher among Caucasians compared with African Americans.

By definition, medulloblastoma arises in the posterior fossa, usually from the cerebellar vermis in the roof of the fourth ventricle, thus presenting as midline tumors (Figure 19-1). As with other PNETs, medulloblastomas have a marked propensity to seed throughout the CSF pathways, with evidence of such metastatic spread occurring in up to 35% of cases at diagnosis[5] (Figure 19-2).

Pathology and Molecular Markers

Histologically, the majority of medulloblastomas (about 80%) are described as having a classical phenotype composed of sheets of generally small round cells with little cytoplasm and frequent mitoses[6] (Figure 19-3). Various degrees of glial or neuronal differentiation may be seen. Cells may be clustered in classic Homer-Wright rosettes. A less common desmoplastic variant typically arises in the cerebellar hemisphere in older children and adolescents (about 5% of tumors in children over 3 years at diagnosis) and may possibly be associated with a better prognosis.[7] This is in contrast to very young children, in whom desmoplasia occurs in up to 50% of medulloblastomas and appears clearly associated with an improved outcome.[8] Varying degrees of anaplasia, which is characterized by cytologic pleomorphism and a high mitotic count, may be seen in medulloblastomas. Widespread and severe anaplasia is observed in about 15% of cases and is associ-

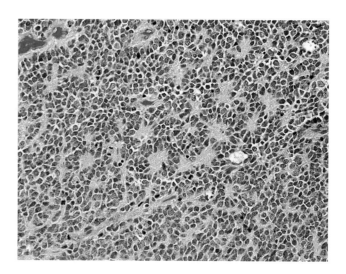

Figure 19-3 Photomicrograph (200x) of classic medulloblastoma with sheets of small primitive tumor cells and numerous Homer Wright (neuroblastic) rosettes, with tumor cells surrounding central collections of neuropil (neuronal processes). **See Plate 45 for color image.**

ated with a poorer prognosis.[6,9,10] The rarer large-cell medulloblastoma accounts for about 5% of cases and appears to be clearly associated with a worse outlook[6] (Figure 19-4).

Based on these reported histologic phenotypes, and the observed differences in their clinical behaviors, the current WHO classification of CNS tumors defines the following histopathological variants of medulloblastoma: (1) classic medulloblastoma, (2) desmoplastic/nodular medulloblastoma, (3) medulloblastoma with extensive nodularity, (4) anaplastic medulloblastoma (if anaplasia is severe and diffuse), and (5) large-cell medulloblastoma.[2]

Recent years have seen significant advances in our understanding of the molecular basis of medulloblastoma development. Although no characteristic cytogenetic or molecular abnormalities have been identified that define medulloblastoma, a series of nonrandom genetic and molecular abnormalities have been revealed, which offer potential for improved disease stratification and/or the identification of novel therapeutic targets. The most prevalent structural abnormality in this disease is isochromosome 17q (loss of the p-arm of chromosome 17 in conjunction with a gain of the associated q-arm; 30% to 50% of cases). *MYC* and *MYCN* represent the most commonly amplified genetic loci, each affecting about 5% of cases, and have been associated with large-cell and anaplastic medulloblastomas. Additional imbalances include losses of chromosomes 8, 9, 10q, 11, 16q, and 17p (each affecting about 30% of cases) and gains of chromosomes 7 and 17q (both in 40% of cases).[11] However, the specific genes targeted by these chromosomal defects remain to be identified in the majority of cases.

Activation of the Wnt/Wingless (Wnt/Wg) and Sonic hedgehog (SHH) developmental cell signaling pathways play significant roles in medulloblastoma. Both pathways are essential in normal neural and cerebellar development[12,13] and become aberrantly activated in subsets of medulloblastomas, by genetic mutation of pathway com-

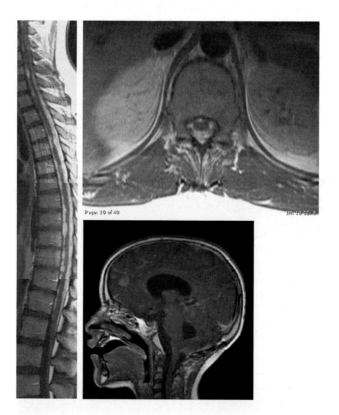

Figure 19-2 Gadolinium-enhanced T1 sagittal and axial images of an MRI demonstrate gross nodular seeding of the neuroaxis from medulloblastoma.

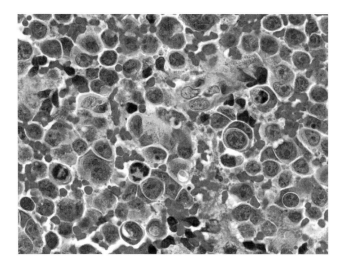

Figure 19-4 Photomicrograph (400x) of large-cell medulloblastoma. The tumor cells are enlarged and the nuclei feature vesicular chromatin and prominent nucleoli. There is also a brisk mitotic index and cell wrapping (tumor cells enveloping one another). **See Plate 46 for color image.**

ponents (Wnt/Wg: mutations in *CTNNB1*, *APC*, or *AXIN1*; SHH: mutations in *PTCH*, *SMO*, or *SUFU*).[11] The recent identification of characteristic gene expression signatures indicates that activation of the Wnt/Wg and SHH pathways defines mutually exclusive subgroups of tumors and occurs in about 15% and 25% of cases, respectively.[14] Sonic hedgehog activation and associated indices (*PTCH* mutation, 9q loss) have been associated with the desmoplastic histopathologic subtype[11] but have also been observed in classic and large-cell/anaplastic tumors.[14] Further studies are now required to clarify this issue. Specific small-molecule inhibitors of the SHH pathway are currently under preclinical development for medulloblastoma therapy.[15]

Wnt/Wg pathway activation defines a unique molecular subgroup of medulloblastoma, which displays distinctive gene expression signatures, patterns of genomic abnormalities, and clinical outcome. Wnt/Wg-active medulloblastomas are exclusively associated with the loss of an entire copy of chromosome 6 in the majority of cases, while pathway activation is independent of chromosome 17 aberrations, the most common chromosomal alterations detected in medulloblastoma.[14,16] Moreover, the Wnt/Wg-active medulloblastoma subgroup displays an idiosyncratic clinical behavior, and β-catenin status has been shown to be an independent marker of favorable clinical outcome (greater than 90% overall survival) across independent clinical trials–based biologic studies.[17,18]

The assessment of Wnt/Wg pathway status highlights the potential utility of molecular markers for the improved therapeutic stratification of medulloblastoma patients. Retrospective analysis of the prognostic significance of molecular defects in medulloblastoma has frequently been limited by the use of small, nonuniformly treated cohorts. Nonetheless, a range of molecular markers with prognostic potential has now been identified in trial-based studies. Factors that have been associated with

a poor prognosis include amplification of the *MYC* oncogene family (*MYC* or *MYCN*),[19] defects of chromosome 17,[19] and expression of the erbB-2 receptor tyrosine kinase.[20] Other defects, such as expression of the *c-myc* oncogene or the *TRKC* neurotrophin receptor, have shown prognostic significance in some studies but have not had demonstrable value in others.[20,21] Initial studies indicate that activation of the SHH pathway or associated defects (ie, 9q loss) do not appear to have prognostic significance.[18,19]

The prospective evaluation of the prognostic importance of these and other markers is a major feature of current medulloblastoma/PNET studies. Alongside the validation of existing markers, the identification of further markers through an enhanced understanding of medulloblastoma pathogenesis remains paramount. In particular, the combined assessment of relationships among molecular, histopathologic, and clinical stratification markers in large clinical trials cohorts will be critical to the development of effective indices for the improved staging of medulloblastoma patients.

Clinical Presentation

The majority of patients with medulloblastoma present with signs and symptoms of raised intracranial pressure due to hydrocephalus following obstruction of the CSF pathways at the level of the fourth ventricle and the aqueduct of Sylvius. Thus headaches, vomiting, lethargy, and drowsiness together with papilledema occur in around 80% of patients at diagnosis. Although many patients present acutely, the diagnosis can often be delayed for several months. Other presenting features include ataxia due to cerebellar involvement and diplopia, cranial nerve palsies, and long tract signs as a result of pressure on or infiltration of the brain stem. Occasionally, patients may present with manifestations of spinal metastases such as back pain or lower limb weakness.

Staging and metastatic evaluation of patients with medulloblastoma or ST-PNET should include both a nonenhanced and contrast-enhanced magnetic resonance imaging (MRI) of the brain and spine, preferably undertaken preoperatively.

The Chang staging classification has been used in most clinical trials testing treatment for medulloblastoma.[22] Evaluation of the primary tumor (Chang T stage) considers the local tumor invasiveness and size; this Chang T-stage system is less commonly utilized in the modern imaging era. M-(metastatic) staging considers tumor spread outside of the primary tumor site.

Prognostic Features

The prognosis for children with medulloblastoma is most closely related to the age of the patient and to the extent of disease at diagnosis. Because of the worse prognosis in very young children and the unacceptable sequelae associated with craniospinal radiotherapy (CSRT), recent therapy in children aged less than 3 to 6 years has focused on the use of so-called Baby Brain protocols as discussed elsewhere in this book. These treatment regimens utilize intensive and/or prolonged administration of chemotherapy in order to delay or avoid the use of radiotherapy and in particular to avoid the use of whole neuraxis radiotherapy.

Numerous studies have failed to demonstrate prognostic significance to the Chang T-staging system.[23–25] In contrast, the presence of metastatic disease at presentation, as diagnosed by the presence of meningeal enhancement on MRI of the brain (Chang stage M2) or spine (Chang stage M3), clearly confers a poor prognosis.[5,26]

A careful metastatic evaluation is critical to the success of the current radiation therapy dose reduction strategy in medulloblastoma. A review of patients registered to the recent North American Children's Oncology Group (COG) A9961 trial has demonstrated an unacceptable failure rate in patients with overlooked M2 or M3 disease upon central radiology review.[27]

The prognostic significance of Chang stage M1 disease, in which tumor cells are found within the CSF without radiologic evidence of metastasis, is less clearly defined, although it is now accepted by both the COG (previously the Children's Cancer Group [CCG] and Pediatric Oncology Group [POG]) and the European SIOP (International Society of Paediatric Oncology) Group that patients with M1 disease have a poorer prognosis than those without evidence of such tumor spread, as shown in studies such as CCG-921.[26] Cerebrospinal fluid taken by lumbar puncture following recovery from surgery has been shown to be more reliable than ventricular CSF for staging purposes.[28]

With regard to local disease, both the COG and SIOP groups accept the prognostic importance of achieving a gross total or near gross total surgical excision, as shown in the CCG-921 study,[23] although this importance was not shown in other studies such as the German HIT-91 study.[29] Residual disease is best demonstrated by comparing the patient's preoperative MRI imaging with that obtained postoperatively. Postoperative imaging is best performed within 72 hours of surgery, after which postoperative changes render interpretation of residual disease difficult.

Thus at the present time, both the North American and European groups define "standard risk" (SIOP) or "average risk" (COG) patients as those over the age of 3 years without evidence of metastatic spread (on MRI and CSF cytology) (M0) *and* having less than or equal to 1.5 cm² (maximum cross-sectional area) of residual disease after surgery. High-risk patients are considered those with less complete resection or patients with evidence of CSF spread (M1 to M3).

Treatment

The standard therapeutic approach for medulloblastoma consists of complete or near complete surgical resection followed by postoperative CSRT. Since Bailey and Cushing first described medulloblastoma, radiation therapy has been a critical component in its management. In their original series, the only survivors were patients who received radiation therapy. The propensity of this tumor to spread by the CSF pathways led to the early adoption of CSRT. In a review by Landberg, the 10-year survival of patients receiving whole CNS radiation therapy was 53%, compared with only 25% and 5% in patients receiving treatment to the posterior fossa and spine or posterior fossa only, respectively.[30] Efforts by the French Society of Pediatric Oncology (SFOP) to eliminate the cranial component of CNS radiation therapy by administering moderate-dose systemic chemotherapy resulted in an unacceptable rate of supratentorial failures and a progression-free survival of only 19%.[31] Craniospinal radiotherapy therefore remains the standard treatment for children with medulloblastoma, except in infants (see Chapter 20).

Until recently, the conventional doses of radiotherapy for all patients were 35 to 36 Gy to the craniospinal axis together with a boost of 18 to 20 Gy to the posterior fossa (total dose 54 to 56 Gy). Using such doses in the absence of chemotherapy, various studies have reported that for nonmetastatic tumors, between 50% and 70% of children are alive and free of progressive disease 5 years from diagnosis, but with lower survival for metastatic cases (see below).[32]

Surgery

Surgery remains a fundamental component of the treatment for medulloblastoma, particularly given the likely prognostic importance of the degree of surgical excision. Modern surgical techniques have allowed complete or near complete tumor resection in a large majority of cases and a reduction in surgical mortality to well under 5%. A particular postoperative problem is the so-called posterior fossa syndrome (also known as the "akinetic mutism" syndrome) occurring in up to 20% of patients and characterized by mutism, limb weakness, cranial nerve palsies, and cerebellar dysfunction. Recovery occurs in most patients, although it may be delayed for many months and, if severe, appears associated with long-term cognitive sequelae.

Radiotherapy

Radiotherapy Techniques

Delivering a homogeneous dose of radiation therapy to the craniospinal axis is one of the more challenging technical aspects of radiation oncology. This challenge is complicated by the need to immobilize children for treatment that can last more than 30 minutes. The classic approach of treatment of the craniospinal axis involves 2 opposed lateral fields treating the brain with a matched posterior field treating the spine. For further details regarding the technical aspects of CSRT, see the relevant chapters on radiation therapy techniques.

There is growing interest in the use of 3-dimensional (3D) conformal radiation therapy for the posterior fossa to reduce the radiation dose to the supratentorial brain and cochlea[33] (Figure 19-5). In addition, there is increasing enthusiasm for using intensity-modulated radiation therapy (IMRT) for treating the posterior fossa. Intensity-modulated radiation therapy has been shown to be associated with better sparing of the critical structures such as the cochlea and supratentorial brain including the hypothalamus and pituitary axis.[34] This benefit may come at the price of a larger volume of brain or other extracranial structures being irradiated at lower doses, the consequences of which remain uncertain. To avoid these risks, a few select centers are approaching the treatment of children with medulloblastoma with proton beam radiation therapy.[35] The unique controllable physical nature of proton beams allows extremely conformal dose distributions without the large volume "integral radiation dose" that accompanies IMRT and to a lesser degree 3D conformal radiation therapy.

In considering the late effects of medulloblastoma radiation therapy, there is currently much interest in the appropriate boost volumes for the primary tumor. Historically, the whole posterior fossa has been irradiated, but it is unclear whether this approach is necessary. Two single-institution pilot series have demonstrated local control rates using a volume limited to the tumor bed comparable to those achieved with whole posterior fossa radiation therapy.[36,37] The SFOP completed a prospective trial of craniospinal radiation therapy followed by a reduced tumor bed boost. Of 48 children evaluable, the 3-year overall and disease-free survival rates were 89% and 81%, respectively. There were no failures in the posterior fossa outside of the reduced target volume boost.[38] The COG is currently testing whether a reduction in treatment volume of the boost can be successfully accomplished without an increased rate in posterior fossa failures.

Finally, in Europe there has been much recent interest in the use of hyperfractionated radiotherapy, using twice-daily fractions that can theoretically increase the dose to tumor without an increase in the late effects to normal nervous tissue. This technique was compared with conventional radiotherapy in the recently completed HIT SIOP PNET-4 randomized controlled trial. The SFOP has evaluated this schedule in standard-risk patients with excellent tumor control results, but the impact on late effects requires more follow-up.[38]

Quality Control of Radiation Therapy

Numerous publications have demonstrated that close attention to the quality of radiation therapy is critical to the successful management of this disease. Incomplete treatment of the brain and spinal axis is associated with an unacceptable rate of treatment failure following radiation therapy. Retrospective series have demonstrated an increased rate of subfrontal and intracranial failures in patients who have shielding of the cribriform plate or middle cranial fossa.[39] In cooperative group trials, the frequency of protocol deviations and their adverse impact on outcome have led to the mandatory central review of radiation therapy and diagnostic imaging in current COG and SIOP studies for medulloblastoma.[40] Computed tomography–based simulation can be both efficient and more accurate in defining the treatment volume.[41] Magnetic resonance images further enhance the ability to target the posterior fossa, tumor bed, and thecal sac.

Delays in completing radiation therapy have also been associated with an increased rate of treatment failure, as demonstrated in the recent SIOP PNET-3 trial, in which the time to complete radiotherapy was found to be an independent prognostic factor.[42]

Chemotherapy

There is now widespread acceptance of the benefit of chemotherapy in the management of medulloblastoma, which is clearly a chemosensitive tumor, as demonstrated in several Phase II studies.

Similar so-called first-generation randomized studies were conducted by the CCG and SIOP in which radiotherapy alone was compared with RT followed by chemotherapy with vincristine, CCNU and prednisone (CCG-942), or CCNU and vincristine (SIOP-1). Both studies showed no statistical differences in survival between the 2 treatment groups as a whole but a clear benefit was seen for a subgroup of patients with high-stage disease. Subsequent studies have explored the timing of chemotherapy in relation to radiotherapy and also the use of new drug combinations in both "high-" and "standard-" risk patients. A variety of different drugs and drug combinations have been investigated in recent Phase III studies, including the platinating drugs (cisplatin and carboplatin), etoposide, and alkylating agents such as cyclophosphamide. With regard to the timing of chemotherapy, studies such as CCG-921 and HIT-91 have suggested a possible detrimental effect of preirradiation chemotherapy when compared with chemotherapy given after radiotherapy; although in each study different pre- and post-irradiation chemotherapy regimens were used. In contrast, the SIOP PNET-3 study showed a significant improvement in 3-year event-free survival (EFS) (79% vs 64%) for patients with standard-risk medulloblastoma

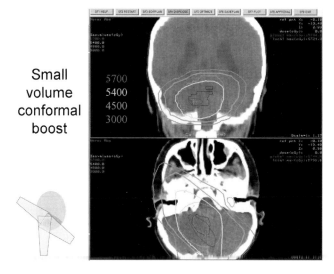

Small volume conformal boost

Figure 19-5 Conformal radiation distribution for a patient with medulloblastoma treated with multiple shaped fields to a limited target volume (cyan contour) defined by the tumor bed with a 1.5-cm margin. Note that the prescribed radiation dose volume spares the cerebrum and the contralateral cochlea. **See Plate 47 for color image.**

treated with moderately intensive preirradiation chemotherapy when compared with those treated with radiotherapy (35 Gy CSRT) alone.[43]

Standard-/Average-Risk Medulloblastoma

Following the "first generation" studies, and recognizing the importance of tumor staging in determining outcome, tumor groups such as CCG, POG, and SIOP have conducted a series of national and international studies in average-/standard-risk medulloblastoma. The two principal aims of these trials were to examine the benefit of chemotherapy given either before or after radiotherapy with the intention of improving survival, and also to explore the potential of reducing the dose of CSRT with the aim of reducing the often devastating neuropsychological and functional sequelae observed in medulloblastoma survivors treated with the previously "standard" doses of whole-brain radiotherapy (35 to 36 Gy).

In the North American POG-8631/CCG-923 study, standard-risk medulloblastoma children were randomized to a CSRT dose of either 36 Gy or 23.4 Gy without chemotherapy in either arm. This study was opened in 1986 and accrued 98 eligible patients prior to its premature closure in 1990 when an excess of relapses was observed in the reduced-dose arm. Long-term follow-up confirmed the original conclusions with a 67% EFS at 5 years for patients treated with standard-dose neuraxis irradiation and 52% for those treated with reduced-dose (p value $= .14$).[44] Investigators in North America continued to explore the use of reduced-dose CSRT, but with the administration of chemotherapy following irradiation. In this respect, the most widely investigated chemotherapeutic combination is cisplatin, CCNU (lomustine), and vincristine introduced in the early 1980s by Packer at the Children's Hospital of Philadelphia. The "Packer" regimen is used in an adjuvant setting following radiotherapy with up to 8 cycles of chemotherapy given every 6 weeks. Excellent initial results using this regimen prompted the initiation of a CCG groupwide study of this chemotherapy following reduced-dose CSRT (23.4 Gy) for standard-risk medulloblastoma. This study, CCG-9892, confirmed the efficacy of this regimen, with a 5-year progression-free survival of 79%.[45] This regimen was carried forward to the recently completed randomized COG study, A9961, which involved the use of reduced-dose craniospinal RT with vincristine, followed by one of two adjuvant chemotherapy arms (CCNU, cisplatin, and vincristine versus cyclophosphamide, cisplatin, and vincristine). For the total cohort of 379 patients, 5-year EFS was 81%, with no significant difference in survival between the two treatment arms.[27] In this respect, the well-recognized long-term side effects of CCNU might be ameliorated by the increased use of cyclophosphamide and a concomitant decrease in the use of CCNU. A further reduction in the dose of CSRT to 18 Gy is being investigated in the current COG study for younger children with average-risk medulloblastoma. The German HIT-91 randomized study also showed a positive effect of maintenance

chemotherapy with the Packer regimen, with patients treated with this regimen having a 3-year progression-free survival of 78%.[29]

The principal toxicities of the Packer regimen are those of CCNU-associated marrow suppression together with nephrotoxicity, and particularly ototoxicity due to cisplatin. In the CCG-9892 study, grades 3 or 4 ototoxicity were noted in 34% of patients, although in the HIT-91 study only 9% of patients receiving maintenance chemotherapy with the Packer regimen experienced these degrees of ototoxicity, probably reflecting different schema for dose modification of cisplatin.

In summary, reduced radiotherapy (23.4 Gy CSRT) with a posterior fossa dose of 54 to 55.8 Gy followed by the Packer regimen or modifications thereof is now generally regarded in both North America and Europe as standard therapy for standard-/average-risk patients, and this treatment forms the basis for forthcoming groupwide trials.

Metastatic Medulloblastoma

As opposed to standard-/average-risk disease (Table 19-1), metastatic medulloblastoma remains a poor-prognosis tumor, and relatively little progress has been made in terms of improving outcome. Standard treatment consists of surgical excision of the primary tumor followed by conventional radiotherapy with doses of radiotherapy of 35 to 36 Gy to the craniospinal axis together with a boost of 18 to 20 Gy to the posterior fossa. In addition, further boosts to sites of metastatic disease are frequently administered.

Chemotherapy is generally accepted as having an important role in the treatment of metastatic medulloblastoma, although the optimal chemotherapy regimen has yet to be defined. Despite the use of chemotherapy, various large, multicenter studies, including the CCG-921 and HIT-91 and PNET-3, have reported survival figures of between 30% and 40% for patients with M2/M3 status at diagnosis.[26,29,46]

More encouraging results in high-risk medulloblastoma have come from a recently completed North American study, POG-9031, in which patients were randomized to preirradiation chemotherapy with cisplatin and etoposide or to immediate radiotherapy followed by the same chemotherapy. Both arms then received identical chemotherapy with vincristine and cyclophosphamide. Five-year EFS was 66.0% in the early chemotherapy arm and 70.0% in the early radiation therapy arm. Five-year overall survival rates were 73.1% and 76.1%, respectively and was over 60% for metastatic patients (Tarbell, personal communication). Among 62 patients with residual disease in the early chemotherapy arm, those who achieved either complete or partial remission ($n = 40$) had improved 5-year EFS, compared with patients who had less than a partial response (72.5% vs 36.4%, p value $= 0.0008$). It is of note, however, that the POG-9031 study used a higher CSRT dose of 40 Gy for patients with metastatic disease with boosts of up to 45 Gy to sites of macroscopic spread. Similarly, encouraging results for metastatic patients were noted in the more recent St Jude Medulloblastoma-96 trial, in which children received 4 cycles of cyclophosphamide-

Table 19-1

Average-/standard-risk disease.

Study	Design	Years of Accrual	CSI Dose (Gy)	Chemotherapy	Number of Patients	Outcomes
CCG 923/ POG 8631[44]	RCT	1986–1990	36 vs 23.4		83	8-yr EFS = 67 vs 52% ($p = 0.141$)
SIOP 2[5]	RCT	1984–1989	35	None	40	5-yr EFS = 60%
			25	None	36	5-yr EFS = 69%
			35	Pre-RT	38	5-yr EFS = 75%
			25	Pre-RT	36	5-yr EFS = 42%
						NS Difference in EFS between RT alone groups
						Worst outcome for pre-RT chemo + reduced-dose RT
SFOP M7[57]	Observational	1985–1988	36 spine	Pre-RT	31	5-yr DFS = 74%
			27 brain			7-yr DFS = 62%
HIT 91[29]	RCT	1991–1997	35.2	Pre-RT vs	158	3-yr EFS = 65% vs
				Post-RT		3-yr EFS = 78%
						($p = 0.03$)
PNET 3[43]	RCT	1992–2000	35	None	89	3-yr EFS = 65%
				Pre-RT	90	3-yr EFS = 79%
						($p = 0.04$)
CCG-9892[45]	Observational	1984–1989	23.4	Post-RT	65	5-yr PFS = 79%
CCG-POG A9961[27]	RCT	1996–2000	23.4	Post-RT A vs	193	5-yr EFS = 81%
			23.4	Post-RT B	186	NS difference between groups.

Abbreviations: RCT, <define?>; RT, radiation therapy; DFS, disease-free survival; EFS, event-free survival; NS, not significant; yr, year; PFS, progression-free survival.

based, dose-intensive chemotherapy following radiotherapy.[18] A 65% 5-year EFS for the 33 patients with M2/M3 disease was observed (Gajjar, personal communication), albeit again in the context of a craniospinal irradiation dose of 39 Gy. The results from both these studies may indicate a dose–response effect for radiotherapy doses above 35 to 36 Gy, although there must be concern with regard to worsening of late neuropsychologic sequelae at such high CSRT doses.

Altered radiotherapy fractionation schedules, such as twice-daily radiotherapy, can theoretically increase the dose to tumor without an increase in the dose to normal nervous tissue. The CCG tested hyperfractionated radiation therapy preceded by 5 months of neoadjuvant chemotherapy for high-risk medulloblastoma (Table 19-2) The disappointing result, with a 3 year EFS of only 46%, may have been related to a delay in the administration of radiation therapy.[47] In contrast, very encouraging data have recently come from the Milan group, using a program of high-dose sequential chemotherapy (methotrexate, etoposide, cyclophosphamide, carbo-

platin) followed by hyperfractionated accelerated radiotherapy in children with metastatic medulloblastoma. For 24 patients, a 3-year disease-free survival of 78% has been reported, and this approach appears certainly worthy of investigation in a multi-institutional study. Current studies are investigating the role of chemotherapy delivered concomitantly with radiotherapy, the use of high-dose chemotherapy with autologous hematopoietic progenitor cell rescue, and altered radiotherapy fractionation schedules.

Supratentorial Primitive Neuroectodermal Tumors

This rare group constitutes around 20% of PNETs and around 2% to 3% of CNS tumors in childhood. The majority of tumors arise in the cerebral hemispheres, principally in the frontal, parietal, and temporal lobes. About 20% arise in the pineal region, where they are known as pineoblastomas. Supratentorial PNETs usually present with symptoms and signs associated with the

Table 19-2

High-risk disease.

Study	Design	Years of Accrual	CSI Dose (Gy)	Chemotherapy	Number of Patients	Outcomes
SFOF M7[57]	Observational	1985–1988	36 spine 27 brain	Pre-RT (8 in 1 + HD-MTX)	37	M+ 7 yr DFS = 45%
SIOP 2[5]	RCT	1984–1989	35	Pre-RT (PCZ, VCR, MTX) vs no pre-RT All high-risk post-RT (CCNU, VCR)	M+ = 29	M+ 5 y EFS ~ 40%
CCG 921[26]	RCT	1986–1992	36	8 in 1 pre- and post-RT vs VCR, CCNU, prednisone post-RT	169 (M+ = 82)	All patients: 5-yr PFS = 45% vs 63% (p = 0.0006) (M1 = 57%, M2+ = 40%)
HIT 91[29]	RCT	1991–1997	35.2	Pre-RT (ifosphamide,etoposide, HD-MTX, cisplatin, cytarabine) vs post-RT (CCNU, VCR, cisplatin)	M1 = 21 M 2/3 = 26	M1 3-yr RFS = 65% M2/3 3-yr RFS = 30%
POG 9031	RCT	1990–1996	40	Arm A: pre-RT (cisplatin, etoposide) Arm B: post-RT (cisplatin, etoposide) Both arms: post-RT consolidation (cyclophosphamide, VCR)	M0 = 113 M1 = 29 M2 = 34 M3 = 32 M4 = 8 M2/3 = 77	Unpublished abstract:[59] Arm A: 5-yr EFS = 66% Arm B: 5-yr EFS = 71% (p = 0.4) M2/3 5-yr EFS = 39%
PNET 3[46]	Observational (for M2/3)	1992–2000	35	Pre-RT (carboplatin, etoposide, cyclophosphamide, VCR)		
St Jude Medullo-blastoma-96[18]	Observational	1996–2003	36 (M1) 39.6 (M2/3)	Post-RT (cisplatin, cyclophosphamide, VCR with stem cell support)	M1 = 9 M2/3 = 33	M1 5-yr EFS = 74% M2/3 5-yr EF = 66% (Gajjar, personal communication)

Abbreviations: DFS, disease-free survival, EFS, event-free survival; RFS, relapse-free survival; RT, radiation therapy; yr, year.

mass effect of the tumor including headaches, seizures, and hemiplegia. Pineoblastoma usually presents with symptoms and signs of hydrocephalus and sometimes Parinaud syndrome. Staging investigations at diagnosis are similar to those for medulloblastoma. Nonpineal ST-PNETs are usually large at presentation, with around half being greater than 5 cm in diameter at diagnosis. A significant minority of patients have metastatic spread at the time of presentation, although the exact proportion is unclear.

Morphologically, ST-PNETs are similar to medulloblastoma, although there is increasing evidence from recent gene expression and comparative genomic hybridization studies to suggest that ST-PNETs are molecularly distinct from their infratentorial counterparts. For example, in a recent study, ST-PNETs were shown to have common losses affecting 1p12-22.1 and 9p, and gains at 19p, but appeared to show a reduced frequency of imbalances involving chromosome 17.[48]

Because of the rarity of ST-PNETs, there have been no large multicenter studies specifically for ST-PNETs; instead, they are generally treated with protocols designed for children with high-risk medulloblastoma. The largest series comes from the SIOP PNET-3, HIT-91, and CCG-921 studies with 66, 64, and 55 patients, respectively.[49–51] Young patients appear to have a particularly poor prognosis, possibly as a result of biologic differences or an underutilization of adequate doses of radiotherapy. The larger series have shown a higher survival for older patients with nonmetastatic pineal tumors (60%-70%) than those with nonpineal ST-PNETs (30%–40%). The reasons for this are unclear but may include earlier presentation and smaller size than nonpineal tumors, due to obstruction of CSF pathways by pineal tumors, or inherent differences in biology or treatment responsiveness. However, the PNET-3 study showed that metastatic pineal disease is a very high risk tumor, with no patients with M2/M3 disease surviving. Other prognostic features for ST-PNETs have not yet been clearly determined. Whereas the CCG-921 showed a detrimental effect of metastatic disease, this effect was not demonstrated in patients entered into the HIT-91 or PNET-3 studies. Likewise, the significance of the extent of surgical resection is unclear.

The generally accepted standard therapy is to remove the tumor as completely as possible, although this may be difficult, and complete resection rates are lower than with medulloblastoma. Craniospinal radiotherapy is delivered with a dose of 35 to 36 Gy, with a boost to the primary tumor that is a particular concern in terms of the potential for severe neurologic damage. This concern may limit the application of an appropriate radiation therapy volume boost to the tumor bed. Chemotherapy is generally administered according to high-risk medulloblastoma protocols.

Late Effects of Therapy

It is now clear that a high proportion of survivors of medulloblastoma have significant long-term sequelae. Although the etiology of these is multifactorial, it is prob-

able that the most important factor in the pathogenesis of these significant sequelae is the dose of CSRT used to treat this disease. Several studies in survivors who have received a whole-brain dose of 35 to 36 Gy have demonstrated marked losses of intelligence quotient of up to 30 points or more, an effect that is most predominant in young children, particularly those less than 7 or 8 years,[52,53] as well as poor general functional outcomes including social and educational difficulties in survivors. Lower CSRT doses such as those used in the CCG study (23.4 Gy) continue to show an adverse affect on intellectual development but not as severe as seen with conventional radiation therapy doses.[54]

The volume irradiated for the boost portion of the radiation therapy may also affect cognitive function. Substantial volumes of the parietal, temporal, and occipital lobes are irradiated during a conventional posterior fossa boost treatment for medulloblastoma. Modern 3D conformal radiation therapy and IMRT techniques are allowing less of the supratentorial brain to receive unnecessary high doses of irradiation.

In addition, the majority of survivors following these doses of CSRT suffer significant growth and endocrine dysfunction, predominantly due to irradiation of the pituitary gland and hypothalamic regions together with the effects of whole-spine radiotherapy.[55]

As mentioned above, both radiation therapy and cisplatin-based chemotherapy may affect the inner ear and result in hearing loss. Attempts are under way to minimize the irradiation dose to the cochlea by using 3D conformal irradiation or IMRT and limiting the boost to the tumor bed rather than the whole posterior fossa.

A systematic evaluation of late effects is a prominent feature of current and proposed North American and European groupwide randomized controlled trials in medulloblastoma.

Relapse

For medulloblastoma, the predominant site of relapse is distant leptomeningeal spread, either alone or in combination with relapse at the primary site. In only approximately 20% of relapsing patients will disease be confined to the posterior fossa. In contrast, the majority of ST-PNETs relapse locally without metastatic disease, implying a need for improved local tumor control.

Using conventional therapy, the prognosis for relapsed PNETs is poor, with fewer than 10% of patients surviving. Over the past 10 to 15 years, however, there is increasing evidence that a number of patients with relapsed medulloblastoma and possibly ST-PNETs may be cured using a strategy based on marrow-ablative dose chemotherapy with bone marrow or peripheral blood hematopoietic progenitor cell rescue. Population-based studies are, however, needed to define the overall impact of this approach in relapsing patients. Patients that appear to particularly benefit from myeloablative chemotherapy include those who relapse locally and those who are able to achieve minimal disease (through surgery or further chemotherapy) at the time of myeloablative chemotherapy.[56,57]

Future Directions

In the current COG study for average-risk medulloblastoma, ACNS0331, all patients are randomized to receive boost irradiation to either whole posterior fossa or tumor bed. Children aged 3 to 7 years are additionally randomized to a CSRT dose of either 18 Gy or 23.4 Gy. All participants will receive adjuvant chemotherapy with a slightly more prolonged regimen than that used in A9961. For the same group of patients, in the recently completed European SIOP Group trial, HIT-SIOP PNET-4, patients were randomized to receive either conventional radiotherapy (23.4 Gy CSRT/posterior fossa boost 54 Gy) or hyperfractionated radiotherapy (1 Gy twice daily) with a dose of 60 Gy to the posterior fossa, with an additional 8 Gy to the tumor bed and 36 Gy to the craniospinal axis. Both groups received identical chemotherapy consisting of 8 weekly doses of vincristine given concomitant with radiotherapy and 8 courses of CCNU, cisplatin, and vincristine following radiotherapy. A critical feature of both studies is the prospective evaluation of a range of biologic markers and the systematic study of late sequelae.[58]

For high-risk patients, the COG has completed a dose escalation trial of carboplatin given concomitantly with daily CSRT for patients with high-risk medulloblastoma and ST-PNET (CCG-99701). The established Phase I dose of carboplatin from this study now forms the basis of a recently opened Phase III randomized trial that will test the addition of 13-cis-retinoic acid along with chemotherapy in maintenance. In Europe, national groups are conducting trials of novel altered irradiation fractionation techniques and of high-dose chemotherapy also in an attempt to improve survival.[59]

Concluding Remarks

Our understanding of the natural history and management of medulloblastoma and ST-PNET continues to evolve. Fortunately, with modern techniques of staging, surgery, radiation therapy, and chemotherapy we are in the pleasant position of de-escalating therapy in low- or average-risk patients in order to reduce the late sequelae of treatment. In many groupwide studies, the acquisition of tumor tissue for molecular analysis has become a high priority, alongside the prospective assessment and validation of combined stratification indices. In the future, we anticipate that therapy for an individual patient will be stratified according to biology that is revealed by detailed analysis of each patient's tumor, alongside clinical and histopathological parameters. Only then will we logically tailor the risk of therapy to the risk posed by the patient's disease.

References

1. Hart MN, Earle KM. Primitive neuroectodermal tumors of the brain in children. *Cancer.* 1973;32(4):890–897.
2. Giangaspero F, Eberhart CG, Haapasalo H, Pietsch T, Wiestler OD, Ellison DW. Medulloblastoma. In: Louis DMN, Ohgaki H, Wiestler OD, Caveneee WK, eds. *WHO Classification of Tumors of the Central Nervous System.* Lyon: IARC Press; 2007:132–140.
3. Pomeroy SL, Tamayo P, Gaasenbeek M, et al. Prediction of central nervous system embryonal tumour outcome based on gene expression. *Nature.* 2002; 415:436–442.
4. McNeil DE, Cote TR, Clegg L, Rorke LB. Incidence and trends in pediatric malignancies. Medulloblastoma/primitive neuroectodermal tumor: A SEER update. *Med Pediatr Oncol.* 2002;39:190–194.
5. Bailey CC, Gnekow A, Wellek S, et al. Prospective randomised trial of chemotherapy given before radiotherapy in childhood medulloblastoma. International Society of Paediatric Oncology (SIOP) and the (German) Society of Paediatric Oncology (GPO): SIOP II. *Med Pediatr Oncol.* 1995;25(3):166–178.
6. Ellison DW. Classifying the medulloblastoma: insights from morphology and molecular genetics. *Neuropathol Appl Neurobiol.* 2002;28:257–282.
7. McManamy CS, Pears J, Weston CL, et al. Nodule formation and desmoplasia in medulloblastomas: defining the nodular/desmoplastic variant and its biological behaviour. *Brain Pathol.* 2007;17:151–164.
8. Rutkowski S, Bode U, Deinlein F, et al. Treatment of early childhood medulloblastoma by postoperative chemotherapy alone. *N Eng J Med.* 2005;352: 978–986.
9. Eberhart CG, Burger PC. Anaplasia and grading in medulloblastomas. *Brain Pathol.* 2003;13:376–385.
10. McManamy CS, Lamont JM, Taylor RE, et al. Morphophenotypic variation predicts clinical behaviour in childhood non-desmoplastic medulloblastomas. *J Neuropath Exp Neurol.* 2003;62:627–632.
11. Ellison DW, Clifford SC, Gajjar A, Gilbertson RJ. What's new in neuro-oncology? recent advances in medulloblastoma. *Eur J Paed Neurol.* 2003;7:53–66.
12. Wechsler-Reya R, Scott MP. The developmental biology of brain tumors. *Ann Rev Neurosci.* 2001;24:385–428.
13. Chenn A, Walsh CA. Regulation of cerebral cortical size by control of cell cycle exit in neural precursors. *Science.* 2002;297:365–369.
14. Thompson MC, Fuller C, Hogg TL, et al. Genomics identifies medulloblastoma subgroups that are enriched for specific genetic alterations. *J Clin Oncol.* 2006;24:1924–1931.
15. Romer JT, Kimura H, Magdaleno S, et al. Suppression of the SHH pathway using a small molecule inhibitor eliminates medulloblastoma in Ptc1(+/–) p53(–/–) mice. *Cancer Cell.* 2004;6:229–240.
16. Clifford SC, Lusher ME, Lindsey JC, et al. Wnt/Wingless pathway activation and chromosome 6 loss characterise a distinct molecular sub-group of medulloblastomas associated with a favourable prognosis. *Cell Cycle.* 2006;5: 2666–2670.
17. Ellison DW, Onilude OE, Lindsey JC, et al. Beta-catenin status predicts a favorable outcome in childhood medulloblastoma. *J Clin Oncol.* 2005;23: 7951–7957.
18. Gajjar A, Chintagumpala M, Ashley D, et al. Risk-adapted craniospinal radiotherapy followed by high-dose chemotherapy and stem-cell rescue in children with newly diagnosed medulloblastoma (St Jude Medulloblastoma-96): long-term results from a prospective, multicentre trial. *Lancet Oncol.* 2006;7: 813–820.
19. Lamont JM, MacManamy CS, Taylor R, et al. Molecular pathological stratification of disease risk in medulloblastoma. *Clin Cancer Research.* 2004;10: 5482–5493.
20. Gajjar A, Hernan R, Kocak M, et al. Clinical, histopathologic, and molecular markers of prognosis: toward a new disease risk stratification system for medulloblastoma. *J Clin Oncol.* 2004;22:984–993.
21. Rutkowski S, von Bueren A, von Hoff K, et al. Prognostic relevance of clinical and biological risk factors in childhood medulloblastoma: results of patients treated in the prospective multicenter trial HIT'91. *Clin Cancer Res.* 2007;13: 2651–2657.
22. Chang CH, Housepian EM, Herbert C. An operative staging system and a megavoltage radiotherapeutic technique for cerebellar medulloblastomas. *Radiology.* 1969;93:1351–1359.
23. Albright AL, Wisoff JH, Zeltzer PM, Boyett JM, Rorke LB, Stanley P. Effects of medulloblastoma resections on outcome in children: a report from the Children's Cancer Group. *Neurosurgery.* 1996;38(2):265–271.
24. Evans AE, Jenkin RD, Sposto R, et al. The treatment of medulloblastoma: results of a prospective randomized trial of radiation therapy with and without CCNU, vincristine, and prednisone. *J Neurosurg.* 1990;72(4):572–582.
25. Packer RJ, Sutton LN, Elterman R, et al. Outcome for children with medulloblastoma treated with radiation and cisplatin, CCNU, and vincristine chemotherapy. *J Neurosurg.* 1994;81(5):690–698.
26. Zeltzer PM, Boyett JM, Finlay JL, et al. Metastasis stage, adjuvant treatment, and residual tumor are prognostic factors for medulloblastoma in children: conclusions from the Children's Cancer Group 921 randomized Phase III study. *J Clin Oncol.* 1999;17(3):832–845.
27. Packer RJ, Gajjar A, Vezina G, et al. Phase III study of craniospinal radiation therapy followed by adjuvant chemotherapy for newly diagnosed average-risk medulloblastoma. *J Clin Oncol.* 2006;24(25):4202–4208.
28. Gajjar A, Fouladi M, Walter AW, et al. Comparison of lumbar and shunt cerebrospinal fluid specimens for cytologic detection of leptomeningeal disease in pediatric patients with brain tumors. *J Clin Oncol.* 1999;17:1825–1828.
29. Kortmann RD, Kuhl J, Timmermann B, et al. Postoperative neoadjuvant chemotherapy before radiotherapy as compared to immediate radiotherapy followed by maintenance chemotherapy in the treatment of medulloblastoma in childhood: results of the German prospective randomized trial HIT '91. *Int J Radiat Oncol Biol Phys.* 2000;46:269–279.
30. Landberg TG, Lindgren ML, Cavallin-Stahl EK, et al. Improvements in the radiotherapy of medulloblastoma, 1946–1975. *Cancer.* 1980;45:670–678.
31. Bouffet E, Bernard JL, Frappaz D, et al. M4 protocol for cerebellar medulloblastoma: supratentorial radiotherapy may not be avoided. *Int J Radiat Onc Biol Phys.* 1992;24(1):79–85.

32. Tarbell NJ, Loeffler JS, Silver B, et al. The change in patterns of relapse in medulloblastoma. *Cancer.* 1991;68(7):1600–1604.

33. Paulino AC, Narayana A, Mohideen M, Jeswani S. Posterior fossa boost in medulloblastoma: an analysis of dose to surrounding structures using 3-dimensional (conformal) radiotherapy. *Int J Radiat Oncol Biol Phys.* 2000;46(2):281–286.

34. Huang E, The BS, Strother DR, et al. Intensity modulated radiation therapy for pediatric medulloblastoma: early report on the reduction of ototoxicity. *Int J Radiat Oncol Biol Phys.* 2002;52:599–605.

35. St. Clair WH, Adams JA, Bues M, et al. Advantage of protons compared to conventional X-ray or IMRT in the treatment of a pediatric patient with medulloblastoma. *Int J Radiat Oncol Biol Phys.* 2004;58(3):727–734.

36. Wolden SL, Dunkel IJ, Souweidane MM, et al. Patterns of failure using a conformal radiation therapy tumor bed boost for medulloblastoma. *J Clin Oncol.* 2003;21:3079–3083.

37. Douglas JG, Barker JL, Ellenbogen RG, Geyer JR. Concurrent chemotherapy and reduced-dose cranial spinal irradiation followed by conformal posterior fossa tumor bed boost for average-risk medulloblastoma: efficacy and patterns of failure. *Int J Radiat Oncol Biol Phys.* 2004;58(4):1161–1164.

38. Carrie C, Muracciole X, Gomez F, et al. Conformal radiotherapy, reduced boost volume, hyperfractionated radiotherapy, and online quality control in standard-risk medulloblastoma without chemotherapy: results of the French M-SFOP 98 protocol. *Int J Radiat Oncol Biol Phys.* 2005;63(3):711–716.

39. Donnal J, Halperin EC, Friedman HS, Boyko OB. Subfrontal recurrence of medulloblastoma. *Am J Neuroradiol.* 1992;13:1617–1618.

40. Carrie C, Hoffstetter S, Gomez F, et al. Impact of targeting deviations on outcome in medulloblastoma: study of the French Society of Pediatric Oncology (SFOP). *Int J Radiat Oncol Biol Phys.* 1999;45(2):435–439.

41. Mah K, Danjoux CE, Manship S, Makhani N, Cardoso M, Sixel KE. Computed tomographic simulation of craniospinal fields in pediatric patients: improved treatment accuracy and patient comfort. *Int J Radial Oncol Biol Phys.* 1998;41(5):997–1003.

42. Taylor RE, Bailey CC, Robinson KJ, et al; United Kingdom Children's Cancer Study Group Brain Tumour Committee; International Society of Paediatric Oncology. Impact of radiotherapy parameters on outcome in the International Society of Paediatric Oncology/United Kingdom Children's Cancer Study Group PNET-3 study of preradiotherapy chemotherapy for M0-M1 medulloblastoma. *Int J Radiat Oncol Biol Phys.* 2004;58(4):1184–1193.

43. Taylor RE, Bailey CC, Robinson K, et al; International Society of Paediatric Oncology; United Kingdom Children's Cancer Study Group. Results of a randomized study of preradiation chemotherapy versus radiotherapy alone for nonmetastatic medulloblastoma: the International Society of Paediatric Oncology/United Kingdom Children's Cancer Study Group PNET-3 Study. *J Clin Oncol.* 2003;21(8):1581–1591.

44. Thomas PR, Deutsch M, Kepner JL, et al. Low-stage medulloblastoma: final analysis of trial comparing standard-dose with reduced-dose neuraxis irradiation. *J Clin Oncol.* 2000;18(16):3004–3011.

45. Packer RJ, Goldwein J, Nicholson HS, et al. Treatment of children with medulloblastomas with reduced-dose craniospinal radiation therapy and adjuvant chemotherapy: a Children's Cancer Group study. *J Clin Oncol.* 1999;17(7):2127–2136.

46. Taylor RE, Bailey CC, Robinson KJ, et al; for the United Kingdom Children's Cancer Study Group (UKCCSG) Brain Tumor Committee. Outcome for patients with metastatic (M2-3) medulloblastoma treated with SIOP/UKCCSG PNET-3 chemotherapy. *Eur J Cancer.* 2005;41(5):727–734.

47. Allen J, Prados M, Mehta M, et al. A Phase I/II study for newly diagnosed high risk PNET consisting of neoadjuvant chemotherapy followed by hyper-fractionated radiotherapy: preliminary results of CCG protocol 9931. *Neuro Oncol.* 1997;247.

48. Pfister S, Remke M, Toedt G, et al. Supratentorial primitive neuroectodermal tumors of the central nervous system frequently harbor deletions of the CDKN2A locus and other genomic aberrations distinct from medulloblastomas. *Genes Chromosomes Cancer.* 2007;46:839–851.

49. Pizer BL, Weston CL, Robinson KJ, et al. Analysis of patients with supratentorial primitive neuro-ectodermal tumours entered into the SIOP/UKCCSG PNET 3 study. *Eur J Cancer.* 2006;42:1120–1128.

50. Timmermann B, Kortmann RD, Kuhl J, et al. Role of radiotherapy in the treatment of supratentorial primitive neuroectodermal tumors in childhood: results of the prospective German brain tumor trials HIT 88/89 and 91. *J Clin Oncol.* 2002;20(3):842–849.

51. Cohen BH, Zeltzer PM, Boyett JM, et al. Prognostic factors and treatment results for supratentorial primitive neuroectodermal tumors in children using radiation and chemotherapy: a Children's Cancer Group randomized trial. *J Clin Oncol.* 1995;13(7):1687–1696.

52. Hoppe-Hirsch E, Renier D, Lellouch-Tubiana A, et al. Medulloblastoma in childhood: progressive intellectual deterioration. *Child's Nerv Syst.* 1990;6(2):60–65.

53. Lannering B, Marky I, Lundberg A, Olsson E. Long-term sequelae after pediatric brain tumors: their effect on disability and quality of life. *Med Pediatr Oncol.* 1990;18(4):304–310.

54. Ris MD, Packer R, Goldwein J, Jones-Wallace D, Boyett JM. Intellectual outcome after reduced-dose radiation therapy plus adjuvant chemotherapy for medulloblastoma: a Children's Cancer Group Study. *J Clin Oncol.* 2001;19:3470–3476.

55. Adan L, Sainte-Rose C, Souberbielle JC, Zucker JM, Kalifa C, Brauner R. Adult height after growth hormone (GH) treatment for GH deficiency due to cranial irradiation. *Med Pediatr Oncol.* 2000;34(1):14–19.

56. Dunkel IJ, Boyett JM, Yates A, et al; Children's Cancer Group. High-dose carboplatin, thiotepa, and etoposide with autologous stem-cell rescue for patients with recurrent medulloblastoma. *J Clin Oncol.* 1998;16(1):222–228.

57. Graham ML, Herndon JE II, Casey JR, et al. High-dose chemotherapy with autologous stem-cell rescue in patients with recurrent and high-risk pediatric brain tumors. *J Clin Oncol.* 1997;15(5):1814–1823.

58. Gentet JC, Bouffet E, Doz F, et al. Preirradiation chemotherapy including "eight drugs in 1 day" regimen and high-dose methotrexate in childhood medulloblastoma: results of the M7 French Cooperative Study. *J Neurosurg.* 1995;82(4):608–614.

59. Tarbell N, Kun L, Freidman H, Kepner J. High stage medulloblastoma: results from pediatric oncology group study 9031. Abstract in *Med Pediatr Oncol.* 2002;39(4):227.

Infant Brain Tumors

J. Russell Geyer and Chantal Kalifa

Introduction

Tumors of the central nervous system (CNS) account for 17% of childhood malignancies, with the highest incidence occurring during the first 5 years of life.[1] Among children less than 1 year at diagnosis, the incidence of CNS tumors exceeds that of acute lymphoblastic leukemia.[2] Although considerable improvement in survival has been achieved in childhood cancer overall and in CNS cancer in older children, little progress has been made in younger children with these tumors. The late effects of therapy are greatest among children treated for CNS tumors at an early age. In addition, it has become increasingly apparent that the biology of brain tumors in very young children is, in some cases, quite different from that seen in older children.

For these reasons, over the past two decades, significant effort has been directed toward designing therapeutic trials for this relatively small group of patients.

Epidemiology

Among children, the incidence of malignant CNS tumors is inversely proportional to age: 4 cases are annually reported per 100 000 children younger than 5 years compared with 2.2 cases per 100 000 among 15- to 20-year-olds.[1] In the first 3 years of life, the rate of CNS tumors in African Americans is one-half to three-quarters of that of Caucasian children, raising the possibility that there may be a delay in diagnosing CNS malignancy.[1]

In the first 3 years of life, ependymomas and medulloblastomas are relatively more frequent than high-grade astrocytomas, which are the most common type of malignancy among older adolescents.[3,4]

In children younger than 12 months, CNS tumors account for 15% of malignancies.[2] Central nervous system tumors increased from 24 per million in the period from 1979 to 1981, to 33 per million in the period from 1989 to 1991 in this age group, and tumors are more commonly located supratentorially (63.9%).[5] The most common histology is astrocytoma, followed by ependymoma and medulloblastoma.[6,7] The recently described atypical teratoid/rhabdoid tumor accounts for some 3% of tumors in this age group.[6]

Neonatal brain tumors account for approximately 7.2% of all neonatal cancer and 0.5% to 11% of all childhood brain tumors.[5] Twenty-one percent of children diagnosed in their first year of life with brain tumors present at 2 months of age or less, 14% in the first month of life.[5] Posterior fossa tumors occurred in only 11% of neonates, but 41% of all pediatric group patients. Neonates with brain tumors most often present with subtle, nonspecific symptoms and rarely with focal findings. More than 50% of patients present with large heads. Focal neurologic changes are infrequent, as are seizures.[5]

Medulloblastoma/Primitive Neuroectodermal Tumors

Medulloblastoma is the prototype of childhood malignant CNS tumors in terms of its curability using radiation therapy, its sensitivity to chemotherapy, and the potentially high price of cure—in terms of neuropsychologic sequelae. The earliest cooperative group studies, which included very young children and utilized craniospinal irradiation, demonstrated that the prognosis for these young children was worse than that for older children, and that the consequences in terms of late effects of cranial irradiation, particularly on cognition, were much greater. Therefore, over the past 2 decades, a number of studies have been undertaken attempting to delay, reduce, or obviate the use of radiation therapy.

Van Eys et al treated 12 children with medulloblastoma between 1976 and 1988 with MOPP (mustargen, oncovin, procarbazine, and prednisone) without radiotherapy, of whom 8 were reported to be long-term survivors.[8]

The Pediatric Oncology Group (Baby POG 1 study) utilized cyclophosphamide and vincristine alternating with cisplatin and etoposide.[9] Children less than 2 years old at diagnosis received 2 years of chemotherapy followed by craniospinal irradiation with a reduced neuraxis dose of 24 Gy, whereas children who were between 24 and 36 months received 1 year of chemotherapy followed by the same regimen of radiation therapy. Sixty-two children with medulloblastoma were entered on study.[9] Gross total surgical resection was performed in 38%. Forty-eight percent demonstrated an objective radiographic response to 2 cycles

Table 20-1

Infant M0 medulloblastoma.

Study	N	Event-Free Survival (%) 3-Yr	Overall Survival 3-Yr
Baby POG1 (8633/8634)[9]	37	38	45
CCG-9921 Regimen A/B[12]	61	39	65
BBSFOP[43]	64	25	70
HIT-SKK 87[19]	28	57	60
HIT-SKK 92[21]	31	68	80
Head Start 1 and 2[22]	24	38	79

Table 20-2

Infant M0 medulloblastoma.

Study	N	Radiation-Free Survival (%) 3-Yr	3-Yr	CSI-Free Survival 3-Yr
Baby POG1 (8633/8634)[9]	37	0	0	0
CCG-9921 Regimen A/B[12]	61	36	26	Na
BBSFOP[43]	64	23	22	62
HIT-SKK 87[19]	28	0	0	0
HIT-SKK 92[21]	31	74	71	74
Head Start 1 and 2[22]	24	50	50	50

of vincristine and cyclophosphamide chemotherapy.[9] The 5-year progression-free survival (PFS) was 31.8%. Progressive disease tended to occur early, with most failures occurring in the first 6 months, and no cases of progressive disease occurred after 2 years of therapy. Overall survival (OS) at 5 years was 40%, and there was no difference in survival by age at diagnosis. The strongest prognostic factor was a gross total resection, with a 60% 5-year survival compared with 32% 5-year survival in those with subtotal resection.[9,10]

The Children's Cancer Group (CCG) study CCG-921 treated 46 children less than 18 months of age with the "8 drugs in 1 day" chemotherapy regimen and proposed delayed irradiation. The 3-year PFS was 22%.[11] In those children with gross total resection and no evidence of metastasis, 30% were reported alive and free of disease. Most of the children with medulloblastoma who were long-term survivors did not receive radiation therapy, by treating physician or parental choice.[11]

In the CCG-9921 study, children less than 36 months were randomized to one of two regimens of chemotherapy (vincristine, cisplatin, cyclophosphamide, and etoposide, Regimen A; versus vincristine, carboplatin, ifosfamide, and etoposide, Regimen B). Maintenance chemotherapy began after the completion of 5 cycles of induction chemotherapy in those children without progressive disease. Children with no residual tumor following induction therapy and no metastatic disease at diagnosis were not to receive radiation therapy unless tumor progression occurred. In the remainder, irradiation was to be delayed until the completion of chemotherapy.[12]

Ninety-two patients with medulloblastoma were entered on study. Seventy-four percent of these had a greater than 90% resection, and 34% had evidence of leptomeningeal dissemination. The combined response rate to chemotherapy was 60%. Overall 1-year event-free survival (EFS) was 52%. The 5-year EFS was 33%, with a 5-year OS of 43%. Eighty-one percent of 5-year survivors did not receive radiotherapy.[12] The 5-year EFS for Regimen A was 38% versus 26% for regimen B, a marginally significant difference.[12] No other variables reached statistical significance, although the presence of metastatic disease, less than complete tumor resection, and young age were each associated with a nominally worse prognosis. In patients with relapsed disease who had not received radiation therapy and subsequently went on to receive irradiation, the 3-year postprogression survival was 28%, compared with zero in those patients who did not receive radiation therapy.[12]

The French Society of Pediatric Oncology Baby Brain Protocol (BB-SFOP) was designed to deliver prolonged postoperative chemotherapy and, if possible, to avoid radiation therapy. Patients were classified into three categories: standard-risk patients with no local residual tumor and no metastasis, high-risk patients with local residual tumor but no metastasis, and high-risk patients with metastasis (with or without local residual tumor). Chemotherapy consisted of alternating cycles of carboplatin and procarbazine, etoposide and cisplatin, vincristine and cyclophosphamide over 16 months. No irradiation was given to patients who were in complete remission at the end of treatment. In the event of progressive disease or relapse, the recommended salvage treatment was the administration of myeloablative chemotherapy including busulfan and thiotepa with autologous hematopoietic cell support, followed by irradiation limited to the site of disease at the time of progression.[13,14]

After 1996, the protocol was modified for high-risk patients. Patients with local residual tumor visible on postoperative imaging (R1M0) received 2 courses of etoposide and carboplatin; peripheral blood hematopoietic cells were harvested, and the myeloablative busulfan and thiotepa combination with autologous hematopoietic cell support was administered.[15] Subsequently, limited posterior fossa irradiation (50 Gy) was administered.[16] Medulloblastoma patients with leptomeningeal dissemination at diagnosis (RxM+) and patients with a primitive neuroectodermal tumor (PNET) other than medulloblastoma were enrolled into a tandem myeloablative chemotherapy regimen with hematopoietic cell support. After 2 courses of etoposide and carboplatin followed by peripheral blood hematopoietic cell harvest, 3 sequential myeloablative courses were given: 2 courses consisted of melphalan, the third of busulfan and thiotepa, each followed by hematopoietic cell rescue.[17] Subsequently, radiation therapy was administered at a dose of 50 Gy to the tumor bed.

Seventy-nine medulloblastoma patients were enrolled. Fifty-eight patients have relapsed and 39 of 58 have received the salvage treatment including the myeloablative busulfan and thiotepa regimen and irradiation to the site of recurrent disease.

Five-year PFS was 29% (18%-44%), 6% (1%-27%), and 13% (4%-38%) in the R0M0, R1M0, and RxM+ groups. Overall survival was 73% (59%-84%), 41% (22%-64%), and 13% (4%-38%) in the R0M0, R1M0, and RxM+ groups, respectively. In those patients with no radiographic evidence of residual disease (R0M0), those in whom the neurosurgeon reported a gross total resection had superior 5-year EFS compared with those in whom residual disease was noted in the operative report (41% vs 0%). In 64 patients without metastasis, radiotherapy-free survival at 3 years was 22% (15%-35%), and craniospinal radiotherapy-free survival was 63%.[18]

Intelligence quotient (IQ) score was available for 33 children at a median interval from diagnosis of 54 months. The mean IQ score was 77% (standard deviation = +/−9), and 14 children had an IQ score of more than 80. For those given only chemotherapy the mean IQ was 91, compared with 72 for those who received high-dose chemotherapy and radiotherapy (RT) at relapse.

Delayed neurotoxic effects of the busulfan and thiotepa regimen and irradiation have been observed: in 25% of patients, transient gadolinium enhancement on brain magnetic resonance imaging (MRI) limited to the irradiated areas of the brain were observed several months after the end of treatment; in some patients, this phenomenon was associated with a worsening of neurologic deficits.

The German study HIT-SKK-87 used procarbazine, ifosfamide, and etoposide, as well as high-dose methotrexate, to delay cranial irradiation. The probability of 5-year EFS was 50%, 60% for patients without evidence of postoperative tumor, and 80% for infants with a complete response to induction.[19,20] In the HIT-SKK-92 study, radiation therapy was replaced, in patients achieving complete responses, with chemotherapy (cyclophosphamide, vincristine, carboplatin, etoposide, and intravenous and intraventricular methotrexate). In children with complete resection, residual tumor, and macroscopic metastases, the 5-year EFS and OS were 82% (standard error (SE)+/−9%) and 93% (SE+/−6%), 50% (SE+/−13%) and 56% (SE+/−14%), and 33% (SE+/−14%) and 38% (SE+/−15%), respectively.[20] Desmoplastic histology was an independent favorable prognostic factor, with an 85% (SE+/−8%) 5-year EFS compared with 34% (SE+/−10%) for those with nondesmoplastic histology.[21]

The Head Start 1 protocol investigated the role of high-dose, marrow-ablative chemotherapy and autologous hematopoietic cell rescue in young children with medulloblastoma. Induction chemotherapy consisted of cyclophosphamide, cisplatin, vincristine, and etoposide.[22] Those without evidence of residual disease after the induction chemotherapy, with or without second surgery, were eligible for myeloablative chemotherapy with hematopoietic cell rescue utilizing carboplatin, etoposide, and thiotepa. Twelve patients younger than 36 months with medulloblastoma were enrolled. Eighty-six percent had a response to induction chemotherapy. The EFS at one year was 69%, and at 2 years was 38%. The OS at 2 years was 62%.[22]

In the successor Head Start 2 study, high-dose methotrexate was added to the induction chemotherapy for patients with metastatic disease, and a complete response rate of 80% was reported for those patients with metastatic medulloblastoma, with an EFS of 51% at 4 years.[23]

In summary, although initial studies in infants with medulloblastoma/PNET utilizing chemotherapy to delay or avoid irradiation resulted in EFS rates substantially inferior to those seen in older children receiving craniospinal irradiation, more recent studies have yielded more encouraging results, particularly in patients with completely resected nonmetastatic tumors. Further, those patients with desmoplastic histology appear to have an excellent outcome without irradiation.

Tumor progression tends to occur early in all reported studies of young children with medulloblastoma/PNET. Approximately two-thirds of recurrences are local, either isolated or in combination with distant recurrences. Approximately one-third are only local, and one-third only distant.[12]

Current strategies in the United States have been influenced by the high rate of local progression noted in previous studies, as well as the development of new advances in radiation therapy technology with the potential of minimizing irradiation-related late effects by more focused radiation therapeutic targeting. The Children's Oncology Group (COG) is evaluating the use of involved-field posterior fossa irradiation following tumor resection and chemotherapy in patients with nonmetastatic disease. The United States Pediatric Brain Tumor Consortium is investigating this approach in combination with intrathecal chemotherapy. European investigators, in contrast, are continuing to explore the use of chemotherapy as the primary modality for completely resected nonmetastatic patients, reserving radiotherapy for those patients with progressive disease or high risk at diagnosis. The role of hematopoietic cell-supported myeloablative chemotherapy, either as primary therapy or at the time of tumor recurrence, continues to be investigated, as does the role of high-dose methotrexate, particularly in the current Head Start 3 study and a recently opened COG trial for young children with metastatic medulloblastoma.

Supratentorial Primitive Neuroectodermal Tumors

As in older children, the approach to the treatment of supratentorial primitive neuroectodermal tumors (ST-PNET) in the very young child has been very similar to that employed for the treatment of children with medulloblastoma. Thirty patients with ST-PNET (which included such entities as cerebral neuroblastoma, ependymoblastoma, and pineoblastoma) were entered on the Baby POG 1 study.[9] Gross total resection was possible in only 8 of these patients.[9] The response rate to chemotherapy (29%) was less than that seen in medulloblastoma.[9] One-year PFS was only 22%, and OS at 3 years was 25%. No patient with pineoblastoma survived.[9,10]

Forty-seven patients with ST-PNET were entered on the CCG-9921 study.[12] Seventy percent were from 12 to 36 months at diagnosis, and 30% were less than 12 months at time of diagnosis. Eighty percent had no evidence of metastatic disease at diagnosis and 60% underwent greater than a 90% resection. Six of 14 patients with measurable postoperative disease responded to initial chemotherapy. The overall PFS was 26% at 1 year and 17% at 5 years, while the overall 5-year survival was 30%.[12]

Twenty-five children with ST-PNET were treated on the BB-SFOP protocol.[24] Four children presented with disseminated leptomeningeal disease. Total resection was performed in 9 patients, subtotal in 9, partial in 3, and a biopsy only in 4 patients. Twenty-four patients progressed or relapsed with a median time of 5.5 months. The 2- and 5-year survivals were 30% and 14%, respectively. At the time of progression, only 4 patients were treated with myeloablative busulfan and thiotepa in addition to irradiation localized to the tumor bed; 2 of these 4 children are reported to be in continuous complete remission.

Twenty-nine children less than 3 years were entered on HIT-SKK87 and HIT-SKK92. Fourteen received RT, while the remainder did not. The 3-year PFS for those patients treated with RT was 24% versus 6% in those without RT, similarly the OS for those receiving RT was 28.6% (5%–52%) versus 6.7% (0%-19%) for those not receiving RT. The authors conclude that RT should be given as a component of primary treatment in this population, though this was not an intent-to-treat design.[25]

Forty-three patients with ST-PNET were entered on Head Start 1 and 2, of whom 20 were younger than 36 months at diagnosis. Patients 6 years and younger were not to receive RT per protocol. Five-year EFS and OS for those less than 36 months was 35% ($\pm$11%) and 40% ($\pm$11%). Age, gender, extent of resection, and metastasis at diagnosis were not statistically associated with survival rate, but pineal location predicted worse outcome than nonpineal location (OS 23% and 50%, respectively). Sixty-three percent of surviving patients had no radiation exposure, and 75% have avoided craniospinal irradiation.[26]

Thus, with the exception of the Head Start program, the outcome of children with ST-PNET is worse than for those with medulloblastoma. In addition, the supratentorial location makes the potential consequence of even conformal radiation therapy to the primary site very worrisome for potential late effects.

Atypical Teratoid Rhabdoid Tumors

The CNS atypical teratoid rhabdoid tumor (AT/RT) was first described in 1987 by Rorke as a tumor distinct from PNETs, with a particularly poor prognosis.[27,28] Recently, the characteristic molecular abnormalities of this tumor have been elucidated.[13,28,29]

The pathology of AT/RT consists of areas of typical rhabdoid cells, each with an eccentric round nucleus and prominent nucleolus. This tumor can also demonstrate areas of primitive neuroepithelial, mesenchymal, and epithelial tissues and is therefore often misdiagnosed as a medulloblastoma or PNET, but also occasionally as a choroid plexus carcinoma or germ cell tumor.[27,28] Atypical teratoid rhabdoid tumors occur in many anatomical sites including the brain, kidneys, and soft tissues.[27]

Rhabdoid tumors are characterized by monosomy 22 or partial deletions of chromosome band 22q11.2, containing the hSNF/INI1 gene.[27,30,31] Homozygous deletions of the entire INI1 gene or loss of 1 allele and mutation of the other copy of the gene have been documented in approximately 85% of rhabdoid tumors.[31,32] INI1 appears to function as a classic tumor suppressor gene.[32] Recently, an immunohistochemical stain utilizing an antibody to INI1 has been described. Of 53 tumors consisting of 20 AT/RT, 10 PNET, and 23 other CNS tumors, no nuclear staining was found in all 20 AT/RT, with most other CNS tumors demonstrating such nuclear staining.[33]

Germline mutations have been reported in patients with sporadic renal and CNS AT/RT.[31,32] When mutations have been reported in patients with sporadic renal and

CNS AT/RT, the parents of these children are rarely carriers of these mutations.[31] Three families with noncarrier parents and 2 or more affected children have been described with the mechanism reported to be gonadal mosaicism.[31] Analysis of blood samples from affected children with somatic mutations is required to rule out a constitutional mutation.[31]

Fifty percent of AT/RT in infancy arise supratentorially.[34] In the posterior fossa, there is a predilection for the cerebello-pontine angle. The tumor can be intra- or extra-axial, often invading adjacent structures, including the meninges. In a database of 42 patients with rhabdoid tumors, the median age at diagnosis was 24 months. Twenty-one percent had metastatic disease, 16 patients were infratentorial, 26 supratentorial, and 48% achieved a complete resection.[35] In the CCG-9921 study, 28 (10%) patients in this study younger than 3 years had rhabdoid tumors. Sixty-four percent were without metastatic disease at diagnosis. Twenty-nine percent were supratentorial, whereas 68% were infratentorial and 64% underwent greater than 90% resection.[12]

Since its recognition as a separate entity, AT/RT has been associated with a poor prognosis. In 55 patients with AT/RT treated on POG trials, the mean postoperative survival was 11 months, with local recurrence as well as metastatic disease common terminal events.[36]

Chemotherapy has been the primary postoperative treatment reported. Although responses to chemotherapy have been documented, such responses are most often transient. In a recently reported United States AT/RT Registry, other modalities of treatment included myeloablative chemotherapy with autologous hematopoietic cell rescue, RT, and intrathecal chemotherapy. There is some evidence that older children do better, though this is confounded by different treatment approaches such as the routine use of craniospinal irradiation in the older child.[31]

Although CNS AT/RT was not recognized as a separate entity in the Baby POG 1 trial, patients with AT/RT have been stratified on subsequent cooperative group infant brain tumor protocols.[35] In the CCG-9921 study, the 1-year and 5-year EFS rates for AT/RT were 32% and 14%, while survival at 5 years was 29%. Response to chemotherapy was noted in this CCG study.[12] There was some evidence that extent of resection was a prognostic factor, but no other variables were associated with significant differences in outcome. In a consensus report, treatment variables that appeared to be more common in AT/RT survivors were complete resection, early RT, and high-dose chemotherapy.[31] In a report of 4 patients treated according to a North American rhabdomyosarcoma regimen for patients with parameningeal or intracranial disease (utilizing vincristine, adriamycin, cisplatin, cyclophosphamide, actinomycin, craniospinal irradiation, and intrathecal chemotherapy), 3 patients were surviving at the time of the report.[37] Subsequently, several other case reports of successful use of this regimen have been published, and a multi-institutional trial evaluating this approach is under way.[31] Alternatively, the Head Start studies have suggested improved outcome for CNS AT/RT with the addition of high-dose methotrexate to the intensive induction regimen, followed by myeloablative chemotherapy with hematopoietic stem cell rescue.[38] A clinical trial utilizing myeloablative chemotherapy and early focal irradiation following radical surgical resection and high-dose methotrexate containing induction chemotherapy is under development in the COG.

Ependymomas

Ependymomas constitute 18% of CNS tumors in children in the first 3 years of life and 19% of those children who are less than 1 year.[3,4,6] As in older children, local control is the predominant problem; metastatic disease at time of diagnosis or recurrence is unusual but may be more frequent than previously recognized in younger children.

As with infants with medulloblastoma, concern regarding the late effects of irradiation led to attempts to delay or obviate irradiation with chemotherapy. Van Eys demonstrated that long-term survival was possible without irradiation, having treated 5 children with ependymoma with MOPP, with long-term survival reported for 2.[8]

Forty-eight children with ependymoma were enrolled in Baby POG 1.[9] Forty-eight percent had complete or partial responses to initial vincristine and cyclophosphamide chemotherapy. As described previously, children less than 24 months at time of diagnosis received 2 years of chemotherapy, and children between 24 and 36 months received 1 year of chemotherapy prior to irradiation. One-year survival was approximately 90% for both groups.[9] However, there was a significant divergence in 5-year survival between the two groups; 25% for the younger children, compared with 63% for the older children. The survival curves diverged beyond 1 year following diagnosis.[39] Other than age, the only prognostic factor was degree of surgical resection. Five-year survival was 66% for total resection, and 25% for subtotal resection.[10,39] It is likely that this difference in survival is directly related to the longer delay to focal irradiation in the younger children, although biologic tumor differences between the younger and older children cannot be excluded. Of note, salvage therapy was poor following irradiation in those children who progressed on chemotherapy.

Seventy-five children with ependymoma were entered on the CCG-9921 study.[12] Twenty percent were less than 1 year, and 80% between 1 and 3 years. Sixteen percent had leptomeningeal disease at initial diagnosis, a proportion much higher than that currently reported for older children in the modern era of MRI. Eighty percent of the tumors were infratentorial, and 80% underwent a greater than 90% resection. The overall response rate among those that were evaluable with postoperative residual disease was 40%. The overall 1-year PFS was 71%, and 5-year EFS was 32%, with a 5-year overall survival of 58%. Among those that had minimal residual disease and were without metastatic disease, the 5-year EFS was 34%, but 5-year OS was 66%. Two-thirds of 5-year event-free survivors did not receive radiotherapy.

There was some evidence that younger age was an unfavorable prognostic factor, as in the POG study, and incomplete resection was also of prognostic significance. The presence of metastatic disease was not statistically significant, although disseminated patients failed at a nominally higher rate.[12]

In the Head Start studies, 29 children younger than 10 years, of whom 22 were younger than 3 years, were treated with induction and myeloablative chemotherapy as described above. Focal RT was administered following chemotherapy to those patients older than 3 years with posterior fossa tumors regardless of age, and to younger children with residual tumor following chemotherapy and second-look surgery. The 5-year EFS and OS from diagnosis were 12% and 38%, respectively.[41]

In an SFOP study, 73 children under 3 years of age were treated with procarbazine, carboplatin, etoposide, cisplatin, vincristine, and cyclophosphamide. No documented responses to chemotherapy greater than 50% were observed. The 4-year PFS was 22%, and the OS 59%. Twenty-three percent were living 4 years following diagnosis without recourse to irradiation. Two factors associated with favorable outcome were supratentorial location and a complete resection.[42]

The United Kingdom Children's Cancer Study Group/International Society of Paediatric Oncology study CNS9204 utilized a similar strategy, treating children younger than 3 years with primary chemotherapy, RT being reserved for those with recurrent tumors. The 5-year EFS for nonmetastatic patients was 41.8% (30%-52%) and OS was 63% (51%-73%). The median age at irradiation was 3.6 years.[43]

The primary site of recurrence in these studies was local.[12,43] Although salvage with RT was poor on the Baby POG 1 study, on the CCG-9921 study patients with recurrent ependymoma receiving irradiation had a 3-year post-progression survival of 46%, compared with 24% in those that did not.

Recognizing the value of postoperative RT, as well as the potential for decreased neurotoxicity with conformal irradiation, a study at St Jude utilized this modality for patients with localized ependymoma.[44] Eighty-eight patients (median age 2.85 ± 4.5 years) received conformal radiotherapy. Patients were categorized according to extent of tumor grade and tumor location. An age-appropriate neurocognitive battery was administered before and serially after RT.

At a median length of follow-up of 38.2 months (± 16.4 months), the 3-year PFS estimate was 75%.[45] Mean scores on all neurocognitive outcomes were stable and within normal limits, with more than half the cohort tested at or beyond 24 months.[44]

The current COG study is evaluating this approach in children greater than 12 months of age at diagnosis. In addition, in this study the utility of chemotherapy in improving the rate of second-look surgery is being investigated. A critical component of this study is the assessment of the cognitive sequelae of involved-field radiation therapy in both the infratentorial and supratentorial areas.

Choroid Plexus Carcinomas

The majority of choroid plexus carcinomas (CPC) occur in very young children. Recent studies have demonstrated inactivation of *INI1* in as many as 73% of CPC, while choroid plexus papillomas do not have the *INI1* mutations.[46] In addition, CPC have occurred in the setting of families with rhabdoid predisposition syndrome caused by germline inactivation of the *INI1* gene.[45]

In a review study of 75 pediatric cases of CPC reported in the literature, the median age at diagnosis was 26 months. In cases with gross total resection, survival was 84%, compared with 18% survival with subtotal resection.[47] In another study, in 11 consecutive children with CPC, the median age at diagnosis was 26 months. Five of 11 children remained in remission, and 4 of these 5 underwent a gross total tumor resection.[48]

Patients with choroid plexus carcinomas have been entered on infant cooperative group trials. In the Baby POG 1 trial, 8 infants with CPC were enrolled: among 4 patients with measurable postoperative disease, 2 responded to initial chemotherapy. Overall, the PFS was 50% at 3 years.[49] Nine patients were treated on the CCG-9921 study, and 5 had progressive disease, 4 of whom have died. The EFS and OS at 3 years are 33% and 63%, respectively. Of the 4 patients who underwent greater than 90% resection and did not have metastatic disease, 2 progressed and the other 2 were alive without disease progression at 5 years.[12]

In summary, the management of infants with choroid plexus carcinomas, beyond the need to attempt a gross total resection, remains unclear. Although responses have been seen following chemotherapy, there is no definitive evidence of the value of this modality in prolonging survival.[50] Also unclear is the relationship between CPC and rhabdoid tumors, both of which share mutations of the *INI1* gene. Finally, the optimal treatment approach to atypical choroid plexus papillomas, which are reported to have a poorer prognosis than pure papillomas when treated with surgical resection alone, remains unknown.

Malignant Gliomas

High-grade astrocytomas occur relatively less frequently in very young children than in older children and adults, and in some studies appear to have a better prognosis. In the Baby POG 1 study, 18 children with malignant gliomas were enrolled: of 10 with residual tumor following surgery, 6 had partial responses to 2 cycles of vincristine and cyclophosphamide chemotherapy. The PFS rate was 54% at 1 year, 43% at 3 years, and the OS was 50% at 5 years. Neither degree of surgical resection, presence or absence of metastasis, nor pathology influenced survival.[9,10,51] On the CCG-9921 study, 9 patients were treated; the 3-year EFS and OS were 33% and 42%, respectively.[12] On CCG 945, 39 children younger than 24 months were entered and treated with "8-in-1" chemotherapy only. Progression-free survival and survival at 3 years were 36% and

51%, respectively.[52] However, on subsequent review, 14 of these tumors were reclassified as low-grade astrocytomas and had a PFS of 43% and OS of 79% at 5 years, so that the EFS for those with centrally reviewed eligible high-grade histology is now less than 25% at 10 years.[53,54]

Late Effects

The adverse effects of RT in infants with brain tumors have driven treatment strategy as much as has poor survival. In one study of children younger than 36 months treated with postoperative craniospinal irradiation and followed over a long period of time, virtually all patients required extra support in school, and of those individuals of working age, only a small minority have obtained employment.[55] In 29 consecutively diagnosed infants and young children treated for medulloblastoma at St Jude who had received postoperative chemotherapy prior to planned irradiation, the median age at diagnosis was 2.6 years. All surviving patients received irradiation either at the time of progression or at the completion of chemotherapy. All patients lost significant cognitive function during and after therapy.[56]

No data from the large cooperative group studies using chemotherapy to delay or avoid RT are yet available to assess the value of this strategy in improving cognitive outcome. However, in one smaller study of 27 children with posterior fossa tumors diagnosed at younger than 36 months, the neurocognitive developmental outcome was positive among those who were treated with surgery and chemotherapy, with minimal declines in performance across time, while those who received cranial RT demonstrated significant neurocognitive and psychosocial deficits.[57] In another study, 10 children having completed the Head Start 1 protocol without irradiation were evaluated at an average of 37 months following myeloablative chemotherapy and hematopoietic cell rescue. The mean scores for the nonirradiated group of children indicate that they perform within the lower average range of overall intelligence. However, this group of children demonstrated significant deficits within the borderline to impaired range on language skills of expressive picture naming and receptive picture vocabulary.[58]

Summary

The poor prognosis, potential for late sequelae, and the often distinctive biology of infant brain tumors have provided the impetus for investigational effort disproportionate to the relatively small number of cases. Several therapeutic trials investigating the potential of chemotherapy to delay or avoid the use of RT have demonstrated the importance of complete surgical resection in a variety of tumor types and have shown that a proportion of young children with malignant brain tumors can be cured without radiotherapy, but that the majority will still develop progressive disease.

Identification of molecular markers of prognosis is crucial for distinguishing those children requiring only chemotherapy, and for developing new strategies of treatment for those at higher risk. Long-term cognitive studies are mandatory to assess the value of these strategies in minimizing late sequelae.

References

1. Bleyer WA. Epidemiologic impact of children with brain tumors. *Child's Nerv Syst.* 1999;15:758–763.
2. Gurney JG, Ross JA, Wall DA, Bleyer WA, Severson RK, Robison LL. Infant cancer in the US: histology-specific incidence and trends, 1973 to 1992. *J Pediatr Hematol Oncol.* 1997;19:428–432.
3. Rickert CH, Paulus W. Epidemiology of central nervous system tumors in childhood and adolescence based on the new WHO classification. *Child's Nerv Syst.* 2001;17:503–511.
4. Dreifaldt AC, Carlberg M, Hardell L. Increasing incidence rates of childhood malignant diseases in Sweden during the period 1960–1998. *Eur J Cancer.* 2004;40:1351–1360.
5. Mazewski CM, Hudgins RJ, Reisner A, Geyer JR. Neonatal brain tumors: a review. *Semin Perinatol,* 1999;23:286–298.
6. Rivera-Luna R, Medina-Sanson A, Leal-Leal C, et al. Brain tumors in children under 1 year of age: emphasis on the relationship of prognostic factors. *Child's Nerv Syst.* 2003;19:311–314.
7. Di Rocco C, Iannelli A, Ceddia A. Intracranial tumors of the first year of life: a cooperative survey of the 1986–1987 Education Committee of the ISPN. *Child's Nerv Syst.* 1991;7:150–153.
8. Ater JL, van Eys J, Woo SY, Moore B III, Copeland DR, Bruner J. MOPP chemotherapy without irradiation as primary postsurgical therapy for brain tumors in infants and young children. *J Neuro-Oncol.* 1997;32:243–252.
9. Duffner PK, Horowitz ME, Krischer JP, et al. Postoperative chemotherapy and delayed radiation in children less than three years of age with malignant brain tumors. *N Engl J Med.* 1993;328:1725–1731.
10. Duffner PK, Horowitz ME, Krischer JP, et al. The treatment of malignant brain tumors in infants and very young children: an update of the Pediatric Oncology Group experience. *Neuro Oncol.* 1999;1:152–161.
11. Geyer JR, Zeltzer PM, Boyett JM, et al. Survival of infants with primitive neuroectodermal tumors or malignant ependymomas of the CNS treated with eight drugs in 1 day: a report from the Children's Cancer Group. *J Clin Oncol.* 1994;12:1607–1615.
12. Geyer JR, et al. Multiagent chemotherapy and deferred radiotherapy in infants with malignant brain tumors: a report from the Children's Cancer Group. *J Clin Oncol.* 2005;23:7621–7631.
13. Boland I, Vassal G, Morizet J, et al. Busulphan is active against neuroblastoma and medulloblastoma xenografts in athymic mice at clinically achievable plasma drug concentrations. *Br J Cancer.* 1999;79:787–792.
14. Kalifa C, Hartmann O, Demeocq F, et al. High-dose busulfan and thiotepa with autologous bone marrow transplantation in childhood malignant brain tumors: a Phase II study. *Bone Marrow Transplant.* 1992;9:227–233.
15. Gentet JC, Doz F, Bouffet E, et al. Carboplatin and VP 16 in medulloblastoma: a Phase II study of the French Society of Pediatric Oncology (SFOP). *Med Pediatr Oncol.* 1994;23:422–427.
16. Vassal G, Hartmann O, Habrand JL, Pico JL, Lemerle J. Enhanced cutaneous radiation effects following high-dose busulfan therapy. *Cancer Chemother Pharmacol.* 1989;23:117–118.
17. Vassal G, Tranchand B, Valteau-Couanet D, et al. Pharmacodynamics of tandem high-dose melphalan with peripheral blood stem cell transplantation in children with neuroblastoma and medulloblastoma. *Bone Marrow Transplant.* 2001;27:471–477.
18. Grill J, Sainte-Rose C, et al. Treatment of medulloblastoma with postoperative chemotherapy alone: an SFOP prospective trial in young children. *Lancet Oncol.* 2005;6(8):573–580.
19. Kühl J, Beck J, Bode U, et al. International Society of Pediatric Oncology, SIOP XXVII meeting. Montevideo, Uruguay, October 10–14, 1995. Abstract O-67. *Med Pediatr Oncol.* 1995;25:250.
20. Schmandt S, Kuhl J. Chemotherapy as prophylaxis and treatment of meningosis in children less than 3 years of age with medulloblastoma. *J Neuro-Oncol.* 1998;38:187–192.
21. Rutkowski S, Bode U, Deinlein F, et al. Treatment of early childhood medulloblastoma by postoperative chemotherapy alone. *N Engl J Med.* 2005;352 (10):978–986.
22. Mason WP, Grovas A, Halpern S, et al. Intensive chemotherapy and bone marrow rescue for young children with newly diagnosed malignant brain tumors. *J Clin Oncol.* 1998;16:210–221.
23. Chi SN, Gardner S, Levy AS, et al. Newly diagnosed high-risk malignant brain tumors with leptomeningeal dissemination in young children: response to "Head Start" induction chemotherapy intensified with high-dose methotrexate. *J Clin Oncol.* 2004;22:4001–4007.
24. Marec-Berard P, Jouvet A, Thiesse P, Kalifa C, Doz F, Frappaz D. Supratentorial embryonal tumors in children under 5 years of age: an SFOP study of treatment with postoperative chemotherapy alone. *Med Pediatr Oncol.* 2002; 38:83–90.
25. Timmermann B, Kortmann RD, Kuhl J, et al. Role of radiotherapy in supratentorial primitive neuroectodermal tumor in young children: results of the

German HIT-SKK87 and HIT-SKK92 trials. *J Clin Oncol.* 2006;24(10):1554–1560.

26. Fangusaro J, Finlay JL, Sposto R, et al. Intensive chemotherapy followed by consolidative myeloablative chemotherapy with autologous hematopoetic cell rescue (AuHCR) in young children with newly-diagnosed supratentorial PNET: a report of the Head Start I and II experience. *Pediatr Blood Cancer.* 2008;50:312–318.

27. Bhattacharjee M, Hicks J, Langford L, et al. Central nervous system atypical teratoid/rhabdoid tumors of infancy and childhood. *Ultrastruct Pathol.* 1997; 21:369–378.

28. Rorke LB, Packer RJ, Biegel JA. Central nervous system atypical teratoid/rhabdoid tumors of infancy and childhood: definition of an entity. *J Neurosurg.* 1996;85:56–65.

29. Biegel JA, Fogelgren B, Wainwright LM, Zhou JY, Bevan H, Rorke LB. Germline INI1 mutation in a patient with a central nervous system atypical teratoid tumor and renal rhabdoid tumor. *Genes Chromosomes Cancer.* 2000; 28:31–37.

30. Biegel JA, Zhou JY, Rorke LB, Stenstrom C, Wainwright LM, Fogelgren B. Germ-line and acquired mutations of INI1 in atypical teratoid and rhabdoid tumors. *Cancer Res.* 1999;59:74–79.

31. Packer RJ, Biegel JA, Blaney S, et al. Atypical teratoid/rhabdoid tumor of the central nervous system: report on workshop. *J Pediatr Hematol Oncol.* 2002; 24:337–342.

32. Biegel JA, Kalpana G, Knudsen ES, et al. The role of INI1 and the SWI/SNF complex in the development of rhabdoid tumors: meeting summary from the workshop on childhood atypical teratoid/rhabdoid tumors. *Cancer Res.* 2002; 62:323–328.

33. Judkins AR, Mauger J, Ht A, Rorke LB, Biegel JA. Immunohistochemical analysis of hSNF5/INI1 in pediatric CNS neoplasms. *Am J Surg Pathol.* 2004; 28:644–650.

34. Hilden JM, Meerbaum S, Burger P, et al. Central nervous system atypical teratoid/rhabdoid tumor: results of therapy in children enrolled in a registry. *J Clin Oncol.* 2004;22:2877–2884.

35. Hilden JM, Watterson J, Longee DC, et al. Central nervous system atypical teratoid tumor/rhabdoid tumor: response to intensive therapy and review of the literature. *J Neuro-Oncol.* 1998;40:265–275.

36. Burger PC, Yu IT, Tihan T, et al. Atypical teratoid/rhabdoid tumor of the central nervous system: a highly malignant tumor of infancy and childhood frequently mistaken for medulloblastoma: a Pediatric Oncology Group study. *Am J Surg Pathol.* 1998;22:1083–1092.

37. Olsen TA, Bayar E, Kosnik E, et al. Successful treatment of disseminated central nervous system malignant rhabdoid tumor. *J Pediatr Hematol Oncol.* 1995;17:71–75.

38. Gardner SL, Asgharzadeh S, Green A, Horn B, McGowage G, Finlay JL. Intensive induction chemotherapy followed by high dose chemotherapy with autologous hematopoietic progenitor cell rescue in young children newly diagnosed with central nervous system atypical teratoid rhabdoid tumors. *Pediatr Blood Cancer.* 2008;51:235–240.

39. Duffner PK, Krischer JP, Sanford RA, et al. Prognostic factors in infants and very young children with intracranial ependymomas. *Pediatr Neurosurg.* 1998;28:215–222.

40. Zacharoulis S, Levy A, Chi SN, et al. Outcome for young children newly diagnosed with ependymoma, treated with intensive induction chemotherapy followed by myeloablative chemotherapy and autologous stem cell rescue. *Pediatr Blood Cancer.* 2007;49(1):34–40.

41. Grill J, Le Deley MC, Gambarelli D, et al. Postoperative chemotherapy without irradiation for ependymoma in children under 5 years of age: a multicenter trial of the French Society of Pediatric Oncology. *J Clin Oncol.* 2001;19: 1288–1296.

42. Grundy RG, Wilne SA, Weston CL, et al. Primary postoperative chemotherapy without radiotherapy for intracranial ependymoma in children: the UKCCSG/SIOP prospective study. *Lancet Oncol.* 2007;8(8):696–705.

43. Merchant TE, Mulhern RK, Krasin MJ, et al. Preliminary results from a Phase II trial of conformal radiation therapy and evaluation of radiation-related CNS effects for pediatric patients with localized ependymoma. *J Clin Oncol.* 2004;22:3156–3162.

44. Gessi M, Giangaspero F, Pietsch T. Atypical teratoid/rhabdoid tumors and choroid plexus tumors: when genetics "surprise" pathology. *Brain Pathol.* 2003;13:409–414.

45. Mueller W, Eum JH, Lass U, et al. No evidence of hSNF5/INI1 point mutations in choroid plexus papilloma. *Neuropathol Appl Neurobiol.* 2004;30:304–307.

46. Fitzpatrick LK, Aronson LJ, Cohen KJ. Is there a requirement for adjuvant therapy for choroid plexus carcinoma that has been completely resected? *J Neuro-Oncol.* 2002;57:123–126.

47. St Clair SK, Humphreys RP, Pillay PK, Hoffman HJ, Blaser SI, Becker LE. Current management of choroid plexus carcinoma in children. *Pediatr Neurosurg.* 1991;17:225–233.

48. Duffner PK, Kun LE, Burger PC, et al. Postoperative chemotherapy and delayed radiation in infants and very young children with choroid plexus carcinomas. The Pediatric Oncology Group experience. *Pediatr Neurosurg.* 1995; 22:189–196.

49. Allen J, Wisoff J, Helson L, Pearce J, Arenson E. Choroid plexus carcinoma: responses to chemotherapy alone in newly diagnosed young children. *J Neuro-Oncol.* 1992;12:69–74.

50. Duffner PK, Krischer JP, Burger PC, et al. Treatment of infants with malignant gliomas: the Pediatric Oncology Group experience. *J Neuro-Oncol.* 1996;28: 245–256.

51. Geyer JR, Finlay JL, Boyett JM, et al. Survival of infants with malignant astrocytomas: a report from the Children's Cancer Group. *Cancer.* 1995;75:1045–1050.

52. Fouladi M, Hunt DL, Pollack IF, et al. Outcome of children with centrally reviewed low-grade gliomas treated with chemotherapy with or without radiotherapy on Children's Cancer Group high-grade glioma study CCG-945. *Cancer.* 2003;98:1243–1252.

53. Batra V, Sposto R, Geyer JR, Allen J, Pollack I, Finlay J. Long-term outcome for children less than six years of age with diagnosis of consensus reviewed high-grade gliomas: a report of the CCG-945 study. *Neuro Oncol.* 2004;6:450.

54. Kiltie AE, Lashford LS, Gattamaneni HR. Survival and late effects in medulloblastoma patients treated with craniospinal irradiation under three years old. *Med Pediatr Oncol.* 1997;28:348–354.

55. Walter AW, Mulhern RK, Gajjar A, et al. Survival and neurodevelopmental outcome of young children with medulloblastoma at St Jude Children's Research Hospital. *J Clin Oncol.* 1999;17:3720–3728.

56. Copeland DR, deMoor C, Moore BD III, Ater JL. Neurocognitive development of children after a cerebellar tumor in infancy: a longitudinal study. *J Clin Oncol.* 1999;17:3476–3486.

57. Sands SA, van Gorp WG, Finlay JL. Pilot neuropsychological findings from a treatment regimen consisting of intensive chemotherapy and bone marrow rescue for young children with newly diagnosed malignant brain tumors. *Child's Nerv Syst.* 1998;14:587–589.

CHAPTER 21

Choroid Plexus Tumors

Johannes E. A. Wolff and Jonathan L. Finlay

Biology

The choroid plexus develops during the eighth week of embryonal development along with the ependymal lining from neuroectodermal stem cells into discrete tissue with epithelial morphology and function. With an incidence of 1 to 3 cases per 10 million people per year,[1] choroid plexus tumors are rare, even when compared with the absolute frequency of other central nervous system (CNS) malignancies of childhood. However, when the small size of the originating tissue is considered, its predilection to cancerous development may be considered to be quite high. In fact, in the neonatal period, choroid plexus tumors are the most prevalent brain tumors. More than half of choroid plexus tumors are diagnosed in the first year of life. To date, it remains unclear why choroid plexus cells tend to develop tumors, but numerous pieces of the puzzle are already known. Choroid plexus tumors were the first experimental model in which virally associated tumor development was investigated. Simian virus 40 (SV40)–infected rodents develop choroid plexus tumors.[2,3] Choroid plexus cells transform in cell culture to a malignant phenotype when infected with SV40.[4] The T antigen of the virus binds to tumor suppressor genes such as *p53* and *pRB*. Involvement of the *p53* tumor suppressor gene is further suggested by the occurrence of cases of choroid plexus carcinoma[5,6] and cases of choroid plexus papilloma in families with Li-Fraumeni syndrome.[7] It remains questionable if SV40 infections are the cause of the majority of choroid plexus tumors in humans. On the one hand, SV40 has been found in high frequency in these tumors,[8–11] while it has not been found in human leukemic cells.[12] The experimental assessment of a causal relationship was in fact accomplished unintentionally; poliomyelitis vaccines had been contaminated for many years with SV40, but no increase in incidence of choroid plexus tumors was subsequently observed.[13,14] The connection might still be true, if the sensitivity of choroid plexus tumors cells is restricted specifically to the prenatal period. On the other hand, the high frequency of SV40 in choroid plexus tumors might only reflect an organotopic viral feature, but the tumors may be related to other causes. A link to the X chromosome is supported by 2 patients with choroid plexus papilloma and Aicardi syndrome.[15,16] *hSNF5/INI1* point mutations are found frequently in choroid plexus carcinoma[17] but not in choroid plexus papilloma.[18] This pathway has been most frequently associated with CNS atypical teratoid/rhabdoid tumors.[19]

Pathology

The 2007 edition of the World Health Organization classification[20] recognized choroid plexus papilloma as grade I, atypical choroid plexus tumors as grade II, and choroid plexus carcinoma as grade III tumors, defined by conventional light microscopy. These tumors may develop from the choroid plexus of the lateral and third ventricles (supratentorially) or from the fourth ventricle (infratentorially). They may rarely also develop wholly within the brain parenchyma. Lateral and third ventricular tumors are more frequent in infants and more frequently highly malignant, while tumors of the fourth ventricle are more common in the older age spectrum, and with a lower-grade histology. The papilloma is typically a well-described papillary intraventricular mass fed by one, or very few, major blood vessels from the choroid plexus or brain adjacent to it. This tumor does not infiltrate the surrounding tissue. On light microscopy, it is composed of delicate fibrovascular connective tissue fronds covered by a single layer of uniform cuboidal to columnar epithelial cells with round or oval, basally situated monomorphic nuclei. Mitotic activity, brain invasion, and necrosis are absent.[20] The carcinoma is fed by numerous blood vessels recruited from the surrounding normal brain tissue. On histology it shows frank signs of malignancy, including nuclear pleomorphism, frequent mitoses, high nuclear-to-cytoplasmic ratios, increased cellular density, blurring of the papillary pattern with poorly structured sheets of tumor cells, necrotic areas, and often diffuse brain invasion.[20] Atypical choroid plexus papillomas have features in between the 2 other entities. The most important differentiating feature from papillomas is the presence of mitoses. With immunohistochemical staining, choroid plexus carcinomas express carcinoembryonic antigen, platelet derived growth factor receptor,[21] and CD44.[22]

Choroid plexus papillomas express more frequently pre-albumin,[23] survivin,[24] and the S100 protein. In one study, average labeling indices with MIB-1, a proliferation marker, were 14% in carcinomas and 3.7% in papillomas.[25] Metastases occur mostly through the cerebrospinal fluid to the spine, to the ventricles or to the subarachnoidal spaces. The tumors metastasize through the bloodstream only rarely, in which case they primarily are reported in the bones or lung parenchyma. The frequency of metastases is higher in infratentorial tumors and in choroid plexus carcinomas. However, numerous reports have also described metastases from papillomas.[26] The development of a tumor from a benign to a more malignant histology has been reported.[27] Furthermore, in the authors' experience, carcinomas treated with aggressive chemotherapy have been found upon second surgical resection of residual tumor to consist entirely of nonmalignant papilloma.

Clinical and Radiographic Diagnosis

Choroid plexus tumors present most frequently with increased intracranial pressure, due to their primarily intraventricular location. Since most of these tumors occur in the first year of life, the most frequent signs are excessive head growth and a distended anterior fontanel. In older patients, headache and vomiting can be the presenting symptoms. Depending upon the tumor location, hemiparesis, cranial nerve pareses, ataxia, seizures, and other signs or symptoms might be also be presenting features. A lumbar puncture must be avoided at least until neuroimaging is completed to rule out hydrocephalus. The tumor appears on brain computed tomography or magnetic resonance imaging studies as a highly contrast-enhancing space-occupying mass in the ventricles or the cerebello-pontine angle. Despite infiltration, the margins of the lesion appear fairly sharp between contrast-enhancing tumor and normal tissue. Differential diagnoses may include echinococcal hydatid cyst,[28] bilateral choroid plexus hyperplasia, and other tumors.[29] Similar to normal choroid plexus, the lesions are positive in sestamibi single-photon emission computed tomography imaging studies.[30] Positron emission tomography can differentiate between papilloma and carcinoma.[31,32]

Treatment

Surgery, irradiation, and chemotherapy have been used to treat choroid plexus tumors. However, the evidence for radiation therapy and chemotherapy is limited. Completeness of surgical resection is considered to be the most significant favorable predictive factor,[33] and it is generally believed that it is of utmost importance to accomplish as complete a resection as is feasible, consistent with preservation of neurologic function. The tumor is known for its associated high risk of intraoperative hemorrhage. Presurgical cerebral angiography and even embolization may be considered for a large lesion that is radiographically suspicious for a choroid plexus

tumor. Intraoperatively, seeking out and ligating the feeder vessel prior to resection has been recommended.[34,35] In case of residual tumor, second surgery, including resection of metastases, is indicated.[36] Once complete resection has been achieved, choroid plexus papilloma rarely recurs, and further treatment is not necessary. For choroid plexus carcinoma, following a gross total resection of tumor and in the setting of no metastatic disease, the need for further therapy is controversial.[37–39] Irradiation has generally proven to offer a survival advantage for children older than 3 years in a retrospective study.[38] The field of irradiation follows recommendation for medulloblastoma, utilizing craniospinal irradiation to 36 Gy, with boost to the primary tumor site to a maximum dose of 59.4 Gy. There is little evidence to support craniospinal irradiation in children younger than 2.5 years; because of the associated significant late sequelae and secondary malignancies, it is not recommended in this age group. Chemotherapy remains the only option after surgery for children with incompletely resectable and/or metastatic choroid plexus carcinoma in this age group. Various chemotherapy protocols have been reported,[33,39–42] predominantly including 2 or more of the drugs vincristine, etoposide, cyclophosphamide, carboplatin, cisplatin, and ifosphamide. The overall response rate is about 20%, but the number of patients reported following treatment with each of these protocols is too small for meaningful comparisons. It is also unclear if these responses translate into better survival. As an additional benefit from chemotherapy, a change in tumor texture has been reported: tumors that were soft, highly vascular, and incompletely resectable prior to chemotherapy became resectable after chemotherapy.[42,43]

The Societé Internationale d'Oncologie Pédiatrique is currently supporting an international study of choroid plexus tumors. All patients with these tumors may be registered on the study, with required central review of pathology. Maximal possible resection including second surgery is recommended for all tumors. World Health Organization grade I histology tumors (papillomas) are followed with observation and imaging evaluation only. The study recommends that grade III tumors (carcinomas) be treated with a prescribed 3-drug chemotherapy protocol, randomizing patients to either a cyclophosphamide-containing or a carboplatin-containing regimen (Figure 21-1). Radiation therapy is recommended for patients older than 3 years with carcinomas.

Prognosis

Depending on the histology and the treatment, the prognosis is very different among choroid plexus tumors. Patients with completely resected choroid plexus papillomas should enjoy almost 100% cure rates without any additional therapy. A metastatic choroid plexus carcinoma, which cannot be resected and is treated with neither irradiation nor chemotherapy, is rapidly fatal. All other cases lie in between those 2 extremes. Completely resected choroid

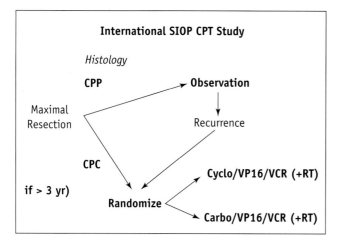

Figure 21-1 International Societé Internationale d'Oncologie Pédiatrique Choroid Plexus Tumours study.

plexus carcinomas, treated with chemotherapy alone or with irradiation in older children, may achieve from 50% to 85% rates of cure. The more frequent situation of a young child younger than 3 years with a partially resected nonmetastatic choroid plexus carcinoma, for whom intensive chemotherapy and other treatment modalities such as delayed surgical resection and possible focal irradiation are planned, should be estimated to have about a 3% to 40% chance of prolonged progression-free survival. The outcome for children with nonresectable metastatic disease has been generally very poor, although there are some anecdotal reports of long-term survivors, usually having been treated with intensive chemotherapy and either initial or delayed craniospinal irradiation. It remains to be demonstrated whether current approaches utilizing myeloablative chemotherapy with autologous hematopoietic cell rescue, as have been utilized with some degree of success in young children with other malignant brain tumors, will benefit young children with incompletely resected or metastatic choroid plexus carcinomas.

References

1. Janisch W, Staneczek W. Primary tumors of the choroid plexus: frequency, localization and age. *Zentralbl Allg Pathol.* 1989;135:235–240.
2. Kirschstein RL, Gerber P. Ependymomas produced after intracerebral inoculation of SV40 into newborn hamsters. *Nature.* 1962;195:299–300.
3. Enjoji M, Iwaki T, Hara H, Sakai H, Nawata H, Watanabe T. Establishment and characterization of choroid plexus carcinoma cell line: connection between choroid plexus and immune systems. *Jpn J Cancer Res.* 1996;87:893–899.
4. Shein HM, Enders JF. Transformation induced by simian virus 40 in human renal cell cultures. *Proc Natl Acad Sci USA.* 1962;48:1164–1172.
5. Garber JE, Burke EM, Lavally BL, et al. Choroid plexus tumors in the breast cancer-sarcoma syndrome. *Cancer.* 1990;66(12):2658–2660.
6. Yuasa H, Tokito S, Tokunaga M. Primary carcinoma of the choroid plexus in Li-Fraumeni syndrome: case report. *Neurosurgery.* 1993;32(1):131–133.
7. Kleihues P, Schauble B, zur Hausen A, Esteve J, Ohgaki H. Tumours associated with p53 germline mutations: a synopsis of 91 families. *Am J Pathol.* 1997;150.1=15.
8. Tabuchi K, Kirsch WM, Van Buskirk JJ. Immunocytochemical evidence of SV 40–related T antigen in two human brain tumours of ependymal origin. *Acta Neurochir (Wien).* 1978;43(3–4):239–249.
9. Bergsagel DJ, Finegold MJ, Butel JS, Kupsky WJ, Garcea R. DNA sequences similar to those of simian virus 40 in ependymomas and choroid plexus tumors of childhood. *N Engl J Med.* 1992;326:988–993.
10. Lednicky JA, Garcea RL, Bergsagel DJ, Butel JS. Natural simian virus 40 strains are present in human choroid plexus and ependymoma tumors. *Virology.* 1995;12:710–717.
11. Martini F, Iaccheri L, Lazzarin L, et al. SV40 early region and large T antigen in human brain tumor, peripheral blood cell, and sperm fluids from healthy individuals. *Cancer Res.* 1996;56:4820–4825.
12. David H, Mendoza S, Konishi T, Miller CW. Simian virus 40 is present in human lymphomas and normal blood. *Cancer Lett.* 2001;162:57–64.
13. Mortimer EA, Lepow ML, Gold E, Robbins FC, Burton GJ, Fraumeni JF. Long-term follow-up of persons inadvertently inoculated with SV40 as neonates. *N Engl J Med.* 1981;305:1517–1518.
14. Carroll-Pankhurst C, Engels EA, Strickler HD, Goedert JJ, Wagner J, Mortimer EA Jr. Thirty-five-year mortality following receipt of SV40-contaminated polio vaccine during the neonatal period. *Br J Cancer.* 2001;85:1295–1297.
15. Hamano K, Matsubara T, Shibata S, et al. Aicardi syndrome accompanied by auditory disturbance and multiple brain tumors. *Brain Dev.* 1991;13:438–441.
16. Trifiletti RR, Incorpora G, Polizzi A, Cocuzza MD, Bolan EA, Parano E. Aicardi syndrome with multiple tumors: a case report with literature review. *Brain Dev.* 1995;17:283–285.
17. Gessi M, Giangaspero F, Pietsch T. Atypical teratoid/rhabdoid tumors and choroid plexus tumors: when genetics "surprise" pathology. *Brain Pathol.* 2003;13:409–414.
18. Mueller W, Eum JH, Lass U, et al. No evidence of hSNF5/INI1 point mutations in choroid plexus papilloma. *Neuropathol Appl Neurobiol.* 2004;30:304–307.
19. Judkins AR, Mauger J, Ht A, Rorke LB, Biegel JA. Immunohistochemical analysis of hSNF5/INI1 in pediatric CNS neoplasms. *Am J Surg Pathol.* 2004;28:644–650.
20. Louis DN, Ohgaki H, Wiestler OD, Cavenee WK, eds. *Pathology and Genetics of Tumours of the Nervous System.* 4th ed. Lyon, France: IARC Press; 2007
21. Nupponen NN, Paulsson J, Jeibmann A, et al. Platelet-derived growth factor receptor expression and amplification in choroid plexus carcinomas. *Mod Pathol.* 2008;21(3):265–270.
22. Varga Z, Vajtai I, Marino S, Schauble B, Yonekawa Y, Aguzzi A. Tubular adenoma of the choroid plexus: evidence for glandular differentiation of the neuroepithelium. *Pathol Res Pract.* 1996;192:840–844.
23. Matsushima T, Inoue T, Takeshita I, Fukui M, Iwaki T, Kitamoto T. Choroid plexus papilloma: an immunohistochemical study with particular reference to the coexpression of prealbumin. *Neurosurgery.* 1988;23:384–389.
24. Altura RA, Olshefski RS, Jiang Y, Boue DR. Nuclear expression of survivin in paediatric ependymomas and choroid plexus tumours correlates with morphologic tumour grade. *Br J Cancer.* 2003;89:1743–1749.
25. Vajtai I, Varga Z, Aguzzi A. MIB-1 immunoreactivity reveals different labeling in low-grade and in malignant epithelial neoplasms of the choroid plexus. *Histopathology.* 1996;29:147–151.
26. Domingues RC, Taveras JM, Reimer P, Rosen B. Foramen magnum choroid plexus papilloma with drop metastases to the lumbar spine. *Am J Neuroradiol.* 1991;12:564–565.
27. Jebmann A, Wrede B, Peters O, Wolff JE, Paulus W, Hasselblatt M. Malignant progression in choroid plexus papillomas. *J Neurosurg.* 2007;107(3 suppl):199–202.
28. Shervani RK, Abrari A, Jayrajpuri ZS, Srivastava VK. Intracranial hydatidosis: report of a case diagnosed on cerebrospinal fluid cytology. *Acta Cytol.* 2003;47:506–508.
29. McIver JI, Link MJ, Giannini C, Cohen-Gadol AA, Driscoll C. Choroid plexus papilloma and meningioma: coincidental posterior fossa tumors: case report and review of the literature. *Surg Neurol.* 2003;60(4):360–365.
30. Wolff JE, Myles, Pinto A, Riegel JE, Angyalfi S, Kloiber R. Detection of choroid plexus carcinoma with Tc-99m sestamibi: case report and review of the literature. *Med Pediatr Oncol.* 2001;36(2):323–325.
31. Sunada I, Tsuyuguchi N, Hara M, Ochi H. 18F-FDG and 11C-methionine PET in choroid plexus papilloma-report of three cases. *Radiat Med.* 2002;20(2):97–100.
32. McEvoy AW, Galloway M, Revesz T, Kitchen ND. Metastatic choroid plexus papilloma: a case report. *J Neuro-Oncol.* 2002;56(3):241–246.
33. Wolff JE, Sajedi M, Brant R, Coppes MJ, Egeler RM. Choroid plexus tumours. *Br J Cancer.* 2002;87:1086–1091.
34. Gupta N, Jay V, Blaser S, Humphreys RP, Rutka JT. Choroid plexus papillomas and carcinomas. In: Youmans JR, ed. *Neurological Surgery: A Comprehensive Reference Guide to the Diagnosis and Management of Neurological Problems.* Philadelphia: Saunders; 1996:2547–2548.
35. Sanford RA, Donahue DJ. Intraventricular tumors. In: Marlin AE, ed. *Intraventricular Tumors.* Philadelphia: Saunders; 1994:31:403–404.
36. Wrede B, Liu P, Ater J, Wolff JE. Second surgery and the prognosis of choroid plexus carcinoma: results of a meta-analysis of individual cases. *Anticancer Res.* 2005;25:4429–4434.
37. Fitzpatrick LK, Aronson LJ, Cohen IQ. Is there a requirement for adjuvant therapy for choroid plexus carcinoma that has been completely resected? *J Neuro-Oncol.* 2002;57:123–126.
38. Wolff JE, Sajedi M, Coppes MJ, Anderson RA, Egeler ME. Radiation therapy and survival in choroid plexus carcinoma. *Lancet.* 1999;353:2126.
39. Wrede B, Liu P, Wolff JE. Chemotherapy improves the survival of patients with choroid plexus carcinoma. *J Neuro-Oncol.* 2007;85(3):345–351.

40. Duffner PK, Kun LE, Burger PC, et al. Postoperative chemotherapy and delayed radiation in infants and very young children with choroid plexus carcinomas: the Pediatric Oncology Group experience. *Pediatr Neurosurg.* 1995; 22:189–196.

41. Allen J, Wisoff J, Helson L, Pearce J, Aronsen E. Choroid plexus carcinoma: responses to chemotherapy alone in newly diagnosed young children. *J Neuro-Oncol.* 1992;12:69–71.

42. Geyer JR, Sposto R, Jennings M, et al; Children's Cancer Group. Multiagent chemotherapy and deferred radiotherapy in infants with malignant brain tumors: a report from the Children's Cancer Group. *J Clin Oncol.* 2005; 23(30):7621–7631.

43. Souweidane MM, Johnson JH Jr, Lis E. Volumetric reduction of a choroid plexus carcinoma using preoperative chemotherapy. *J Neuro-Oncol.* 1999; 43(2):167–171.

Germ Cell Tumors of the Central Nervous System

Eric Bouffet, Blanca Diez, and Stewart J. Kellie

Introduction

Germ cell tumors of the central nervous system (CNS) are a heterogeneous group of tumors that constitute approximately 3% of primary pediatric CNS tumors in Europe and the United States but a far higher percentage in Japan and Taiwan. These tumors commonly develop within the suprasellar or pineal regions but may also be found in the basal ganglia, spinal cord, or nonmidline structures. These tumors occur most commonly in the first and second decades of life and demonstrate a higher incidence in males compared to females.

Mounting evidence of the sensitivity of CNS germ cell tumors to chemotherapy has sparked international controversy concerning treatment design. Recently completed and current clinical trials seek to maximize survival and minimize adverse treatment-related toxicities and late sequelae by carefully refining risk group and prognostic

classifications, treatment intensity, and defining the roles of surgery, radiation therapy, and chemotherapy.

The aim of this chapter is to review the clinical features of CNS germ cell tumors, to explore areas of diagnostic difficulty, and to examine the evidence underscoring international debate about optimal treatment. The chapter also aims to examine the contemporary clinical and therapeutic hypotheses being tested in Europe and North America, in order to provide insight into current controversies in this important area.

Incidence and Epidemiology

One of the most striking characteristics of CNS germ cell tumors is the evidence of a significantly higher incidence in Asian countries compared with Western countries (Figure 22-1). These tumors account for less than 3% of all intracranial malignancies before age 20 in the West, but

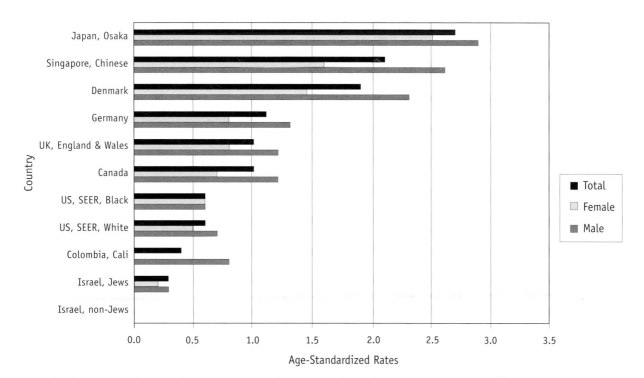

Figure 22-1 International variation in intracranial germ cell tumors (ages 0–14). Age-standardized rates (per million).

compose up to 9% to 15% of all primary brain tumors in children in East Asia, reflecting a 3- to 4-fold higher incidence than in the West.[1,2]

In the United States, the Surveillance, Epidemiology, and End Results program data suggest a steady increase in the average annual incidence between 1975 and 1995.[3] The reason for this increase in incidence is not clear, but it may be due in part to previous underreporting.

The primary CNS germ cell tumors affect mostly teenagers and young adults with a median age at diagnosis of 13 to 15 years according to published series or data from registries. Male predominance is consistent throughout all registries. The age distribution of pure germinomas and the remaining group of "mixed malignant germ cell tumors" (otherwise called "nongerminomatous germ cell tumors") is illustrated in Figures 22-2 and 22-3. Overall, the male-to-female ratio of CNS germ cell tumors is 2 to 1 to 2.5 to 1; however, this sex predilection is influenced by tumor location within the CNS, with most pineal region tumors occurring in boys (male-to-female ratios ranging from 5.5 to 12.6), and tumors in the suprasellar region are reported to be within a range from slightly more common in girls up to 2.4 times more common in boys. The nongerminomatous germ cell tumors are more common in boys than are pure germinomas.[4–8]

Pathology

Germ cell tumors arising in the CNS are homologues of germinal neoplasms arising in the gonads and at other extragonadal sites. Most of the current classifications of germ cell tumors arising in either gonadal or extragonadal locations are modifications of Teilum's concepts[9] (Figure 22-4). Approximately 50% to 65% of CNS germ cell tumors are pure germinomas. Intracranial germ cell tumors often demonstrate mixed histological features, with only germinomas and teratomas likely to be seen in "pure" form, so that features of mixed germ cell tumors are evident in approximately 30% of cases. Mixed germ cell tumors demonstrate a range of combinations, including germinoma, teratoma (mature or immature), yolk sac tumor, embryonal carcinoma, and choriocarcinoma. Thus, the commonly used term "nongerminomatous germ cell tumors" to describe those tumors other than pure germinomas is a misnomer and should perhaps be replaced by the more accurate "mixed malignant germ cell tumors."

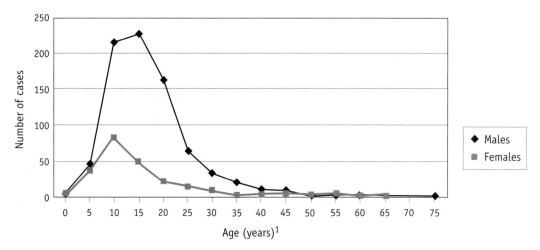

Figure 22-2 Intracranial germinoma: Age at diagnosis.

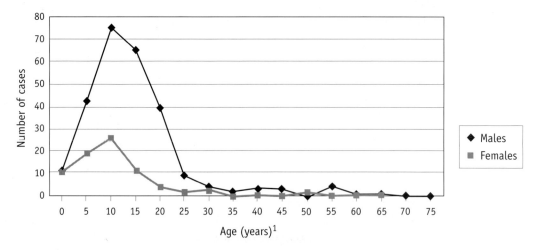

Figure 22-3 Intracranial nongerminomatous germ cell tumors: Age at diagnosis.

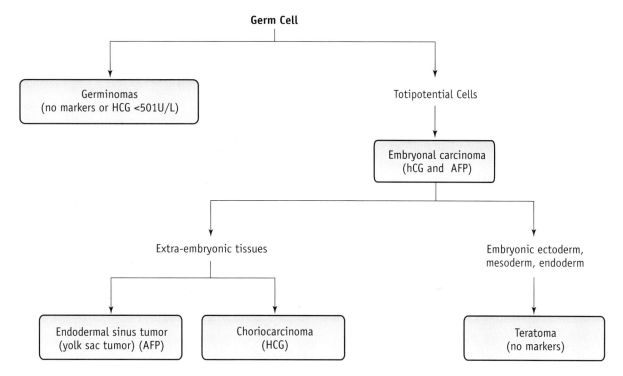

Germ Cell

Germinomas
(no markers or HCG <501U/L)

Totipotential Cells

Embryonal carcinoma
(hCG and AFP)

Extra-embryonic tissues

Embryonic ectoderm,
mesoderm, endoderm

Endodermal sinus tumor
(yolk sac tumor) (AFP)

Choriocarcinoma
(HCG)

Teratoma
(no markers)

Figure 22-4 Classification scheme of germ cell tumors, based on Teilum's classification. AFP, alpha-fetoprotein; HCG, human chorionic gonadotropin.

Immunohistochemical studies may be necessary to identify the various tissue elements accurately, and characteristic staining patterns are described in Table 22-1.

Most European and North American investigators segregate malignant CNS germ cell tumors into only 2 therapeutic categories—germinomas and a heterogeneous group called "nongerminomatous germ cell tumors." Japanese researchers commonly stratify patients into 3 therapeutic groups, thus complicating interregional analysis of outcomes.[10]

Diagnosis and Staging of Central Nervous System Germ Cell Tumors

Tissue Diagnosis Versus Indirect Evidence

The necessity of obtaining tumor tissue for histopathologic diagnosis of CNS germ cell tumors is controversial in patients with raised serum or cerebrospinal fluid (CSF)

tumor markers (alpha-fetoprotein, AFP, or the beta subunit of human chorionic gonadotropin, βHCG) and neuroimaging evidence of a midline brain tumor. There is a broad consensus among investigators associated with European and North American CNS germ cell tumor trials that these patients can be successfully managed without a neurosurgical procedure to obtain tissue, because current therapeutic approaches are uniform among patients with abnormally elevated CSF or serum tumor markers.

Some Japanese protocols rely on histopathology in patients with evidence of elevated tumor markers because patients are stratified into 1 of 3 risk strata at diagnosis based on the tissue elements seen in patients with mixed germ cell tumors.[10] There is wide consensus that tissue for diagnosis should be obtained from patients with neuroimaging evidence of a CNS tumor without evidence of elevated tumor markers. Exceptions to this rule include patients with characteristic neuroimaging features associated with low

Table 22-1

Immunohistochemical profiles of central nervous system germ cell tumors.

	Alpha-fetoprotein	Human Chorionic Gonadotropin	Human Placental Lactogen	Placental Alkaline Phosphatase	Cytokeratins
Germinoma	−	+/−	−	++++	−
Teratoma	+	−	−	−	+
Yolk sac tumor	++++	−	−	+/−	+
Embryonal carcinoma	−/+	−/+	−	+	+++
Choriocarcinoma	−	++++	+	+/−	+

levels of HCGβ secretion (less than 50 IU/ml) in CSF or serum[11-13] and in patients with bifocal tumors involving the pineal gland and the suprasellar region; the latter appearance is highly suggestive of bifocal pure germinoma.[14]

Prognostic Staging/Risk Classification

Central nervous system germ cell tumors can disseminate throughout the neuraxis via the CSF pathways, and comprehensive staging investigations, including magnetic resonance imaging (MRI) scans of both the brain and the spine, and CSF cytology, are essential for determining extent of disease, estimating prognosis, and planning treatment, particularly when focal radiation therapy is planned. Table 22-2 represents one example of a comprehensive risk classification of CNS germ cell tumors used widely in Japan and North America.

Cerebrospinal fluid collection is mandatory, except where contraindicated by the presence of hydrocephalus or other risk factors for cerebral herniation. Cerebrospinal fluid should be submitted for cytological examination for evidence of tumor cells and also for assays for tumor biomarkers. Concentrations of AFP and βHCG in serum and CSF often do not correlate predictably.[15] Comparisons between ventricular and lumbar CSF biomarkers have not been systematically studied to date.

Bifocal Central Nervous System Germ Cell Tumors

Fifteen percent to 25% of CNS germ cell tumors, mostly germinomas, present with bifocal tumors located in the pineal gland and suprasellar region.[14] No agreement exists about the treatment of patients with these tumors. Some investigators regard bifocal disease as evidence of metastatic disease warranting craniospinal axis irradiation in addition to chemotherapy, whereas others regard bifocal disease a unique variant of loco-regional disease warranting, at most, regional irradiation.

Identifying Malignancy: The Role of Tumor Markers

One of the most significant issues to be clarified during the initial patient evaluation is to determine whether malignant elements are present within the germ cell tumor. Traditionally, histopathologic examination or the identification of tumor marker excretion in serum or CSF is mandatory; however, AFP and βHCG can be raised in a variety of unrelated circumstances that may create diagnostic uncertainty (Table 22-3).

Alpha-fetoprotein is synthesized by yolk sac cells and is a marker of yolk sac (otherwise known as endodermal sinus) elements in a germ cell tumor, while βHCG is associated with choriocarcinoma cells or syncytiotrophoblastic giant cells. Tumors with mixed histology often are associated with an elevation of AFP and/or βHCG. Mature teratomas and pure germinomas do not usually secrete tumor markers. However, some germinomas with syncytiotrophoblastic elements may secrete relatively low levels of βHCG (conventionally stated as being less than 50 mIU/ml) and still be broadly categorized within the "germinoma" category[11-13] (Table 22-4).

Alpha-fetoprotein is a major physiologic plasma protein in the developing fetus, synthesized from all 3 fetal layers, reaching a peak concentration at around 15 weeks of gestation and declining thereafter.[17] Physiologic concentrations of AFP in infants do not reach "adult" normal levels until about 8 months of age.[18] These high, but physiologic, levels can confuse the evaluation of infants with suspected CNS germ cell tumors, and care is required to not misinterpret an apparently elevated serum AFP con-

Table 22-2
Risk classification of intracranial germ cell tumors.

	Standard Risk	Intermediate Risk	High Risk
Tumor pathology	Pure germinoma Mature teratoma	Germinoma with syncytiotrophoblastic giant cells Multifocal germinoma Immature teratoma Germinoma with immature teratoma	Choriocarcinoma Yolk sac tumor Embryonal carcinoma Mixed germ cell tumor with above elements
Metastatic disease	Localized, nonmetastatic	Localized, nonmetastatic	Disseminated disease (MRI/CSF cytology)
Serum markers	Negative	AFP negative HCGβ < 50 mIU/ml	Elevated βHCG and AFP HCGβ > 50 mIU/ml
CSF markers	Negative	HCGβ < 50 mIU/ml	HCGβ > 50 mIU/ml and/or AFP positive

Abbreviations: CSF, cerebrospinal fluid; βHCG, beta human chorionic gonadotropin; AFP, alpha-fetoprotein; MRI, magnetic resonance imaging.

Table 22-3

Raised alpha-fetoprotein and beta-human chorionic gonadotropin in nonmalignant conditions.[a]

Raised alpha-fetoprotein (AFP) in nonmalignant conditions

Hepatic pathology
- Extrahepatic biliary atresia
- Neonatal hepatitis
- Viral hepatitis, acute or chronic
- Liver cirrhosis
- Liver abscess

Hereditary disorders
- Hereditary AFP persistence
- Ataxia telangiectasia
- Hereditary tyrosinaemia, type 1

Other
- Systemic lupus erythematosus
- Hirschsprung disease
- Infancy

Raised βHCG in nonmalignant disorders

- Very uncommon
- Chronic renal insufficiency
- Systemic lupus erythematosus

[a]Adapted from Schneider et al.[16]

Table 22-4
Tumor marker secretion.

	AFP	HCG	PLAP
Germinoma	−	(+)/−	+
Embryonal carcinoma	+	+/−	−
Yolk sac tumor	++	−	−
Choriocarcinoma	−	++	−
Teratoma: Mature	−	−	−
Immature	+/−	−	−
Mixed germ cell tumor	+/−	+/−	+/−

Abbreviations: AFP, alpha-fetoprotein; HCG; human chorionic gonadotropin; (+), HCG concentrations < 50 mIU/ml are considered to be consistent with the diagnosis of germinoma in patients with normal AFP concentrations; PLAP, placental alkaline phosphatase.

centration as a marker of malignancy. More recently, physiologic levels of CSF AFP have been determined in normal infants, demonstrating that adult "normal" values in CSF are not achieved until at least beyond 2 to 3 months of corrected gestational age[19] (Figure 22-5).

Clinical Presentation of Central Nervous System Germ Cell Tumors

Initial signs and symptoms of CNS germ cell tumors are influenced by location, size, extent of pituitary dysfunction, and the presence or absence of hydrocephalus. Pineal tumors are mostly associated with manifestations of increased cranial pressure due to obstruction of the cerebral aqueduct, and Parinaud's ocular signs due to involvement of the tectal plate.

Tumors located in the suprasellar compartment often present with endocrinopathy, particularly diabetes insipidus and visual disturbances.[5–7] Diabetes insipidus is a common presenting feature of suprasellar tumors but can also occasionally be observed in patients with pineal region tumors without neuroimaging evidence of overt suprasellar disease.[20] It is postulated that, in such cases,

diabetes insipidus is related to radiographically occult infiltration of the infundibulum. Diabetes insipidus is not specific for CNS germ cell tumors. In children, diabetes insipidus associated with absence of the physiologic posterior pituitary bright spot on MRI, and occasionally thickening of the pituitary stalk, may suggest Langerhans cell histiocytosis, which should be considered a part of the differential diagnosis in patients without evidence of gross tumor.

Treatment

The efficacy of cisplatin-containing combination chemotherapy in patients with metastatic gonadal germ cell tumors and the sensitivity of these tumors to radiation therapy have been recognized since the 1970s. These observations have contributed to renewed interest in defining optimal treatment strategies for children and adults with CNS germ cell tumors, although there is no international consensus on an optimal treatment strategy. A range of chemotherapy combinations has been used.

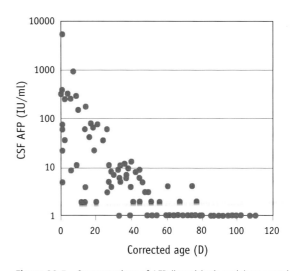

Figure 22-5 Concentrations of AFP (logarithmic scale) measured in CSF of normal infants, corrected for gestational age at birth (d, days).

The availability and documented efficacy of cisplatin-containing chemotherapy regimens served to refocus the therapeutic debate on the relative importance of radiation therapy and/or chemotherapy on survival and quality of life in patients with germinoma in whom very high survival rates were reported following craniospinal irradiation alone. In contrast, the overall cure rate among patients with the nongerminomatous mixed malignant germ cell tumors was poor following treatment with radiation therapy only. Evidently, optimal therapy of CNS germ cell tumors must be considered according to various subgroups. Patients with mature or immature teratomas without evidence of malignancy are unlikely to benefit from either chemotherapy or radiation therapy; surgical resection remains the mainstay of treatment for these patients. Because of the midline location of these tumors and proximity to the suprasellar region and hypothalamus, attempts at surgical resection are often associated with significant morbidity.[2,21]

The relative contributions of radiation therapy and chemotherapy remain a topic of debate, particularly in the treatment of highly curable CNS germinomas.

Central Nervous System Germinomas

Surgery

There is wide consensus among neurosurgeons and oncologists that definitive histological diagnosis of tumor marker–negative CNS tumors is required. However, evidence supporting the extent of surgery in the management of these lesions is limited, and evidence that the extent of resection influences the outcome is lacking.[22,23] Endoscopic surgical biopsy is increasingly important in the management of patients with CNS germ cell tumors, particularly when tumor markers are negative at the time of diagnosis. The endoscopic neurosurgical procedure may be extended to include a third ventriculostomy for the correction of hydrocephalus, the sampling of CSF for tumor cell cytology and tumor markers, in addition to biopsy of the primary tumor for histopathologic diagnosis.[24,25]

Radiation Therapy Only

High survival rates can be achieved among patients with germinomas treated with craniospinal irradiation alone.[26,27] Until recently, craniospinal irradiation has been regarded as the standard of care by many investigators. Historically, the irradiation doses used were comparable to the high doses used in patients with medulloblastoma. In the German protocol MAKEI (Maligne Keimzelltumoren) 86 protocols, a craniospinal dose of 36 Gy was given followed by a boost of 14 Gy to the tumor site. The high cure rates observed with these doses prompted a study examining the efficacy and toxicity of a reduced craniospinal dose of 30 Gy and, more recently, 24 Gy in a clinical trial sponsored by the Societé Internationale d'Oncologie Pédiatrique (SIOP).[23] In a study from the St Jude Children's Research Hospital, the authors reported a 100% event-free survival (EFS) at a median follow-up of 69 months in 12 patients treated with a median craniospinal irradiation dose of 25.2 Gy and a median total primary tumor site dose of 50.4 Gy.[28]

The efficacy of lower craniospinal irradiation doses has been demonstrated,[29] and the possibility of offering reduced-volume irradiation without chemotherapy has been proposed by several authors for patients with localized germinoma.[30,31]

Rogers et al have reported a metaanalysis of radiation therapy and outcome for patients with CNS germinomas. They found that the recurrence rate after whole-brain or whole-ventricular irradiation was 7.6%, compared with 3.8% after craniospinal irradiation. There was no predilection for isolated spinal metastases (2.9% vs 1.2%). The authors concluded that reduced-volume irradiation plus a boost should replace craniospinal irradiation in patients receiving radiation therapy only.[31]

Ogawa et al, reporting the Japanese experience with craniospinal irradiation, expressed a similar view that patients without evidence of metastatic disease may require only involved field irradiation.[30] Thorough perioperative extent of disease staging using MRI and CSF examinations suggests that the incidence of metastatic germinoma is approximately 10%, lower than previously reported, and the risk of isolated spinal relapse reported in the literature is low.[32] The use of radiation therapy alone has been associated with an unusual incidence of extra-CNS relapses.[23] Similar findings have been reported in medulloblastoma patients using craniospinal irradiation as the only treatment modality.[33]

Local field irradiation (either whole-brain irradiation or more limited irradiation volume) is advocated by some authors for localized tumors.[34,35] Evidence supporting whole-brain irradiation is limited and is expected to be associated with more widespread white matter changes, particularly in younger patients. A link between irradiation-associated white matter volume loss and neurocognitive decline has been observed, particularly involving educational skills mediated by attention disorders.[36]

Several authors have emphasized the risk of local recurrence associated with the use of limited field, focal irradiation.[34,37] The best results have been reported with the use of whole-ventricular irradiation, including the tumor bed, the third and lateral ventricles including the sellar and pineal regions.[10] Rogers et al noted the endoscopic discovery of plaques of regionally disseminated disease in the region of the third ventricle at the time of third ventriculostomy, which remained undetectable on MRI scanning. These findings illustrate one of the limitations of staging and scanning investigations in the detection of regional or disseminated disease in patients with this type of disease and underscore the need for careful radiation therapy planning.[31]

Combination Chemotherapy and Radiation Therapy

Germinomas are highly sensitive to chemotherapy (Figure 22-6). Cyclophosphamide, cisplatin, carboplatin, and etoposide have demonstrated activity in patients with newly diagnosed and recurrent tumors.[28,38–40] Accordingly, chemotherapy has been included in modern treat-

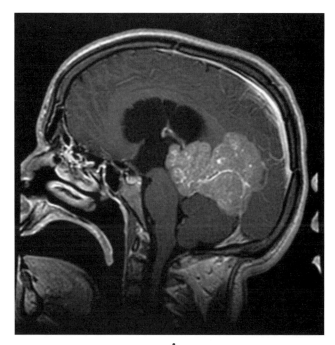

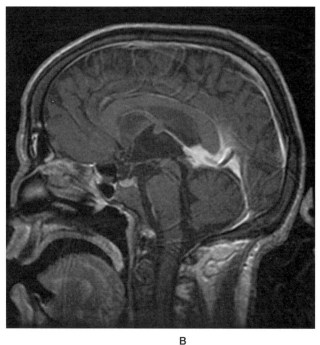

Figure 22-6 Chemosensitivity of germinoma. (A) Pineal region germinoma at diagnosis. (B) Tumor shrinkage after 2 courses of chemotherapy according to the SIOP protocol.

ment protocols for germinoma, with the objective of reducing the volume and the dose of irradiation without compromising overall rates of survival.

Using a combination of carboplatin, etoposide, and ifosfamide as initial therapy, followed by a focal irradiation at a dose of 40 Gy, Baranzelli reported a 93.3% EFS and 100% overall survival at 32 months in a group of 29 patients.[41] A follow-up from the same group reporting on 57 patients reconfirmed these results.[22] Others have reported outcomes of newly diagnosed patients receiving lower regional doses

of irradiation. Sawamura treated 17 patients with 4 cycles of cisplatin and etoposide followed by 24 Gy focal irradiation. Three patients with evidence of germinoma with metastases within the CNS received craniospinal irradiation. At a median follow-up of 24 months, 16 out of 17 patients were alive without recurrence.[42] Recently, the French and the SIOP group reviewed the pattern of relapse in the group of patients treated with focal irradiation and chemotherapy.[43] This review showed that a significant number of relapses occurred in the vicinity of the primary tumor, particularly within the ventricular region.[44] The authors concluded that whole–ventricular field irradiation should be the "standard" approach for patients with non-metastatic germinoma.

Adjuvant Chemotherapy Only

The rationale for the use of chemotherapy in patients with CNS germinomas is based on the success of relatively simple chemotherapy comprising vinblastine, bleomycin, and cisplatin that improved the outcome of males with disseminated gonadal germ cell tumors from less than 10% to more than 57%. The refinement of this approach using high-dose cisplatin and carboplatin, and the replacement of vinblastine with etoposide, further increased survival rates to 60% to 90%.[47–49]

The largest chemotherapy-only experience in CNS germinomas is found in the First and Second International CNS Germ Cell Tumor Study Group reports.[45–47] In the First study, 45 patients with germinomas received 4 cycles of carboplatin (500 mg/m^2/day, days 1 and 2), etoposide (150 mg/m^2/day, days 1 to 3) and bleomycin (15 mg/m^2/day, day 3) following diagnosis. Patients who achieved a complete radiographic and tumor marker response after the first 4 cycles received 2 more identical cycles. Those with less than a complete response received 2 additional cycles in which chemotherapy was intensified by the addition of cyclophosphamide (65 mg/kg), but without radiation therapy. Complete remissions were observed in 37 of 45 patients (82%); however, 4 patients died in complete remission, and only 19 of the 45 patients remain free of relapse or progression without radiotherapy at a median follow-up of 31 months. Nineteen of 22 relapsed patients could be salvaged with radiation therapy with or without further chemotherapy, but the 2-year overall survival for patients with germinoma was only 84%.

The Second study used an intensified chemotherapy induction, including the substitution of carboplatin with cisplatin and the addition of high-dose cyclophosphamide.[48] The regimen previously used in the First study (carboplatin, etoposide, and bleomycin) was alternated with the cisplatin/cyclophosphamide combination after induction to maximize the probability of achieving a lasting complete remission and also to decrease the toxicity profile, particularly the cumulative ototoxicity and nephrotoxicity of cisplatin and the cumulative hematologic toxicity of carboplatin. Nineteen patients with germinoma were enrolled, ranging in age from 1 to 24 years, (median, 14 years). Nine had diabetes insipidus. All 11 patients with residual postoperative disease assessable for response achieved a complete remission. With a median follow-up of 6.5 years, 8 out of 19 patients (42%) remain in first remission without irradiation and another 3 patients are in stable second or subsequent remissions. However, 3 of the 9 patients with diabetes insipidus died of treatment-related toxicities. The Second study experience of treatment-related mortality and significant auditory, renal, and pulmonary late effects highlighted the hazards of intensive cisplatin or bleomycin chemotherapy, particularly in patients with diabetes insipidus.

Mixed Malignant ("Nongerminomatous") Germ Cell Tumors

Surgery

The therapeutic impact of surgery in the treatment of the CNS mixed malignant germ cell tumors has not been clearly defined. The need for surgery or even biopsy to establish the diagnosis of these tumors is highly questionable in patients with elevated AFP or HCGβ and MRI evidence of an intracranial tumor. In addition, a biopsy yielding a small specimen may not be representative of the potentially mixed germ cell tumor elements present. For these reasons, diagnostic biopsy is not commonly advocated in the evaluation of these patients, at least in Western protocols, and their management is essentially based on chemotherapy and irradiation.

A significant proportion of CNS mixed malignant germ cell tumors contain tumor elements that are less responsive to chemotherapy and/or irradiation. Several retrospective reviews, most of them from East Asian authors, have suggested that initial macroscopic total resection may improve the outcome of patients with these tumors.[7,49] Increasing evidence supports a role for delayed surgical resection in patients with residual radiographic abnormalities following treatment. Resection of a residual mass in these patients typically yields fibrosis, necrosis, or either mature or immature teratoma.[50]

Although the benefit of delayed surgery on overall long-term survival has not been clearly established, most contemporary protocols recommend second-look surgery for these patients with negative markers but residual radiographic abnormalities after initial chemotherapy (Figure 22-7).

A small proportion of these tumors can exhibit a paradoxical response to chemotherapy, with falling tumor markers contrasting with an enlargement of the primary tumor. Surgery is the treatment of choice for this complication, commonly known as the "growing teratoma syndrome" (Figure 22-8). Surgical resection in these circumstances usually shows mature or immature teratoma alone.[51] The recognition of this unusual entity is important to avoid confusion with progressive malignancy, because the outcome of these patients is generally excellent.

Radiation Therapy Only

Central nervous system nongerminomatous germ cell tumors are relatively resistant to irradiation and are asso-

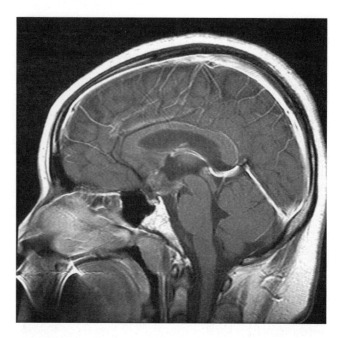

Figure 22-7 Suprasellar nongerminomatous germ cell tumor (initial HCGβ > 6000 IU/l). Residual tumor after completion of treatment with chemotherapy and focal irradiation. Resection of the residual mass may be associated with significant surgical morbidity. In this case, the decision was made to consider careful observation. No evidence of progression was observed after 36 months.

ciated with a relatively poor outcome following treatment with focal or craniospinal irradiation alone. Five-year survival rates for patients with these tumors treated with irradiation alone range from 0% to 33%.[33,52,53] These disappointing results and the significant breakthrough in survival observed when chemotherapy and irradiation are combined serve to explain why irradiation alone has been abandoned for patients with CNS nongerminomatous germ cell tumors.

Combination Chemotherapy and Radiation Therapy

The first reported trial involving a combination of chemotherapy and irradiation for newly diagnosed CNS nongerminomatous germ cell tumors was conducted in Japan in the early 1980s.[54] Chemotherapy comprising cisplatin, etoposide, and bleomycin was administered after irradiation, and the 2-year overall survival among 30 patients was 68%. Most current protocols for these tumors use chemotherapy before irradiation. Chemotherapy agents used are similar to those employed for the treatment of germinoma. Several prospective trials have documented a high response to "germ cell" chemotherapy, and the efficacy of platinum-containing regimens in the nongerminomatous germ cell tumors is well established.[39,55]

The Societé Française d'Oncologie Pédiatrique (SFOP) has reported a 100% response rate in a group of 27 patients receiving a carboplatin-based combination carboplatin-etoposide alternating with ifosfamide-etoposide.[56] The SIOP protocol uses a cisplatin-based combination (cisplatin-etoposide-ifosfamide) with similar results.[57] However, the use of cisplatin in patients with endocrine deficits, particu-

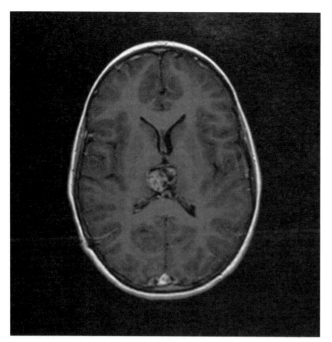

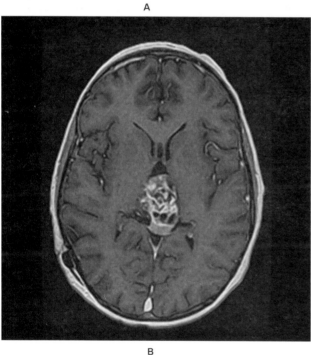

Figure 22-8 Growing teratoma syndrome. (A) Pineal nongerminomatous germ cell tumor with AFP secretion. (B) increase in size of the tumor after 2 courses of chemotherapy despite normalization of AFP. At resection, histology showed immature teratoma with high proliferation rate (MIB-1 proliferation index of ≈15%–20%).

larly diabetes insipidus, may be associated with significant risk of toxicity.[48] Bleomycin is a potentially toxic drug, and its continued use in patients with germ cell tumors is questioned. There is no evidence that bleomycin contributes significantly to the overall survival of patients with CNS nongerminomatous germ cell tumors.

Comparisons with historical data have shown that the combination of chemotherapy and irradiation has significantly improved survival rates in patients with CNS nongerminomatous germ cell tumors. However, the optimal irradiation dose and treatment volumes remain controversial. Several authors advocate a craniospinal irradiation dose of 36 Gy for nonmetastatic CNS nongerminomatous germ cell tumors.[3,13,53,57] In the German MAKEI study, 22 patients initially treated with chemotherapy received 36 Gy craniospinal irradiation with an additional 18 Gy tumor boost.[58] The EFS of these patients was 75% at a mean follow-up of 42 months. Although the efficacy of craniospinal volume irradiation has not been tested in the setting of a randomized study, craniospinal irradiation is still widely regarded as the standard irradiation for these patients.

The experience of the SFOP and SIOP suggest that focal irradiation is associated with similar results in patients with nonmetastatic nongerminomatous germ cell tumors.[56,59] The SIOP reported a significant correlation between the level of AFP at the time of diagnosis and the risk of treatment failure. Patients with an AFP greater than 1000 IU/l in the serum or the CSF demonstrated significantly poorer event-free and overall survival.[60] These findings have been confirmed by others.[61]

Chemotherapy Alone

Four prospective studies of chemotherapy without irradiation for CNS nongerminomatous germ cell tumors have been published.[54,61–63] The SFOP used 1 of 2 different protocols comprising vinblastine, bleomycin, carboplatin, etoposide, and ifosfamide or etoposide, carboplatin, and ifosfamide between 1988 and 1992.[62] Patients were irradiated if there was residual tumor on neuroimaging at the end of chemotherapy. All 18 patients achieved complete tumor marker response after 3 cycles of chemotherapy. Despite this impressive response rate, 12 out the 13 non-irradiated patients ultimately relapsed. The authors concluded that irradiation was required in addition to chemotherapy, even in patients who achieved a dramatic response to initial chemotherapy.

Matsukato reported the experience of the Japanese CNS Germ Cell Tumor Study Group in which an intensive induction with cisplatin, bleomycin, and vinblastine was followed by a maintenance program using the same agents.[54] The author reported a 70% response rate to chemotherapy and a 67.7% survival rate at 2 years in 30 patients, comparing favorably with historical data.

Using the same clinical research design as for germinoma patients, the First International CNS Germ Cell Tumor Study also treated 26 newly diagnosed patients with CNS nongerminomatous germ cell tumors.[63] The complete radiographic and tumor marker response rate was 81%. Four patients progressed during chemotherapy, and 9 ultimately relapsed. The overall survival at 2 years was 62%. Four patients died of toxicity-related events in first complete remission. Interestingly, 9 of 26 patients were free of disease progression or relapse without the use of radiotherapy after a median follow-up period of 31 months. Six of the 13 patients with progressive or relapsed disease were retrieved with further treatment. These observations provided optimism that, at least in a subset of patients with CNS nongerminomatous germ cell tumors, cure could potentially be achieved without the use of radiation therapy.

The Second International CNS Germ Cell Tumor Study enrolled 20 patients with nongerminomatous germ cell tumors.[61] Patients who did not achieve a complete remission after 4 treatment courses underwent second-look surgery and/or irradiation. Sixteen of 17 patients assessable for response after 2 courses of treatment achieved a complete or partial response. With a median follow-up of 6.3 years, 14 of 20 patients were free of disease. Eight of these 14 patients were in first remission, including 3 who received local irradiation in violation of the protocol requirements, and 6 patients were in durable second or third complete remission after further chemotherapy and/or irradiation. The 5-year event-free and overall survivals were 36% and 75%, respectively. The overall survival in this study compares favorably with the outcome of similar groups of patients published by European and Japanese investigators. All patients in this study had histologic and/or tumor marker evidence of nongerminomatous malignant elements of embryonal carcinoma, yolk sac tumor, or choriocarcinoma.

Management of Relapse of Central Nervous System Germ Cell Tumors

Timing of Relapse

The median time to relapse among patients with CNS germinoma and the nongerminomatous germ cell tumors varies considerably. Central nervous system germinoma is more likely to be associated with late recurrences, in contrast to the more common observation of relatively early recurrences in patients with nongerminomatous germ cell tumors.[22,56,64] Sawamura reported a median time to recurrence of 37 months in a retrospective review of 15 patients with recurrent germinoma.[42] In the French experience, the median time to relapse in these patients was 27 months, compared with 11 months in patients with CNS nongerminomatous germ cell tumors.

Influence of Prior Treatment on Outcome Following Relapse

The outcome of patients experiencing relapse of CNS germ cell tumors is strongly influenced by their initial management. Patients receiving initial treatment with chemotherapy only, particularly patients with germinoma, can often be successfully salvaged with craniospinal irradiation alone.[65] Merchant reported 8 patients with germinoma initially enrolled on the First International CNS Germ Cell Tumor Study. These patients were successfully retreated at the time of recurrence with high-dose cyclophosphamide followed by craniospinal irradiation. All patients were alive and free of disease at a median follow-up of 24 months. Similar results were reported by Shibamoto using craniospinal irradiation alone or craniospinal irradiation followed by adjuvant chemotherapy.[66]

The ability to salvage patients treated initially with combined modality therapy is less certain. The cumulative irradiation doses in patients initially treated with craniospinal irradiation is limited by the risk of cumulative radiotherapy-related toxicity.[67]

Role of Myeloablative Chemotherapy with Hematopoietic Cell Rescue at Recurrence

Increasing evidence suggests that patients relapsing after receiving irradiation-containing therapy may still respond to chemotherapy. In a recent report on 21 patients with recurrent CNS germ cell tumors, Modak et al reported promising results using a thiotepa-based myeloablative chemotherapy regimen followed by bone marrow or peripheral hematopoietic cell rescue.[68] Seventeen patients received chemotherapy prior to myeloablative chemotherapy in an effort to reduce tumor burden. Eight patients achieved a partial response, 8 achieved a complete response, and 1 patient had stable disease. At the time of the report, 7 out of 8 patients with recurrent germinoma survived without evidence of disease at a median follow-up of 48 months, and 4 of 12 patients with recurrent nongerminomatous germ cell tumors survived without evidence of disease at a median follow-up of 35 months in the latter group. Similar results have been reported by the SFOP group in a preliminary report.[69] These results have significant implications, not only for the management of patients at the time of recurrence. They suggest that myeloablative chemotherapy may be considered for poor responders to initial chemotherapy in newly diagnosed patients with CNS nongerminomatous germ cell tumors, in order to consolidate remission and potentially improve survival.

Late Effects and Quality of Life

Many factors impact upon the long-term outcome of these patients, including endocrine deficits, visual disturbance, and hydrocephalus that are primarily related to the mass effect of tumor. Most patients with suprasellar tumors develop multiple endocrine deficits, such as diabetes insipidus, central hypocorticoidism, hypothyroidism, hypogonadism, and growth hormone deficiency.[30]

Authors favoring the role of craniospinal irradiation as a "standard" treatment for germinoma and as a part of combined modality treatment of nongerminomatous germ cell tumors argue that the degree of cognitive impairment and other irradiation effects are less severe in this population, because CNS germ cell tumors tend to occur more commonly in postpubertal adolescent patients. St Jude Children's Research Hospital reported no significant differences at a median follow-up of 69 months between pre- and postirradiation full-scale, verbal, and performance intelligence quotient (IQ) scores among 12 patients with germinoma treated with craniospinal irradiation.[70] Another report from Oka with longer follow-up (161 months) was more disconcerting, reporting significant intellectual decline in 50% of patients.[71]

Kieffer-Renaut reported the neurocognitive outcome of 16 patients treated in the SFOP study with chemotherapy followed by focal irradiation at a dose of 40 Gy for germinoma and 55 Gy for nongerminomatous germ cell tumors. Nine patients had tumors located in the pineal area, and 7 patients had tumors in the suprasellar region. Kieffer-Renaut reported no difference in the intellectual outcome with tumor site. All patients demonstrated normal intellectual functioning, despite evidence of moderate memory impairment.[72] In a retrospective review of 12 patients treated with focal (7 patients) or craniospinal irradiation (5 patients), Mabbott reported an average IQ of 98.[73] Language, spelling, reading, mathematics, visual-perceptual ability, and executive functioning were intact, but speed sequencing was poor. Poorer attention was observed for patients treated with craniospinal compared with focal irradiation. Pineal tumors were associated with memory impairments relative to suprasellar tumors.

In the First International CNS Germ Cell Tumor Study experience, survivors had an increased risk of adverse quality of life and neuropsychologic functioning.[74] These late effects were worse in younger patients, in patients with CNS nongerminomatous germ cell tumors compared with CNS germinomas, and in patients treated with radiation therapy. Parents of children 18 years and younger at the time of testing (median, 6.1 years after diagnosis) who received irradiation reported significantly lower self-esteem in addition to limitations in their roles at school and with friends because of emotional or behavioral problems.

Future Directions of International Cooperative Group Trials

Children's Oncology Group (United States)

Germinoma

The current Children's Oncology Group (COG) study for CNS germinoma consists of a randomized clinical trial to test the hypothesis that the addition of preirradiation chemotherapy will permit a response-based reduction in irradiation treatment volume and doses and therefore achieve a reduction in neurocognitive deficits, compared with children randomized to receive higher-dose irradiation without chemotherapy. The study is expected to accrue 225 patients over 5 years, and the patterns of recurrence may provide valuable insights into the potential risks of limited-volume irradiation.

Patients with pathologically confirmed germinoma with negative AFP and serum or CSF βHCG levels below 50 mIU/mL will be eligible for randomization. The radiation doses and treatment volumes are determined by extent of disease at presentation and treatment regimen. Patients with localized disease randomized to receive irradiation receive only 24 Gy whole ventricular irradiation with a 21 Gy boost to the primary site. Patients with metastatic disease receive a craniospinal dose of 24 Gy, and a 21 Gy boost to sites of measurable disease.

Patients without metastatic disease, (M0), randomized to preirradiation treatment arm who achieve a complete remission after 2 cycles of chemotherapy receive a further 2 courses of chemotherapy followed by 30 Gy to the involved field only.

Nongerminomatous Germ Cell Tumors

The current COG study of CNS nongerminomatous germ cell tumors is aimed at improving the progression-free and overall survival among patients with these tumors by increasing the complete or partial response rate using 3 courses of carboplatin and etoposide alternating with 3 courses of ifosfamide and etoposide followed by 36 Gy craniospinal irradiation including an involved field boost of an additional 20 Gy. Patients demonstrating a poor tumor response with persisting tumor maker elevation receive consolidation with myeloablative thiotepa and etoposide and peripheral hematopoietic cell rescue followed by craniospinal irradiation.

The aim of the future SIOP CNS Germ Cell Tumor 2 study is to demonstrate that better EFS rates can be achieved with therapies tailored according to specific risk factors. This protocol is intended to pilot therapeutic strategies and compare their outcome with those of historical controls from patients on the SIOP CNS Germ Cell Tumor 96 study. Study questions in the diagnostic subgroups are: (1) Can EFS be increased in patients with germinoma by better staging (lower proportion of misclassified patients), optimized chemotherapy, and modified radiotherapy? (2) Can the EFS be increased in patients with nongerminomatous germ cell tumors by intensification of chemotherapy? In this protocol, patients with nonmetastatic low-risk germinoma who are in complete remission after 4 courses of chemotherapy will receive modified low-dose irradiation as compared with previous studies. Patients with metastatic germinoma will be treated with low-dose craniospinal irradiation without chemotherapy. Patients with nongerminomatous germ cell tumors will be stratified according to risk factors (metastatic status, age, and level of AFP secretion). All patients will receive the same induction (3 courses of cisplatin, etoposide, and ifosfamide). Patients with high-risk features will then proceed to myeloablative chemotherapy with peripheral hematopoietic cell rescue. Patients above 5 years will receive irradiation, either focal in patients with localized disease or craniospinal in case of metastatic spread.

References

1. Committee of Brain Tumor Registry of Japan. Report of Brain Tumor Registry of Japan (1969–1996). *Neurol Med Chir (Tokyo)*. 2003;43(suppl 1–7):1–111.
2. Balmaceda C, Modak S, Finlay J. Central nervous system germ cell tumors. *Semin Oncol*. 1998;25(2):243–250.
3. Ries LAG, Eisner MP, Kosary CL, et al, eds. *SEER Cancer Statistics Review, 1975–2001*. Bethesda, MD: National Cancer Institute; 2004. http://seer.cancer.gov/csr/1975_2001/.
4. Bouffet E, Brown C, Bartels U, Hyder D, McLaughlin J. Epidemiology of intracranial germ cell tumours (IGCT): lessons from registries and published series. *Proc 1st Int Symp CNS Germ Cell Tumors* [abstract O-2]. 2003.
5. Hoffman HJ, Otsubo H, Hendrick EB, et al. Intracranial germ-cell tumors in children. *J Neurosurg*. 1991;74(4):545–551.
6. Jennings MT, Gelman R, Hochberg F. Intracranial germ-cell tumors: natural history and pathogenesis [review]. *J Neurosurg*. 1985;63(2):155–167.
7. Matsutani M, Sano K, Takakura K, et al. Primary intracranial germ cell tumors: a clinical analysis of 153 histologically verified cases. *J Neurosurg*. 1997;86(3):446–455.
8. Ho DM, Liu HC. Primary intracranial germ cell tumor: pathologic study of 51 patients. *Cancer*. 1992;70(6):1577–1584.
9. Teilum G. Classification of endodermal sinus tumor (mesoblastoma vitellinum) and so-called "embryonal carcinoma" of the ovary. *Acta Pathol Microbiol Scand*. 1965;64(4):407–429.
10. Matsutani M; Japanese Pediatric Brain Tumor Study Group. Combined chemotherapy and radiation therapy for CNS germ cell tumors: the Japanese experience. *J Neuro-Oncol*. 2001;54(3):311–316.

11. Utsuki S, Oka H, Tanaka S, Tanizaki Y, Fujii K. Long-term outcome of intracranial germinoma with hCG elevation in cerebrospinal fluid but not in serum. *Acta Neurochir (Wien).* 2002;144(2):1151–1154.

12. Uematsu Y, Tsuura Y, Miyamoto K, Itakura T, Hayashi S, Komai N. The recurrence of primary intracranial germinomas: special reference to germinoma with STGC (syncytiotrophoblastic giant cell). *J Neuro-Oncol.* 2002;13(3):247–256.

13. Shibamoto Y, Takahashi M, Sasai K. Prognosis of intracranial germinoma with syncytiotrophoblastic giant cells treated by radiation therapy. *Int J Radiat Oncol Biol Phys.* 1997;37(3):505–510.

14. Sugiyama K, Uozumi T, Kiya K, et al. Intracranial germ-cell tumor with synchronous lesions in the pineal and suprasellar regions: report of six cases and review of the literature. *Surg Neurol.* 1992;38(2):114–120.

15. Seregni E, Massimino M, Nerini Molteni S, et al. Serum and cerebrospinal fluid human chorionic gonadotropin (hCG) and alpha-fetoprotein (AFP) in intracranial germ cell tumors. *Int J Biol Markers.* 2002;17(2):112–118.

16. Schneider DT, Calaminus G, Göbel U. Diagnostic value of alpha 1-fetoprotein and beta-human chorionic gonadotropin in infancy and childhood. *Pediatr Hematol Oncol.* 2001;18(1):11–26.

17. Gitlin D, Perricelli A, Gitlin GM. Synthesis of α-fetoprotein by liver, yolk sac, and gastrointestinal tract of the human conceptus. *Cancer Res.* 1972;32(5):979–982.

18. Wu JT, Book L, Sudar K. Serum alpha fetoprotein (AFP) levels in normal infants. *Pediatr Res.* 1981;15(1):50–52.

19. Coakley J, Kellie SJ, Nath A, Munas A, Cooke-Yarborough C. Interpretation of alpha-fetoprotein concentrations in cerebrospinal fluid of infants. *Ann Clin Biochem.* 2005;42(1):24–29.

20. Reddy AT, Wellons JC III, Allen JC, et al. Refining the staging evaluation of pineal region germinoma using neuroendoscopy and the presence of preoperative diabetes insipidus. *Neuro Oncol.* 2004;6(2):127–133.

21. Oi S, Matsumoto S. Controversy pertaining to therapeutic modalities for tumors of the pineal region: a worldwide survey of different patient populations. *Child's Nerv Syst.* 1992;8(6):332–336.

22. Bouffet E, Baranzelli MC, Patte C, et al. Combined treatment modality for intracranial germinomas: results of a multicentre SFOP experience. Société Francaise d'Oncologie Pediatrique. *Br J Cancer.* 1999;79(7–8):1199–1204.

23. Bamberg M, Kortmann RD, Calaminus G, et al. Radiation therapy for intracranial germinoma: results of the German cooperative prospective trials MAKEI 83/86/89. *J Clin Oncol.* 1999;17(8):2585–2592.

24. Gangemi M, Maiuri F, Colella G, Buonamassa S. Endoscopic surgery for pineal region tumors. *Minim Invasive Neurosurg.* 2001;44(2):70–73.

25. Oi S, Shibata M, Tominaga J, et al. Efficacy of neuroendoscopic procedures in minimally invasive preferential management of pineal region tumors: a prospective study. *J Neurosurg.* 2000;93(2):245–253.

26. Maity A, Shu, H-KG, Janss A, et al. Craniospinal radiation in the treatment of biopsy-proven intracranial germinomas: twenty-five years' experience in a single center. *Int J Radiat Oncol Biol Phys.* 2004;58(4):1165–1170.

27. Huh SJ, Shin KH, Kim IH, Ahn YC, Ha SW, Park CI. Radiotherapy of intracranial germinomas. *Radiother Oncol.* 1996;38(1):19–23.

28. Allen JC, Kim JH, Packer RJ. Neoadjuvant chemotherapy for newly diagnosed germ-cell tumors of the central nervous system. *J Neurosurg.* 1987;67(1):65–70.

29. Schoenfeld, GO, Amdur RJ, Schmalfuss IM, et al. Low-dose prophylactic craniospinal radiotherapy for intracranial germinoma. *Int J Radiat Oncol Biol Phys.* 2006;65(2):481–485.

30. Ogawa K, Shikama N, Toita T, et al. Long-term results of radiotherapy for intracranial germinoma: a multi-institutional retrospective review of 126 patients. *Int J Radiat Oncol Biol Phys.* 2004;58(3):705–713.

31. Rogers SJ, Mosleh-Shirazi MA, Saran FH. Radiotherapy of localized intracranial germinoma: time to sever historical ties? *Lancet Oncol.* 2005;6(7):509–519.

32. Brada M, Rajan B. Spinal seeding in cranial germinoma. *Br J Cancer.* 1990;61(2):339–340.

33. Kunschner LJ, Kuttesch J, Hess K, Yung WK. Survival and recurrence factors in adult medulloblastoma: the M. D. Anderson Cancer Center experience from 1978 to 1998. *Neuro Oncol.* 2001;3(3):167–173.

34. Aoyama H, Shirato H, Kakuto Y, et al. Pathologically-proven intracranial germinoma treated with radiation therapy. *Radiother Oncol.* 1998;47(2):201–205.

35. Borg M. Germ cell tumours of the central nervous system in children—controversies in radiotherapy. *Med Pediatr Oncol.* 2003;40(6):367–374.

36. Mulhern RK, Merchant TE, Gajjar A, Reddick WE, Kun LE. Late neurocognitive sequelae in survivors of brain tumours in childhood. *Lancet Oncol.* 2004;5(7):399–408.

37. Timmerman RD, Patel D, Boaz JC, Goldman J, Jakacki RI. Patterns of failure after induction of chemotherapy followed by consolidative radiation therapy for children with central nervous system germinoma. *Med Pediatr Oncol.* 2003;41(6):564–566.

38. Allen JC, DaRosso RC, Donahue B, Nirenberg A. A Phase II trial of preirradiation carboplatin in newly diagnosed germinoma of the central nervous system. *Cancer.* 1994;74(3):940–944.

39. Robertson PL, DaRosso RC, Allen JC. Improved prognosis of intracranial non-germinoma germ cell tumors with multimodality therapy. *J Neuro-Oncol.* 1997;32(1):71–80.

40. Buckner JC, Peethambaram PP, Smithson WA, et al. Phase II trial of primary chemotherapy followed by reduced-dose radiation for CNS germ cell tumors. *J Clin Oncol.* 1999;17(3):933–940.

41. Baranzelli MC, Patte C, Bouffet E, et al. Nonmetastatic intracranial germinoma: the experience of the French Society of Pediatric Oncology. *Cancer.* 1997;80(9):1792–1797.

42. Sawamura Y, Shirato H, Ikeda J, et al. Induction chemotherapy followed by reduced-volume radiation therapy for newly diagnosed central nervous system germinoma. *J Neurosurg.* 1998;88(1):66–72.

43. Aoyama H, Shirato H, Ikeda J, Fujieda K, Miyasaka K, Sawamura Y. Induction chemotherapy followed by low-dose involved-field radiotherapy for intracranial germ cell tumors. *J Clin Oncol.* 2002;20(3):857–865.

44. Alapetite C, Ricardi U, Saran F, et al. Whole ventricular irradiation in combination with chemotherapy in intracranial germinoma: the consensus of the SIOP CNS GCT Study Group. *Med Pediatr Oncol.* 2002;39(4):248.

45. Nichols CR, Williams SD, Loehrer PJ, et al: Randomized study of cisplatin dose intensity in advanced germ cell tumors: a Southeastern and Southwest Oncology Group protocol. *J Clin Oncol.* 1991;9(7):1163–1172.

46. Pinkerton CR, Broadbent V, Horwich A, et al. "JEB": a carboplatin based regimen for malignant germ cell tumors in children. *Br J Cancer.* 1990;62(2):257–262.

47. Bajorin DF, Sarosdy MF, Pfister DG, et al. Randomized trial of etoposide and cisplatin versus etoposide and carboplatin in patients with good-risk germ cell tumors: a multiinstitutional study. *J Clin Oncol.* 1993;11(4):598–606.

48. Kellie SJ, Boyce H, Dunkel IJ, et al. Intensive cisplatin and cyclophosphamide-based chemotherapy without radiotherapy for intracranial germinomas: failure of a primary chemotherapy approach. *Pediatr Blood Cancer.* 2004;43(2):126–133.

49. Ogawa K, Toita T, Nakamura K, et al. Treatment and prognosis of patients with intracranial nongerminomatous malignant germ cell tumors: a multiinstitutional retrospective analysis of 41 patients. *Cancer.* 2003;98(2):369–376.

50. Weiner HL, Lichtenbaum RA, Wisoff JH, et al. Delayed surgical resection of central nervous system germ cell tumors. *Neurosurgery.* 2002;50(4):727–733.

51. O'Callaghan AM, Katapodis O, Ellison DW, Theaker JM, Mead GM. The growing teratoma syndrome in a nongerminomatous germ cell tumor of the pineal gland: a case report and review. *Cancer.* 1997;80(5):942–947.

52. Dearnaley DP, A'Hern RP, Whittaker S, Bloom HJ. Pineal and CNS germ cell tumors: Royal Marsden Hospital experience 1962–1987. *Int J Radiat Oncol Biol Phys.* 1990;18(4):773–781.

53. Wolden SL, Wara WM, Larson DA, Prados MD, Edwards MS, Sneed PK. Radiation therapy for primary intracranial germ-cell tumors. *Int J Radiat Oncol Biol Phys.* 1995;32(4):943–949.

54. Matsukado Y, Abe H, Tanaka R, et al. Cisplatin, vinblastine and bleomycin (PVB) combination chemotherapy in the treatment of intracranial malignant germ cell tumors: a preliminary report of a phase II study—The Japanese Intracranial Germ Cell Tumor Study Group. *Gan No Rinsho.* 1986;32(11):1387–1393.

55. Kida Y, Kobayashi T, Yoshida J, Kato K, Kageyama N. Chemotherapy with cisplatin for AFP-secreting germ-cell tumors of the central nervous system. *J Neurosurg.* 1986;65(4):470–475.

56. Baranzelli MC, Patte C, Bouffet E, et al. Carboplatin-based chemotherapy (CT) and focal irradiation (RT) in primary cerebral germ cell tumors (GCT): a French Society of Pediatric Oncology (SFOP) experience. *Proc Am Soc Clin Oncol.* 1999;18:140a.

57. Calaminus G, Andreussi L, Garre ML, Kortmann RD, Schober R, Gobel U. Secreting germ cell tumors of the central nervous system (CNS): first results of the cooperative German/Italian pilot study (CNS sGCT). *Klin Padiatr.* 1997;209(4):222–227.

58. Calaminus G, Bamberg M, Baranzelli MC, et al. Intracranial germ cell tumors: a comprehensive update of the European data. *Neuropediatr.* 1994;25(1):26–32.

59. Calaminus G, Nicholson JC, Alapetite C, et al. Malignant CNS germ cell tumor: interim analysis after 5 years of SIOP CNS GCT 96 [abstract]. *Med Pediatr Oncol.* 2002;39(4):227.

60. Calaminus G, Alapetite C, Frappaz, et al. Malignant CNS germ cell tumor: interim analysis after 5 years of SIOP CNS GCT 96 [abstract O–15]. *Proc 1st Int Symp CNS Germ Cell Tumors.* Kyoto; 2003.

61. Kellie SJ, Boyce H, Dunkel IJ, et al. Primary chemotherapy for intracranial nongerminomatous germ cell tumors: results of the second international CNS germ cell study group protocol. *J Clin Oncol.* 2004;22(5):846–853.

62. Baranzelli MC, Patte C, Bouffet E, et al. An attempt to treat pediatric intracranial alphaFP and betaHCG secreting germ cell tumors with chemotherapy alone: SFOP experience with 18 cases. Societe Française d'Oncologie Pediatrique. *J Neuro-Oncol.* 1998;37(3):229–239.

63. Balmaceda C, Heller G, Rosenblum M, et al. Chemotherapy without irradiation—a novel approach for newly diagnosed CNS germ cell tumors: results of an international cooperative trial. The First International Central Nervous System Germ Cell Tumor Study. *J Clin Oncol.* 1996;14(11):2908–2915.

64. Sawamura Y, Ikeda JL, Tada M, Shirato H. Salvage therapy for recurrent germinomas in the central nervous system. *Br J Neurosurg.* 1999;13(4):376–381.

65. Merchant TE, Davis BJ, Sheldon JM, Leibel SA. Radiation therapy for relapsed CNS germinoma after primary chemotherapy. *J Clin Oncol.* 1998;16(1):204–209.

66. Shibamoto Y, Sasai K, Kokubo M, Hiraoka M. Salvage radiation therapy for intracranial germinoma recurring after primary chemotherapy. *J Neuro-Oncol.* 1999;44(2):181–185.
67. Ono N, Isobe I, Uki J, Kurihara H, Shimizu T, Kohno K. Recurrence of primary intracranial germinomas after complete response with radiotherapy: recurrence patterns and therapy. *Neurosurgery.* 1994;35(4):615–620.
68. Modak S, Gardner S, Dunkel IJ, et al. Thiotepa-based high-dose chemotherapy with autologous stem-cell rescue in patients with recurrent or progressive CNS germ cell tumors. *J Clin Oncol.* 2004;22(10):1934–1943.
69. Bouffet E, Baranzelli MC, Patte C, et al. High-dose etoposide and thio-TEPA for recurrent malignant intracranial germ cell tumours [abstract]. *Med Pediatr Oncol.* 2000;35(3):177.
70. Merchant TE, Sherwood SH, Mulhern RK, et al. CNS germinoma: disease control and long-term functional outcome for 12 children treated with craniospinal irradiation. *Int J Radiat Oncol Biol Phys.* 2000;46(5):1171–1176.
71. Oka H, Kawano N, Tanaka T, et al. Long-term functional outcome of suprasellar germinomas: usefulness and limitations of radiotherapy. *J Neuro-Oncol.* 1998;40(2):185–190.
72. Kieffer Renaux V, Pirou V, Patte C, et al. Neuropyschological profile of children treated with chemotherapy and local irradiation for an intracranial malignant germ cell tumor [abstractO-62]. *Proc 1st Int Symp CNS Germ Cell Tumors.* Kyoto; 2003.
73. Mabbott D, Guger S, Kennedy K, Bouffet E, Spiegler B. Neurocognitive status in children after treatment of tumours of the third ventricle. 11th biennal Canadian Neuro-oncology Meeting. *Can J Neurol Sci.* 2004;(suppl):16.
74. Sands SA, Kellie SJ, Davidow AL, et al. Long-term quality of life and neuropsychologic functioning for patients with CNS germ-cell tumors: from the First International CNS Germ-Cell Tumor Study. *Neuro Oncol.* 2001;3(3):174–183.

Neuroblastoma

Howard M. Katzenstein and Susan L. Cohn

Introduction

Neuroblastoma is a biologically heterogeneous tumor with a broad spectrum of clinical behavior.[1] Spontaneous regression occurs in some infants, while tumors in older children may sometimes differentiate into benign ganglioneuromas.[2] Almost all patients with localized tumors can be cured with surgery alone, regardless of the extent of tumor resection.[3] In addition, most infants with disseminated disease have favorable outcomes following treatment with chemotherapy and surgery.[4,5] In contrast, the majority of children older than 18 months with advanced-stage neuroblastoma die from progressive disease despite intensive multimodality therapy.[6] This clinical diversity correlates closely with numerous clinical and biological factors including tumor stage, patient age, tumor histology, and genetic tumor abnormalities.[7,8] However, the molecular basis underlying the variability in tumor growth, clinical behavior, and responsiveness to therapy remains largely unknown.

Incidence

Neuroblastoma is the second most common pediatric solid tumor and is the most common tumor in children less than one year of age. This tumor is derived from neural crest cells, and it most commonly arises in the adrenal medulla or paraspinal sympathetic ganglia. It comprises 8-10% of all pediatric malignancies. There are approximately 600 new cases of neuroblastoma in the United States each year, with a prevalence of approximately 1 case per 7,000 births and a slight predominance in males and Caucasians.[9] The median age at diagnosis is 22 months of age with one-third of patients diagnosed in the first year of life and 90% of children diagnosed before 5 years of age. Occasionally patients can be diagnosed in adolescence and young adulthood and have an indolent course with poor overall survival.

Epidemiology and Pathogenesis

No environmental influences or parental exposures that significantly impact disease occurrences have been identified. Although neuroblastoma usually occurs sporadically, in 1-2% of cases there is a family history and in rare cases neuroblastoma can occur with other disorders of neural crest tissue, implicating a genetic etiology.[10] Considerable biological and clinical heterogeneity is observed within the familial cases, although more than half of the offspring of survivors of familial neuroblastoma will develop tumors.[11] The occurrence of neuroblastoma with Hirschsprung disease and/or congenital central hypoventilation syndrome led to the discovery of the first bonified neuroblastoma predisposition gene *PHOX2B*.[12,13] *PHOX2B* mutations are almost exclusive to cases with associated neurocristopathies and are not detected in somatically acquired tumors. More recently, germline mutations in the anaplastic lymphoma kinase (*ALK*) gene have been identified in patients with familial neuroblastoma.[14] Somatic mutations in the *ALK* gene have also been detected in a subset of primary neuroblastomas and cell lines.[14,15] Functional studies demonstrate that many of the *ALK* mutations represent gain-of-function alleles that can sustain key signaling pathways and are, therefore, likely to be valid therapeutic targets for ALK inhibitors.[15] In addition to the *ALK* gene, which is located on chromosome 2, a common genetic variation at chromosome band 6p22 has been shown to be associated with susceptibility to neuroblastoma in a genomewide association study.[16] In this study, patients with neuroblastoma who were homozygous for the risk alleles at 6p22 were more likely to have high-risk features and poor outcome.

Clinical Presentation

Presenting signs and symptoms of children with neuroblastoma are quite variable and reflect both the location of the primary tumor and the extent of disease. Primary tumors are located in the abdomen in approximately two-thirds of patients, slightly more than half of which are located within an adrenal gland. Tumors may also originate in the thorax, pelvis, neck, or elsewhere along the sympathetic chain. Metastatic disease is observed in approximately 70% of all newly diagnosed patients, particularly in children older than one year, and most commonly involves spread of tumor to cortical bone, bone marrow, lymph nodes, liver, and skin. Dissemination of disease to the parenchyma of either the brain (Figure 23-1) or lung is a rare occurrence. Patients with localized disease are often asymptomatic, while children with metastatic disease typically appear ill at presentation with systemic symptoms including fever, malaise, anemia, and bone pain secondary to tumor dissemination. Metastatic disease to the orbit may manifest as proptosis or orbital ecchymoses and is commonly mistaken for child abuse. Patients with paraspinal tumors (Figure 23-2) may present with signs of spinal cord compression including paraplegia, bowel and bladder dysfunction, or weakness. Horner syndrome is sometimes observed in individuals with cervical or apical thoracic masses. Infants may present with profound hepatomegaly from metastatic deposits that may result in respiratory distress and organ compromise. Several paraneoplastic syndromes may also be seen at presentation, including opsoclonus/myoclonus/ataxia. Rarely, tumor secretion of vasoactive intestinal peptide can result in profuse, watery diarrhea. Excessive catecholamine secretion, which occurs in 90% to 95% of patients, may rarely result in hypertension, tachycardia, headache, sweating, and flushing, although hypertension is more commonly associated with tumor compression of the renal vasculature.

Diagnostic Evaluation

The International Neuroblastoma Staging System (INSS), which was initially developed in 1986 and subsequently revised in 1993,[17] has been implemented worldwide (Table 23-1). According to INSS criteria, the diagnosis of neuroblastoma can be made either by characteristic histolopathologic evaluation of tumor tissue, or by the presence of tumor cells in a bone marrow aspirate/biopsy and elevated levels of urinary catecholamines. Specific requirements for staging include bilateral bone marrow aspirations and biopsies, computed tomography of the body (excluding the head if clinically not indicated), bone scintigraphy, and meta-iodobenzylguanadine (mIBG) scintigraphy (Figure 23-3).[17] Meta-iodobenzylguanadine is a catecholamine analogue that is selectively taken up in

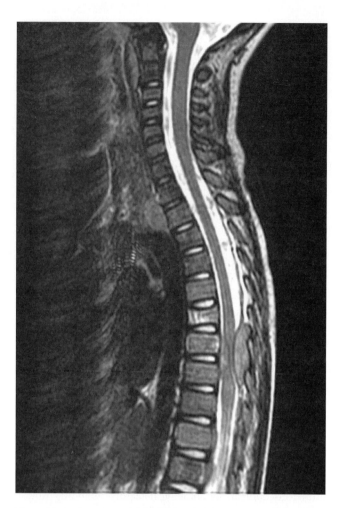

Figure 23-2 Tumor mass in the epidural space at T7 and T8 that effaces the thecal sac, invades the spinal canal, displaces the spinal cord, and causes severe cord compression. There is marked heterogeneity of marrow signal throughout the vertebral bodies at all levels representing diffuse metastases.

neuroblastoma tumor tissue and is positive in approximately 85% of patients. Recent studies have suggested that the radiographic response to therapy evaluated by mIBG imaging can be predictive of outcome and may be used to guide therapeutic decisions.[18,19] Magnetic resonance imaging may be helpful in evaluating the extent of intraspinal disease in patients with dumbbell tumors and/or cord compression. The role of positron emission tomography in neuroblastoma has not yet been established.

Laboratory Studies

Elevated serum ferritin (>142 ng/ml), lactic dehydrogenase (>1500 IU/L), and neuron-specific enolase (>100 ng/ml) have all been associated with an adverse prognosis in neuroblastoma.[20] Determination of urine catecholamine excretion by analysis of spot urine samples for vanillylmandelic acid (VMA) and homovanillic acid (HVA) may help confirm the diagnosis and may also be useful as a noninvasive method to monitor tumor response to therapy. A diagnostic ratio of HVA to VMA >1 has also been associated with an adverse prognosis.[21]

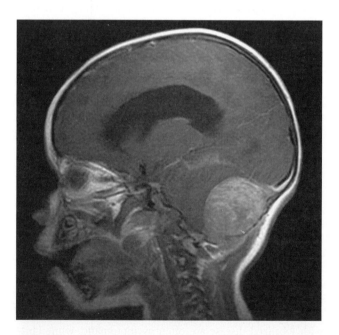

Figure 23-1 Large extra-axial neuroblastoma centered within the posterior fossa causing surrounding mass effect and obstructive hydrocephalus.

Table 23-1

International neuroblastoma staging system.[a]

Stage 1	Localized tumor with complete gross excision, with or without microscopic residual disease. Representative ipsilateral lymph nodes negative for tumor microscopically (nodes attached to and removed with the primary tumor may be positive).
Stage 2A	Localized tumor with incomplete gross excision: representative ipsilateral nonadherent lymph nodes negative for tumor microscopically.
Stage 2B	Localized tumor with or without complete gross excision with ipsilateral nonadherent lymph nodes positive for tumor. Enlarged contralateral lymph nodes must be negative microscopically.
Stage 3	Unresectable unilateral tumor infiltrating across the midline[b] with or without regional lymph node involvement; localized unilateral tumor with contralateral regional lymph node involvement; or midline tumor with bilateral extension by infiltration (unresectable) or by lymph node involvement.
Stage 4	Any primary tumor with dissemination to distant lymph nodes, bone, bone marrow, liver, skin and/or other organs (except as defined in 4S).
Stage 4S	Localized primary tumor (as defined by stage 1, 2A, or 2B) with dissemination limited to skin, liver, and or bone marrow[c] (limited to infants < 1 year)

[a] Reprinted with permission from Brodeur GM, Pritchard J, Berthold F, et al.[17]

[b] The midline is defined as the vertebral column. Tumors originating on one side and crossing the midline must infiltrate to or beyond the opposite side of the vertebral column.

[c] Marrow involvement in stage 4S should be minimal—ie, < 10% of total nucleated cells identified as malignant on bone marrow biopsy or on marrow aspirate. More extensive marrow involvement would be considered to be stage 4. The mIBG scan (if performed) should be negative in the marrow.

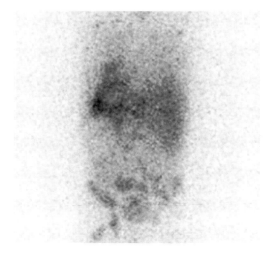

Figure 23-3 —123 mIBG scan demonstrating uptake within an abdominal neuroblastoma as well as metastatic disease to the pelvis, and proximal left femur (posterior view).

Biologic Studies

Histology

Neuroblastoma is a member of the family of small, round, blue cell tumors of childhood and can be further identified by immunohistochemical staining of neuronal markers such as synaptophysin and neuron-specific enolase. Neuroblastic tumors include neuroblastomas, ganglioneuroblastomas (including the nodular subtype), and ganglioneuromas. In 1984 Shimada and colleagues devised a histopathologic classification schema that is predictive of clinical behavior.[22] Tumors are classified as favorable or unfavorable depending upon the degree of neuroblast differentiation, Schwannian stroma content, mitosis-karyorhexis index, and age at diagnosis. The International Neuroblastoma Pathology Classification system, a modification of the Shimada system, was established in 1999, and the prognostic significance of this system has been confirmed.[7] Although it remains unknown why unfavorable histology tumors are more clinically aggressive, amplification of the *MYCN* oncogene is strongly associated with unfavorable histology.[23,24]

MYCN Oncogene

MYCN amplification (> 10 copies) occurs in approximately 20% of primary neuroblastoma tumors and is strongly associated with the presence of metastatic disease and poor prognosis.[25,26] These observations suggest that the *MYCN* oncogene (located on the short arm of chromosome 2) critically contributes to the clinically aggressive behavior of high-risk neuroblastoma tumors, and laboratory studies support this hypothesis.[27] *MYCN* amplification is observed in approximately 30% to 40% of patients with advanced-stage disease. In contrast, only 5% to 10% of patients with localized disease are *MYCN* amplified. *MYCN* amplification status is an inherent biologic property of neuroblastoma tumor cells and does not usually change during the course of treatment as a sign of chemoresistance.

A role for *MYCN* in neuroblastoma pathogenesis is further supported by studies demonstrating neuroblastoma tumor development in transgenic mice with targeted expression of *MYCN*.[28] Although *MYCN* amplification clearly identifies a subset of neuroblastomas with highly malignant behavior, *MYCN* gain (defined as 1-4 extra copies of the *MYCN* gene relative to chromosome 2 copy number) does not appear to be associated with clinical outcome.[29,30] Furthermore, the clinical significance of *MYCN* expression in children with neuroblastoma remains controversial.[31,32] The reason for the discordant results may, in part, be due to disparities in patient populations, as the proportion of infants younger than 1 year, of patients with advanced-stage disease, and of children with *MYCN*-amplified tumors differs in the various series. Recently, high levels of *MYCN* expression were found not to be predictive of worse outcome in a retrospective analysis of patients with advanced-stage disease and normal *MYCN* copy number.[33] Thus, the precise role, if any, that *MYCN* plays in nonamplified tumors remains unknown.

Tumor Cell Ploidy

A number of studies have shown that cellular DNA content in neuroblastoma tumor cells is predictive of outcome, particularly in infants younger than 1 year.[34–36] Hyperdiploidy, mostly in near-triploid constitution, is mainly observed in low-stage tumors of infants and is associated with excellent long-term survival. In contrast, diploidy in this age group often is associated with early treatment failure.[23,35] Although a correlation exists between diploidy and *MYCN* amplification, each factor has been validated as an independent prognostic variable.[23,34] Ploidy in children older than 2 years does not appear to be prognostic and is not currently used to guide therapy.

Chromosome Abnormalities

Both gain and loss of genetic material are commonly detected in neuroblastoma cell lines and primary tumors. The most common genetic abnormality in primary neuroblastoma is gain of 17q genetic material. This genetic abnormality is strongly associated with high-risk features and adverse outcome.[37] Consistent areas of chromosomal loss include chromosome band 1p36, 11q23, and 14q23-qter.[8] A strong correlation exists between the allelic loss of 1p and high-risk neuroblastoma features, including older age, metastatic disease, *MYCN* amplification, and unfavorable outcome.[38] Two large independent studies have shown that although deletion of 1p is associated with unfavorable outcome in univariate analysis, this factor is not prognostic after adjusting for *MYCN* copy number.[39] In contrast, Caron and colleagues reported that loss of 1p was predictive of unfavorable outcome, independent of *MYCN* amplification.[40] Recently, a large Children's Cancer Group (CCG) study has shown that 1p deletion independently predicts for a decreased event-free survival (EFS) but not overall survival. Recently, *CHD5*, a chromatin remodeling gene, has been identified as a candidate 1p36.31 neuroblastoma tumor suppressor gene.[42] Although homozygous genetic inactivation of *CHD5* was not identified, strong promoter methylation of the remaining allele in 1p-deleted neuroblastoma lines was seen, resulting in virtually absent CHD5 expression. Forced expression of CHD5 in neuroblastoma cell lines causes dramatic suppression of clonogenicity and tumorigenicity. Consistent with its role as a tumor suppressor, high CHD5 expression was strongly associated with favorable outcome in an analysis of 101 neuroblastoma tumors.

In contrast to 1p loss of heterozygosity (LOH), 11q LOH and 14q LOH are inversely correlated with *MYCN* amplification.[43,44] Univariate analysis revealed no survival disadvantage for patients whose tumors had 11q genetic loss. However, within the cohort of patients with normal *MYCN* copy number tumors, 11q LOH was associated with a significant decrease in overall survival probability. The clinical relevance of 14q LOH is not clear.

Neurotrophins and Neurotrophin Receptors

The Trk family of tyrosine kinases are critical mediators of neutrophin signaling and play an essential role in normal neuronal development.[45] Differential expression of these neurotrophin receptors is highly associated with the variable biologic and clinical characteristics of neuroblastoma.[46] *TrkA* expression is inversely related to disease stage and *MYCN* amplification status,[47] and accordingly, high *TrkA* expression is associated with favorable prognosis.[48] Similar to *TrkA*, *TrkC* is also highly expressed in biologically favorable neuroblastomas.[46] Conversely, *TrkB* is expressed primarily in advanced-stage tumors that are *MYCN* amplified,[49] whereas it is expressed at low levels or in a truncated form in biologically favorable tumors.[46] Trk receptor targeting and modulation of Trk expression are being explored as novel therapeutic alternatives.

Multidrug Resistance

The multidrug resistance-associated protein (MRP) has been associated with an adverse outcome in tumors with high level of MRP expression and appears to denote a drug-resistant phenotype.[50,51] High levels of MRP expression are correlated with *MYCN* amplification,[52] and a recent study has shown that the *MRP1* gene is directly regulated by MYCN.[53] In contrast, the significance of the multidrug resistance gene (*MDR1*) in neuroblastoma is unclear and remains controversial.

Minimal Residual Disease

The detection of minimal residual disease in both the peripheral blood and bone marrow of children with neuroblastoma has been performed using a variety of methods. The identification of residual tumor cells in samples of blood and bone marrow during therapy has been shown to be prognostic and predicts a cohort of patients at increased risk of relapse.[54] The optimal method and timing during the course of therapy to assess minimal residual disease have yet to be determined.

Prognostic Factors

Stage and Age

Table 23-2 lists the clinical and biologic prognostic factors for patients with neuroblastoma. As with most malignancies, stage of disease is a powerful prognostic factor in neuroblastoma,[55] and several retrospective analyses have

Table 23-2

Prognostic factors in neuroblastoma.

Prognostic Factor	Favorable	Unfavorable
Clinical Factors		
Stage	1, 2, 4S	3, 4
Age	<365 days	>365 days
Tumor Markers		
Ferritin	Low	High
LDH	Low	High
NSE	Low	High
Histology	Favorable	Unfavorable
Biologic Factors		
MYCN oncogene	Normal copy	Amplified
DNA index	>1.0 (Hyperdiploid)	1.0 (Diploid)
Chromosome 1p	Normal	Deletion
Chromosome 11q	Normal	Deletion
Chromosome 17q	Normal	Gain
TrkA expression	High	Low
TrkC expression	High	Low
TrkB expression		High/FL

Abbreviations: LDH, lactic dehydrogenase; NSE, neuron-specific enolase; FL, full-length; MRP, multidrug resistance-associated protein.

confirmed the clinical relevance of the INSS.[56,57] The "special" stage of 4S identified by Evans is limited to infants younger than 1 year and is defined as a stage 1 or 2 primary tumor with metastatic spread limited to liver, skin, and <10% of bone marrow. Age at diagnosis remains the only other independent clinical prognostic factor. For all stages of disease beyond localized tumors, infants younger than 12 months have significantly better disease-free survival than older children with equivalent stages of disease.[58] Recently, studies have suggested that toddlers between 12 and 18 months of age with disseminated disease and favorable tumor biology have an excellent outcome following intensive multimodality therapy.[59,60] These observations suggest that these toddlers may not require intensive myeloablative therapy with hematopoietic stem cell rescue to achieve remission and may respond well to the moderate-dose chemotherapy regimen that is currently used to treat infants with stage 4 disease. To test this hypothesis, the Children's Oncology Group is currently conducting an intermediate-risk clinical trial in which toddlers with favorable biology stage 3 and 4 tumors are being treated with 8 cycles of moderate-dose chemotherapy.

Risk Group Classification

Although modern treatment strategies are tailored according to patient risk, the current approaches to risk stratification vary greatly throughout the world. The COG neuroblastoma risk stratification system is based on an international risk grouping system.[61] In the COG, patients are assigned into low-, intermediate-, and high-risk categories based upon analysis of age at diagnosis, INSS stage, histopathology, *MYCN* amplification status, and DNA index (Table 23-3). However, because the definition of risk is defined differently in other cooperative groups, it is not possible to directly compare the results of clinical trials conducted in different regions of the world. The International Neuroblastoma Risk Group (INRG) classification system was developed to establish a consensus approach for pre-treatment risk stratification.[62] Survival tree regression analyses testing the prognostic significance of 13 factors in 8,800 patients were performed, and the most highly statistically significant and clinically relevant factors were included in the risk group schema. A new staging system (INRG Staging System) based on clinical criteria and tumor imaging was developed for the INRG Classification System.[63] It is anticipated that by defining homogenous pre-treatment patient cohorts, the INRG classification system will greatly facilitate the comparison of risk-based clinical trials conducted in different regions of the world and the development of international collaborative studies.

Treatment

Low-Risk Disease

Low-risk patients require minimal therapy.[64] Previous Pediatric Oncology Group (POG) and CCG studies have shown that treatment with surgery alone results in survival rates of >95% for patients with stage 1 disease.[3,65] The management of the infrequent patient with stage 1 or 2 disease with *MYCN* amplification remains controversial.[3,66] Although patients with *MYCN*-amplified stage 1 tumors have significantly worse EFS and survival rates, a subset may achieve long-term remission following surgery alone.[65,66] These rare cases require continued prospective evaluation to clarify optimal management.

A high rate of spontaneous regression is seen in infants with stage 4S neuroblastoma, and high survival rates have been reported in 4S infants whose tumors lack *MYCN* amplification.[67,68] However, a significant number of 4S infants die within the first month of life from rapidly progressive disease despite favorable tumor biology, and the genetic factors that contribute to this clinical behavior are unknown. Interestingly, in contrast to what has been reported in the POG experience, Tonini and colleagues reported that in the Italian experience, favorable outcomes were also seen in infants with *MYCN*-amplified stage 4S neuroblastoma.[69]

Newborns with small adrenal masses constitute another particularly favorable cohort of patients.[70,71] Recently, trials of expectant observation have been reported for newborns with adrenal masses, and to date, virtually all tumors in these patients have decreased in size or resolved spontaneously.[72,73] These observations suggest that newborns with small or cystic, localized neuroblastomas can be safely observed with a low risk of progression to advanced-stage disease. Currently, the COG has an ongoing clinical

Table 23-3
Children's Oncology Group: Neuroblastoma risk-group schema.*

Stage	Age	MYCN	Ploidy	Histology	Other	Risk Group
1						Low
2A/2B		NA			> 50% resect	Low
		NA			< 50% resect	Inter.
		NA			Bx only	Inter.
		Amp				High
3	< 547 d	NA				Inter.
	≥ 547 d	NA		FH		Inter.
		Amp				High
	≥ 547	NA		UH		High
4	< 365 d	Amp				High
	< 365 d	NA				Inter.
	365–< 547 d	Amp				High
	365–< 547 d		DI = 1			High
	365–< 547 d			UH		High
	365–< 547 d	NA	DI > 1	FH		Inter.
	≥ 547 d					High
4S	< 365 d	NA	DI > 1	FH	Asymptomatic	Low
	< 365 d	NA	DI = 1			Inter.
	< 365 d	Missing	Missing	Missing		Inter.
	< 365 d	NA			Symptomatic	Inter.
	< 365 d	NA		UH		Inter.
	< 365 d	Amp				High

*Reprinted with permission from the Children's Oncology Group (COG).

trial in which neonates with asymptomatic small adrenal masses are being observed.

Excellent outcome is also seen in patients with stages 2A and 2B disease. Four-year EFS and survival rates of $81\% \pm 4\%$ and $98\% \pm 1.5\%$, respectively, were reported in previous CCG studies following treatment with surgery alone.[3] In POG studies, localized disease that was not completely resected (analogous to INSS Stage 2A) was treated with surgery and chemotherapy. Estimated 3-year survival for patients with hyperdiploid tumors that lacked MYCN amplification was 96%.[4] Similarly, excellent outcome for patients with localized neuroblastoma (defined as INSS stages 1, 2, and 3) was seen in the French NBL 90 Study.[74] These findings support the reduction in therapy approach that was tested in the recently completed COG low-risk study. The overall objective of the COG low-risk study was to preserve the excellent survival rate for patients with low-risk neuroblastoma by using surgery as the primary treatment approach, thereby minimizing the risks of acute and long-term chemotherapy-related morbidity for the majority of these patients. The use of chemotherapy is indicated for symptomatic low-risk patients with spinal cord compression, patients with invasive local-region tumors that can not be resected, and patients with stage 4S disease with organ dysfunction.

Intermediate-Risk Disease

In previous POG studies, treatment for infants with regional and metastatic disease was stratified by MYCN amplification and tumor cell ploidy. Infants with hyperdiploid tumors were treated with cyclophosphamide and doxorubicin, whereas infants with diploid tumors received cisplatin and teniposide after an initial course of cyclophosphamide plus doxorubicin.[4] The most recent analysis of patients enrolled on that study demonstrates estimated 11-year survival rates of $94\% \pm 5\%$ and $52\% \pm 16\%$ for patients with hyperdiploid versus diploid tumors.[75] A survival rate of $71\% + .7\%$ was reported in a prospective CCG trial in which infants with regional and metastatic disease were treated with a 4-drug chemotherapy regimen, surgery, and local radiation to residual disease.[5] Infants with tumors that lacked *MYCN* amplification had a 93% ± 4% 3-year EFS, whereas those with amplified *MYCN* tumors had a 10% ± 7% 3-year EFS ($p < 0.0001$). These results emphasize the clinical significance of neuroblastoma tumor biology.

Excellent survival rates have been reported in patients older than 1 year with favorable biology regional tumors following treatment with surgery and chemotherapy.[76,77] However, the use of adjuvant therapy for patients with regional disease has been challenged in a single-institution study in which 88% of patients with INSS stages 2B and 3 tumors that lacked *MYCN* amplification survived without disease progression following surgery alone.[78] These observations suggest that for the majority of patients with biologically favorable regional tumors, chemotherapy may be safely reduced or eliminated. In an effort to avoid associated acute and long-term complications while maintaining high cure rates, adjuvant chemotherapy and radiotherapy have been reduced in the recently completed COG intermediate-risk study. Intermediate-risk patients with favorable biology tumors were treated with a short course of chemotherapy (4 cycles), while intermediate-risk patients with unfavorable biology received a longer course of chemotherapy (8 cycles). The current Children's Oncology Group intermediate-risk clinical trial is testing a further reduction in therapy strategy in patients with favorable biology disease. In this study, treatment is being stratified by the status of chromosome 1p and 11q in addition to *MYCN* status, tumor cell ploidy, and tumor histology.

High-Risk Disease

Survival for children with high-risk disease has improved modestly during the past 20 years, although cure rates remain low.[6,79,80] This improvement is thought to be due to intensification of induction chemotherapy, megatherapy consolidation, and improved supportive care.[81] Cisplatin, etoposide, cyclophosphamide, and doxorubicin are the backbone of high-risk neuroblastoma chemotherapy. Dose intensity has been shown to correlate strongly with both response and progression-free survival, and response rates between 70% and 80% have been seen with intensive multiagent induction regimens.[6,82] Furthermore, several single-armed studies have suggested that intensification of consolidation therapy with autologous stem cell transplantation following myeloablative doses of chemotherapy with or without total body irradiation (TBI) also contributes to improved overall survival.[79,83] A report from the European Group for Blood and Marrow Transplant of 1070 myeloablative procedures followed by stem cell rescue indicated that survival at 2 years posttransplant was 49%, and 5-year survival was 33%.[84] More recently, the superiority of myeloablative therapy and autologous bone marrow transplant over conventional dose chemotherapy has been definitively demonstrated in a randomized study conducted by the CCG.[6] In this study, 3-year EFS was significantly better for patients randomized to the transplant arm than for patients randomized to continuous chemotherapy (34% + 4% vs 22% + 4%, respectively, $p = 0.034$).

In an effort to further dose-intensify consolidation therapy, some investigators have treated patients with tandem cycles of high-dose therapy in conjunction with stem cell rescue. A single-arm trial of peripheral blood stem cell (PBSC)–supported tandem transplantation for high-risk neuroblastoma patients demonstrated that tandem transplant was feasible in this patient cohort, and that toxicity was acceptable.[85] The estimated 3-year EFS rate from the date of diagnosis was promising at 58% (90% confidence interval, 40%-72%). Another pilot study utilized 3 cycles of high-dose therapy with PBSC rescue.[86] With a median of 32 months follow-up, the estimated 3-year EFS rate from the time of diagnosis on that study was 57% ± 11%.

Unfortunately, despite intensive multimodality treatment, more than 50% of children with high-risk disease will relapse due to drug-resistant residual disease.[6] Eradication of refractory microscopic disease remains one of the most significant challenges in the treatment of high-risk neuroblastoma. In an effort to treat chemotherapy-resistant tumor cells, the differentiating agent 13-*cis*-retinoic acid (RA) has been administered to high-risk patients following completion of consolidation therapy. A recently completed CCG study demonstrated that the administration of 13-*cis*-RA in the setting of minimal residual disease was clinically effective and resulted in improved 3-year EFS.[6] Preliminary data suggest that other biologic agents may also be clinically effective in the setting of minimal residual disease.

Surgery

Surgery is an integral part of neuroblastoma therapy. Diagnostic biopsies are critical for diagnosis and for obtaining sufficient tumor for biologic studies that help to guide risk-based therapy. However, the effectiveness of modern chemotherapy and the identification of favorable risk groups allow for more serious consideration of surgical intervention to avoid potential surgical morbidity. Sampling of nonadherent intracavitary lymph nodes is recommended for accurate staging. However, the sacrifice of vital organs should be avoided. The impact of surgical resection of the primary tumor on outcome in patients with high-risk metastatic disease remains controversial.[87,88]

Radiotherapy

The role of radiotherapy in neuroblastoma treatment is not entirely defined despite the fact that neuroblastoma is clearly a radiosensitive tumor. Patients with low- and intermediate-risk disease usually can be cured without radiotherapy. The use of radiotherapy is often considered only in stage 4S patients with compromising hepatomegaly and patients with spinal cord compression, although the benefit in these settings is unclear. For the high-risk cohort of patients, TBI has been previously incorporated in myeloablative regimens but without any significant improvement in overall outcome. More recently, reports have suggested that radiotherapy (21–34 Gy) to the primary tumor site is effective in decreasing the incidence of local tumor recurrence in patients following myeloablative therapy.[89,90] The role of radiotherapy to metastatic sites that either resolve or remain persistent, especially with continued mIBG positivity, is not defined.

Treatment of Spinal Cord Compression

Approximately 7% to 15% of patients present with paraspinal tumors that extend through vertebral foramina either with or without associated spinal cord compression.[91] Prompt resolution of spinal cord compression may prevent the development of permanent neurologic impairment in these children. Current therapeutic strategies to relieve spinal cord compression include surgical resection either with or without laminectomy, chemotherapy, and radiation therapy.[92,93] The optimal treatment approach for cord decompression, however, remains unknown. In a retrospective review of the POG experience, similar rates of neurologic recovery were observed in symptomatic patients following treatment with chemotherapy or laminectomy, although more orthopedic sequelae were observed in the children treated with laminectomy.[94] Plantaz and colleagues similarly reported that chemotherapy effectively relieved neurologic symptoms from cord compression due to neuroblastoma.[95] Taken together, these results support a primary medical approach for the initial treatment of children with intraspinal neuroblastoma, particularly in those patients with prolonged symptomatology (>1 week). Laminectomy may be reserved for those patients who progress following the initiation of chemotherapy or who present with paralysis of extremely short duration (<24–48 hours).

Treatment of Opsoclonus/ Myoclonus Syndrome

The opsoclonus/myoclonus syndrome that occurs coincident with neuroblastoma in about 4% of patients is believed to be immune mediated and may consist of random, dysconjugate eye movements, abnormal muscle jerks, and ataxia. Although approximately 60% of patients will respond to adrenocorticotropic hormone or corticosteroid therapy, most patients will have recurrences of their neurologic symptoms and will experience developmental delay or mental retardation despite the fact that these tumors are typically associated with a more favorable prognosis.[96] Several retrospective studies suggest that the administration of chemotherapy may improve the long-term neurologic outcome of this group of patients, including patients with low-risk disease who would typically be expected to be cured of their disease with surgical resection alone.[97] There have also been several case reports indicating good responses to treatment with intravenous gamma globulin.[98] Recently, the COG has designed a prospective study to determine if the addition of intravenous gamma globulin to chemotherapy and steroids will improve the neurologic outcome for patients with neuroblastoma and coincident opsoclonus/ myoclonus syndrome.

Relapsed and Refractory Disease

Treatment and prognosis for patients with recurrent disease are based upon the initial risk classification, initial therapy, extent of recurrence, and tumor biology. Some low- and intermediate-risk patients who develop recurrence may be treated with surgical resection alone if the tumor has been entirely re-excised. Patients who do not have a complete resection following recurrence are treated with chemotherapy. Intermediate-risk patients with extensive recurrence and/or unfavorable biology are candidates for aggressive high-risk therapeutic approaches.

Patients who initially had high-risk disease and have either refractory disease or recurrent disease post myeloablative therapy have an extremely poor outcome and are rarely curable.[99] These patients should be considered for Phase I and II trials and other novel therapeutic approaches.

Experimental Therapies

Cytotoxic Agents

Responses to topotecan, a topoisomerase I inhibitor, have been observed in patients with refractory or recurrent neuroblastoma.[100] Combination therapy with topotecan plus cyclophosphamide or carboplatin has also been shown to have activity against recurrent neuroblastoma.[101,102] Based on these promising results, 2 cycles of dose-intensive topotecan in combination with cyclophoshamide have been incorporated into the induction regimen of the current Children's Oncology Group high-risk clinical trial. The COG is currently evaluating the clinical efficacy of another topoisomerase I inhibitor, irinotecan in combination with temozolamide.

Retinoids

Retinoids are natural and synthetic derivatives of vitamin A. Treatment with all trans-RA and 13-cis-RA induces neuroblastoma differentiation in vitro, down-regulates MYCN mRNA expression, and leads to a sustained arrest of tumor cell proliferation.[103–105] These laboratory observations prompted the development of clinical trials designed to test the clinical utility of 13-cis-RA in children with relapsed neuroblastoma. In Phase I and II trials, the overall activity of 13-cis-RA in patients with high tumor burden was disappointing.[106,107] However, as mentioned above, in a subsequent randomized Phase III study, 13-cis-RA was shown to improve 3-year EFS when it was administered to patients with minimal residual disease following completion of consolidation therapy.[6] Thus, 13-cis-RA appears to be most effective in the setting of minimal residual disease.

The synthetic retinoid fenretinide (4-HPR) has also been shown to inhibit neuroblastoma growth in vitro, and it is highly active against RA-resistant neuroblastoma cell lines.[105] In contrast to 13-cis-RA and all trans-RA, 4-HPR induces apoptosis and necrosis.[108] Furthermore, a recent report indicates that 4-HPR may also inhibit neuroblastoma-induced angiogenesis.[109] Phase I and II trials are being conducted to determine the clinical activity of this compound against neuroblastoma.

Immunotherapy

Another promising approach for the treatment of multidrug resistant microscopic disease is targeted immunotherapy, which exploits tumor selectivity and has minimal cross-resistance and overlapping toxicities with chemotherapy. Disialoganglioside (GD2) is particularly suitable for immunotherapy because it is expressed at a high density in human neuroblastoma tumors.[110] Several anti-GD2 monoclonal antibodies have been developed and tested in clinical trials.[111] Initial studies were performed with murine monoclonal antibodies (3F8 and 14G.2a), and more recently, a human-murine chimeric antibody (ch14.18) has been developed and tested.[112] Therapeutic responses have been observed in Phase I and Phase II studies with both the murine and chimeric antibodies.[113,114] In small series of patients, therapeutic responses have been reported with radiolabeled I[131]-3F8 antibody (8-28 mCi/kg) followed by autologous bone marrow rescue.[112]

In an effort to enhance response rates, cytokines have been combined with anti-GD2 antibodies to increase antibody-dependent cellular cytotoxicity (ADCC). Granulocyte-macrophage colony-stimulating factor (GM-CSF) has been shown to increase leukocyte number and enhance their anti-GD2 mediated ADCC[26], and therapeutic responses have been observed in trials using ch14:18 anti-GD2 antibody plus GM-CSF in patients with recurrent/refractory neuroblastoma.[111] Interleukin-2 has also been shown to augment lymphocyte-mediated ADCC.[115] Enhancement of natural killer cell activity by IL-2 has been observed in some patients treated with the combination of anti-GD2 and IL-2.[116] The COG is currently conducting a randomized Phase III trial that has been designed to determine if the addition of ch14:18 anti-GD2 antibody and cytokines to 13-cis-RA in the setting of minimal residual disease will improve the outcome of high-risk neuroblastoma patients.

Other targeted immunotherapy studies are being conducted with cytokine-modified neuroblastoma cells, cytotoxic T lymphocytes, modified dendritic cells, and recombinant IL-2.[117] Interleukin-2 has been infused following myeloablative therapy and stem cell rescue in several small series.[118] To target delivery of cytokine therapy and achieve more effective concentrations of IL-2 in the tumor microenvironment, a hu14:18-IL2 fusion protein has recently been generated.[119] Preclinical studies have demonstrated that this fusion protein induces a cellular immune response that results in inhibited tumor growth. A recent COG Phase II study testing the hu14:18-IL2 fusion protein in relapsed neuroblastoma patients has been completed, which demonstrated responses in patients with only mIBG and/or bone marrow disease but not in patients with bulky disease.

Radioiodinated Meta-iodobenzylguanadine

Radioiodinated mIBG has been used to target delivery of radiotherapy, and responses have been observed.[120] Prom-

ising results have also been reported with combination radiolabeled mIBG and myeloablative chemotherapy followed by autologous stem cell rescue.[121] Additional clinical trials are ongoing in North America and Europe that are hoped to determine the optimal dose, schedule, and timing of mIBG therapy. These trials also seek to determine if mIBG can improve the survival of high-risk patients and whether it is feasible to deliver such therapy to a large cooperative group population.

Antiangiogenic Therapy

Angiogenesis plays an important role in the growth and metastasis of malignant tumors.[122] In neuroblastoma, high-level expression of angiogenesis activators and high tumor vascularity have been shown to correlate with advanced-stage disease, whereas low vascular tumor density correlates with localized disease and favorable outcome.[123,124] Furthermore, preclinical studies have demonstrated that antiangiogenic agents effectively inhibit neuroblastoma growth in vivo and that the optimal response may be in the setting of minimal residual disease.[125] These observations suggest that angiogenesis inhibitors may be effective in the treatment of patients with highly vascular neuroblastoma tumors. Phase I studies testing a number of angiogenesis inhibitors are ongoing.

Late Effects

The long-term effects of modern neuroblastoma therapy have not been fully established. Low- and intermediate-risk therapy, as currently designed, is not expected to result in significant long-term sequelae, with the exception of patients with the opsoclonus/myoclonus syndrome who often have long-term neurologic and developmental problems and patients with spinal cord compression who may develop scoliosis post laminectomy.

Patients with high-risk disease often have many long-term therapy-related complications, including psychosocial problems, growth problems, secondary malignancies, and ototoxicity.

Screening

Screening for neuroblastoma has been evaluated in North America, Japan, and Germany. Data from all of these studies demonstrate that the neuroblastoma tumors identified by screening urine samples are associated with favorable stage and tumor biology.[126] Population-based studies have demonstrated that screening results in an increase in the incidence of neuroblastoma in infants, but there has not been a decrease in the rate of occurrence in older children nor a decrease in mortality rates. Thus, there is no clear benefit for neuroblastoma screening in the first year of life, and most programs have been abandoned.

Summary

Although substantial progress has been made in the treatment of children with low- and intermediate-risk neuroblastoma, cure rates for high-risk patients remain dismal.

Research aimed at discovering new genes and pathways critical to neuroblastoma tumorigenesis and drug resistance should be prioritized in an effort to identify new targets for therapeutic strategies. The hope is that further development of innovative, biologically based treatment approaches will prove to be effective in the treatment of neuroblastoma and result in improved survival of children with clinically aggressive neuroblastoma.

References

1. Brodeur GM, Maris JM. Neuroblastoma. In: Pizzo PA, Poplack DG, eds. *Principles and Practice of Pediatric Oncology*. 4th ed. Philadelphia: Lippincott-Raven; 2001:895–937.
2. D'Angio GJ, Evans AE, Koop CE. Special pattern of widespread neuroblastoma with a favourable prognosis. *Lancet*; 1971;1(7708):1046–1049.
3. Perez CA, Matthay KK, Atkinson JB, et al. Biological variables in the outcome of stages I and II neuroblastoma treated with surgery as primary therapy: a Children's Cancer Group study. *J Clin Oncol*. 2000;18:18–26.
4. Bowman LC, Castleberry RP, Cantor A, et al. Genetic staging of unresectable or metastatic neuroblastoma in infants: a Pediatric Oncology Group Study. *J Natl Cancer Inst*. 1997;89:373–380.
5. Schmidt ML, Lukens JN, Seeger RC, et al. Biologic factors determine prognosis in infants with stage IV neuroblastoma: a prospective Children's Cancer Group Study. *J Clin Oncol*. 2000;18:1260–1268.
6. Matthay KK, Villablanca JG, Seeger RC, et al. Treatment of high-risk neuroblastoma with intensive chemotherapy, radiotherapy, autologous bone marrow transplantation, and 13-*cis*-retinoic acid. *N Engl J Med*. 1999;341:1165–1173.
7. Shimada H, Ambros IM, Dehner LP, et al. The International Neuroblastoma Pathology Classification (the Shimada System). *Cancer*. 1999;86:364–372.
8. Maris JM, Matthay KK. Molecular biology of neuroblastoma. *J Clin Oncol*. 1999;17:2226–2279.
9. Brodeur GM, Maris JM Neuroblastoma In Pizzo PA, Poplack DG, eds. *Principles and Practice of Pediatric Oncology*. 4th ed. Philadelphia. Lipincott-Raven; 2001:895–937.
10. Maris JM, Kyemba SM, Rebbeck TR, et al. Familial prediposition to neuroblastoma does not map to chromosome band 1p36. *Cancer Res*. 1996;56:3421–3425.
11. Kurshner BH, Gilbert F, Helson L Familial neuroblastoma. Case reports, literature review, and etiologic conderations. *Cancer*. 1986;57:1887–1893.
12. Mosse YP, Lauderslager M, Khazi D, et al. Germline PHOX2B mutation in hereditary neuroblastoma. *AM J Hum Genet*. 2004;75:727–730.
13. Trochet D, Bourdeaut F, Janoueix-Lerosey I, et al. Germline mutations of the paired-like homeobox 2B (PHOX2B) gene in neuroblastoma. *Am J Hum Genet*. 2004;74:761–764.
14. Mosse YP, Laudenslager M, Longo L, et al. Identification of ALK as a major familial neuroblastoma predisposition gene. *Nature*. in press.
15. George RE, Sanda T, Hanna M, et al. Activating mutations in the *ALK* tyrosine kinase provide a therapeutic target in neuroblastoma. *Nature*. in press.
16. Maris JM, Mosse YP, Bradfield JP, et al. Chromosome 6p22 locus associated with clinically aggressive neuroblastoma. *N Engl J Med*. 2008;358:2585–2593.
17. Brodeur GM, Pritchard J, Berthold F, et al. Revisions of the international criteria for neuroblastoma diagnosis, staging, and response to treatment. *J Clin Oncol*. 1993;11:1466–1477.
18. Matthay KK, Edeline V, Lumbroso J, et al. Correlation of early metastatic response by 123I-metaiodobenzylguanidine scintigraphy with overall response and event-free survival in stage IV neuroblastoma. *J Clin Oncol*. 2003;21:2486–2491.
19. Katzenstein HM, Cohn SL, Shore RM, et al. Scintigraphic response by 123I-metaiodobenzylguanidine scan correlates with event-free survival in high-risk neuroblastoma. *J Clin Oncol*. 2004;22:3909–3915.
20. Riley RD, Heney D, Jones D, et al. A systematic review of molecular and biological tumor markers in neuroblastoma. *Clin Cancer Res*. 2004;10:4–12.
21. Kushner BH, LaQuaglia MP, Kramer K, Cheung NK. Radically different treatment recommendations for newly diagnosed neuroblastoma: pitfalls in assessment of risk. *J Pediatr Hematol Oncol*. 2004;26:35–39.
22. Shimada H, Chatten J, Newton WA Jr, et al. Histopathologic prognostic factors in neuroblastic tumors: definition of subtypes of ganglioneuroblastoma and an age-linked classification of neuroblastomas. *J Natl Cancer Inst*. 1984; 73:405–416.
23. Cohn SL, Rademaker AW, Salwen HR, et al. Analysis of DNA ploidy and proliferative activity in relation to histology and N-*myc* amplification in neuroblastoma. *Am J Pathol*. 1990;136:1043–1052.
24. Shimada H, Stram DO, Chatten J, et al. Identification of subsets of neuroblastomas by combined histopathologic and N-*myc* analysis. *J Natl Cancer Inst*. 1995;87:1470–1476.
25. Brodeur GM, Seeger RC, Schwab M, Varmus HE, Bishop JM. Amplification of N-*myc* in untreated human neuroblastomas correlates with advanced disease stage. *Science*. 1984;224:1121–1124.
26. Seeger RC, Brodeur GM, Sather H, et al. Association of multiple copies of the N-*myc* oncogene with rapid progression of neuroblastomas. *N Engl J Med*. 1985;313:1111–1116.
27. Schweigerer L, Breit S, Wenzel A, Tsunamoto K, Ludwig R, Schwab M. Augmented *MYCN* expression advances the malignant phenotype of human neuroblastoma cells: evidence for induction of autocrine growth factor activity. *Cancer Res*. 1990;50:4411–4416.
28. Weiss WA, Aldape K, Mohapatra G, Feuerstein BG, Bishop JM. Targeted expression of *MYCN* causes neuroblastoma in transgenic mice. *Embo J*. 1997; 16(11):2985–2995.
29. Spitz R, Hero B, Skowron M, Ernestus K, Berthold F. *MYCN*-status in neuroblastoma: characteristics of tumours showing amplification, gain, and non-amplification. *Eur J Cancer*. 2004;40(18):2639–2642.
30. Cohn SL, Tweddle DA. *MYCN* amplification remains prognostically strong 20 years after its "clinical debut." *Eur J Cancer*. 2004;40(18):2639–2642.
31. Bordow SB, Norris MD, Haber PS, Marshall GM, Haber M. Prognostic significance of *MYCN* oncogene expression in childhood neuroblastoma. *J Clin Oncol*. 1998;16:3286–3294.
32. Chan HSL, Gallie BL, DeBoer G, et al. MYCN protein expression as a predictor of neuroblastoma prognosis. *Clin Cancer Res*. 1997;3:1699–1706.
33. Cohn SL, London WB, Huang D, et al. *MYCN* expression is not prognostic of adverse outcome in advanced-stage neuroblastoma with nonamplified *MYCN*. *J Clin Oncol*. 2000;18:3604–3613.
34. Look AT, Hayes FA, Shuster JJ, et al. Clinical relevance of tumor cell ploidy and N-*myc* gene amplification in childhood neuroblastoma: a Pediatric Oncology Group study. *J Clin Oncol*. 1991;9:581–591.
35. Look AT, Hayes FA, Nitschke R, McWilliams NB, Green AA. Cellular DNA content as a predictor of response to chemotherapy in infants with unresectable neuroblastoma. *N Engl J Med*. 1984;311:231–235.
36. Taylor SR, Locker J. A comparative analysis of nuclear DNA content and N-*myc* gene amplification in neuroblastoma. *Cancer*. 1990;65:1360–1366.
37. Bown N, Cotterill S, Lastowska M, et al. Gain of chromosome arm 17q and adverse outcome in patients with neuroblastoma. *N Engl J Med*. 1999;340: 1954–1961.
38. Fong CT, Dracopoli NC, White PS, et al. Loss of heterozygosity for the short arm of chromosome 1 in human neuroblastomas: correlation with N-*myc* amplification. *Proc Natl Acad Sci USA*. 1989;86:3753–3757.
39. Maris JM, White PS, Beltinger CP, et al. Significance of chromosome 1p loss of heterozygosity in neuroblastoma. *Cancer Res*. 1995;55:4664–4669.
40. Caron H, van Sluis P, de Kraker J, et al. Allelic loss of chromosome 1p as a predictor of unfavorable outcome in patients with neuroblastoma. *N Engl J Med*. 1996;334:225–230.
41. Maris JM, Weiss MJ, Guo C, et al. Loss of heterozygosity at 1p36 independently predicts for disease progression, but not decreased overall survival probability in neuroblastoma patients: a Children's Cancer Group Study. *J Clin Oncol*. 2000;18:1888–1899.
42. Fujita T, Igarashi J, Okawa ER, et al. CHD5, a tumor suppressor gene deleted from 1p36.31 in neuroblastomas. *J Natl Cancer Inst*. 2008;100:940–949.
43. Guo C, White PS, Weiss MJ, et al. Allelic deletion at 11q23 is common in *MYCN* single copy neuroblastomas. *Oncogene*. 1999;18:4948–4957.
44. Thompson PM, Seifried BA, Kyemba SM, et al. Loss of heterozygosity for chromosome 14q in neuroblastoma. *Med Pediatr Oncol*. 2001;36:28–31.
45. Barbacid, M. Neurotrophic factors and their receptors. *Curr Opin Cell Biol*. 1995;7:148–155.
46. Brodeur GM, Nakagawara A, Yamashiro DJ, et al. Expression of *TrkA*, *TrkB* and *TrkC* in human neuroblastomas. *J Neuro-Oncol*. 1997;31:49–55.
47. Nakagawara A, Arima M, Azar CG, Scavarda NJ, Brodeur GM. Inverse relationship between *trk* expression and N-*myc* amplification in human neuroblastomas. *Cancer Res*. 1992;52:1364–1368.
48. Nakagawara A, Arima-Nakagawara M, Scavarda NJ, Azar CG, Cantor AB, Brodeur GM. Association between high levels of expression of the *TRK* gene and favorable outcome in human neuroblastoma. *N Engl J Med*. 1993;328: 847–854.
49. Nakagawara A, Azar CG, Scavarda NJ, Brodeur GM. Expression and function of *TRK-B* and *BDNF* in human neuroblastomas. *Mol Cell Biol*. 1994;14:759–767.
50. Norris MD, Bordow SB, Marshall GM, Haber PS, Cohn SL, Haber, M. Expression of the gene for multidrug-resistance-associated protein and outcome in patients with neuroblastoma. *N Engl J Med*. 1996;334:231–238.
51. Haber M, Bordow SB, Gilbert J, et al. Altered expression of the *MYCN* oncogene modulates *MRP* gene expression and response to cytotoxic drugs in neuroblastoma cells. *Oncogene*. 1999;18:2777–2782.
52. Bordow SB, Haber M, Madafiglio J, Cheung B, Marshall GM, Norris MD. Expression of the multidrug resistance-associated protein (MRP) gene correlates with amplification and overexpression of the N-*myc* oncogene in childhood neuroblastoma. *Cancer Res*. 1994;54:5036–5040.
53. Manohar CF, Bray JA, Salwen HR, et al. MYCN-mediated regulation of the MRP1 promoter in human neuroblastoma. *Oncogene*. 2004;23:753–762.
54. Seeger RC, Reynolds CP, Gallego R, Stram DO, Gerbing RB, Matthay KK. Quantitative tumor cell content of bone marrow and blood as a predictor of outcome in stage IV neuroblastoma: a Children's Cancer Group Study. *J Clin Oncol*. 2000;18:4067–4076.
55. Evans AE, D'Angio GJ, Propert K, Anderson J, Hann H-WL. Prognostic factors in neuroblastoma. *Cancer*. 1987;59:1853–1859.

56. Haase GM, Atkinson JB, Stram DO, Lukens JN, Matthay KK. Surgical management and outcome of locoregional neuroblastoma: comparison of the Children's Cancer Group and the international staging systems. *J Pediatr Surg.* 1995;30:289–294.
57. Castleberry RP, Shuster JJ, Smith EI. The Pediatric Oncology Group experience with the International Staging System criteria for neuroblastoma. Member Institutions of the Pediatric Oncology Group. *J Clin Oncol.* 1994;12(11):2378–2381.
58. Evans AE, D'Angio GJ, Randolph J. A proposed staging for children with neuroblastoma. Children's Cancer Study Group A. *Cancer.* 1971;27(2):374–378.
59. George R, London WB, Maris JM, Cohn SL, Diller L, Look AT. Age as a continuous variable in predicting outcome for neuroblastoma patients with metastatic disease: impact of tumor biological features. *Proc Am Soc Clin Oncol.* 2003;22.
60. Schmidt ML, Lal A, Seeger R, Maris JM, Shimada H, O'Leary M, Gerbing R, Matthay K. Favorable prognosis for patients age 12–18 months with stage 4 MYCN-nonamplified neuroblastoma. *Proc Am Soc Clin Oncol.* 2003;22.
61. Castleberry RP, Pritchard J, Ambros P, et al. The International Neuroblastoma Risk Groupings (INRG): a preliminary report. *Eur J Cancer.* 1997;33:2113–2116.
62. Cohn SL, Pearson ADJ, London WB, et al. The International Neuroblastoma Risk Group (INRG) Classification System. *J Clin Oncol.* 2008.
63. Monclair T, Brodeur GM, Ambros PF, et al. The International Neuroblastoma Risk Grouping (INRG) staging system. *J Clin Oncol.* 2008.
64. Nitschke R, Smith EI, Shochat S, et al. Localized neuroblastoma treated by surgery: a Pediatric Oncology Group study. *J Clin Oncol.* 1988;6:1271–1279.
65. Alvarado CS, London WB, Look AT, et al. Natural history and biology of stage A neuroblastoma: a Pediatric Oncology Group study. *J Pediatr Hematol Oncol.* 2000;22:197–205.
66. Cohn SL, Look AT, Joshi VV, et al. Lack of correlation of N-myc gene amplification with prognosis in localized neuroblastoma: a Pediatric Oncology Group study. *Cancer Res.* 1995;55:721–726.
67. Katzenstein HM, Bowman LC, Brodeur GM, et al. Prognostic significance of age, MYCN oncogene amplification, tumor cell ploidy, and histology in 110 infants with stage D(S) neuroblastoma: the Pediatric Oncology Group experience. A Pediatric Oncology Group Study. *J Clin Oncol.* 1998;16:2007–2017.
68. Nickerson HJ, Matthay KK, Seeger RC, et al. Favorable biology and outcome of stage IV-S neuroblastoma with supportive care or minimal therapy: a Children's Cancer Group study. *J Clin Oncol.* 2000;18:477–486.
69. Tonini GP, Boni L, Pession A, et al. MYCN oncogene amplification in neuroblastoma is associated with worse prognosis, except in stage 4s: the Italian experience with 295 children. *J Clin Oncol.* 1997;15:85–93.
70. Ho PT, Estroff JA, Kozakewich H, et al. Prenatal detection of neuroblastoma: a ten-year experience from the Dana-Farber Cancer Institute and Children's Hospital. *Pediatrics.* 1993;92:358–364.
71. Saylors RL, Cohn SL, Morgan ER, Brodeur GM. Prenatal detection of neuroblastoma by fetal ultrasonography. *Am J Pediatr Hematol Oncol.* 1994;16:356–360.
72. Holgersen LO, Subramanian S, Kirpekar M, Mootabar H, Marcus JR. Spontaneous resolution of antenatally diagnosed adrenal masses. *J Pediatr Surg.* 1996;31:153–155.
73. Yamamoto K, Hanada R, Kikuchi A, et al. Spontaneous regression of localized neuroblastoma detected by mass screening. *J Clin Oncol.* 1998;16:1265–1269.
74. Rubie H, Hartmann O, Michon J, et al; for the Societe Française d'Oncologie Pediatrique N-myc gene amplification is a major prognostic factor in localized neuroblastoma: results of the French NBL 90 Study. *J Clin Oncol.* 1997;15:1171–1182.
75. Bagatell R, Rumcheva P, London WB, et al. Outcomes of children with intermediate-risk neuroblastoma after treatment stratified by MYCN status and tumor cell ploidy. *J Clin Oncol.* 2005;23(34):8819–8827.
76. Matthay KK, Perez C, Seeger RC, et al. Successful treatment of Stage III neuroblastoma based on prospective biologic staging: a Children's Cancer Group Study. *J Clin Oncol.* 1998;16:1256–1264.
77. Strother D, van Hoff J, Rao PV, et al. Event-free survival of children with biologically favourable neuroblastoma based on the degree of initial tumour resection: results from the Pediatric Oncology Group. *Eur J Cancer.* 1997;33:2121–2125.
78. Kushner BH, Cheung N-KV, LaQuaglia MP, et al. Survival from locally invasive or widespread neuroblastoma without cytotoxic therapy. *J Clin Oncol.* 1996;14:373–381.
79. Philip T, Zucker JM, Bernard JL, et al. Improved survival at 2 and 5 years in the LMCE1 unselected group of 72 children with stage IV neuroblastoma older than 1 year of age at diagnosis: is cure possible in a small subgroup? *J Clin Oncol.* 1991;9:1037–1044.
80. Matthay KK, Castleberry RP. Treatment of advanced neuroblastoma: the US experience. In: Brodeur GM, Sawada T, Tsuchida Y, Voute PA, eds. *Neuroblastoma.* Amsterdam: Elsevier Science BV; 2000:417–436.
81. Cheung NK, Heller G. Chemotherapy dose intensity correlates strongly with response, median survival, and median progression-free survival in metastatic neuroblastoma. *J Clin Oncol.* 1991;9:1050–1058.
82. Kushner BH, LaQuaglia MP, Bonilla MA, et al. Highly effective induction therapy for stage 4 neuroblastoma in children over 1 year of age. *J Clin Oncol.* 1994;12:2607–2613.
83. Kushner BH, O'Reilly RJ, Mandell LR, Gulati SC, LaQuaglia M, Cheung NK. Myeloablative combination chemotherapy without total body irradiation for neuroblastoma. *J Clin Oncol.* 1991;9:274–279.
84. Philip T, Ladenstein R, Lasset C, et al. 1070 myeloablative megatherapy procedures followed by stem cell rescue for neuroblastoma: 17 years of European experience and conclusions. European Group for Blood and Marrow Transplant Registry Solid Tumour Working Party. *Eur J Cancer.* 1997;33:2130–2135.
85. Grupp SA, Stern JW, Bunin N, et al. Tandem high-dose therapy in rapid sequence for children with high-risk neuroblastoma. *J Clin Oncol.* 2000;18:2567–2575.
86. Kletzel M, Katzenstein HM, Haut PR, et al. Treatment of high-risk neuroblastoma with triple-tandem high-dose therapy and stem-cell rescue: results of the Chicago Pilot II Study. *J Clin Oncol.* 2002;20:2284–2292.
87. Adkins ES, Sawin R, Gerbing RB, London WB, Matthay KK, Haase GM. Efficacy of complete resection for high-risk neuroblastoma: a Children's Cancer Group Study. *J Pediatr Surg.* 2004;39(6):931–936.
88. La Quaglia MP, Kushner BH, Su W, et al. The impact of gross total resection on local control and survival in high-risk neuroblastoma. *J Pediatr Surg.* 2004;39:412–417.
89. Bradfield SM, Douglas JG, Hawkins DS, Sanders JE, Park JR. Fractionated low-dose radiotherapy after myeloablative stem cell transplantation for local control in patients with high-risk neuroblastoma. *Cancer.* 2004;100:1268–1275.
90. Haas-Kogan DA, Swift PS, Selch M, et al. Impact of radiotherapy for high-risk neuroblastoma: a Children's Cancer Group study. *Int J Radiat Oncol Biol Phys.* 2003;56:28–39.
91. Hoover M, Bowman LC, Crawford SE, et al. Long-term outcome of patients with intraspinal neuroblastoma. *Med Pediatr Oncol.* 1999;32:353–359.
92. Hayes FA, Thompson EI, Hvizdala E, O'Connor D, Green AA. Chemotherapy as an alternative to laminectomy and radiation in the management of epidural tumor. *J Pediatr.* 1984;104:221–224.
93. Raffel C. Spinal cord compression by epidural tumors in childhood. *Neurosurg Clin North Am.* 1992;3:925–930.
94. Katzenstein HM, Kent PM, London WB, Cohn SL. Treatment and outcome of 83 children with intraspinal neuroblastoma: the Pediatric Oncology Group experience. *J Clin Oncol.* 2001;19:1047–1055.
95. Plantaz D, Rubie H, Michon J, et al. The treatment of neuroblastoma with intraspinal extension with chemotherapy followed by surgical removal of residual disease. *Cancer.* 1996;78:311–319.
96. Koh PS, Raffensperger JG, Berry S, et al. L. Long-term outcome in children with opsoclonus-myoclonus and ataxia and coincident neuroblastoma. *J Pediatr.* 1994;125:712–716.
97. Russo C, Cohn SL, Petruzzi MJ, de Alarcon PA. Long-term neurologic outcome in children with opsoclonus-myoclonus associated with neuroblastoma: a report from the Pediatric Oncology Group. *Med Pediatr Oncol.* 1997;28:284–288.
98. Petruzzi MJ, de Alarcon PA. Neuroblastoma-associated opsoclonus-myoclonus treated with intravenously administered immune globulin G. *J Pediatr.* 1995;127:328–329.
99. Lau L, Tai D, Weitzman S, Grant R, Baruchel S, Malkin D. Factors influencing survival in children with recurrent neuroblastoma. *J Pediatr Hematol Oncol.* 2004;26:227–232.
100. Nitschke R, Parkhurst J, Sullivan J, Harris MB, Bernstein M, Pratt C. Topotecan in pediatric patients with recurrent and progressive solid tumors: a Pediatric Oncology Group phase II study. *J Pediatr Hematol Oncol.* 1998;20:315–318.
101. Saylors RL, Stine KC, Sullivan J, et al; the Pediatric Oncology Group. Cyclophosphamide plus topotecan in children with recurrent or refractory solid tumors: a Pediatric Oncology Group phase II study. *J Clin Oncol.* 2001;19:3463–3469.
102. Athale UH, Stewart C, Kuttesch JF, et al. Phase I study of combination topotecan and carboplatin in pediatric solid tumors. *J Clin Oncol.* 2002;20:88–95.
103. Sidell, N. Retinoic acid-induced growth inhibition and morphologic differentiation of human neuroblastoma cells in vitro. *J Natl Cancer Inst.* 1982;68:589–596.
104. Thiele CJ, Reynolds CP, Israel MA. Decreased expression of N-myc precedes retinoic acid-induced morphological differentiation of human neuroblastoma. *Nature.* 1985;313:404–406.
105. Reynolds CP, Lemons RS. Retinoid therapy of childhood cancer. *Hematol Oncol Clin North Am.* 2001;15(5):867–910.
106. Finklestein JZ, Krailo MD, Lenarsky C, et al. 13-cis-retinoic acid (NSC 122758) in the treatment of children with metastatic neuroblastoma unresponsive to conventional chemotherapy: report from the Children's Cancer Study Group. *Med Pediatr Oncol.* 1992;20(4):307–311.
107. Villablanca JG, Khan AA, Avramis VI, et al. Phase I trial of 13-cis-retinoic acid in children with neuroblastoma following bone marrow transplantation. *J Clin Oncol.* 1995;13:894–901.
108. Lovat PE, Ranalli M, Annichiarrico-Petruzzelli M, et al. Effector mechanisms of fenretinide-induced apoptosis in neuroblastoma. *Exp Cell Res.* 2000;260:50–60.
109. Ribatti D, Alessandri G, Baronio M, et al. Inhibition of neuroblastoma-induced angiogenesis by fenretinide. *Int J Cancer.* 2001;94:314–321.
110. Wu ZL, Schwartz E, Seeger R, Ladisch S. Expression of GD2 ganglioside by untreated primary human neuroblastomas. *Cancer Res.* 1986;46:440–443.

111. Cheung N-KV, Yu AL. Immunotherapy of neuroblastoma. In: Brodeur GM, Sawada T, Tsuchida Y, Voute PA, eds., *Neuroblastoma*. Amsterdam: Elsevier Science; 2000:541–560.
112. Cheung NK, Kushner BH, Kramer K. Monoclonal antibody-based therapy of neuroblastoma. *Hematol Oncol Clin North Am*. 2001;15:853–866.
113. Handgretinger R, Baader P, Dopfer R, et al. A phase I study of neuroblastoma with the anti-ganglioside GD2 antibody 14.G2a. *Cancer Immunol Immunother*. 1992;35:199–204.
114. Yu AL, Uttenreuther-Fischer MM, Huang CS. Phase I trial of a human-mouse chimeric anti-disialoganglioside monoclonal antibody ch14.18 in patients with refractory neuroblastoma and osteosarcoma. *J Clin Oncol*. 1998;16: 2169–2180.
115. Munn DH, Cheung NK. Interleukin-2 enhancement of monoclonal antibody-mediated cellular cytotoxicity against human melanoma. *Cancer Res*. 1987; 47:6600–6605.
116. Frost JD, Hank JA, Reaman GH, et al. A phase I/IB trial of murine monoclonal anti-GD2 antibody 14.G2a plus interleukin-2 in children with refractory neuroblastoma: a report of the Children's Cancer Group. *Cancer*. 1997;80:317–333.
117. Haight AE, Bowman LC, Ng CY, Vanin EF, Davidoff AM. Humoral response to vaccination with interleukin-2-expressing allogeneic neuroblastoma cells after primary therapy. *Med Pediatr Oncol*. 2000;35:712–715.
118. Pardo N, Marti F, Fraga G, et al. High-dose systemic interleukin-2 therapy in stage IV neuroblastoma for one year after autologous bone marrow transplantation: pilot study. *Med Pediatr Oncol*. 1996;27:534–539.
119. Becker JC, Varki N, Gillies SD, Furukawa K, Reisfeld RA. An antibody-interleukin 2 fusion protein overcomes tumor heterogeneity by induction of a cellular immune response. *Proc Natl Acad Sci USA*. 1996;93:7826–7831.
120. Matthay KK, DeSantes K, Hasegawa B, et al. Phase I dose escalation of 131I-metaiodobenzylguanidine with autologous bone marrow support in refractory neuroblastoma. *J Clin Oncol*. 1998;16:229–236.
121. Yanik GA, Levine JE, Matthay KK, et al. Pilot study of iodine-131-metaiodobenzylguanidine in combination with myeloablative chemotherapy and autologous stem-cell support for the treatment of neuroblastoma. *J Clin Oncol*. 2002;20:2142–2149.
122. Folkman J. What is the evidence that tumors are angiogenesis dependent? *J Natl Cancer Inst*. 1990;82:4–6.
123. Meitar D, Crawford SE, Rademaker AW, Cohn SL. Tumor angiogenesis correlates with metastatic disease, N-*myc* amplification, and poor outcome in human neuroblastoma. *J Clin Oncol*. 1996;14:405–414.
124. Eggert A, Ikegaki N, Kwiatkowski J, Zhao H, Brodeur GM, Himelstein BP. High-level expression of angiogenic factors is associated with advanced tumor stage in human neuroblastomas. *Clin Cancer Res*. 2000;6:1900–1908.
125. Katzenstein HM, Rademaker AW, Senger C, Salwen H, Nguyen N, Cohn SL. Effectiveness of the angiogenesis inhibitor TNP-470 in reducing the growth of human neuroblastoma in nude mice inversely correlates with tumor burden. *Clin Cancer Res*. 1999;5:4273–4278.
126. Woods WG, Gao RN, Shuster JJ, et al. Screening of infants and mortality due to neuroblastoma. [see comment]. *N Engl J Med*. 2002;346:1041–1046.

Renal Tumors

Paul E. Grundy, Jeffrey S. Dome, John Kalapurakal, Elizabeth J. Perlman, and Michael L. Ritchey

Introduction

Wilms tumor, the most common primary malignant renal tumor of childhood, is a model of success of the collaborative multidisciplinary approach to treatment of a childhood tumor and the utility of sequential clinical trials. Careful prospective observation and retrospective analyses have also led to refinements in surgical technique, staging and radiation therapy, optimization of chemotherapy, and identification of prognostic factors. Together, these advances in knowledge have resulted in a dramatic improvement in the prognosis for most patients using therapy targeted to the risk of relapse.

Incidence and Epidemiology

Wilms tumor represents about 6% of childhood cancers, with a total incidence in the United States of about 500 cases per year, and represents over 90% of all childhood renal tumors. The incidence rate is slightly higher for Black populations, but substantially lower in Asians, both nationally and internationally.[1] For reasons yet unknown, the tumor presents at an earlier age among boys, with the mean age at diagnosis for those with unilateral disease being 41.5 months, compared with 46.9 months among girls. The mean age at diagnosis for those who present with bilateral disease is 29.5 months for boys and 32.6 months for girls.[2]

Two percent to 4% of Wilms tumors occur as part of one of several rare congenital syndromes. About 1% of patients have the Wilms tumor, Aniridia, Genitourinary malformation, mental Retardation (WAGR) syndrome, which results from a germline deletion of the *WT1* gene at chromosome 11p. Less common is the Denys-Drash syndrome (DDS), with pseudohermaphroditism, degenerative renal disease (glomerulonephritis or nephrotic syndrome), and Wilms tumor associated with mutations within the *WT1* gene. All of the *WT1*-associated syndromes carry a high risk of the development of Wilms tumor.[3] Beckwith-Wiedemann syndrome (BWS), which includes macroglossia, omphalocele, and visceromegaly, with or without hemihypertrophy, is associated with a lesser but still significant risk of Wilms tumor, perhaps 5%

to 10%, although it is being increasingly well defined that this risk varies depending on the underlying molecular defect.[3] Wilms tumor has been reported in a similar overgrowth syndrome called the Simpson-Golabi-Behmel syndrome, which results from deletion of the *GPC3* gene. Homozygous mutations of the *BRCA2* gene in patients with Fanconi anemia group D also seem clearly related to Wilms tumorigenesis in a small subset of Wilms patients.

No consistent significant correlations between environmental exposures for Wilms tumor patients or their parents have been identified. It is likely, then, that genetic risk factors are of greater consequence for the development of Wilms tumor than are environmental risk factors.

Molecular Biology

Although initially thought to involve a single tumor suppressor gene, it is now clear that several genetic events contribute to Wilms tumorigenesis.[4] *WT1*, the first gene identified in the development of Wilms tumor, remains the most fully characterized. Children with the WAGR syndrome have heterozygous germline deletions at chromosome 11p13, usually detectable cytogenetically, which encompass both *PAX6*, the gene responsible for aniridia, and *WT1*. The WT1 protein regulates the expression of other genes, many of which are involved in cell growth, differentiation, and apoptosis. It remains unclear, however, which of these genes are functionally important for tumorigenesis, although involvement of the Wnt signaling pathway is suggested by the discovery that activating mutations of the β-catenin gene are found in more than half the Wilms tumors with *WT1* mutation.

In most Wilms tumors associated with the WAGR syndrome, loss of both *WT1* alleles is required for tumor development, as expected for a classic tumor suppressor gene. Specific alterations to only one allele may also contribute to abnormal cell growth. Patients with DDS harbor constitutional point mutations in only one *WT1* allele. Most germline DDS mutations are single-base-pair mutations, and the abnormal protein product is thought to disrupt the function of the normal gene product. However, tumor tissues from patients with DDS show mutations of both *WT1* alleles, suggesting that single mutations that interfere with genitourinary development are not necessarily sufficient for tumor formation. Despite clear evidence for the involvement of *WT1* in the etiology of some Wilms tumors, mutations of *WT1* have only been found in about 10% of sporadic Wilms tumors, proving that additional genes are involved in at least some Wilms tumors.

WTX, located on the X chromosome, has recently been reported to be inactivated by mutation in about 30% of Wilms tumors.[5] No case in this series had mutations in both *WT1* and *WTX*, and intriguingly, it has now been demonstrated that *WTX* is a major component of the Wnt signaling pathway and serves as a negative regulator of the β-catenin protein. Genotype-phenotype correlations have not been reported, and constitutional or inherited mutations have not been documented.

Historically, the second Wilms tumor locus to be identified, often referred to as *WT2,* maps to the same region of chromosome 11p15.5 as BWS. This region has multiple imprinted genes that are preferentially expressed from either the maternal or paternal alleles. Although the precise pathogenetic link between *WT2* and Wilms tumorigenesis is undefined, a key gene appears to be the growth factor *IGF2*. In normal cells, *IGF2* is expressed only from the paternal allele. Various genetic or epigenetic mechanisms leading to expression of *IGF2* from both alleles are commonly found in Wilms tumor. Genetic or epigenetic alterations to *WT2* are commonly observed in Wilms tumors but probably are not sufficient themselves for tumorigenesis.[6]

Familial predisposition to Wilms tumor is rare, and only about 1% to 2% of all cases have a positive family history. In fact, a survey of 191 offspring of 99 patients with unilateral Wilms tumor did not identify a single case of cancer. Constitutional mutations of the *WT1* gene have been implicated in only a few Wilms tumor families and rarely in unilateral tumor patients without congenital anomalies.[7] Two familial loci have been mapped, *FWT1* on chromosome 17q, and *FWT2,* on chromosome 19q.[8] Some families do not exhibit linkage to *WT1, FWT1,* or *FWT2,* and so the existence of yet additional Wilms tumor loci must be assumed. Although work continues on a research basis, practical genetic testing for most families is not available.[9] True estimates of the risks in offspring of Wilms tumor patients await long-term follow-up studies of offspring from survivors.

Additional tumor-suppressor or tumor-progression genes may lie on chromosomes 16q and 1p, as evidenced by loss of heterozygosity (LOH) for these regions in subsets of Wilms tumors. Patients classified by tumor-specific loss of 1p and 16q have significantly worse relapse-free and overall survival rates, so these genes may affect the behavior of the tumor rather than be etiologic. Nevertheless, this molecular genetic assay may now be clinically useful as a prognostic marker.[10]

Mutations of the *p53* tumor-suppressor gene have also been reported in a few Wilms tumors. A striking association between *p53* mutation and the anaplastic histology compared with favorable histology suggests that mutation of this gene may underlie the anaplastic phenotype.[11]

Taken together, these data suggest that Wilms tumor is characterized by alterations in multiple genes that may regulate cell growth, differentiation, or proliferative potential. It is likely that Wilms tumors are heterogeneous and involve different combinations of genetic defects.

Pathology

Most Wilms tumors are unilateral lesions, although 7% are bilateral and 12% are multifocal. Most Wilms tumors are unilateral lesions, although 7% are bilateral and 12% are multifocal. Wilms tumors are usually sharply demarcated, spherical masses with a "pushing" border relative to the renal parenchyma and a fibrous pseudocapsule. This appearance contrasts with most other malignant renal tumors, the majority of which have infiltrative borders. Cysts are also common, however, and the texture may vary from soft and friable to firm, depending on the predominant histological differentiation.[12]

Microscopically, the classic nephroblastoma consists of varying proportions of 3 cell types, blastemal, stromal, and epithelial. Not all specimens are triphasic, however, and the monophasic patterns often present diagnostic difficulties. Monophasic blastemal Wilms tumor must be differentiated from other small, round, blue cell tumors such as neuroblastoma, primitive neuroepithelial tumor, and lymphoma. Monophasic undifferentiated stromal Wilms tumor may simulate primary sarcomas such as clear cell sarcoma of the kidney, congenital mesoblastic nephroma, or synovial sarcoma. Purely tubular and papillary variants may at times be difficult to distinguish from papillary renal cell carcinoma and metanephric adenoma.

The absence of anaplastic nuclear changes allows classification of Wilms tumor as "favorable histology" (FH). Anaplasia, which may be focal or diffuse, is characterized by the presence of markedly enlarged nuclei with a diameter more than 3 times that of neighboring cells, and the presence of multipolar or obviously polyploid mitotic figures.[13] Focal anaplasia is restricted to circumscribed regions of the tumor. Diffuse anaplasia is considered to exist when anaplastic changes are not circumscribed, or in any extrarenal site. Because anaplasia adversely impacts on the prognosis, diffuse more so than focal, meticulous documentation and photographs should be part of the pathologic examination.[12]

Nephrogenic rests are precursor lesions to Wilms tumor.[14] They are composed of abnormally persistent embryonal nephroblastic tissue with small clusters of blastemal cells, tubules, or stromal cells. Intralobar nephrogenic rests, which tend to be situated deep within the renal lobe, are commonly stroma-rich and intermingle with the adjacent renal parenchyma. Perilobar nephrogenic rests (PLNR), located at the periphery of the kidney, are usually subcortical, sharply demarcated, and contain predominantly blastema and tubules. The term *nephroblastomatosis* is used to refer to the presence of multiple nephrogenic rests. Occasionally, diffuse overgrowth of PLNR may produce a thick "rind" of tissue that enlarges the kidney but preserves its original shape. Only a small number of nephrogenic rests develop into a Wilms tumor, which is typically spherical and develops a pseudocapsule separating it from the original nephrogenic rest. Some rests may become hyperplastic, with dramatic enlargement, while preserving the shape of the preceding rest. It may be extremely difficult to differentiate this type of tumor from a Wilms tumor unless the interface between the rest and the adjacent normal kidney is present within the sample. Hyperplastic nephrogenic rests may completely regress or differentiate following the administration of chemotherapy. The majority of nephrogenic rests become dormant or involute spontaneously. Nevertheless, children in whom nephrogenic rests are identified in the nephrectomy specimen are at increased risk of developing additional Wilms tumor(s) and are generally recommended to be followed for such an occurrence in the contralateral kidney until the age of 8 years.

Clear cell sarcoma of the kidney (CCSK) is not a variant of Wilms tumor. The name is based on the staining characteristics of the predominant cell type that commonly demonstrates clear cytoplasm. The tumor has a propensity for bone and brain metastases and requires treatment distinct from FH Wilms tumor. Although the classic histologic appearance of CCSK is distinctive, many tumors show epithelioid, spindling, myxoid, and other variants that can be confusing.[15]

Rhabdoid tumor of the kidney (RTK) is a highly malignant tumor previously not distinguished from Wilms tumor. The name derives from the prominently acidophilic cytoplasm, resembling rhabdomyoblasts. There are no ultrastructural or other features of skeletal muscle, however, and the cell of origin is unknown. Patients with RTK at times also develop separate primary tumors of the brain, variously called atypical teratoid or rhabdoid tumors. Like renal rhabdoid tumors, the brain tumors are now known to have mutations or deletions of the *INI1* gene on chromosome 22q.

Renal cell carcinomas (RCC) constitute approximately 6% of pediatric renal tumors. Pediatric papillary RCC represent the counterpart to adult papillary RCC and are thought to be the most common type. Translocation RCC, accounting for approximately 20% of pediatric RCC, contain translocations involving the *TFE3* gene at chromosome Xp11.2. These tumors are composed of cells with voluminous clear cytoplasm often arranged in papillary or tubular formation.[16]

Renal medullary carcinoma may affect individuals with sickle cell trait and is associated with very poor prognosis. Patients typically present at an advanced stage with metastatic disease.[17] Approximately 30% of pediatric RCC cannot be classified according to the new World Health Organization criteria.

Clinical Presentation

Most children with Wilms tumor are generally well at presentation and seek medical attention because of abdominal swelling or because a family member has felt an abdominal mass. Other frequent presenting symptoms include abdominal pain, gross or microscopic hematuria, and fever.

On physical examination, a Wilms tumor is usually palpable as a nontender distinct flank mass, uncommonly crossing the midline. A varicocele, particularly if persistent when supine, may be associated with the presence of a tumor thrombus in the renal vein or inferior vena cava (IVC). Hypertension is not infrequent. It is also important to specifically note any signs of Wilms tumor–associated syndromes such as aniridia, genitourinary abnormalities such as hypospadias and cryptorchidism, partial or complete hemihypertrophy, macroglossia, and omphalocele.

Diagnostic Evaluation

Initial evaluation should include complete blood count, tests of coagulation, renal function, serum calcium, urinalysis, and imaging studies. Significant elevation of the serum calcium may occur in association with rhabdoid tumor or congenital mesoblastic nephroma. Acquired von Willebrand disease occurs in about 8% of patients and could result in surgical bleeding.

Imaging studies are necessary to establish the presence of a renal tumor and a normally functioning contralateral kidney, to assess the contralateral kidney for tumor, to document the patency of the IVC, and to assess the lungs for metastatic disease.

An abdominal ultrasound (US) examination is usually performed first. Contrast-enhanced computed tomography (CT) of the abdomen provides further detail and allows evaluation of extension of the tumor into adjacent structures, although evidence of invasion of the liver on CT is often found at surgical exploration to represent hepatic compression rather than invasion. Careful attention should be paid to the contralateral kidney for focal abnormalities that may be nephrogenic rests or Wilms tumor, because the presence of bilateral lesions will alter the surgical and therapeutic approach. It is important that the CT scan include a supine view of the abdomen following contrast injection for planning and review of radiation therapy. Magnetic resonance imaging (MRI) of the abdomen may be used in place of CT. Magnetic resonance imaging may be useful in differentiating actively proliferating lesions from sclerosing rests, but this remains to be well defined.[18]

The patency of the IVC may be demonstrated relatively inexpensively using Doppler US. Whether CT is as sensitive in this regard is not known. When tumor is identified within the IVC, the proximal extent of the thrombus must be established prior to surgery because sudden death has been reported at laparotomy following dislodgement of unsuspected intravascular tumor.

Chest CT should be obtained to identify pulmonary metastases. Computed tomography is more sensitive than conventional chest radiography but identifies some lesions that are not metastases, suggesting the need for lung biopsy. Such studies are recommended before surgery because the interpretation of postoperative imaging studies is often confounded by effusions and atelectasis. Also, diagnostic thorocentesis in the case of an effusion or lung biopsy can be planned in conjunction with the nephrectomy if indicated.

A radionuclide bone scan and radiographic skeletal survey should be obtained postoperatively on all children with CCSK and on all Wilms tumor patients with pulmonary or hepatic metastases who have symptoms suggestive of bone metastasis. A bone scan should also be undertaken as part of the initial workup of RCC because after lung, bone is the most common site of distant metastasis. Brain imaging by MRI or CT should be obtained on all children with CCSK, RTK, or with RCC because they are associated with intracranial metastases or second primary malignant brain tumors.

Classification and Staging

The malignant renal tumors are classified first by histology as Wilms tumor, clear cell sarcoma, rhabdoid tumor, or RCC. The histologic finding of anaplasia continues to be the most important determinant of prognosis and further divides Wilms tumors into an FH category versus anaplastic, focal, or diffuse, as described above. All renal tumors except the RCCs are classified by the same staging system, which utilizes the results of the imaging studies and both surgical and pathologic findings at nephrectomy. The current staging system as used by the Children's Oncology Group (COG) is outlined below.

In *stage I* disease, the tumor is limited to the kidney and is completely resected. The renal capsule has an intact outer surface. The tumor is not ruptured or biopsied prior to removal. The vessels of the renal sinus are not involved.

In *stage II* disease, the tumor extends beyond the capsule of the kidney but is completely resected with no evidence of tumor at or beyond the margins of resection. The blood vessels outside the renal parenchyma, including those of the renal sinus, may contain tumor. Although previously classified as stage II, biopsy or operative local spillage of the tumor is now classified as stage III.

In *stage III* disease, residual tumor (gross or microscopic) is present but confined to the abdomen, including: unresectable or incompletely resected primary tumor, lymph node metastases, positive surgical margins, biopsy or tumor spillage before or during surgery, or transected tumor thrombus.

In *stage IV* disease, there are hematogenous metastases (lung, liver, bone, or brain), or lymph node metastases outside the abdominopelvic region.

In *stage V* disease, bilateral renal involvement is present at diagnosis. Each side is then staged according to the above criteria (I-III) at the time of nephrectomy.

The Societé Internationale d'Oncologie Pédiatrique (SIOP) uses a very similar staging system, although importantly, staging is most frequently determined on the nephrectomy specimen obtained after 4 to 6 weeks of chemotherapy. It cannot be stressed enough that although the same staging terminology is used, pre- and postchemotherapy stage are not equivalent.[19] The SIOP classification now uses stage in addition to histologic features of the postchemotherapy tumor. Thus, low-risk Wilms tumors are those that are completely necrotic, high-risk Wilms tumors are blastemal predominant, and the remaining tumors, the majority, are deemed intermediate risk. Stage I low-risk Wilms tumors are not given any postoperative chemotherapy, and high-risk tumors receive an intensified course of chemotherapy.

No other factors are currently used for classification or treatment stratification in North America, but several are under study. The combination of age younger than 2 years at diagnosis with a stage I tumor weighing less than 550 gm defines a group of patients with very low risk of recurrence in whom the possibility of treatment reduction will be examined.[20] Patients whose tumors have LOH 1p and 16q have a worse prognosis, stage for stage, and the benefits of treatment intensification need to be determined.

Treatment and Prognosis
Surgery

Surgical resection is the initial treatment for most children with Wilms tumor because it allows accurate surgicopathologic staging as described above, which is essential to determine the appropriate chemotherapy regimen and the need for radiation therapy. Intraoperative events that can have an adverse impact on patient survival include tumor spill or rupture that is associated with an increased risk of local abdominal relapse,[21] incomplete removal, and surgical complications.

The tumor should be removed by radical or modified radical nephrectomy using a transperitoneal approach to the tumor to allow inspection of the regional lymph nodes, a very important criterion for staging.[21] After the peritoneal cavity is entered, thorough exploration of the abdominal cavity is carried out to assess the liver, regional lymph nodes, and other evidence of tumor spread. Although selective sampling of nodes is necessary for accurate staging, formal retroperitoneal lymph node dissection is not recommended. It is not necessary to mobilize and inspect the contralateral kidney if there is no evidence of lesions on CT or MRI.

Nephrectomy should be deferred and chemotherapy used first, if complete tumor removal would require excision of all or parts of adjoining organs that might be invaded, because such procedures are associated with an increased risk of significant surgical complications.[22] Inoperability should be decided at surgery, though. Preoperative imaging can overestimate local tumor extension because these tumors often compress and adhere to adjacent structures without frank invasion. However, if the lesion can be completely removed, wedge resection of an infiltrated portion of the liver is advisable because this converts a stage III tumor to stage II with minimal morbidity. Likewise, attempts at primary surgical excision of the tumor with vena caval extension at or above the liver should not be undertaken.[22] Prenephrectomy chemotherapy should be administered to such patients because it often makes the standard transabdominal approach subsequently feasible (Figure 24-1), avoiding thoracoabdominal incisions, cardiac bypass, and the other maneuvers necessary to extract the tumor without embolizing.

Preoperative chemotherapy is also advisable in selected other children including occasional patients with massive tumors that are judged to pose too great a risk for surgical removal. Although this approach may reduce the compli-

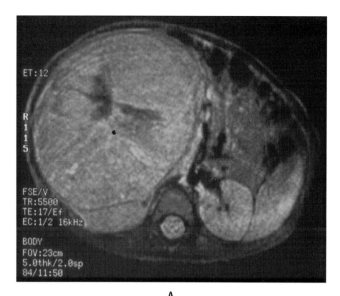

A

B

Figure 24-1 Computed tomography images taken pre (A) and post (B) chemotherapy showing a tumor that was judged intraoperatively to be initially safely unresectable. The postchemotherapy image shows a dramatic reduction in size of the tumor, which facilitated the surgical removal of the tumor.

cation rate,[23] it does not result in improved survival rates.[24] Prevailing North American practice is initial nephrectomy because treatments can best be modulated in their intensity according to accurate histopathologic and staging criteria that are obscured by preoperative treatment. Thus, children should still undergo initial exploration to establish the diagnosis by biopsy and to assess operability because imaging studies alone may result in misdiagnosis and both under- and overstaging. Definitive resection should be completed once there is an adequate reduction in the size of the tumor, usually at week 6, because the majority of response will have occurred by then. Failure of the tumor to shrink could be due to predominance of skeletal muscle or benign elements, and a second-look procedure to confirm persistent tumor may be necessary.[25]

The treatment of children with bilateral tumors must be individualized. The 2 goals of therapy are to eradicate all of the tumor and to preserve as much normal renal tissue as possible, with the hope of decreasing the significant risk of chronic renal failure among these children.[26] Primary excision of the tumor masses should not be attempted, but rather patients should be given preoperative chemotherapy to maximize the possibility of successful partial nephrectomy. In fact, when imaging studies are consistent with a diagnosis of Wilms tumor, biopsy is not recommended given the very narrow differential diagnosis, the difficulty in interpretation of such biopsies, and the resultant classification as stage III. Reevaluation by imaging is performed at about week 6 to determine whether there has been sufficient response of the tumors to allow tumor resection with preservation of a substantial amount of normal renal tissue. Failure to shrink may be due to persistence of skeletal muscle or differentiated elements rather than persistent viable or anaplastic tumor,[27] so a second-look procedure, including at least a biopsy, is recommended at this time. Partial nephrectomy or wedge resection of the kidney should be considered, but only if complete tumor resection with negative margins can be obtained and part of either or both kidneys can be salvaged.

Radiotherapy

Wilms tumor of FH is a very radiosensitive tumor. National Wilms Tumor Study (NWTS) trials 1 through 3 demonstrated that use of irradiation could be eliminated in children with stage I or II FH tumors and that for stage III tumors, only 10.80 Gy was required when combined with 3-drug chemotherapy.[28–30] Abdominal radiation is used for all stages of anaplastic Wilms tumor, CCSK, and RTK. Abdominal irradiation should be delivered within 14 days of nephrectomy.[31]

Current recommendations for radiation therapy for pediatric renal tumors are shown in Table 24-1. Megavoltage x-rays (4-6 MV) are recommended for irradiation. The recommended daily dose/fraction is 1.5 to 1.8 Gy. The use of immobilization devices and CT simulation is essential for accurate treatment planning and delivery.

For abdominal irradiation, the tumor bed (flank) is defined as the kidney and its associated lesion as they are visualized on preoperative imaging studies. The irradiation portal is always extended across the midline medially to include the entire vertebral column. The field is extended as needed to include the paraaortic chains when paraaortic nodes are found to be involved. The portal for whole-abdominal irradiation includes all the peritoneal surfaces and extends from the domes of the diaphragm to the inferior margins of the obturator foramina.

In NWTS 1-5, whole-lung irradiation (WLI) to 12 Gy has been recommended for children with pulmonary metastases visible on chest radiographs. The value of WLI in patients with pulmonary metastasis identified only on CT scans but not on chest radiographs is not clearly established and is currently under study in the COG. The entire thoracic cavity is irradiated without shielding, except for the humeral heads. The field extends from the apex of the lung to the posterior inferior recesses of the costophrenic sulci with a margin of at least 1 cm.

Table 24-1
Radiation therapy dosing guidelines.

Clinical Criteria	Radiation Dose and Field
Stage I-II FH Wilms tumor	None
Stage I-II FA or DA Wilms tumor or CCSK	10.5 Gy flank
Stage III FH Wilms tumor or CCSK	10.5 Gy flank
• cytology positive ascites or pre-operative rupture	10.5 Gy whole abdomen
• residual gross disease >3 cm	10.8 Gy boost to residual tumor
Stage III DA	20 Gy flank or whole abdomen as above for stage III FH
Stage I-III RTK	
Lung metastases	12 Gy whole lung
Brain metastases	30.6 Gy whole brain, or
	20 Gy whole brain + 10-15 Gy IMRT or stereotactic boost to tumor
Liver metastases	19.8 Gy whole liver
Bone metastases	25–30 Gy to the lesion plus 3 cm margin
Lymph node metastases	19.8 Gy to lymph nodes
Recurrent abdominal Wilms tumor	
• <12 months of age	12.6-18 Gy tumor plus margin
• ≥12 months of age	21.6 Gy if previous radiation dose ≤10.8 Gy
• gross residual tumor after surgery	Up to 9 Gy boost to residual tumor

Abbreviations: FH, Favorable histology; FA, focal anaplasia; DA, diffuse anaplasia; CCSK, clear cell sarcoma of the kidney; RTK, rhabdoid tumor of the kidney; IMRT, intensity modulated radiation therapy.

For children who have liver metastases at diagnosis, only those with unresectable tumors are irradiated. Liver tolerance is approached by the doses recommended, especially since dactinomycin and doxorubicin are radiation enhancing, and careful monitoring of liver function tests is recommended. Metastases to lymph nodes, brain, bone, or other areas are treated similarly to the liver, although with higher doses for the brain and bone (Table 24-1). The entire bone need not be irradiated for skeletal metastases.

Irradiation in children with bilateral tumors is used for those who fail to achieve an adequate response to chemotherapy or for those with residual disease following surgical resection. Localized irradiation can be used when surgical margins of resection are microscopically positive in spite of surgical attempts at renal-sparing surgery.

All patients with anaplastic Wilms tumor, CCSK, and RTK, regardless of stage, are recommended to receive postoperative abdominal irradiation.

Chemotherapy

The National Wilms Tumor Study Group (NWTSG) in North America and SIOP in Europe have used similar chemotherapy regimens, but their treatment approaches are fundamentally different in that the NWTSG recommends initial nephrectomy whereas SIOP advocates preoperative chemotherapy. Both approaches yield excellent outcomes for patients with FH Wilms tumor.[32,33] Initial nephrectomy allows for greater consideration of surgical, pathologic, and biologic factors in determining optimal patient-specific therapy, whereas the use of postchemotherapy nephrectomy allows response of the tumor to chemotherapy to be considered in determining subsequent therapy.[34]

The fourth National Wilms Tumor Study (NWTS-4) demonstrated that single-dose dactinomycin and doxorubicin produce less hematologic toxicity than the previous standard regimens,[35] can be administered at less cost,[36] and result in equivalent outcomes.[33] The same study also demonstrated that approximately 6 months of chemotherapy resulted in equivalent outcomes as the previously standard 15 months of treatment.[37]

The treatment regimens that were used in NWTS-5 are shown in Table 24-2. Patients younger than 12 months should receive 50% of the usual dose of any chemotherapeutic agent because of excessive toxicity when previously treated with full doses. Unpublished results suggest that these regimens provide a reasonable standard of care.

Patients with bilateral Wilms tumor should be given preoperative chemotherapy. Traditionally, initial treatment for stage I or II FH tumors has been with a 2-drug regimen including vincristine and actinomycin-D (Table 24-2). Those with more-extensive disease at diagnosis, or whose tumors fail to respond adequately, have been treated with doxorubicin in addition (Table 24-2).

Table 24-2

Standard treatment regimens.

Stage	Histology	Regimen	0	1	2	3	4	5	6	7	8	9	10	11	12	13	14	15	16	17	18	19	20	21	22	23	24
I-II	FH	EE4A	A			A			A			A			A			A			A						
				V	V	V	V	V	V	V	V	V	V		V*			V*			V*						
I I-IV III-IV	DA FA FH	DD4A	A			D			A			D			A			D*			A			D*			A
				V	V	V	V	V	V	V	V	V	V		V*			V*			V*			V*			V*
I-IV II-IV	CCSK DA	I	D			C			D			C			D			C			D			C			D
									C*						C*						C*						C*
						E						E						E						E			
				V	V		V	V		V	V		V	V	V*			V*			V*			V*			V*

Abbreviations: FH, favorable histology Wilms tumor; FA, focal anaplastic Wilms tumor; DA, diffuse anaplastic Wilms tumor; CCSK, clear cell sarcoma of the kidney; A, actinomycin D (1.35 mg/m², max 2.3 mg); D, doxorubicin (45 mg/m²); D*, doxorubicin (30 mg/m²); C, cyclophosphamide (440 mg/m²/d × 3); C*, cyclophosphamide (440 mg/m²/d × 5); E, etoposide (100 mg/m²/day × 5); V, vincristine (1.5 mg/m², max 2 mg); V*, vincristine (2.0 mg/m², max 2 mg).

If one chooses prenephrectomy chemotherapy for an inoperable unilateral tumor, the current standard treatment is as for a stage III tumor. Following surgical resection, usually about week 6, patients should continue on treatment until they have completed their planned regimen. Radiation therapy is given postoperatively to all patients.

On NWTS-5, patients with stage I focal or diffuse anaplastic Wilms tumor were treated with the 2-drug protocol, regimen EE-4A, based on the excellent outcomes for this patient group on previous studies.[33] However, outcomes were not as favorable as on previous studies. Future studies will therefore evaluate the benefit of adding doxorubicin and radiation therapy to the treatment of patients with stage I focal or diffuse anaplastic Wilms tumor. Stage II to IV tumors with focal anaplasia may also be treated with regimen DD4A, but NWTS-5 sought to improve the outcomes for patients with stages II to IV diffuse anaplastic Wilms tumor by adding cyclophosphamide/etoposide (regimen I). The regimen was well tolerated and provides a reasonable guideline for the treatment of patients with stages II to IV anaplastic Wilms tumor.

Clear cell sarcoma of the kidney patients in NWTS-5 were also treated with regimen I because the use of doxorubicin is particularly effective for this histology.[15] Preliminary results suggest that outcomes compare favorably to those of NWTS-4, and regimen I is therefore recommended as an appropriate treatment regimen for all patients with CCSK.

The outcome for children with RTK has been very poor using regimens used for the treatment of Wilms tumor, including those on NWTS-5 treated with carboplatin/etoposide alternating with cyclophosphamide. Case reports of successful outcome for metastatic RTK after ifosfamide/carboplatin/etoposide (ICE) chemotherapy alternating with vincristine/doxorucibin/cyclophosphamide are encouraging.[38,39]

Historically, patients with RCC were not included in cooperative group trials for pediatric renal tumors, so knowledge of treatment regimens is based only on retrospective case series and literature reviews. Like adult RCC, pediatric RCC is not very chemosensitive, and complete surgical resection remains the mainstay of therapy, although children with RCC and local lymph node involvement may have better outcomes than their adult counterparts.

Because most recurrences occur within 2 years of diagnosis in the lungs and pleura, tumor bed, and liver and less frequently in the bone, brain, and distant lymph nodes, follow-up every 3 months for 2 years is indicated. Lung metastases are best seen on CT, but chest x-ray may be adequate for clinical purposes because earlier detection of pulmonary relapse has not been demonstrated to improve outcomes. Either abdominal US or CT is adequate to detect infradiaphragmatic relapses. Only patients who present with hematogenous metastasis (brain, lung, liver, and bone) at initial diagnosis require specific ongoing evaluation of the affected sites. Consideration should be given to longer follow-up for clear cell sarcoma patients because relapses are known to occur for as long as 5 years post diagnosis.

In children with any of the Wilms tumor–predisposing syndromes, or with nephrogenic rests in one or both kidneys, ultrasonography of the remaining kidney is performed for a longer period, at least until age 7, because the opposite kidney continues to be at risk for several years.

Therapy at Relapse

Favorable prognostic factors at the time of recurrence include no prior treatment with doxorubicin, relapse more than 12 months after diagnosis, and intra-abdominal relapse in a patient not previously treated with abdominal irradiation.[40,41] Children in this more favorable group should be treated aggressively with doxorubicin, vincristine, cyclophosphamide, and etoposide (regimen I) (Table 24-2) because as many as 70% achieve 3-year event-free survival.[42] Although surgical excision of pulmonary metastases has not been demonstrated to improve outcome, surgical biopsy should be considered to confirm recurrent disease histologically. Several highly effective chemotherapy combinations, including ICE, cyclophosphamide/etoposide, and carboplatin/etoposide, are considered first-line treatment for recurrent disease.[43]

It has been suggested that high-dose chemotherapy with stem cell rescue should be employed in the management of those patients with adverse prognostic factors at the time of relapse,[44–47] although it remains unproven whether stem cell transplant is more efficacious and/or less toxic than conventional chemotherapy.

Outcomes

Recent estimates of survival outcomes for children with renal tumors treated following NWTS-5 protocols are shown in Table 24-3.

Because Wilms tumor is usually a curable malignancy, it is essential to limit iatrogenic sequelae. The NWTSG experience suggests that serious renal dysfunction, though, is not common in patients with unilateral Wilms tumor and an apparently normal contralateral kidney, being identified in only 0.25% of more than 5000 patients.[26] Most instances of renal failure occur in children with bilateral disease in whom the most common cause of renal failure was bilateral nephrectomy followed by radiation-induced damage. It is noteworthy, however, that many of these children with unilateral Wilms tumor are still young. They therefore remain at risk for renal deterioration, and indeed, patients have been described with proteinuria and hypertension developing 10 to 20 years after nephrectomy. A group of patients that is particularly vulnerable to late-onset renal failure are those with WAGR syndrome who have a cumulative risk of renal failure approaching 30%.[48]

Cardiac complications are most frequent in those treated with doxorubicin and radiation, although the risks may be lower with current use of lower doses of doxorubicin.[49] The same may be said for second malignant neoplasms,[50] and therefore patients should be followed long term for both issues. Complications during pregnancy also occur in irradiated female survivors who should probably receive specialized pregnancy care because of

Table 24-3

Survival outcomes on NWTS-5.

Disease/Stage	# Patients	4-yr Relapse Free Survival %	4-yr Overall Survival %
FH Wilms Tumor[a]			
Stage I	233	91.5	97.0
Stage II	490	81.4	97.6
Stage III	432	88.7	94.8
Stage IV	192	74.6	86.3
Stage V	98	58.4	79.1
FA Wilms Tumor[b]			
Stage I	10	67.5	88.9
Stage II	5	80.0	80.0
Stage III	8	87.5	100
Stage IV	1	0	0
DA Wilms Tumor[c]			
Stage I	19	68.4	78.9
Stage II	23	82.6	81.5
Stage III	43	68.3	72.0
Stage IV	15	33.3	33.3
CCSK[a]			
Stage I	8	100	100
Stage II	20	89.2	93.8
Stage III	27	81.7	88.6
Stage IV	4	37.5	100
RTK[a]			
Stage I-IV	18	16.7	16.7
RCC			
Stage I			92.4
Stage II			84.6
Stage III			72.7
Stage IV			13.9

[a] Figures are unpublished results of fully evaluable patients on NWTS-5.

[b] Dome JS, Cotton CA, Perlman EJ, et al.[52]

[c] Figures represent percentage of patients alive from an extensive literature review.

higher risk of premature delivery.[51] More precise estimates of risks will become available through the ongoing Wilms Tumor Late Effects Study. It is important that children treated for Wilms tumor are examined regularly by a physician who is familiar with the natural history of the disease and complications of therapy.

Summary

Major progress has been made in the management of Wilms tumor in children. More than 85% of patients can be cured by current therapies. The most important imme-

diate need is for new prognostic markers to distinguish those patients who require more effective therapy for cure from those who could potentially be cured without agents that are associated with adverse sequelae, such as radiation and doxorubicin. Without such classifiers and considering the generally high frequency of cure, it will be difficult to conduct traditional randomized trials because of the large accrual required to measure small differences in outcome.

The efficacy of chemotherapeutic agents other than anthracyclines in combination with vincristine and dactinomycin for the initial treatment of patients with a higher risk of relapse must be studied. Combinations currently being studied in relapsed patients, including cyclophosphamide/etoposide and carboplatinum/etoposide, show promise. Even more so, novel effective agents are required for the therapy of advanced-stage anaplastic Wilms tumors and RTK, the prognosis for which remains dismal.

Other issues that need to be carefully evaluated include the use of renal-sparing surgical procedures in the management of patients with bilateral Wilms tumor and those with conditions known to predispose to the development of metachronous Wilms tumor.

Evolving understanding of the genesis of Wilms tumor at the genetic level may allow an increased ability to identify individuals at highest risk for development of the disease, including those within a family segregating the tumor, and or within the subsets of children with a Wilms tumor–predisposing condition.

Acknowledgment

The authors thank the investigators of the COG and the many pathologists, surgeons, pediatricians, radiation therapists, and other health professionals who managed the children entered on the NWTS.

References

1. Stiller CA, Parkin DM. Geographic and ethnic variations in the incidence of childhood cancer. *Br Med Bull.* 1996;52:682–703.
2. Breslow N, Olshan A, Beckwith JB, Green DM. Epidemiology of Wilms tumor. *Med Pediatr Oncol.* 1993;21:172–181.
3. Scott RH, Walker L, Olsen OE, et al. Surveillance for Wilms tumour in at-risk children: pragmatic recommendations for best practice. *Arch Dis Child.* 2006; 91:995–999.
4. Dome JS, Coppes MJ. Recent advances in Wilms tumor genetics. *Curr Opin Pediatr.* 2002;14(1):5–11.
5. Rivera M, Kim WJ, Wells J, et al. An X chromosome gene, *WTX,* is commonly inactivated in Wilms tumor. *Science.* 2007;315:642–645.
6. DeBaun MR, Niemitz EL, McNeil E, Brandenburg SA, Lee MP, Feinberg AP. Epigenetic alterations of H19 and LIT1 distinguish patients with Beckwith-Wiedemann syndrome with cancer and birth defects. *Am J Hum Gen.* 2002; 70(3):604–611.
7. Diller L, Ghahremani M, Morgan J, et al. Constitutional WT1 mutations in Wilms' tumor patients. *J Clin Oncol.* 1998;16(11):3634–3640.
8. McDonald JM, Douglass EC, Fisher R, et al. Linkage of familial Wilms' tumor predisposition to chromosome 19 and a two-locus model for the etiology of familial tumors. *Cancer Res.* 1998;58(7):1387–1390.
9. Hawkins MM, Winter DL, Burton HS, Potok MH. Heritability of Wilms' tumor. *J Natl Cancer Inst.* 1995;87(17):1323–1324.
10. Grundy P, Breslow N, Li S, et al. The relationship between loss of heterozygosity for chromosomes 1p and 16q and prognosis in Wilms tumor: a report from the National Wilms Tumor Study Group. *J Clin Oncol.* 2005;23(29): 7312–7321.
11. Bardeesy N, Falkoff D, Petruzzi M-J, et al. Anaplastic Wilms' tumour, a subtype displaying poor prognosis, harbours p53 gene mutations. *Nat Genet.* 1994;7:91–97.
12. Perlman EJ. Pediatric renal tumors: practical updates for the pathologist. *Pediatr Dev Pathol.* 2005;7(3):320–338.
13. Zuppan CW, Beckwith JB, Luckey DW. Anaplasia in unilateral Wilms tumor: a report from the National Wilms Tumor Study Pathology Center. *Hum Pathol.* 1988;19:1199–1209.
14. Beckwith JB. Precursor lesions of Wilms tumor: clinical and biological implications. *Med Pediatr Oncol.* 1993;21:158–168.
15. Argani P, Perlman EJ, Breslow N, et al. Clear cell sarcoma of the kidney (CCSK): a review of 351 cases from the National Wilms Tumor Study Group Pathology Center. *Am J Surg Pathol.* 2000;24:4–18.
16. Geller JI, Dome JS. Local lymph node involvement does not predict poor outcome in pediatric renal cell carcinoma. *Cancer.* 2004;101(7):1575–1583.
17. Swartz MA, Karth J, Schneider DT, Rodriguez R, Beckwith JB, Perlman EJ. Renal medullary carcinoma: clinical, pathologic, immunohistochemical, and genetic analysis with pathogenetic implications. *Urology.* 2002;60(6):1083–1089.
18. Gylys-Morin V, Hoffer FA, Kozakewich H, Shamberger RC. Wilms tumor and nephroblastomatosis: imaging characteristics at gadolinium-enhanced MR imaging. *Radiology.* 1993;188:517–521.
19. Vujanic G, Sandstedt B, Harms D, Kelsey A, Leuschner I, DeKraker J. Revised International Society of Pediatric Oncology (SIOP) working classification of renal tumors of childhood. *Med Pediatr Oncol.* 2002;38:79–82.
20. Green DM, Breslow NE, Beckwith JB, et al. Treatment with nephrectomy only for small, stage I/favorable histology Wilms' tumor: a report from the National Wilms' Tumor Study Group. *J Clin Oncol.* 2001;19(17):3719–3724.
21. Shamberger RC, Guthrie KA, Ritchey ML, et al. Surgery-related factors and local recurrence of Wilms tumor in National Wilms Tumor Study–4. *Ann Surg.* 1999;229(2):292–297.
22. Ritchey ML, Shamberger RC, Haase G, Horwitz JR, Bergemann T, Breslow NE. Surgical complications after primary nephrectomy for Wilms' tumor: report from the National Wilms' Tumor Study Group. *J Amer Coll Surg.* 2001; 192(1):63–68.
23. Godzinski J, Tournade MF, DeKraker J. Rarity of surgical complications after postchemotherapy nephrectomy for nephroblastoma: experience of the International Society of Paediatric Oncology: trial and study "SIOP-9." *Eur J Pediatr Surg.* 1998;8:83–96.
24. De Kraker J, Pein F, Graf N, et al. The SIOP nephroblastoma trial and study 93–01 results and consequences [abstract]. *Med Pediatr Oncol.* 2001; 37(3):192.
25. Ritchey ML, Pringle KC, Breslow NE, et al. Management and outcome of inoperable Wilms tumor: a report of National Wilms Tumor Study–3. *Ann Surg.* 1994;220(5):683–690.
26. Ritchey ML, Green DM, Thomas PRM, et al. Renal failure in Wilms' tumor patients: a report from the National Wilms' Tumor Study Group. *Med Pediatr Oncol.* 1996;26:75–80.
27. Weirich A, Leuschner I, Harms D. Clinical impact of histologic subtypes in localized non-anaplastic nephroblastoma treated according to the trial and study SIOP-9/GPOH. *Ann Oncol.* 2001;12:311–319.
28. D'Angio GJ, Evans AE, Breslow N, et al. The treatment of Wilms' tumor. *Cancer.* 1976;38:633–646.
29. D'Angio GJ, Evans AE, Breslow N, et al. The treatment of Wilms' tumor: results of the second National Wilms' Tumor Study. *Cancer.* 1981;47:2302–2311.
30. Thomas PRM, Tefft M, Compaan PJ, Norkool P, Breslow NE, D'Angio GJ. Results of two radiotherapy randomizations in the Third National Wilms' Tumor Study (NWTS-3). *Cancer.* 1991;68:1703–1707.
31. Kalapurakal JA, Li SM, Breslow NE, et al. Influence of radiation therapy delay on abdominal tumor recurrence in patients with favorable histology Wilms' tumor treated on NWTS-3 and NWTS-4: a report from the National Wilms' Tumor Study Group. *Int J Radiat Oncol Biol Phys.* 2003;57(2):495–499.
32. Tournade MF, Com-Nougue C, Voute PA, et al. Results of the sixth International Society of Pediatric Oncology Wilms' Tumor Trial and Study: a risk-adapted therapeutic approach in Wilms' tumor. *J Clin Oncol.* 1993;11:1014–1023.
33. Green DM, Breslow NE, Beckwith JB, et al. Comparison between single-dose and divided-dose administration of dactinomycin and doxorubicin for patients with Wilms' tumor: a report from the National Wilms' tumor study group. *J Clin Oncol.* 1998;16(1):237–245.
34. Bergeron C, Graf N, van Tintern H, et al. From results of SIOP-nephroblastoma-93-01 study to SIOP nephroblastoma 2001 study (abstract). *Med Pediatr Oncol.* 2003;41(4):289.
35. Green DM, Breslow NE, Evans I, et al. The effect of chemotherapy dose intensity on the hematological toxicity of the treatment for Wilms' tumor: a report of the National Wilms Tumor Study. *Am J Pediatr Hematol Oncol.* 1994;16: 207–212.
36. Green DM, Breslow NE, Evans I, et al. Relationship between dose schedule and charges for treatment on National Wilms' Tumor Study-4: a report from the National Wilms' Tumor Study Group. *J Natl Cancer Inst Monographs.* 1995;19:21–25.
37. Green DM, Breslow NE, Beckwith JB, et al. Effect of duration of treatment on treatment outcome and cost of treatment for Wilms' tumor: a report from the National Wilms' Tumor Study Group. *J Clin Oncol.* 1998;16(12):3744–3751.
38. Waldron PE, Rodgers BM, Kelly MD, Womer RB. Successful treatment of a patient with a stage IV rhabdoid tumor of the kidney: case report and review. *J Pediatr Hematol Oncol.* 1999;21(1):53–57.
39. Wagner L, Hill DA, Fuller C, et al. Treatment of metastatic rhabdoid tumor of the kidney. *J Pediatr Hematol Oncol.* 2002;24(5):385–388.
40. Grundy P, Breslow NE, Green DM, Sharples K, Evans A, D'Angio GJ. Prognostic factors of children with recurrent Wilms tumor: results from the second and third National Wilms Tumor Study. *J Clin Oncol.* 1989;7:638–647.
41. Dome JS, Liu T, Krasin M, et al. Improved survival for patients with recurrent Wilms tumor: the experience at St. Jude Children's Research Hospital. *J Pediatr Hematol Oncol.* 2002;24(3):192–198.
42. Green DM, Cotton CA, Malogolowkin M, et al. Treatment of Wilms tumor relapsing after initial treatment with vincristine and actinomycin D: a report from the National Wilms Tumor Study Group. *Pediatr Blood Cancer.* 2007;48 (5):493–499.
43. Malogolowkin M, Cotton CA, Green DM, et al. Treatment of Wilms tumor relapsing after initial treatment with vincristine, actinomycin D, and doxorubicin. A report from the National Wilms Tumor Study Group. *Pediatr Blood Cancer.* 2008;50(2):236–241.

44. Garaventa A, Hartmann O, Bernard JL, et al. Autologous bone marrow transplantation for pediatric Wilms' tumor: the experience of the European Bone Marrow Transplantation Solid Tumor Registry. *Med Pediatr Oncol.* 1994;22: 11–14.

45. Pein F, Michon J, Valteau-Couanet D, et al. High-dose melphalan, etoposide, and carboplatin followed by autologous stem-cell rescue in pediatric high-risk recurrent Wilms' tumor: a French Society of Pediatric Oncology Study. *J Clin Oncol.* 1998;16(10):3295–3301.

46. Kremens B, Gruhn B, Klingebiel T, et al. High-dose chemotherapy with autologous stem cell rescue in children with nephroblastoma. *Bone Marrow Transplant.* 2002;30:893–898.

47. Campbell AD, Cohn SL, Reynolds M, et al. Treatment of relapsed Wilms' tumor with high-dose therapy and autologous hematopoietic stem-cell rescue: the experience at Children's Memorial Hospital. *J Clin Oncol.* 2004; 22(14):2885–2890.

48. Breslow NE, Takashima JR, Ritchey ML, Strong LC, Green DM. Renal failure in the Denys-Drash and Wilms; tumor-aniridia syndromes. *Cancer Res.* 2000; 60(15):4030–4032.

49. Green DM, Breslow NE, Moksness J, D'Angio GJ. Congestive heart failure following initial therapy for Wilms tumor (abstract). *AACR.* 1998;161A.

50. Breslow NE, Takashima JR, Whitton JA, Moksness J, D'Angio GJ, Green DM. Second malignant neoplasms following treatment for Wilms' tumor: a report from the National Wilms' Tumor Study Group. *J Clin Oncol.* 1995;13(8): 1851–1859.

51. Green DM, Peabody EM, Nan B, Peterson S, Kalapurakal JA, Breslow NE. Pregnancy outcome after treatment for Wilms tumor: a report from the National Wilms Tumor Study Group. *J Clin Oncol.* 2002;20(10):2506–2513.

52. Dome JS, Cotton CA, Perlman EJ, et al. Treatment of anaplastic histology Wilms' tumor: results from the fifth National Wilms' Tumor Study. *J Clin Oncol.* 2006;24(15):2352–2358.

Soft-Tissue Sarcomas

William H. Meyer, Timothy P. Cripe, and Michael C. G. Stevens

Introduction

The soft tissue sarcomas are a heterogeneous group of malignant connective tissue tumors that arise in soft tissue sites throughout the body. These sarcomas typically have a normal mesenchymal tissue counterpart including: striated muscle (rhabdomyosarcoma [RMS]), fibrous connective tissue (fibrosarcomas), fat cells (liposarcomas), smooth or nonstriated muscle (leiomyosarcomas), blood vessels (angiosarcomas and malignant hemangiopericytoma), synovial tissue (synovial sarcoma), and cartilage (chondrosarcomas). In addition, the malignant peripheral nerve sheath tumors are included with the soft tissue sarcomas. Extraosseous Ewings tumor shares the same biologic features with Ewings tumor of bone and is discussed in the chapter on bone sarcomas. In children, the most common soft tissue sarcoma is RMS. All the other sarcomas are individually rare and often grouped together as nonrhabdomyosarcoma soft tissue sarcomas (NRSTS).

Incidence/Epidemiology

The soft tissue sarcomas represent 7.4% of all cancer cases in the 0- to 19-year age group. The annual incidence in the United States is 11.0 per million, with 850 to 900 cases reported annually;[1] the incidence rate is the same in Europe. The incidence rates for soft tissue sarcomas vary by age, gender, and race. Rhabdomyosarcoma is most common in younger children, with approximately 350 new cases reported yearly in the United States. Rhabdomyosarcoma comprises well more than half of all soft tissue sarcomas in the 0- to 9-year age group. During the first decade of life, the incidence rates are quite stable for those older than 1 year at approximately 10 per million. However, the incidence rate for soft tissue sarcomas in infants younger than 1 year is 15.2 per million, attributed to a higher incidence of NRSTS, particularly infantile fibrosarcoma and malignant hemangiopericytoma. In the 10- to 14- and 15- to 19-year age groups, the NRSTS as a group represent 70% and 77% of all soft tissue sarcoma diagnoses, respectively. Incidence rates for males tend to be slightly higher than for females in all age groups and histologic subtypes. Black children also have slightly

higher incidence rates. The reasons for these differences remain unknown.

Most soft tissue sarcomas develop in children without any recognized predisposing risk factor. Although RMS has been reported in association with neurofibromatosis type 1 (NF-1),[2,3] Beckwith-Wiedemann syndrome,[4,5] Li-Fraumeni syndrome,[6,7] cardio-facio-cutaneous syndrome,[8] Costello syndrome,[9,10] a variety of congenital anomalies,[11] and parental use of cocaine and marijuana,[12] the vast majority of cases appear to be sporadic. Nonrhabdomyosarcoma soft tissue sarcomas, specifically malignant peripheral nerve sheath tumors, may arise in benign neurofibromas in people with NF-1.[13,14] Children with hereditary retinoblastoma (who harbor germline Rb mutations) are at increased risk for development of sarcomas.[15] Nonrhabdomyosarcoma soft tissue sarcomas may also occur in sites of prior irradiation. Children infected with the human immunodeficiency virus may develop leiomyosarcomas; these children often have the Epstein-Barr virus, which may contribute to the pathogenesis of this soft tissue sarcoma.[16]

Pathology and Molecular Pathogenesis
Rhabdomyosarcoma

The hallmark for diagnosis of RMS is evidence of skeletal muscle differentiation. Occasionally, cross-striations characteristic of skeletal muscle or plump rhabdomyoblasts are noted.[17] However, muscle-related immunohistochemical stains (myogenin, MyoD, muscle specific actin, myoglobin, and or desmin) are often required to differentiate this tumor from the other small, round, blue cell neoplasms that occur in children and adolescents.[18–20] In addition, molecular analysis for detection of translocations and other gene expression markers is becoming increasingly important.[21–23] Appropriate examination of tumor specimens is critical for accurate diagnosis and triage of tumor specimens.[24] Rhabdomyosarcomas are classified using the modified International Classification.[25]

Embryonal RMS is the most common histologic variant, representing more than half of all RMS cases. These tumors are characterized by primitive spindle cells, often with myxoid areas. The botryoid variant of embryonal RMS typically arises in hollow organs and presents as a grapelike, protruding mass. This variant is typified by subepithelial condensation of tumor cells (cambium layer).

Alveolar histology tumors are less common, constituting 25% to 40% of RMSs. These tumors are more common in adolescents and in extremity tumors. Histologically, alveolar tumors are composed of round or oval noncohesive tumor cells that form "alveolar" spaces surrounded by a framework of fibrous septae. A solid variant of alveolar histology is also characterized by the presence of typical cytological features without alveolar spaces.[26] Myogenin and MyoD1 typically have higher expression in alveolar histology tumors than in other RMSs.[27]

Contemporary theory of cancer pathogenesis ascribes 5 distinct functional characteristics to all cancer cells: resistance to normal extracellular signals that inhibit cell growth, independence from external growth signals (autocrine growth), ability to divide indefinitely (immortalization), evasion of programmed cell death (apoptosis) that might otherwise be triggered by genetic mutations and other cell stresses, and the ability to grow a vascular supply (angiogenesis).[28,29] As is the case for many cancers, dysregulated expression of genes and/or proteins involved in each of these abilities has been identified for RMS and other soft tissue sarcomas. Figure 25-1 shows an extensive list of dysregulated genes or pathways that have been found in these cancers or cell lines derived from them, but many others will likely be discovered, and only a subset probably play a role in a particular patient's cancer. Mouse models suggest that disruption of cell-signaling pathways involving the tumor suppressors p53 and Rb, in combination with aberrant c-Met signaling, is a seminal event during the development of RMS.[30]

The fact that multiple cellular functions can be altered by a single dysregulated "master" transcription factor, and therefore that cancer development may not require the

acquisition of multiple mutations over many years, may explain why such cancers as RMS occur early in life. During myogenesis, the developmental transcription factor PAX3 is expressed in muscle precursor cells as they migrate from axial somites to limb buds. The closely related PAX7 is expressed in postnatal satellite muscle cells that grow, divide, migrate, and differentiate to form new myocytes in response to muscle damage. Thus, these transcription factors are associated with induction of growth and migration of immature muscle cells. It is not surprising, then, that they are reactivated in RMS. The chromosomal translocations t(2;13) and t(1;13) fuse the DNA-binding domain of PAX3 or PAX7, respectively, to the activation domain of a ubiquitous transcription factor, FOXO1a (formerly FKHR); these translocations are pathognomonic for the alveolar type of RMS[31–34] and may be detected in paraffin-embedded tissue using fluorescent in situ hybridization analysis.[35] Similarly, ectopic PAX7 expression is characteristic of embryonal RMS,[36] suggesting the muscle satellite cell as its origin. PAX3, PAX7, and/or PAX3/7-FOXOa1 have been shown to directly up-regulate proteins involved in several of the required cancer characteristics (see asterisks in Figure 25-1), including one of the critical signaling pathways in RMSs, c-Met. Chromosomal translocations and the resulting expression of novel hybrid proteins may play similar roles in other sarcomas.

Nonrhabdomyosarcoma Soft Tissue Sarcomas

The NRSTS occurring in children typically have a similar histologic appearance to their counterpart that develops in adults although, in some cases, biologic behavior differs. Histologic grading of NRSTS is important for assessment of prognosis in some diagnostic subtypes. In the United States, these tumors are graded using a modification of the National Cancer Institute's tumor grading system that recognizes the features of certain sarcomas that occur uniquely in children.[37] Other appropriate grading systems exist, including the French Federation of Cancer Centers Sarcoma Group system.[38]

A number of specific cytogenetic abnormalities are found in various subtypes of NRSTS (Table 25-1) that may provide opportunities to better understand their pathogenesis.

Clinical Presentation

Rhabdomyosarcoma is among the most heterogeneous of all cancers: it can occur anywhere and is not associated with any organ or body site; it is not even limited to muscle. Rather, RMS has been reported to arise in any of a number of unusual locations, including mucosal-lined cavities (ear, nose, mouth, larynx, bladder, and vagina), meninges, parotid gland, ovary, fallopian tube, female breast, testes, spermatic cord, penis, conjunctiva, lungs, gastrointestinal tract, biliary tract, kidney, bone marrow (where it can mimic leukemia), skin, and even bone. Parenchymal brain and spinal cord RMS lesions are usually metastases. Despite the

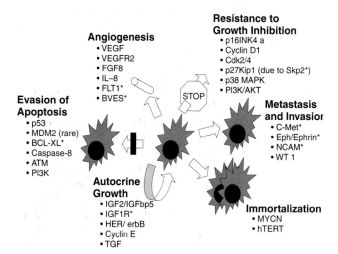

Figure 25-1 The five required characteristics of all cancer cells, including sarcomas. Effector molecules for each characteristic have been identified for rhabdomyosarcoma and other soft tissue sarcomas. Up arrows indicate up-regulated gene or protein expression, while down arrows indicate down-regulated expression, mutation or deletion, or evidence of a disrupted pathway. The asterisks indicate genes for which there is evidence of transcriptional regulation by PAX3, PAX7, and/or PAX3/7-FKHR.

Table 25-1

Characteristic cytogenetic abnormalities in NRSTS.

Tumor Type	Chromosomal Abnormalities	Fusion Product
Extraosseous PNET/Ewing sarcoma	t(11;22)(q24;q12)	EWS-FLI1
	t(21;22)(q22;q12)	EWS-ERG
	t(7;22)(p22;q12)	EWS-ETV1
	t(17;22)(q12;q12)	EWS-E1AF
	t(2;22)(q33;q12)	FEV-EWS
Fibrosarcoma (infantile)	t(12;15;)(p13;q25)	ETV6-NTRK3 (TEL-TRKC)
Synovial sarcoma	t(X;18)(p11;q11)	SYT-SSX1, SYT-SSX2
Alveolar soft part sarcoma	t(X;17)(p11.2;q25)	ASPL-TFE3
Desmoplastic small round cell tumor	t(11;22)(p13;q12)	EWS-WT1
Clear cell sarcoma (malignant melanoma of soft parts)	t(12;22)(q13;q12)	EWS-ATF1
Malignant peripheral nerve sheath tumor	10p, 11q, 17q, 22q	
Leiomyosarcoma	12q, 1p, 6q, 11p, 22q	

numerous possible locations, the most common sites for primary RMS are head and neck including orbit (~40% of cases), genitourinary system (~20%), and extremities (~20%; see Figure 25-2).[39–44]

Interestingly, in some locations there is a predilection for one of the two major histologic subtypes of RMS (Figure 25-2). Although the alveolar type occurs in ~20% to 40% of cases overall, it is rarely found in orbital[45,46] and paratesticular tumors (<10%),[47,48] more commonly found in extremity and bone marrow primaries (70%),[49,50] and almost exclusively found in cases arising in the female breast (96%).[51] Overall, extremity lesions account for the most cases of alveolar RMS.

At diagnosis, 85% of RMS cases are localized to the primary site, with no evidence of distant spread. Of the 15% of cases with metastatic disease, nearly 40% have spread to the lungs, with metastases to bone marrow, lymph nodes, and/or bone found in ~30% of cases (Figure 25-3).[52]

The age of onset for RMS also varies widely; however, the vast majority of cases occur in childhood. Age is also loosely related to site of disease. In the female genitourinary tract, for example, lesions are most common in the vagina during early childhood, the cervix during adolescence and reproductive years, and the uterus post menopause. Extremity RMS is most commonly seen in adolescence.

Because RMS can arise anywhere, the presenting symptoms vary widely. Like many cancers, RMS often presents as a painless mass, most typically as superficial head and neck, extremity, paratesticular, and truncal lesions. However, other symptoms may be present and are largely the result of the location of disease due to compression or invasion of adjacent structures. For example, orbit tumors typically cause proptosis and esotropia, whereas nasopharyngeal and paranasal tumors may cause airway obstruction with snoring, sinusitis, epistaxis, pain, and cranial

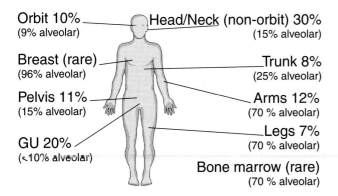

Figure 25-2 Presenting site distribution and histology association for rhabdomyosarcoma. The percentage of cases for each region are shown, as well as the relative incidence of alveolar histology.

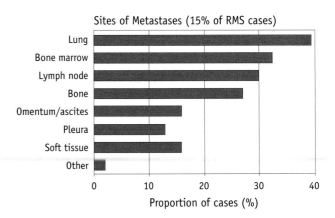

Figure 25-3 Sites of metastatic disease at diagnosis for rhabdomyosarcoma.

nerve palsies. Bladder and prostate tumors present with hematuria, urinary obstruction, and constipation. Mucosal cavity tumors may protrude from the orifice. Thus, both the location and the symptoms of RMS are protean.

Diagnostic Evaluation

An open surgical biopsy is preferred for diagnosis in order to provide sufficient material for histopathological interpretation as well as for additional cytogenetic and for molecular biologic studies; these studies are increasingly helpful in differential diagnosis and important in prognostic stratification.

Precise definition of the locoregional extension of disease and detailed assessment of potential metastatic sites are mandatory before planning therapy. Pretreatment investigations may vary depending on the primary site and clinical presentation but should include the following for all patients.

- Complete physical examination, with a precise definition of tumor site and size, and a careful assessment of regional lymph nodes.
- Laboratory studies, including complete blood count, evaluation of liver and renal function, serum electrolytes, and coagulation parameters.
- Magnetic resonance imaging (MRI) and/or computed tomography (CT) scan of the primary lesion, with 3-dimensional measurement if possible. Ultrasound evaluation may be particularly important in the assessment of genitourinary and other pelvic tumors. During follow-up it is important to be consistent with the imaging modality used at diagnosis.
- Chest x-ray and chest CT.
- Bone marrow aspiration and trephine biopsy is advised in all patients. Bilateral sampling should be performed for patients with evidence of node or distant metastases and for all those with alveolar histology.
- Radioisotope bone scan is generally recommended although the chance of a positive result in patients without other evidence of metastatic disease is very small. It should be included if symptoms indicate.
- Positron emission tomography imaging is being investigated as a staging tool and for assessment of response to therapy.

Other complementary investigations appropriate to the primary site include:

- Parameningeal head and neck: brain MRI and/or CT scan and cerebrospinal fluid (CSF) cytology. Magnetic resonance imaging is superior to CT in defining soft tissue and intracranial extension, but bone destruction is more accurately defined on CT.
- Genitourinary: MRI or CT ± ultrasound of retroperitoneum. Cystourethroscopy with biopsy for bladder or prostate tumors.
- Limbs: MRI or CT scan ± ultrasound of regional lymph nodes and retroperitoneum for lower extremity. Many

protocols require biopsy of regional nodes for all patients with extremity primary tumors. Sentinel node biopsy may be useful.[53] Computed tomography or MRI of the brain may be considered because brain metastases seem more commonly associated with extremity primaries, although studies have shown a very low incidence for asymptomatic brain metastases unless the primary tumor is in the head and neck region.[54]

- Paratesticular: The routine use of retroperitoneal lymph node sampling is controversial. Lymph node sampling is rarely performed in Europe, where emphasis is placed principally on clinical/radiological evaluation, but it is used selectively in North America, specifically for high-risk patients (age > 10 years, primary tumors > 5 cm). Imaging must include the draining nodes in the paraaortic region.
- Trunk: spinal MRI if neurologic signs of medullary compression are present.

Classification and Staging

Rhabdomyosarcoma

All international collaborative studies stratify treatment strategies for RMS according to risk groups defined by key prognostic factors. Although minor differences emerge between different analyses, the principal determinants of prognosis are *site, stage and group, pathology,* and *age.*[55]

Site of primary tumor has a major impact on survival. Site is associated with a number of factors including the speed of presentation, likelihood of regional nodes, distant metastatic disease (Figure 25-4), association with favorable or unfavorable pathologic subtype, and ease of surgical resectability. The most favorable sites are the orbit, genitourinary non-bladder prostate, and nonparameningeal head and neck locations.

Extent of disease is one of the most important predictors for outcome in children with RMS. Since the inception of cooperative group studies conducted by the Intergroup Rhabdomyosarcoma Study (IRS) Group, a

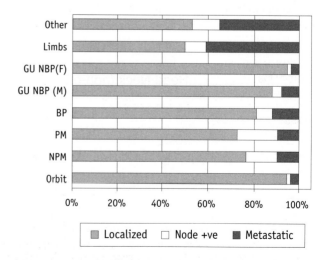

Figure 25-4 Extent of disease for different primary tumor sites (rhabdomyosarcoma).

clinical grouping system has been used to assess the extent of tumor (Table 25-2).[39] Clinical group is determined by the surgical resectability of the primary tumor and presence of metastatic disease. In current U.S. studies, a pretreatment staging system is mandated, using modification of the International Union Against Cancer TNM staging system (Table 25-3) that accounts for the prognostic significance of tumor primary site.[56,57]

The principal determinant of poor prognosis from the pathologic perspective is the presence of alveolar subtype,[55,58,59] both in its classical form and as the solid variant.[26] The presence of alveolar subtype is universally recognized as an adverse feature and is associated with a significantly more aggressive clinical course and, specifi-

cally, a higher risk of distant metastatic disease both at diagnosis and at relapse.

More recently, age has emerged as an important prognostic variable.[60] Patients older than 10 years at diagnosis fare less well. The IRS data suggest that infants younger than 1 year have a less favorable outcome, although this result was not replicated in the European experience.

Patients with completely excised tumors (Group I), those with tumors arising in favorable sites (stage 1), and those without regional node involvement (N_0) consistently have the most favorable outcomes. Patients with metastatic disease (Group IV, stage 4), including those of all ages for those with alveolar histology tumors and those older than 10 years with embryonal RMS, have

---

Table 25-2
IRS clinical grouping classification.

Group I: **Localized disease, completely resected**

(Regional nodes not involved—lymph node biopsy or dissection is required except for head and neck lesions)

  a. Confined to muscle or organ of origin

  b. Contiguous involvement—infiltration outside the muscle or organ of origin, as through fascial planes.

Group II: **Total gross resection with evidence of regional spread**

  a. Grossly resected tumor with microscopic residual disease

  b. Regional disease with involved nodes, completely resected with no microscopic residual.

  c. Regional disease with involved nodes, grossly resected, but with evidence of microscopic residual and/or histologic involvement of the most distal regional node (from the primary site) in the dissection.

NOTATION: The presence of microscopic residual disease makes this group different from 2b, and nodal involvement makes this group different from Group 2a.

Group III: **Incomplete resection with gross residual disease**

  a. After biopsy only

  b. After gross or major resection of the primary (>50%)

Group IV: **Distant metastatic disease present at onset**

(Lung, liver, bones, bone marrow, brain, and distant muscle and nodes)

Table 25-3
Intergroup Rhabdomyosarcoma Study modified TNM pretreatment.

Stage	Sites	T	Size	N	M
1	Favorable	T_1 or T_2	a or b	N_0 or N_1 or N_x	M_0
2	Unfavorable	T_1 or T_2	a	N_0 or N_x	M_0
3	Unfavorable	T_1 or T_2	a	N_1	M_0
		b	N_0 or N_1 or N_x	M_0	
4	All	T_1 or T_2	a or b	N_0 or N_1	M_1

Definitions: *Tumor:* T_1, confined to anatomic site of origin; T_2, extension and/or fixation to surrounding tissues. *Size:* a, ≤5 cm in diameter; b, >5 cm in diameter. *Regional nodes:* N_0, regional nodes not clinically involved; N_1, regional nodes clinically involved; N_x, clinical status of regional nodes unknown. *Metastasis:* M_0, no distant metastasis; M_1, metastasis present.

the poorest outcomes. Children's Oncology Group protocols for RMS assign patients to 1 of 3 risk groups (Table 25-4). These protocols also provide specific guidelines for local tumor control by site that are required to maximize local tumor control while attempting to minimize late effects of therapy. European studies have used very similar risk stratification (Table 25-5) schemes to assign therapy, although strategies for local control have varied, particularly in the Societé Internationale Oncologie Pédiatrique (SIOP) Malignant Mesenchymal Tumors (MMT) studies, in which a more selective approach has been taken to the use of radiotherapy.[61,62]

Table 25-4

Children's Oncology Group protocol risk assignment: D series of studies.[a]

Risk Group	Histology	Group/Stage	Proportion of Patients (%)
Low	Embryonal	Group I/II	
		Group III, Stage 1	30
Intermediate	Embyronal	Group III, Stage 2, 3	55
	Alveolar	Group IV (under age 10 years)	
		Groups I-III	
High	Embryonal	Group IV (> 10 yrs)	15
	Alveolar	Group IV (all ages)	

[a] The above grid shows the risk assignment for the D series (D9602, D9802, and D9803 studies). For the series of COG rhabdomyosarcoma studies initiated in 2004 and 2005, all patients with metastatic disease regardless of histology will be classified as high risk, moving the subset of patients younger than 10 years with metastatic embryonal histology tumors from intermediate risk to high risk.

Table 25-5

European Pediatric Soft Tissue Sarcoma Group protocol risk assignment.

Risk Group	Subgroups	Pathology	IRS Group	Site	Node Stage	Size and Age
Low Risk	A	Favorable	I	Any	N0	Favorable
Standard Risk	B	Favorable	I	Any	N0	Unfavorable
	C	Favorable	II, III	Favorable	N0	Any
	D	Favorable	II, III	Unfavorable	N0	Favorable
High Risk	E	Favorable	II, III	Unfavorable	N0	Unfavorable
	F	Favorable	II, III	Any	N1	Any
	G	Unfavorable	I, II, III	Any	N0	Any
Very High Risk	H	Unfavorable	I, II, III	Any	N1	Any

Pathology:

Favorable = all embryonal, spindle cell, botryoid RMS, and RMS NOS (not otherwise specified)

Unfavorable = all alveolar tumors (including the solid-alveolar variant)

Site:

Favorable = orbit, genitourinary nonbladder prostate (ie, paratesticular and vagina/uterus) and nonparameningeal (PM) head and neck

Unfavorable = all other sites (parameningeal, extremities, genitourinary bladder/prostate and "other site")

Node stage

According to the TNM classification

N0 = no clinical or pathological nodal involvement

N1 = clinical or pathological nodal involvement

Size and Age:

Favorable = Tumour size (maximum dimension) < 5cm *and* Age > 1 year and < 10 years

Unfavorable = all others (ie, Size > 5 cm *or* Age ≤ 1 or ≥ 10 years)

Nonrhabdomyosarcoma Soft Tissue Sarcomas

Nonrhabdomyosarcoma soft tissue sarcomas in childhood have been generally staged using the same criteria as developed for RMS. However, the most important prognostic variables are tumor grade, size, extent of resection, and presence of metastatic disease.[63] Treatment stratification and prognosis are strongly correlated with the extent of tumor resection.

Treatment and Prognosis

Rhabdomyosarcoma

The substantial improvements in outcome for children and adolescents with RMS have been attained using a multidisciplinary approach to therapy. Initial assessment by a multimodality team, including a surgical subspecialist and radiation oncologist, is crucial for appropriate treatment planning. Because micrometastatic but clinically undetectable disease exists in most patients, multiagent chemotherapy is required. In most settings, specific measures for local tumor control are also mandatory. Successive improvements in outcome have occurred since the initiation of cooperative group studies. The percentage of patients alive at 5 years from diagnosis has increased: 55% on IRS-I,[39] 63% on IRS-II,[40] 69% on IRS-III,[41] and 73% on IRS-IV.[42] Children of all ethnic backgrounds have benefited.[64] In Europe, studies have been conducted by three cooperative groups—SIOP MMT Group, CWS (German Cooperative Group), and Italian Cooperative Group—with similar improvements in outcome (5-year overall survival rates 69%-71%),[44,62] although treatment approaches and philosophies have shown some important differences.

To minimize the risk of recurrence, all studies have stressed immediate tumor resection for most tumor sites when possible without major functional or cosmetic sequelae, followed by adjuvant chemotherapy. Patients that can have the tumor completely excised (Group I) generally have the most favorable outcome; for embryonal tumors, adequate surgical resection avoids the need for local irradiation. Tumors that are not completely excised (Groups II and III) typically have received local irradiation in U.S. studies. In Europe, particularly in the MMT studies, concerns regarding the late effects of irradiation have led to a more selective approach to the use of additional local therapy in patients who achieve complete remission (CR) with chemotherapy with or without surgery, particularly at certain tumor sites (eg, orbit).[45,65] The following sections provide an overview of chemotherapy, local control measures, and site-specific treatment modifications.

Chemotherapy

Several chemotherapy agents have activity against RMS. Vincristine, cyclophosphamide, dactinomycin,[39,40] doxorubicin,[66] ifosfamide,[67] and etoposide are among the most active agents and are part of many multiagent treatment approaches. Although some other agents have demonstrated some activity, including melphalan,[68,69] cisplatin,[70,71] and methotrexate,[72] they do not have any role

in frontline therapy because of additive toxicity and the lack of proven benefit. In North America combinations of vincristine, dactinomycin, and, for higher-risk children, cyclophosphamide are the primary agents.[42] The IRS-IV randomly allocated patients to vincristine/dactinomycin/cyclophosphamide (VAC) or 2 experimental arms, where ifosfamide was substituted for cyclophosphamide (VAI) and etoposide substituted for dactinomycin.[42] All 3 arms of this trial had similar outcome, with no benefit for the ifosfamide-containing treatments. Thus, in North America, VAC continues to be the treatment of choice for more advanced stage/group patients. Ifosfamide, however, remains the alkylating agent of choice in all European studies.

The treatment paradigm for recently completed studies and the new generation of studies in North America recognizes 3 risk groups (Table 25-4). The low-risk group represents about 30% of the patient population and includes only patients with embryonal histology tumors, those with Group I or II tumors, or those who are Group III, stage 1. This group of children has an estimated long-term survival of 93% to 94%. Approximately 55% of patients with RMS have intermediate-risk disease. This group includes all those with nonmetastatic (ie, Groups I-III) alveolar and undifferentiated histology tumors, as well as those with the more advanced embryonal histology tumors (Group III, stage 2 or 3). In the previous series of Children's Oncology Group (COG) studies, patients with Group IV embryonal tumors younger than 10 years at diagnosis were also included in this group. The long-term failure-free survival for the intermediate-risk group is about 64%. Those at highest risk of treatment failure include all patients with metastatic alveolar (Group IV, stage 4) tumors, about 15% to 20% of the population, with a predicted survival of less than 30%. All previous European studies have used similar stratifications to allocate patients to different risk groups, hence to treatment regimens of varying intensity and complexity. A new European intergroup study for patients with nonmetastatic RMS identifies 4 risk groups (Table 25-5). Patients in the most favorable group are highly selected and account for only 6% to 8% of this total population. These patients have Group I embryonal tumors and favorable age (< 10 years) and tumor size (< 5 cm). The standard-risk group includes all other patients with embryonal Group I tumors, those with embryonal Group II and III tumors at favorable sites, and those with tumors at unfavorable sites who have favorable age and tumor size (approximately 35% of patients). The high-risk group (50%-55% patients) includes patients with other embryonal Group II or III tumors and unfavorable age and tumor size, all those with embryonal node positive tumors, and those with all alveolar tumors, unless they are also node positive. This latter small group of patients is considered to be very high risk and will be treated in the same fashion as those with metastatic disease.

The approach to patients with low-risk RMS attempts to maintain excellent cure rates while decreasing the burden of care. The recently completed COG cooperative group trial used vincristine and dactinomycin for the most favorable risk subset, with the addition of cyclophosphamide (2.2 g/m²/dose) reserved for the subgroup with more extensive disease. Patients with microscopic (Group II) or gross residual (Group III) disease received local irradiation. The outcome for this group is excellent, with 97% 3-year overall survival; however, many children who were cured received substantial exposure to cyclophosphamide (28.6 g/m²). The European approach to treating these lower-risk patients uses significantly less aggressive therapy and lower total exposures to alkylating agents. In future European studies, those in the most favorable group will receive only vincristine and dactinomycin for a period of 22 weeks, while those in the standard-risk group will commence standard therapy with IVA. Alkylating agent exposure will be reduced in those who receive radiotherapy as local therapy (cumulative ifosfamide dose will range between 24 and 54 g/m²). A current COG trial is testing whether substantial dose reductions, including limiting the total cumulative cyclophosphamide exposure to 4 g/m², will maintain excellent cure rates and decrease the morbidity of therapy.

The intermediate-risk group of patients with RMS requires a more aggressive therapy approach. Based on the results of IRS-IV, VAC has remained the gold standard for therapy in North America. However, a pilot study of dose intensification of cyclophosphamide failed to show any advantage of very high dose administration.[73] Phase II studies in relapsed patients and previously untreated patients at highest risk of treatment failure have demonstrated that the combination of topotecan/cyclophosphamide is active against rhabdomyosarcoma.[74,75] Building on these Phase II results, a recently completed randomized COG study tested whether the addition of topotecan/cyclophosphamide to VAC improved outcome; preliminary analysis failed to demonstrate improvement in outcome for those receiving topotecan and cyclophosphamide. Recent parallel European studies undertaken by SIOP and by the German and Italian groups have compared an intensified 6-drug combination first used in treatment of patients with stage 4 disease (IVA with carboplatin, epirubicin, and etoposide) with standard-therapy IVA in the SIOP studies, and VAIA—IVA plus doxorubicin—in the German-Italian study). Preliminary results show no overall benefit, so the high-risk group of nonmetastatic patients in the new European protocol will be entered into a randomized strategy that will explore: (a) the value of early intensification with anthracycline (comparing standard IVA with VAIA and (b) a duration of therapy question. Treatment duration has always been shorter in European studies compared with IRS/COG studies, and patients who achieve CR after conventional therapy will be randomized to stop therapy or to continue with a 6-month maintenance phase using a novel combination of vinorelbine and oral cyclophosphamide.[76]

The outcome for children with metastatic rhabdomyosarcoma remains poor.[77,78] The IRS and subsequent COG trials in North America have used Phase II windows, followed by VAC therapy for patients at highest risk of treatment failure. This approach has permitted the identification of several active single agents and combinations, including ifosfamide/etoposide,[69] ifosfamide/doxorubicin,[79] vincristine/melphalan,[69] topotecan,[80] topotecan/cyclophosphamide,[75] irinotecan, and irinotecan/vincristine,[81] and amply demonstrated the predictive nature of rhabdomyosarcoma human xenograft models.[68,82,83] However, a brief window of an active agent or combination followed by VAC has had little impact on outcome.[78] Single-institution and small consortium trials using dose-intensive therapies, often with autologous stem cell reinfusions, have also had little impact for these advanced-stage patients.[84] A previous European intergroup study confirmed no evidence of survival benefit for consolidation in CR of high-dose chemotherapy, with stem cell support, in patients with metastatic RMS.[85] New and innovative approaches will be required to improve the outcome for children with metastatic RMS.

Surgery

Complete surgical excision obviates the need for other local control measures in children with embryonal RMS. Wide and complete resection with a surrounding envelope of normal tissue should be considered whenever possible. Where feasible, pretreatment re-excision may be advisable to ensure complete tumor excision.[86,87] However, RMS often arises in sites where complete excision is not technically possible or would result in unacceptable loss of function, so the majority of patients commence therapy after incomplete excision or biopsy alone. Although not routinely recommended, initial tumor debulking may have some value in selected patients.[88] Typically, complete excision is not considered for tumors arising in the orbit,[45,46] most genitourinary sites,[89–94] parameningeal sites,[95] and some other sites.[96,97] The recent IRS/COG studies have minimized initial surgery in an attempt at bladder preservation; however, not all patients will maintain normal bladder function with this approach.[98] In North American studies, sampling of draining regional nodes is mandatory for tumors arising in extremity sites and in boys older than 10 years with paratesticular primary tumors.[47,49,99,100] In selected primary tumor sites, second-look or delayed primary tumor resections may also be considered.

Radiation Therapy

Local irradiation is indicated for most children and adolescents with RMS. In North America, local irradiation is recommended for patients with incompletely resected or gross residual (Groups II and III) embryonal histology tumors, irrespective of response to chemotherapy, and for all those with alveolar histology tumors. However, local irradiation to high doses (up to 50.4 Gy depending upon site and response to other therapy) risks significant long-term side effects, especially in young children.[101–103] Timing of irradiation has varied in the IRS series of studies. For most patient groups, protocols delayed local irradiation until at least week 12, except for patients with parameningeal primary tumors with evidence of intracranial extension, for whom early institution of irradiation is indicated. Timing of irradiation may be important for this tumor site.[104,105] The new COG intermediate-risk trial uses this experience to test the early use of local irradiation for all patient groups, in an attempt to improve local disease control. Because of the concern with late effects, the European approach has attempted to minimize the initial exposure to irradiation, not using local radiotherapy in many patient groups, and anticipating a higher local failure rate with effective salvage for patients who develop recurrent disease. There is evidence that it is feasible to avoid irradiation in a subset of patients who show complete response to chemotherapy with or without surgery, although it is difficult to clearly identify these patients at diagnosis.[62]

There is no evidence that accelerated or hyperfractionated radiation techniques add value.[106] However, newer techniques,[107] including a limited role for brachytherapy, particularly in the management of female nonbladder genitourinary tract tumors, may decrease the late side effects of irradiation.

Approach to Recurrent Disease

Most children who develop recurrent RMS have a dismal prognosis, with 5-year survival from relapse of about 10%, particularly if recurrence is metastatic or arises locally within a previous radiotherapy field.[108,109] A small group (less than 20% of all relapses in IRS/COG studies) with locally recurrent, embryonal histology tumors that were Group I at initial diagnosis and those with botryoid histology tumors have about a 50% chance of salvage. There was no consistent approach to therapy for these children and adolescents in IRS studies, making treatment recommendations impossible. In previous SIOP studies, higher local relapse rates were associated with the less frequent use of radiation as part of primary therapy, but consistent relapse guidelines, incorporating mandatory irradiation as local therapy, have achieved higher salvage rates in patients with local relapse.

To better define a rational approach and identify new agents that may have activity in RMS, the COG used a standardized approach for all those at first recurrence, testing 2 different schedules of irinotecan/vincristine and alternating combinations of cyclophosphamide/doxorubicin (with tirapazamine) and ifosfamide/etoposide. The role of high-dose therapy with stem cell rescue is unproven for recurrent RMS.

Nonrhabdomyosarcoma Soft Tissue Sarcomas

Few children and adolescents with NRSTS have been the subject of prospective clinical trials.[63,110–114] As a consequence, therapy for these tumors is less well defined, and in most settings clinicians have adopted treatment approaches designed for RMS. This may not be appropriate, and the roles of local radiotherapy and chemotherapy are more controversial. With the exception of, for example, infantile fibrosarcoma[115,116] and haemangiopericytoma,[117,118] there is little evidence that the biologic characteristics of tumors more frequently encountered in adult practice are significantly different when diagnosed in childhood.

Surgery is the mainstay of effective therapy for NRSTS tumors, and every effort should be made to completely excise the primary tumor with clear tumor margins. Those patients with completely excised low-grade tumors or high-grade tumors smaller than 5 cm have a favorable outcome with survival exceeding 85%. Typically, no other therapy beyond complete tumor excision is required. For patients with high-grade tumors and positive tumor resection margins, local adjuvant irradiation (either external beam and/or brachytherapy) is usually indicated. Because patients with low-grade tumors are at lower risk of recurrence and can almost always be salvaged, irradiation is usually not indicated as part of the initial therapy.[63]

Children and adolescents with high-grade NRSTS tumors that are larger than 5 cm and those with unresectable, localized disease have an intermediate prognosis; about half will survive long-term.[113] Patients with unresectable tumors are often offered a trial of chemotherapy on a neoadjuvant basis, while the management of patients with the same pathologic subtype by medical oncologists emphasizes local control (surgery and radiotherapy) with more selective use of chemotherapy. There is, however, evidence for the chemosensitivity of many NRSTS, but it is not clear whether this translates into a survival advantage. The role of chemotherapy in unresectable synovial sarcoma is better defined.[119,120] Adjuvant chemotherapy is more controversial and has had only modest benefit in adults with high-grade sarcomas.[121] In spite of the limited data available, many centers approach these patients with combination chemotherapy, usually ifosfamide and doxorubicin, and local irradiation.[122–124] Children and adolescents with metastatic NRSTS have a dismal long-term outlook; fewer than 10% will survive 5 years from diagnosis. Although ifosfamide/doxorubicin combination therapy can be attempted, the response rate is well under 50%, and early introduction of novel therapy approaches is warranted.

Experimental Therapy

Experimental therapies can be broadly divided into pharmaceutical and biologic ones. Pharmaceutical agents currently in development and testing for soft tissue sarcomas include conventional chemotherapeutic agents that lack specificity, targeting cellular processes common to all dividing cells, but which may have selective activity for certain cancers. These agents include such agents as newer-generation vinca alkaloids (eg, vinorelbine), camptothecins (irinotecan), and nucleoside analogues (eg, gemcitibine). Other agents are under development that target specific molecules or signal pathways, including the IGF/mTOR (insulin growth factor/mammalian target of rapamycin) pathway, in the cell. In addition to these small molecular inhibitors, protein and gene therapy approaches are being pursued to also target these molecules and pathways. Both pharmaceutical and biologic agents include those that target angiogenesis, signal transduction pathways, apoptotic pathways, differentiation pathways, gene transcription, mediators of cell invasion and metastasis, and cell cycle functions. Agents that sensitize a cell to chemotherapy or radiotherapy and those that cause cytopathic effects (oncolytic viruses) are also being evaluated.

Definition of Best Therapy: Controversies and Uncertainties

Protocols for treatment of RMS can be confusing and their results difficult to integrate, partly due to the use of different staging systems and partly because the complexity of prognostic variables often results in a relatively large number of possible treatment choices. International collaborations have begun to ensure that the staging systems and definition of factors used to determine treatment allocation will be more consistent in the future. There remain, however, some philosophical differences in the approach to therapy, particularly toward the method and timing of local treatment, and, most specifically, to the place of radiotherapy in guaranteeing local control for patients who may achieve complete remission with chemotherapy, with or without significant surgery. Local relapse rates are generally higher in the SIOP studies than those elsewhere, although the SIOP experience has also made it clear that a significant number of patients who relapse may be cured with alternative treatment. In this context, overall survival (rather than disease-free or progression-free survival) becomes the most important criterion for measuring outcome. However, overall survival should also be linked to a measure of the "cost" of survival that takes into account the total burden of therapy experienced by an individual patient, including that received for relapse if appropriate, and the predicted late sequelae that may result.

Chemotherapy

The VAC combination remains the gold standard in North America for the treatment of RMS, while there is consistent use of ifosfamide in European studies and no evidence to show that one is superior to the other. It is likely that acute toxicity profile, ease of administration, the need for hematopoietic growth factors (eg, granulocyte colony-stimulating factor G-CSF) support and long-term sequelae will ultimately be the criteria that distinguish between them.

The use of doxorubicin in RMS is controversial. Doxorubicin was evaluated in a number of IRS group studies without any indication of significant advantage for its addition to VAC. However, recent data from an "upfront" window study of doxorubicin in newly diagnosed patients with high-risk metastatic RMS performed in France have confirmed a response rate of 65%, and a new European intergroup study will explore the value of doxorubicin as early intensification when added to VAI.[125] A new COG study for patients with metastatic disease also uses doxorubicin in a dose-compression phase of treatment.

Radiotherapy

The evidence from European studies that it may be possible to delay or avoid local therapy in some children who would otherwise receive radiation therapy requires further evaluation.[45] Most especially, there is a need to define such favorable patients at the outset so as to reduce the risk of relapse in those for whom this strategy would not be suitable. Children's Oncology Group studies have mandated radiotherapy in more patients, and a new intermediate-risk study will test the early use of irradiation.

Doses of radiation therapy have, somewhat pragmatically, been tailored to age with reduced doses in younger children, although there is no defined threshold below which late effects can be avoided and yet tumor control can still be achieved. The CWS group has explored the use of reduced radiation dose in children who demonstrate better response to chemotherapy (32 vs 54 Gy) and has also explored the delivery of (lower-dose) radiation prior to delayed surgery. Children's Oncology Group studies are also testing reductions in radiotherapy dose. The possibility of further reducing radiation dose must remain a target for future investigation.

Long-Term Outcome and Late Effects of Therapy

All elements of treatment can contribute to significant late sequelae. The majority of children with RMS are very young, and 40% of tumors occur in the head and neck, where the need for radiotherapy creates special concern.[101,126] Exenteration for orbital tumors is, fortunately, rarely required and is usually performed only when disease recurs after radiotherapy. Nevertheless, those who receive radiotherapy experience important late sequelae including cataract, dry eye, orbital hypoplasia, and pituitary insufficiency.[127] Radiation therapy at other sites may cause significant bone and soft tissue hypoplasia, maximal in those treated at a young age.

Historically, only about 50% of children with bladder or prostate RMS retain their bladder after successful treatment, and a significant minority of these have a degree of bladder dysfunction. Due to improved surgical and conformal radiotherapy techniques, bladder salvage rates may be better in more recent studies[98] but associated with long-term morbidity in some patients.[97] The value of retroperitoneal lymph node dissection as part of staging procedures for paratesticular RMS is controversial; clinicians in Europe have tended to consider this procedure unnecessary, particularly as bilateral sampling may cause intestinal obstruction, loss of ejaculatory function, and lymphedema of the leg.[128] The policy of the COG studies has varied in recent years, and modified retroperitoneal node dissection is now used in patients older than 10 years.

Chemotherapy is also associated with significant sequelae in some patients, and the use of alkylating agents and anthracycline drugs is of particular concern in relation to the risks of gonadal toxicity, cardiotoxicity, and second malignancy.[129] The use of ifosfamide as the alkylating agent component of chemotherapy for soft tissue sarcoma in Europe is well established but remains controversial. There is concern about the renal toxicity profile of ifosfamide, although the incidence of significant nephrotoxicity is very low when the cumulative dose is less than approximately 60 g/m^2. Data are not yet available to confirm whether ifosfamide is less damaging to gonadal function than cyclophosphamide. Other chemotherapy-induced late effects depend on specific drug exposures and interaction with other forms of therapy. For example, there has been concern about neurotoxicity when intrathecal chemotherapy is delivered in conjunction with cranial radiotherapy for parameningeal tumors.

All survivors of cancer in childhood are at risk both for very late recurrence of the primary tumor and of second malignancy, although the reported cumulative incidence in survivors of RMS is reassuringly low.[130] Radiotherapy is the dominant risk factor, but there is a compound effect from concurrent exposure to chemotherapy, and there is concern that rates might rise in patients treated with more recent, higher-dose multiagent chemotherapy schedules.

Prospective evaluation of all survivors is required in order to document the frequency and functional significance of the sequelae of all types of therapy.

Summary

The soft tissue sarcomas in children and adolescents are a histologically and biologically heterogeneous group of tumors. Rhabdomyosarcoma is curable in about 70% of patients; however, cure rate is highly dependent upon extent of disease and histologic subtype. Multidisciplinary therapy is required. The challenge for these patients is maximizing cure rates while minimizing the sometimes substantial side effects of curative therapy. The NRSTS are as a group more common than RMS, occurring more often in adolescents. Surgery is the primary therapy modality for most of these patients; however, many will require a multidisciplinary approach to therapy. Newer approaches to therapy are required for those with metastatic disease.

References

1. Ries LAG, Smith MA, Gurney JG, et al.. *Cancer Incidence and Survival Among Children and Adolescents: United States SEER Program 1975–1995.* (NIH Pub. No. 99-4649). Bethesda, MD: National Cancer Institute, SEER Program; 1999.
2. Yang P, Grufferman S, Khoury MJ, et al. Association of childhood rhabdomyosarcoma with neurofibromatosis type I and birth defects. *Genet Epidemiol.* 1995;12:467–474.
3. Sung L, Anderson JR, Arndt C, et al. Neurofibromatosis in children with Rhabdomyosarcoma: a report from the Intergroup Rhabdomyosarcoma study IV. *J Pediatr.* 2004;144:666–668.
4. Smith AC, Squire JA, Thorner P, et al. Association of alveolar rhabdomyosarcoma with the Beckwith-Wiedemann syndrome. *Pediatr Dev Pathol.* 2001; 4:550–558.
5. Cohen PR, Kurzrock R. Miscellaneous genodermatoses: Beckwith-Wiedemann syndrome, Birt-Hogg-Dube syndrome, familial atypical multiple mole melanoma syndrome, hereditary tylosis, incontinentia pigmenti, and supernumerary nipples. *Dermatol Clin.* 1995;13:211–229.
6. Malkin D, Li FP, Strong LC, et al. Germ line p53 mutations in a familial syndrome of breast cancer, sarcomas, and other neoplasms. *Science.* 1990;250: 1233–1238.
7. Carnevale A, Lieberman E, Cardenas R. Li-Fraumeni syndrome in pediatric patients with soft tissue sarcoma or osteosarcoma. *Arch Med Res.* 1997;28: 383–386.
8. Bisogno G, Murgia A, Mammi I, Strafella MS, Carli M. Rhabdomyosarcoma in a patient with cardio-facio-cutaneous syndrome. *J Pediatr Hematol Oncol.* 1999;21:424–427.
9. Hennekam RC. Costello syndrome: an overview. *Am J Med Genet.* 2003; 117C:42–48.
10. Gripp KW, Scott CIJ, Nicholson L, et al. Five additional Costello syndrome patients with rhabdomyosarcoma: proposal for a tumor screening protocol. *Am J Med Genet.* 2002;108:80–87.
11. Ruymann FB, Maddux HR, Ragab A, et al. Congenital anomalies associated with rhabdomyosarcoma: an autopsy study of 115 cases. A report from the Intergroup Rhabdomyosarcoma Study Committee (representing the Children's Cancer Study Group, the Pediatric Oncology Group, the United Kingdom Children's Cancer Study Group, and the Pediatric Intergroup Statistical Center). *Med Pediatr Oncol.* 1988;16:33–39.
12. Grufferman S, Schwartz AG, Ruymann FB, Maurer HM. Parents' use of cocaine and marijuana and increased risk of rhabdomyosarcoma in their children. *Cancer Causes Control.* 1993;4:217–224.
13. Korf BR. Malignancy in neurofibromatosis type 1. *Oncologist.* 2000;5:477–485.
14. Shearer P, Parham D, Kovnar E, et al. Neurofibromatosis type I and malignancy: review of 32 pediatric cases treated at a single institution. *Med Pediatr Oncol.* 1994;22:78–83.
15. Hawkins MM, Draper GJ, Kingston JE. Incidence of second primary tumours among childhood cancer survivors. *Br J Cancer.* 1987;56:339–347.
16. McClain KL, Leach CT, Jenson HB, et al. Association of Epstein-Barr virus with leiomyosarcomas in children with AIDS. *N Engl J Med.* 1995;332:12–18.
17. Horn RC Jr, Enterline HT. Rhabdomyosarcoma: a clinicopathological study and classification of 39 cases. *Cancer.* 1958;11:181–199.
18. Parham DM, Webber B, Holt H, Williams WK, Maurer H. Immunohistochemical study of childhood rhabdomyosarcomas and related neoplasms: results of an Intergroup Rhabdomyosarcoma study project. *Cancer.* 1991;67:3072–3080.
19. Cessna MH, Zhou H, Perkins SL, et al. Are myogenin and myoD1 expression specific for rhabdomyosarcoma? a study of 150 cases, with emphasis on spindle cell mimics. *Am J Surg Pathol.* 2001;25(9):1150–1157.
20. Kumar S, Perlman E, Harris CA, Raffeld M, Tsokos M. Myogenin is a specific marker for rhabdomyosarcoma: an immunohistochemical study in paraffin-embedded tissues. *Mod Pathol.* 2000;13:988–993.
21. Schaaf GJ, Ruijter JM, van Ruissen F, et al. Full transcriptome analysis of rhabdomyosarcoma, normal, and fetal skeletal muscle: statistical comparison of multiple SAGE libraries. *Faseb J.* 2005;19:404–406.
22. Davicioni E, Finckenstein FG, Shahbazian V, et al. Identification of a PAX-FKHR gene expression signature that defines molecular classes and determines the prognosis of alveolar rhabdomyosarcomas. *Cancer Res.* 2006;66: 6936–6946.
23. Lae M, Ahn EH, Mercado GE, et al. Global gene expression profiling of PAX-FKHR fusion-positive alveolar and PAX-FKHR fusion-negative embryonal rhabdomyosarcomas. *J Pathol.* 2007;212:143–151.
24. Qualman SJ, Bowen J, Parham DM, Branton PA, Meyer WH. Protocol for the examination of specimens from patients (children and young adults) with rhabdomyosarcoma. *Arch Pathol Lab Med.* 2003;127:1290–1297.
25. Newton WAJ, Gehan EA, Webber BL, et al. Classification of rhabdomyosarcomas and related sarcomas: pathologic aspects and proposal for a new classification—an Intergroup Rhabdomyosarcoma Study. *Cancer.* 1995;76:1073–1085.
26. Parham DM, Shapiro DN, Downing JR, Webber BL, Douglass EC. Solid alveolar rhabdomyosarcomas with the t(2;13): report of two cases with diagnostic implications. *Am J Surg Pathol.* 1994;18:474–478.
27. Morotti RA, Nicol KK, Parham DM, et al. An immunohistochemical algorithm to facilitate diagnosis and subtyping of rhabdomyosarcoma: the Children's Oncology Group experience. *Am J Surg Pathol.* 2006;30:962–968.
28. Hanahan D, Weinberg RA. The hallmarks of cancer. *Cell.* 2000;100:57–70.
29. Hahn WC, Weinberg RA. Rules for making human tumor cells. *N Engl J Med.* 2002;347:1593–1603.
30. Cavenee WK. Muscling in on rhabdomyosarcoma. *Nat Med.* 2002;8:1200–1201.
31. Barr FG, Galili N, Holick J, et al. Rearrangement of the PAX3 paired box gene in the paediatric solid tumour alveolar rhabdomyosarcoma. *Nat Genet.* 1993; 3:113–117.
32. Barr FG, Chatten J, D'Cruz CM, et al. Molecular assays for chromosomal translocations in the diagnosis of pediatric soft tissue sarcomas. *JAMA.* 1995; 273:553–557.
33. Biegel JA, Nycum LM, Valentine V, Barr FG, Shapiro DN. Detection of the t(2;13)(q35;q14) and PAX3-FKHR fusion in alveolar rhabdomyosarcoma by fluorescence in situ hybridization. *Genes Chromosomes Cancer.* 1995;12:186–192.
34. Barr FG. Gene fusions involving PAX and FOX family members in alveolar rhabdomyosarcoma. *Oncogene.* 2001;20:5736–5746.
35. Nishio J, Althof PA, Bailey JM, et al. Use of a novel FISH assay on paraffin-embedded tissues as an adjunct to diagnosis of alveolar rhabdomyosarcoma. *Lab Invest.* 2006;86:547–556.
36. Tiffin N, Williams RD, Shipley J, Pritchard-Jones K. PAX7 expression in embryonal rhabdomyosarcoma suggests an origin in muscle satellite cells. *Br J Cancer.* 2003;89:327–332.
37. Parham DM, Webber BL, Jenkins JJ, Cantor AB, Maurer HM. Nonrhabdomyosarcomatous soft tissue sarcomas of childhood: formulation of a simplified system for grading. *Mod Pathol.* 1995;8:705–710.
38. Coindre JM, Terrier P, Bui NB, et al. Prognostic factors in adult patients with locally controlled soft tissue sarcoma: a study of 546 patients from the French

Federation of Cancer Centers Sarcoma Group. *J Clin Oncol.* 1996;14:869–877.

39. Maurer HM, Beltangady M, Gehan EA, et al. The Intergroup Rhabdomyosarcoma Study-I: a final report. *Cancer.* 1988;61:209–220.
40. Maurer HM, Gehan EA, Beltangady M, et al. The Intergroup Rhabdomyosarcoma Study-II. *Cancer.* 1993;71:1904–1922.
41. Crist W, Gehan EA, Ragab AH, et al. The Third Intergroup Rhabdomyosarcoma Study. *J Clin Oncol.* 1995;13:610–630.
42. Crist WM, Anderson JR, Meza JL, et al. Intergroup Rhabdomyosarcoma Study-IV: results for patients with nonmetastatic disease. *J Clin Oncol.* 2001;19:3091–3102.
43. Pappo AS, Shapiro DN, Crist WM, Maurer HM. Biology and therapy of pediatric rhabdomyosarcoma. *J Clin Oncol.* 1995;13:2123–2139.
44. Koscielniak E, Harms D, Henze G, et al. Results of treatment for soft tissue sarcoma in childhood and adolescence: a final report of the German Cooperative Soft Tissue Sarcoma Study CWS-86. *J Clin Oncol.* 1999;17:3706–3719.
45. Oberlin O, Rey A, Anderson J, et al. Treatment of orbital rhabdomyosarcoma: survival and late effects of treatment—results of an international workshop. *J Clin Oncol.* 2001;19:197–204.
46. Kodet R, Newton WAJ, Hamoudi AB, et al. Orbital rhabdomyosarcomas and related tumors in childhood: relationship of morphology to prognosis—an Intergroup Rhabdomyosarcoma Study. *Med Pediatr Oncol.* 1997;29:51–60.
47. Raney RBJ, Tefft M, Lawrence WJ, et al. Paratesticular sarcoma in childhood and adolescence: a report from the Intergroup Rhabdomyosarcoma Studies I and II, 1973–1983. *Cancer.* 1987;60:2337–2343.
48. Leuschner I, Newton WAJ, Schmidt D, et al. Spindle cell variants of embryonal rhabdomyosarcoma in the paratesticular region: a report of the Intergroup Rhabdomyosarcoma Study [published erratum appears in *Am J Surg Pathol.* 1993;17(8):858]. *Am J Surg Pathol.* 1993;17:221–230.
49. Neville HL, Andrassy RJ, Lobe TE, et al. Preoperative staging, prognostic factors, and outcome for extremity rhabdomyosarcoma: a preliminary report from the Intergroup Rhabdomyosarcoma Study IV (1991–1997). *J Pediatr Surg.* 2000;35:317–321.
50. Andrassy RJ, Corpron CA, Hays D, et al. Extremity sarcomas: an analysis of prognostic factors from the Intergroup Rhabdomyosarcoma Study III. *J Pediatr Surg.* 1996;31:191–196.
51. Hays DM, Donaldson SS, Shimada H, et al. Primary and metastatic rhabdomyosarcoma in the breast: neoplasms of adolescent females: a report from the Intergroup Rhabdomyosarcoma Study. *Med Pediatr Oncol.* 1997;29:181–189.
52. Breneman JC, Lyden E, Pappo AS, et al. Prognostic factors and clinical outcomes in children and adolescents with metastatic rhabdomyosarcoma: a report from the Intergroup Rhabdomyosarcoma Study IV. *J Clin Oncol.* 2003;21:78–84.
53. McMulkin HM, Yanchar NL, Fernandez CV, Giacomantonio C. Sentinel lymph node mapping and biopsy: a potentially valuable tool in the management of childhood extremity rhabdomyosarcoma. *Pediatr Surg Int.* 2003;19:453–456.
54. Spunt SL, Anderson JR, Teot LA, et al. Routine brain imaging is unwarranted in asymptomatic patients with rhabdomyosarcoma arising outside of the head and neck region that is metastatic at diagnosis: a report from the Intergroup Rhabdomyosarcoma Study Group. *Cancer.* 2001;92:121–125.
55. Meza JL, Anderson J, Pappo AS, Meyer WH. Analysis of prognostic factors in patients with nonmetastatic rhabdomyosarcoma treated on Intergroup Rhabdomyosarcoma Studies III and IV: the Children's Oncology Group. *J Clin Oncol.* 2006;24:3844–3851.
56. Lawrence WJ, Gehan EA, Hays DM, Beltangady M, Maurer HM. Prognostic significance of staging factors of the UICC staging system in childhood rhabdomyosarcoma: a report from the Intergroup Rhabdomyosarcoma Study (IRS-II). *J Clin Oncol.* 1987;5:46–54.
57. Lawrence WJ, Anderson JR, Gehan EA, Maurer H. Pretreatment TNM staging of childhood rhabdomyosarcoma: a report of the Intergroup Rhabdomyosarcoma Study Group. Children's Cancer Study Group. Pediatric Oncology Group. *Cancer.* 1997;80:1165–1170.
58. Hays DM, Newton WJ, Soule EH, et al. Mortality among children with rhabdomyosarcomas of the alveolar histologic subtype. *J Pediatr Surg.* 1983;18:412–417.
59. Anderson JR, Link M, Qualman S, Maurer HM, Crist WM. Improved outcome for patients (pts) with embryonal (EMB) histology (HIST) but not alveolar HIST rhabdomyosarcoma (RMS): results from Intergroup Rhabdomyosarcoma Study-IV (IRS-IV) [abstract]. *Proc Annu Meet Am Soc Clin Oncol.* 1998;17:526a.
60. Joshi D, Anderson JR, Paidas C, et al. Age is an independent prognostic factor in rhabdomyosarcoma: a report from the Soft Tissue Sarcoma Committee of the Children's Oncology Group. *Pediatr Blood Cancer.* 2004;42:64–73.
61. Flamant F, Rodary C, Rey A, et al. Treatment of non-metastatic rhabdomyosarcomas in childhood and adolescence: results of the second study of the International Society of Paediatric Oncology: MMT84. *Eur J Cancer.* 1998;34:1050–1062.
62. Stevens MC, Rey A, Bouvet N, et al. Treatment of nonmetastatic rhabdomyosarcoma in childhood and adolescence results of the Third Study of the International Society of Paediatric Oncology—SIOP Malignant Mesenchymal Tumor 89. *J Clin Oncol.* 2005;23:2618–2628.
63. Spunt SL, Poquette CA, Hurt YS, et al. Prognostic factors for children and adolescents with surgically resected nonrhabdomyosarcoma soft tissue sarcoma: an analysis of 121 patients treated at St Jude Children's Research Hospital. *J Clin Oncol.* 1999;17:3697–3705.
64. Baker KS, Anderson JR, Lobe TE, et al. Children from ethnic minorities have benefited equally as other children from contemporary therapy for rhabdomyosarcoma: a report from the Intergroup Rhabdomyosarcoma Study Group. *J Clin Oncol.* 2002;20:4428–4433.
65. Stevens MC. Treatment for childhood rhabdomyosarcoma: the cost of cure. *Lancet Oncol.* 2005;6:77–84.
66. Pratt CB, Shanks EC. Doxorubicin in treatment of malignant solid tumors in children. *Am J Dis Child.* 1974;127:534–536.
67. Pappo AS, Etcubanas E, Santana VM, et al. A phase II trial of ifosfamide in previously untreated children and adolescents with unresectable rhabdomyosarcoma. *Cancer.* 1993;71:2119–2125.
68. Horowitz ME, Etcubanas E, Christensen ML, et al. Phase II testing of melphalan in children with newly diagnosed rhabdomyosarcoma: a model for anticancer drug development. *J Clin Oncol.* 1988;6:308–314.
69. Breitfeld PP, Lyden E, Beverly RR, et al. Ifosfamide and etoposide are superior to vincristine and melphalan for pediatric metastatic rhabdomyosarcoma when administered with irradiation and combination chemotherapy: a report from the Intergroup Rhabdomyosarcoma Study Group. *Am J Pediatr Hematol Oncol.* 2001;23:225–233.
70. Baum ES, Gaynon P, Greenberg L, Krivit W, Hammond D. Phase II trial cisplatin in refractory childhood cancer: Children's Cancer Study Group Report. *Cancer Treat Rep.* 1981;65:815–822.
71. Nitschke R, Starling KA, Vats T, Bryan H. Cis-diamminedichloroplatinum (NSC-119875) in childhood malignancies: a Southwest Oncology Group study. *Med Pediatr Oncol.* 1978;4:127–132.
72. Pappo AS, Bowman LC, Furman WL, et al. A phase II trial of high-dose methotrexate in previously untreated children and adolescents with high-risk unresectable or metastatic rhabdomyosarcoma. *J Pediatr Hematol Oncol.* 1997;19:438–442.
73. Spunt SL, Smith LM, Ruymann FB, et al. Cyclophosphamide dose intensification during induction therapy for intermediate-risk pediatric rhabdomyosarcoma is feasible but does not improve outcome: a report from the Soft Tissue Sarcoma Committee of the Children's Oncology Group. *Clin Cancer Res.* 2004;10:6072–6079.
74. Saylors RL, Stine KC, Sullivan J, et al. Cyclophosphamide plus topotecan in children with recurrent or refractory solid tumors: a Pediatric Oncology Group Phase II study. *J Clin Oncol.* 2001;19:3463–3469.
75. Walterhouse DO, Lyden ER, Breitfeld PP, et al. Efficacy of topotecan and cyclophosphamide given as a Phase II window in children with newly diagnosed metastatic rhabdomyosarcoma: a report from the Soft Tissue Sarcoma Committee of the Children's Oncology Group. *J Clin Oncol.* 2004;22:1398–1403.
76. Casanova M, Ferrari A, Bisogno G, et al. Vinorelbine and low-dose cyclophosphamide in the treatment of pediatric sarcomas: pilot study for the upcoming European Rhabdomyosarcoma Protocol. *Cancer.* 2004;101:1664–1671.
77. Carli M, Colombatti R, Oberlin O, et al. European intergroup studies (MMT4-89 and MMT4-91) on childhood metastatic rhabdomyosarcoma: final results and analysis of prognostic factors. *J Clin Oncol.* 2004;22:4735–4742.
78. Lager JJ, Lyden ER, Anderson JR, et al. Pooled analysis of phase II window studies in children with contemporary high-risk metastatic rhabdomyosarcoma: a report from the Soft Tissue Sarcoma Committee of the Children's Oncology Group. *J Clin Oncol.* 2006;24:3415–3422.
79. Sandler E, Lyden E, Ruymann F, et al. Efficacy of ifosfamide and doxorubicin given as a phase II "window" in children with newly diagnosed metastatic rhabdomyosarcoma: a report from the Intergroup Rhabdomyosarcoma Study Group. *Med Pediatr Oncol.* 2001;37:442–448.
80. Pappo AS, Lyden E, Breneman J, et al. Up-front window trial of topotecan in previously untreated children and adolescents with metastatic rhabdomyosarcoma: an Intergroup Rhabdomyosarcoma Study. *J Clin Oncol.* 2001;19:213–219.
81. Pappo AS, Lyden E, Breitfeld P, et al. Two consecutive phase II window trials of irinotecan alone or in combination with vincristine for the treatment of metastatic rhabdomyosarcoma: the Children's Oncology Group. *J Clin Oncol.* 2007;25:362–369.
82. Houghton PJ, Cheshire PJ, Hallman JD2, et al. Efficacy of topoisomerase I inhibitors, topotecan and irinotecan, administered at low dose levels in protracted schedules to mice bearing xenografts of human tumors. *Cancer Chemother Pharmacol.* 1995;36:393–403.
83. Furman WL, Stewart CF, Poquette CA, et al. Direct translation of a protracted irinotecan schedule from a xenograft model to a phase I trial in children. *J Clin Oncol.* 1999;17:1815–1824.
84. Weigel BJ, Breitfeld PP, Hawkins D, Crist WM, Baker KS. Role of high-dose chemotherapy with hematopoietic stem cell rescue in the treatment of metastatic or recurrent rhabdomyosarcoma. *J Pediatr Hematol Oncol.* 2001;23:272–276.
85. Carli M, Colombatti R, Oberlin O, et al. High-dose melphalan with autologous stem-cell rescue in metastatic rhabdomyosarcoma. *J Clin Oncol.* 1999;17:2796–2803.
86. Hays DM, Lawrence WJ, Wharam M, et al. Primary reexcision for patients with 'microscopic residual' tumor following initial excision of sarcomas of trunk and extremity sites. *J Pediatr Surg.* 1989;24:5–10.

87. Cecchetto G, Guglielmi M, Inserra A, et al. Primary re-excision: the Italian experience in patients with localized soft-tissue sarcomas. *Pediatr Surg Int.* 2001;17:532–534.

88. Raney RB, Stoner JA, Walterhouse DO, et al. Results of treatment of fifty-six patients with localized retroperitoneal and pelvic rhabdomyosarcoma: a report from the Intergroup Rhabdomyosarcoma Study-IV, 1991–1997. *Pediatr Blood Cancer.* 2004;42:618–625.

89. Lobe TE, Wiener E, Andrassy RJ, et al. The argument for conservative, delayed surgery in the management of prostatic rhabdomyosarcoma. *J Pediatr Surg.* 1996;31:1084–1087.

90. Hays DM, Raney RB, Jr., Lawrence W, Jr., et al. Primary chemotherapy in the treatment of children with bladder-prostate tumors in the Intergroup Rhabdomyosarcoma Study (IRS-II). *J Pediatr Surg.* 1982;17:812–820.

91. Filipas D, Fisch M, Stein R, et al. Rhabdomyosarcoma of the bladder, prostate or vagina: the role of surgery. *BJU Int.* 2004;93:125–129.

92. Andrassy RJ, Wiener ES, Raney RB, et al. Progress in the surgical management of vaginal rhabdomyosarcoma: a 25-year review from the Intergroup Rhabdomyosarcoma Study Group. *J Pediatr Surg.* 1999;34:731–734.

93. Andrassy RJ, Hays DM, Raney RB, et al. Conservative surgical management of vaginal and vulvar pediatric rhabdomyosarcoma: a report from the Intergroup Rhabdomyosarcoma Study III. *J Pediatr Surg.* 1995;30:1034–1036.

94. Arndt CA, Donaldson SS, Anderson JR, et al. What constitutes optimal therapy for patients with rhabdomyosarcoma of the female genital tract? *Cancer.* 2001;91:2454–2468.

95. Raney RB, Meza J, Anderson JR, et al. Treatment of children and adolescents with localized parameningeal sarcoma: experience of the Intergroup Rhabdomyosarcoma Study Group protocols IRS-II through -IV, 1978–1997. *Med Pediatr Oncol.* 2002;38:22–32.

96. Lawrence WJ, Hays DM. *Surgical Lessons from the Intergroup Rhabdomyosarcoma Study.* Natl Cancer Inst Monogr. 1981:159–163.

97. Ferrer FA, Isakoff M, Koyle MA. Bladder/prostate rhabdomyosarcoma: past, present and future. *J Urol.* 2006;176:1283–1291.

98. Arndt C, Rodeberg D, Breitfeld PP, et al. Does bladder preservation (as a surgical principle) lead to retaining bladder function in bladder/prostate rhabdomyosarcoma? Results from intergroup rhabdomyosarcoma study iv. *J Urol.* 2004;171:2396–2403.

99. Wiener ES, Lawrence W, Hays D, et al. Retroperitoneal node biopsy in paratesticular rhabdomyosarcoma. *J Pediatr Surg.* 1994;29:171–177.

100. Wiener ES, Anderson JR, Ojimba JI, et al. Controversies in the management of paratesticular rhabdomyosarcoma: is staging retroperitoneal lymph node dissection necessary for adolescents with resected paratesticular rhabdomyosarcoma? *Semin Pediatr Surg.* 2001;10:146–152.

101. Raney RB, Asmar L, Vassilopoulou-Sellin R, et al. Late complications of therapy in 213 children with localized, nonorbital soft-tissue sarcoma of the head and neck: a descriptive report from the Intergroup Rhabdomyosarcoma Studies (IRS)-II and -III. IRS Group of the Children's Cancer Group and the Pediatric Oncology Group. *Med Pediatr Oncol.* 1999;33:362–371.

102. Raney RB, Anderson JR, Kollath J, et al. Late effects of therapy in 94 patients with localized rhabdomyosarcoma of the orbit: report from the Intergroup Rhabdomyosarcoma Study (IRS)-III, 1984–1991. *Med Pediatr Oncol.* 2000;34:413–420.

103. Estilo CL, Huryn JM, Kraus DH, et al. Effects of therapy on dentofacial development in long-term survivors of head and neck rhabdomyosarcoma: the Memorial Sloan-Kettering Cancer Center experience. *J Pediatr Hematol Oncol.* 2003;25:215–222.

104. Michalski JM, Meza J, Breneman JC, et al. Influence of radiation therapy parameters on outcome in children treated with radiation therapy for localized parameningeal rhabdomyosarcoma in Intergroup Rhabdomyosarcoma Study Group trials II through IV. *Int J Radiat Oncol Biol Phys.* 2004;59:1027–1038.

105. Smith SC, Lindsley SK, Felgenhauer J, Hawkins DS, Douglas JG. Intensive induction chemotherapy and delayed irradiation in the management of parameningeal rhabdomyosarcoma. *J Pediatr Hematol Oncol.* 2003;25:774–779.

106. Donaldson SS, Meza J, Breneman JC, et al. Results from the IRS-IV randomized trial of hyperfractionated radiotherapy in children with rhabdomyosarcoma: a report from the IRSG. *Int J Radiat Oncol Biol Phys.* 2001;51:718–728.

107. Wolden SL, La TH, LaQuaglia MP, et al. Long-term results of three-dimensional conformal radiation therapy for patients with rhabdomyosarcoma. *Cancer.* 2003;97:179–185.

108. Pappo AS, Anderson JR, Crist WM, et al. Survival after relapse in children and adolescents with rhabdomyosarcoma: a report from the Intergroup Rhabdomyosarcoma Study Group. *J Clin Oncol.* 1999;17:3487–3493.

109. Mazzoleni S, Bisogno G, Garaventa A, et al. Outcomes and prognostic factors after recurrence in children and adolescents with nonmetastatic rhabdomyosarcoma. *Cancer.* 2005;104:183–190.

110. Pratt CB, Pappo AS, Gieser P, et al. Role of adjuvant chemotherapy in the treatment of surgically resected pediatric nonrhabdomyosarcomatous soft tissue sarcomas: a Pediatric Oncology Group Study. *J Clin Oncol.* 1999;17:1219–1226.

111. Walter AW, Shearer PD, Pappo AS, et al. A pilot study of vincristine, ifosfamide, and doxorubicin in the treatment of pediatric non-rhabdomyosarcoma soft tissue sarcomas. *Med Pediatr Oncol.* 1998;30:210–216.

112. Pappo AS, Devidas M, Jenkins J, et al. Vincristine (V), ifosfamide (I), doxorubicin (D), and G-CSF (G) for pediatric unresected metastatic non-rhabdomyosarcomatous soft tissue sarcomas (NRSTS): a Pediatric Oncology Group (POG) study [abstract]. *Proc Annu Meet Am Soc Clin Oncol.* 2001;20:378a.

113. Spunt SL, Hill DA, Motosue AM, et al. Clinical features and outcome of initially unresected nonmetastatic pediatric nonrhabdomyosarcoma soft tissue sarcoma. *J Clin Oncol.* 2002;20:3225–3235.

114. Pratt CB, Maurer HM, Gieser P, et al. Treatment of unresectable or metastatic pediatric soft tissue sarcomas with surgery, irradiation, and chemotherapy: a Pediatric Oncology Group study. *Med Pediatr Oncol.* 1998;30:201–209.

115. Rubin BP, Chen CJ, Morgan TW, et al. Congenital mesoblastic nephroma t(12;15) is associated with ETV6-NTRK3 gene fusion: cytogenetic and molecular relationship to congenital (infantile) fibrosarcoma. *Am J Pathol.* 1998;153:1451–1458.

116. Knezevich SR, McFadden DE, Tao W, Lim JF, Sorensen PH. A novel ETV6-NTRK3 gene fusion in congenital fibrosarcoma. *Nat Genet.* 1998;18:184–187.

117. Rodriguez-Galindo C, Ramsey K, Jenkins JJ, et al. Hemangiopericytoma in children and infants. *Cancer.* 2000;88:198–204.

118. Ferrari A, Casanova M, Bisogno G, et al. Hemangiopericytoma in pediatric ages: a report from the Italian and German Soft Tissue Sarcoma Cooperative Group. *Cancer.* 2001;92:2692–2698.

119. Okcu MF, Munsell M, Treuner J, et al. Synovial sarcoma of childhood and adolescence: a multicenter, multivariate analysis of outcome. *J Clin Oncol.* 2003;21:1602–1611.

120. Pappo AS, Fontanesi J, Luo X, et al. Synovial sarcoma in children and adolescents: the St Jude Children's Research Hospital experience. *J Clin Oncol.* 1994;12:2360–2366.

121. Tierney JF, Mosseri V, Stewart LA, Souhami RL, Parmar MK. Adjuvant chemotherapy for soft-tissue sarcoma: review and meta-analysis of the published results of randomised clinical trials. *Br J Cancer.* 1995;72:469–475.

122. Patel SR, Vadhan-Raj S, Burgess MA, et al. Results of two consecutive trials of dose-intensive chemotherapy with doxorubicin and ifosfamide in patients with sarcomas. *Am J Clin Oncol.* 1998;21:317–321.

123. von Mehren M. New therapeutic strategies for soft tissue sarcomas. *Curr Treat Options Oncol.* 2003;4:441–451.

124. Demetri GD, Elias AD. Results of single-agent and combination chemotherapy for advanced soft tissue sarcomas: implications for decision making in the clinic. *Hematol Oncol Clin North Am.* 1995;9:765–785.

125. Bergeron C, Thiesse P, Rey A, et al. Revisiting the role of doxorubicin in the treatment of rhabdomyosarcoma: an up-front window study in newly diagnosed children with high-risk metastatic disease. *Eur J Cancer.* 2008;44:427–431.

126. Wharam MDJ, Foulkes MA, Lawrence WJ, et al. Soft tissue sarcoma of the head and neck in childhood: nonorbital and nonparameningeal sites: a report of the Intergroup Rhabdomyosarcoma Study (IRS)-I. *Cancer.* 1984;53:1016–1019.

127. Heyn R, Ragab A, Raney RB, Jr., et al. Late effects of therapy in orbital rhabdomyosarcoma in children: a report from the Intergroup Rhabdomyosarcoma Study. *Cancer.* 1986;57:1738–1743.

128. Wiener EW, Anderson JR, Ojimba JI, et al. Controversies in the management of paratesticular rhabdomyosarcoma: is staging retroperitoneal lymph node dissection necessary for adolescents with resected paratesticular rhabdomyosarcoma? *Sem Pediatr Surg.* 2001;10:146–152.

129. Punyko JA, Mertens AC, Gurney JG, et al. Long-term medical effects of childhood and adolescent rhabdomyosarcoma: a report from the childhood cancer survivor study. *Pediatr Blood Cancer.* 2005;15:643–653.

130. Sung L, Anderson JR, Donaldson SS, et al. Late events occurring five years or more after successful therapy for childhood rhabdomyosarcoma: a report from the Soft Tissue Sarcoma Committee of the Children's Oncology Group. *Eur J Cancer.* 2004;40:1878–1885.

Pediatric Systemic Germ Cell Tumors

Roger H. Giller

Introduction

Germ cell tumors are a diverse family of neoplasms sharing a common origin from primordial cells involved in gametogenesis. These tumors arise at various primary sites and with a range of histologic subtypes. This chapter will review the biology and treatment of germ cell tumors of low malignant potential (mature teratomas), tumors of intermediate malignant potential (immature teratomas), and the varied forms of germ cell cancer (germinoma, embryonal carcinoma, yolk sac tumor [endodermal sinus tumor], choriocarcinoma, malignant germ cell tumors of mixed histology) that occur during infancy, childhood, and adolescence.

The heterogeneity of germ cell neoplasms challenges the pathologist and pediatric oncologist to properly classify each tumor and its malignant potential. Highly effective chemotherapy regimens for pediatric germ cell malignancies exist, but some germ cell tumor variants can be cured without chemotherapy. Thus, optimal patient stratification and development of risk-adjusted therapy are important aims of current clinical trials. Finally, newer insights into the biology of pediatric germ cell tumors may point the way to better, targeted treatments.

Epidemiology

Malignant germ cell tumors arising outside the central nervous system (CNS) represent 2% to 4% of all pediatric cancers, based upon several large surveys conducted in the United States, Great Britain, Belgium, and Denmark.[1–4] Data from the National Cancer Institute's Surveillance, Epidemiology, and End Results program indicate an annual incidence of 8.0 cases of germ cell cancer per million population younger than 20 years.[5] This figure breaks down to an incidence of 6.4 cases per million per year for malignant germ cell tumors arising in the ovaries and testes and 1.6 for tumors occurring at nongonadal sites. The incidence of mature teratomas is less well defined. Sacrococcygeal germ cell tumors, mature teratomas in 80% of cases, have been estimated to occur in 1 in every 35,000 live births.[6] Using these incidence figures one can predict that approximately 600 cases of malignant germ cell cancer will occur annually

in children and adolescents among a total population of approximately 75 million younger than 20 years in the United States. An additional 100 cases of congenital sacrococcygeal mature teratoma can be expected to occur annually in the United States among a total of approximately 4 million live births.

Following childhood, there is a steep increase in the incidence of both testicular and ovarian germ cell cancers in adolescents and young adults.[5,7] Interestingly, the increased incidence of testicular germ cell cancer during adolescence and young adulthood is less pronounced in African American as opposed to Caucasian males.

Although the incidence of cancer in infancy is low relative to the remainder of childhood, malignant germ cell tumors represent a larger fraction of those seen. In two series of neonatal cancers, malignant germ cell tumors represented approximately 6% and 2%, respectively.[8,9] In another survey of malignant neoplasms in children younger than 1 year, germ cell cancers represented 7.3% of the total.[10]

Both mature and malignant germ cell tumors occur more frequently in girls than boys younger than 14 years.[5,11] This female predominance derives from the greater frequency of sacrococcygeal mature teratoma in females, and from the more common occurrence of germ cell malignancy in the ovary as opposed to the testicle during childhood. In contrast, during adolescence and young adulthood, males suffer a greater incidence of germ cell cancer due to the higher frequency of testicular germ cell cancer beyond childhood.

Cryptorchidism, which occurs in about 1 in 500 men, has been identified as a risk factor for subsequent development of testicular germ cell cancer. Batata et al have reported that the probability of testicular cancer developing in an undescended testicle is 30 to 50 times greater than in a normally descended testicle.[12] Testicular cancer developed in these patients between 15 and 62 years, with a median age at diagnosis of 32 years. Thus, the oncogenic effects of congenital cryptorchidism are expressed only after a prolonged latency period. Of note was that germ cell cancers were more prone to develop in both the cryptorchid testicles and the normally descended contralateral testicles. Correction of the cryptorchidism by orchiopexy, hormonal therapy, or spontaneous descent of the testicle did not appear to ameliorate the increased risk of cancer in these patients completely. A more recent, large, retrospective study in Sweden examined whether age at surgical correction of cryptorchidism influenced subsequent risk for developing testicular cancer. Patients who underwent orchiopexy were identified through the Swedish Hospital Discharge Register and followed for occurrence of testicular cancer through the Swedish Cancer Registry. The study confirmed increased risk of testicular cancer in all those with cryptorchidism; however, it found that this risk could be more than halved by carrying out corrective orchiopexy prior to 13 years of age.[13]

Population studies have indicated that the incidence of testicular cancer in the United States has been rising over time in adolescents and adults.[14] Preliminary evidence has also suggested that the incidence of mature and malignant germ cell tumors has also been rising in some pediatric populations over the past 30 years.[5] To evaluate the possible influence of environmental factors on development of adult testicular cancer, Brown et al carried out a case-controlled epidemiologic study of pre- and postnatal factors.[15] In their analysis, low birth weight (< 5 pounds) was associated with a 12-fold increase in the risk of subsequent testicular germ cell cancer. Lesser but statistically significant increases in risk were also associated with maternal bleeding or spotting during pregnancy, and with maternal exposure to sedative medications, alcohol, or irradiation. In contrast, more recent studies in pediatric populations have failed to show any strong epidemiologic associations with exogenous female hormone exposure during pregnancy, parental or child exposure to pesticides or other environmental toxins, parental cigarette smoking or alcohol consumption, or maternal passive smoke exposure.[16–18] Thus, while prenatal factors may influence subsequent development of testicular germ cell cancer during adolescence and early adulthood, similar associations with childhood germ cell tumors have not been found.

Tumor Biology

Embryology

During embryonic development, primordial germ cells initially are found at 3 to 4 weeks of gestation extraembryonically in the wall of the yolk sac near the allantois[19] (Figure 26-1). Also at that time, the gonads begin to develop within the 4 week old embryo as a pair of longitudinal structures, the genital ridges, on each side of the midline. From their site of origin in the yolk sac wall, the primordial germ cells migrate upward along the dorsal mesentery of the hindgut, traveling in the midline until they reach the level of the genital ridges. Lateral migration then occurs so that by the sixth week of development, the primordial germ cells move into the gonadal ridges. During this period of germ cell migration, the genital ridges extend from the cervical to the lumbar levels of the developing vertebral column. The gonad continues its development in this position and subsequently descends to its final position in the scrotum or pelvis. The occurrence of germ cell tumors at extragonadal, midline sites may be explained by aberrant patterns of migration and persistence of germ cells in ectopic sites such as the pineal, mediastinum, retroperitoneum, or sacrococcygeal region. Viable germ cells remaining in these locations, as well as those cells that reach their final destination in the ovary or testis, may give rise to germ cell neoplasms at any of these sites. If the concept of aberrant germ cell migration is indeed correct, it would help explain the fact that 65% to 70% of pediatric germ cell tumors occur at extragonadal sites. That germ cell tumors do in fact arise from primordial germ cells is further supported by recent studies of genetic imprinting patterns in the tumors.[20,21] This link likewise is substantiated by novel cell-surface antigens expressed on both normal spermatogonia and germ cell neoplasms.[22]

Critical to the embryonic journey of the developing germ cell is the interaction between the *c-kit* receptor on its surface and the graded presence of its ligand, stem cell factor, in tissues along its course of migration. In animal models, this interaction appears to guide migration, prevent apoptosis, and enhance proliferation of the maturing germ cell as it moves toward the gonad.[23] It follows that disturbances in *c-kit*/stem cell factor interactions could be involved in aberrant primordial germ cell migration postulated in germ cell tumor development.

Oncogenesis

The events that explain neoplastic alteration of germ cells remain incompletely understood. It was believed, at one time, that teratomas represented the frustrated development of a conjoined twin. However, two theories concerning the cellular events that promote germ cell tumor formation have currently evolved based on more recent laboratory observations.[24]

Initially, during the 1950s, inbred mouse strains were developed with a high incidence of spontaneous teratocarcinoma. Cells from these tumors were used to establish transplantable cell culture lines. When these anaplastic teratocarcinoma cells were injected intraperitoneally into secondary hosts, three morphologically distinct cell types and patterns of growth were identified—those resembling the visceral yolk sac, others consistent with mesenchymal connective tissue, as well as cells similar to those of human embryonal carcinoma. Pierce et al further demonstrated the multipotentiality of the murine teratocarcinoma lines by injecting the cells subcutaneously into syngeneic mice.[25] The teratocarcinoma cells produced both malignant and

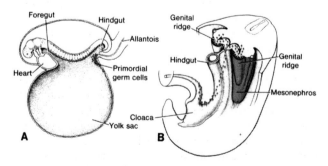

Figure 26-1 (A) Origin of embryonic germ cells. (B) Migration of embryonic germ cells. Reproduced with permission from Langman J. *Medical Embryology*. 4th ed. Baltimore: Lippincott Williams & Wilkins; 1981.

benign structures. The origin of this wide variety of tumor types from a single multipotential cell was confirmed in subsequent experiments using transfer of single embryonal carcinoma cells.[26]

Based on the above observations, Teilum and colleagues proposed a scheme for the histogenesis of germ cell tumors[27] (Figure 26-2). In their view, tumors of pluripotent germ cells may initially follow two courses of differentiation. Along one path are the germinomas (seminoma, dysgerminoma), which bear histopathologic resemblance to primordial germ cells. Along the other pathway are tumors demonstrating histologic patterns similar to those of normal intra- and extraembryonic structures. Teilum postulated that the least differentiated of these later tumors are the embryonal carcinomas, while subsequent differentiation yields the malignant variants of yolk sac tumor and choriocarcinoma on the one hand, and mature teratomas on the other.

The first of the theories of oncogenesis contends that the malignant potential of germ cells is under the exogenous control of microenvironmental signals. Key support for this theory is the work of Brinster, who carried out experiments in which blastocysts harvested from ovulating female mice were injected in vitro with mouse teratocarcinoma cells, then transferred to syngeneic "foster mothers."[28] The offspring from these hybrid embryos developed into normal, tumor-free adult mice. Moreover, these animals were chimeric, derived from both the benign and the malignant parent cells. The signals causing the malignant germ cells to revert to a benign phenotype have not been fully characterized; however, a number of features of the differentiation process have been established. First, the differentiation process is site specific—that is, it occurs only when the malignant cells are injected into the blastocele, the cavity of the blastocyst. Second, the tumorogenecity of the teratocarcinoma cells is lessened in proportion to the time period they are exposed to the differentiating influences of the blastocyst. Finally, these influences are tissue specific in that they affect only teratocarcinoma cells and are unable to exert this influence on leukemia, melanoma, or sarcoma cells.

The second theory concerning the etiology of germ cell tumors suggests that somatic cell mutation is the central event in the process. Support for this concept is derived from family histories of germ cell tumors among first-degree relatives, the association of germ cell tumors with congenital anomalies, the more frequent occurrence of germ cell cancers in individuals with constitutional chromosome abnormalities such as Klinefelter and Down syndromes, and demonstration of specific, recurring cytogenetic abnormalities in human germ cell tumors.[29–41]

The heterogeneous cell types often found within a single germ cell tumor raise questions concerning the validity of theories postulating a single genetic mutational event in the etiology of these tumors. However, the theories of microenvironmental control and somatic cell mutation need not be mutually exclusive. For example, it is conceivable that an initial mutational event predisposes to oncogenesis, while local microenvironmental factors within a given tissue influence the phenotypic and biologic characteristics ultimately expressed by the tumor.

Genetic Factors

There is now abundant evidence suggesting that genetic factors have a primary role in the etiology of germ cell tumors. The first suggestion that heritable factors were involved in causation of germ cell tumors came from an observation that patients with these tumors reported a high incidence of twinning in their families.[36] However, this association could not be confirmed by others. Family clusters of malignant germ cell tumors have also been reported in father-son pairs, siblings, twins, mothers and daughters, and even across three generations in one family.[33–36] A case-control study showed that 6 of 269 testicular cancer patients and only 1 of 259 control subjects had a first-degree relative with testicular cancer, a relative risk of 5.6 for second testicular germ cell cancers developing in male family members of index cases.[36] In addition, synchronous or metachronous bilateral testicular germ cell tumors have been noted in up to 6% of adult males with testicular cancer.[37–39] These observations support the view that genetic or environmental influences predispose multiple germ cells within individual patients and close family members to undergo malignant transformation.

In children, Sakashita et al noted congenital anomalies, including retrocaval ureter, diverticulum of the bladder, Down syndrome, and inguinal hernia in 4 of 25 children with testicular germ cell tumors.[40] Mann et al also identified congenital defects in 17% of 126 children with malignant germ cell tumors at various sites.[30] Although inconclusive, these observations suggest that there may be some genetic or environmental linkage between germ cell tumors in children and congenital anomalies.

Klinefelter syndrome, a disorder in males with a 47 XXY karyotype, has been associated with testicular and extragonadal germ cell tumors, the latter typically located in the mediastinum or CNS.[31,32] The bulk of tumors in patients with Klinefelter syndrome occur during adolescence and early adulthood. In addition, children with 46 XY gonadal dysgenesis (Swyer syndrome), a familial condition characterized by female phenotype and hypoplastic gonads, are predisposed to develop germ cell neoplasms.[42] The increased risk of tumor that children affected by Swyer syndrome experience may also extend to their siblings who are unaffected by gonadal dysgenesis.[43]

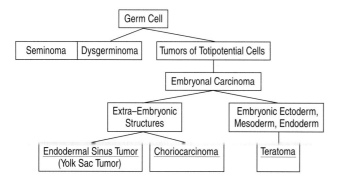

Figure 26-2 Proposed histogenesis of germ cell tumors. Reproduced with permission from Teilum G. Special tumors of ovary and testis and related extragonadal lesions: Comparative pathology and histological identification. 2nd ed. Philadelphia: J.B. Lippincott Company; 1976.

Using newer techniques for chromosome analysis, such as fluorescent in situ hybridization (FISH) and comparative genomic hybridization, a specific karyotypic abnormality, isochromosome 12p [i(12p)] can be identified in the vast majority of adult germ cell cancers studied.[41] This marker chromosome, composed of 2 copies of 12p from the same parental origin, represents an overall gain of material on the short arm of chromosome 12. The i(12p) may be an early and potentially causal event in the genesis of adult germ cell cancers. This supposition derives from the fact that the i(12p) has been found by FISH in intratubular germ cell neoplasia, a precursor lesion of adult testicular cancer.[44]

Pediatric germ cell tumors have distinct cytogenetic differences from their adolescent and adult counterparts. In striking contrast to adult germ cell malignancies, pediatric germ cell cancers occurring prior to puberty rarely demonstrate i(12p).[45,46] Thus, i(12p) is not commonly found in tumors of the sacrococcyx and infantile testis, which occur during early childhood. However, in pubertal and postpubertal adolescents, malignant germ cell tumors arising in the testis, ovary, and extragonadal sites regularly demonstrate the i(12p).

Malignant germ cell tumors of the infant testis are nearly all yolk sac tumors. They are typically diploid or tetraploid and show several recurring cytogenetic abnormalities, including deletion of 1p and 6q and gains of 1q, chromosome 3, and chromosome 21. Malignant germ cell tumors of the pubertal and postpubertal testis and ovary are generally aneuploid and often show the i(12p) as well as deletions of 1p and gains of 1q and chromosomes 3, 8, 14, and 21. In contrast, pure mature and immature teratomas generally have normal karyotypes.[45,46]

The above cytogenetic features suggest that gain of genetic material at 1q and via i(12p) and loss of heterozygosity at 1p and 6q may be involved in the molecular pathogenesis of germ cell cancers. Recently, overexpression of the homeobox transcription factor gene *NANOG*, located on 12p, has been implicated in the molecular pathogenesis of i(12p) positive germ cell malignancies.[47] Likewise, the *RUNX3* gene, lost via the 1p36 deletion, has been proposed as a possible tumor suppressor gene involved in germ cell tumor pathogenesis.[48] Studies of gene expression profiles in germ cell tumors have suggested additional candidate genes to explore as potential etiologic factors in tumorigenesis.[41]

In murine models, inactivation of the *dead end* gene via the *Ter* mutation causes primordial germ cell loss. When expressed in the 129 mouse strain, the *Ter* mutation predisposes to testicular germ cell cancer development as well, possibly modeling pediatric testicular tumors.[49] The *Ter* mutation may act through a novel tumorigenic effect on RNA editing.

Serum Tumor Markers

Serum biochemical markers are particularly useful in the diagnosis and monitoring of germ cell tumors. The most valuable of these markers are α-fetoprotein (AFP) and the beta subunit of human chorionic gonadotropin (βHCG).

Yolk sac tumors produce AFP, while choriocarcinomas elaborate βHCG. In some instances, embryonal carcinoma may secrete AFP and/or βHCG, although generally in far smaller amounts than yolk sac tumors and choriocarcinomas (Table 26-1). Germinomas and mature teratomas are not associated with elevations of serum AFP or βHCG. The presence of an elevated AFP or βHCG in patients diagnosed with pure mature teratoma suggests that the tumor may contain undetected foci of yolk sac tumor or choriocarcinoma and that further tumor sampling should be considered for effective risk stratification and optimal treatment planning. In a recent series of children younger than 16 years with malignant germ cell tumors, serum AFP was elevated in 87% of patients, while βHCG was increased in 10%.[30]

Alpha-fetoprotein is a glycoprotein of approximately 70 kiloDalton molecular weight that is normally produced in the fetal yolk sac, liver, and gastrointestinal tract.[50] Synthesis of AFP begins in the liver of the developing embryo at approximately 6 weeks' gestation. It becomes the major serum protein of the human fetus, reaching levels of 3 mg/ml at the twelfth week of gestation and subsequently declining to the normal adult range of less than approximately 15 ng/ml by 8 months of age postnatally. Due to the physiologic changes in serum AFP levels, this marker is difficult to utilize as an indicator of residual or recurrent germ cell tumor in infants younger than 6 months. Wu et al have reported a large series of serum AFP levels in normal neonates and infants that describes the physiologic changes in AFP levels that occur over the first year of life[51] (Table 26-2). Beyond 4 months of age, AFP half-life settles in the 5- to 7-day range. This rate of AFP elimination has been confirmed in older infants and adults following complete resection of localized, AFP-producing germ cell tumors.

While serum AFP levels are elevated in many adults and children with malignant germ cell tumors, such elevation is not specific for germ cell tumors. A variety of other conditions, including hepatoblastoma, gastrointestinal tract malignancies, ataxia telangiectasia, hereditary tyrosinemia, and other nonmalignant liver diseases such as viral hepatitis, can produce elevated AFP levels.

Human chorionic gonadotropin is a glycoprotein of approximately 45 kiloDalton molecular weight that is composed of 2 distinct polypeptide subunits designated *alpha* and *beta*. The alpha subunit of HCG is identical in

Table 26-1
Serum markers of germ cell tumors.

Histology	AFP	βHCG
Germinoma	−	−
Embryonal carcinoma	+/−	+/−
Yolk sac tumor	++++	−
Choriocarcinoma	−	++++
Teratoma		
Mature	−	−
Immature	−	−

Table 26-2
Serum AFP in normal infants at various ages.[a]

Age	Number of Samples	Mean ± S.D. (ng/ml)
Premature	11	134,734 ± 41,444
Newborn	55	48,406 ± 34,718
Newborn–2 weeks	16	33,113 ± 32,503
2 weeks–1 month	43	9,452 ± 12,610
1 month	12	2,654 ± 3,080
2 months	40	323 ± 278
3 months	5	88 ± 87
4 months	31	74 ± 56
5 months	6	46.5 ± 19
6 months	9	12.5 ± 9.8
7 months	5	9.7 ± 7.1
8 months	3	8.5 ± 5.5

[a]*Source:* Wu JT, Book L, Sudar K. Serum alpha fetoprotein (AFP) levels in normal infants. *Pediatr Res.* 1981;15:50–52.

amino acid sequence to other trophic hormones including luteinizing hormone, follicle-stimulating hormone, and thyrotropin. In contrast, the beta subunit of HCG is unique in its amino acid composition and thus lends itself to detection by specific antibody in immunoassays.[52] The metabolic half-life of the whole HCG molecule is approximately 30 hours. Serum βHCG levels are markedly elevated in choriocarcinoma or mixed germ cell cancers in which choriocarcinoma represents a significant portion of the tumor. More modest elevations of serum βHCG also

may occur in embryonal carcinoma. Furthermore, occasional patients with metastatic germinoma demonstrate modest elevations of serum βHCG. These elevations do not necessarily reflect presence of a choriocarcinomatous component but rather the presence of βHCG-secreting syncytiotrophoblastic cells within a pure germinoma. In addition, increased serum βHCG levels are also present in pregnancy, with hepatic tumors in children, and in cancers of the breast, stomach, and pancreas in adults.

The value of monitoring serum AFP and βHCG levels has been demonstrated in both adult and pediatric series.[53–55] When the serum AFP and βHCG levels decline at half-lives of 5 to 7 days and less than or equal to 3 days, respectively, in response to therapy, improved disease-free survival can be anticipated (Figure 26-3A,B). Conversely, if the serum markers decline with a prolonged half-life or increase after a tumor has shown an initial response to therapy, refractory or recurrent disease can be expected. Nevertheless, improvement in marker studies must be interpreted cautiously as a measure of complete response in germ cell cancer, given the possible presence of germ cell elements that do not produce serum markers. Additionally, it is recognized that upon initiation of chemotherapy in patients with sizeable tumor burdens, there may be a brief, transient increase in serum tumor marker levels due to rapid tumor lysis and marker release into the blood. This phenomenon can be misleading when assessing tumor response during the initial weeks of treatment in some patients.

Other serum biochemical markers of germ cell neoplasms have been evaluated with respect to their utility as initial diagnostic and prognostic tools, and as follow-up measures for persistent or recurrent tumor. Lactate dehydrogenase isoenzyme-1 (LDH-1), while not specific for germ cell tumors, has value as a prognostic measure in adults.[56] Other serum markers such as neuron-specific

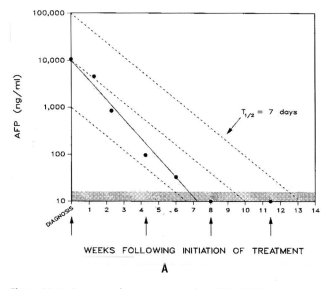
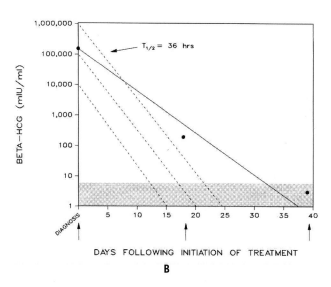

Figure 26-3 Response of serum tumor markers (AFP, βHCG) to chemotherapy. (A) 3-year-old female with a bulky unresectable stage III mediastinal yolk sac tumor that invaded the inferior vena cava and right atrium. (B) 14-year-old female with a stage IV ovarian choriocarcinoma with extensive, unresectable retroperitoneal tumor and multiple pulmonary metastases. Both patients received cisplatin vinblastine, etoposide, and bleomycin combination chemotherapy. In both cases tumor markers normalized following 2 cycles of chemotherapy. Second-look surgeries after 4 cycles of treatment showed only residual fibrotic debris. Both patients survive disease-free at greater than 2 years from diagnosis.

enolase, placental alkaline phosphatase (PLAP), pregnancy-specific β-glycoprotein, human placental lactogen, placental cystine aminopeptidase, carcinoembryonic antigen, α-1-antitrypsin, ferritin, and fibronectin have all undergone preliminary studies but have yet to gain an established place in clinical practice.[57–59] Recent analyses of pediatric data from France have suggested that the degree of serum AFP elevation at diagnosis was helpful in identifying patients with localized tumors at higher risk of eventual treatment failure.[60] In contrast, analysis of a cohort of children with stage I to IV extragonadal tumors from the recent Pediatric Oncology Group/Children's Cancer Group (POG/CCG) intergroup study did not find a correlation between serum AFP level and prognosis, albeit in a somewhat different patient population and with a different treatment approach.[61]

Pathology

Differential Diagnosis and Classification

Gonadal and extragonadal germ cell tumors may be of mature, immature, or malignant histology.[62–71] A useful system of classification for pediatric germ cell tumors is shown in Table 26-3. In the ovary and testis, germ cell tumors must be distinguished from the gonadal stromal tumors arising from the sex cords and stroma of the developing gonad. Granulosa cell and theca cell tumors of the ovary and Sertoli cell and Leydig cell tumors of the testis are examples of these latter tumors. A larger portion of malignant ovarian neoplasms are epithelial in origin after age 15 years. These non–germ cell malignancies include adenocarcinoma, cystadenocarcinoma, malignant endometrioid tumors, clear-cell tumors, Brenner tumors, and undifferentiated carcinomas. Rhabdomyosarcoma of the paratesticular tissues and ovarian or testicular infiltration by leukemia or non-

Table 26-3

Classification of pediatric germ cell tumors.

I. Germinoma (Dysgerminoma, Seminoma)
II. Teratoma
   A. Mature
   B. Immature
III. Embryonal Carcinoma
IV. Yolk Sac Tumor (Endodermal Sinus Tumor)
V. Choriocarcinoma
VI. Gonadoblastoma
VII. Malignant Germ Cell Tumor of Mixed Histology

Hodgkin lymphoma must also be considered in the differential diagnosis of germ cell tumors. Immunohistochemical stains of tumor tissue can be helpful in establishing an accurate diagnosis (Table 26-4).

Histopathology

Teratoma (Mature, Immature)

Teratomas are tumors composed of multiple tissues foreign to the anatomic site at which they occur. The ectopic location of the tumor distinguishes teratomas from hamartomas. Teratomas typically contain tissues derived from more than 1 of the 3 embryonic germ layers (ectoderm, mesoderm, and endoderm). Within teratomas, the ectodermal layer may give rise to squamous epithelium and neuroglial elements; neoplastic mesoderm may produce bone, cartilage, and/or muscle, while endoderm may form mucous glands and gastrointestinal and respiratory tissues. The component tissues of teratomas show poor organization and varying degrees of maturation. Tumors may be

Table 26-4

Immunohistochemistry of malignant germ cell tumors.[a]

Histology	Antibody					
	PLAP[b]	NSE	LCA	CK	AFP	βHCG
Germinoma	53/61[c] (87)[d]	51/61 (84)	0/61 (0)	6/61 (10)	0/61 (0)	3/61 (5)
Embryonal carcinoma	49/57 (86)	46/57 (81)	0/57 (0)	54/57 (97)	19/57 (33)	12/57 (21)
Yolk sac tumor	10/19 (53)	13/19 (68)	0/19 (0)	19/19 (100)	14/19 (74)	0/19 (0)
Choriocarcinoma	13/24 (54)	11/24 (46)	0/24 (0)	24/24 (100)	0/24 (0)	24/24 (100)

[a]*Source:* Niehans GA, Manivel C, Copland GT, Scheithauer BW, Wick MR. Immunohistochemistry of germ cell and trophoblastic neoplasms. *Cancer.* 1988;62:1113–1123.

[b]Abbreviations: PLAP, placental alkaline phosphatase; NSE, neuron-specific enolase; LCA, leukocyte common antigen; CK, cytokeratin; AFP, alpha-fetoprotein; βHCG, beta subunit of human chorionic gonadotropin.

[c]Number of specimens positive out of total examined.

[d]Percent positive.

solid or contain one or more cysts (Figures 26-4A,B). Based upon their aberrant locations, disorganized structure, asynchronous maturation, and malignant potential, teratomas are considered true neoplasms.

Teratomas can be divided into three histologic categories based upon their microscopic features: mature teratomas, immature teratomas, and teratomas with malignant elements. Mature teratomas are composed exclusively of well-differentiated tissues that are commonly arranged in an organoid manner. These tumors are most commonly located in the ovary and sacrococcygeal region. Microscopically, the simplest forms of mature teratoma are composed of nests of cartilage, mucous, squamous or transitional epithelium-lined cysts, and smooth muscle. Some tumors show more complex organization with abortive attempts to form intestine, brain, eye, pancreas, teeth, salivary glands, and other organs. The malignant potential of mature teratomas is illustrated by the reports of Altman and others, concerning the natural history of mature teratomas in the sacrococcygeal region.[11] These studies suggest that delayed recognition and surgical excision, and lack of surgical coccygectomy, permit remaining tumor cells to undergo malignant degeneration.

Immature teratomas are tumors of intermediate malignant potential. The basis on which to predict the malignant potential of these tumors remains controversial. Thurlbeck and Scully presented a system of pathologic grading of immature teratomas, subsequently modified by others.[70,71] Based upon their microscopic appearance, these tumors can be placed into one of four grades between 0 and 3. As can be seen in Table 26-5, the grading system is based in large part upon the degree and maturity of neuroepithelial tissues present within the tumor (Figure 26-5). This grading system may be more predictive of the biologic behavior of immature teratomas in adults. In adults, immature teratomas are most commonly observed in the ovary. In a retrospective review, Gershenson et al[72] found that 15 of 16 patients treated with surgery alone developed recurrent disease. In contrast, only 3 of 21 patients managed with postoperative chemotherapy developed recurrent tumor. In this series it appeared that only those patients with stage I, grade 0-I disease could be managed successfully with surgery alone. These retrospective findings in adults contrast with prospective study results from the recent POG/CCG intergroup trial, in which 69 of 73 patients (93%) with pure immature teratomas survived event-free at 3 years from diagnosis with surgery alone and irrespective of tumor grading.[73] These findings suggest that similar prospective

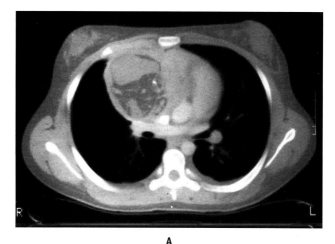

A

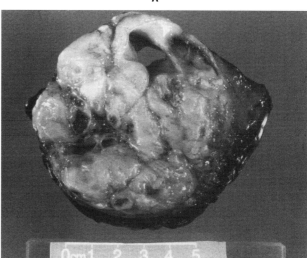

B

Figure 26-4 Benign teratoma of the anterior mediastinum in a 13-year-old girl. (A) CT scan demonstrating variable tissue density within the tumor. (B) Gross tumor anatomy showing cystic cavities.

clinical trials are warranted in adults with pure immature teratomas.

Teratomas may contain one or more malignant germ cell components (germinoma, yolk sac tumor, embryonal carcinoma, choriocarcinoma), in addition to mature or immature elements. Tumors with these features fall within the category of malignant germ cell tumors of mixed histology (Table 26-3). The behavior of these mixed tumors corresponds to the typical behavior of the most malignant

Table 26-5

Pathologic grading of immature teratomas.[62,70,71]

Grade	Histologic Characteristics
0	Differentiated somatic elements. Mature foci of neuroglia, if present.
1	Occasional foci of immature somatic elements. Absent or rare immature neuroepithelium.
2	Moderate amount of immature neuroepithelium with or without other immature somatic elements.
3	Frequent foci (consecutive microscopic fields) of immature tissue with or without neuroepithelial components.

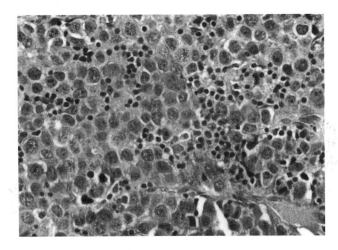

Figure 26-5 Histopathology of a sacrococcygeal grade 1 immature teratoma with neuroepithelial elements occurring in a 2-year-old female. H&E stain, 40x.

element, and aggressive treatment, including chemotherapy, is generally required to achieve a satisfactory long-term outcome.

Mature and immature teratomas typically do not stain for either AFP or βHCG, nor are serum levels of these markers typically elevated. If AFP or βHCG is identified in the tumor tissue or serum, one should be suspicious of the occult presence of yolk sac tumor or choriocarcinoma and anticipate that these tumors might behave in a malignant fashion. The large size of many teratomas, the inhomogeneous distribution of tumor elements, and the prognostic importance of finding malignant components underscore the need for extensive sampling of teratomas in order to determine their histologic pattern with confidence. Nonetheless, occasional pure mature and immature teratomas are indeed found to stain for AFP. In these cases, such staining is usually associated with identifiable areas of hepatoid or gastrointestinal epithelial differentiation.

Germinoma

Germinoma is a generic term encompassing seminoma of the testis, dysgerminoma of the ovary, and germinoma of extragonadal sites. Regardless of the primary site, the histology of these neoplasms is the same. Therefore, use of the term germinoma permits an appropriate simplification of prior schemes.

Germinoma of the testis, in contrast to yolk sac and other germ cell tumors, generally occurs in an older population. In a series of 115 patients with testicular germ cell tumors, Brawn found that pure seminoma represented only 6% of testicular tumors in patients younger than 20 years, whereas it represented 80% of tumors in patients older than 40 years.[68] According to Teilum's theory of germ cell differentiation, germinomas are viewed as a unipotential neoplastic variant (Figure 26-2). Thus, the totipotential capabilities of the germ cell tumor precursors may decline with aging and thereby favor the occurrence of germinomas in older patients.

Overall, germinomas represent approximately 12% of the malignant germ cell tumors in children and adoles-

cents and 4% to 5% of all germ cell neoplasms in this age group.[30,65–67] The ovary, anterior mediastinum, and pineal and suprasellar areas of the brain are the most common locations for germinoma in the pediatric age group. Germinomas are often found as a component of mixed germ cell neoplasms. Elevation of the serum AFP in a patient with "histologically pure" germinoma indicates the presence of occult yolk sac or embryonal elements. On occasion, mild elevations of serum βHCG may occur in association with syncytiotrophoblastic proliferation in patients with pure seminoma. However, marked elevation of the serum βHCG level should prompt a careful search for choriocarcinoma within the tumor. Germinoma is the usual malignant histology found in undescended testes and dysgenetic gonads and may be seen in association with gonadoblastoma, a benign germ cell variant.

Histologically, germinomas contain a relatively uniform cell population composed of sheets of large hexagonal or round cells resembling the primitive germ cells of the embryo. Tumor cells are eosinophilic with a clear or finely granular cytoplasm enclosed by a delicate cell membrane (Figure 26-6). Nuclei are spherical. Nuclear chromatin is granular, and one or two distinct nucleoli are typically present. Mitotic figures are rare. The tumor stroma is composed of a delicate fibrovascular network with varying amounts of lymphocytic infiltration. Histochemical stains of tumor cells may reveal glycogen in the cytoplasm. Immunohistochemical stains typically are positive for PLAP (Table 26-4). In pure testicular seminoma, stains for AFP and βHCG are characteristically negative, although on rare occasions staining for βHCG may be positive when syncytiotrophoblastic proliferation is present.

Embryonal Carcinoma

Based upon the scheme of Teilum (Figure 26-2), embryonal carcinoma is the most undifferentiated of the nonseminomatous germ cell tumors. According to this view, embryonal carcinoma cells can be considered the stem cells, which upon further differentiation give rise to teratoma, yolk sac tumor, choriocarcinoma, or mixtures thereof. Thus, the cells

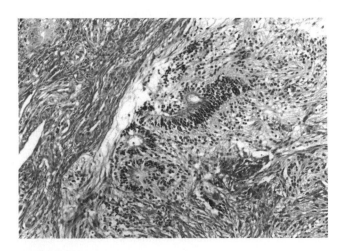

Figure 26-6 Histopathology of mediastinal germinoma occurring in an 18-year-old male. H&E stain, 100x.

of embryonal carcinoma may give rise to tumors that mimic either embryonic tissues (teratomas) or extraembryonic structures (yolk sac tumors, choriocarcinomas).

Embryonal carcinomas represent approximately 8% of cases of malignant germ cell tumors in children and adolescents.[30,65–67] This figure indicates the fraction of tumors that are "pure" embryonal carcinomas; however, elements of embryonal carcinoma are also commonly found in mixed germ cell tumors. Embryonal carcinomas can be found in the full range of primary sites where germ cell tumors typically occur, including the gonads, the CNS, and other extragonadal sites.

Grossly, embryonal carcinomas have a malignant appearance with grayish-white color, granular consistency, areas of necrosis and hemorrhage, and little evidence of encapsulation. Histologically, the tumor is composed of cells with clear cytoplasm and a primitive epithelial appearance (Figure 26-7). Embryonal carcinomas often contain papillary, glandular, or solid foci and, at times, may prove difficult to differentiate from germinomas and yolk sac tumors.

Immunohistochemical staining can often be of help in establishing the diagnosis of embryonal carcinoma. These tumors typically do not stain for either AFP or βHCG, while the converse is true for yolk sac tumors and choriocarcinomas. In instances where embryonal carcinomas do stain for these markers, staining is generally light. Moreover, serum levels of AFP and βHCG should be normal or only modestly increased to confidently arrive at a diagnosis of "pure" embryonal carcinoma. As with other germ cell neoplasms, careful histologic sampling is essential to arrive at a proper pathologic diagnosis.

Yolk Sac Tumor

Yolk sac tumor, also termed endodermal sinus tumor, is the most common malignant germ cell neoplasm of children and adolescents, representing 55% of selected case series.[30,65–67] The ovary, testicle, and sacrococcygeal region are the most common primary sites of origin. Malignant yolk sac elements also are common components of mixed germ cell cancers.

Grossly, yolk sac tumors have a gray to yellow-tan color with areas of necrosis and cyst formation. These tumors tend to be quite friable and frequently infiltrate surrounding soft tissues. Histopathologically, four microscopic patterns have been described—pseudopapillary or festoon, reticular, polyvessicular vitelline, and solid. The pseudopapillary arrangement is the classic microscopic pattern. This variant is often associated with perivascular arrays of tumor cells called Schiller-Duval bodies (Figure 26-8A,B). Many yolk sac tumors contain eosinophilic intra- and extracellular hyaline bodies, which stain positive for glycogen. Most yolk sac tumors are strongly positive for AFP by immunostaining methods and produce marked elevations of serum AFP levels (Tables 26-1 and 26-4). Pure yolk sac tumors never stain for or produce elevated serum levels of βHCG.

Choriocarcinoma

Along with yolk sac tumors, choriocarcinomas represent an extraembryonic form of differentiation of neoplastic totipotential germ cells. "Pure" choriocarcinoma is an uncommon germ cell malignancy during childhood and adolescence. The tumor may occur in two settings, gestational and nongestational, each with a distinct natural history and therapeutic responsiveness. Gestational choriocarcinoma arises from the placenta. The period of greatest risk for this tumor is between the ages of 15 and 19 years.[74] Gestational choriocarcinoma may also give rise to congenital choriocarcinoma in the neonate, typically presenting with multiple, miliary metastases to the infant's visceral organs.[75]

Nongestational choriocarcinoma may occur in gonadal, CNS, and other extragonadal primary sites. It represents fewer than 1% of germ cell cancers in children and adolescents.[30,65–67] Choriocarcinoma is a highly malignant neoplasm and, in some series, when found in pure form or as a component of a mixed germ cell neoplasm, imparted a poorer prognosis.[76,77] The adverse impact of high serum βHCG levels on survival in adults with germ cell cancer supports the prognostic importance of choriocarcinoma.[78,79] The tumor has a high propensity to disseminate

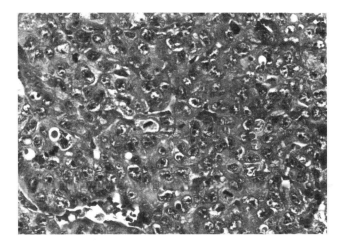

Figure 26-7 Histopathology of an embryonal carcinoma in a 12-year-old female with stage IV ovarian disease. H&E stain, 100x.

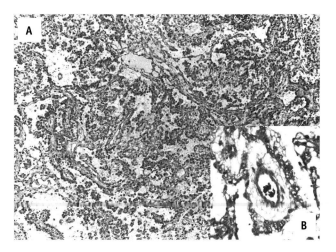

Figure 26-8 Histopathology of a stage III mediastinal yolk sac tumor in a 3-year-old female. (A) H&E stain, 16x. (B) Higher-power view demonstrating a Schiller-Duval body; H&E stain, 40x.

early in its course, leading many patients to present with pulmonary or CNS metastases.[80] Males with choriocarcinoma may develop gynecomastia, and girls may have precocious breast development, due to high serum levels of chorionic gonadotropins secreted by the tumor, which in turn prompt estrogen production.[81–83]

Grossly, choriocarcinomas are small primary tumors showing hemorrhage and necrosis. Microscopically, the tumor is composed of two principal elements—cytotrophoblasts and syncytiotrophoblasts. Cytotrophoblasts are large, round cells with clear cytoplasm while syncytiotrophoblasts are even larger, multinucleated cells with vaculated cytoplasm and dark, dense nuclei (Figure 26-9). These cell types commonly surround vascular sinusoids mimicking placental vessels. Syncytiotrophoblasts characteristically stain positive for βHCG by immunoperoxidase techniques, and patients with these tumors likewise have elevations of their serum βHCG levels. Both cytotrophoblastic and syncytiotrophoblastic elements must be identified to establish a diagnosis of choriocarcinoma. This is noteworthy because some germinomas have occasional scattered syncytiotrophoblastic cells alone and should not be considered to contain choriocarcinoma.

Malignant Germ Cell Tumors of Mixed Histology
These tumors may be composed of mature and/or immature teratoma along with one or more of the malignant germ cell tumor types or may be made up exclusively of malignant elements of varied types. Mixed malignant tumors are sometimes referred to as "teratocarcinomas" or "malignant teratomas." Because this terminology is confusing, it would be best to eliminate these diagnoses and instead identify such tumors as malignant germ cell neoplasms of mixed histology with precise indication of which germ cell elements are present. Tumors of mixed histology represent approximately 23% of the pediatric germ cell cancers.[30,65–67] Again, extensive histologic sampling and the application of immunohistochemical stains play important roles in accurately identifying the various tumor elements.

Gonadoblastoma
Gonadoblastomas are low-grade neoplasms that occur almost exclusively in dysgenetic gonads. In 75% of cases, the karyotypes of affected individuals are either 46 XY (male pseudohermaphrodite) or 46 XY/45 XO.[83] In both these states, individuals have gonadal dysgenesis. Overall, it is estimated that 25% of patients with gonadal dysgenesis will develop germ cell neoplasia, usually gonadoblastoma or germinoma.[84] Although gonadoblastomas exhibit indolent behavior clinically, approximately 20% of patients will harbor an associated germ cell cancer in the ipsilateral or contralateral gonad. Gonadoblastomas are encapsulated yellow-tan tumors that may have fine calcifications on gross inspection. Microscopically, the tumor is composed of primordial germ cells surrounded by stromal elements resembling Sertoli cells.

Clinical Features

Germ cell tumors in children may initially present with signs and symptoms directly related to the primary tumor, such as an externally visible mass, as in sacrococcygeal teratomas during infancy, or complaints related to tumor compression such as pain, constipation, urinary obstruction, or respiratory embarrassment. Gonadal masses may lead to torsion of the ovary or testicle and produce a surgical emergency due to pain and vascular compromise. In other instances, patients may present with signs and symptoms of metastatic disease. Examples of presentations related to metastases include respiratory complaints from extensive pulmonary parenchymal infiltration, bone pain or pathologic fracture, and right upper quadrant pain or obstructive jaundice due to hepatic or perihepatic tumor dissemination. Occasional patients may develop a paraneoplastic syndrome of gynecomastia or isosexual precocious puberty secondary to βHCG production by tumors containing choriocarcinoma elements.[81–83]

To ensure a proper initial evaluation and surgical approach, it is important to consider germ cell tumors in the differential diagnosis of masses in the pelvis, testicle, ovary, retroperitoneum, mediastinum, hypothalamus, and pineal gland. Consideration of germ cell tumors during the initial evaluation of masses at these sites will allow for appropriate preoperative laboratory studies, such as baseline levels of tumor markers (AFP, βHCG, LDH), and imaging studies to determine extent of local and metastatic disease. This approach will also help the surgeon determine the optimal operative procedure for initial diagnosis and treatment. For example, in a patient with an unresectable abdominal or pelvic primary tumor and extensive metastatic disease, biopsy of a superficial bone lesion would incur lower surgical morbidity, allow earlier initiation of chemotherapy, and permit less-complicated delayed resection of the primary tumor following shrinkage with chemotherapy. In contrast, suspicion of a malignant testicular tumor should prompt

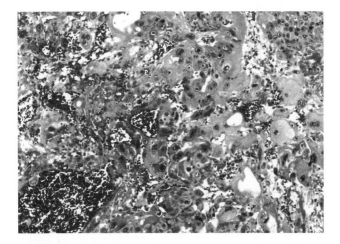

Figure 26-9 Histopathology of a stage IV ovarian choriocarcinoma in a 14-year-old female. H&E stain, 40x.

radical inguinal orchiectomy rather than a transscrotal testicular biopsy.

Germ cell malignancies may have a rapid growth rate and display highly aggressive behavior. Thus, the initial evaluation of patients suspected of having these tumors should be done expeditiously. Because germ cell tumors occur in such a wide variety of locations and display highly varied biologic behavior, the unique aspects of tumors occurring at specific primary sites will be reviewed in greater detail below.

Presentation and Initial Evaluation

Extragonadal Sites

Sacrococcyx   The sacrococcygeal region is the most common site at which germ cell tumors develop in children, representing 34% of cases in selected large pediatric series.[64–66] Among tumors at this site, 54% are mature teratomas, 14% are immature teratomas, and 30% are of frankly malignant histology. The occurrence of sacrococcygeal germ cell tumors is largely restricted to early childhood. In the large series reported by Malogolowkin et al from the Children's Hospital of Los Angeles, 82% (55 of 67) of germ cell tumors in the sacrococcygeal region occurred in children younger than 2 years.[66] Moreover, 70% (55 of 78) of all germ cell tumors in children younger than 2 years involved the sacrococcyx. In contrast, in this same series only 4% (2 of 51) of germ cell tumors in children and adolescents 10 years of age and older occurred in the sacrococcygeal region. Finally, sacrococcygeal germ cell tumors are more common in females, representing between 64% and 74% of tumors at this site in 3 reported series.[11,64,66]

Interestingly, the biologic behavior of germ cell tumors appears to be influenced by both the tumor topography within the pelvis and the age of the patient at diagnosis. In this regard, Altman et al reported a series of 398 cases of sacrococcygeal germ cell tumor.[11] The frequency of malignant histology for tumors diagnosed before the age of 2 months was approximately 10%. In contrast, in infants older than 2 months, malignant histologies were identified in 67% of males and 48% of females. In Altman's series, tumors were also categorized based upon the presence or absence of an externally visible sacrococcygeal mass and the degree of intrapelvic and intra-abdominal tumor extension (Figure 26-10). In general, tumors with a greater degree of internal extension more frequently exhibited malignant behavior. One explanation for this observation might be that internal location leads to delays in diagnosis, thereby permitting a longer interval during which malignant transformation may occur. The relative frequency, rates of metastasis, and mortality for each of the 4 sacrococcygeal tumor types described by Altman et al are indicated in Figure 26-10.

Ninety percent of sacrococcygeal germ cell tumors in infants present with an externally visible mass (types I, II, and III). Although simple observation suggests the diagnosis in most cases, it is essential for surgical planning to determine the extent of intrapelvic and intra-abdominal disease. Thus, rectal examination and diagnostic imaging

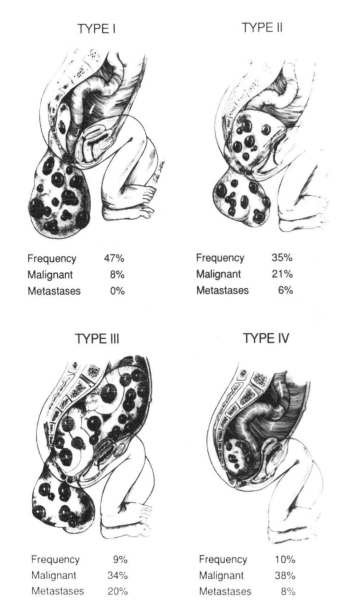

TYPE I		TYPE II	
Frequency	47%	Frequency	35%
Malignant	8%	Malignant	21%
Metastases	0%	Metastases	6%

TYPE III		TYPE IV	
Frequency	9%	Frequency	10%
Malignant	34%	Malignant	38%
Metastases	20%	Metastases	8%

Figure 26-10   Anatomic variants of sacrococcygeal germ cell tumors. Data and illustrations used with permission from Altman RP, Randolph JG, Lilly JR. Sacrococcygeal teratoma: American Academy of Pediatrics Surgical Section Surgery—1973. *J Pediatr Surg*. 1974;9:389–398.

studies such as computerized tomographic (CT) scanning, magnetic resonance imaging, and ultrasound are important components of the initial evaluation. In type IV lesions where no external tumor is evident, the need for rectal examination and diagnostic imaging is commonly suggested by a recent history of constipation, urinary obstruction, urinary urgency or frequency, lower back or pelvic pain, lower extremity weakness, or sensory disturbance due to tumor compression of normal structures.

Germ cell tumors are among the diagnoses that must be considered in infants and children presenting with masses over the caudal spine. Other diagnoses such as lipomeningocele, lipoma, meningocele, mixed neural masses, hemangioma, bone malformation, rectal duplication, abscess, malignant bone sarcoma, and epidermal cyst also must be considered. Internal presacral masses that must be differentiated from germ cell tumors in the sacrococcygeal area include chordoma, neuroblastoma, lymphoma, bone sarcoma, gastrointestinal tract carcinoma, ependymoma, glioma, Schwannoma, anterior meningocele, and pilonidal cyst.[85]

Mediastinum Approximately 4% of germ cell tumors arise in the mediastinum.[64-66] These tumors are typically located in the anterior, superior region of the mediastinum, often originating from the thymus gland. Germ cell neoplasms arising from the pericardium, heart, and lung have also been reported. Mediastinal germ cell neoplasms occur more commonly in males than females at a ratio of approximately 2 to 1.[64,66] In the series by Malogolowkin et al, mediastinal germ cell tumors were most frequently seen in children 10 years and older, representing 6 of 51 tumors in that age group.[66] Interestingly, none of the 59 tumors in children 2 to 9 years were found in the mediastinum, and only 2 of 78 tumors in children younger than 2 years occurred there. Tumors of mature, immature, and malignant histology may be encountered in the mediastinum. Other neoplasms that must be distinguished from mediastinal germ cell tumors include thymomas, lymphomas, lymphangiomas, and chest wall sarcomas. Bronchial or enteric cysts, thymic cysts, ectopic thyroid tissue, and inflammatory adenopathy due to sarcoidosis, collagen vascular disease, or infections such as histoplasmosis may also need to be considered in the differential diagnosis.

Cough, wheezing, shortness of breath, and pain are common presenting features of these tumors. In contrast, thoracic germ cell tumors also may be entirely asymptomatic and are sometimes found incidentally on chest radiographs performed for other purposes.

Chest radiographs demonstrate mediastinal germ cell tumors as radiodense, rounded masses that may contain calcifications due to the presence of bone fragments or teeth. Computed tomography scans of the chest are useful to demonstrate the relationship of the tumor to adjacent normal structures and may demonstrate the presence of cystic cavities and areas of varied attenuation indicative of the different tissues that may be present in teratomas (Figure 26-4A). Baseline laboratory evaluations should include serum tumor markers (AFP, βHCG, LDH). Again, preoperative metastatic evaluation may prove helpful in guiding the surgical approach.

Other, Non–Central Nervous System Extragonadal Sites Approximately 5% of germ cell tumors in children arise in the abdomen.[64-66] The majority of these abdominal tumors occur in the retroperitoneum; however, germ cell neoplasms have also been reported to arise from the stomach, liver, mesentery, omentum, peritoneum, and abdominal wall. Most abdominal germ cell tumors occur in children younger than 4 years. Mature teratomas, immature teratomas, and malignant germ cell tumors all occur at this site.

Approximately 6% of germ cell tumors in selected series arise in the head and neck. Most of these tumors occur in children younger than 1 year and are often con-

genital. Masses arising from the palate, thyroid gland, tongue, parotid gland, pharynx, maxilla, nose, and occipital bone have been reported.[64-66] Almost all of the lesions are mature teratomas; however, cases of malignant yolk sac tumors arising in the lip and in the buccal tissues of the cheek have been reported.

Germ cell tumors of the uterus, vagina, prostate, bladder, and umbilical cord have also been described in infants, children, and adolescents.

Central Nervous System Primary CNS germ cell tumors are typically located in the pineal or suprasellar regions.[86] They constitute from 0.5% to 3.4% of all CNS neoplasms. In combined pediatric series, CNS sites account for 7% of all the germ cell tumors encountered.[64-66] In the series reported by Packer et al from the Children's Hospital of Philadelphia, germ cell tumors accounted for 8 of 234 (3.4%) of all histologically proven primary intracranial neoplasms.[86] Evaluation and management of CNS germ cell tumors are covered elsewhere in this book.

Gonadal Sites

Ovary The ovary is the second most common site of pediatric germ cell tumors, constituting approximately 30% of cases in combined series.[64-66] Of germ cell neoplasms occurring at this site in children and adolescents, 69% are mature teratomas, 5% are immature teratomas, and 26% display malignant histology.[65,66,87] Ovarian tumors are unusual in children younger than 2 years. In the series by Malogolowkin et al, only 2 of 73 ovarian germ cell tumors occurred in children younger than 2 years, while 37 cases occurred in children between 2 and 9 years, and 34 cases were reported in children 10 years and older.[66] Mature teratomas occur in all the pediatric age groups; however, malignant ovarian germ cell neoplasms are uncommon below the age of 7 years. The relative frequency of germ cell tumors at ovarian sites accounts for much of the 2 to 1 female to male preponderance among all germ cell tumors. Among the reported malignant ovarian germ cell tumors in pediatric patients, the following histologies are encountered: germinoma (38%), yolk sac tumor (18%), embryonal carcinoma (2%), choriocarcinoma (1%), and malignant tumors of mixed histology (40%).

Abdominal pain is the most common presenting complaint of girls with ovarian tumors. Onset of pain may be acute due to torsion of a pendulous ovarian tumor upon its Fallopian tube stalk. Torsion was, in fact, the presenting feature in 16 of 66 ovarian germ cell tumors in one European series.[88] Rupture of a necrotic area of tumor may also precipitate acute complaints of pain. This sudden onset of pain may mimic appendicitis. Other children may come to medical attention due to increasing abdominal girth or appreciation of an abdominal mass by a parent. Malignant germ cell neoplasms producing high levels of βHCG may lead to isosexual precocious puberty. The constellation of increasing lower abdominal girth and elevated serum and urine βHCG can, on rare occasions, be confused with pregnancy. Under these circumstances, ultrasound should help separate the two possibilities.

Tumors of germ cell origin constitute approximately 81% of malignant ovarian tumors in children.[87,89] Of the remaining cases of malignant tumors, epithelial carcinomas represent 7%, sex cord-stromal tumors (theca-granulosa cell, Sertoli-Leydig cell, and unclassified) 5% to 6%, and other histologies 5%. Numerous benign entities, including appendicitis, ovarian cyst, tubal pregnancy, and pelvic abscess, also enter into the differential diagnosis of ovarian germ cell tumors in children and adolescents.

Testicle   Approximately 10% of all pediatric germ cell tumors occur in the testicle, roughly one-third the frequency of tumors at ovarian and sacrococcygeal primary sites.[64–66] Of testicular germ cell tumors in children, 39% are mature teratomas, 3% are immature teratomas, and 58% contain malignant elements. Among the malignant pediatric germ cell tumors, pure yolk sac cancer is the dominant histologic variant, representing 97% of cases of germ cell cancer from the Pediatric Testicular Tumor Registry of the American Urologic Association.[90] Malignant germ cell tumors of mixed histology accounted for the remaining 3% of cases in this series. Almost all testicular germ cell cancers in children occur in those younger than 3 years.[5,30] The incidence of testicular germ cell tumors then sharply rises during adolescence and young adulthood. Unlike ovarian germ cell cancers and testicular germ cell malignancy in adults, bilaterality of infantile testicular yolk sac cancer is rare, occurring in fewer than 1% of cases.[91]

Among childhood testicular tumors, the various germ cell neoplasms account for approximately 80% of cases.[90] Other testicular neoplasms occurring during childhood and adolescence include the gonadal stromal tumors (Leydig cell, Sertoli cell, granulosa cell) (8%), adnexal tumors such as rhabdomyosarcoma (6%), tumors of supporting testicular tissues such as fibrosarcoma (2%), and leukemia or lymphoma (1%). Non-neoplastic entities that must be considered in the differential diagnosis include hydrocele, hematocele, hernia, and torsion of a normal testicle. Factors predisposing to testicular germ cell cancer include cryptorchidism, Klinefelter syndrome, and gonadal dysgenesis, as previously discussed.

Most patients present with a slowly enlarging testicular mass.[92] Unless there is a complication such as torsion or tumor necrosis, pain is usually not a feature. Occasional patients may present with abdominal swelling due to nodal metastases or malignant ascites, inguinal lymphadenopathy, abdominal pain, or symptoms of distant metastases such as respiratory difficulty or bone pain. Isosexual precocious puberty may develop in boys with βHCG-secreting choriocarcinomas. Gynecomastia may also occur with βHCG-secreting tumors.[81,83]

Physical examination reveals testicular enlargement. The presence of a hydrocele should not decrease one's suspicion that a testicular tumor is present; as many as 25% of testicular tumors may be associated with hydrocele.[93] When children enter adolescence, it is important to begin teaching boys the proper method for testicular self-examination. Given the frequency of testicular can-

cer, self-examination is an important skill for young adult males to develop.

Ultrasonography can be extremely effective in detecting tumors of the testicle and adnexal structures. Use of this modality by an experienced urologist or radiologist can provide reassurance that a testicular mass is not associated with a hydrocele. If a testicular tumor is identified, ultrasonography and CT scanning of the abdomen should be obtained to identify any macroscopic nodal or hepatic metastases. Serum tumor markers, particularly AFP, but also βHCG and LDH, should be obtained preoperatively and followed carefully after surgical resection to exclude the presence of occult metastatic disease. If pathologic evaluation of the testicle produces a diagnosis of germ cell cancer, the metastatic workup should be completed by obtaining a chest radiograph and chest CT scan to rule out pulmonary disease. In the case of yolk sac tumors, serial measurements of the serum AFP need to be followed carefully to be certain the level is declining with the proper half-life of 5 to 7 days. Slow fall-off in the serum AFP level or subsequent rise of the marker suggests the presence of residual or recurrent disease.[92]

Sites of Malignant Tumor Dissemination

Approximately 20% of malignant germ cell tumors in children are associated with distant metastases at the time of diagnosis.[30] An additional 25% of patients have locally advanced and surgically unresectable primary tumors, often with direct tumor infiltration of surrounding tissues or intracavitary seeding by malignant cells. Such advanced-stage disease is common in tumors arising from the sacrococcyx, ovary, mediastinum, and retroperitoneum. In contrast, advanced disease is quite uncommon in children with germ cell cancer of the testis.[30,91]

Tumor dissemination occurs in several different ways: by local extension, by intracavitary seeding (particularly within the abdomen, pelvis, and CNS), by lymphatic pathways, and by bloodborne spread. Common sites of metastases in children with germ cell cancer include the lungs, the liver, and the regional lymph nodes. Intracavitary spread may involve the omentum, the bowel, the spleen, the diaphragm, and the pelvic organs. Bones may occasionally be involved by direct extension or hematogenous metastasis. Interestingly, despite the extensive hematogenous dissemination that can occur in patients with germ cell cancer, the marrow is rarely involved.[30,67,94]

Staging

There has been a lack of a uniformly agreed upon and applied staging system for pediatric germ cell cancer. This predicament can make comparisons of different clinical trials problematic. The varied sites at which germ cell malignancies arise in children have made development of a single, comprehensive staging system difficult. Therefore, many investigators currently favor site-specific staging systems. The staging systems used in the current Children's Oncology Group (COG) germ cell tumor trials are shown in Table 26-6. Of note, for testicular germ cell

Table 26-6

Staging of pediatric germ cell cancers.

TESTICULAR GERM CELL TUMORS

Stage	Extent of Disease
I	Limited to testis (testes), completely resected by high inguinal orchiectomy; no clinical, radiographic, or histologic evidence of disease beyond the testes. Patients with normal or unknown tumor markers at diagnosis must have a negative ipsilateral retroperitoneal node sampling to confirm stage I disease if radiographic studies demonstrate lymph nodes >2 cm.
II	Transscrotal biopsy; microscopic disease in scrotum or high in spermatic cord (<5 cm from proximal end). Failure of tumor markers to normalize or decrease with an appropriate half-life.
III	Retroperitoneal lymph node involvement, but no visceral or extra-abdominal involvement lymph nodes >4 cm by CT or >2 cm and <4 cm with biopsy proof.
IV	Distant metastases, including liver.

OVARIAN GERM CELL TUMORS

Stage	Extent of Disease
I	Limited to ovary (peritoneal evaluation negative). No clinical, radiographic, or histologic evidence of disease beyond the ovaries.
II	Microscopic residual (peritoneal evaluation negative). Failure of tumor markers to normalize or decrease with appropriate half-life.
III	Lymph node involvement (metastatic nodule); gross residual or biopsy only; contiguous visceral involvement (omentum, intestine, bladder); peritoneal evaluation positive for malignancy.
IV	Distant metastases, including liver.

EXTRAGONADAL GERM CELL TUMORS

Stage	Extent of Disease
I	Complete resection at any site; coccygectomy for sacrococcygeal site; negative tumor margins.
II	Microscopic residual; lymph nodes negative.
III	Regional lymph node involvement with metastatic disease, or gross residual or biopsy only with regional lymph nodes negative or positive.
IV	Distant metastases, including liver.

tumors, the staging system is modified to incorporate serum tumor markers as an alternative to retroperitoneal lymph node dissection. This approach was adopted because the incidence of AFP-producing yolk sac tumors is high, while the occurrence of retroperitoneal lymph node metastases is low in young children who develop these tumors.

Prognostic Features and Risk Stratification in Pediatric Germ Cell Cancer

Since the advent of effective platinum-based chemotherapy for germ cell cancer in adults, greater emphasis has been placed on the identification of features that separate patients into subgroups at high, intermediate, and low risk for treatment failure. The International Germ Cell Consensus Classification (IGCC) provides a scheme using these features to risk-stratify adult patients with malignant germ cell tumors.[95] By this system, approximately 56%, 28%, and 16% of adult patients with nonseminomatous germ cell tumors are assigned to the good, intermedi-

ate, and poor prognosis categories, respectively, based on site(s) of primary tumor and metastatic disease as well as height of serum tumor markers. Good-prognosis patients, who enjoy an approximately 90% event-free survival (EFS), are those with testicular or retroperitoneal primary tumors, no extranodal, nonpulmonary metastases, and low serum tumor markers. In contrast, poor-prognosis patients have only about 40% EFS and can be distinguished based on a mediastinal primary site, nonpulmonary visceral metastases, or extreme serum tumor marker elevation (AFP, βHCG, LDH). Pure germinomas are classified separately in the IGCC as to their prognosis. The IGCC system is now widely used to assign adult germ cell cancer patients for clinical trials of risk-adjusted therapy. After initiation of therapy, failure of serum tumor markers (AFP, βHCG) to fall with an appropriate half-life portends a worse outcome.[96]

Factors predictive of treatment outcome have also been identified for pediatric germ cell cancers. Although of great importance in designing ideal therapy for children with these tumors, one must remember that prognostic features identified in any given study are dependent on the overall effectiveness of the treatment applied. Thus, all useful studies of prognostic features must focus on patients treated in the modern era of platinum-based chemotherapy. Among clinical factors, the site of the primary tumor appears to have an impact even when differing chemotherapy regimens are utilized. Specifically, gonadal tumors have a more favorable outcome than tumors at nongonadal sites.[30,60,94] Mediastinal primary site among the extragonadal tumors further defines an adverse prognostic group.[61] The CCG report of findings by Ablin et al also identified age greater than 11 years as an adverse prognostic indicator.[97] Interestingly, in the CCG study, effective chemotherapy appeared to abrogate the effect of metastatic disease at diagnosis on outcome compared to pre–platinum era results. As noted for adults, the rate of tumor response also is an important variable in children with germ cell cancer. Thus, in the CCG series, the presence of active malignant disease by imaging studies, positive serum tumor markers, or histopathology at second-look surgery at week 18 following two 9-week cycles of chemotherapy, strongly correlated with poorer long-term survival.[97]

A review of pediatric intergroup germ cell data from the recently reported POG/CCG trials (1990–96) did not support full use of the adult IGCC system for risk stratification in younger patients.[98] Data from 210 male patients, for whom data were complete, were analyzed. Mediastinal primary site and serum AFP levels greater than 10 000 ng/ml were the only two prognostic factors that adversely impacted EFS and overall survival. None of the other factors listed in the IGCC for adults—site of metastasis, level of serum βHCG, or LDH—were of prognostic significance in this pediatric cohort. These analyses, as well as data from these trials suggesting improved EFS in extragonadal tumors with more aggressive chemotherapy, have been used to build a risk stratification scheme for the current generation of COG germ cell tumor clinical trials.

Associations of Germ Cell Neoplasms with Other Disorders

The association of congenital anomalies, cryptorchidism, XY gonadal dysgenesis (androgen insensitivity syndrome), and Klinefelter syndrome with germ cell tumors has been discussed above. Associations between germ cell malignancy and second neoplasms have also been described. Nichols and others have described the association of hematologic neoplasia with mediastinal germ cell cancers in 16 men.[99] Patients developed either acute myeloid leukemia (AML) or myelodysplastic syndrome (MDS) as their second neoplasm. The median time from the diagnosis of mediastinal germ cell cancer to the recognition of the hematologic neoplasia was 6 months, with a range of 0 to 122 months. Interestingly, this association was not found for germ cell tumors arising at other sites and thus was not felt to be a consequence of exposure to platinum-based chemotherapy. In multiple cases, the same marker chromosome, isochromosome (12p), was

identified both in the germ cell tumor and in leukemic blasts, suggesting a common cell of origin for both neoplasms. Most leukemias were of the acute megakaryocytic subtype, not a common subtype of therapy-associated AML. Therapeutic outcome was poor. Overall risk of leukemia was estimated to be 1 in 17 for adults with non-seminomatous germ cell malignancies. Similar cases have been reported in children with germ cell tumors.[100]

True therapy-associated AML and MDS have been seen in association with chemotherapy with or without radiotherapy in pediatric germ cell tumor patients.[100] Several of the pediatric patients had cytogenetic findings, such as MLL rearrangement and monosomy 7, typical of therapy-induced leukemias. Moreover, in 5 of 6 cases in this series the patients' primary tumors did not originate in the mediastinum. The Indiana group also identified a cohort of 14 males who developed low-grade spindle cell tumors between 0 and 8½ years after the initial diagnosis of a germ cell malignancy.[101] The authors speculated that some of the cases might represent outgrowth of a spindle cell component of yolk sac tumor selected out by chemotherapy.

Therapy

Surgery

Complete resection is the ultimate goal of surgery for all pediatric germ cell tumors. For mature or immature teratomas, an aggressive surgical approach is required because tumor remnants may replicate or produce enlarging cysts and cause recurrent symptoms from tumor compression. Moreover, residual tumor may undergo malignant transformation or contain in situ malignant elements capable of proliferating and producing cancerous tumor recurrence.[11,69,73,102,103] Except in instances where serum tumor markers or the presence of metastatic disease indicate malignancy, the surgeon may have few preoperative clues as to whether the germ cell tumor at hand is mature or malignant. In other instances, such as when an ovarian tumor undergoes torsion, appendicitis may be the principal consideration, and the surgeon may not anticipate tumor at all preoperatively. Due to these uncertainties, all potential germ cell tumors should be treated as malignant at the time of initial surgery.

For malignant germ cell neoplasms, if the primary tumor is resectable without major operative risk, this should be accomplished at the initial surgery. For stage I disease, high rates of cure can be achieved with surgery alone in infants with testis tumors.[90–93] The same strategy now is being explored for tumors of the ovary and sacrococcyx.[104–107]

If a malignant primary tumor is large and invades adjacent structures or surrounds major blood vessels, the risk of surgical morbidity with an extensive procedure may be excessive. Given the availability of highly effective chemotherapy, under these circumstances it is preferable to biopsy the lesion, treat with chemotherapy initially, and follow with delayed surgery to resect any residual tumor. In occasional cases where primary surgical resection has been deferred, chemotherapy alone induces a complete response with resolution of all tumor masses by imaging studies along with normalization of serum tumor markers. In such instances, there may be no need for a second surgical procedure.

In malignant tumors, where masses remain following induction chemotherapy, the residual tissue may be composed of fibrosis, mature or immature teratoma, persistent malignant elements, or combinations thereof. Therefore, when feasible, residual tumor at both primary and metastatic sites should be surgically removed. These "second look" procedures permit excision of any residual malignant elements, determine the need for further chemotherapy, and eliminate the possibility of residual mature teratoma undergoing malignant degeneration or causing local problems from regrowth of benign tumor cysts.[108–110] Special surgical considerations that apply to germ cell neoplasms at specific sites are discussed below.

Sacrococcyx

Germ cell tumors at this site require resection of the coccyx along with the tumor mass to prevent recurrence. In the series reported by Hawkins et al, all 4 patients with sacrococcygeal mature teratomas who underwent tumor resection without coccygectomy suffered local recurrence of yolk sac cancer between 1 and 31 months following their initial surgery.[69] The survey data reported by Altman et al indicate that 367 of 395 (93%) infants with sacrococcygeal germ cell neoplasms were able to undergo complete tumor resection at their initial surgeries.[11] In type I and II lesions, complete tumor removal can generally be achieved by a sacrococcygeal or caudal approach, while for type IV lesions a transabdominal surgical approach is required, and for type III lesions with large internal and external tumor components, a combined abdominosacral approach is necessary in most instances (Figure 26-10). In cases where extensive malignant tumor infiltrates pelvic bones or encases the bowel, bladder, and/or vagina, an initial biopsy can be taken and definitive surgical extirpation can be delayed until a chemotherapeutic response has been achieved. Where extensive metastases are present, biopsy of a more superficial metastatic lesion may carry a lower operative risk than pelvic surgery.

For stage I malignant sacrococcygeal germ cell tumors, surgery plus adjuvant chemotherapy has been the standard approach. However, preliminary data suggest that surgery alone may cure the majority of patients and that it may be tenable to reserve chemotherapy for the minority of children who recur.[102] This concept awaits further study in a prospective clinical trial.

Ovary

The surgeon must first attempt to determine whether an ovarian mass is neoplastic or nonneoplastic in order to select the appropriate surgical approach.[89] The likely etiology of an ovarian mass can be assessed preoperatively by ultrasound or CT scan. Serum should be obtained preoperatively for determinations of AFP, βHCG, and LDH levels. At laparotomy, the involved ovary should be carefully inspected to determine the appropriate surgical procedure to perform. Benign ovarian cysts, which constitute as many as 50% of ovarian masses, are located on the surface of the ovary, appear transparent, and contain clear fluid surrounded by a thin membrane.[111] Simple benign ovarian cysts can be managed by drainage without removal of the ovary. Cyst fluid should be sent for cytologic examination. Any solid components within the mass should raise suspicion of malignancy and mandate removal of the entire involved ovary. True neoplasms may contain one or more cysts; therefore, identification of cystic components within a mass by itself does not rule out the possibility of germ cell malignancy, immature teratoma, mature teratoma, or other ovarian neoplasms.

For staging, peritoneal washings and samples of ascitic fluid should be sent for cytologic evaluation immediately upon opening the abdominal cavity.[112] The entire peritoneal surface should be examined for the presence of implants, with particular attention paid to the surfaces of the liver and the inferior aspects of both diaphragms. Pelvic and periaortic lymph nodes should be inspected and biopsied. If malignancy is suspected, a unilateral oophorectomy or salpingo-oophorectomy should be performed. The presence of spontaneous tumor rupture or spillage following handling of the tumor at surgery should be noted. Omentectomy is generally performed for staging purposes. The pelvic organs should also be carefully inspected and biopsied where disease extension or seeding is suspected. The surgical findings and procedures should be detailed in the operative note, to aid in subsequent staging if the patient is found to have a malignant tumor. The surgeon should interpret frozen section reports with caution, because extensive sampling and immunohistologic stains may be required to demonstrate the malignant elements within germ cell tumors of mixed histology. Since malignant tumors of similar histology may be found in the contralateral ovary in as many as 10% to 15% of patients, the opposite ovary should be carefully inspected and, if suspicious, bivalved and biopsied.[112] If tumor is discovered in the contralateral ovary, bilateral oophorectomy should be considered. In cases where an ovarian tumor is encountered unexpectedly, as during laparotomy for suspected appendicitis, an appropriate abdominal incision should be made to permit thorough exploratory laparotomy and complete tumor resection.

For patients with stage I malignant ovarian germ cell tumors, surgical excision has generally been supplemented with adjuvant chemotherapy.[30,113] However, recent experience in French and German trials suggests that the majority of pediatric patients with stage I ovarian tumors can be successfully treated by surgery and observation.[104–106] In aggregate, these studies showed EFS of 67% in 39 girls managed in this manner. Of the 13 patients who recurred, 12 were salvaged with platinum-based chemotherapy, resulting in 97.4% overall survival, a result comparable to that achieved when all patients receive upfront adjuvant chemotherapy. The current COG trial, AGCT0132, is testing whether surgery and observation for stage I ovarian tumors can confirm the European experience.

Testicle

When a testicular tumor is suspected based on physical examination and ultrasound, and a general evaluation does not suggest testicular infiltration by hematologic malignancy, high inguinal orchiectomy should be performed.[92] The vast majority of children with testicular germ cell cancers have disease that is localized to the testicle.[90–93] Thus, radical inguinal orchiectomy is the preferred initial surgical procedure. This approach is generally curative in children with yolk sac tumors and avoids the unnecessary risks of residual spermatic cord disease and tumor local spill or dissemination that may accompany transscrotal testicular biopsy.

In the recommended procedure for germ cell tumors of the testis, an inguinal incision is made exposing the external oblique fascia. The fascia is opened and the spermatic cord is isolated all the way up to the level of the internal inguinal ring. The spermatic cord can be secured with a vascular clamp to prevent the theoretical risk of dislodging tumor cells into the circulation by manipulating the testicle. The testis is then delivered into the wound and, if inspection reveals the suspected tumor mass, the testicle and the extra-abdominal spermatic cord are resected in their entirety. If inguinal lymphadenopathy is present, it should be biopsied. If the tumor is adherent to scrotal soft tissues, a hemiscrotectomy should be carried out.

Whether it is necessary to carry out retroperitoneal lymph node dissection for staging purposes in young children with testicular yolk sac tumors has been a matter of controversy in the past. This issue arose from the fact that 40% to 60% of adult patients with malignant, nonseminomatous germ cell tumors of the testicle have nodal metastases at the time of presentation. Thus, in adult men, retroperitoneal lymph node dissection is often a useful diagnostic procedure for nonseminomatous germ cell tumors that guides subsequent treatment and may also have some therapeutic benefit. Unfortunately, radical retroperitoneal lymph node dissection can be associated with significant operative morbidity, including damage to renal blood vessels, loss of a kidney, lymphocele, chylous ascites, lymphedema, ejaculatory dysfunction, and azoospermia.

The same methods of retroperitoneal lymph node examination and resection used in adults may be appropriate in pubertal and postpubertal patients who develop testicular germ cell cancer, because their natural history is more akin to that of adults. However, there is now general consensus that retroperitoneal lymph node dissection for detection of occult nodal disease is not indicated in the younger child with testicular germ cell cancer. This opinion is based upon the finding that only between 4% and 14% of children subjected to this procedure were found to have lymph nodes positive for tumor.[90,91,93] Thus, if retroperitoneal lymph node dissection were used uniformly in children with disease that appeared clinically localized to the testis, approximately 90% of these patients would undergo the procedure unnecessarily. Moreover, with careful follow-up and current chemotherapy approaches, relapsing patients can be salvaged using chemotherapy in nearly all cases.[92,113,114]

Inguinal orchiectomy and observation are now the preferred management for infants and young children with clinical stage I testicular germ cell cancer. Because virtually all malignancies in this age group are yolk sac tumors, the serum AFP can be an extremely helpful surveillance tool, paying special attention to the elevated normal range in infants younger than 8 months (Table 26-2). Using this approach in 63 patients, the POG/CCG intergroup trial found a 6-year EFS of 78%. All patients who recurred were salvaged by platinum-based chemotherapy, yielding a 6-year overall survival rate of 100%.[92,113] Similar results have been reported in smaller studies.[30,114]

Mediastinum

As mentioned earlier, most germ cell tumors at this site are located in the anterior superior compartment of the mediastinum. Smaller, well-circumscribed lesions can generally be resected through a unilateral thoracotomy incision; however, complete resection of large masses may require median sternotomy. Some malignant germ cell tumors may invade or surround vital mediastinal structures, precluding initial complete surgical resection. Under these circumstances, adequate biopsies should be obtained and definitive surgery deferred until response to chemotherapy has been achieved. Whether mature or immature teratoma or malignant germ cell tumor, invaded or adherent contiguous tissue should be resected along with the primary tumor mass where possible. Recent publications by Billmire et al[108] and Schneider et al[109] analyzing the POG/CCG and the German MAKEI mediastinal germ cell cancer experiences, respectively, suggest that complete tumor resection, either initially or delayed until after induction chemotherapy, may be critical for cure. Thus, aggressive surgery for tumors at this site is advocated.

Radiotherapy

Radiotherapy can play a key role in curative treatment of CNS germ cell tumors and of germinomas (seminoma, dysgerminoma) at any site. Other nonseminomatous germ cell malignancies are radiosensitive; however, since the advent of highly active platinum-based chemotherapy, the use of radiotherapy in the primary treatment of these tumors has not been found to improve cure rates.[30]

Outside the CNS, germinomas are quite uncommon in children and adolescents. When these tumors do occur, they are generally found in the ovary or mediastinum. Germinomas are highly radiosensitive and, in many instances, curable with this modality alone. Bjorkholm et al reported a series of 60 women and girls with ovarian germinomas treated at the Karolinska Hospital in Stockholm between 1927 and 1984.[115] Nineteen of the patients were younger than 20 years at diagnosis. Treatment consisted of surgery along with radiotherapy to affected areas of the abdomen and pelvis as well as routine treatment of ipsilateral iliac and paraaortic lymph nodes up to the level of T12. By carefully designing the treatment fields, the contralateral ovary could frequently be spared significant irradiation exposure, and successful pregnancy was subsequently possible. Sixty percent of the patients had completely resected tumors (FIGO stage Ia or Ib), while 40% of patients had microscopic or gross residual tumor (FIGO stages Ic to IV). Actuarial survival was 83% at 5 years, with 70% of patients surviving without disease recurrence. Moreover, since the introduction of megavoltage equipment in 1963, all patients with ovarian germinomas achieved long-term survival regardless of stage. The authors acknowledged that the need for adjuvant radiotherapy in patients with completely resected stage I tumors merits further study.

In 1985 Lee et al reported their results of primary radiotherapy for treatment of mediastinal germinoma in six young men 25 to 30 years of age.[116] Treatment consisted of 30 Gy to 35 Gy to the entire mediastinum and both supraclavicular fossae. One patient also received chemotherapy as part of his primary treatment. Outcome was favorable, with 5 of 6 patients alive without recurrence after a minimum of 3 years of follow-up. One patient in the group recurred with a solitary bone metastasis one year following diagnosis and again became free of disease following local radiotherapy.

Weinblatt and Ortega reported a series of 9 girls with ovarian germinomas.[117] Four of the patients had stage Ia or Ib disease and were treated with surgery alone; they remained free of disease from 6 to 11 years following diagnosis, suggesting that adjuvant radiotherapy may not be required for completely resected ovarian germinomas in the pediatric age group. The remaining patients had stage III disease and were treated with varying combinations of surgery, irradiation, and chemotherapy. Three of these 5 survived long-term without disease, one apparently cured with a combination of VAC (vincristine, actinomycin D, and cyclophosphamide) chemotherapy and second-look surgery. The authors suggest that primary chemotherapy might be used to limit the need for extensive surgery and irradiation. Platinum-based chemotherapy is now recognized to be highly active in germinomas. Thus, this strategy merits continued investigation as an alternative to radiotherapy, particularly in children and adolescents, because it offers the possibility of sparing pelvic and reproductive organs, preserving bone growth, and diminishing the risk of second malignant neoplasms.

The radiosensitivity and curability of testicular germinomas in adults has also been well demonstrated in several case series.[118] The usual treatment approach involves removal of the involved testicle via a high inguinal approach and 25 Gy to 30 Gy irradiation to the ipsilateral iliac lymph nodes and periaortic chain. Additional treatment is sometimes given to the left renal hilum for left testicular tumors and to the inguinal region for cases of spermatic cord involvement or tumors involving an undescended testicle. Prophylactic radiotherapy to the mediastinum does not appear to be of benefit.[119] Recently, in a randomized trial, single-dose adjuvant carboplatin treatment has been shown to produce equivalent relapse-free survival rates compared with adjuvant nodal irradiation (20 Gy to 30 Gy) in stage I adult testicular germinoma.[120] Finally, surgical resection followed by surveillance also is viewed as an appropriate option for patients with stage I testicular germinoma, given the limited 15% to 20%

recurrence risk and the high rate of salvage by chemotherapy and/or irradiation.[121]

No clear-cut role for radiotherapy in primary treatment of germ cell cancers apart from germinomas and CNS tumors has been established. However, it is clear that nonseminomatous germ cell malignancies can be sensitive to irradiation at doses of 45 Gy to 55 Gy.[109] Therefore, radiotherapy may be useful in palliative or salvage therapy for patients with resistant or recurrent disease.

Chemotherapy

Mature Teratomas

Mature teratomas are curable by surgical resection alone. Chemotherapy has no known role in the treatment of this neoplasm. As reviewed above, complete surgical resection, including coccygectomy for sacrococcygeal tumors, successfully prevents local recurrence of mature teratoma elements as well as local or metastatic recurrence of germ cell elements that have undergone malignant transformation.

Immature Teratomas

Until recently, the place of chemotherapy in the treatment of immature teratomas (histologic grade I-III) has been poorly defined. This uncertainty arose from retrospective observations in adult patients that localized immature teratomas, particularly those classified as histologic grade III, often recurred as malignant germ cell tumors of either embryonal or yolk sac histology.[71,72,122] For the pediatric age group, this matter has been clarified greatly by the recent POG/CCG intergroup trial.[73] In that study, patients with pure immature teratomas, irrespective of histologic grade, were treated with complete resection and observation without adjuvant chemotherapy. Seventy-three patients with immature teratomas of ovaries, testes, and extragonadal sites were enrolled. Three-year EFS was 93%, indicating excellent success with surgery alone regardless of histologic grade. Five of the 73 patients experienced malignant recurrence of their tumors. Of these 5 patients, 4 were salvaged with subsequent platinum-based chemotherapy. Additional observations included somewhat higher rates of recurrence for tumors arising at extragonadal primary sites, for tumors that, on central review, showed microscopic foci of yolk sac tumor, as well as for patients with serum AFP elevation at diagnosis.

Adult patients with pure immature teratomas await future prospective clinical trials to better define optimal treatment. Strict surgical guidelines and central pathology review are needed to best carry out such trials.

Peritoneal seeding with neuroepithelial elements from immature teratomas, so called gliomatosis peritonei, is not by itself an indication for chemotherapy, since these nodules typically undergo spontaneous regression and rarely, if ever, become malignant.[123]

Malignant Germ Cell Tumors

Lessons from Adult Germ Cell Cancer Therapy

Adult testicular cancer is the most common and extensively studied form of germ cell malignancy. Consequently, testicular cancer in adults has served as a model for the development of treatment for germ cell cancers at other sites and in the pediatric age group. Although modeling these therapies after those developed for adult testicular cancer has certainly been helpful, treatments used for adult testicular cancer have not uniformly produced comparable benefits in tumors arising in the ovary or at extragonadal sites. Moreover, it may be hazardous to completely generalize treatment results in adults to those anticipated in children, due to the differing frequencies of tumor sites and histologies in the two age groups as well as possible differences in underlying tumor biology.

The first suggestion that systemic chemotherapy might have value in treatment of germ cell malignancies arose from studies of gestational choriocarcinoma.[124] Studies of germ cell tumors at other sites followed and showed major (complete and partial, CR + PR) responses in the range of 30% to 60% with a variety of single agents, including methotrexate, chlorambucil, bleomycin, vinblastine, vincristine, cyclophosphamide, and actinomycin D.[125-128]

In the late 1950s combination chemotherapy for treatment of testicular germ cell malignancies was introduced. In 1960, Li and colleagues reported a 20% complete response rate to a combination of methotrexate, chlorambucil, and actinomycin D in men with disseminated testicular cancer.[129] Subsequent studies confirmed a 50% to 70% overall response rate (CR + PR) to these agents in men with testicular cancer.[130,131] In addition, marked activity of this drug combination was noted in four patients with malignant ovarian germ cell tumors, including two patients aged 8 and 13 years.[132] The VAC regimen was also found to produce occasional CRs in men with disseminated testicular cancer.[133] These exciting results suggested that further refinements in combination chemotherapy might produce cures of these tumors.

In the 1970s, studies by Samuels and colleagues using vinblastine and bleomycin in combination were particularly encouraging.[134,135] They based their use of this combination on data documenting antitumor activity of each agent alone and on the theory that they might demonstrate synergy. They reasoned that mitotic arrest induced by vinblastine and cycle-specific killing of tumor cells blocked at the G2-M interphase by bleomycin would enhance cytoreduction. Using this combination, CRs were achieved in 33% to 65% of patients. The highest response rates were seen when bleomycin was administered as a continuous infusion.[134]

The discovery of cisplatin and its introduction into clinical trials was the next major advance in the development of effective chemotherapy for germ cell malignancies. As a single agent in nonseminomatous testicular germ cell tumors, cisplatin induced CRs in approximately 50% of patients, with an additional 20% achieving objective PRs.[136] In addition, at the doses used, cisplatin was only mildly myelosuppressive. This feature made cisplatin an ideal drug to employ in combination with vinblastine and bleomycin, which caused more marrow suppression.

At the Memorial Sloan-Kettering Cancer Center, the VAB regimen (vinblastine, actinomycin D, and bleomycin) was used in combination with cisplatin (VAB-2). The VAB-1 regimen, which used vinblastine, actinomycin D, and bleomycin without cisplatin, produced only 14% CRs and 22% PRs.[137] The VAB-2 regimen with cisplatin added to the 3-drug backbone achieved greater success, yielding 60% CRs and 36% PRs in 25 men with metastatic nonseminomatous testicular cancer.[138]

In 1977 Einhorn and Donohue reported the successful treatment of men with disseminated testicular germ cell cancer using the PVB regimen (cisplatin, vinblastine, bleomycin; Table 26-7).[139] In 47 evaluable patients, PVB chemotherapy alone produced 74% CRs and 26% PRs.

Table 26-7
Platinum-based chemotherapy regimens.

Regimen	Drug	Dosage	Interval & Duration
PVB[139]	Cisplatin	20 mg/m²/day IV, days 1-5	Q3 Wks × 3-4 cycles
	Vinblastine	0.2 mg/kg/day IV, days 1 & 2	Q3 Wks × 3-4 cycles
	Bleomycin	30 units IV, begin day 2, then …	Weekly × 12 doses
"Adult" BEP[142,157]	Cisplatin	20 mg/m²/day IV, days 1-5	Q3 Wks × 3-4 cycles
	Etoposide	100 mg/m²/day IV, days 1-5	Q3 Wks × 3-4 cycles
	Bleomycin	30 units IV, begin day 2, then …	Weekly × 9-12 doses
COG PEB[113]	Cisplatin	20 mg/m²/day IV, days 1-5	Q3 Wks × 4-6 cycles
	Etoposide	100 mg/m²/day IV, days 1-5	Q3 Wks × 4-6 cycles
	Bleomycin	15 units/m² IV, day 1	Q3 Wks × 4-6 cycles
UKCCG JEB[114]	Carboplatin	600 mg/m² IV, day 2	Q3-4 Wks × 4-6 cycles
	Etoposide	120 mg/m²/day IV, days 1-3	Q3-4 Wks × 4-6 cycles
	Bleomycin	15 units/m² IV, day 3	Q3-4 Wks × 4-6 cycles

An additional 5 patients with PRs following chemotherapy were rendered free of disease following second-look surgery, yielding an 85% CR rate overall with combined modality induction therapy. Long-term follow-up of patients with testicular cancer treated using various PVB regimens at the University of Indiana showed durability of these CRs, with 64% of patients alive and free of disease at a median of 8.5 years from diagnosis.[140]

Careful analysis of patients with disseminated testicular cancer treated on the PVB studies also demonstrated the benefit of postinduction or so-called second-look surgery for residual primary and metastatic tumor masses. In 24 patients with radiographic evidence of residual tumor, 7 had pathologic evidence of residual malignancy. In those patients found to have persistent malignant elements at postinduction surgery, 2 additional cycles of PVB were given. This approach of delayed resection of residual tumor coupled with postoperative chemotherapy for those with residual malignant tumor increased disease-free survival to approximately 80%.[141]

The introduction of etoposide and recognition of its single-agent activity in germ cell cancers plus its probable synergy with cisplatin spawned development of the BEP regimen (bleomycin, etoposide, cisplatin; Table 26-7). Trials of BEP chemotherapy in adult males with testicular cancer have shown high response rates for both nonseminomatous germ cell tumors and germinomas. Williams et al reported the outcomes of a randomized clinical trial of 261 men with disseminated germ cell tumors in which cisplatin and bleomycin were combined with either vinblastine or etoposide.[142] Among 244 patients evaluated for treatment response, 74% of those receiving PVB and 83% of those receiving BEP achieved disease-free status. Among patients with high tumor volume, BEP proved significantly more effective in producing CRs, 77% versus 61%. In addition, the etoposide-containing regimen produced less toxicity, particularly with respect to neuromuscular side effects such as paresthesias, abdominal cramps, and myalgias. Further evaluation of the BEP regimen found that 3 cycles of therapy produced equivalent disease-free survival with less toxicity than 4 cycles in men with favorable-prognosis disseminated nonseminomatous germ cell cancer of the testis.[143]

In spite of the dramatic successes of VAB/cisplatin, PVB, and BEP chemotherapy in disseminated testicular cancer in adults, comparable results have been more difficult to achieve for certain other groups of adult patients with germ cell cancer, including those with ovarian primaries, extragonadal primaries, and high-risk features such as extremely high tumor markers and/or metastatic disease to sites other than lung or lymph nodes. For those patients, these chemotherapy regimens have produced long-term disease-free survival in only 30% to 75% of cases.[95,144,145]

Other platinum-based combination chemotherapy regimens have demonstrated similar antitumor activity to that of VAB/cisplatin, PVB, and BEP in adults with germ cell cancer. Preliminary data concerning carboplatin, etoposide, and bleomycin (JEB) in combination suggested similar antitumor activity to BEP, with fewer renal and neurologic toxicities. However, randomized trials of JEB versus BEP showed inferior CR rates and EFS with the carboplatin regimen. Attempts to substitute carboplatin for cisplatin, eliminate bleomycin, or to reduce treatment to fewer than 3 cycles have yielded inferior outcomes in randomized trials.[146-149]

Surgery and irradiation, as discussed above, have historically been the mainstays of treatment for germinomas. More recently, platinum-based regimens have also demonstrated a high degree of activity in this group of germ cell tumors.[144,150-153] Thus, chemotherapy may be appropriately used to manage metastatic germinoma as well as for cytoreduction of locoregional disease for which extensive surgery and wide field radiotherapy would otherwise be required. Recently, in a randomized trial of adjuvant therapy in men with clinical stage I testicular germinoma, a single cycle of carboplatin chemotherapy was equivalent to standard ipsilateral pelvic/abdominal nodal irradiation with respect to relapse-free survival.[120] In addition, the patients treated with adjuvant chemotherapy developed fewer second primary tumors in the contralateral testis than those in the irradiated group, suggesting an overall advantage to adjuvant carboplatin. Surgery followed by surveillance is also an option in stage I testicular germinoma, producing approximately 85% EFS. Chemotherapy proved effective in retrieving patients who relapsed following surgery alone.[121]

Considerable effort is now being directed toward developing therapies to improve outcome for patients at high risk of initial treatment failure and those with refractory or recurrent disease. These efforts generally have followed two differing tacks, either dose escalation of previously employed agents to overcome tumor resistance or the addition of new agents with single-agent activity against germ cell cancer to a conventional dose backbone.

It has long been recognized that germ cell tumors exhibit a steep dose-response curve to platinum compounds. In 1984 the Southwest Oncology Group reported a randomized trial of two PVB regimens in adults with advanced testicular cancer.[154] In that study, cisplatin administered at a dose of 120 mg/m^2 compared with 75 mg/m^2 per cycle produced higher complete response and survival rates. In addition, Ozols and colleagues found that escalation of cisplatin to 200 mg/m^2 (40 mg/m^2/day for 5 days) administered in 3% saline to prevent nephrotoxicity was capable of producing responses in patients with disease refractory to conventional-dose cisplatin.[155] The principle of cisplatin dose escalation was then tested in a randomized trial of initial therapy for high-risk patients.[156] In that study, patients received either conventional-dose PVB or a combination of high-dose cisplatin (200 mg/m^2) along with vinblastine, bleomycin, and etoposide. Treatment with the high-dose regimen produced an increased complete remission rate (88% vs 67%) and resulted in a lower rate of relapse (17% vs 41%). Disease-free survival was also significantly improved in patients randomized to receive the high-dose platinum regimen (68% vs 33%). The Southeastern and Southwest Oncology Groups subsequently collaborated in a randomized study of two BEP regimens using either standard-dose cisplatin (20 mg/m²/day for 5 days) or high-dose cisplatin (40 mg/m²/day for 5 days) for patients with poor-prognosis germ cell cancers.[157] In contrast to the study by Ozols,[156] these groups found that doubling the dose of cisplatin in the BEP regimen increased toxicity without improving disease-free survival. Neither study clearly addressed whether the incorporation of both high-dose cisplatin and vinblastine in the BEP regimen could improve the results of standard BEP therapy.

In general, the integration of additional established agents into frontline chemotherapy regimens for poor-prognosis advanced adult germ cell cancer has failed to produce improvements in EFS compared with the now standard BEP regimen. This has generally been the case whether a single additional agent has been added to the BEP backbone or alternating, non–cross-resistant chemotherapy combinations have been used as a means to integrate a wider variety of agents into the chemotherapy regimen.[158–161] One strategy currently being investigated in England tests the concept that treatment failure may be due to rapid tumor recovery with tumor regrowth occurring when chemotherapy pulses are delivered every 21 to 28 days. In this Phase II trial, using a more "metronomic" schedule, multiagent chemotherapy with cisplatin, carboplatin, bleomycin, and vincristine is delivered weekly for the initial 6 weeks of treatment, followed by 3 cycles of BEP. Preliminary results suggest improved outcomes in poor-risk patients, such as those with mediastinal primary tumors, with a 3-year overall survival of 77%.[162] A randomized trial comparing this strategy with conventional BEP has recently been opened.

High-dose, potentially myeloablative chemotherapy with autologous hematopoietic stem cell transplant (AHSCT) has also been investigated during frontline therapy to consolidate initial responses to conventional-dose chemotherapy. This approach is based on success using high-dose chemotherapy in patients with recurrent malignant germ cell tumors. In particular, escalation of etoposide and carboplatin to maximal tolerated doses can overcome resistance to these agents in some patients in spite of resistance to conventional doses of etoposide and cisplatin. Cross-resistance of tumors to both cisplatin and carboplatin appears common; thus it is likely that dose escalation is the key factor in generating responses in cisplatin-resistant patients. Phase II trials have suggested potential benefit from such an approach. Despite the apparent promise of high-dose chemotherapy with AHSCT in frontline therapy, a recent Phase III randomized trial testing this strategy versus conventional BEP alone failed to show benefit in the transplant arm.[163]

Among newer agents, ifosfamide, paclitaxel, gemcitabine, and oxaliplatin have been evaluated in Phase II studies and have activity as single agents in germ cell cancers refractory to frontline PVB or PEB treatment.[164–167] The newer agents have subsequently been combined in multiagent salvage regimens. These efforts as well as potential biologically targeted treatment strategies have been recently reviewed.[168] Of the newer chemotherapy combinations, oxaliplatin/gemcitabine, oxaliplatin/irinotecan, and oxali-

platin/paclitaxel have shown some promise in limited Phase II trials.

For adults with relapsed or refractory nonseminomatous germ cell cancer, depending on prognostic features, 25% to 75% can be salvaged using alternative conventional dose chemotherapy regimens combined with local control measures and, in some cases, consolidation by high-dose chemotherapy with AHSCT.[160,161,168] Recent analyses suggest probable value to double tandem transplants as opposed to a single consolidative transplant for salvage treatment.[169]

Chemotherapy for Children and Adolescents with Germ Cell Cancer

Early Studies

The chemotherapy approaches developed for children and adolescents with malignant germ cell tumors have drawn heavily upon data from therapeutic trials in adults. Based upon the natural history of germ cell cancer in the pediatric age group, multiagent chemotherapy can be recommended in the initial treatment plan for all patients with malignant germ cell tumors with the exception of (1) young children with stage I testicular yolk sac tumors, who can generally be cured by inguinal orchiectomy alone, and (2) older children and adolescents with localized germinomas who can be rendered tumor-free with nonmutilating surgery, possibly followed by adjuvant limited-field radiotherapy or platinum-based chemotherapy. Elimination of chemotherapy in initial management of malignant stage I ovarian and sacrococcygeal tumors is being actively investigated in prospective pediatric trials.

Single-agent chemotherapy trials involving children with germ cell cancer have convincingly demonstrated the activity of cisplatin and high-dose cyclophosphamide, even in patients with refractory or recurrent disease.[67,170,171] More limited data exist for carboplatin and ifosfamide but nonetheless suggest activity of these two agents as well.[172,173] Trials of methotrexate, anthracyclines (doxorubicin, daunorubicin), and even etoposide suggest little activity of these agents in refractory disease.[67,174] As with all Phase II studies, results must be interpreted with caution because data in refractory disease may not be generalizable to untreated tumors, the optimal dosage and scheduling of the agent may not have been utilized, and potential synergy with other active agents cannot be evaluated.

In 1983 Sawada et al reported significant activity of both PVB and VAC against human yolk sac tumors heterotransplanted into nude mice.[175] Preclinical studies such as these concerning the predominant histologic type of germ cell cancer in pediatric patients, along with the encouraging results of treatment trials in men with testicular cancer, laid the groundwork for studies of VAC and platinum-based chemotherapy in children and adolescents.

In 1984 Flamant and colleagues reported a series of 35 pediatric patients with malignant germ cell tumors with either advanced locoregional disease (stage III) or distant metastases (stage IV).[176] Treatment consisted of partial resection of the primary tumor, retroperitoneal lymphadenectomy in selected patients with testicular disease, then chemotherapy with alternating cycles of actinomycin D, cyclophosphamide with or without methotrexate, and vincristine, doxorubicin, bleomycin, plus cisplatin at 100 mg/m^2 as a single dose. Patients received 6 cycles of chemotherapy. Three patients in the group received local radiotherapy to residual tumor. The results from this series were compared with a group of historical controls matched for stage, histology, and site but treated with different chemotherapy consisting of methotrexate, actinomycin D, cyclophosphamide with or without doxorubicin, plus local radiotherapy. The patients in the more contemporary series achieved decidedly better disease-free survival compared with the historical controls, 60% versus 10% at 25 months following diagnosis. Clinically significant nephrotoxicity, ototoxicity, and pulmonary toxicity occurred in approximately 10% of patients on the new regimen. There was one death from bleomycin-related pulmonary fibrosis. This report suggested that the inclusion of vincristine, cisplatin, and bleomycin in the chemotherapy regimen was instrumental in producing improved disease-free survival. It also indicated that vincristine might have efficacy comparable to that of vinblastine and that radiotherapy was not a major contributor to long-term disease-free survival.

In 1986 Pinkerton et al followed the above report with a paper confirming the efficacy of platinum-based regimens in pediatric germ cell cancers.[177] This series included 13 patients with stage II to IV disease, 7 with gonadal and 6 with extragonadal primary sites. Surgical resection was done where possible. Chemotherapy was nonuniform but emphasized the use of cisplatin in all cases. The chemotherapy regimens used were PVB alone ($n = 3$), PEB ($n = 7$), PVB plus PEB ($n = 1$), VAC plus PVB ($n = 1$), and VAC plus PEB ($n = 1$). Patients received from 4 to 7 cycles of chemotherapy. Cisplatin was administered as a single dose of 100 mg/m^2/cycle and bleomycin as a single dose of 15 mg/m^2/cycle. Complete responses were achieved in 12 of the 13 patients with a PR occurring in the remaining patient. Eleven of 13 patients (85%) remained free of disease with follow-up of 11 to 42 months. Second-look surgical procedures were carried out in 5 patients due to the presence of a persistent mass on follow-up imaging studies. Four of the surgical procedures showed no evidence of disease, while in one patient a small nidus of residual malignant cells was removed, producing a surgical complete remission. Although this series lacked a control group and utilized nonuniform chemotherapy regimens, it again demonstrated the substantial activity of platinum-based chemotherapy regimens in pediatric germ cell cancer. Nephrotoxicity, hypomagnesemia, ototoxicity, and subclinical pulmonary toxicity were observed; however, the results suggested that severe pulmonary toxicity might be avoided without loss of therapeutic effect by decreasing the frequency of bleomycin administration.

Mann et al reported the results of sequential studies of pediatric germ cell cancers conducted by the United Kingdom Children's Cancer Study Group (UKCCSG) between 1979 and 1987.[30] A total of 122 patients formed the basis of this report, including 64 patients who received chemotherapy as a part of their initial treatment, 14 who received chemotherapy for recurrences after initial surgery with or without local radiotherapy, and 44 patients with localized disease managed with surgery alone. Unlike most prior studies, patients with germinomas ($n = 5$) and immature teratomas ($n = 11$) were considered eligible. By protocol guidelines, patients with stage I testicular primary tumors were managed with inguinal orchiectomy alone, while all other patients received chemotherapy as an adjunct to initial surgery. Four different drug regimens were tested: low-dose VAC, high-dose VAC with or without doxorubicin, PVB, and BEP. Favorable results were found with the high-dose VAC, PVB, and BEP chemotherapy regimens, producing 5-year disease-free survival rates of 87%, 67%, and 84%, respectively. In contrast, the low-dose VAC regimen produced only 8% survival at 5 years. Survival also varied dependent on the site of the primary tumor. Testicular tumors, most of which were stage I and managed with surgery alone, were rarely fatal, permitting 96% 5-year survival. Patients with ovarian primaries also fared well, with 78% survival at 5 years. In contrast, patients with sacrococcygeal or thoracic primary sites had 5-year survival rates of only 48% and 40%, respectively. Radiotherapy delivered to sites of localized residual disease produced transient tumor responses but did not appear to have an impact on overall survival. The toxicity profiles observed in these series were most notable for fatal bleomycin pulmonary fibrosis in 3 patients treated with the PVB regimen, which included 15 weekly doses of bleomycin. Interestingly, no life-threatening pulmonary toxicity was observed in patients receiving the BEP regimen in which bleomycin was administered only once every 3 weeks, generally for a total of only 5 doses. In summary, this report suggested that high-dose VAC and BEP produced high rates of survival with acceptable toxicity. The high-dose VAC regimen had the disadvantages of more frequent although salvagable tumor recurrences, a longer total duration of therapy, and the potential late effects of sterility and second malignant neoplasms related to cyclophosphamide exposure. In contrast, BEP produced more durable CRs, required a shorter duration of treatment, and offered the potential for less sterility and second malignancy. Still, BEP had the undesirable side effects of nephrotoxicity and ototoxicity.

In 1991 Ablin and colleagues from the Children's Cancer Study Group in the United States reported the results of CCG-861, a chemotherapy trial in 93 children with selected germ cell cancers.[97] Patients with tumors of nonseminomatous histology at ovarian ($n = 30$) and extragonadal ($n = 63$) sites were treated. Those with testicular primaries, germinomas, or immature teratomas were excluded. Patients with both localized and advanced stages of disease were eligible. Treatment consisted of initial surgery followed by two 9-week cycles of PVB with actinomycin D, cyclophosphamide, and doxorubicin. During the induction chemotherapy phase, cisplatin was administered at 60 mg/m^2/dose once per cycle. At week 18 of the induction period, a second-look surgical procedure was carried out to identify and resect residual disease. Patients with residual disease that could not be completely resected at second surgery received radiotherapy to the sites of known or suspected tumor. Maintenance chemotherapy, consisting of 1 course of cisplatinum, 4 of bleomycin, 6 of doxorubicin, and 9 more courses of vinblastine, cyclophosphamide, and actinomycin D, was given to all patients for total treatment duration of 2 years.

The CCG-861 trial reported 49% 4-year EFS, which broke down to 63% EFS in patients with ovarian primaries and 42% EFS for those with nongonadal tumors. At a glance, the outcome reported in this study appears inferior to that found in some of the pediatric series described above. However, this outcome may be partially explained by the heavy skewing of the patient population toward those with nongonadal primary tumors, a factor now known to independently worsen prognosis. In contrast, the lower EFS might also have been due in part to an underemphasis of cisplatin in the chemotherapy program, which used low individual doses and infrequent administration.

Contemporary Risk-Adjusted Therapy

The pediatric studies reviewed above helped to establish the relative risk of treatment failure based on tumor histology, primary site, and stage of disease. These observations have led to subsequent and ongoing investigations in which treatment intensity has been adjusted for these risk factors. Thus, patients with pure mature teratomas and pure immature teratomas regardless of site, and young children with stage I malignant testicular tumors, are allocated to the lowest risk stratum, because they have greater than 80% EFS with complete surgical resection alone. In contrast, patients with metastatic extragonadal nonseminomatous malignant tumors fall into the highest risk category, since EFS of around 70% is achievable only with aggressive combined surgical and chemotherapy approaches. Table 26-8 shows the risk stratification used in current COG clinical trials for nonseminomatous germ cell tumors.

Using the type of risk stratification described above, in the 1990s the CCG and the POG collaborated in a set of intergroup studies. POG 9048/CCG 8891 tested therapies for immature teratomas and localized malignant tumors, and POG 9049/CCG 8882 studied treatment of patients with higher-risk disease based on their primary site and stage at presentation. In POG 9048/CCG 8891, patients with pure immature teratomas and stage I malignant testicular tumors were treated with surgery alone.[73,92] This approach provided excellent outcomes while minimizing chemotherapy exposure, as reviewed above. Patients with stage II malignant testis tumors, those with stage I chemotherapy-naïve testis tumors after recurrence as stage II tumors, and girls with stage I and II malignant ovarian tumors received 4 cycles of "standard-dose" PEB chemotherapy (Table 26-7). The 74 patients treated in this fashion had a 6-year EFS of 95%. By primary site and stage for the chemotherapy treated groups, EFS was 100% for stage II testicular disease ($n = =17$), 95% for stage I ovarian tumors ($n = =41$), and 88% for stage II ovarian tumors ($n = 16$). Two patients of the 74 ultimately died from recurrent disease, and 1 died of secondary AML. Another PEB-treated patient with an ovarian tumor developed secondary AML and survived free of recurrence following an AHSCT. No toxic deaths occurred, and ototoxicity, renal dysfunction, and pulmonary toxicity were minimal using this "standard-dose" PEB regimen.[113]

The POG 9049/CCG 8882 study for higher risk and advanced stage nonseminomatous pediatric germ cell cancers was a randomized trial that investigated the efficacy of cisplatin dose escalation.[94] In this study, the therapeutic potential of "high-dose" cisplatin (40 mg/m^2/day for 5 days; high-dose PEB) was compared with "standard-dose" cisplatin (20 mg/m^2/day for 5 days; standard-dose PEB). Both the high-dose and standard-dose PEB regimens used the same dosing of etoposide and bleomycin. Patients younger than or equal to 21 years with stage III or IV gonadal (ovary, $n = 74$; testis, $n = 60$) tumors or stage I to IV extragonadal tumors ($n = 165$) were eligible. Following initial surgery, patients received 4 cycles of their assigned chemotherapy regimen. If residual tumor was found on post-induction imaging, second-look surgery was undertaken. Those with malignant elements in the resected residual received an additional 2 cycles of their initial chemotherapy. Analysis of disease outcome showed significant improvement in 6-year EFS in 149 patients receiving high-dose PEB versus the 150 who received standard-dose PEB (90% vs 80%; $p = 0.03$). Overall survival (high-dose PEB 92%; standard-dose PEB 86%) showed a similar trend as EFS for the 2 chemotherapy regimens but did not reach statistical significance ($p = 0.18$). Tumor-related deaths were more common after standard-dose PEB (14 vs 2), while toxic deaths, all from infection, were more frequent with high-dose PEB (6 vs 1). Severe ototoxicity was markedly higher in patients treated on the high-dose PEB arm of the study.

Several pediatric trials in Europe have examined whether carboplatin could effectively replace cisplatin in germ cell cancer treatment and thereby reduce the rates of ototoxicity and nephrotoxicity. This question remains unresolved to date. The UKCCSG investigated a carboplatin, etoposide, bleomycin regimen ("JEB"; Table 26-7) and found EFS of 85% in stage III tumors and 78% in stage IV disease, similar outcomes to those seen in the above POG/CCG intergroup trials.[114] Of note, the UK trials employed a carboplatin dose of 600 mg/m^2. This dose is significantly higher than that used in French pediatric germ cell cancer trials, which found that carboplatin

Table 26-8

Children's Oncology Group risk strata for pediatric germ cell cancers.

Risk Stratum	Primary Site	Stage
Low	Testis	I
	Ovary	I
Intermediate	Testis	II, III, IV
	Ovary	II, III, IV
	Extragonadal	I, II
High	Extragonadal	III, IV

at 400 mg/m² per cycle resulted in inferior outcomes compared with their standard-dose cisplatin regimens.[178]

Results of the above POG/CCG intergroup trials and various European reports have led to a number of new questions currently under examination in ongoing COG studies. Among these questions is whether the strategy of surgery alone with surveillance and chemotherapy rescue for relapsing patients can safely be expanded to girls with stage I malignant ovarian tumors. In addition, for patients with higher-stage gonadal primary tumors and early-stage extragonadal tumors, the new studies are investigating whether a reduction in standard-dose PEB therapy can retain high EFS. Finally, for those with advanced-stage extragonadal tumors where more aggressive chemotherapy appeared to improve EFS but resulted in concerning numbers of toxic deaths and frequent severe ototoxicity, intensification of standard-dose PEB by addition of cyclophosphamide is being explored.

Although great strides have been made in understanding the biology, natural history, and treatment of pediatric germ cell tumors, numerous questions worthy of further investigation remain. Among the challenges for future investigators is the design of pediatric studies of sufficient size, possibly international in scope, to better define prognostic risk groups and further optimize treatment approaches. Finally, studies of pediatric germ cell tumor biology have the potential to identify new therapeutic targets and move the paradigm away from exclusive use of cytotoxic chemotherapy toward less-toxic, molecularly targeted treatments.

Late Effects of Therapy

Contemporary management of infants, children, and adolescents with germ cell tumors results in 70% to 100% survival with very low risk of tumor recurrence beyond 2 years from initial diagnosis. Given this high rate of recurrence-free survival, it has become increasingly important to recognize the nature and frequency of late complications of present treatment strategies in young patients. This information can help to better guide and test new risk-adjusted approaches.

Surprisingly, only a limited amount is known about late effects seen following treatment of pediatric germ cell tumors. One exception to this is the clear dose-related frequency of severe and long-lasting hearing loss noted in the POG 9049/CCG 8882 trial comparing high-dose PEB with standard-dose PEB therapy.[94] Severe ototoxicity was recognized in 14% of patients treated with high-dose PEB as compared with none in those receiving standard-dose PEB. Reporting of ototoxicity by research staff at participating centers was believed to underestimate the true frequency of hearing loss due to problems in interpreting audiograms and grading abnormalities. To better determine ototoxicity risk, Li et al reviewed a subset of audiograms from this study employing more stringent grading criteria.[179] This analysis found that 67% of patients who received high-dose PEB versus 10.5% of patients on the standard-dose PEB arm suffered hearing loss of sufficient severity to

require hearing aids. Additional findings in this report, which analyzed a total of 153 children aged 6 months to 18 years with germ cell tumors as well as other cancer diagnoses, included added risk for cisplatin-associated hearing loss in patients younger than 5 years and after larger individual and cumulative doses. In contrast, severe renal or pulmonary toxicity was infrequent (less than 8%) on POG 9049/CCG 8882, irrespective of treatment arm. The lower frequency of acute and chronic lung toxicity in pediatric versus adult germ cell cancer treatment trials likely is related to the more limited use of bleomycin in most pediatric regimens.

The emphasis on platinum agents, etoposide, and sometimes alkylators such as cyclophosphamide and ifosfamide makes secondary leukemia a potential concern in children treated for germ cell malignancies. Indeed, true therapy-associated AML has been reported in association with chemotherapy with or without radiotherapy in pediatric germ cell tumor patients.[100] In most of these patients, cytogenetic findings typical of therapy-induced leukemias (*MLL* rearrangement, monosomy 7) were identified. In this European cohort, the Kaplan-Meier estimates of the cumulative incidence of therapy-associated AML after 10 years was 1% for patients treated with chemotherapy and 4.2% for patients treated with combined chemotherapy and irradiation. Of note, no secondary solid tumors were identified on follow-up of the study patients.

Long-term follow-up of adults treated for germ cell malignancies has identified a variety of other potential long-term sequelae of treatment. These include fertility issues; renal dysfunction; hypertension; vascular occlusive events involving the coronary, cerebral, or peripheral vascular circulation; abnormal lipid profiles; and peripheral neuropathies.[180,181] While these and other toxicities have not yet been carefully evaluated in children following germ cell tumor therapy, the growing number of long-term survivors merit monitoring. Reductions in therapy for low- and intermediate-risk patient groups offer the potential for reduced long-term complications and are among the goals of current clinical trials in pediatric germ cell cancer treatment. In contrast, for the high-risk patient group, maintaining therapeutic intensity while modulating ototoxicity by judicious selection of chemotherapeutic agents and their doses is being tested. Finally, growing understanding of germ cell tumor biology offers the hope of changing treatment paradigms away from traditional cytotoxic agents and toward more biologically targeted therapies, thereby offering the possibility of fewer long-term treatment-associated toxicities.

References

1. Stewart AM. Cancers in juveniles. *Proc Roy Soc Med.* 1969; 62;16–20.
2. Young JL, Miller RW. Incidence of malignant tumors in U.S. children. *J Pediatr.* 1975;86:254–258.
3. Young JL, Gloeckler Ries L, Silverberg E, Horm JW, Miller RW. Cancer incidence, survival and mortality for children younger than age 15 years. *Cancer.* 1986;58:598–602.
4. Brown PD, Hertz H, Olsen JH, Yssing M, Scheibel E, Jensen OM. Incidence of childhood cancer in Denmark 1943–1984. *Int J Epidemiol.* 1989;18:546–555.
5. Surveillance, Epidemiology End Results (SEER); http://seer.cancer.gov.
6. Berry CL, Keeling J, Hilton L. Teratoma in infancy and childhood: a review of 91 cases. *J Pathol.* 1969;98:241–252.

7. Spitz MR, Sider JG, Pollack ES, Lynch HK, Newell GR. Incidence and descriptive features of testicular cancer among United States whites, blacks and hispanics, 1973–1982. *Cancer.* 1986;58:1785–1790.

8. Crom DB, Wilimas JA, Green AA, Pratt CB, Jenkins JJ, Behm FG. Malignancy in the neonate. *Med Pediatr Oncol.* 1989;17:101–104.

9. Campbell AN, Chan HSL, O'Brien A, Smith CR, Becker LE. Malignant tumours in the neonate. *Arch Dis Child.* 1987;62:19–23.

10. Neira L, Ninane J, Verbruggen B, Vermylen C, Cornu G. Malignancies in children less than one year old. Relative incidence and survival [abstract]. *Med Pediatr Oncol.* 1989;17:323.

11. Altman RP, Randolph JG, Lilly JR. Sacrococcygeal teratoma: American Academy of Pediatrics Surgical Section Surgery—1973. *J Pediatr Surg.* 1974;9:389–398.

12. Batata MA, Chu FC, Hilaris BS, Whitmore WF, Golbey RB. Testicular cancer in cryptorchids. *Cancer.* 1982;49:1023–1030.

13. Pettersson A, Richiardi L, Nordenskjold A, Kaijser M, Akre O. Age at surgery for undescended testis and risk of testicular cancer. *N Engl J Med.* 2007;356:1835–1841.

14. Brown LM, Pottern LM, Hoover RN, Devesa SS, Aselton P, Flannery JT. Testicular cancer in the United States: trends and incidence and mortality. *Int J Epidemiol.* 1986;15:164–170.

15. Brown LM, Pottern LM, Hoover RN. Prenatal and perinatal risk factors for testicular cancer. *Cancer Res.* 1986;46:4812–4816.

16. Chen Z, Robison L, Giller R, et al. Risk of childhood germ cell tumors in association with parental smoking and drinking. *Cancer.* 2005;103(5):1064–1071.

17. Chen Z, Robison L, Giller R, et al. Environmental exposure to residential pesticides, chemicals, dusts, fumes, and metals, and risk of childhood germ cell tumors. *Int J Hyg Environ Health.* 2006;209(1):31–40.

18. Shankar S, Davies S, Giller R, et al. In utero exposure to female hormones and germ cell tumors in children. *Cancer.* 2006;106(5):1169–1177.

19. Langman J. *Medical Embryology.* 4th ed. Baltimore: Williams & Wilkins; 1981.

20. Bussey KJ, Lawce HJ, Himoe E, et al. SNRPN methylation patterns in germ cell tumors as a reflection of primordial germ cell development. *Genes Chromosomes Cancer.* 2001;32(4):342–352.

21. Schneider DT, Schuster AE, Fritsch MK, et al. Multipoint imprinting analysis indicates a common precursor cell for gonadal and nongonadal pediatric germ cell tumors. *Cancer Res.* 2001;61(19):7268–7276.

22. Looijenga LH, Stoop H, de Leeuw HP, et al. POU5F1 (OCT3/4) identifies cells with pluripotent potential in human germ cell tumors. *Cancer Res.* 2003;63(9):2244–2250.

23. de Felici M. Regulation of primordial germ cell development in the mouse. *Int J Dev Biol.* 2000;44:575–580.

24. Loehrer PJ, Sledge GW, Einhorn LH. Heterogeneity among germ cell tumors of the testis. *Semin Oncol.* 1985;12:304–316.

25. Pierce GB, Dixon JL, Verny EL. Teratocarcinogenic and tissue-forming potentials of the cell types comprising neoplastic embryoid bodies. *Lab Invest.* 1960;9:583–602.

26. Kleinsmith LJ, Pierce GB. Multipotentiality of single embryonal carcinoma cells. *Cancer Res.* 1964;24:1544–1548.

27. Teilum G. *Special Tumors of Ovary and Testis and Related Extragonadal Lesions: Comparative Pathology and Histological Identification.* 2nd ed. Philadelphia: Lippincott; 1976.

28. Brinster RL. The effect of cells transferred into mouse blastocysts on subsequent development. *J Exp Med.* 1974;140:1049–1056.

29. Fuller DB, Plenk HP. Malignant testicular germ cell tumors in a father and two sons. *Cancer.* 1986;58:955–958.

30. Mann JR, Pearson D, Barrett A, Faafat F, Barnes JM, Wallendszus KR. Results of the United Kingdom Children's Cancer Study Group's malignant germ cell tumor studies. *Cancer.* 1989;63:1657–1667.

31. Nichols CR, Heerema NA, Palmer C, Loehrer PJ, Williams SD, Einhorn LH. Klinefelter's syndrome associated with mediastinal germ cell neoplasms. *J Clin Oncol.* 1987;5:1290–1294.

32. Arens A, Marcus D, Engelberg S, Findler G, Goodman RM, Passwell JH. Cerebral germinomas and Klinefelter syndrome. *Cancer.* 1988;61:1228–1231.

33. Trentini GP, Palmieri B. An unusual case of gonadic germinal tumor in a brother and sister. *Cancer.* 1974;33:250–255.

34. Liber AF. Ovarian cancer in mother and 5 daughters. *Arch Pathol.* 1950;42:280–290.

35. Jackson SM. Ovarian dysgerminoma in three generations. *J Med Genet.* 1967;4:112–113.

36. Tollerud DJ, Blattner WA, Fraser MC, et al. Familial testicular cancer and urogenital developmental anomalies. *Cancer.* 1985;55:1849–1854.

37. Cockburn AG, Vugrin D, Batata M, Hadju S, Whitmore WF. Second primary germ cell tumors in patients with seminoma of the testis. *J Urol.* 1983;130:357–359.

38. Dieckmann KP, Boeckmann W, Brosig W, Jonas D, Bauer HW. Bilateral testicular germ cell tumors; report of nine cases and review of the literature. *Cancer.* 1986;57:1254–1258.

39. Patel SR, Richardson RL, Kvols L. Synchronous and metachronous bilateral testicular tumors: Mayo Clinic Experience. *Cancer.* 1990;65:1–4.

40. Sakashita S, Koyanagi T, Tsuji I, Arikado K, Matsuno T. Congenital anomalies in children with testicular germ cell tumor. *J Urol.* 1980;124:889–891.

41. Houldsworth J, Korkola JE, Bosl GJ, Chaganti RS. Biology and genetics of adult male germ cell tumors. *J Clin Oncol.* 2006;24(35):5512–5518.

42. Teter J, Boczkowski K. Occurrence of tumors in dysgenetic gonads. *Cancer.* 1967;20:1301–1310.

43. Kingsbury AC, Frost F, Cookson WOCM. Dysgerminoma, gonadoblastoma, and testicular germ cell neoplasia in phenotypically female and male siblings with 46 XY genotype. *Cancer.* 1987;59:288–291.

44. Oosterhuis JW, Castedo SMMJ, deJone B, et al. Karyotyping and DNA flow cytometry of an orchidoblastoma. *Cancer Genet Cytogenet.* 1988;36:7–11.

45. Bussey KJ, Lawce HJ, Olson SB, et al. Chromosome abnormalities of eighty-one pediatric germ cell tumors: sex-, age-, site-, and histopatholgy-related differences—a Children's Cancer Group study. *Genes Chromosomes Cancer.* 1999;25:134–146.

46. Schneider DT, Schuster AE, Fritsch MK, et al. Genetic analysis of childhood germ cell tumors with comparative genomic hybridization. *Klin Padiatr.* 2001;213(4):204–211.

47. Hart AH, Hartley L, Parker K, et al. The pluripotency homeobox gene *NANOG* is expressed in human germ cell tumors. *Cancer.* 2005;104(10):2092–2098.

48. Kato N, Tamura G, Fukase M, Shibuya H, Motoyama T. Hypermethylation of the *RUNX3* gene promoter in testicular yolk sac tumor of infants. *Am J Pathol.* 2003;163(2):387–391.

49. Youngren KK, Coveney D, Peng X, et al. The Ter mutation in the dead end gene causes germ cell loss and testicular germ cell tumours. *Nature.* 2005;435(19):360–364.

50. Gitlin D, Pserricelli A. Synthesis of serum albumin, prealbumin, alpha-fetoprotein, alpha-1-antitrypsin and transferrin by the human yolk sac. *Nature.* 1970;228:995–997.

51. Wu JT, Book L, Sudar K. Serum alpha fetoprotein (AFP) levels in normal infants. *Pediatr Res.* 1981;15:50–52.

52. Vaitukatis JL, Braunstein GD, Ross GT. A radioimmunoassay which specifically measures human chorionic gonadotropin in the presence of human luteinizing hormone. *Am J Obstet Gynecol.* 1972;113:751–758.

53. Walhof CM, Van Sonderen LV, Voute PA, Delemarre JFM. Half-life of alpha-fetoprotein in patients with a teratoma, endodermal sinus tumor, or hepatoblastoma. *Pediatr Hematol Oncol.* 1988;5:217–227.

54. Fizazi K, Culine S, Kramar A, et al. Early predicted time to normalization of tumor markers predicts outcome in poor-prognosis nonseminomatous germ cell tumors. *J Clin Oncol.* 2004;22(19):3868–3876.

55. Geller NL, Gosl GJ, Chan EYW. Prognostic factors for relapse after complete response in patients with metastatic germ cell tumors. *Cancer.* 1989;63:440–445.

56. Kinumaki H, Takeuchi H, Nakamura K, Ohmi K, Bessho F, Kobayashi N. Serum lactate dehydrogenase isoenzyme-1 in children with yolk sac tumor. *Cancer.* 1985;56:178–181.

57. Kuzmits R, Schernthaner G, Krisch K. Serum neuron-specific enolase: a marker for response to therapy in seminoma. *Cancer.* 1987;60:1017–1021.

58. Niehans GA, Manivel C, Copland GT, Scheithauer BW, Wick MR. Immunohistochemistry of germ cell and trophoblastic neoplasms. *Cancer.* 1988;62:1113–1123.

59. Javadpour N. Tumor markers in testicular cancer: an update. *Prog Clin Biol Res.* 1985;203:141–154.

60. Baranzelli MC, Kramar A, Bouffet E, et al. Prognostic factors in children with localized malignant nonseminomatous germ cell tumors. *J Clin Oncol.* 1999;17:1212–1218.

61. Marina N, London WB, Frazier AL, et al. Prognostic factors in children with extragonadal malignant germ cell tumors: a Pediatric Intergroup study. *J Clin Oncol.* 2006;24:2544–2548.

62. Dehner LP. Gonadal and extragonadal germ cell neoplasms: teratomas in childhood. In: Finegold M, ed. *Pathology of Neoplasia in Children and Adolescents.* Philadelphia: Saunders; 1986.

63. Sesterhenn IA, Davis CJ. Pathology of germ cell tumors of the testis. *Cancer Control.* 2004;11(6):374–387.

64. Bale PM, Painter DM, Cohen D. Teratomas in childhood. *Pathology.* 1975;7:209–218.

65. Marsden HB, Birch JM, Swindell R. Germ cell tumours of childhood: a review of 137 cases. *J Clin Pathol.* 1981;34:879–883.

66. Malogolowkin MH, Mahour GH, Krailo M, Ortega JA. Germ cell tumors in infancy and childhood: a 45 year experience. *Pediatr Pathol.* 1990;10:231–241.

67. Brodeur GM, Howarth CB, Pratt CB, Caces J, Hustu HO. Malignant germ cell tumors in 57 children and adolescents. *Cancer.* 1981;48:1890–1898.

68. Brawn PN. The origin of germ cell tumors of the testis. *Cancer.* 1983;51:1610–1614.

69. Hawkins EP, Finegold MJ, Hawkins HK, Krischer JP, Starling KA, Weinberg A. Nongerminomatous malignant germ cell tumors in children: a review of 89 cases from the Pediatric Oncology Group, 1971–1984. *Cancer.* 1986;58:2579–2584.

70. Thurlbeck WW, Scully RE. Solid teratoma of the ovary: a clinicopathologic analysis of nine cases. *Cancer.* 1960;13:804–811.

71. Norris HI, Zirkin HI, Benson WL. Immature (malignant) teratoma of the ovary: a clinical and pathologic study of 58 cases. *Cancer.* 1976;37:2359–2372.

72. Gershenson DM, del Junco G, Silva EG, Copeland LJ, Wharton JT, Rutledge FN. Immature teratoma of the ovary. *Obstet Gynecol.* 1986;68:624–629.

73. Marina NM, Cushing B, Giller R, et al. Complete surgical excision is effective treatment for children with immature teratomas with or without malignant elements: a Pediatric Oncology Group/Children's Cancer Group Intergroup study. *J Clin Oncol.* 1999;17:2137–2143.

74. Hayashi K, Bracken MB, Freeman DH, Hellenbrand K. Hydatidiform mole in the United States (1970–1977): a statistical and theoretical analysis. *Am J Epidemiol.* 1982;115:67–77.

75. Witzleben CL, Bruninga G. Infantile choriocarcinoma: a characteristic syndrome. *J Pediatr.* 1968;73:374–378.

76. Birch R, Williams S, Cone A, et al. Prognostic factors for favorable outcome in disseminated germ cell tumors. *J Clin Oncol.* 1986;4:400–407.

77. Stoter G, Sylvester R, Sleijfer DT, et al. Multivariate analysis of prognostic factors in patients with disseminated nonseminomatous testicular cancer: results from a European organization for research on treatment of cancer multiinstitutional phase III study. *Cancer Res.* 1987;47:2714–2718.

78. Droz JP, Kramar A, Ghosn M, et al. Prognostic factors in advanced nonseminomatous testicular cancer: a multivariate logistic regression analysis. *Cancer.* 1988;62:564–568.

79. International Germ Cell Cancer Collaborative Group. International Germ Cell Consensus Classification: a prognostic factor-based staging system for metastatic germ cell cancers. *J Clin Oncol.* 1997;15:594–603.

80. Rustin GJS, Newlands ES, Bagshawe KD, Begent RHJ, Crawford SM. Successful management of metastatic and primary germ cell tumors in the brain. *Cancer.* 1986;57:2108–2113.

81. Stepanas AV, Samaan NA, Schultz PN, Holoyne PY. Endocrine studies in testicular tumor patients with and without gynecomastia: a report of 45 cases. *Cancer.* 1978;41:369–376.

82. Hansen JR, Cook JS, Afifi AK, Janovick J, Conn PM, Tsalikian E. Peripheral isosexual precocious puberty in a girl with a primary intracranial chorionic gonadotropin-secreting tumor [abstract #492]. *Pediatr Res.* 1989;25:85A.

83. Welch WR, Robboy SJ. Abnormal sexual development: a classification with emphasis on pathology and neoplastic conditions. In: Kogan SJ, Hafex ESF, eds. *Pediatric Andrology.* Boston: Martinus Hijhoff; 1981:71–85.

84. Manuel M, Katayama KP, Jones HW. The age of occurrence of gonadal tumors in intersex patients with a Y chromosome. *Am J Obstet Gynecol.* 1976;124:293–300.

85. Lemire RJ, Graham CB, Beckwith JB. Skin-covered sacrococcygeal masses in infants and children. *J Pediatr.* 1971;79:948–954.

86. Packer RJ, Sutton LN, Rosenstock JG, et al. Pineal region tumors of childhood. *Pediatrics.* 1984;74:97–102.

87. Adkins JC, Jaffe R. Tumors of the female genital tract in children. In: Broecker BH, Klein FA, eds. *Pediatric Tumors of the Genitourinary Tract.* New York: Alan R. Liss; 1988:207–228.

88. de Backer A, Madern GC, Oosterhuis JW, Hakvoort-Cammel F, Hazebroek F. Ovarian germ cell tumors in children: a clinical study of 66 patients. *Pediatr Blood Cancer.* 2006;46(4):459–464.

89. Ehren IM, Mahour GH, Isaacs H. Benign and malignant ovarian tumors in children and adolescents: a review of 63 cases. *Am J Surg.* 1984;147:339–344.

90. Kaplan GW, Cromie WC, Kelalis PP, Silber I, Tank ES. Prepubertal yolk sac testicular tumors: report of the testicular tumor registry. *J Urol.* 1988;140:1109–1112.

91. Green DM. The diagnosis and treatment of yolk sac tumors in infants and children. *Cancer Treat Rev.* 1983;10:265–288.

92. Schlatter M, Rescorla F, Giller R, et al. Excellent outcome in patients with stage I germ cell tumors of the testes: a study of the Children's Cancer Group/Pediatric Oncology Group. *J Pediatr Surg.* 2003;38(3):319–324.

93. Exelby PR. Testicular cancer in children. *Cancer.* 1980;45:1803–1809.

94. Cushing B, Giller R, et al. Randomized comparison of combination chemotherapy with etoposide, bleomycin, and either high-dose or standard dose cisplatin in children and adolescents with high risk malignant germ cell tumors: a Pediatric Intergroup study (POG9049 and CCG8882). *J Clin Oncol.* 2004;22(13):2691–2700.

95. International Germ Cell Cancer Collaborative Group. International Germ Cell Consensus Classification: a prognostic factor-based staging system for metastatic germ cell cancers. *J Clin Oncol.* 1997;15:594–603.

96. Mazumdar M, Bajorin DF, Bacik J, Higgins G, Motzer RJ, Bosl GJ. Predicting outcome to chemotherapy in patients with germ cell tumors: the value of the rate of decline of human chorionic gonadotrophin and alpha-fetoprotein during therapy. *J Clin Oncol.* 2001;19:2534–2541.

97. Ablin AR, Krailo MD, Ramsay NKC, et al. Results of treatment of malignant germ cell tumors in 93 children: a report from the Children's Center Study Group. *J Clin Oncol.* 1991;9:1782–1792.

98. Frazier AL, Olson T, Giller R, et al. Outcome of childhood malignant nonseminomatous germ cell tumors (MGCT) according to adult International Germ Cell Classification System (IGCCC) [abstract #3226]. *Proc Am Soc Clin Oncol.* 2003.

99. Nichols CR, Roth BJ, Heerema N, Griep J, Tricot G. Hematologic neoplasia associated with primary mediastinal germ-cell tumors. *N Engl J Med.* 1990; 322:1425–1429.

100. Schneider DT, Hilgenfeld E, Schwabe D, et al. Acute myelogenous leukemia after treatment for malignant germ cell tumors in children. *J Clin Oncol.* 1999;17(10):3326–3333.

101. Ulbright RM, Michael H, Loehrer PJ, Donohue JP. Spindle cell tumors resected from male patients with germ cell tumors. *Cancer.* 1990;65:148–156.

102. Huddard SN, Mann JR, Robinson K, et al. Sacrococcygeal teratoma: the UK Children's Cancer Study Group's experience. I. Neonatal. *Pediatr Surg Int.* 2003;19(1–2):47–51.

103. Rescorla FJ, Sawin RS, Coran AG, Dillon PW, Azizkhan RG. Long-term outcome for infants and children with sacrococcygeal teratoma: a report from the Children's Cancer Group. *J Pediatr Surg.* 1998;33:171–176.

104. Gobel U, Schneider DT, Calaminus G, Haas RJ, Schmidt P, Harms D. Germcell tumors in childhood and adolescence. GPOH MAKEI and the MAHO study groups. *Ann Oncol.* 2000;11:263–271.

105. Baranzelli MC, Bouffett E, Quintana E, Portas M, Thyss A, Patte C. Nonseminomatous ovarian germ cell tumours in children. *Eur J Cancer.* 2000;36:376–383.

106. Baranzelli MC, Flamant F, De Lumley L, Le Gall E, Lejars O. Treatment of non-metastatic, non-seminomatous malignant germ-cell tumours in childhood: experience of the "Societ Francaise d'Oncologie Pediatrique" MGCT 1985–1989 study. *Med Pediatr Oncol.* 1993;21:395–401.

107. Dark GG, Bower M, Newlands ES, Paradinas F, Rustin GJ. Surveillance policy for stage I ovarian germ cell tumors. *J Clin Oncol.* 1997;15(2):620–624.

108. Billmire D, Vinocur C, Rescorla F, et al. Malignant mediastinal germ cell tumors: an Intergroup study. *J Pediatr Surg.* 2001;36:18–24.

109. Schneider DT, Calaminus G, Reinhard H, et al. Primary mediastinal germ cell tumors in children and adolescents: results of the German cooperative group protocols MAKEI 83/86, 89, 93. *J Clin Oncol.* 2000;18:832–839.

110. Rescorla F, Billmire D, Stolar C, et al. The effect of cisplatin dose and surgical resection in children with malignant germ cell tumors at the sacrococcygeal region: a pediatric Intergroup trial (POG 9049/CCG 8882). *J Pediatr Surg.* 2001;36:12–17.

111. Towne BH, Mahour GH, Woolley MM, Isaacs H. Ovarian cysts and tumors in infancy and childhood. *J Pediatr Surg.* 1975;10:311–320.

112. Billmire D, Vinocur C, Rescorla F, et al; Children's Oncology Group (COG). Outcome and staging evaluation in malignant germ cell tumors of the ovary in children and adolescents: an Intergroup study. *J Pediatr Surg.* 2004;39:424–429.

113. Rogers PC, Olson TA, Cullen JW, et al. Pediatric Oncology Group 9048; Children's Cancer Group 8891. Treatment of children and adolescents with stage II testicular and stages I and II ovarian malignant germ cell tumors: a pediatric Intergroup study—Pediatric Oncology Group 9048 and Children's Cancer Group 8891. *J Clin Oncol.* 2004;22:3563–3569.

114. Mann JR, Raafat F, Robinson K, et al. The United Kingdom Children's Cancer Study Group's second germ cell tumor study: carboplatin, etoposide and bleomycin are effective treatment for children with malignant extracranial germ cell tumors, with acceptable toxicity. *J Clin Oncol.* 2000;18:3809–3818.

115. Bjorkholm E, Lundell M, Gyftodimos A, Silfversward C. Dysgerminoma: the Radiuhemmet series. *Cancer.* 1990;65:38–44.

116. Lee YM, Jackson SM. Primary seminoma of the mediastinum: Cancer Control Agency of British Columbia experience. *Cancer.* 1985;55:450–452.

117. Weinblatt ME, Ortega JA. Treatment of children with dysgerminoma of the ovary. *Cancer.* 1982;49:2608–2611.

118. Jones RH, Vasey PA. Part I: testicular cancer—management of early disease. *Lancet Oncol.* 2003;4:730–737.

119. Sommer K, Brockmann WP, Hubener KH. Treatment results and acute and late toxicity of radiation therapy for testicular seminoma. *Cancer.* 1990;66:259–263.

120. Oliver RT, Mason MD, Mead GM, et al. Radiotherapy versus single-dose carboplatin in adjuvant treatment of stage I seminoma: a randomized trial. *Lancet.* 2005;366:293–300.

121. Martin J, Chung P, Warde P. Treatment options, prognostic factors and selection of treatment in stage I seminoma. *Onkologie.* 2006;29:554–555.

122. Malogolowkin MH, Ortega JA, Krailo M, et al. Immature teratomas: identification of patients at risk for malignant recurrence. *J Natl Cancer Inst.* 1989; 81:870–874.

123. Favara BE, Franciosi RA. Ovarian teratoma and neuroglial implants on the peritoneum. *Cancer.* 1973;31:678–682.

124. Li MC, Hertz R, Spencer DB. Effect of methotrexate on choriocarcinoma and chorioadenoma. *Proc Soc Exp Biol Med.* 1956;93:361–366.

125. Kennedy BJ. Mithramycin therapy in advanced testicular neoplasms. *Cancer.* 1970;26:755–766.

126. Merrin CE, Murphy GP. Metastatic testicular carcinoma: single agent chemotherapy (actinomycin D) in treatment. *NY State J Med.* 1974;74(4):654–657.

127. Blum RH, Carter S, Agre K. A clinical review of bleomycin: a new antineoplastic agent. *Cancer.* 1973;31:903–914.

128. Samuels ML, Howe CD. Vinblastine in the management of testicular cancer. *Cancer.* 1970;25:1009–1017.

129. Li MC, Whitmore WF, Golbey R, Grabstald H. Effects of combined drug therapy on metastatic cancer of the testis. *JAMA.* 1960;174:1291–1299.

130. Ansfield FJ, Korbitz BC, Davis HL, Ramirez G. Triple drug therapy in testicular tumors. *Cancer.* 1969;24:442–446.

131. MacKenzie AR. Chemotherapy of metastatic testis cancer: results in 154 patients. *Cancer.* 1966;19:1369–1376.

132. Wider JA, Marshall JR, Bardin CW, Lipsett MB, Ross GT. Sustained remissions after chemotherapy for primary ovarian cancers containing choriocarcinoma. *N Engl J Med.* 1969;280:1439–1442.

133. Jacobs EM. Combination chemotherapy of metastatic testicular germinal cell tumors and soft part sarcomas. *Cancer.* 1970;25:324–332.

134. Samuels ML, Johnson EE, Holoye PY. Continuous intravenous bleomycin therapy with vinblastine in stage III testicular neoplasia. *Cancer Chemother Rep.* 1975;59(3):563–570.

135. Samuels ML, Lanzotti VJ, Holoye PY, Boyle LE, Smith TL, Johnson DE. Combination chemotherapy in germinal cell tumors. *Cancer Treat Rev.* 1976;3:185–204.
136. Torti FM, Lum BL. Management of disseminated testicular cancer. In: Javadpour N, ed. *Principles and Management of Testicular Cancer.* New York: Thieme; 1986:258–294.
137. Cvitkovic E, Cheng E, Whitmore WF, Golbey RB. Germ cell tumor chemotherapy update [abstract #C-232]. *Proc Am Soc Clin Oncol.* 1977;18:324.
138. Cheng E, Cvitkovic E, Wittes RE, Golbey RB. Germ cell tumors II: VAB II in metastatic testicular cancer. *Cancer.* 1978;42:2162–2168.
139. Einhorn LH, Donohue J. Cis-diamminedichloroplatinum, vinblastine, and bleomycin combination chemotherapy in disseminated testicular cancer. *Ann Intern Med.* 1977;87:293–298.
140. Roth BJ, Greist A, Kubilis PS, Williams SD, Einhorn LH. Cisplatin-based combination chemotherapy for disseminated germ cell tumors: long-term follow-up. *J Clin Oncol.* 1988;6:1239–1247.
141. Mandelbaum I, Yaw PB, Einhorn LH, Williams SD, Rowland RG, Donahue JP. The importance of one-stage median sternotomy and retroperitoneal node dissection in disseminated testis cancer. *Ann Thorac Surg.* 1983;36:524–528.
142. Williams SD, Birch R, Einhorn LH, Irwin L, Greco FA, Loehrer PJ. Treatment of disseminated germ-cell tumors with cisplatin, bleomycin and either vinblastine or etoposide. *N Engl J Med.* 1987;316:1435–1440.
143. Einhorn LH, Williams SD, Loehrer PJ, et al. Evaluation of optimal duration chemotherapy in favorable-prognosis disseminated germ cell tumors: a Southeastern Cancer Study Group protocol. *J Clin Oncol.* 1989;7:387–391.
144. Gershenson DM. Management of ovarian germ cell tumors. *J Clin Oncol.* 2007;25:2938–2943.
145. Nichols CR, Saman S, Williams SD, et al. Primary mediastinal nonseminomatous germ cell tumors: a modern single institution experience. *Cancer.* 1990;65:1641–1646.
146. Bajorin DF, Sarosdy MF, Pfister DG, et al. Randomized trial of etoposide and cisplatin versus etoposide and carboplatin in patients with good-risk germ cell tumors: a multiinstitutional study. *J Clin Oncol.* 1993;11:598–606.
147. Horwich A, Sleijfer DT, Fossa SD, et al. Randomized trial of bleomycin, etoposide, and cisplatin compared with bleomycin, etoposide, and carboplatin in good-prognosis metastatic nonseminomatous germ cell cancer: a multi-institutional Medical Research Council/European Organization for Research and Treatment of Cancer trial. *J Clin Oncol.* 1997;15:1844–1852.
148. de Wit R, Stoter G, Kaye SB, et al. Importance of bleomycin in combination chemotherapy for good-prognosis testicular nonseminoma: a randomized study of the European Organization for Research and Treatment of Cancer Genitourinary Tract Cancer Cooperative Group. *J Clin Oncol.* 1997;15:1837–1843.
149. Loehrer PJ, Johnson D, Elson P, Einhorn LH, Trump D. Importance of bleomycin in favorable-prognosis disseminated germ cell tumors: an Eastern Cooperative Oncology Group trial. *J Clin Oncol.* 1995;13:470–476.
150. Loehrer PJ, Birch R, Williams SD, Greco FA, Einhorn LH. Chemotherapy of metastatic seminoma: the Southeastern Cancer Study Group experience. *J Clin Oncol.* 1987;5:1212–1220.
151. Gershenson DM, Wharton JT, Kline RC, Larson DM, Kavanagh JJ, Rutledge FN. Chemotherapeutic complete remission in patients with metastatic ovarian dysgerminoma: potential for cure and preservation of reproductive capacity. *Cancer.* 1986;58:2594–2599.
152. Bokemeyer C, Kollmannsberger C, Stenning S, et al. Metastatic seminoma treated with either single agent carboplatin or cisplatin-based combination chemotherapy: a pooled analysis of two randomized trials. *Br J Cancer.* 2004;91:683–687.
153. Gholam D, Fizazi K, Terrier-Lacombe MJ, Jan P, Culine S, Theodore C. Advanced seminoma—treatment results and prognostic factors for survival after first-line, cisplatin-based chemotherapy and for patients with recurrent disease: a single-institution experience in 145 patients. *Cancer.* 2003;98:745–752.
154. Samson MK, Rivkin SE, Jones SE, et al. Dose-response and dose-survival advantage for high versus low-dose cisplatin combined with vinblastine and bleomycin in disseminated testicular cancer: a Southwest Oncology Group study. *Cancer.* 1984;53:1029–1035.
155. Ozols RF, Corden BJ, Jacob J, Wesley MN, Ostchega Y, Young RC. High-dose cisplatin in hypertonic saline. *Ann Intern Med.* 1984;100:19–24.
156. Ozols RF, Ihde DC, Linehan M, Jacob J, Ostchega Y, Young RC. A randomized trial of standard chemotherapy vs a high-dose chemotherapy regimen in the treatment of poor prognosis nonseminomatous germ-cell tumors. *J Clin Oncol.* 1988;6:1031–1040.
157. Nichols CR, Williams SD, Loehrer PJ, et al. Randomized study of cisplatin dose intensity in poor-risk germ cell tumors: a Southeastern Cancer Study Group and Southwest Oncology Group protocol. *J Clin Oncol.* 1991;9:1163–1172.
158. Nichols CR, Catalano PJ, Crawford ED, Vogelzang NJ, Einhorn LH, Loehrer PJ. Randomized comparison of cisplatin and etoposide and either bleomycin or ifosfamide in treatment of advanced disseminated germ cell tumors: an Eastern Cooperative Oncology Group, Southwest Oncology Group, and Cancer and Leukemia Group B study. *J Clin Oncol.* 1998;16:1287–1293.
159. Kaye SB, Mead GM, Fossa S, et al. Intensive induction-sequential chemotherapy with BOP/VIP-B compared with treatment with BEP/EP for poor-prognosis metastatic nonseminomatous germ cell tumor: a Randomized Medical Research Council/European Organization for Research and Treatment of Cancer study. *J Clin Oncol.* 1998;16:692–701.
160. Sirohi B, Huddart R. The management of poor-prognosis, non-seminomatous germ-cell tumours. *Clin Oncol (R Coll Radiol).* 2005;17(7):543–552.
161. Kondagunta GV, Motzer RJ. Chemotherapy for advanced germ cell tumors. *J Clin Oncol.* 2006;24:5493–5502.
162. Christian JA, Huddart RA, Norman A, et al. Intensive induction chemotherapy with CBOP/BEP in patients with poor prognosis germ cell tumors. *J Clin Oncol.* 2003;21:871–877.
163. Motzer RJ, Nichols CJ, Margolin KA, et al. Phase III randomized trial of conventional-dose chemotherapy with or without high-dose chemotherapy and autologous hematopoietic stem-cell rescue as first-line treatment for patients with poor-prognosis metastatic germ cell tumors. *J Clin Oncol.* 2007;25:247–256.
164. Wheeler BM, Loehrer PJ, Williams SD, Einhorn LH. Ifosfamide in refractory male germ cell tumors. *J Clin Oncol.* 1986;4:28–34.
165. Motzer RJ, Bajorin DF, Schwartz LH, et al. Phase II trial of paclitaxel shows antitumor activity in patients with previously treated germ cell tumors. *J Clin Oncol.* 1994;12:2277–2283.
166. Bokemeyer C, Gerl A, Schoffski P, et al. Gemcitabine in patients with relapsed or cisplatin-refractory testicular cancer. *J Clin Oncol.* 1999;17:512–516.
167. Kollmannsberger C, Rick O, Derigs HG, et al. Activity of oxaliplatin in patients with relapsed or cisplatin-refractory germ cell cancer: a study of the German Testicular Cancer Study Group. *J Clin Oncol.* 2002;20:2031–2037.
168. Kollmannsberger C, Nichols C, Bokemeyer C. Recent advances in management of patients with platinum-refractory testicular germ cell tumors. *Cancer.* 2006;106:1217–1226.
169. Einhorn LH, Williams SD, Chamness A, Brames MJ, Perkins SM, Abonour R. High-dose chemotherapy and stem-cell rescue for metastatic germ-cell tumors. *N Engl J Med.* 2007;357:340–348.
170. Pratt CB, Hayes A, Green AA, et al. Pharmacokinetic evaluation of cisplatin in children with malignant solid tumors: a phase II study. *Cancer Treat Rep.* 1981;65:1021–1026.
171. Allen JC, Kim JH, Packer RJ. Neoadjuvant chemotherapy for newly diagnosed germ-cell tumors of the central nervous system. *J Neurosurg.* 1987;67:65–70.
172. Ettinger LJ, Gaynon PS, Krailo MD, et al. A phase II study of carboplatin in children with recurrent or progressive solid tumors: a report from the Children's Cancer Group. *Cancer.* 1994;73:1297–1301.
173. Pratt CB, Etcubanas E, Goren MP, et al. Clinical studies of ifosfamide/mesna at St Jude Children's Research Hospital, 1983–1988. *Semin Oncol.* 1989;16:51–55.
174. Kung F, Hayes FA, Krischer J, et al. Clinical trial of etoposide (VP-16) in children with recurrent malignant solid tumors: a phase II study from the Pediatric Oncology Group. *Invest New Drugs.* 1988;3:31–36.
175. Sawada M, Matsui Y, Okudaira Y. Chemotherapy of human yolk sac tumor heterotransplanted in nude mice. *J Natl Cancer Inst.* 1983;71:1221–1225.
176. Flamant F, Schwartz L, Delons E, Caillaud JM, Hartmann O, Lemerle J. Nonseminomatous malignant germ cell tumors in children. *Cancer.* 1984;54:1687–1691.
177. Pinkerton CR, Pritchard J, Spitz L. High complete response rate in children with advanced germ cell tumors using cisplatin-containing combination chemotherapy. *J Clin Oncol.* 1986;4:194–199.
178. Baranzelli MC, Bouffet E, Quintana E, Portas M, Thyss A, Patte C. Non-seminomatous ovarian germ cell tumours in children. *Eur J Cancer.* 2000;36:376–383.
179. Li Y, Womer RB, Silber JH. Predicting cisplatin ototoxicity in children: the influence of age and the cumulative dose. *Eur J Cancer.* 2004;40:2445–2451.
180. Efstathiou E, Logothetis CJ. Review of late complications of treatment and late relapse in testicular cancer. *J Natl Compr Cancer Netw.* 2006;4:1059–1070.
181. Gershenson DM, Miller AM, Champion VL, et al. Reproductive and sexual function after platinum-based chemotherapy in long-term ovarian germ cell tumor survivors: a Gynecologic Oncology Group study. *J Clin Oncol.* 2007;25:2792–2797.

Pediatric Osteosarcoma

Neyssa Marina, Richard Gorlick, and Stefan Bielack

Introduction

This chapter will describe recent advances in the diagnosis, biology, and therapy of osteosarcoma, a rare bone cancer. Although we have made significant progress in the diagnosis and management of patients with this tumor, not much progress has been made understanding its pathogenesis and biologic behavior. Additionally, as cure rates have improved, therapy-related complications have become of increasing concern. Therefore, the challenge over the next few decades will be to develop strategies to better understand the biology and behavior of this tumor, so that we can develop targeted therapy as well as strategies to minimize the long-term impact of treatment.

Incidence and Epidemiology

Bone lesions in children include benign, metastatic (ie, from neuroblastoma, lymphoma, and rhabdomyosarcoma), and primary bone malignancies (the focus of this chapter).[1,2] In general, primary malignant bone tumors in children are rare, with an estimated 8.7 per million in patients younger than 20 years, representing 650 to 700 new bone cancer patients a year in the United States.[3] Primary bone tumors are the sixth most common malignant neoplasm in children; in adolescents and young adults, they are the third most frequent neoplasms, following only leukemias and lymphomas.[3] The two most common primary bone tumors are osteosarcoma (400 cases per year in the United States) and Ewing sarcoma (200 cases per year in the United States).[4,5] Other primary bone tumors include chondrosarcoma and non-Hodgkin lymphoma of bone, which are considerably rarer.

Osteosarcoma has a bimodal age distribution, with a first peak during the second decade of life (during the adolescent growth spurt; modal age: 16 years in girls and 18 in boys) and a second peak in older adults. Boys are affected more frequently in most series,[3–6] and the incidence in black children is slightly higher than in whites. It is extremely rare before 5 years of age.

Etiology and Pathogenesis

Although the etiology and pathogenesis of osteosarcoma is poorly understood, some have utilized its age of onset to generate hypotheses. The peak incidence coincides with a period of rapid bone growth, suggesting a correlation between rapid bone growth and the evolution of this cancer. For osteosarcoma, other evidence supporting this relationship includes the higher incidence of osteosarcoma in large dog breeds as compared with smaller breeds,[7] and the earlier peak age in girls as compared with boys, corresponding to their earlier growth spurt.[8] However, a recent study focusing on a single breed of large dogs failed to find an association within that group between height and the development of osteosarcoma.[9] In addition, although initial evidence suggested a higher incidence in tall people compared with short people, this finding has not been confirmed in all studies. A large recently published study concluded that osteosarcoma occurs more frequently in patients with tall stature.[10] Radiation exposure and Paget disease are well-documented risk factors for osteosarcoma, which can also occur as a secondary malignancy, usually following the use of ionizing radiation. However, since the latency for secondary osteosarcomas is long, this is most likely not relevant to most de novo osteosarcoma patients.[1,2,4,5]

Molecular Biology

There is now a large amount of information regarding the molecular biology of bone tumors. Generally, the genetic alterations in sarcomas fall into two categories: (1) reciprocal translocations with balanced karyotypes and alterations of tumor suppressor gene pathways, and (2) complex unbalanced karyotypes with alterations of the p53 and retinoblastoma (Rb) pathways.[11] In sarcomas with reciprocal translocations, these genetic alterations are central to the tumor's pathogenesis. Ewing sarcoma is representative of the former category, and osteosarcoma of the latter category.

Osteosarcoma is believed to arise from osteoblasts.[4,5] Despite the complexity of the karyotypes and the absence of characteristic reciprocal translocations, numerous, nonrandom chromosomal abnormalities are usually present in osteosarcoma. Many studies describe cytogenetic abnormalities in this tumor, and the majority of these are clonally abnormal, with heterogeneity even within the same patient.[12] The majority of osteosarcoma samples (58%) have marker chromosomes (structurally abnormal chromosomes in which no part is identified). Ring chromosomes (7%) accompanied by multiple numerical (65%) and structural (72%) abnormalities are also frequently observed.[12,13] There is also evidence of genomic amplification (homogeneously staining regions or double minutes) in more than one-third of cases. Common numerical abnormalities include: gains of chromosome 1; loss of chromosomes 9, 10, 13, and/or 17; and partial or complete loss of the long arm of chromosome 6.[14–17] Frequent structural abnormalities include rearrangements of chromosomes 11, 19, and 20.[12,13,18,19]

The p53 and Rb tumor suppressor pathways are clearly involved in the pathogenesis of osteosarcoma. Most tumor samples have inactivation of the Rb and p53 tumor suppressor pathways, and about 3% of patients with sporadic osteosarcoma harbor germline mutations in p53.[20,21] In studies of osteosarcoma, a number of loci have loss of heterozygosity (3q, 13q, 17p, 18q), including the locations of the *Rb* and *p53* tumor suppressor genes.[22,23] Interestingly, retinoblastoma survivors have an increased incidence of second malignancies, the majority of which are osteosarcoma.[24–27] In the hereditary form of retinoblastoma, germline mutations of the *Rb* gene are common, likely forming the basis for the increased frequency of secondary cancers, since the rate of second malignancies in survivors of unilateral sporadic retinoblastoma is much less. Germline mutations in the *p53* gene can also lead to a high risk of malignant tumor formation, including osteosarcoma (Li-Fraumeni syndrome).[28] The p53 gene product in normal cells increases in response to DNA damage and directs the cell to either stop progression through the cell cycle or undergo apoptosis.[14,15] The Rb gene product likewise regulates cell cycle progression.[16,17,29] Although germline mutations of either *p53* or the *Rb* gene are rare, these genes are altered in the majority of osteosarcoma tumor samples.[30,31] Other altered oncogenes in osteosarcoma tumor cells include amplifications of the product of the murine double minute 2 gene and cyclin-dependent kinase 4.[32,33] Amplification of the 12q13 region (containing MDM2 and CDK4) or INK4A deletion can affect both the p53 and Rb pathways, and indeed these alterations seldom coexist with *Rb* or *p53* alterations.[20,32,33] Although it is clear that alterations in tumor suppressor genes and oncogenes are necessary to produce osteosarcomas, it is not clear which of these events occurs first.[20]

The complex unbalanced karyotypes that characterize osteosarcoma may reflect its pathogenesis. Karyotypic complexity may reflect chromosomal fusion-bridge-breakage cycles resulting from advanced telomere erosion. A potential etiology of this chromosomal instability is telomere dysfunction, as has been implicated in epithelial cancers.[34] Telomeres are nucleoprotein structures that cap chromosome ends and serve at least 3 protective functions: preventing recognition of chromosomes as damaged DNA, preventing chromosomal end-to-end fusions and recombinations, and accommodating the loss of DNA that occurs with each round of replication. Normal human somatic cells have finite proliferative capacity, and telomere length is one of the checkpoints that determines when a cell stops dividing.[35,36] Cells bypass this checkpoint by activating mechanisms that lengthen telomeres, a central feature of cancer cells. About 85% of cancers activate an enzyme called telomerase, which lengthens telomeres, and the other 15% of cancers use a recombination-based method called alternative telomere lengthening.[37,38] Unlike most cancers, at least 50% of osteosarcoma samples are dependent upon the alternative telomere-lengthening mechanism to maintain telomeres.[39–41] The alternative telomere-lengthening and telomerase mechanisms are different means to the same end, but they are not equivalent. Telomerase-dependent osteosarcoma cell lines have short telomeres with a minor range of length, whereas alternative telomere-lengthening-dependent osteosarcoma cell lines have long telomeres with great heterogeneity in length.[42] The alternative telomere-lengthening cell lines also have greater genetic instability and more translocations than the telomerase-positive cell lines.[39]

Other authors suggest that osteosarcomas may have a viral etiology based on the fact that bone sarcomas can be induced in selected animals by viruses.[43,44] For example, hamsters injected with cell-free extracts of human osteosarcoma develop osteosarcomas,[45] and some human osteosarcomas contain SV40-like sequences. SV40, a DNA polyomavirus, consists of 3 major nonstructural proteins: the small T antigen (enhances the ability of large T antigen to transform cells), the smaller T antigen (function unknown), and the large T antigen (assists in viral replication, interacts with *p53* and *Rb*, and promotes cell proliferation by inhibiting *p53* function).[46] A 1996 study showed that 11 of 18 osteosarcoma samples had evidence of incorporated SV40 DNA;[46] a 1998 study showed no correlation between the presence of SV40 and *p53* or *Rb* mutation status;[47] and a 1997 study showed that 50% of osteosarcoma samples had incorporated SV40 DNA from each of the 4 regions of the viral genome.[48,49] However, there are no convincing data that viruses are a major etiologic factor in osteosarcoma.

Pathology

Osteosarcoma has a broad spectrum of histologic appearances, which have in common the proliferation of malignant mesenchymal cells and the production of osteoid and/or bone by tumor cells.[4,5] The amount of osteoid and/or bone production varies greatly both between tumors and within an individual tumor, and thus identification of diagnostic osteoid may require extensive sampling. Chondroid and fibrous matrix may also be present, reflecting the mesenchymal origin of the malignant cells and their consequent ability to differentiate in various cell types. Conventional osteosarcoma is a primary intramedullary high-grade sarcoma and constitutes the vast majority of osteosarcoma in children and adolescents. The current World Health Organization (WHO) classification of osteosarcoma recognizes 3 major subtypes of conventional osteosarcoma: osteoblastic, chondroblastic, and fibroblastic, reflecting the predominant type of matrix in the tumor.[14] In addition to conventional osteosarcoma and its subtypes, the WHO classification recognizes additional histologic variants, including telangiectatic, small cell osteosarcoma, secondary, parosteal, periosteal, low-grade central, and high-grade surface.[50,51] The diagnosis of osteosarcoma is typically made based on its histologic appearance using routine light microscopy.

Clinical Presentation

Most patients with osteosarcoma present with pain and swelling of the involved region, which precedes diagnosis by an average of approximately 2 months.[52,53] Pain can be intermittent at first but becomes continuous with tumor progression. A typical misinterpretation that often leads to considerable diagnostic delays is to attribute pain caused by osteosarcoma to recent trauma. A palpable mass or swelling of the involved region is detectable only several weeks after the onset of pain. In some cases, there is loss of motion of the neighboring joints. In rare instances, particularly in patients with osteolytic tumors, a pathological fracture is the first sign of disease. Systemic symptoms, such as weight loss or shortness of breath, are notoriously late to develop and are signs of advanced metastatic disease. Death from osteosarcoma is usually due to pulmonary insufficiency caused by lung metastases.

Although osteosarcoma can occur in any bone, it is most common in the metaphysis of long bones. The most common primary sites are the distal femur, proximal tibia, and proximal humerus,[1,54–56] with approximately 50% originating around the knee area.[1,54,55] About 10% of patients present with tumors in the axial skeleton, most commonly the pelvis.[57] About 15% to 20% of patients present with radiographic metastases most commonly to the lung,[58,59] but metastases can also develop in bone, lymph nodes, and rarely brain.[60,61]

Diagnostic Evaluation

Imaging Studies

The evaluation of a patient with suspected osteosarcoma begins with a full history, physical examination, and plain radiographs. A variety of imaging studies must be performed to completely evaluate the patient with a suspected bone tumor. An accurate description of the local extent of the primary tumor is essential, and a meticulous search for primary metastases is warranted. Later, the response to induction chemotherapy is also of interest, and during follow-up, imaging studies are performed to detect local and/or systemic recurrences.

Primary Tumor

Conventional radiography and magnetic resonance imaging (MRI) are complementary methods to evaluate the primary tumor.[62,63] Plain radiographs are mainly helpful to describe osseous changes. Osteosarcomas can present with osteoblastic, osteolytic, or mixed appearances on conventional radiographs. They often have a soft tissue component, in which patchy calcifications resulting from new bone formation or spiculae (thin, centrifugal lines of reactive calcifications that form a radial or "sunburst"' pattern) may be observed. A triangular area of periosteal calcification in the border region of tumor and healthy tissue is known as Codman triangle (Figure 27-1). Magnetic

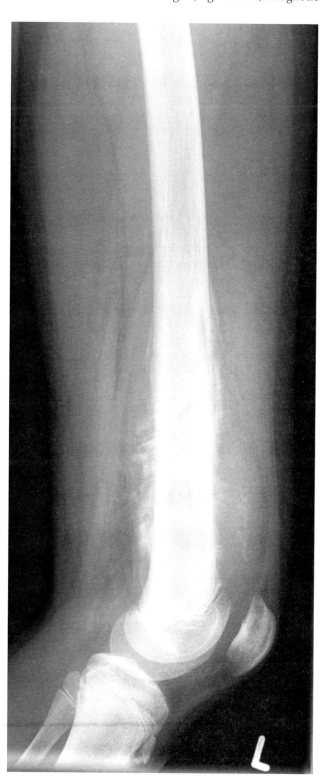

Figure 27-1 Conventional radiograph of an osteosarcoma of the left distal femur in a 12-year-old female.

resonance imaging is the best modality to assess the soft tissue component; its relation to surrounding tissues, vessels, and nerves; and its intramedullary extension (Figure 27-2).[62,63] The exact description of the tumor's anatomy on MRI is essential for safe surgery. The region assessed by MRI should include the whole involved bone as well as the neighboring joints, so as to not miss skip lesions (intramedullary tumor foci without direct contact to the primary lesion). Computed tomography (CT), angiography, and other radiological methods are of minor importance compared with plain radiographs and MRI and are reserved for specific questions.

Systemic Staging

A metastatic workup is essential because one of the most important prognostic factors appears to be the presence of metastatic disease at initial diagnosis.[53] If present, metastases usually involve the lung or, less frequently, distant bones, while other sites are almost never affected in patients without lung or bone metastases.[64] The search for metastases must therefore focus on the lungs and include the skeleton. All patients with osteosarcoma must have evaluation by chest radiographs (Figure 27-3) and a high-resolution CT scan of the thorax (Figure 27-4).[65] The latter adds considerable sensitivity and must be interpreted with a high index of suspicion. Lung metastases from osteosarcoma typically present as round opacities, often in the periphery of the pulmonary parenchyma, and may be calcified. Metastases to distant bones are searched for by a 3-phase 99m-Technetium bone scan. Bone scans will also show the primary tumor and ossifying metastases located outside of the skeleton (Figure 27-5). Other methods, such as positron emission tomography (PET), do not reliably add to the staging information gathered by the methods discussed above.

Routine Laboratory Tests

A variety of laboratory tests are required before interdisciplinary treatment is started. Most of these are tests directed toward assessing organ function and general health prior to the initiation of treatment, because there are no specific laboratory tests for osteosarcoma. Evaluations performed prior to chemotherapy initiation include a complete blood count and differential, blood group typing, tests for serum electrolytes, creatinine and (estimated) creatinine clearance, bilirubin, transaminases, a coagulation profile, and hepatitis and human immunodeficiency virus testing. In many patients, alkaline phosphatase levels in serum are elevated, and whether this is a sign of increased bone turnover or of enzyme secreted by the tumor cells themselves is not known. High alkaline phosphatase serum levels have been associated with inferior outcomes.[66,67] To a lesser extent, the same holds true for lactate dehydrogenase.[66,68] Because chemotherapy treatment for osteosarcoma can result in cardiac and auditory dysfunction, patients should also have baseline assessment with echocardiogram or multiple gated acquisition scan as well as an audiogram.

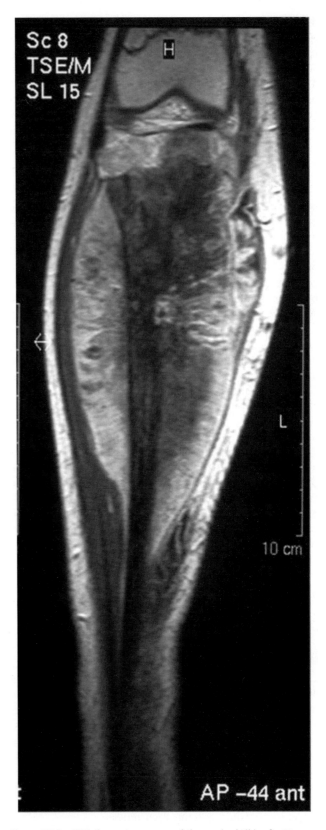

Figure 27-2 MRI of an osteosarcoma of the proximal tibia of a 15-year-old female.

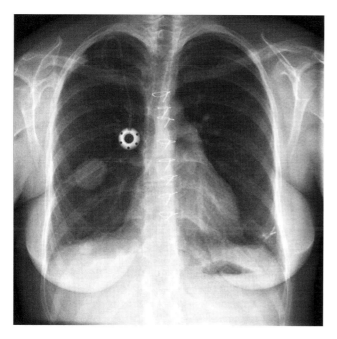

Figure 27-3 Chest X-ray with pulmonary metastases from osteosarcoma.

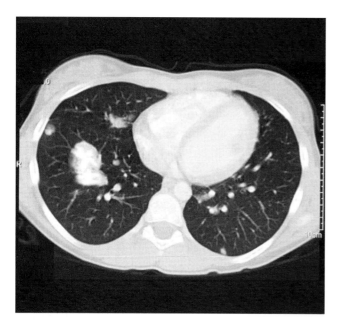

Figure 27-4 CT scan of the chest with multiple pulmonary metastases from osteosarcoma.

Evaluating Tumor Response to Induction Chemotherapy

Information about the expected response of an osteosarcoma to preoperative chemotherapy will influence the plane of resection and thereby help decide which type of surgery to use. Serial dynamic MRI, serial quantitative bone scans, and serial PET scans can all be used to predict response with a relatively high accuracy, but none of these methods are infallible.[69–72]

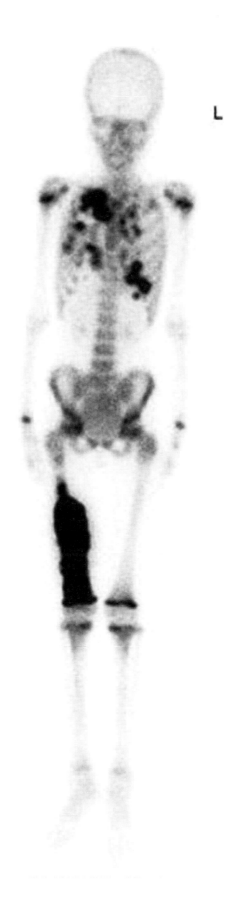

Figure 27-5 99m Tc Bone scan in a patient with an osteosarcoma of the right distal femur and additional avid tracer uptake in ossifying lung metastases.

Imaging During Follow-Up

The search for recurrences must again center on the lungs. Serial x-rays or CT scans of the chest are the methods of choice. Most investigators will also evaluate the former primary site at regular intervals. This is done by x-rays or other appropriate methods, which may differ between individuals depending on the type of reconstructive procedure performed. Local recurrences are, however, much rarer than lung metastases, and, other than these, often point to themselves by pain or swelling, so that the yield of routine follow-up imaging of the former primary site is much lower than that of pulmonary monitoring. The same holds true for the search for metastases to distant bones. Most centers therefore do not include regular bone scans into their routine follow-up program. A suggestion for follow-up investigations that is based on current European and American protocols is depicted in Table 27-1.

Classification and Staging

For many years, the Musculoskeletal Tumor Society staging system (MSTS) developed by Enneking et al has been the one most widely used.[73] The MSTS system distinguishes between 2 grades of malignancy (low grade, stage I; high grade, stage II). Added to this is a suffix that describes the local extension of the primary tumor (intracompartmental, A; extracompartmental, B). Tumors extending beyond the cortex are considered extracompartmental, while metastatic tumors are regarded as stage III.[73] The vast majority of osteosarcomas are classified as stage IIB in this system.

Previous editions of the TNM classification have not achieved widespread compliance, because they did not add much to the description of bone sarcomas. The new sixth edition of the International Union Against Cancer (UICC) stage grouping, however, seems better adapted to the biological situation encountered in osteosarcoma than its predecessors. It distinguishes between small (≤ 8 cm, T1) and large primaries (> 8cm, T2) and also allows classification of discontinuous tumors in the primary bone site ("skip" metastases, T3). Distant metastases can be classified as pulmonary (M1a) or as involving other sites (M1b) (Table 27-2). Reminiscent of the MSTS system, the UICC stage grouping again includes the grade of malignancy (high or low) for the definition of tumor stages (Table 27-3).[74]

Treatment and Prognosis

Surgical Biopsy

Most patients with bone tumors undergo diagnostic biopsies using an incisional or core biopsy, and the biopsy site is usually determined by assessment of the extent of local disease and the relation of the tumor to critical structures such as the neurovascular bundle. It is strongly recommended that the biopsy be performed by the surgeon who will be performing the definitive resection so that the biopsy tract can be excised *en bloc* with the planned surgical resection.[75]

Definitive Surgery

The management of all patients with bone tumors requires a multidisciplinary team approach. Surgical management has evolved into a complex field, and the approach used varies depending on tumor type, location,

---

Table 27-1

Recommended follow-up for osteosarcoma patients.[a]

| Time Point | Tumor Directed | | Late Effects |
	Primary Site	Metastases	
Baseline	Plain film & CT/MRI	Chest x-ray & CT	Echocardiogram, audiogram, liver & kidney function, hepatitis B/C, & HIV serology
Year 1 & 2	Plain film q 4 months	Chest x-ray q 6-12 weeks	Echocardiogram q 1-2 years, audiogram,[b] liver,[b] & kidney[b] function
Year 3 & 4	Plain film q 4 months	Chest x-ray q 2-4 months	Echocardiogram q 1-2 years[c]
Years 5-10	If clinical suspicion[d]	Chest x-ray q 6 months[d]	Echocardiogram q 2-4 years[c]
> 10 years	If clinical suspicion	Metastases reported as late as 2 decades post treatment. Discuss with patient whether to continue chest x-ray q 6-12 months	Echocardiogram q 2-4 years[c]

[a]Every clinic visit must include detailed history and physical examination. Many institutions will add complete blood counts. Evaluate any site of unexplained pain or swelling. Although chest CT is optional, it should always be performed if chest radiograph shows metastasis or is inconclusive. Add consultation with orthopedic surgery and physical therapy as indicated. Offer fertility testing for males. Additional investigations may be indicated.

[b]Need not be repeated if normal at 1 year.

[c]Longer interval if normal function and post pubertal at diagnosis.

[d]Some groups recommend continued annual radiographs of the primary site until year 10.

Table 27-2

International Union Against Cancer TNM classification for malignant bone tumors.

	T (Primary Tumor)	N (Regional Lymph Nodes)	M (Distant Metastases)
X	Cannot be assessed	Cannot be assessed	Cannot be assessed
0	No evidence of primary tumor	No regional lymph node metastases	No distant metastases
1	≤8 cm in greatest dimension	Regional lymph node metastases	Distant metastases 1a–Lung
2	>8 cm in greatest dimension		1b–Other distant sites
3	Discontinuous tumors at the primary bone site		

Table 27-3

International Union Against Cancer stage grouping.

Stage	T (Primary Tumor)	N (Regional Lymph nodes)	M (Distant Metastases)	Grade of Malignancy
IA	1	0	0	Low
IB	2	0	0	Low
IIA	1	0	0	High
IIB	2	0	0	High
III	3	0	0	Any
IVA	Any	0	1a	Any
IVB	Any	N1.	Any	Any
	Any	Any	M1b	Any

extent of disease, and age of the patient. In most situations, surgical therapy for osteosarcoma occurs after the administration of preoperative therapy. Following surgical recovery, postoperative treatment involves the use of postoperative chemotherapy. The goal of resection is to perform an *en bloc* resection with adequate margins because marginal resections increase the risk of local recurrence.[76] The use of multiagent chemotherapy has allowed equivalent outcomes for patients receiving amputation and limb-salvage surgery. Therefore, limb salvage has become the standard of care except in situations where it is impossible to obtain clear margins. It is important to remember that obtaining adequate margins is the goal of the surgical resection and should never be sacrificed.

The development of expandable endoprostheses has allowed the use of limb-sparing surgeries in younger patients.[77–80] As with any reconstruction in the skeletally immature patient, the construct must be dynamic so that it facilitates skeletal growth. Patients with tumors of the pelvis or the axial skeleton present a difficult situation because obtaining adequate margins is not always possible.[81,82] As with other osteosarcoma patients, outcome is dependent on the degree of resection,[53] and a recent study demonstrates that patients who are able to undergo complete resection have outcomes that are not inferior to those of patients with extremity osteosarcoma.[83,84]

Chemotherapy

The outcome of patients with osteosarcoma was poor before the use of multiagent chemotherapy, with 2-year survival rates of 15% to 20%.[54,55,85,86] Most patients appear to have microscopic metastases at diagnosis, because 80% to 90% will develop metastases to the lung following treatment with surgical resection and/or radiotherapy.[54,55,85,86] The most active chemotherapy agents include cisplatin,[87–89] doxorubicin,[90,91] high-dose methotrexate,[92–95] and most recently ifosfamide,[96] alone or combined with etoposide.[97]

Although early nonrandomized trials suggested that systemic chemotherapy improved the outcome for osteosarcoma patients when compared with historical controls,[98–102] some investigators were concerned that the improved outcome resulted from patient selection, earlier diagnosis (staging with CT), or improved surgical techniques.[103,104] In the early 1980s investigators at the Mayo Clinic carried out the first randomized trial of adjuvant chemotherapy for osteosarcoma[105] and reported a disease-free survival of 40% with no difference among treatment groups, suggesting the natural history had changed. Two subsequent randomized prospective studies established the importance of adjuvant chemotherapy in the treatment of patients with nonmetastatic osteosarcoma.[106,107] Patients receiving chemotherapy had a significant survival advantage over those treated with surgery and observation (2-year disease-free survival of 66% vs 17%).[107] In both studies, the outcome of patients treated with observation was no different than that of patients treated in the 1970s, confirming that the natural history of the disease had not changed.

The concept of preoperative chemotherapy introduced by Rosen[108,109] offered the possibility of developing an endoprosthesis for limb-salvage procedures as well as early treatment of micrometastases. It also allowed for the evaluation of histologic response to chemotherapy, which has become a strong predictor of outcome.[108,110–112] A potential concern with this approach was that delayed tumor removal would lead to chemotherapy resistance. However, a randomized Pediatric Oncology Group study revealed equivalent outcome for patients receiving adjuvant and neoadjuvant therapy.[113] The use of preoperative therapy has become the standard of care given its advantages facilitating tumor removal and allowing evaluation of response to chemotherapy. Although investigators at Memorial Sloan-Kettering Cancer Center reported improved outcome when postoperative therapy was adjusted following a poor histologic response,[114] longer follow-up failed to confirm this improvement,[66] and other investigators have been unable to reproduce these results.[110,111] Although the intensification of preoperative therapy increases the number of good responders, in this setting histologic response loses its predictive value.[115] Therefore, although histologic response remains a strong prognostic factor, attempts to improve outcome by increasing the number of good responders or adjusting postoperative therapy for poor responders have been largely unsuccessful.

The Cooperative Osteosarcoma Study Group (COSS), including centers in Germany, Austria, and Switzerland, has performed a series of studies since 1977 incorporating chemotherapy and surgical resection. The investigators have also recognized the value of histologic response[116] and on COSS-82 attempted to spare patients the toxic cisplatin effects by administering it only as salvage following a poor histologic response.[110] Unfortunately, this approach was unsuccessful, and patients with a poor histologic response had a 4-year metastases-free survival of 41%. The investigators concluded that it was not possible to omit the use of the very active drug pair cisplatin and doxorubicin. The COSS's best results are based on the use of methotrexate, cisplatin, doxorubicin, and ifosfamide, with a 10-year survival of 71%.[117] Although the administration of intra-arterial cisplatin offers multiple theoretical advantages,[118,119] a nonrandomized COSS study showed no advantage to administration of intra-arterial cisplatin in the context of multiagent chemotherapy.[120]

Meanwhile, investigators from the United Kingdom and European centers have participated in a series of studies over the past 20 years under the auspices of the European Osteosarcoma Intergroup. Based on a randomized trial that did not show a survival advantage to administration of 3-drug therapy (methotrexate, cisplatin, and doxorubicin),[121,122] these investigators have used a backbone of 6 cycles of cisplatin and doxorubicin as their standard treatment.[123] Intensification of therapy by administering this combination every 2 weeks did not improve outcome.[123]

Therefore, the standard treatment for patients with nonmetastatic osteosarcoma, although variable, would definitely include the use of cisplatin and doxorubicin with the addition of high-dose methotrexate by various groups, including COG, COSS, Scandinavia Sarcoma Group (SSG),

and the study from the Rizzoli Orthopedic Institute. Ifosfamide is generally included in the treatment of patients by COSS, SSG, and the investigators from the Rizzoli Orthopedic Institute. Because the survival of patients with osteosarcoma appears to have plateaued, it is apparent that to improve outcome further and to prove that limited improvements are possible, randomized trials involving a large number of patients will be needed, and therefore European and North American investigators have agreed to collaborate for future trials as part of the European and American Osteosarcoma Study Group, EURAMOS.

Based on the promising activity of ifosfamide[124] with or without etoposide[97] in patients with metastatic osteosarcoma, and the encouraging results from a nonrandomized study from the Rizzoli Orthopedic Institute suggesting that addition of this drug pair improves the outcome for patients with a poor histologic response,[125] EURAMOS investigators have agreed on evaluating the addition of this drug pair to standard postoperative therapy for patients with a poor histologic response. Secondary to concerns regarding toxicity for patients with a good histologic response, EURAMOS investigators have decided not to evaluate ifosfamide and etoposide in patients with a good histologic response. Investigators from SSG have reported encouraging results with the use of interferon[126] following surgical resection. The development of a long-acting interferon preparation with fewer side effects has prompted interest in evaluating this agent. Therefore, patients with a good histologic response are randomized to the administration of interferon following standard 3-drug therapy. This trial, which is ongoing, has already accrued more than 1000 patients and is the largest osteosarcoma trial to date.

Radiotherapy

The prognosis for patients with osteosarcoma was poor before the use of systemic chemotherapy.[107] Treatment with surgery and/or radiotherapy resulted in 2-year survival of 15% to 20%.[54,55,85,86] In general, surgery with wide margins is the best option for local control, and patients unable to undergo complete resection have a poor outcome.[57,82–84] Therapeutic alternatives for patients who are unable or refuse to have surgery are limited, and although a recent report suggests that a small number of patients can be cured without radical surgery,[127] the standard of care involves the use of multiagent therapy and radical surgery. Recent data also suggest that the administration of radiotherapy may be useful in patients treated with multiagent therapy who are unable to undergo complete resection or who have microscopic residual following attempted resection.[84,128] The use of samarium-153 ethylene diamine tetramethylene phosphonate[129,130] also appears to be effective, although the role of these two modalities is not well defined and needs further evaluation in controlled clinical trials.

Supportive Care

Along with the therapeutic advances in cancer management, a number of agents have been developed to help ameliorate chemotherapy- and tumor-related toxicities.

The introduction of serotonin-antagonists[131-133] has dramatically improved the quality of life of cancer patients, because it has dramatically reduced chemotherapy-induced emesis. This agent alone or combined with dexamethasone[134] has become the standard of care with the use of emetogenic chemotherapy. Other agents used in the management of osteosarcoma patients include the use of opioids for pain control and the use of growth factors. The latter agents have decreased the incidence and duration of neutropenia as well as decreased the length of hospitalization.[135,136]

Relapse

Unfortunately, the prognosis for patients with recurrent osteosarcoma remains poor, and only about one-quarter survive 5 years or more.[137-141] Time to relapse[141,142] and tumor burden[138,141,142] correlate with postrelapse outcome. As is the case for patients with newly diagnosed tumors, complete resection is an essential component of curative second-line therapy, and long-term survival is only possible in these patients.[137-142] Although retrieval chemotherapy can lead to marked responses, its impact on survival is more limited than during first-line therapy.[140-142] Several studies have shown a correlation between the administration of chemotherapy and longer survival in patients who did not achieve a second surgical remission.[140-142] The role of "adjuvant" chemotherapy in patients who achieve a second surgical remission is still controversial.[140-142] Accordingly, there is no consensus concerning the type or number of drugs or the duration of treatment. It seems reasonable to employ agents that have not been used during first-line therapy. Relatively high response rates have, for instance, been reported for the combination of high-dose ifosfamide and etoposide.[143] High-dose chemotherapy with autologous peripheral blood stem cell transplantation was unsuccessful in the few reported series.[144-146] The participation of patients with relapsed osteosarcoma in clinical trials should be strongly encouraged so that the role of retrieval therapy is better defined.

Experimental Therapy

There is a clear need for newer effective agents for patients with osteosarcoma, especially those who present with metastatic disease or develop disease recurrence. These patients are candidates for participation in clinical trials of novel agents. Monoclonal antibodies directed against osteosarcoma may prove useful as treatment. Trastuzumab, a target against epidermal growth factor receptor type-2, is currently under investigation in patients with metastatic osteosarcoma because it appears that patients with metastases express HER-2.[147] Monoclonal antibodies specific for the ganglioside GD2, a cell surface antigen expressed by human neuroblastomas, also recognizes human osteosarcomas and could be considered for therapy.[148] Other biologic approaches including the use of inhaled granulocyte macrophage colony-stimulating factor are under investigation for patients with isolated lung metastases following therapy completion.[149] Insulin-like growth factor I is expressed on osteosarcoma cells, suggesting that growth hormone antagonists may be effective.[150] Bone-seeking isotopes such as samarium-153 ethylene diamine tetramethlene phosphonate may allow the delivery of extremely high doses of local irradiation, perhaps providing an appropriate treatment approach for sites of mineralized disease.[129] Investigation of new agents such as gemcitabine,[151] trimetrexate, and imatinib is also an active area of research in osteosarcoma.

Definition of Best Therapy

The standard treatment for patients with nonmetastatic osteosarcoma, although variable, would include an open biopsy to establish the diagnosis. This would be followed by neoadjuvant therapy including cisplatin and doxorubicin[121-123] with the addition of high-dose methotrexate[152] by COG, COSS, SSG, and investigators from the Rizzoli Orthopedic Institute. Ifosfamide[117] is generally included in the treatment of patients by investigators from the Rizzoli Orthopedic Institute, and a recent French trial reported better histological response to preoperative therapy for patients who received high-dose methotrexate coupled with ifosfamide and etoposide, as compared with patients receiving high-dose methotrexate and doxorubicin.[153] Following about 10 weeks of neoadjuvant therapy, patients proceed to surgical ablation. Because researchers have been unable to alter the outcome of poor responders by altering postoperative therapy, continuation of postsurgical therapy with the same agents used preoperatively appears warranted other than in the context of a controlled clinical trial. Patients who present with metastatic disease at diagnosis have a worse outcome,[58,64,154] and long-term cure is obtained only with aggressive approaches to achieve complete resection of all disease sites. The enrollment of those patients in clinical trials is also essential in order to identify new agents with activity.

Long-Term Outcome (Side Effects of Therapy)

Many former osteosarcoma patients will become long-term survivors with current interdisciplinary therapy and are therefore at risk for long-term sequelae. Functional and cosmetic consequences are related to the site and extent of disease as well as the type of surgery performed. Amputations and especially rotationplasty are considered mutilating procedures, but they may result in limb function similar to that observed following limb-salvage procedures.[155] Ablative surgery is usually definitive, while attempted limb salvage may be followed by the need for revisions for periprosthetic infection, loosening, fracture, or prosthetic wear. Expandable prostheses implanted into young, skeletally immature patients require multiple revisions for lengthening the extremity although there are newer self-expanding prostheses.

Chemotherapy can lead to life-threatening late effects in a small minority of patients.[53] Many osteosarcoma protocols include high cumulative doxorubicin doses, so anthracycline-induced cardiomyopathy is a risk.[156,157] Lifelong cardiac follow-up with serial echocardiograms is generally recommended. Secondary malignancies will develop in approximately 3% of patients within the first 10 years following treatment.[158] Both the mutagenic side effects of cytostatic treatment and individual predisposition contribute to the development of second cancers. Other chemotherapy-related late effects are rarely life threatening but may still have a considerable impact on an individual patient's everyday life. For instance, high-frequency hearing loss secondary to cisplatin is frequent, and some patients will require hearing aids.[159,160] Most males and some females will develop sterility if high cumulative ifosfamide doses are employed. Rarely, cisplatin and ifosfamide may produce renal dysfunction manifested as changes in glomerular filtration rate,[161,162] hypomagnesemia,[93] or proximal tubular damage.[163,164]

Summary

The outcome for patients with osteosarcoma has dramatically improved with the use of multiagent chemotherapy and surgical resection.[53,107,117] The most important prognostic factors are the presence of metastases, histologic response, and the ability to perform a complete resection.[53] Further progress in the treatment of these patients will require a better understanding of the biology of these tumors. Collection of tumor samples at the time of diagnosis provides an opportunity to assess biologic factors in these patients. Gene arrays are an active area of investigation attempting to identify genes that are important in tumor progression or the presence of metastases. Continued progress will likely require international collaboration.

References

1. Link MP, Eilber F. Osteosarcoma. In: Pizzo PA, Poplack DG, eds. *Principles and Practice of Pediatric Oncology*. Philadelphia: Lippincott-Raven; 1997:889–920.
2. Rosen G, Forscher CA, Mankin HJ, et al. Neoplasms of bone and soft tissue: bone tumors. In: Bast RCJ, Kufe DW, Pollock RE, et al, eds. *Cancer Medicine*. 5th ed. Hamilton, BC: Decker; 2000:1870–1902.
3. Gurney JG, Swensen AR, Bulterys M. Malignant bone tumors. In: Ries LAG, Smith MA, Gurney JG, et al, eds. Cancer incidence and survival among children and adolescents: United States SEER Program 1975–1995. Bethesda, MD: National Cancer Institute, SEER Program; 1999:99–110.
4. Huvos A. *Bone Tumors: Diagnosis, Treatment and Prognosis*. Philadelphia: W. B. Saunders; 1991.
5. Dorfman HD, Czerniak B. Bone cancers. *Cancer*. 1995;75:203–210.
6. Dahlin DC, Unni KK. Osteosarcoma. In: Dahlin DC, Unni KK, eds. *Bone Tumors. General Aspects and Data on 8542 Cases*. Springfield, IL: Charles C Thomas; 1986:269–307.
7. Tjalma RA. Canine bone sarcoma: estimation of relative risk as a function of body size. *J Natl Cancer Inst*. 1966;36:1137–1150.
8. Price C. Primary bone-forming tumours and their relationship to skeletal growth. *J Bone Joint Surg Br*. 1958;40:574–593.
9. Cooley DM, Beranek BC, Schlittler DL, et al. Endogenous gonadal hormone exposure and bone sarcoma risk. *Cancer Epidemiol Biomarkers Prev*. 2002;11:1434–1440.
10. Cotterill SJ, Wright CM, Pearce MS, et al. Stature of young people with malignant bone tumors. *Pediatr Blood Cancer*. 2004;42:59–63.
11. Borden EC, Baker LH, Bell RS, et al. Soft tissue sarcomas of adults: state of the translational science. *Clin Cancer Res*. 2003;9:1941–1956.
12. Bridge JA, Nelson M, McComb E, et al. Cytogenetic findings in 73 osteosarcoma specimens and a review of the literature. *Cancer Genet Cytogenet*. 1997; 95:74–87.
13. Sandberg AA, Bridge JA. Updates on the cytogenetics and molecular genetics of bone and soft tissue tumors: osteosarcoma and related tumors. *Cancer Genet Cytogenet*. 2003;145:1–30.
14. Diller L, Kassel J, Nelson CE, et al. p53 functions as a cell cycle control protein in osteosarcomas. *Mol Cell Biol*. 1990;10:5772–5781.
15. Lane DP. Cancer: p53, guardian of the genome. *Nature*. 1992;358:15–16.
16. Harris H. Malignant tumours generated by recessive mutations. *Nature*. 1986; 323:582–583.
17. Huang HJ, Yee JK, Shew JY, et al. Suppression of the neoplastic phenotype by replacement of the RB gene in human cancer cells. *Science*. 1988;242:1563–1566.
18. Raymond AK, Ayala AG, Knuutila S. Conventional osteosarcoma. In Kleihues P, Sobin L, Fletcher C, et al, eds. *WHO Classification of Tumours: Pathology and Genetics of Tumours of Soft Tissue and Bone*. Lyon, France: IARC Press; 2002:267–269.
19. Bayani J, Zielenska M, Pandita A, et al. Spectral karyotyping identifies recurrent complex rearrangements of chromosomes 8, 17, and 20 in osteosarcomas. *Genes Chromosomes Cancer*. 2003;36:7–16.
20. Ladanyi M, Gorlick R. Molecular pathology and molecular pharmacology of osteosarcoma. *Pediatr Pathol Mol Med*. 2000;19:391–413.
21. Toguchida J, Yamaguchi T, Dayton SH, et al. Prevalence and spectrum of germline mutations of the p53 gene among patients with sarcoma. *N Engl J Med*. 1992;326:1301–1308.
22. Kruzelock RP, Hansen MF. Molecular genetics and cytogenetics of sarcomas. *Hematol Oncol Clin North Am*. 1995;9:513–540.
23. Kruzelock RP, Murphy EC, Strong LC, et al. Localization of a novel tumor suppressor locus on human chromosome 3q important in osteosarcoma tumorigenesis. *Cancer Res*. 1997;57:106–109.
24. Meadows AT, Strong LC, Li FP, et al. Bone sarcoma as a second malignant neoplasm in children: influence of radiation and genetic predisposition. *Cancer*. 1980;46:2603–2606.
25. Smith LM, Donaldson SS, Egbert PR, et al. Aggressive management of second primary tumors in survivors of hereditary retinoblastoma. *Int J Radiat Oncol Biol Phys*. 1989;17(3):499–505.
26. Draper GJ, Sanders BM, Kingston JE. Second primary neoplasms in patients with retinoblastoma. *Br J Cancer*. 1986;53:661–671.
27. Abramson DH, Ellsworth RM, Kitchin FD, et al. Second nonocular tumors in retinoblastoma survivors: are they radiation-induced? *Ophthalmology*. 1984; 91:1351–1355.
28. Friend SH, Bernards R, Rogelj S, et al. A human DNA segment with properties of the gene that predisposes to retinoblastoma and osteosarcoma. *Nature*. 1986;323:643–646.
29. Murphree AL, Benedict WF. Retinoblastoma: clues to human oncogenesis. *Science*. 1984;223:1028–1033.
30. Miller CW, Aslo A, Tsay C, et al. Frequency and structure of p53 rearrangements in human osteosarcoma. *Cancer Res*. 1990;50:7950–7954.
31. Toguchida J, Yamaguchi T, Ritchie B, et al. Mutation spectrum of the p53 gene in bone and soft tissue sarcomas. *Cancer Res*. 1992;52:6194–6199.
32. Ladanyi M, Cha C, Lewis R, et al. MDM2 gene amplification in metastatic osteosarcoma. *Cancer Res*. 1993;53:16–18.
33. Wei G, Lonardo F, Ueda T, et al. CDK4 gene amplification in osteosarcoma: reciprocal relationship with INK4A gene alterations and mapping of 12q13 amplicons. *Int J Cancer*. 1999;80:199–204.
34. Artandi SE, Chang S, Lee SL, et al. Telomere dysfunction promotes non-reciprocal translocations and epithelial cancers in mice. *Nature*. 2000;406:641–645.
35. Bodnar AG, Ouellette M, Frolkis M, et al. Extension of life-span by introduction of telomerase into normal human cells. *Science*. 1998;279:349–352.
36. Harley CB. Telomere loss: mitotic clock or genetic time bomb? *Mutat Res*. 1991;256:271–282.
37. Shay JW, Bacchetti S. A survey of telomerase activity in human cancer. *Eur J Cancer*. 1997;33:787–791.
38. Bryan TM, Englezou A, Dalla-Pozza L, et al. Evidence for an alternative mechanism for maintaining telomere length in human tumors and tumor-derived cell lines. *Nat Med*. 1997;3:1271–1274.
39. Scheel C, Schaefer KL, Jauch A, et al. Alternative lengthening of telomeres is associated with chromosomal instability in osteosarcomas. *Oncogene*. 2001; 20:3835–3844.
40. Aue G, Muralidhar B, Schwartz HS, et al. Telomerase activity in skeletal sarcomas. *Ann Surg Oncol*. 1998;5:627–634.
41. Sangiorgi L, Gobbi GA, Lucarelli E, et al. Presence of telomerase activity in different musculoskeletal tumor histotypes and correlation with aggressiveness. *Int J Cancer*. 2001;95:156–161.
42. Chang S, Khoo CM, Naylor ML, et al. Telomere-based crisis: functional differences between telomerase activation and ALT in tumor progression. *Genes Dev*. 2003;17:88–100.
43. Finkel MP, Biskis BO, Jinkins PB. Virus induction of osteosarcomas in mice. *Science*. 1966;151:698–701.
44. Friedlaender GE, Mitchell MS. A virally induced osteosarcoma in rats: a model for immunological studies of human osteosarcoma. *J Bone Joint Surg Am*. 1976;58:295–302.
45. Finkel MP, Biskis BO, Farrell C. Osteosarcomas appearing in Syrian hamsters after treatment with extracts of human osteosarcomas. *Proc Natl Acad Sci USA*. 1968;60:1223–1230.
46. Carbone M, Rizzo P, Procopio A, et al. SV40-like sequences in human bone tumors. *Oncogene*. 1996;13:527–535.
47. Mendoza SM, Konishi T, Miller CW. Integration of SV40 in human osteosarcoma DNA. *Oncogene*. 1998;17:2457–2462.
48. Lednicky JA, Stewart AR, Jenkins JJ III, et al. SV40 DNA in human osteosarcomas shows sequence variation among T-antigen genes. *Int J Cancer*. 1997; 72:791–800.
49. Heinsohn S, Scholz RB, Weber B, et al. SV40 sequences in human osteosarcoma of German origin. *Anticancer Res*. 2000;20:4539–4545.
50. Matsuno T, Okada K, Knuutila S. Telangiectatic osteosarcoma. In: Fletcher CDM, Unni KK, Mertens F, eds. *WHO Classification of Tumours: Pathology and*

Genetics of Tumours of Soft Tissue and Bone. Lyons, France: IARC Press; 2002: 271–272.

51. Kalil R, Bridge JA. Small cell osteosarcoma. In: Fletcher CDM, Unni KK, Mertens F, eds. *WHO Classification of Tumours: Pathology and Genetics of Tumours of Soft Tissue and Bone.* Lyons, France: IARC Press; 2002:273–274.

52. Pollock BH, Krischer JP, Vietti TJ. Interval between symptom onset and diagnosis of pediatric solid tumors. *J Pediatr.* 1991;119:725–732.

53. Bielack SS, Kempf-Bielack B, Delling G, et al. Prognostic factors in high-grade osteosarcoma of the extremities or trunk: an analysis of 1,702 patients treated on neoadjuvant cooperative osteosarcoma study group protocols. *J Clin Oncol.* 2002;20:776–790.

54. Weinfeld MS, Dudley HR. Osteogenic sarcoma: a follow-up study of the ninety-four cases observed at the Massachusetts General Hospital from 1920 to 1960. *J Bone Joint Surg Am.* 1962;44A:269–276.

55. Dahlin DC, Coventry MB. Osteogenic sarcoma: a study of six hundred cases. *J Bone Joint Surg Am.* 1967;49:101–110.

56. Dahlin DC, Unni KK. Osteosarcoma of bone and its important recognizable varieties. *Am J Surg Pathol.* 1977;1:61–72.

57. Estrada-Aguilar J, Greenberg H, Walling A, et al. Primary treatment of pelvic osteosarcoma: report of five cases. *Cancer.* 1992;69:1137–1145.

58. Meyers PA, Heller G, Healey JH, et al. Osteogenic sarcoma with clinically detectable metastasis at initial presentation. *J Clin Oncol.* 1993;11:449–453.

59. Kaste SC, Pratt CB, Cain AM, et al. Metastases detected at the time of diagnosis of primary pediatric extremity osteosarcoma at diagnosis: imaging features. *Cancer.* 1999;86:1602–1608.

60. Jeffree GM, Price CH, Sissons HA. The metastatic patterns of osteosarcoma. *Br J Cancer.* 1975;32:87–107.

61. Marina NM, Pratt CB, Shema SJ, et al. Brain metastases in osteosarcoma: report of a long-term survivor and review of the St Jude Children's Research Hospital experience. *Cancer.* 1993;71:3656–3660.

62. Sanders TG, Parsons TW III. Radiographic imaging of musculoskeletal neoplasia. *Cancer Control.* 2001;8:221–231.

63. Saifuddin A. The accuracy of imaging in the local staging of appendicular osteosarcoma. *Skeletal Radiol.* 2002;31:191–201.

64. Kager L, Zoubek A, Potschger U, et al. Primary metastatic osteosarcoma: presentation and outcome of patients treated on neoadjuvant Cooperative Osteosarcoma Study Group protocols. *J Clin Oncol.* 2003;21:2011–201.

65. Picci P, Vanel D, Briccoli A, et al. Computed tomography of pulmonary metastases from osteosarcoma. The less poor technique. A study of 51 patients with histological correlation. *Ann Oncol.* 2001;12:1601–1604.

66. Meyers PA, Heller G, Healey J, et al. Chemotherapy for nonmetastatic osteogenic sarcoma: the Memorial Sloan-Kettering experience [see comments]. *J Clin Oncol.* 1992;10:5–15.

67. Bacci G, Picci P, Ferrari S, et al. Prognostic significance of serum alkaline phosphatase measurements in patients with osteosarcoma treated with adjuvant or neoadjuvant chemotherapy. *Cancer.* 1993;71:1224–1230.

68. Bacci G, Ferrari S, Sangiorgi L, et al. Prognostic significance of serum lactate dehydrogenase in patients with osteosarcoma of the extremities. *J Chemother.* 1994;6:204–210.

69. van der Woude HJ, Bloem JL, Hogendoorn PC. Preoperative evaluation and monitoring chemotherapy in patients with high-grade osteogenic and Ewing's sarcoma: review of current imaging modalities. *Skeletal Radiol.* 1998;27:57–71.

70. Franzius C, Bielack S, Flege S, et al. Prognostic significance of (18)F-FDG and (99m)Tc-methylene diphosphonate uptake in primary osteosarcoma. *J Nucl Med.* 2002;43:1012–1017.

71. Hawkins DS, Rajendran JG, Conrad EU III, et al. Evaluation of chemotherapy response in pediatric bone sarcomas by [F-18]-fluorodeoxy-D-glucose positron emission tomography. *Cancer.* 2002;94:3277 3284.

72. Brisse H, Ollivier L, Edeline V, et al. Imaging of malignant tumours of the long bones in children: monitoring response to neoadjuvant chemotherapy and preoperative assessment. *Pediatr Radiol.* 2004.

73. Enneking WF, Spanier SS, Goodman MA. A system for the surgical staging of musculoskeletal sarcoma. *Clin Orthop.* 1980:106–120.

74. Sobin LH, Wittekind C. *UICC TNM Classification of Malignant Tumors.* 6th ed. New York: Wiley; 2002.

75. Mankin HJ, Mankin CJ, Simon MA. The hazards of the biopsy, revisited. Members of the Musculoskeletal Tumor Society. *J Bone Joint Surg Am.* 1996; 78:656–663.

76. Gherlinzoni F, Picci P, Bacci G, et al. Limb sparing versus amputation in osteosarcoma: correlation between local control, surgical margins and tumor necrosis: Istituto Rizzoli experience. *Ann Oncol.* 1992;3(suppl 2P):S23–S27.

77. Finn HA, Simon MA. Limb-salvage surgery in the treatment of osteosarcoma in skeletally immature individuals. *Clin Orthop.* 1991:108–118.

78. Grimer RJ, Belthur M, Carter SR, et al. Extendible replacements of the proximal tibia for bone tumours. *J Bone Joint Surg Br.* 2000;82:255–260.

79. Ward WG, Yang RS, Eckardt JJ. Endoprosthetic bone reconstruction following malignant tumor resection in skeletally immature patients. *Orthop Clin North Am.* 1996;27:493–502.

80. Eckardt JJ, Kabo JM, Kelley CM, et al. Expandable endoprosthesis reconstruction in skeletally immature patients with tumors. *Clin Orthop.* 2000:31–01.

81. Flege S, Kevric M, Ewerbeck V, et al. Axial osteosarcoma: local surgical control is still of paramount importance in the age of interdisciplinary therapy. *Sarcoma.* 2001:233.

82. Fahey M, Spanier SS, Vander Griend RA. Osteosarcoma of the pelvis: a clinical and histopathological study of twenty-five patients. *J Bone Joint Surg Am.* 1992;74:321–330.

83. Bielack SS, Wulff B, Delling G, et al. Osteosarcoma of the trunk treated by multimodal therapy: experience of the Cooperative Osteosarcoma study group (COSS). *Med Pediatr Oncol.* 1995;24:6–12.

84. Ozaki T, Flege S, Kevric M, et al. Osteosarcoma of the pelvis: experience of the Cooperative Osteosarcoma Study Group. *J Clin Oncol.* 2003;21:334–341.

85. Friedman MA, Carter SK. The therapy of osteogenic sarcoma: current status and thoughts for the future. *J Surg Oncol.* 1972;4:482–510.

86. Marcove RC, Mike V, Hajek JV, et al. Osteogenic sarcoma under the age of twenty-one: a review of one hundred and forty-five operative cases. *J Bone Joint Surg Am.* 1970;52:411–423.

87. Ochs JJ, Freeman AI, Douglass HO, et al. cis-Dichlorodiammineplatinum (II) in advanced osteogenic sarcoma. *Cancer Treat Rep.* 1978;62:239–245.

88. Gasparini M, Rouesse J, van Oosterom A, et al. Phase II study of cisplatin in advanced osteogenic sarcoma. European Organization for Research on Treatment of Cancer Soft Tissue and Bone Sarcoma Group. *Cancer Treat Rep.* 1985; 69:211–213.

89. Baum ES, Gaynon P, Greenberg L, et al. Phase II trail cisplatin in refractory childhood cancer: Children's Cancer Study Group Report. *Cancer Treat Rep.* 1981;65:815–822.

90. Pratt CB, Shanks EC. Doxorubicin in treatment of malignant solid tumors in children. *Am J Dis Child.* 1974;127:534–536.

91. Cortes EP, Holland JF, Wang JJ, et al. Amputation and adriamycin in primary osteosarcoma. *N Engl J Med.* 1974;291:998–1000.

92. Jaffe N, Frei E, Traggis D, et al. Adjuvant methotrexate and citrovorum-factor treatment of osteogenic sarcoma. *N Engl J Med.* 1974;291:994–997.

93. Hayes FA, Green AA, Senzer N, et al. Tetany: a complication of cis-Dichlorodiamminoeplatinum (II) therapy. *Cancer Treat Rep.* 1979;63:547–548.

94. Pratt CB, Howarth C, Ransom JL, et al. High-dose methotrexate used alone and in combination for measurable primary or metastatic osteosarcoma. *Cancer Treat Rep.* 1980;64:11–20.

95. Pratt CB, Roberts D, Shanks EC, et al. Clinical trials and pharmacokinetics of intermittent high-dose methotrexate: "leucovorin rescue" for children with malignant tumors. *Cancer Res.* 1974;34:3326–3331.

96. Harris MB, Cantor AB, Goorin AM, et al. Treatment of osteosarcoma with ifosfamide: comparison of response in pediatric patients with recurrent disease versus patients previously untreated: a Pediatric Oncology Group study. *Med Pediatr Oncol.* 1995;24:87–92.

97. Goorin AM, Harris MB, Bernstein M, et al. Phase II/III trial of etoposide and high-dose ifosfamide in newly diagnosed metastatic osteosarcoma: a Pediatric Oncology Group trial. *J Clin Oncol.* 2002;20:426–433.

98. Pratt C, Shanks E, Hustu O, et al. Adjuvant multiple drug chemotherapy for osteosarcoma of the extremity. *Cancer.* 1977;39:51–57.

99. Pratt CB, Rivera G, Shanks E, et al. Combination chemotherapy for osteosarcoma. *Cancer Treat Rep.* 1978;62:251–257.

100. Sutow WW, Gehan EA, Dyment PG, et al. Multidrug adjuvant chemotherapy for osteosarcoma: interim report of the Southwest Oncology Group Studies. *Cancer Treat Rep.* 1978;62:265–269.

101. Sutow WW, Sullivan MP, Fernbach DJ, et al. Adjuvant chemotherapy in primary treatment of osteogenic sarcoma: a Southwest Oncology Group study. *Cancer.* 1975;36:1598–1602.

102. Goorin AM, Frei E III, Abelson HT. Adjuvant chemotherapy for osteosarcoma: a decade of experience. *Surg Clin North Am.* 1981;61:1379–1389.

103. Taylor WF, Ivins JC, Pritchard DJ, et al. Trends and variability in survival among patients with osteosarcoma: a 7-year update. *Mayo Clin Proc.* 1985;60: 91–104.

104. Carter SK. Adjuvant chemotherapy in osteogenic sarcoma: the triumph that isn't? *J Clin Oncol.* 1984;2:147 148.

105. Edmonson JH, Green SJ, Ivins JC, et al. A controlled pilot study of high-dose methotrexate as postsurgical adjuvant treatment for primary osteosarcoma. *J Clin Oncol.* 1984;2:152–156.

106. Eilber F, Giuliano A, Eckardt J, et al. Adjuvant chemotherapy for osteosarcoma: a randomized prospective trial. *J Clin Oncol.* 1987;5:21–26.

107. Link MP, Goorin AM, Miser AW, et al. The effect of adjuvant chemotherapy on relapse-free survival in patients with osteosarcoma of the extremity. *N Engl J Med.* 1986;314:1600–1606.

108. Rosen G, Marcove RC, Caparros B, et al. Primary osteogenic sarcoma: the rationale for preoperative chemotherapy and delayed surgery. *Cancer.* 1979; 43:2163–2177.

109. Rosen G, Murphy ML, Huvos AG, et al. Chemotherapy, en bloc resection, and prosthetic bone replacement in the treatment of osteogenic sarcoma. *Cancer.* 1976;37:1–11.

110. Winkler K, Beron G, Delling G, et al. Neoadjuvant chemotherapy of osteosarcoma: results of a randomized cooperative trial (COSS-82) with salvage chemotherapy based on histological tumor response. *J Clin Oncol.* 1988;6: 329–337.

111. Provisor AJ, Ettinger LJ, Nachman JB, et al. Treatment of nonmetastatic osteosarcoma of the extremity with preoperative and postoperative chemotherapy: a report from the Children's Cancer Group. *J Clin Oncol.* 1997;15:76–84.

112. Bacci G, Picci P, Ruggieri P, et al. Primary chemotherapy and delayed surgery (neoadjuvant chemotherapy) for osteosarcoma of the extremities. The Istituto Rizzoli Experience in 127 patients treated preoperatively with intravenous methotrexate (high versus moderate doses) and intraarterial cisplatin. *Cancer.* 1990;65:2539–2553.

113. Goorin AM, Schwartzentruber DJ, Devidas M, et al. Presurgical chemotherapy compared with immediate surgery and adjuvant chemotherapy for

nonmetastatic osteosarcoma: Pediatric Oncology Group Study POG-8651. *J Clin Oncol*. 2003;21:1574–1580.

114. Rosen G, Caparros B, Huvos AG, et al. Preoperative chemotherapy for osteogenic sarcoma: selection of postoperative adjuvant chemotherapy based on the response of the primary tumor to preoperative chemotherapy. *Cancer.* 1982;49:1221–1230.

115. Meyers PA, Gorlick R, Heller G, et al. Intensification of preoperative chemotherapy for osteogenic sarcoma: results of the Memorial Sloan-Kettering (T12) protocol. *J Clin Oncol*. 1998;16:2452–2458.

116. Winkler K, Beron G, Kotz R, et al. Neoadjuvant chemotherapy for osteogenic sarcoma: results of a Cooperative German/Austrian study. *J Clin Oncol*. 1984; 2:617–624.

117. Fuchs N, Bielack SS, Epler D, et al. Long-term results of the co-operative German-Austrian-Swiss osteosarcoma study group's protocol COSS-86 of intensive multidrug chemotherapy and surgery for osteosarcoma of the limbs. *Ann Oncol*. 1998;9:893–899.

118. Jaffe N, Knapp J, Chuang VP, et al. Osteosarcoma: intra-arterial treatment of the primary tumor with cis-diammine-dichloroplatinum II (CDP). Angiographic, pathologic, and pharmacologic studies. *Cancer.* 1983;51:402–407.

119. Jaffe N, Robertson R, Ayala A, et al. Comparison of intra-arterial cis-diamminedichloroplatinum II with high-dose methotrexate and citrovorum factor rescue in the treatment of primary osteosarcoma. *J Clin Oncol*. 1985;3: 1101–1104.

120. Winkler K, Bielack S, Delling G, et al. Effect of intraarterial versus intravenous cisplatin in addition to systemic doxorubicin, high-dose methotrexate, and ifosfamide on histologic tumor response in osteosarcoma (study COSS-86). *Cancer.* 1990;66:1703–1710.

121. Souhami RL, Craft AW, Van der Eijken JW, et al. Randomised trial of two regimens of chemotherapy in operable osteosarcoma: a study of the European Osteosarcoma Intergroup. *Lancet*. 1997;350:911–917.

122. Bramwell VH, Burgers M, Sneath R, et al. A comparison of two short intensive adjuvant chemotherapy regimens in operable osteosarcoma of limbs in children and young adults: the first study of the European Osteosarcoma Intergroup. *J Clin Oncol*. 1992;10:1579–1591.

123. Lewis IJ, Nooij M; Intergroup ftEO. Chemotherapy at standard or increased dose intensity in patients with operable osteosarcoma of the extremity: A randomised controlled trial conducted by the European Osteo Sarcoma Intergroup (ISRCTN 86294690). *Proc Am Soc Clin Oncol*. Chicago: Lippincott, Williams & Wilkins; 2003.

124. Harris MB, Gieser P, Goorin AM, et al. Treatment of metastatic osteosarcoma at diagnosis: a Pediatric Oncology Group Study. *J Clin Oncol*. 1998;16:3641–3648.

125. Bacci G, Picci P, Ferrari S, et al. Primary chemotherapy and delayed surgery for nonmetastatic osteosarcoma of the extremities: results of 164 patients preoperatively treated with high doses of methotrexate followed by cisplatin and doxorubicin. *Cancer.* 1993;72:3227–3238.

126. Strander H, Bauer HC, Brosjo O, et al. Long-term adjuvant interferon treatment of human osteosarcoma: a pilot study. *Acta Oncol*. 1995;34:877–880.

127. Jaffe N, Carrasco H, Raymond K, et al. Can cure in patients with osteosarcoma be achieved exclusively with chemotherapy and abrogation of surgery? *Cancer.* 2002;95:2202–2210.

128. Machak GN, Tkachev SI, Solovyev YN, et al. Neoadjuvant chemotherapy and local radiotherapy for high-grade osteosarcoma of the extremities. *Mayo Clin Proc*. 2003;78:147–155.

129. Anderson PM, Wiseman GA, Dispenzieri A, et al. High-dose samarium-153 ethylene diamine tetramethylene phosphonate: low toxicity of skeletal irradiation in patients with osteosarcoma and bone metastases. *J Clin Oncol*. 2002; 20:189–196.

130. Franzius C, Bielack S, Flege S, et al. High-activity samarium-153–EDTMP therapy followed by autologous peripheral blood stem cell support in unresectable osteosarcoma. *Nuklearmedizin*. 2001;40:215–220.

131. Alvarez O, Freeman A, Bedros A, et al. Randomized double-blind crossover ondansetron-dexamethasone versus ondansetron-placebo study for the treatment of chemotherapy-induced nausea and vomiting in pediatric patients with malignancies. *J Pediatr Hematol Oncol*. 1995;17:145–150.

132. Cohen IJ, Zehavi N, Buchwald I, et al. Oral ondansetron: an effective ambulatory complement to intravenous ondansetron in the control of chemotherapy-induced nausea and vomiting in children. *Pediatr Hematol Oncol*. 1995; 12:67–72.

133. Kaasa S, Kvaloy S, Dicato MA, et al. A comparison of ondansetron with metoclopramide in the prophylaxis of chemotherapy-induced nausea and vomiting: a randomized, double-blind study. International Emesis Study Group. *Eur J Cancer*. 1990;26:311–314.

134. Peterson C, Hursti TJ, Borjeson S, et al. Single high-dose dexamethasone improves the effect of ondansetron on acute chemotherapy-induced nausea and vomiting but impairs the control of delayed symptoms. *Support Care Cancer*. 1996;4:440–446.

135. Furman WL, Fairclough D, Cain AM, et al. Use of GM-CSF in children after high-dose chemotherapy. *Med Pediatr Oncol Suppl*. 1992;2:26–30.

136. Anglin P, Strauss BA, Brandwein JM. Prevention of chemotherapy-induced neutropenia using G-CSF with VACOP-B: a case report. *Leuk Lymphoma*. 1993;11:469–472.

137. Goorin AM, Delorey MJ, Lack EE, et al. Prognostic significance of complete surgical resection of pulmonary metastases in patients with osteogenic sarcoma: analysis of 32 patients. *J Clin Oncol*. 1984;2:425–431.

138. Meyer WH, Schell MJ, Kumar AP, et al. Thoracotomy for pulmonary metastatic osteosarcoma: an analysis of prognostic indicators of survival. *Cancer.* 1987;59:374–379.

139. Tabone MD, Kalifa C, Rodary C, et al. Osteosarcoma recurrences in pediatric patients previously treated with intensive chemotherapy. *J Clin Oncol*. 1994; 12:2614–2620.

140. Saeter G, Hoie J, Stenwig AE, et al. Systemic relapse of patients with osteogenic sarcoma: prognostic factors for long term survival. *Cancer.* 1995; 75:1084–1093.

141. Ferrari S, Briccoli A, Mercuri M, et al. Postrelapse survival in osteosarcoma of the extremities: prognostic factors for long-term survival. *J Clin Oncol*. 2003; 21:710–715.

142. Kempf-Bielack B, Bielack S, Jürgens H, et al. Osteosarcoma relapse after combined modality therapy: An analysis of unselected patients in the Cooperative Osteosarcoma Study Group (COSS). *J Clin Oncol* 2005;23:559–568.

143. Gentet JC, Brunat-Mentigny M, Demaille MC, et al. Ifosfamide and etoposide in childhood osteosarcoma: a phase II study of the French Society of Paediatric Oncology. *Eur J Cancer*. 1997;33:232–237.

144. Colombat P, Biron P, Coze C, et al. Failure of high-dose alkylating agents in osteosarcoma. Solid Tumors Working Party. *Bone Marrow Transplant*. 1994; 14:665–666.

145. Sauerbrey A, Bielack S, Kempf-Bielack B, et al. High-dose chemotherapy (HDC) and autologous hematopoietic stem cell transplantation (ASCT) as salvage therapy for relapsed osteosarcoma. *Bone Marrow Transplant*. 2001;27: 933–937.

146. Fagioli F, Aglietta M, Tienghi A, et al. High-dose chemotherapy in the treatment of relapsed osteosarcoma: an Italian sarcoma group study. *J Clin Oncol*. 2002;20:2150–2156.

147. Gorlick R, Huvos AG, Heller G, et al. Expression of HER2/erbB-2 correlates with survival in osteosarcoma. *J Clin Oncol*. 1999;17:2781–2788.

148. Heiner JP, Miraldi F, Kallick S, et al. Localization of GD2-specific monoclonal antibody 3F8 in human osteosarcoma. *Cancer Res*. 1987;47:5377–5381.

149. Rao RD, Anderson PM, Arndt C, et al. Aerosolized granulocyte macrophage colony-stimulating factor (GM-CSF) therapy in metastatic cancer. *Am J Clin Oncol*. 2003;26:493–498.

150. Pollak M, Sem AW, Richard M, et al. Inhibition of metastatic behavior of murine osteosarcoma by hypophysectomy. *J Natl Cancer Inst*. 1992;84:966–971.

151. Merimsky O, Meller I, Flusser G, et al. Gemcitabine in soft tissue or bone sarcoma resistant to standard chemotherapy: a phase II study. *Cancer Chemother Pharmacol*. 2000;45:177–181.

152. Meyers PA, Schwartz CL, Bernstein M, et al. Addition of ifosfamide and muramyl tripeptide to cisplatin, doxorubicin and high-dose methotrexate improves event free survival (EFS) in localized osteosarcoma (OS). *Proc Am Soc Clin Oncol*. 2001;20:1463a.

153. Le D, Guinebretière G, et al. SFOP OS94: a randomised trial comparing preoperative high-dose methotrexate plus doxorubicin to high-dose methotrexate plus etoposide and ifosfamide in osteosarcoma patients. *Eur J Cancer*. 2007;43:752–761.

154. Marina NM, Pratt CB, Rao BN, et al. Improved prognosis of children with osteosarcoma metastatic to the lung(s) at the time of diagnosis [published erratum appears in *Cancer*. 1993;71(9):2879]. *Cancer.* 1992;70:2722–2727.

155. Hosalkar HS, Dormans JP. Limb sparing surgery for pediatric musculoskeletal tumors. *Pediatr Blood Cancer*. 2004;42:295–310.

156. Goorin AM, Chauvenet AR, Perez-Atayde AR, et al. Initial congestive heart failure, six to ten years after doxorubicin chemotherapy for childhood cancer. *J Pediatr*. 1990;116:144–147.

157. Lipshultz SE, Lipsitz SR, Mone SM, et al. Female sex and higher drug dose as risk factors for late cardiotoxic effects of doxorubicin therapy for childhood cancer. *N Engl J Med*. 1995;332:1738–1743.

158. Aung L, Gorlick RG, Shi W, et al. Second malignant neoplasms in long-term survivors of osteosarcoma: Memorial Sloan-Kettering Cancer Center Experience. *Cancer.* 2002;95:1728–1734.

159. Brock PR, Bellman SC, Yeomans EC, et al. Cisplatin ototoxicity in children: a practical grading system. *Med Pediatr Oncol*. 1991;19:295–300.

160. Schaefer SD, Post JD, Close LG, et al. Ototoxicity of low- and moderate-dose cisplatin. *Cancer.* 1985;56:1934–1939.

161. Gonzalez-Vitale JC, Hayes DM, Cvitkovic E, et al. The renal pathology in clinical trials of cis-platinum (II) diamminedichloride. *Cancer.* 1977;39: 1362–1371.

162. Hayes DM, Cvitkovic E, Golbey RB, et al. High dose cis-platinum diammine dichloride: amelioration of renal toxicity by mannitol diuresis. *Cancer.* 1977; 39:1372–1381.

163. Marina NM, Poquette CA, Cain AM, et al. Comparative renal tubular toxicity of chemotherapy regimens including ifosfamide in patients with newly diagnosed sarcomas. *J Pediatr Hematol Oncol*. 2000;22:112–118.

164. Pratt CB, Meyer WH, Jenkins JJ, et al. Ifosfamide, Fanconi's syndrome, and rickets. *J Clin Oncol*. 1991;9:1495–1499.

Ewing Sarcoma Family of Tumors

Jeffrey A. Toretsky, Heinrich Kovar, Michael Paulussen, R. Lor Randall, Andreas Schuck, Lisa A. Teot, Heribert Juergens, and Mark Bernstein

Introduction

The Ewing Sarcoma Family of Tumors (ESFT) is the second most frequent primary malignant bone cancer, after osteosarcoma, diagnosed in patients younger than 20 years. It is slightly more common in males (55 male: 45 female). The most common age of diagnosis is the second decade of life, although 20% to 30% of cases are diagnosed in younger children, and in one series approximately 20% were diagnosed in patients older than 20 years. The disease is more common in Caucasians than Asians and especially African Americans, or Africans, in whom the disease is rare.[1,2]

Presentation

Local pain is the most common presenting symptom in patients with ESFT. The pain can be intermittent and variable in intensity.[3] Because the majority of ESFT patients are in their second decade of life and physically active, pain is often mistaken for "bone growth" or injuries resulting from sport or everyday activities. Pain may be accompanied by paresthesia in some cases. Pain as the initial symptom may be followed by a palpable mass. The duration of symptoms prior to the definitive diagnosis can be weeks to months, or rarely even years, with a median of 3 to 9 months.[3–5] Pain without a history of trauma consistent with the symptoms, pain lasting longer than a month, and/or pain continuing at night should prompt imaging studies. Slight or moderate fever and other nonspecific symptoms are more common in more advanced and/or metastatic stages. About one-quarter of patients have metastatic disease at initial presentation.[3–6]

Tumor growth will eventually lead to a visible or palpable swelling of the affected site. The tumor bulk, however, may be indiscernible for a long time in patients with pelvic, chest wall, or femoral tumors. Because ESFT may arise in virtually any bone and from soft tissue, additional symptoms may vary depending on the affected site. Spinal cord compression by a vertebral body tumor requires emergency intervention, either laminectomy or chemo- or radiotherapy following biopsy. Patients with chest wall or pelvic primaries may experience significant complaints only at a very late stage.

On initial physical examination, tendonitis is often an initial diagnosis in adolescent or adult patients, while hip inflammation and osteomyelitis are often suspected in younger children.[3] In patients with metastatic disease, non-specific symptoms such as malaise and fever may resemble symptoms of septicemia. Such patients sometimes also experience loss of appetite and weight. Children younger than 5 years may thus present a constellation of symptoms similar to those of disseminated neuroblastoma, although ESFT is uncommon in children younger than 5 years.

No blood, serum, or urine test can specifically identify ESFT. Nonspecific signs of tumor or inflammation may be noted, such as an elevated erythrocyte sedimentation rate, moderate anemia, or leukocytosis. Elevated levels of serum lactate dehydrogenase (LDH) correlate with tumor burden and for this reason with inferior outcome.

Most ESFTs occur in bones, and their locations tend to differ from those usually noted for osteosarcoma. Flat bones of the axial skeleton are relatively more commonly affected by ESFT, and in long bones ESFTs tend to arise from the diaphyseal rather than the metaphyseal portion. The most common primary locations of ESFTs are the pelvic bones, the long bones of the lower extremities, and the bones of the chest wall (Figure 28-1). Primary metastases in lungs, bone, bone marrow, or a combination of sites are detectable in about 25% of patients. Metastases to lymph nodes or other sites like liver or central nervous system are rare.

When an osseous lesion is suspected, a radiograph in two planes should be part of the initial diagnostic evaluation. Tumor-related osteolysis, detachment of the periosteum from the bone (Codman triangle), and calcification in soft tissue tumor masses suggest the diagnosis of a malignant bone tumor. Osteomyelitis may present a pattern similar to ESFT on plain radiograph. Diaphyseal location suggests an ESFT, as compared with the metaphyseal location more common in osteosarcoma. Magnetic resonance imaging (MRI) provides the most precise definition of local disease, including intramedullary extension and any involvement of neurovascular structures (Figure 28-2).[3,7–10]

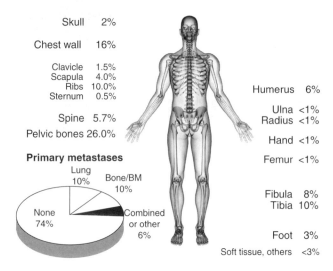

Skull 2%
Chest wall 16%
Clavicle 1.5%
Scapula 4.0%
Ribs 10.0%
Sternum 0.5%
Spine 5.7%
Pelvic bones 26.0%
Humerus 6%
Ulna <1%
Radius <1%
Hand <1%
Femur <1%
Fibula 8%
Tibia 10%
Foot 3%
Soft tissue, others <3%

Primary metastases
Lung 10%
Bone/BM 10%
None 74%
Combined or other 6%

Figure 28-1 Primary tumor sites in Ewing Sarcoma. Data based on 1426 patients from (EI)CESS trials.

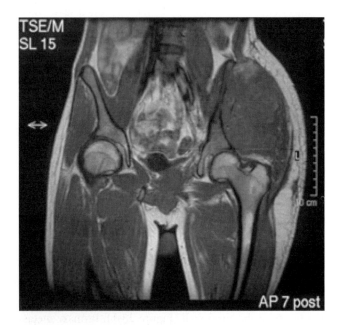

Figure 28-2 Pelvic Ewing Sarcoma, MRI.

Pathophysiology

There are no known causes of ESFT, and therefore cases are thought to be sporadic. However, family members of ESFT patients have an increased incidence of neuroecto-dermal and stomach malignancies.[11] Growth parameters such as height and weight have not been linked to the development of ESFTs.[12] Ewing Sarcoma has occurred as a second neoplasm, although the exact incidence is unknown.

Arguments for both neuronal and epithelial origins of ESFTs have been advanced. Ewing Sarcoma has generally been considered to derive from a neuroectodermal cell, possibly a postganglionic cholinergic neuron.[13] Alternatively, mesenchymal bone marrow cells demonstrate ESFT

phenotypic features when transfected with an EWS-FLI1 construct, which may indicate their potential as the "normal homologue of ESFT."[14,15]

The translocation t(11;22)(q24;q12), or another in a series of related translocations, occurs in greater than 95% of ESFTs. Some argue that such a translocation is pathognomonic and is both necessary and sufficient for a diagnosis of ESFT. The classic t(11;22)(q24;q12) translocation joins the 5′ portion of the ESFT (*EWS*) gene located on chromosome 22 to the 3′ portion of an *ets*-family gene, FLI1 (*Friend Leukemia Insertion*), located on chromosome 11.[16] The rearrangement results in the translocation of the 3′ portion of the fli1 (*Friend leukemia virus integration site 1*) gene from chromosome 11 to the 5′ portion of the ESFT gene ews on chromosome 22 (Figure 28-3). It occurs in about 75% of ESFT patients.

In most of the remaining cases, variant translocations are observed, always involving chromosomes 22q12 and either 21q22 (10% of ESFTs) or 7p22, 17q12, and 2q36 (fewer than 1% of ESFTs each). In the rare variant translocations ews is fused to genes closely related to *FLI1*, either *ERG, E1AF/ETV4/PEA3, ETV1/ER81,* or *FEV.* These variant translocations frequently occur as either complex or interstitial chromosomal rearrangements and are therefore difficult to diagnose by conventional cytogenetics. Additional structural chromosome changes can be observed in ESFTs.[17–19]

The EWS-FLI1 fusion transcript encodes a 68-kDa protein with two primary domains. The EWS domain is a potent transcriptional activator, while the FLI1 domain contains a highly conserved *ets* DNA-binding domain. The EWS-FLI1 fusion protein thus acts as an aberrant transcription factor and transforms mouse fibroblasts. To effect this transformation, both the EWS and FLI1 functional domains must be intact.[20] In addition, the IGF-I receptor (IGF-IR) is required for EWS-FLI1 to transform fibroblasts.[21] When the expression level of EWS-FLI1 is reduced by antisense RNA or antisense oligonucleotides, ESFT cell lines die and tumors in nude mice regress.[22–24]

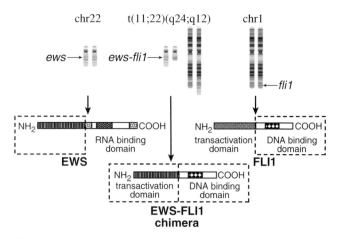

Figure 28-3 The reciprocal translocation between chromosomes 11 and 22 results in the formation of an *EWS-FLI1* fusion gene on the abnormal chromosome 22 that codes for a chimeric transcription factor with the N-terminal transcriptional regulatory domain deriving from EWS and the ETS specific DNA binding domain derived from FLI1.

These studies have established the critical nature of the EWS-FLI1 transcript to ESFT cells and its role as a therapeutic target. Effective strategies for reducing the activity of EWS-FLI1 in ESFT patients through novel delivery systems of small interfering (si) RNA are in development.[25,26] Early investigations of EWS-FLI1-induced transformation of mouse fibroblasts demonstrated that not all fibroblasts could be equally transformed. The fibroblasts that were transformable were immortalized and were found to lack some component of the G1 checkpoint, most often p16(INK4a).[27] Approximately 25% of ESFTs from patients have been shown to lack some component of the G1 checkpoint, either p16, p15, p14, p53, or p21.[28] The role of the loss of these checkpoint genes on patient survival is discussed in the section on prognosis.

Biopsy, Pathology, and Molecular Pathology

As for other malignant diseases, the definitive diagnostic test is the biopsy. Although the diagnosis can be made by fine needle aspiration biopsy or by core needle biopsy, the most adequate sampling is achieved by open biopsy. The initial biopsy is usually incisional rather than excisional, and usually from the soft tissue extension of the primary bone mass, except in the rare case of a small lesion in an expendable bone such as the proximal fibula. The biopsy incision is usually longitudinal, so as to not violate tissue flap planes and neurovascular structures. A longitudinal incision can thus facilitate eventual complete excision and limb salvage, if surgery is to be the primary mode of local control. The biopsy is best performed by an experienced orthopedic oncologist, especially by one working as part of a multidisciplinary oncology team.[29] Frozen section to confirm the adequacy of the tissue sample is essential, and the tissue should be rapidly sent while fresh, prior to fixation, to the pathology department so that subsequent molecular genetic assays and tissue banking can be performed.

Ewing Sarcoma encompasses tumors with a spectrum of histologic appearances and ultrastructural and immunohistochemical features. Classic ESFT, as first described by James Ewing in 1921,[30] is composed of a monotonous population of small, round cells with high nuclear to cytoplasmic ratios arrayed in sheets (Figure 28-4A). The cells have scant, faintly eosinophilic to amphophilic cytoplasm, indistinct cytoplasmic borders, and round nuclei with evenly distributed, finely granular chromatin and inconspicuous nucleoli (Figure 28-4B).[31–33] Mitotic activity is usually low. Cytoplasmic glycogen, which appears as periodic acid-Schiff positive diastase-digestible granules, is usually present.

Strong expression of the cell-surface glycoprotein p30/32^{MIC2} (CD99) is characteristic of ESFT, and strong, diffuse membrane staining in a "chainmail pattern" is present in 95% to 100% of ESFTs with one or more of the monoclonal antibodies to this antigen, including O13, 12E7, and HBA71 (Figure 28-4C).[34–36] High expression of CD99 has been found to correlate with the presence of a classic or variant ESFT chromosomal translocation.[37–39] In addition,

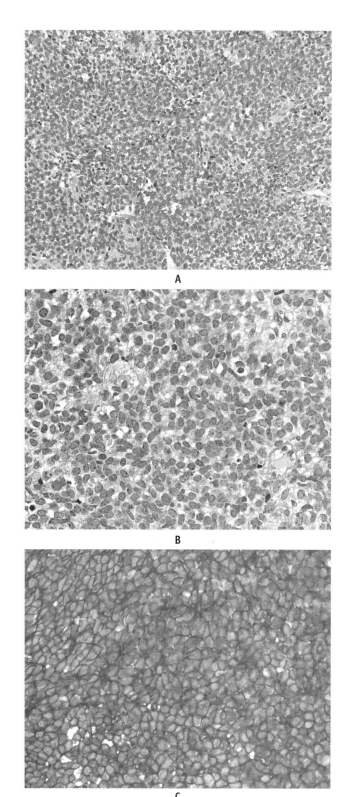

Figure 28-4 (A) Histologic and immunohistochemical features of Ewing Sarcoma/pPNET: Classic Ewing Sarcoma appears as sheets of monotonous, round cells. (Hematoxylin and eosin, original magnification X200). (B) Histologic and immunohistochemical features of Ewing Sarcoma/pPNET: The cells have scanty cytoplasm and round nuclei with evenly distributed finely granular chromatin and inconspicuous nucleoli. (Hematoxylin and eosin, original magnification X400). (C) Histologic and immunohistochemical features of Ewing Sarcoma/pPNET: Strong, diffuse membrane staining is observed with the O13 monoclonal antibody to p30/32^{MIC2}. (Immunoperoxidase, original magnification X400). **See Plates 48-50 for color images.**

ESFT is immunoreactive for vimentin.[40–42] More differentiated ESFTs (peripheral primitive neuroectodermal tumors, pPNET) may also show immunohistochemical evidence of neural differentiation, staining for neuron-specific enolase (NSE), S-100 protein, Leu-7, and/or PgP 9.5.[43] Ewing Sarcoma is immunoreactive for cytokeratins in up to 20% of cases, with diffuse immunoreactivity for cytokeratins noted in up to 10% of cases.[44]

Because the histologic and immunophenotypic features of ESFTs overlap to varying degrees with the other small, round cell tumors of childhood, an expanded panel of immunohistochemical studies may be necessary to exclude other entities. Like ESFT, neuroblastoma is immunoreactive for NSE, S-100, and Leu-7, but in contrast to the pPNET variant of ESFT, it is negative for vimentin and immunoreactive for neurofilament protein. Like ESFT, lymphoblastic lymphoma is strongly immunoreactive for CD99 in a membrane pattern, but unlike the former, lymphoblastic lymphoma is also immunoreactive for leukocyte common antigen (CD45) and/or TdT and other lymphoid markers. Rhabdomyosarcoma may also be immunoreactive with antibodies to CD99; however, staining is usually focal, weak, and cytoplasmic, and in contradistinction to ESFT, rhabdomyosarcoma is immunoreactive for myogenin, myoD1, desmin, and actin. The distinction between poorly differentiated small cell synovial sarcoma and poorly differentiated ESFT may be difficult in some cases. Although synovial sarcoma is immunoreactive for cytokeratin and/or EMA, poorly differentiated small cell variants may be immunoreactive for CD99 in a membrane pattern and show only focal, weak staining for cytokeratin, thus mimicking poorly differentiated ESFT.

Molecular genetic studies, using fluorescent in situ hybridization and/or reverse transcriptase–polymerase chain reaction (RT-PCR), are valuable adjuncts for the evaluation of undifferentiated small, round cell tumors of childhood, particularly in cases with indeterminate histologic and/or immunohistochemical features. Detection of characteristic translocations by these methods may allow for definitive diagnosis of ESFT, rhabdomyosarcoma, and synovial sarcoma.[45,46] Distinction between these tumors is critical, because their treatments are significantly different.

With the availability of molecular tools to confirm unambiguously the presence of EWS-ETS gene rearrangements, the spectrum of ESFT-related neoplasms has recently been expanded to include rare CD99[MIC2]-positive extraskeletal tumors in various anatomic sites including kidney,[47–51] breast,[48] gastrointestinal tract,[52–55] prostate,[56] endometrium,[57] lung,[51] adrenal gland,[58] and meninges.[59] Although ESFTs typically arise during adolescence, there is also an increasing number of adults being diagnosed with a CD99[MIC2] and EWS-ETS positive small, round cell tumor. The oldest patient reported to date was 77 years old.[60–61]

Staging

Diagnostic staging at presentation must include an appropriate search and staging for metastases, which will be detected in about 25% of patients (Table 28-1). The most common metastatic sites are the lungs and the pleural space, the skeletal system, and the bone marrow, or combinations thereof. Locoregional lymph node involvement is rare. Imaging studies should include computed tomography scan of the chest to document or exclude intrathoracic metastases and 99m-Technetium whole-body radionuclide bone scans to search for skeletal metastases. Fluorine-18 fluorodeoxyglucose positron emission tomography (FDG-PET) has recently proven to be a highly sensitive screening method for detection of bone metastases in ESFTs.[62] However, the specificity was only 73% in one series. The exact role of FDG-PET imaging in the management of ESFT remains to be defined. The use of FDG-PET may also be of value in delineating the initial response to therapy as shown by change in the standard uptake value (SUV). Perhaps more important, the measured SUV after induction chemotherapy may predict outcome.[62]

Microscopically detectable bone marrow metastases occur in fewer than 10% of patients and are associated with a poor prognosis.[63] Since tumor cells may be focally distributed in bone marrow, bone marrow samples should

Table 28-1
Staging investigations at diagnosis.

Investigation	Primary Tumor Site	Staging for Metastases
Radiograph in two planes, whole bone with adjacent joints	+	at suspicious sites
MRI and/or CT, affected bone(s) and adjacent joints	+	at suspicious sites
Biopsy: material for histology and molecular biology	+	at suspicious sites
Thoracic CT (lung window)		+
Bone marrow biopsy and aspirates: microscopy (molecular biology still investigational)		+
Whole-body 99m-technetium bone scan	+	+
FDG-PET	+*	+*

Abbreviations: MRI, magnetic resonance imaging; CT, computed tomography; FDG-PET, fluorine-18 fluorodeoxyglucose positron emission tomography; +, mandatory; +*, indicated, if available.

be harvested from multiple sites, conventionally both posterior iliac crests. Aspirates or trephine biopsies are analyzed by light microscopy. If the tumor is of pelvic origin, an aspirate or trephine may contain tumor from the primary site and not reflect metastatic disease. The prognostic relevance of detection of micrometastatic disease by RT-PCR in the absence of overt bone marrow metastases is under current evaluation in prospective studies. Preliminary results from retrospective analyses seem to indicate that RT-PCR detection of ESFT-specific RNA in the bone marrow at diagnosis[64,65] and persistence of such findings despite adequate chemotherapy[66] may be related to an inferior outcome.

Current Treatment

Before the era of chemotherapy, fewer than 10% of patients with ESFTs survived, despite the well-known radiosensitivity of this tumor.[67,68] Patients commonly died of metastases within two years, indicating the need for systemic treatment.[67] With the use of modern multimodal therapeutic regimens including combination chemotherapy, surgery, and radiotherapy, cure rates of 50% and more can be achieved.[69–83] The treatment of ESFT patients worldwide is organized in cooperative trials, aiming to improve treatment outcome further.

Prognostic Features

A number of prognostic features correlate with ultimate outcome for patients with ESFT. Overall survival in patients with ESFT is 60%. For patients with localized disease it approaches 70%. Those patients with isolated pulmonary metastases have a slightly better outcome (approximately 30% survive) when compared with those with bone or bone marrow metastases at initial diagnosis (20% or fewer).[77,82,84] The presence of metastatic disease at initial presentation has been reproducibly the most significant adverse prognostic factor in the treatment of patients with ESFT despite aggressive chemotherapy.[77] The prognostic factors that have been repeatedly evaluated in multiple clinical trials include age at diagnosis, sex, serum LDH levels, size and location of tumor, and neural differentiation. In early ESFT studies, the most reproducible prognostic factor in patients with localized disease was tumor volume. In general, larger tumors (often axial, volume > 200 ml) had a poorer prognosis and correlated with other poor prognostic factors. Aggressive multiagent chemotherapy as well as effective local management has somewhat reduced the prognostic value of such indices. Most studies show a trend to improved survival in patients who are younger (less than 10 or 15 years) but not all reports are in agreement.[82] In contrast, there has been some question as to the outcome of the limited number of infants with ESFTs. A recent retrospective evaluation of infants with ESFT identified 14 infants (age < 12 months) enrolled over a 25-year period. Their outcome was similar to that of older children.[61] Persistence of ESFT-specific RNA in bone marrow after treatment may also be unfavorable.[63]

Molecular features holding great promise for separating standard- from high-risk patients with localized disease are p53 mutation or the homozygous deletion of p16/p14ARF. In a retrospective analysis cohort of 60 patients who received 5-drug therapy, tumors in 13% had confirmed p53 mutation. No patients whose tumor had a p53 mutation survived beyond 2 years from diagnosis. The same cohort demonstrated 13% whose tumor had homozygous p16/p14ARF deletion, which also predicted for poor survival in both univariate and multivariate analysis.[85]

Many additional molecular markers have begun to be evaluated as prognostic indicators in patients with ESFT. Several of these include translocation breakpoint regions and other chromosomal abnormalities. Among individual patients the t(11;22) may result from the fusion of different exons from EWS and FLI1 to form the fusion message. The most common combination is the EWS exon 7 fused to FLI1 exon 6 (type 1 translocation), which occurs in approximately 50% to 64% of ESFTs. Retrospective analyses have suggested that patients who have localized tumors with the 7/6 fusion may have a 70% 4-year survival, while patients with the other variants had a 20% 4-year survival.[86] The more recent cohort of 60 patients reported from Memorial Sloan-Kettering Cancer Center (MSKCC) showed a trend that did not reach statistical significance between patients whose tumors expressed type 1 versus the other translocations.[85] The prognostic value of translocation type is the subject of ongoing prospective evaluation. Loss of chromosome 1p36 has been associated with poor prognosis in patients with localized disease.[17] Additional abnormalities, including +8 and +12, may portend a better prognosis.[17]

Local Therapy

Cure of ESFT can be achieved only with both chemotherapy and local control measures. Current treatment schedules favor primary induction chemotherapy, followed by local therapy and then further adjuvant chemotherapy. For several decades, radiotherapy was regarded as the standard local treatment modality; contemporary orthopedic surgery, however, is aimed at preservation of function and improved limb salvage without compromising survival rates.[87–90] In planning the optimal local therapy, an interdisciplinary approach involving experts experienced in this field is essential. The efficacy of this approach has been shown in 2 consecutive European trials by the reduction of local recurrences following the institution of centralized counseling regarding local therapy, including radiation therapy.[91] Local treatment should be individually adapted depending upon the site and size of the tumor, the anatomical structures near the tumor, the patient's age, and individual preference.

Surgical Treatment of Ewing Sarcoma

In general, patients with an isolated, resectable tumor after induction chemotherapy should have the tumor treated with surgery alone. Preoperative radiotherapy may be necessary to avoid an intralesional resection (Table 28-2).

Table 28-2

Enneking classification of surgical intervention.

Intralesional resection	Tumor opened during surgery, or surgical field contaminated, or microscopic or macroscopic residual disease.
Marginal resection	Tumor removed en bloc, however, resection through the pseudocapsule of the tumor; microscopic residual disease likely.
Wide resection	Tumor and its pseudocapsule removed en bloc, surrounded by healthy tissue, within the tumor-bearing compartment.
Radical resection	The whole tumor-bearing compartment is removed en bloc, eg, above-knee amputation in lower leg tumor.

When a negative surgical margin is obtained following preoperative irradiation, results are comparable to those achieved with negative margin surgery for more amenable lesions. In Children's Oncology Group protocols, negative margins are defined as bony margins of at least 1 cm, with a 2 to 5 cm margin recommended. In soft tissue, at least 5 mm in fat or muscle is required, with 2 mm through fascial planes, with the margin being through noninflammatory tissue.

When surgery is planned, limb salvage is almost always attempted, although there remain a small number of lesions for which either limb salvage surgery or irradiation would lead to an unsatisfactory orthopedic result, and in whom amputation is warranted.

Types of Reconstruction The main reconstructive options include autogenous bone grafts, structural bone allografts (intercalary or osteoarticular), and metallic endoprosthetics. Allografts and endoprosthetics may also be used as part of a composite reconstruction. Autogenous bone grafts may be vascularized (eg, fibula). The technique employed is a function of the location of the tumor, age of the patient, and types of adjuvant therapies that will be employed (ie, chemotherapy and/or radiation). Infection, nonunion, and fracture may complicate the surgery, especially since patients will be receiving continuing chemotherapy and possibly radiotherapy.[92–94]

Generally, after induction (neoadjuvant) chemotherapy, a preoperative follow-up assessment of the tumor must be performed. The response to chemotherapy can be assessed by dynamic MRI. Positron emission tomography and thallium may also provide useful information.[62,95–99] In certain cases, an individual who was a questionable candidate for limb salvage may be eligible after induction chemotherapy. Patients who remain borderline candidates following induction chemotherapy may be considered for preoperative radiotherapy. If the margins are certain to be inadequate at the preoperative staging evaluation, then amputation is the only available surgical option.

Because ESFTs are radiosensitive, radiation may be used instead of or in addition to surgery.

Radiotherapy
Indications for Radiotherapy
To date, there has been no randomized trial comparing local therapy modalities. Therefore, the question as to which modality, radiotherapy or surgery, is preferred for local therapy in ESFT has been a matter of debate for some time. From retrospective analyses of several groups, the impression has been that local control is improved when surgery is possible.[90,100,101] These data are usually confounded by the fact that there is a selection bias favoring patients in whom surgery is possible. Several European and North American collaborative trials have been performed. Overall, local control rates range from 53% to 93%, with the poorer results usually reported in the earlier series.[75,76,78,102,103]

Definitive Radiotherapy Patients who receive radiotherapy as the only local therapy modality usually represent an unfavorable group of patients. They frequently present with large tumors, or tumors in unfavorable locations (eg, vertebral tumors), or both, making radiotherapy difficult but surgery impossible. In a recent analysis of 1058 patients with localized ESFT treated in the European Intergroup Cooperative ESFT Studies (EICESS) trials, 266 patients had radiotherapy alone. Local or combined local and systemic failures in this subgroup occurred in 26% of patients,[90,100] which was worse than the recurrence rate following surgery with or without radiotherapy (4%-10%). It was not possible to define a subgroup of patients in whom the use of radiotherapy alone achieved the same local control rate as surgery. Even for the favorable subgroup of patients with small extremity tumors, local control with surgery was better than with definitive radiotherapy. Therefore, when marginal or wide resection is possible, surgery should be performed.

In contrast, debulking procedures do not improve local control and are associated with additional unnecessary morbidity. In the experience of the European Cooperative ESFT Studies (CESS) and the EICESS trials, patients who had an intralesional resection followed by radiotherapy had the same local control rate as patients who had radiotherapy alone.[90,100] Therefore, if only a debulking procedure is possible, surgery should not be included as part of local control. Rather, definitive radiotherapy should be administered.

Radiation Dose and Fractionation In order to control ESFTs, a radiation dose above 40 Gy is necessary. In the St Jude's Children's Research Hospital experience with the use of lower radiation doses, a high rate of local recurrence was observed.[102] A clear dose response correlation at doses above 40 Gy has not yet been established. For definitive radiotherapy, doses between 55 and 60 Gy, most frequently not exceeding 55.8 Gy, are usually given. When surgery precedes or follows radiotherapy, the doses range between 45 Gy and 55 Gy depending on the individual risk factors (ie, resection margins and response). It is uncertain whether irradiation of the site of completely resected lesions that demonstrate a poor histologic response is of benefit. European investigators recommend such irradiation, whereas it is not incorporated in North American protocols. There has been no controlled trial addressing this issue.

Usually conventional fractionation with daily fractions of 1.8 Gy to 2 Gy is given. In the CESS 86 and EICESS 92 trials, hyperfractionated radiotherapy with twice daily doses of 1.6 Gy was also applied; after 22.4 Gy a 10-day break was scheduled to permit the administration of chemotherapy. There has been no detectable difference in local control between the 2 different fractionation groups.[104]

Target Volume Definition and Treatment Planning

In a randomized trial, the treatment of the whole tumor-bearing compartment showed no better results than radiation to the tumor and an additional safety margin.[103] Therefore, the planning target volume is defined as the initial tumor extent on MRI with an additional longitudinal margin of at least 2 to 3 cm and lateral margins of 2 cm in long bones. If doses of more than 45 Gy are used, a shrinking field technique is applied. In patients with an axial tumor site, a minimum of a 2 cm safety margin around the initial tumor extent must be employed. In tumors protruding into preformed cavities (ie, thorax, pelvis) without infiltration, the residual intracavitary tumor volume following chemotherapy is used for treatment planning. Surgically contaminated areas, scars, and drainage sites must be included in the radiation fields. Circumferential irradiation of extremities should be avoided in order to reduce the risk of lymphedema. In growing children, growth plates must be considered. They should either be fully included in the radiation field or not be included at all. A dose gradient through the epiphysis results in asymmetric growth and may lead to functional deficits. Similarly, vertebral bodies should be either fully included or spared from the radiation field.

Three-dimensional conformal radiotherapy should be given in patients with ESFT. In selected cases—for example, in vertebral tumors—intensity modulated radiotherapy or proton therapy may be beneficial.

Chemotherapy

The first reports of drug treatment of ESFT stem from the 1960s. In 1962 Sutow and Pinkel independently published reports on the use of cyclophosphamide for ESFT.[105,106] With Hustu's publication on the combination of cyclophosphamide, vincristine, and radiotherapy that resulted in sustained responses in 5 patients, the era of modern multimodality treatment of ESFT began.[70] Results

of selected Phase III studies in Ewing Sarcoma are listed in Table 28-3.

In brief, in 1974 Rosen from the MSKCC published the first results of a trial of radiotherapy given with a 4-drug regimen consisting of vincristine, actinomycin D, cyclophosphamide, and doxorubicin (VACD) used in combination rather than sequentially, leading to long-term survival in 12 patients with ESFT.[72] The VACD regimen then became a standard therapy in numerous clinical trials. The first Intergroup ESFT Study IESS-I showed the superiority of the VACD 4-drug regimen over a 3-drug VAC regimen (without doxorubicin), in terms of effectiveness of local control (96% vs 86%) and event-free survival (EFS) (60% vs 24%).[75] On the basis of excellent Phase II results achieved with the combination of ifosfamide and etoposide (IE),[114–116] Pediatric Oncology Group–Children's Cancer Group (POG-CCG) study INT-0091 randomized VACD versus VACD-IE. The VACD arm achieved 54% 5-year EFS in patients with localized disease, as compared with 69% EFS in the experimental arm with addition of IE.[82] Therefore, in North America, the 5-drug alternating regimen is considered standard. There have been parallel investigations in Europe. The ongoing Euro-ESFT study includes induction vincristine-ifosfamide-doxorubicin-etoposide for all patients with newly diagnosed ESFT.[117]

Contemporary investigations include the recently completed Children's Oncology Group study, AEWS 0031, that used the strategy of interval compression, with therapy administered every 2 weeks in the experimental arm as compared with every 3 weeks in the standard arm. Time-dose intensity of all drugs was thus increased, perhaps interacting in a favorable way with cell cycle kinetics of the malignant cell population. Interval compression was successfully achieved in a preceding limited institution pilot study.[118] Recently analyzed information from the groupwide study (AEWS 0031) supports its feasibility. In addition, the compressed arm showed an advantage in EFS, 76% vs 65% at 4 years ($p = 0.029$) and in overall survival, 91% vs 85% at 4 years ($p = 0.026$, unpublished data, R. Womer). The next randomized Children's Oncology Group study will incorporate vincristine, topotecan, and cyclophosphamide containing cycles for one-half of patients, on the basis of encouraging classic and window Phase II studies.[119,120] This study will be preceded by a pilot study examining the feasibility of interval compression of the regimen containing vincristine, topotecan, and cyclophosphamide, because compressed regimens will be used, given the superiority of the compressed arm of AEWS 0031 as compared with the standard-timing arm.

Another treatment intensification strategy in ESFT is high-dose chemotherapy with autologous hematopoietic stem cell rescue (HDT).[121] Due to the considerable toxicity of this approach, most studies investigate HDT for very high risk patients, most commonly those with metastatic disease at diagnosis, or following recurrence.[84,122–124] Part of the ongoing EUROpean Ewing tumour Working Initiative of National Groups 1999 (Euro-EWING) 99 study is a controlled, randomized study of HDT for patients with large primary tumors locally treated with both surgery and irra-

Table 28-3

Treatment results in selected clinical studies of localized Ewing Sarcoma.

Study	Schedule	Patients	5-year EFS	p§	Comments
IESS studies					
IESS-I [1973–1978][75]	VAC	342	24%	VAC/VAC + WLI: 0.001	Value of D
	VAC + WLI		44%	VAC/VACD: 0.001	Benefit of WLI?
	VACD		60%	VAC + WLI/VACD: 0.05	
IESS-II [1978–1982][76]	VACD-HD	214	68%	0.03	Value of aggressive cytoreduction
	VACD-MD		48%		
First POG–CCG (INT-0091) [1988–1993][82]	VACD	200	54%	0,005	Value of combination IE in localized disease, no benefit in metastatic disease
	VACD + IE	198	69%		
Second POG–CCG [1995–1998][107]	VCD + IE 48 weeks	492	75% (3 years)	0.57	No benefit of dose-time compression
	VCD + IE 30 weeks		76% (3 years)		
Memorial Sloan-Kettering					
T2 [1970–1978][108]	VACD (adjuvant)	20	75%		After local therapy only, cumulative dose of D up to 600 mg/m²
P6 [1990–1995][109]	HD-CVD + IE	36	77% (2 years)		C dose escalation 4.2g/m²/course
P6 [1991–2001][81]	HD-CVD + IE	68	localized: 81% (4 years); metastatic: 12% (4 years)		Good results in localized disease, poor outcome in metastatic patients
St Jude studies					
ES-79 [1978–1986][110]	VACD	52	82% <8 cm (3 years); 64% ≥8 cm (3 years)		Tumor size as prognostic factor
ES-87 [1987–1991][111]	Therapeutic window with IE VCDIE × 3	26	Clinical responses in 96%		Combination IE effective
EW-92 [1992–1996][112]	VCD/IE Intensific.	34	78% (3 years)		Tumor size (≥ 8 cm) loses prognostic relevance with more intensive treatment
ROI Bologna/Italy					
REN-3 [1991–1997][139]	VDC + VIA + IE	157	71%		Surgery in 78% of patients
SFOP/France					
EW-88 [1988–1991][79]	VD + VD/VA	141	58%		Histological response better predictor of outcome comparable to tumor volume
SSG/Scandinavia					
SSG IX [1990–1999][113]	VID + PID	88	58% (metastases-free survival); 41%		70% overall survival after 5 years
UKCCSG/MRC studies					
ET-1 [1978–1986][5]	VACD	120	Extr. 52%; Axial 38%; Pelvic 13%		Tumor site as the most important prognostic factor
ET-2 [1987–1993][78]	VAID	201	62%; Extr. 73%; Axial 55%; Pelvic 41%		Importance of the administration of high-dose alkylating agents (I)
CESS studies					
CESS-81 [1981–1985][74]	VACD	93	<100 ml 80%; ≥100 ml 31% (both 3 yrs); Viable tumor >10%: 79%; >10%: 31% (both 3 yrs)		Tumor volume (≥100 ml) and histological response are prognostic factors
CESS-86 [1986–1991][80]	<100 ml (SR): VACD; ≥100 ml (HR): VAID	301	52% (10 years); 51% (10 years)		Intensive treatment with I for high-risk patients. Tumor volume (≥200 ml) and histologic response as prognostic factor
EICESS studies (CESS + UKCCSG)					
EICESS-92 [1992–1999] (EICESS group, personal communication, May 2004)	SR: VAID/VACD	155	68%/61%	0.8406	Stage, histologic response, type of local therapy as prognostic factors; randomized comparisons^ns
	HR: VAID/EVAID	326	51%/61%	0.2141	

§ p-Values are given only for trials comparing randomized treatment arms.

Abbreviations: EFS, event-free survival; NA, not available; A, actinomycin D; D, doxorubicin; E, etoposide, I, ifosfamide; P, cisplatinum; V, vincristine; WLI, whole lung irradiation; HD, high-dose; MD, moderate-dose; SR, standard risk; HR, high risk; ns, not significant.

diation, or small primary tumors (volume < 200 ml) and an unfavorable histologic or radiologic response to induction chemotherapy (arm R2loc). Accrual is ongoing.[117] Due to the intrinsic risk of using high-dose therapy, such efforts should be strictly limited to the setting of controlled clinical trials.[125,126]

Metastatic Disease

At initial diagnosis, approximately 25% of ESFT patients present with clinically detectable metastases in the lung and/or in bone and/or in bone marrow. The presence of metastatic disease is the most important adverse prognostic factor.[63,77,82,127] Patients with isolated lung metastases have been shown to have a better prognosis than those with extrapulmonary metastases; however, survival is still disappointing.[63,128] Bilateral pulmonary irradiation at a dose of 14 to 20 Gy was reported to improve the outcome of patients with pulmonary disease.[129–132] The Children's Oncology Group has joined the Euro-EWING randomized study comparing standard therapy including pulmonary irradiation with high-dose therapy using busulfan and melphalan followed by stem cell reinfusion for patients with initially isolated pulmonary metastatic disease (study arm R2pulm).[117]

Solitary or circumscribed bony metastases should be irradiated to doses of 40 to 50 Gy, in addition to local therapy to the primary site, and ESFT-directed chemotherapy. However, the survival rates of patients with multiple bony metastases are reported to be below 20%.[63,81,127] The discouraging results of treatment of metastatic disease have led to more aggressive approaches including myeloablative high-dose therapy with stem cell rescue. Conclusive results are pending, but preliminary data are discouraging.[84,124]

Alternate approaches include the targeting of the tumor vasculature. Angiogenesis, the generation of new blood vessels, is crucial to the progression of malignant disease.[133] These new blood vessels are sensitive to low-dose chemotherapy given over an extended period of time ("metronomic chemotherapy").[134,135] In ESFT, the EWS-FLI1 oncogene product may function as a transcriptional activator for vascular endothelial growth factor (VEGF). This pathway may thus present a particularly attractive target in ESFT. The Children's Oncology Group has nearly completed a pilot study, AEWS 02P1, examining the tolerability of a background of low-dose vinblastine and celecoxib[136] therapy incorporated into a standard 5-drug regimen (vincristine-doxorubicin-cyclophosphamide alternating with ifosfamide-etoposide).

Treatment of Recurrent Disease

Improved multimodal therapeutic regimens that combine more intensive systemic treatment with chemotherapy, improved surgical approaches, and advanced radiotherapy planning have led to a reduced frequency of recurrent disease, in particular, of local recurrence.[74,137] Nevertheless, 30% to 40% of patients still experience recurrent disease either locally, distantly, or combined. Such patients have a

dismal prognosis. Those with primary metastatic disease have a higher risk of relapse than those with initially localized disease, and recurrence is frequently earlier in those with initially metastatic disease.[77,137] The likelihood of long-term survival after recurrence is less than 20% to 25%.[138–140] The timing and type of recurrence are important prognostic factors.[134] Patients with early relapse, within the first 2 years following initial diagnosis, have a poorer prognosis with 4% to 8.5% 5-year survival. Those with later recurrence experience a 23% to 35% 5-year survival.[141,142] Recurrence may be very late, as compared with most other pediatric and adolescent cancers. A report from the Dana-Farber Cancer Institute described 82 patients initially diagnosed and treated with localized (60 patients) or metastatic (22 patients) ESFT between 1971 and 1988. Thirty-one patients survived at least 5 years from diagnosis, of whom 5 subsequently developed recurrent disease at 5.7, 6.7, 6.9, 9.3, and 17.1 years.[143] Simultaneous local and distant recurrences have been observed to be associated with more aggressive disease with earlier recurrence and poorer outcome.[78,138,140,141,144]

Patients with suspected recurrence should be evaluated appropriately to assess the extent of the local recurrence and the presence of metastatic disease and to plan treatment strategies. The majority of patients with local treatment failure have concomitant distant gross or microscopic disease. Detection of metastases with diagnostic imaging including CT, total body MRI, PET with 18F-deoxyglucose, and Tc-methylene diphosphonate bone scans is recommended. However, the images may be difficult to interpret due to prior therapy.

There is no established treatment regimen for these patients. Salvage treatment includes multiagent chemotherapy, local control measures with radiotherapy and surgery, or a combination of these as appropriate.

Patients with local recurrence are usually treated with surgery and further chemotherapy.[141] Recurrent distant disease involving the lungs or bones occurs in more than 50% of patients presenting with local recurrence and mandates further chemotherapy.[63,74,76,131,138,145,146] Patients with a single pulmonary nodule appear to benefit from additional whole-lung irradiation and have better outcomes, especially if the recurrence is late, more than 2 years following the primary diagnosis.[131]

Chemotherapy options are limited and dependent on the patient's prior treatment and possible impaired function of vital organs—eg, heart and kidneys. Agents that are considered for combination therapy are chosen to potentiate each other's activity and circumvent the emergence of drug resistance. These regimens have included combinations of topoisomerase I or topoisomerase II inhibitors with alkylating agents and, in addition, several myeloablative high-dose consolidation therapy regimens with and without total body irradiation (TBI).

Ifosfamide and etoposide have been shown to be active agents in Phase II studies,[114–116] although many patients will already have received these agents as part of their primary therapy. Topotecan in combination with cyclophosphamide produced responses in approximately 35% of patients with recurrent ESFT.[119–120] Temozolomide in combination with irinotecan has also shown promising activity, with 1 complete, 3 partial, and 3 minor responses in 14 patients who could be evaluated, with a median duration of response of 30 weeks, in a series from 4 institutions.[147] Further study of this combination is planned. The combination of gemcitabine and docetaxel has shown unexpectedly good activity in leiomyosarcoma, and will be investigated in some recurrent sarcomas, including recurrent Ewing Sarcoma. Both in vitro and anecdotal clinical evidence support this development in the context of a controlled clinical trial. In the pilot study, 2 patients with Ewing Sarcoma were among the 35 patients treated. One patient showed a partial response and the other, stable disease.[148] High-dose consolidation therapy with melphalan and etoposide with hyperfractionated TBI with or without carboplatin, followed by autologous stem-cell reinfusion, despite initial response, has failed to result in long-term remission in the treatment of early relapse.[84,149,150] Results from a hematopoietic stem cell transplantation regimen using combinations of active alkylating agents including busulfan and melphalan seem more encouraging and may improve the prognosis.[114,151] However, the role of stem cell transplantation in the treatment of patients with recurrent disease remains under discussion. Further studies to define the best approach for these patients are needed.[84,121,142,149]

Results of treatment of recurrent disease are still unsatisfactory. Whenever possible the patient should be included in organized clinical trials. New drug combinations offering a durable therapeutic benefit are yet to be established. Molecular research and better understanding of ESFT cell biology with its interplay regulating cell growth, apoptosis, differentiation, genomic integrity, and treatment resistance are needed to enrich the limited portfolio of active agents.

Targeted Therapy

Since the EWS-ETS fusion protein is unique to ESFT and present in almost all cases, it, or critical gene products regulated by the fusion protein, represent ideal tumor-specific targets. Experimentally, proof of principle has been obtained by both antisense and RNA interference studies that demonstrated that modulation of EWS-FLI1 expression results in growth inhibition of ESFTs in vitro and in vivo.[22-24,26,152-154] The clinical use of antisense RNA oligonucleotides or small inhibitory RNAs is impeded by the difficulty of efficiently delivering nucleic acids into disseminated tumor cells. One possible method to achieve this goal may be the inclusion of oligonucleotides (stabilized as phosphorothioates) into nanocapsules or nanospheres. This approach has been successfully applied to stop ESFT growth in xenotransplanted nude mice.[154,155] An alternative approach to targeting EWS-FLI1 is through its protein-protein interactions. Since transcription occurs in a multiprotein complex, the potentially novel 3-dimensional shape of EWS-FLI1 would present unique and targetable protein domains.[156] Key protein interactions have been discovered for EWS-FLI1, and these might be amenable to small-molecule disruption.[157-160]

CD99[MIC2] may represent another promising candidate for targeted therapy in ESFT. Although neither a ligand for CD99[MIC2] nor the mechanisms by which this antigen is involved in ESFT are known, in vitro studies on cell lines demonstrated that CD99[MIC2] binding and silencing by specific antibodies induces rapid tumor cell death, enhanced by combination with conventional chemotherapeutic drugs. In vivo studies have been restricted to athymic mice subcutaneously xenografted with an ESFT cell line and indicated reduced ESFT growth upon anti-CD99[MIC2] treatment.[161] However, there is no direct homolog of CD99[MIC2] in mice, and thus toxicity of anti-CD99[MIC2] treatment cannot be assessed in this model. Because of high-level expression of CD99[MIC2] in hematopoietic stem cells and several cell types in the gonads and the pancreas in humans, clinical trials using anti-CD99[MIC2] antibodies have not yet been attempted.

As noted above, VEGF may be a downstream target activated by EWS-FLI1. An open Children's Oncology Group protocol is examining the randomized addition of the anti-VEGF antibody bevacizumab to a backbone regimen of vincristine, topotecan, and cyclophosphamide for patients with a first recurrence of ESFT. Therapeutic antibodies that specifically block the interaction of IGF with the IGF-IR are currently undergoing development by 8 different pharmaceutical companies.[162] The monoclonal antibody, SCH 717454, has considerable activity against ESFT.[163] Human Phase I trials are under way and have produced encouraging results in patients with ESFT.

Late Effects

Late effects can be grouped into two major categories: orthopedic outcome, based on the location of the primary tumor and the surgery or radiotherapy used in its therapy, and overall outcome, based on the symptoms initially caused by the disease as well as the entire therapeutic package. Preservation of the hand in patients with upper extremity primaries is associated with an improved functional outcome and better self-image. Orthopedic outcome for patients with lower extremity lesions can be quite satisfactory even if distal amputation is required. Limb salvage procedures using massive internal prostheses or bone allografts can be complicated by late prosthetic failure or infection, requiring reoperation and, sometimes, delayed amputation.

Radiation therapy can be complicated by growth disturbances of both bone and soft tissue. In addition, irradiation can induce second cancers, most frequently osteosarcoma. This is dose related, with a significant increase in rate at administered doses above 40 Gy. In contrast, an increased rate of osteosarcoma has been reported after as little as 10 Gy. Moreover, the onset may be late.[164-166] Similarly, chemotherapy has been associated with induced malignancy. There has been a 1% to 2% rate of secondary leukemia following a sequence of protocols for ESFT, usually within 3 years of initial diagnosis. The IESS trial that compared VDC with VDCIE showed no difference in second malignancies between therapeutic arms, suggesting that, in the dose and schedule employed, the addition of etoposide did not independently increase the risk of second malignancy.[82] In contrast, it is notable that arm C of the CCG/POG intergroup study (INT 0091) designed for patients with disease metastatic at diagnosis, in which very high cumulative doses of ifosfamide (140 g/m²) and cyclophosphamide (17.6 g/m²) were prescribed, also demonstrated a very high rate of therapy-related leukemia with 6 patients diagnosed among the 60 treated, a cumulative incidence of approximately 11%.[167] Also, exposure to etoposide has been linked to the occurrence of second malignancy in a different series of patients that implicated high-dose therapy even more strongly.[168] There may be a threshold or stepwise effect, with a low rate of induced leukemia with conventional dose treatment, but a much higher rate at the high cumulative doses prescribed in arm C.

Other complications of chemotherapy are agent dependent.[169] Briefly, anthracyclines, including doxorubicin, induce a dose-related cardiomyopathy. Protocol doses are therefore usually limited to less than a lifetime total of 450 mg/m². In addition, administration is often either prolonged over a 48-hour period or, if given as a short intravenous bolus, preceded by the cardioprotectant dexrazoxane, in those jurisdictions in which it is available. Thoracic irradiation that includes the heart can augment the cardiotoxicity of anthracyclines. Doxorubicin is sometimes stopped at the lower cumulative dose of 300 mg/m² if thoracic irradiation is to be given. The alkylating agents cyclophosphamide and ifosfamide are associated with infertility, especially male infertility, so that sperm cryopreservation should be offered to postpubertal boys prior to the institution of chemotherapy. When the technology is better developed, ovarian cryopreservation should similarly be offered to females. Irradiation is sterilizing. Shielding of the testes and transposition of the ovaries should be considered when appropriate. In addition, ifosfamide can cause a persistent renal tubular electrolyte loss and, less commonly, a decrease in glomerular function, again in a dose-dependent fashion.

Despite these concerns, the overall functioning of survivors of ESFT is reasonably good.[170] There is frequent need for medical services among survivors, however, so that ensuring adequate follow-up and the provision of adequate resources are necessary.[171]

Summary and Conclusions

Ewing Sarcoma family tumors are the second most frequent primary bone cancer, usually affecting patients in the second and third decades of life. Patients presenting with localized disease have an approximately two-thirds chance of being cured. Those whose disease is initially metastatic have a much worse outcome. Those with isolated pulmonary metastases experience an approximately 30% EFS, whereas those with more widespread disease, usually involving bone or bone marrow, have a less than 20% chance of cure with currently available therapy. Patients whose disease has recurred share this grim out-

look. Advances in understanding the biology of ESFT have led to increased knowledge concerning the underlying molecular basis of disease, as yet insufficient to have led to the new therapeutic approaches required to cure those with currently refractory disease, and to cure all with fewer short- and long-term toxicities.

Acknowledgment

We thank Gabriela Perazza for assistance with the preparation of the manuscript.

References

1. Gurney JG, Swensen AR, Bulterys M. Malignant bone tumors. In: Ries LAG, Smith MA, Gurney JG, et al, eds. *Cancer Incidence and Survival among Children and Adolescents: United States SEER Program 1975–1995.* Volume Pub. No. 99–4649. Bethesda, MD: NIH; 1999:99–110.
2. Hense HW, Ahrens S, Paulussen M, et al. [Descriptive epidemiology of Ewing's tumor—analysis of German patients from (EI)CESS 1980–1997]. *Klin Padiatr.* 1999;211(4):271–275.
3. Widhe B, Widhe T. Initial symptoms and clinical features in osteosarcoma and Ewing Sarcoma. *J Bone Joint Surg Am.* 2000;82(5):667–674.
4. Sneppen O, Hansen LM. Presenting symptoms and treatment delay in osteosarcoma and Ewing Sarcoma. *Acta Radiol Oncol.* 1984;23(2–3):159–162.
5. Craft AW, Cotterill SJ, Bullimore JA, Pearson D. Long-term results from the first UKCCSG Ewing's Tumour Study (ET-1). United Kingdom Children's Cancer Study Group (UKCCSG) and the Medical Research Council Bone Sarcoma Working Party. *Eur J Cancer.* 1997;33(7):1061–1069.
6. Ferrari S, Bertoni F, Mercuri M, et al. Ewing Sarcoma of bone: relation between clinical characteristics and staging. *Oncol Rep.* 2001;8(3):553–556.
7. Henk CB, Grampp S, Wiesbauer P, et al. [Ewing Sarcoma. Diagnostic imaging]. *Radiologe.* 1998;38(6):509–522.
8. Tateishi U, Gladish GW, Kusumoto M, et al. Chest wall tumors: radiologic findings and pathologic correlation: part 2. Malignant tumors. *Radiographics.* 2003;23(6):1491–1508.
9. Frouge C, Vanel D, Coffre C, et al. The role of magnetic resonance imaging in the evaluation of Ewing Sarcoma: a report of 27 cases. *Skeletal Radiol.* 1988; 17(6):387–392.
10. Cohen MD, Weetman RM, Provisor AJ, et al. Efficacy of magnetic resonance imaging in 139 children with tumors. *Arch Surg.* 1986;121(5):522–529.
11. Novakovic B, Goldstein AM, Wexler LH, Tucker MA. Increased risk of neuroectodermal tumors and stomach cancer in relatives of patients with Ewing Sarcoma [see comments]. *J Natl Cancer Inst.* 1994;86(22):1702–1706.
12. Buckley JD, Pendergrass TW, Buckley CM, et al. Epidemiology of osteosarcoma and Ewing Sarcoma in childhood: a study of 305 cases by the Children's Cancer Group. *Cancer.* 1998;83(7):1440–1448.
13. McKeon C, Thiele CJ, Ross RA, et al. Indistinguishable patterns of proto oncogene expression in two distinct but closely related tumors: Ewing Sarcoma and neuroepithelioma. *Cancer Res.* 1988;48(15):4307–4311.
14. Riggi N, Suva ML, Stamenkovic I. Ewing Sarcoma-like tumors originate from EWS-FLI-1-expressing mesenchymal progenitor cells. *Cancer Res.* 2006; 66(19):9786.
15. Tirode F, Laud-Duval K, Prieur A, et al. Mesenchymal stem cell features of Ewing Sarcoma. *Cancer Cell.* 2007;11(5):421–429.
16. Delattre O, Zucman J, Plougastel B, et al. Gene fusion with an ETS DNA-binding domain caused by chromosome translocation in human tumours. *Nature.* 1992;359(6391):162–165.
17. Hattinger CM, Rumpler S, Strehl S, et al. Prognostic impact of deletions at 1p36 and numerical aberrations in Ewing Sarcoma. *Genes Chromosomes Cancer.* 1999;24(3):243–254.
18. Hattinger CM, Potschger U, Tarkkanen M, et al. Prognostic impact of chromosomal aberrations in Ewing tumours. *Br J Cancer.* 2002;86(11):1763–1769.
19. Maurici D, Perez-Atayde A, Grier HE, et al. Frequency and implications of chromosome 8 and 12 gains in Ewing Sarcoma. *Cancer Genet Cytogenet.* 1998;100(2):106–110.
20. May WA, Gishizky ML, Lessnick SL, et al. Ewing Sarcoma 11;22 translocation produces a chimeric transcription factor that requires the DNA-binding domain encoded by FLI1 for transformation. *Proc Natl Acad Sci USA.* 1993; 90(12):5752–5756.
21. Toretsky JA, Kalebic T, Blakesley V, et al. The insulin-like growth factor-I receptor is required for EWS/FLI-1 transformation of fibroblasts. *J Biol Chem.* 1997;272(49):30822–30827.
22. Ouchida M, Ohno T, Fujimura Y, et al. Loss of tumorigenicity of Ewing Sarcoma cells expressing antisense RNA to EWS-fusion transcripts. *Oncogene.* 1995;11(6):1049–1054.
23. Tanaka K, Iwakuma T, Harimaya K, et al. EWS-Fli1 antisense oligodeoxynucleotide inhibits proliferation of human Ewing Sarcoma and primitive neuroectodermal tumor cells. *J Clin Invest.* 1997;99(2):239–247.

24. Toretsky JA, Connell Y, Neckers L, Bhat NK. Inhibition of EWS-FLI-1 fusion protein with antisense oligodeoxynucleotides. *J Neuro-Oncol.* 1997;31(1–2): 9–16.

25. Chansky HA, Barahmand-Pour F, Mei Q, et al. Targeting of EWS/FLI-1 by RNA interference attenuates the tumor phenotype of Ewing Sarcoma cells in vitro. *J Orthop Res.* 2004;22(4):910–917.

26. Dohjima T, Lee NS, Li H, et al. Small interfering RNAs expressed from a Pol III promoter suppress the EWS/Fli-1 transcript in an Ewing Sarcoma cell line. *Mol Ther.* 2003;7(6):811–816.

27. Deneen B, Denny CT. Loss of p16 pathways stabilizes EWS/FLI1 expression and complements EWS/FLI1 mediated transformation. *Oncogene.* 2001; 20(46):6731–6741.

28. Kovar H, Jug G, Aryee DN, et al. Among genes involved in the RB dependent cell cycle regulatory cascade, the p16 tumor suppressor gene is frequently lost in the Ewing family of tumors. *Oncogene.* 1997;15(18):2225–2232.

29. Mankin HJ, Mankin CJ, Simon MA. The hazards of the biopsy, revisited. Members of the Musculoskeletal Tumor Society. *J Bone Joint Surg Am.* 1996; 78(5):656–663.

30. Ewing J. Diffuse endothelioma of bone. *Proc NY Pathol Soc.* 1921;21:17–24.

31. Horowitz ME, Tsokos MG, DeLaney TF. Ewing Sarcoma. *CA Cancer J Clin.* 1992;42(5):300–320.

32. Tsokos M. Peripheral primitive neuroectodermal tumors. Diagnosis, classification, and prognosis. *Perspect Pediatr Pathol.* 1992;16:27–98.

33. Dehner LP. Primitive neuroectodermal tumor and Ewing Sarcoma. *Am J Surg Pathol.* 1993;17(1):1–13.

34. Fellinger EJ, Garin-Chesa P, Su SL, et al. Biochemical and genetic characterization of the HBA71 Ewing Sarcoma cell surface antigen. *Cancer Res.* 1991; 51(1):336–340.

35. Ramani P, Rampling D, Link M. Immunocytochemical study of 12E7 in small round-cell tumours of childhood: an assessment of its sensitivity and specificity. *Histopathology.* 1993;23(6):557–561.

36. Weidner N, Tjoe J. Immunohistochemical profile of monoclonal antibody O13: antibody that recognizes glycoprotein p30/32MIC2 and is useful in diagnosing Ewing Sarcoma and peripheral neuroepithelioma. *Am J Surg Pathol.* 1994;18(5):486–494.

37. Ambros IM, Ambros PF, Strehl S, et al. MIC2 is a specific marker for Ewing Sarcoma and peripheral primitive neuroectodermal tumors. Evidence for a common histogenesis of Ewing Sarcoma and peripheral primitive neuroectodermal tumors from MIC2 expression and specific chromosome aberration. *Cancer.* 1991;67(7):1886–1893.

38. Ladanyi M, Lewis R, Garin-Chesa P, et al. EWS rearrangement in Ewing Sarcoma and peripheral neuroectodermal tumor. Molecular detection and correlation with cytogenetic analysis and MIC2 expression. *Diagn Mol Pathol.* 1993;2(3):141–146.

39. Desmaze C, Zucman J, Delattre O, et al. Interphase molecular cytogenetics of Ewing Sarcoma and peripheral neuroepithelioma t(11;22) with flanking and overlapping cosmid probes. *Cancer Genet Cytogenet.* 1994;74(1):13–18.

40. Navarro S, Cavazzana AO, Llombart-Bosch A, Triche TJ. Comparison of Ewing Sarcoma of bone and peripheral neuroepithelioma. An immunocytochemical and ultrastructural analysis of two primitive neuroectodermal neoplasms. *Arch Pathol Lab Med.* 1994;118(6):608–615.

41. Lizard-Nacol S, Lizard G, Justrabo E, Turc-Carel C. Immunologic characterization of Ewing Sarcoma using mesenchymal and neural markers. *Am J Pathol.* 1989;135(5):847–855.

42. Dierick AM, Roels H, Langlois M. The immunophenotype of Ewing Sarcoma. An immunohistochemical analysis. *Pathol Res Pract.* 1993;189(1):26–32.

43. Shanfield RI. Immunohistochemical analysis of neural markers in peripheral primitive neuroectodermal tumor (pPNET) without light microscopic evidence of neural differentiation. *Appl Immunohistochem Mol Morphol.* 1997;5: 78–86.

44. Gu M, Antonescu CR, Guiter G, et al. Cytokeratin immunoreactivity in Ewing Sarcoma: prevalence in 50 cases confirmed by molecular diagnostic studies. *Am J Surg Pathol.* 2000;24(3):410–416.

45. Ladanyi M, Bridge JA. Contribution of molecular genetic data to the classification of sarcomas. *Hum Pathol.* 2000;31(5):532–538.

46. Hill DA, O'Sullivan MJ, Zhu X, et al. Practical application of molecular genetic testing as an aid to the surgical pathologic diagnosis of sarcomas: a prospective study. *Am J Surg Pathol.* 2002;26(8):965–977.

47. Marley EF, Liapis H, Humphrey PA, et al. Primitive neuroectodermal tumor of the kidney—another enigma: a pathologic, immunohistochemical, and molecular diagnostic study. *Am J Surg Pathol.* 1997;21(3):354–359.

48. Sezer O, Jugovic D, Blohmer JU, et al. CD99 positivity and EWS-FLI1 gene rearrangement identify a breast tumor in a 60-year-old patient with attributes of the Ewing family of neoplasms. *Diagn Mol Pathol.* 1999;8(3):120–124.

49. Sheaff M, McManus A, Scheimberg I, et al. Primitive neuroectodermal tumor of the kidney confirmed by fluorescence in situ hybridization. *Am J Surg Pathol.* 1997;21(4):461–468.

50. Kuroda M, Urano M, Abe M, et al. Primary primitive neuroectodermal tumor of the kidney. *Pathol Int.* 2000;50(12):967–972.

51. Mikami Y, Nakajima M, Hashimoto H, et al. Primary pulmonary primitive neuroectodermal tumor (PNET): a case report. *Pathol Res Pract.* 2001;197(2): 113–119; discussion 121–112.

52. Kie JH, Lee MK, Kim CJ, et al. Primary Ewing Sarcoma of the suodenum: a case report. *Int J Surg Pathol.* 2003;11(4):331–337.

53. Tokudome N, Tanaka K, Kai MH, et al. Primitive neuroectodermal tumor of the transverse colonic mesentery defined by the presence of EWS-FLI1 chimeric mRNA in a Japanese woman. *J Gastroenterol.* 2002;37(7):543–549.

54. Shek TW, Chan GC, Khong PL, et al. Ewing Sarcoma of the small intestine. *J Pediatr Hematol Oncol.* 2001;23(8):530–532.

55. Maesawa C, Iijima S, Sato N, et al. Esophageal extraskeletal Ewing Sarcoma. *Hum Pathol.* 2002;33(1):130–132.

56. Colecchia M, Dagrada G, Poliani PL, et al. Primary primitive peripheral neuroectodermal tumor of the prostate: immunophenotypic and molecular study of a case. *Arch Pathol Lab Med.* 2003;127(4):e190–193.

57. Sinkre P, Albores-Saavedra J, Miller DS, et al. Endometrial endometrioid carcinomas associated with Ewing Sarcoma/peripheral primitive neuroectodermal tumor. *Int J Gynecol Pathol.* 2000;19(2):127–132.

58. Kato K, Kato Y, Ijiri R, et al. Ewing Sarcoma family of tumor arising in the adrenal gland—possible diagnostic pitfall in pediatric pathology: histologic, immunohistochemical, ultrastructural, and molecular study. *Hum Pathol.* 2001;32(9):1012–1016.

59. Dedeurwaerdere F, Giannini C, Sciot R, et al. Primary peripheral PNET/Ewing Sarcoma of the dura: a clinicopathologic entity distinct from central PNET. *Mod Pathol.* 2002;15(6):673–678.

60. Cheung CC, Kandel RA, Bell RS, et al. Extraskeletal Ewing Sarcoma in a 77-year-old woman. *Arch Pathol Lab Med.* 2001;125(10):1358–1360.

61. van den Berg H, Dirksen U, Ranft A, Jurgens H. Ewing Sarcoma in infants. *Pediatr Blood Cancer.* 2007.

62. Hawkins DS, Schuetze SM, Butrynski JE, et al. [18F]Fluorodeoxyglucose positron emission tomography predicts outcome for Ewing Sarcoma. *J Clin Oncol.* 2005;23(34):8828–8834.

63. Paulussen M, Ahrens S, Burdach S, et al. Primary metastatic (stage IV) Ewing tumor: survival analysis of 171 patients from the EICESS studies. European Intergroup Cooperative Ewing Sarcoma Studies. *Ann Oncol.* 1998;9(3):275–281.

64. Zoubek A, Ladenstein R, Windhager R, et al. Predictive potential of testing for bone marrow involvement in Ewing tumor patients by RT-PCR: a preliminary evaluation. *Int J Cancer.* 1998;79(1):56–60.

65. Schleiermacher G, Peter M, Oberlin O, et al. Increased risk of systemic relapses associated with bone marrow micrometastasis and circulating tumor cells in localized Ewing tumor. *J Clin Oncol.* 2003;21(1):85–91.

66. Avigad S, Cohen IJ, Zilberstein J, et al. The predictive potential of molecular detection in the nonmetastatic Ewing family of tumors. *Cancer.* 2004;100(5): 1053–1058.

67. Ewing J. Further report of endothelial myeloma of bone. *Proc NY Pathol Soc.* 1924;24:93–100.

68. Jenkin RD. Ewing Sarcoma a study of treatment methods. *Clin Radiol.* 1966; 17(2):97–106.

69. Phillips RF, Higinbotham NL. The curability of Ewing's endothelioma of bone in children. *J Pediatr.* 1967;70(3):391–397.

70. Hustu HO, Holton C, James D, Jr., Pinkel D. Treatment of Ewing Sarcoma with concurrent radiotherapy and chemotherapy. *J Pediatr.* 1968;73(2):249–251.

71. Sutow WW, Vietti TJ, Fernbach DJ, et al. Evaluation of chemotherapy in children with metastatic Ewing Sarcoma and osteogenic sarcoma. *Cancer Chemother Rep.* 1971;55(1):67–78.

72. Rosen G, Wollner N, Tan C, et al. Proceedings: Disease-free survival in children with Ewing Sarcoma treated with radiation therapy and adjuvant four-drug sequential chemotherapy. *Cancer.* 1974;33(2):384–393.

73. Gasparini M, Barni S, Lattuada A, et al. Ten years experience with Ewing Sarcoma. *Tumori.* 1977;63(1):77–90.

74. Jurgens H, Exner U, Gadner H, et al. Multidisciplinary treatment of primary Ewing Sarcoma of bone: a 6-year experience of a European Cooperative Trial. *Cancer.* 1988;61(1):23–32.

75. Nesbit ME, Jr., Gehan EA, Burgert EO, Jr., et al. Multimodal therapy for the management of primary, nonmetastatic Ewing Sarcoma of bone: a long-term follow-up of the First Intergroup study. *J Clin Oncol.* 1990;8(10):1664–1674.

76. Burgert EO, Jr., Nesbit ME, Garnsey LA, et al. Multimodal therapy for the management of nonpelvic, localized Ewing Sarcoma of bone: intergroup study IESS-II. *J Clin Oncol.* 1990;8(9):1514–1524.

77. Cotterill SJ, Ahrens S, Paulussen M, et al. Prognostic factors in Ewing's tumor of bone: analysis of 975 patients from the European Intergroup Cooperative Ewing Sarcoma Study Group. *J Clin Oncol.* 2000;18(17):3108–3114.

78. Craft A, Cotterill S, Malcolm A, et al. Ifosfamide-containing chemotherapy in Ewing Sarcoma: the Second United Kingdom Children's Cancer Study Group and the Medical Research Council Ewing's Tumor Study. *J Clin Oncol.* 1998; 16(11):3628–3633.

79. Oberlin O, Deley MC, Bui BN, et al. Prognostic factors in localized Ewing's tumours and peripheral neuroectodermal tumours: the third study of the French Society of Paediatric Oncology (EW88 study). *Br J Cancer.* 2001; 85(11):1646–1654.

80. Paulussen M, Ahrens S, Dunst J, et al. Localized Ewing tumor of bone: final results of the cooperative Ewing Sarcoma Study CESS 86. *J Clin Oncol.* 2001; 19(6):1818–1829.

81. Kolb EA, Kushner BH, Gorlick R, et al. Long-term event-free survival after intensive chemotherapy for Ewing's family of tumors in children and young adults. *J Clin Oncol.* 2003;21(18):3423–3430.

82. Grier HE, Krailo MD, Tarbell NJ, et al. Addition of ifosfamide and etoposide to standard chemotherapy for Ewing Sarcoma and primitive neuroectodermal tumor of bone. *N Engl J Med.* 2003;348(8):694–701.

83. Bacci G, Forni C, Longhi A, et al. Long-term outcome for patients with non-metastatic Ewing Sarcoma treated with adjuvant and neoadjuvant chemotherapies: 402 patients treated at Rizzoli between 1972 and 1992. *Eur J Cancer.* 2004;40(1):73–83.

84. Meyers PA, Krailo MD, Ladanyi M, et al. High-dose melphalan, etoposide, total-body irradiation, and autologous stem-cell reconstitution as consolidation therapy for high-risk Ewing Sarcoma does not improve prognosis. *J Clin Oncol*. 2001;19(11):2812–2820.

85. Huang HY, Illei PB, Zhao Z, et al. Ewing Sarcomas with p53 mutation or p16/p14ARF homozygous deletion: a highly lethal subset associated with poor chemoresponse. *J Clin Oncol*. 2005;23(3):548–558.

86. De Alava E, Kawai A, Healey JH, et al. EWS-FLI1 fusion transcript structure is an independent determinant of prognosis in Ewing's Sarcoma. *J Clin Oncol*. 1998;16:1248–1255.

87. Aparicio J, Munarriz B, Pastor M, et al. Long-term follow-up and prognostic factors in Ewing Sarcoma: a multivariate analysis of 116 patients from a single institution. *Oncology*. 1998;55(1):20–26.

88. Carrie C, Mascard E, Gomez F, et al. Nonmetastatic pelvic Ewing Sarcoma: report of the French society of pediatric oncology. *Med Pediatr Oncol*. 1999; 33(5):444–449.

89. Bacci G, Ferrari S, Bertoni F, et al. Prognostic factors in nonmetastatic Ewing Sarcoma of bone treated with adjuvant chemotherapy: analysis of 359 patients at the Istituto Ortopedico Rizzoli. *J Clin Oncol*. 2000;18(1):4–11.

90. Schuck A, Ahrens S, Paulussen M, et al. Local therapy in localized Ewing Sarcoma: results of 1058 patients treated in the CESS 81, CESS 86, and EICESS 92 trials. *Int J Radiat Oncol Biol Phys*. 2003;55(1):168–177.

91. Dunst J, Sauer R, Burgers JM, et al. Radiation therapy as local treatment in Ewing Sarcoma: results of the Cooperative Ewing Sarcoma Studies CESS 81 and CESS 86. *Cancer*. 1991;67(11):2818–2825.

92. Gebhardt MC, Jaffe K, Mankin HJ. Bone allografts for tumors and other reconstructions in children. In: Langlais F, Tomeno B, eds. *Limb Salvage: Major Reconstructions in Oncologic and Nontumoral Conditions*. Berlin: Springer-Verlag; 1991:561–572.

93. Shapiro MS, Endrizzi DP, Cannon RM, Dick HM. Treatment of tibial defects and nonunions using ipsilateral vascularized fibular transposition. *Clin Orthop*. 1993(296):207–212.

94. Ozaki T, Hillmann A, Wuisman P, Winkelmann W. Reconstruction of tibia by ipsilateral vascularized fibula and allograft: 12 cases with malignant bone tumors. *Acta Orthop Scand*. 1997;68(3):298–301.

95. Schulte M, Brecht-Krauss D, Werner M, et al. Evaluation of neoadjuvant therapy response of osteogenic sarcoma using FDG PET. *J Nucl Med*. 1999;40 (10):1637–1643.

96. van der Woude HJ, Bloem JL, Hogendoorn PC. Preoperative evaluation and monitoring chemotherapy in patients with high-grade osteogenic and Ewing Sarcoma: review of current imaging modalities. *Skeletal Radiol*. 1998;27(2): 57–71.

97. Sato O, Kawai A, Ozaki T, et al. Value of thallium-201 scintigraphy in bone and soft tissue tumors. *J Orthop Sci*. 1998;3(6):297–303.

98. Reddick WE, Bhargava R, Taylor JS, et al. Dynamic contrast-enhanced MR imaging evaluation of osteosarcoma response to neoadjuvant chemotherapy. *J Magn Reson Imaging*. 1995;5(6):689–694.

99. Imbriaco M, Yeh SD, Yeung H, et al. Thallium-201 scintigraphy for the evaluation of tumor response to preoperative chemotherapy in patients with osteosarcoma. *Cancer*. 1997;80(8):1507–1512.

100. Schuck A, Hofmann J, Rube C, et al. Radiotherapy in Ewing Sarcoma and PNET of the chest wall: results of the trials CESS 81, CESS 86 and EICESS 92. *Int J Radiat Oncol Biol Phys*. 1998;42(5):1001–1006.

101. Sailer SL, Harmon DC, Mankin HJ, et al. Ewing Sarcoma: surgical resection as a prognostic factor. *Int J Radiat Oncol Biol Phys*. 1988;15(1):43–52.

102. Arai Y, Kun LE, Brooks MT, et al. Ewing Sarcoma: local tumor control and patterns of failure following limited-volume radiation therapy. *Int J Radiat Oncol Biol Phys*. 1991;21(6):1501–1508.

103. Donaldson SS, Torrey M, Link MP, et al. A multidisciplinary study investigating radiotherapy in Ewing Sarcoma: end results of POG #8346. Pediatric Oncology Group. *Int J Radiat Oncol Biol Phys*. 1998;42(1):125–135.

104. Dunst J, Jurgens H, Sauer R, et al. Radiation therapy in Ewing Sarcoma: an update of the CESS 86 trial. *Int J Radiat Oncol Biol Phys*. 1995;32(4):919–930.

105. Sutow WW, Sullivan MP. Cyclophosphamide therapy in children with Ewing Sarcoma. *Cancer Chemother Rep*. 1962;23:55–60.

106. Pinkel D. Cyclophosphamide in children with cancer. *Cancer*. 1962;15:42–49.

107. Granowetter 2001 *Med Pediatr Oncol*. 37:172

108. Rosen G, Juergens H, Caparros B, Nirenberg A, et al. Combination chemotherapy (T-6) in the multidisciplinary treatment of Ewing's sarcoma. *Natl Cancer Inst Monogr*. 1981;(56), 289–299.

109. Kushner BH, Meyers PA, Gerald WL, Healey JH, et al. Very-high-dose short-term chemotherapy for poorrisk peripheral primitive neuroectodermal tumors, including Ewing sarcoma, in children and young adults. *J Clin Oncol*. 1995;13(11), 2796–2804.

110. Hayes FA, Thompson EI, Meyer WH, Kun L, et al. Therapy for localized Ewing's sarcoma of bone. *J Clin Oncol*, 1989;7(2), 208–213.

111. Meyer WH, Kun L, Marina N, Roberson P, Parham D, et al. Ifosfamide plus etoposide in newly diagnosed Ewing's sarcoma of bone. *J Clin Oncol*. 1992;10(11), 1737–1742.

112. Marina NM, Pappo AS, Parham DM, Cain, AM, et al. Chemotherapy dose-intensification for pediatric patients with Ewing's family of tumors and desmoplastic small round-cell tumors: a feasibility study at St. Jude Children's Research Hospital. *J Clin Oncol*. 1999;17(1), 180–190.

113. Elomaa I, Blornqvist CP, Saeter G, Akerman M, et al. Five-year results in Ewing's sarcoma. The Scandinavian Sarcoma Group experience with the SSG IX protocol. *Eur J Cancer*. 2000:36(7), 875–880.

114. Kung FH, Pratt CB, Vega RA, et al. Ifosfamide/etoposide combination in the treatment of recurrent malignant solid tumors of childhood: a Pediatric Oncology Group Phase II study. *Cancer*. 1993;71(5):1898–1903.

115. Miser JS, Kinsella TJ, Triche TJ, et al. Ifosfamide with mesna uroprotection and etoposide: an effective regimen in the treatment of recurrent sarcomas and other tumors of children and young adults. *J Clin Oncol*. 1987;5(8): 1191–1198.

116. Pratt CB, Luo X, Fang L, et al. Response of pediatric malignant solid tumors following ifosfamide or ifosfamide/carboplatin/etoposide: a single hospital experience. *Med Pediatr Oncol*. 1996;27(3):145–148.

117. Euro-E.W.I.N.G. Study Committee. Euro-E.W.I.N.G. 99 Study Manual: EUROpean Ewing Tumor Initiative of National Groups Ewing Tumor Studies 1999. 1999.

118. Womer RB, Daller RT, Fenton JG, Miser JS. Granulocyte colony stimulating factor permits dose intensification by interval compression in the treatment of Ewing Sarcomas and soft tissue sarcomas in children. *Eur J Cancer*. 2000; 36(1):87–94.

119. Kushner BH, Kramer K, Meyers PA, et al. Pilot study of topotecan and high-dose cyclophosphamide for resistant pediatric solid tumors. *Med Pediatr Oncol*. 2000;35(5):468–474.

120. Saylors RL III, Stine KC, Sullivan J, et al. Cyclophosphamide plus topotecan in children with recurrent or refractory solid tumors: a Pediatric Oncology Group phase II study. *J Clin Oncol*. 2001;19(15):3463–3469.

121. Ladenstein R, Lasset C, Pinkerton R, et al. Impact of megatherapy in children with high-risk Ewing's tumours in complete remission: a report from the EBMT Solid Tumour Registry. *Bone Marrow Transplant*. 1995;15(5):697–705.

122. Kinsella TJ, Glaubiger D, Diesseroth A, et al. Intensive combined modality therapy including low-dose TBI in high-risk Ewing Sarcoma Patients. *Int J Radiat Oncol Biol Phys*. 1983;9(12):1955–1960.

123. Burdach S, Jurgens H, Peters C, et al. Myeloablative radiochemotherapy and hematopoietic stem-cell rescue in poor-prognosis Ewing Sarcoma. *J Clin Oncol*. 1993;11(8):1482–1488.

124. Kushner BH, Meyers PA. How effective is dose-intensive/myeloablative therapy against Ewing Sarcoma/primitive neuroectodermal tumor metastatic to bone or bone marrow? The Memorial Sloan-Kettering experience and a literature review. *J Clin Oncol*. 2001;19(3):870–880.

125. Pinkerton CR. Intensive chemotherapy with stem cell support-experience in pediatric solid tumours. *Bull Cancer*. 1995;82(suppl 1):61s–65s.

126. Meyers PA. High-dose therapy with autologous stem cell rescue for pediatric sarcomas. *Curr Opin Oncol*. 2004;16(2):120–125.

127. Cangir A, Vietti TJ, Gehan EA, et al. Ewing Sarcoma metastatic at diagnosis. Results and comparisons of two intergroup Ewing Sarcoma studies. *Cancer*. 1990;66(5):887–893.

128. Sandoval C, Meyer WH, Parham DM, et al. Outcome in 43 children presenting with metastatic Ewing Sarcoma: the St Jude Children's Research Hospital experience, 1962 to 1992. *Med Pediatr Oncol*. 1996;26(3):180–185.

129. Bizer VA, Timukhina VN, Afanasova NV. [Programs for the radiation and drug treatment of metastases of Ewing Sarcoma to the lungs in children.] *Med Radiol (Mosk)*. 1983;28(11):8–12.

130. Dunst J, Paulussen M, Jurgens H. Lung irradiation for Ewing Sarcoma with pulmonary metastases at diagnosis: results of the CESS-studies. *Strahlenther Onkol*. 1993;169(10):621–623.

131. Paulussen M, Ahrens S, Craft AW, et al. Ewing's tumors with primary lung metastases: survival analysis of 114 (European Intergroup) Cooperative Ewing Sarcoma Studies patients. *J Clin Oncol*. 1998;16(9):3044–3052.

132. Whelan JS, Burcombe RJ, Janinis J, et al. A systematic review of the role of pulmonary irradiation in the management of primary bone tumours. *Ann Oncol*. 2002;13(1):23–30.

133. Folkman J. Anti-angiogenesis: new concept for therapy of solid tumors. *Ann Surg*. 1972;175(3):409–416.

134. Vacca A, Iurlaro M, Ribatti D, et al. Antiangiogenesis is produced by nontoxic doses of vinblastine. *Blood*. 1999;94(12):4143–4155.

135. Klement G, Huang P, Mayer B, et al. Differences in therapeutic indexes of combination metronomic chemotherapy and an anti-VEGFR-2 antibody in multidrug-resistant human breast cancer xenografts. *Clin Cancer Res*. 2002; 8(1):221–232.

136. Fosslien E. Molecular pathology of cyclooxygenase-2 in neoplasia. *Ann Clin Lab Sci*. 2000;30(1):3–21.

137. Ahrens S, Hoffmann C, Jabar S, et al. Evaluation of prognostic factors in a tumor volume-adapted treatment strategy for localized Ewing Sarcoma of bone: the CESS 86 experience. Cooperative Ewing Sarcoma Study. *Med Pediatr Oncol*. 1999;32(3):186–195.

138. Bacci G, Picci P, Ferrari S, et al. Neoadjuvant chemotherapy for Ewing Sarcoma of bone: no benefit observed after adding ifosfamide and etoposide to vincristine, actinomycin, cyclophosphamide, and doxorubicin in the maintenance phase—results of two sequential studies. *Cancer*. 1998;82(6):1174–1183.

139. Klingebiel T, Pertl U, Hess CF, et al. Treatment of children with relapsed soft tissue sarcoma: report of the German CESS/CWS REZ 91 trial. *Med Pediatr Oncol*. 1998;30(5):269–275.

140. Ozaki T, Hillmann A, Hoffmann C, et al. Significance of surgical margin on the prognosis of patients with Ewing Sarcoma. A report from the Cooperative Ewing Sarcoma Study. *Cancer*. 1996;78(4):892–900.

141. Rodriguez-Galindo C, Billups CA, Kun LE, et al. Survival after recurrence of Ewing Sarcoma: the St Jude Children's Research Hospital experience, 1979–1999. *Cancer.* 2002;94(2):561–569.

142. Burdach S. Treatment of advanced Ewing Sarcoma by combined radiochemotherapy and engineered cellular transplants. *Pediatr Transplant.* 2004;8 Suppl 5:67–82.

143. McLean TW, Hertel C, Young ML, et al. Late events in pediatric patients with Ewing Sarcoma/primitive neuroectodermal tumor of bone: the Dana-Farber Cancer Institute/Children's Hospital experience. *J Pediatr Hematol Oncol.* 1999;21(6):486–493.

144. Shankar AG, Pinkerton CR, Atra A, et al. Local therapy and other factors influencing site of relapse in patients with localised Ewing Sarcoma. United Kingdom Children's Cancer Study Group (UKCCSG). *Eur J Cancer.* 1999;35(12):1698–1704.

145. Nesbit ME, Jr., Perez CA, Tefft M, et al. Multimodal therapy for the management of primary, nonmetastatic Ewing Sarcoma of bone: an Intergroup Study. *Natl Cancer Inst Monogr.* 1981(56):255–262.

146. Bacci G, Mercuri M, Longhi A, et al. Neoadjuvant chemotherapy for Ewing's tumour of bone: recent experience at the Rizzoli Orthopaedic Institute. *Eur J Cancer.* 2002;38(17):2243–2251.

147. Wagner LM, McAllister N, Goldsby RE, et al. Temozolomide and intravenous irinotecan for treatment of advanced Ewing Sarcoma. *Pediatr Blood Cancer.* 2007;48(2):132–139.

148. Leu KM, Ostruszka LJ, Shewach D, et al. Laboratory and clinical evidence of synergistic cytotoxicity of sequential treatment with gemcitabine followed by docetaxel in the treatment of sarcoma. *J Clin Oncol.* 2004;22(9):1706–1712.

149. Burdach S, Meyer-Bahlburg A, Laws HJ, et al. High-dose therapy for patients with primary multifocal and early relapsed Ewing's tumors: results of two consecutive regimens assessing the role of total-body irradiation. *J Clin Oncol.* 2003;21(16):3072–3078.

150. Frohlich B, Ahrens S, Burdach S, et al. [High-dosage chemotherapy in primary metastasized and relapsed Ewing Sarcoma. (EI)CESS]. *Klin Padiatr.* 1999;211(4):284–290.

151. Hawkins D, Barnett T, Bensinger W, et al. Busulfan, melphalan, and thiotepa with or without total marrow irradiation with hematopoietic stem cell rescue for poor-risk Ewing-Sarcoma-Family tumors. *Med Pediatr Oncol.* 2000;34(5):328–337.

152. Kovar H, Ban J, Pospisilova S. Potentials for RNAi in sarcoma research and therapy: Ewing Sarcoma as a model. *Semin Cancer Biol.* 2003;13(4):275–281.

153. Kovar H, Aryee DN, Jug G, et al. EWS/FLI-1 antagonists induce growth inhibition of Ewing tumor cells in vitro. *Cell Growth Differ.* 1996;7(4):429–437.

154. Lambert G, Bertrand JR, Fattal E, et al. EWS fli-1 antisense nanocapsules inhibits Ewing Sarcoma-related tumor in mice. *Biochem Biophys Res Commun.* 2000;279(2):401–406.

155. Maksimenko A, Malvy C, Lambert G, et al. Oligonucleotides targeted against a junction oncogene are made efficient by nanotechnologies. *Pharm Res.* 2003;20(10):1565–1567.

156. Uren A, Tcherkasskaya O, Toretsky JA. Recombinant EWS-FLI1 oncoprotein activates transcription. *Biochemistry.* 2004;43(42):13579–13589.

157. Bertolotti A, Melot T, Acker J, et al. EWS, but not EWS-FLI-1, is associated with both TFIID and RNA polymerase II: interactions between two members of the TET family, EWS and hTAFII68, and subunits of TFIID and RNA polymerase II complexes. *Mol Cell Biol.* 1998;18(3):1489–1497.

158. Kim S, Denny CT, Wisdom R. Cooperative DNA binding with AP-1 proteins is required for transformation by EWS-Ets fusion proteins. *Mol Cell Biol.* 2006;26(7):2467–2478.

159. Petermann R, Mossier BM, Aryee DN, et al. Oncogenic EWS-Fli1 interacts with hsRPB7, a subunit of human RNA polymerase II. *Oncogene.* 1998;17(5):603–610.

160. Toretsky JA, Erkizan V, Levenson A, et al. Oncoprotein EWS-FLI1 activity is enhanced by RNA helicase A. *Cancer Res.* 2006;66(11):5574–5581.

161. Scotlandi K, Baldini N, Cerisano V, et al. CD99 engagement: an effective therapeutic strategy for Ewing Sarcoma. *Cancer Res.* 2000;60(18):5134–5142.

162. Feng Y, Dimitrov DS. Monoclonal antibodies against components of the IGF system for cancer treatment. *Curr Opin Drug Discovery Devel.* 2008;11(2):178–185.

163. Kolb EA, Gorlick R, Houghton PJ, et al. Initial testing (stage 1) of a monoclonal antibody (SCH 717454) against the IGF-1 receptor by the pediatric preclinical testing program. *Pediatr Blood Cancer.* 2008.

164. Kuttesch JF Jr, Wexler LH, Marcus RB, et al. Second malignancies after Ewing Sarcoma: radiation dose-dependency of secondary sarcomas. *J Clin Oncol.* 1996;14(10):2818–2825.

165. Dunst J, Ahrens S, Paulussen M, et al. Second malignancies after treatment for Ewing Sarcoma: a report of the CESS-studies. *Int J Radiat Oncol Biol Phys.* 1998;42(2):379–384.

166. Le Vu B, de Vathaire F, Shamsaldin A, et al. Radiation dose, chemotherapy and risk of osteosarcoma after solid tumours during childhood. *Int J Cancer.* 1998;77(3):370–377.

167. Bhatia S, Krailo MD, Chen Z, et al. Therapy-related myelodysplasia and acute myeloid leukemia after Ewing Sarcoma and primitive neuroectodermal tumor of bone: A report from the Children's Oncology Group. *Blood.* 2007;109(1):46–51.

168. Paulussen M, Ahrens S, Lehnert M, et al. Second malignancies after Ewing tumor treatment in 690 patients from a cooperative German/Austrian/Dutch study. *Ann Oncol.* 2001;12(11):1619–1630.

169. Friedman DL, Meadows AT. Late effects of childhood cancer therapy. *Pediatr Clin North Am.* 2002;49(5):1083–1106.

170. Nagarajan R, Neglia JP, Clohisy DR, et al. Education, employment, insurance, and marital status among 694 survivors of pediatric lower extremity bone tumors: a report from the childhood cancer survivor study. *Cancer.* 2003;97(10):2554–2564.

171. Fuchs B, Valenzuela RG, Inwards C, et al. Complications in long-term survivors of Ewing Sarcoma. *Cancer.* 2003;98(12):2687–2692.

Childhood Hepatic Tumors

Marcio H. Malogolowkin, Piotr Czauderna, Hector L. Monforte, Giorgio Perilongo, and
Jorge A. Ortega

Introduction

Primary hepatic malignancies in children and adolescents are rare. Hepatoblastomas account for greater than two-thirds of all hepatic malignancies in infants and young children, while hepatocellular carcinomas (HCCs) are more commonly encountered in older children and adolescents. Other hepatic malignancies are even more infrequent in children and adolescents. This chapter will emphasize the two most common tumors, focusing especially on their similarities and differences, as well as describing the most common liver sarcomas, undifferentiated embryonal sarcoma of the liver (UESL) and biliary rhabdomyosarcoma (RMS).

Incidence

Malignant hepatic tumors account for 1.1% of all malignancies in children. The incidence of hepatic tumors in children and adolescents is 0.5 to 2.5 cases per 10^6 children at risk, and approximately two-thirds of these are malignant tumors.[1] Table 29-1 shows the distribution of hepatic tumors, benign and malignant, according to age.[2,3]

In a review of 1256 cases of primary hepatic tumors of childhood, Weinberg and Finegold[4] found that hepato-

blastoma accounted for 43% of them, HCCs for 23%, while 13% were benign vascular tumors, 6% mesenchymal hamartomas (MHs), 6% sarcomas, 2% adenomas, 2% focal nodular hyperplasia, and 5% other tumors.

The vast majority of cases of hepatoblastoma occur during infancy and early childhood, with less than 5% of the diagnosed cases being in children older than 4 years. The mean age at diagnosis for patients with hepatoblastoma is 16 months;[3] however, a few cases of hepatoblastoma in adults have been reported.[5,6] There is a slight predominance of males diagnosed with hepatoblastoma, with a male-to-female ratio ranging between 1.4 to 1.0 and 2.0 to 1.0.[3,4,7] According to the Surveillance, Epidemiology, and End Results data, the incidence of hepatoblastoma in North America has increased by approximately 5% per year in the past 20 years.[8] Kenney et al reported that the incidence of primary liver tumors in infants younger than 1 year has increased from 2% in the 1970s to approximately 4% in the 1980s.[9] A similar increase has been seen in the United Kingdom, as reported by the Manchester Tumor Registry.[10]

Hepatocellular carcinomas are seen more often in children older than 10 years, and they represent the most common primary hepatic malignant tumor in adolescents. Rarely, HCCs have been reported in infants.[3,11] Similarly

Table 29-1

Primary hepatic tumors in children.

Age	Benign	Malignant
0-3 years	Hemangioendothelioma	Hepatoblastoma
	Hamartoma	Rhabdoid tumor
	Teratomas	Yolk sac tumor
		Rhabdomyosarcoma
3-12 years	Angiolipoma	Hepatocellular carcinoma
		Undifferentiated sarcoma
		Angiosarcoma
>12 years	Adenomas	Hepatocellular carcinoma (fibrolamellar)
	Cystic adenoma of biliary tree	Leiomyosarcoma
		Lymphoma

to hepatoblastoma, HCC has a prevalence in males compared with females, with the exception of the fibrolamellar variant, which has a similar incidence in males and females.[12] Chronic infection with hepatitis B virus is the leading cause of HCC in children, adolescents, and young adults in Asia and Africa. However, in Western countries, fewer than a third of the adolescent or young adult patients diagnosed with HCC have an identifying cause such as hepatitis or other inflammatory liver disease.[13,14] This is in marked contrast to older adults, in whom almost 90% of cases of HCC are cirrhosis related, or secondary to viral infection or alcohol consumption.[15] The prevention of a carrier state in children through a universal program of hepatitis B immunization has shown a dramatic decrease in chronic hepatitis B virus prevalence, and a decline in the rates of HCC in Taiwan among children younger than 15 years.[16]

Undifferentiated embryonal sarcoma of the liver represents about 0.004 to 0.01% of all the soft tissue sarcomas.[17] Embryonal rhabdomyosarcoma (ERMS), although being the most common soft tissue sarcoma representing 50% of all soft tissue tumors (STS) and 4% to 8% of all pediatric cancers, very rarely arises in the liver.[18] Among North American Intergroup Rhabdomyosarcoma Study (IRS) data collected by Ruymann, RMS of the biliary tree represented 0.8% all ERMS cases.

Undifferentiated embryonal sarcoma affects predominantly older children and adolescents; 90% of cases occur between 6 and 15 years of age.[17,19,20] In contrast, ERMS tends to occur in younger children (generally younger than 5 to 6 years). In UESL, a very slight male preponderance has been noted.

It has been hypothesized that UESL represents a malignant counterpart of MH, and indeed cases of UESL developing within MH have been described, but other researchers have questioned this relationship.[19,21,22] Because MH develops at a younger age than UESL, it

might indeed represent a precursor lesion to it. Also, the behavior of MH itself can be variable and sometimes aggressive.

Unlike UESL, RMS is a biliary tree tumor that arises mainly from extrahepatic bile ducts, including gallbladder and the ampulla of Vater, with growth extending into the liver. Rhabdomyosarcomas of intrahepatic biliary ducts are exceedingly rare. Occasionally, RMS may develop within a choledochal cyst.[23]

Biology and Predisposing Conditions

Hepatic malignant neoplasms have been associated with different genetic syndromes as well as with many environmental factors (Table 29-2).

Children with Beckwith-Wiedemann syndrome (BWS) and hemihypertrophy (HH) are at higher risk of embryonal tumor development such as ERMS, Wilms tumor, adrenal carcinoma, as well as hepatoblastoma.[24] Beckwith-Wiedemann syndrome and HH are most likely within a spectrum of similar disorders. Beckwith-Wiedemann syndrome and HH are considered *overgrowth syndromes*. The frequency of embryonal tumors in BWS is 1000-fold higher than in the normal population; about 2% of all hepatoblastomas are affected by BWS or HH. According to the North American BWS Registry, the relative risk for these patients of developing hepatoblastoma is 2280 times than for other embryonal tumors.[25] A disrupting expression of some maternally derived genes regulating cell growth located in the 11p15 locus—a complex imprinting region—causing an overexpression of the paternally derived genes has been postulated as the genetic defects underlying the etiology of the disease.[24,26,27] The condition is known as loss of imprinting, meaning the loss of preferential parental origin-specific gene expression, and can involve either abnormal expression of the normally silent allele, leading to a bi-allelic expression, or silencing of the

Table 29-2

Risk factors associated with liver tumors in children, adolescents, and young adults.

	Hepatoblastoma	Hepatocellular Carcinoma
Congenital abnormalities	• Familial polyposis • Gardner syndrome • Beckwith-Wiedemann syndrome • Hemihypertrophy	• Hereditary tyrosinemia • Biliary cirrhosis • Glycogen storage diseases • α-1 antitrypsin deficiency • Hemochromatosis • Ataxia telangiectasia
Environment factors	• Fetal alcohol syndrome • Prematurity and prolonged parenteral nutrition • Oral contraceptives • Oral gonadotropins • Parental exposure to metal, petroleum products, paint	• Hepatitis B & C • Alcohol consumption • Anabolic steroids • Aflatoxin • Carcinogens (pesticides, vinyl chloride, Thorotrast)

normally expressed allele, leading to epigenetic silencing of the locus. Uni-parental disomy, maternal balanced chromosomal translocations or inversions, paternal imbalanced duplication, and loss of insulin-like growth factor II (IGF2) or mutation of p57 gene are the genetic alterations commonly described in BWS. The biological effect of these changes is a net increase of IGF2, an autocrine and paracrine growth factor, the mitogenic effects of which are mediated by signaling through the IGF1 receptor. The causative role of IGF2 in tumor progression has been repeatedly documented. The possible role of IGF2 in allowing cells to escape apoptosis has been proposed. Two other imprinted genes located at the 11p15 locus have been proposed to cooperate with the IGF2 gene: the cyclin-dependent kinase inhibitor (CDKN1 formerly called p57 gene),[28] with a putative inhibitor effect on cell growth, and the H19 gene,[29,30] which share with the IGF2 gene the regulatory sequence, with a reciprocal pattern of imprinting. Loss of imprinting of IGF2 indeed was reported in hepatoblastoma, sometimes in association with loss of imprinting of the H19 gene, which is also found in cases of Wilms tumor.[31] The WT1 gene, located on chromosome 11p13, which seems to be specifically involved in renal development, is, as anticipated, distinct from these 11p15 BWS genes, which seem to have a broader organ effect favoring the development of different tumors: ERMS, hepatoblastoma, and adrenal carcinoma. In brief, disturbances in the expression of the cell growth regulatory gene complex located in the 11p15 region ultimately lead to aberrant growth development during organogenesis, which favors tumor development. Loss of heterozygosity at the 11p15 locus has been documented also in sporadic hepatoblastoma. Simpson-Golabin-Behmel syndrome is a rare and complex congenital overgrowth syndrome that has overlapping clinical features with BWS and also predisposes affected individuals to the risk of embryonal tumor development, including hepatoblastoma. Simpson-Golabin-Behmel syndrome is an X-linked syndrome, which appears to arise from point mutations or deletions within the glypican 3-gene at the Xq26 locus. The glypican 3-gene is a member of a multigene family encoding for a class of molecules that have been found to play an essential role in development by modulating cell responses to growth factors and morphogens.

The association between familial adenomatous polyposis (FAP) and hepatoblastoma was initially documented by Kingston et al in 1982 and later confirmed by others.[32–34] Familial adenomatous polyposis is caused by a germline mutation of the adenomatous poliposis coli (APC) gene localized to chromosome 5.[35] With the exception of hepatoblastoma, this mutation has not been reported in other embryonal tumors.[36] Alteration in the degradation of β-catenin, which is regulated by the APC gene, is frequently detected in hepatoblastoma. A recent study has demonstrated that at least half of the cases of hepatoblastoma are associated with mutation of the β-catenin gene.[36,37] The significance of this finding is still under investigation.

The frequent association between reported hepatoblastoma cases and genetic cancer syndromes suggests that this tumor may result from a possible genetic mutation of chromosomes 11p or 5q.[38]

Trisomies of chromosome 18 have been detected in many patients with hepatoblastoma.[39–42] Tumor karyotypes have often revealed the presence of extra chromosomes or trisomies at times associated with other structural changes.[43,44] Within the same tumor, multiple clones with different types of trisomies can be observed, suggesting a clonal evolution with gain of extra chromosomes. Trisomies 2 and 20 are the most commonly found abnormalities associated with hepatoblastoma, and each has been found as the only karyotype abnormality, suggesting that they represent early stages in tumor evolution. Trisomy 8 has also been reported in association with hepatoblastoma, but it is found less frequently than chromosomes 2 and 20.[45]

Schneider et al reported the translocation t(1;4) (q12, q34) for the first time in 4 male patients with advanced hepatoblastoma.[46] Other investigators have also detected this translocation.[45,47,48] In all cases, this translocation was associated with other chromosomal abnormalities including trisomies 2, 8, and 20.

Prader-Willi syndrome has been reported in association with hepatoblastoma.[49] Although the p53 mutation (Li-Fraumeni syndrome) has been associated with hepatoblastoma, it does not seem to be a predisposing factor for its development.[50]

Epidemiological studies have suggested an association between prematurity and the development of hepatoblastomas.[51–53] Ikeda et al reported that in Japan, hepatoblastoma accounts for 58% of all cancers observed in premature infants weighing less than 1000 grams at birth.[54,55] Tanimura also noted that there is an inverse relationship between the risk for the development of hepatoblastoma and birth weight. According to this study, the relative risk for developing hepatoblastoma is 15.64 in newborns weighing less than 1000 grams, compared with 2.53 for those between 1000 and 1500 grams and 1.21 for those weighing more than 2000 grams.[56] Feusner and Ribons have confirmed the increased incidence of hepatoblastoma in premature infants in North America.[51,57,58] However, the factors associated with prematurity that may predispose to the development of hepatoblastoma have yet to be identified. Different environmental factors, such as fetal alcohol syndrome[9] and maternal use of contraceptives,[59,60] have been associated with the development of hepatoblastoma. In an epidemiologic study of 70 children with hepatoblastoma and 75 case-matched controls, Buckley et al[61] demonstrated an association between tumor development and maternal occupational exposure to metals, petroleum products, paints, and pigments. However, paternal exposure to metals was the only factor significantly associated with the development of tumor.

Hepatocellular carcinomas are frequently associated with hereditary metabolic diseases that lead to hepatic cirrhosis, such as hereditary tyrosinemia,[62] glycogen storage disease type I,[63] Alagille syndrome,[64] and α-antitrypsin deficiency.[65] The prolonged use of androgens in patients with Fanconi anemia has been associated with the development of both benign as well as malignant hepatic tumors.[66] Ataxia telangiectasia syndrome has also been associated with the development of HCC.

Recent publications have summarized the vast data now available on the genetic and molecular pathogenesis of human HCC.[67–69] Briefly, the development of HCC is a slow, multistep process associated with changes in genomic expression that lead to alterations of the hepatocellular phenotype and the appearance and progression of tumor. The development of HCC may take many years, and it starts in the setting of chronic hepatitis or cirrhosis with destruction of hepatocytes and inflammatory changes that alter the matrix and the microenvironment of the liver.

Hepatocellular carcinoma as a second malignant neoplasm has been reported following abdominal radiotherapy for treatment for Wilms tumor, as well as following the use of methotrexate for the treatment of acute lymphoblastic leukemia.[70,71]

In UESL, there is a pattern of cytogenetic alterations described similar to that in other pediatric sarcomas. Consistent molecular changes, such as tumor-specific translocations, have been described that may result in gene fusions—for example, EWS/FLI1 or EWS/ERG.[72,73] Also, translocations involving 19q13 have been found both in mesenchymoma and UESL.[74] Because the 19q region is also involved in other sarcomas, it is possible that these changes activate some oncogenes or inactivate tumor-suppressor genes located in this region. Complex genetic alterations in the form of chromosomal amplifications (1q, 5p, and 8p) and deletions have also been found in UESL.[22] Most UESLs are diploid; aneuploidy may be associated with a more malignant behavior, although observations are limited.[75]

Clinical Presentation

At the time of diagnosis, the majority of children with hepatic tumors present with an asymptomatic abdominal mass in the right upper quadrant that is frequently palpated by a parent or by the pediatrician. These masses are occasionally associated with abdominal distention (Table 29-3). Patients with hepatoblastoma usually present with an asymptomatic mass, whereas patients with HCC frequently present with constitutional symptoms such as anorexia, weight loss, and abdominal pain as well as vomiting.[7,38] Jaundice is generally rare in patients with pediatric liver tumors, with the exception of some cases of HCC as well as the rare cases of biliary-tree ERMS.

Occasionally, males with hepatoblastoma may present with precocious puberty secondary to the abnormal secretion of the β subunit of human chorionic gonadotropin (HCGβ).[76–79]

Congenital anomalies such as Meckel diverticulum, congenital absence of adrenal glands, and renal abnormalities have been rarely associated with the development of hepatoblastoma. The presence of a certain degree of osteopenia at the time of diagnosis is seen in a number of patients with hepatoblastoma.[80] This finding disappears with treatment, but it can be severe in up to 20% to 30% of patients, occasionally associated with back pain, refusal to walk, and radiographic evidence of pathological fractures and compression fractures of vertebral bodies.

In patients with HCC associated with preexisting inflammatory or metabolic diseases, signs of hepatic cirrhosis are frequent and include hepatosplenomegaly as well as cutaneous telangiectasis.

Hemoperitoneum secondary to tumor rupture has been reported;[81] however, this condition has rarely been seen in children.

Metastases to the lung occur in up to 20% to 30% of patients at the time of diagnosis for patients with hepatoblastoma and HCC. Peritoneal implants (especially in HCC), extension into adjacent intraabdominal structure, and spread to distant lymph nodes, bones, bone marrow, and the central nervous system can be occasionally identified.[82,83]

Clinical symptoms of liver sarcomas are not specific and include the presence of an abdominal mass (which may be painful), fever, and occasionally vomiting and weight loss. Despite the commonly large size of the tumors in UESL, jaundice is rarely present; however, biliary obstruction and jaundice are prominent symptoms of ERMS evolving from the extrahepatic biliary tree. In one case of primary liver ERMS, a paraneoplastic syndrome in the form of hypertrophic osteopathy was described.[84] Both UESL and primary liver ERMS tend to metastasize to lungs, albeit infrequently.[83]

Table 29-3

Clinical characteristics of pediatric liver tumors at diagnosis.

Characteristic	Hepatoblastoma	Hepatocellular Carcinoma
Abdominal tumor	Frequent	Frequent
Abdominal distention	Frequent	Frequent
Anorexia	Rare	Occasional
Weight loss	Rare	Occasional
Nausea and vomiting	Rare	Frequent
Jaundice	Rare	25%
Splenomegaly	Occasional	Frequently associated with cirrhosis
Preexistent condition		Frequent

Diagnostic Evaluation

Laboratory Investigations

The initial evaluation should include a complete hematological analysis (Table 29-4). A mild normochromic, normocytic anemia can be seen, as well as thrombocytosis and occasionally polycythemia secondary to extrarenal secretion of erythropoietin. Thrombocytosis with platelet counts exceeding 500000 per cu mm are observed in more than 80% of children with hepatoblastoma and less frequently in patients with HCC. Thrombocytosis is frequently associated with an increased secretion of thrombopoietin,[85,86] or due to intratumoral synthesis of interleukin-6.[87] The liver enzymes and alkaline phosphatase may be elevated in some patients with HCC but are frequently normal in those with hepatoblastoma. Hyperbilirubinemia is found in fewer than 5% of patients with hepatoblastoma and in 25% of those with HCC. There is no correlation between elevation of bilirubin or hepatic enzyme levels and prognosis of patients with liver tumors.

The serum α-fetoprotein (AFP) is the most sensitive tumor marker for the diagnosis and clinical evaluation of hepatic tumors in children.[88,89] Alpha-fetoprotein is a glycoprotein initially found in the fetus starting during the fourth week of gestation; it is originally produced in the yolk sac and the liver, and then from the eleventh week only the liver produces it. Alpha-fetoprotein synthesis peaks during the fourteenth week of gestation, gradually declining to normal adult levels (3-20 ng/ml) within 6 months after birth.[90,91] The half-life of AFP is between 5 and 7 days.

Alpha-fetoprotein levels are almost always elevated in children with hepatoblastoma and elevated in 50% to 60% of children with HCC.[91-93] Alpha-fetoprotein levels are usually much higher in hepatoblastoma than in HCC. Alpha-fetoprotein levels in patients with fibrolamellar HCC are usually within normal ranges. Rarely, patients with benign liver tumors, such as hamartomas and hemangioendotheliomas, can present with elevated AFP levels, leading to erroneous diagnoses if the pathologic confirmation of tumor is not obtained.

Alpha-fetoprotein is an excellent biologic marker to determine tumor activity. Following complete surgical resection of hepatoblastoma, the AFP level declines exponentially to normal, according to its half-life. An increase in AFP level frequently precedes the detection of tumor recurrence.[94-97] VanTornout et al demonstrated that the magnitude of decline of AFP levels following diagnosis is the most important prognostic factor for patients with unresectable or metastatic hepatoblastoma.[93] This finding may therefore facilitate early detection of an inadequate tumor response to chemotherapy and allow for introduction of therapeutic modifications prior to tumor progression. However, further studies are necessary to confirm this hypothesis.

Patients with hepatoblastoma and low AFP levels (less than 100 ng/ml) at diagnosis had a worse outcome in a German hepatoblastoma cooperative study[98] as well as in the SIOPEL 2 study of the International Liver Tumors Study Group of SIOP (International Society of Pediatric Oncology), suggesting a more aggressive behavior of these tumors and a higher risk for treatment failure.[99]

The use of lectin-affinity immuno-electrophoresis has been proposed to differentiate AFP produced by the tumor (based upon structural microheterogeneity in the carbohydrate moiety of the molecule) from AFP physiologically produced during hepatic regeneration or in response to inflammatory stimuli.[96]

Beta-human chorionic gonadotropin is abnormally elevated in those cases presenting with isosexual pseudo-precocious puberty.[100,101] Elevated urinary cystathionine levels have been reported in children with hepatoblastoma, but this test is rarely used in the diagnostic workup of children with hepatic tumors.[102] Serum cholesterol can be elevated in children with hepatoblastoma or HCC,[103-106] while levels of ferritin and carcino-embryonic antigen may be elevated in some patients with HCC. The fibrolamellar variant of hepatocellular carcinoma can be associated with an abnormality of the vitamin B12 binding protein, which can occasionally be used to monitor disease status and response to therapy.[92,107] Screening for viral hepatitis (B and C) should be performed in all patients.

Radiologic Investigations

Radiologic investigations are required to determine intrahepatic and intraabdominal tumor extension, the relation-

---

Table 29-4

Diagnostic evaluation of hepatic tumors.

Infants and Children Younger Than 4 Years

- Complete hematologic evaluation
- Liver function tests
  - Transaminases
  - Bilirubin
  - Alkaline phosphatase
  - Cholesterol
- α-Fetoprotein
- β-Human chorionic gonadotropin

Children Older Than 4 Years and Adolescents

- Complete hematologic evaluation
- Liver function tests
  - Transaminases
  - Bilirubin
  - Alkaline phosphatase
  - Cholesterol
- α-Fetoprotein
- Carcino embryonic antigen
- Hepatitis B and C
- Vitamin B12 binding protein

ship of the liver tumor to the complex vascular anatomy of the liver, and the presence of distant metastases. Abdominal ultrasound, contrast-enhanced spiral computed tomography (CT) scan, and magnetic resonance imaging (MRI) are diagnostic tools used to study tumor extension. Instead of establishing the superiority of one technique over others, it is usually recommended that one should rely on the locally existing expertise and on the multidisciplinary evaluation of radiologic findings to study tumor extension carefully.

Plain radiographs of the abdomen frequently demonstrate the presence of a right upper quadrant mass, and calcifications may be noted in approximately 6% of malignant hepatic tumors.[108] Ultrasonography is a reliable and noninvasive imaging technique in establishing the presence of an intrahepatic mass. It aids in differentiating solid from cystic masses, and in determining the presence and degree of vascular involvement.[109,110] Computed tomography scanning including the chest is the most commonly used imaging study to determine both local and distant extent of tumor involvement. The presence of multiple lesions or portal hypertension may suggest the diagnosis of hepatocellular carcinoma.[111,112] Due to the multiplanar nature of MRI, this technique is rapidly replacing the CT scan as a predictor of tumor resectability.[113]

Positron emission tomography is a new, not widely available, option that might prove particularly useful in staging of the disease and detection of recurrence in patients with rising serum AFP levels and negative standard imaging; however, very few contradictory reports exist.[114,115]

Arteriography has been used to help surgeons map the liver vasculature in planning for surgery; however, MRI or magnetic resonance angiography or helical angioCT are increasingly being used for this purpose. Although gallium scanning is infrequently used in the diagnosis of liver tumors, it may aid in distinguishing between regenerating nodules of cirrhosis and tumors, since the regenerating nodules are frequently gallium negative.

Imaging methods used for the study of liver sarcomas are similar to those for hepatoblastoma and HCC. The sonographic appearance of UESL varies from a cystic, hypoechoic mass with multiple echogenic septae to a largely echogenic mass with multiple small cysts.[20,116] In biliary ERMS, abdominal ultrasound usually demonstrates the presence of a solid mass within the hepatic hilum. On CT, UESL usually appears as a large, hypodense mass with multiple septations and with occasionally large areas of solid tissue within a mass, or as a peripheral solid lesion.[19,20] The abundant myxoid matrix of the tumor explains the low attenuation seen on CT.[116] On T1-weighted MR images, UESL is predominantly hypointense and heterogeneous with focal areas of increased signal intensity, while the T2-weighted images reveal a hyperintense mass that contains hypointense septae.[20] For the assessment of biliary ERMS, MR cholangiopancreatography (MRCP), also called MRI cholangiography or cholangioresonance study, is of particular value.[18,117] However, imaging of intrahepatic biliary ERMS may be very challenging.[117] Other imaging techniques applicable to biliary ERMS, albeit more invasive, include endoscopic retrograde cholangiopancreatography or, in case of jaundice, percutaneous transhepatic cholangiography. Percutaneous transhepatic cholangiography can be done in an ultrasound-guided manner. Cholangiography usually shows a bizarre filling defect due to the tumor and visualizes smaller intrahepatic ducts better than MRCP.[117] Overall radiological characteristics of UESL may resemble those of MH with a tendency to be more solid; the age of the patient can be a distinguishing factor, because UDS is very rare below the age of 5 years, while MH usually presents in infants and very young children.[19] However, cystic-like lesions may occasionally be found within hemangioendothelioma, HCC, angiosarcoma, and intrahepatic lymphoma.

Metastatic lesions to the liver are frequently seen in many common malignancies of children and adolescents, such as neuroblastoma, Wilms tumor, and germ cell tumor. However, these lesions are rarely associated with clinical symptoms and are found by imaging studies during the evaluation of extent of disease (staging).

Tumor Staging

The use of a staging system that facilitates the separation of patients into distinct clinical groups is essential to determine prognosis and plan therapy. In North America, the most widely used staging system is based upon the extent of tumor and surgical resectability (Table 29-5).[95,118,119] The International Society of Pediatric Oncology, however, has developed a preoperative

---

Table 29-5

Pediatric Oncology Group staging of hepatoblastoma.

- Stage I (favorable histology) tumors are those that are completely resected and have a typical histology of a purely fetal histologic pattern with a low mitotic index (< 2 per 10 high-power fields).

- Stage I (other histology) tumors are completely resected tumors with a histologic picture other than purely fetal with low mitotic index.

- Stage II tumors are grossly resected tumors with evidence of microscopic residual disease. Resected tumors with preoperative (intraoperative) rupture are classified as stage II.

- Stage III (unresectable) tumors are those that are considered by the attending surgeon to be not resectable without undue risk to the patient. This includes partially resected tumors with measurable tumor left behind. Lymph node involvement is considered to constitute stage III disease.

- Stage IV tumors are those that present with measurable metastatic disease to lungs or other organs.

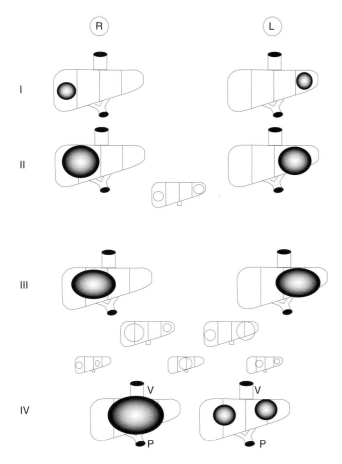

Figure 29-1 PRETEXT system. V, extension into the vena cava and/or all three hepatic veins; P, extension into the main portal vein and/or both left and right portal branches; R, right; L, left.

staging system (<u>Pre</u>-<u>t</u>reatment <u>e</u>valuation of <u>t</u>umor <u>ext</u>ension: PRETEXT). The PRETEXT system relies on radiologic staging, using the main hepatic and portal veins to identify the number of liver sectors involved by tumor.[120,121] In the PRETEXT system, the liver is divided into 4 sectors—an anterior and a posterior sector on the right and a medial and a lateral sector on the left (see Figure 29-1). In this way, 4 PRETEXT categories are identified. Tumors are classified as PRETEXT I when 3 adjoining sectors are free and only 1 is involved by the tumor; as PRETEXT II when 2 adjoining sectors are free and 2 involved; as PRETEXT III when just 1 sector is free and 3 involved (or 2 nonadjoining sectors are free), and PRETEXT IV when there are no tumor-free sectors. Intraabdominal extension of the tumor beyond the liver is indicated by "V" in the case of extension into the vena cava and/or all 3 hepatic veins; "P" in the case of extension into the main trunk and/or both left and right branches of the portal vein; "E" in the case of extrahepatic extension other than "P" and "V"; and "M" when distant metastases are detected. The prognostic value of the system has been proven in the SIOPEL 1 study; the system is additionally useful for predicting operability and the type of resection anticipated.

In a recent article, Aronson et al[122] discussed the accuracy, reproducibility, and predictive value of the PRETEXT staging system from the SIOP Liver Tumor Study Group used for patients enrolled on the SIOPEL-1 study. In this article, the authors also compared the PRETEXT system in a retrospective manner with 2 alternative systems: the system used by the American-based Children's Oncology Group (COG; formerly the Children's Cancer Study Group/Pediatric Oncology Group [POG]) and the conventional TNM system, previously used by the German cooperative hepatoblastoma trials, and concluded that the PRETEXT staging system was superior to the COG staging system for predicting survival. In a review of this manuscript, Meyers et al[123] supported the conclusion that the PRETEXT system is a wonderful tool for predicting resectability and even survival in the subgroup of patients who successfully complete neoadjuvant chemotherapy; however, they pointed out that due to flaws in the study design, one should be careful in accepting the conclusion in regards to the comparison of staging systems. Further research is necessary to evaluate the predictive value of PRETEXT in all patients with hepatoblastoma.

There is no uniformly accepted staging system for HCC, especially so in patients with liver cirrhosis in which not only the tumor itself but additional patient factors, such as the Child-Pugh class (degree of liver compensation, hyperbilirubinemia, presence of ascites, hypoalbuminemia) have to be taken into account. The classical TNM system, although the oldest, does not seem to be particularly well suited to HCC. Most adult groups use the Okuda system, Barcelona score, or Cancer of the Liver Italian Program scale.[124] In children with noncirrhotic HCC, traditional hepatoblastoma staging systems are used (eg, PRETEXT). It is obvious that a single unique international staging system is needed in order to permit a comparison between the results obtained by different therapeutic protocols.

Pathology

The pediatric surgical pathologist has multiple responsibilities in the diagnosis and management of pediatric liver disease. The diversity of tumor-like lesions and tumors occurring in children and adolescents represents a broad spectrum of conditions.

This section approaches malignant hepatic tumors in children and adolescents by a morphologic approach. Although the discussion will focus on the 4 most common malignancies (hepatoblastoma, hepatocellular carcinoma HCC, UESL, and ERMS), other benign and malignant conditions in pediatric practice will be discussed briefly as they are necessarily considered in the morphologic differential diagnosis. Ancillary procedures will be discussed as these (when warranted) are used to support or validate a specific diagnosis. The greatest ultimate responsibility that the pathologist has is not only to render a final diagnosis, but also to exclude any and every other tumor and tumor-like lesion known to occur in the liver, either as primary or metastatic/systemic disease.

Handling and Management of Tissue by the Pathologist

During the biopsy procedures, a critical immediate role for the pathologist, of paramount importance to the patient, clinician, and surgeon, is determining adequacy of tissue material for diagnosis, depending on the final or differential diagnosis rendered during intraoperative frozen section consultation.

A factor often overlooked is the potential of underlying metabolic liver disease as a background for development of hepatic neoplasia. This situation requires special prompt tissue handling for ultrastructural studies as well as archival of uninvolved liver tissue, snap-frozen for enzymatic or molecular genetic assays.

Biopsy Specimens and/or Tumor Section Samples for Intraoperative Consultation

The participation of the pathologist during biopsy of a suspected malignancy includes frozen section diagnosis for the establishment of a working differential diagnosis and determination of the need for additional biopsy material, depending on the quality of diagnostic material. Depending on the type of tumor, frozen tissue is secured for any pertinent ancillary procedures in addition to the formalin-fixed, paraffin-embedded tissue; the latter is adequate for immunohistochemistry and fluorescence in situ hybridization (FISH) studies. The advantage of this approach is that the pathologist can verify that the sample submitted includes material representative of tumor. Cytogenetic analysis, when warranted, requires a sterile tissue sample placed in cell culture medium, which can in turn be used for karyotyping and FISH on whole nuclei or on metaphase spreads.

Tumor Resection

Resected malignant tumor specimens include: tumorectomy with margin of uninvolved liver, segmentectomy, hepatic lobectomy, extended lobectomy, tri-segmentectomy, and liver explant in the case of transplantation. Radical resection specimen blocks may potentially include the liver and biliary tree as well as porta hepatis lymph nodes, or adherent diaphragm and adjacent contiguously involved structures.

It is imperative that the pathologist receives surgical pathology specimens intact, preferably in the operating room. The initial assessment includes documentation with the surgeon as to the extent of the resected specimen and issues of intraoperative assessment of the hepatic parenchymal, biliary tree, and other margins as warranted. Ideally, the specimens should be cut immediately, by making serial sections of the whole specimen in a plane that will *best* demonstrate the topography of the tumor and its relationships to the liver and adjacent structures when present. It is desirable to cut specimens in an anatomic plane, either a coronal plane, which correlates well with MRI studies, or a transverse plane, which correlates with CT scan appearance. The gross description in the surgical pathology report and tumor sampling should reflect a "written photograph" of the specimen so that the individual reading the report obtains a clear mental image of the specimen. Required assessments are: the type of specimen, the size and weight of the specimen, measurement of the tumor in 3 dimensions, the size of the parenchymal margin, the integrity of the Glisson capsule or extracapsular extension (surface or porta hepatis soft tissues, gallbladder), the extent of viable-appearing tumor (particularly following chemotherapy or embolization), gross texture characteristics, topographic distribution of the tumor (circumscribed, multifocal, permeative, encapsulated, extrahepatic extension, vascular invasion, and so on), heterologous elements or cysts present, and areas of hemorrhage and/or necrosis. Other critical descriptors include the extent of tumor and its relationship to the surgical margins of resection, including measurements of the distance between the edge of the tumor and the surgical margin. Presence or absence of regional nodes and/or other structures with measurements and gross characteristics are also required. Finally, description of the appearance of the uninvolved adjacent liver is of great importance.

Tumor Diagnosis

Epithelial or Epithelioid Cell Tumors

The better-differentiated liver cell tumors recapitulate the cord or trabecular architecture of the liver, usually thicker than one cell (infants have cords composed of 2 cells), delimiting sinusoidal spaces, and lined by endothelial cells. Depending on cell size, growth pattern, and nuclear or cytoplasmic atypia, the differential diagnosis includes the following entities:

1. *Hepatic Adenomas:* These tumors are single or multiple, sometimes pedunculated and prone to rupture, grossly circumscribed, firm, fleshy, pale (when showing fatty change) (Figure 29-2A,B), brown, or bile stained. They are expansile, compressing the adjacent liver and perhaps showing encapsulation, but by definition, no evidence of permeation into the adjacent hepatic cords or vascular invasion is to be found (Figure 29-2C). Occasional adenomas with cytologic atypia can be seen, particularly in those associated with increased serum steroid levels.

2. *Focal Nodular Hyperplasia:* These tumors are intrahepatic, small or large, and may be pedunculated; grossly and sometimes apparent by imaging is a central stellate scar (Figure 29-3). They are nonencapsulated liver cell proliferations that include portal (bile duct, vessel) structures, allowing distinction from adenomas, which lack portal structures, and from macro-regenerative nodules by the lack of underlying disease in the adjacent liver. Nodular regenerative hyperplasia may occasionally form tumor-like lesions.

3. *Hepatoblastoma (Fetal, Embryonal, Macro-Trabecular):* While the traditional classification is still in place, criteria for diagnosis of hepatoblastoma tumors must follow strict guidelines.[125] Epithelial hepatoblastomas are single, massive, or multifocal, usually extensively infiltrative, non-encapsulated tumor; gross features include fleshy homogeneous friable tumors with hemorrhage and necrosis. Microscopically

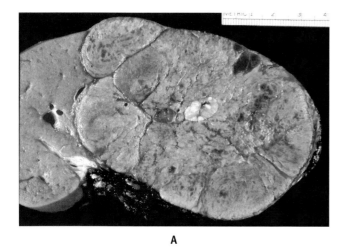

A

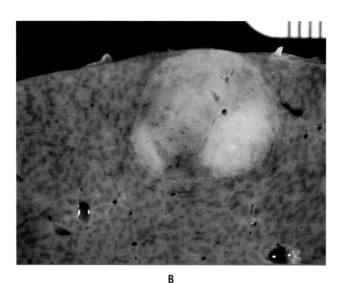

B

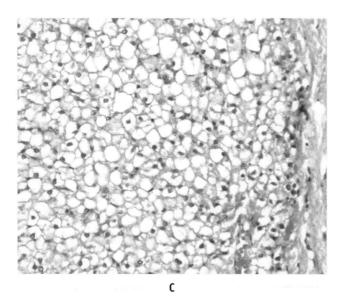

C

Figure 29-2 (A) Large hepatic adenoma showing circumscribed borders and lobulated homogeneous appearance. (B) Circumscribed subcapsular adenoma showing pallor, usually related to fatty change. (C) Photomicrograph of hepatic adenoma with clear cells due to fatty accumulation. **See Plate 51 for color image of (C).**

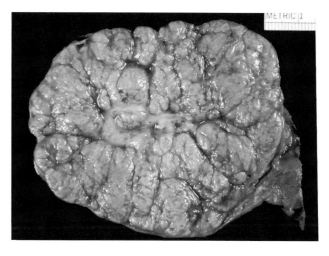

Figure 29-3 Focal nodular hyperplasia with stellate scar in the central region.

they are composed of intermediate-sized, eosinophilic, finely granular polygonal cells (fetal pattern) or sometimes clear cells, which may be pure or more commonly mixed with less-differentiated, primitive- (embryonal-) appearing cells also growing in cords, but with a high nuclear to cytoplasmic ratio and hyperchromasia. Bile production in cytoplasm may be seen (Figure 29-4A-E). These tumors may show extramedullary hematopoiesis, organoid growth, and pseudo-canalicular formations. Recently described hepatoblastoma with "cholangioblastic features" by their morphology and expression of cytokeratin 19 are yet another example of multiphenotypic features of hepatoblastoma.[126] The use of immunohistochemistry in the workup and diagnosis of hepatoblastoma is limited because it shares positive immuno-phenotypic features with its closest mimicker, HCC.[127] Hepatoblastoma and HCC both express hepatocyte paraffin 1 (HepPar1) in a cytoplasmic pattern and CEA in a canalicular pattern. When warranted, HepPar1 and CEA appear to be useful in separating endodermal sinus tumor and metastatic carcinomas to the liver. Various markers are expressed in both HBL and HCC; vimentin appears to be less frequently positive in HBL. The recent documentation of C-Kit expression in the membrane of fetal HBL and in the cytoplasm of embryonal HBL cells supports the notion that these are derived from pluripotent stem-like cells.[128,129]

4. *Hepatocellular Carcinoma:* Hepatocellular carcinoma tumors can vary from small ($>$2-5 cm encapsulated tumor or with focally infiltrative borders) to massive, and can also be multifocal or diffuse. Hepatocellular carcinoma is usually a diffusely infiltrative tumor with morphology ranging from well differentiated to anaplastic and giant cell tumor.[130] HCC cells are typically larger than those of normal liver and of hepatoblastoma cells. These cells also have defined borders; large, round, uniform nuclei, and distinct, conspicuous nucleoli. HCC can have various growth patterns including cords and trabecular, macro-trabecular, pseudo-glandular, scirrhous (with sclerotic fibrous tissue), among others. All variants of HCC infiltrate the underlying vasculature of the liver (Figure 29-5A,B). The fibrolamel416lar variant is characterized by

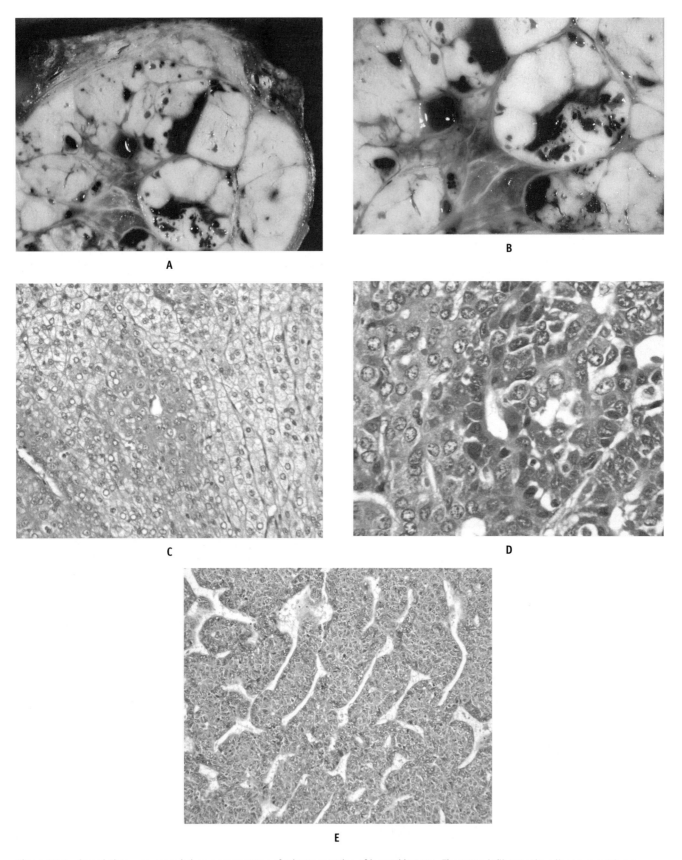

Figure 29-4 (A and B) Low-power and close-up appearance of primary resection of hepatoblastoma. The tumor infiltrates the adjacent parenchyma (upper) and is a lobulated, relatively homogeneous fleshy mass. (C) Morphology of fetal hepatoblastoma showing uniform population of neoplastic hepatocytes with distinct cell borders. Some have clear cytoplasm; other areas show slight nuclear enlargement. (D) Embryonal hepatoblastoma adjacent to fetal component, showing increased nucleo-cytoplasmic ratio and embryonal morphology. The tumor is recognizable as hepatoblastoma, given its recapitulation of trabecular morphology. (E) Macrotrabecular pattern composed of thick multicellular cords defining sinusoidal spaces. **See Plates 52-54 for color images for (C), (D), and (E).**

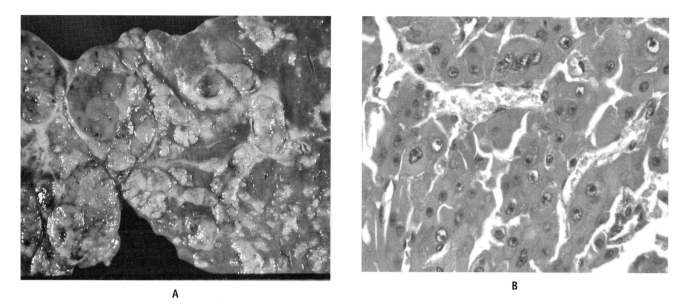

Figure 29-5 (A) Macroscopic appearance of disseminated hepatocellular carcinoma shows extensive vascular permeation, invasion into hepatic veins, and focal bile production. (B) Morphology of relatively well differentiated HCC showing large polygonal cells and abundant cytoplasm, large nuclei, and distinct nucleoli, delimiting sinusoidal spaces. **See Plate 55 for color image of (B).**

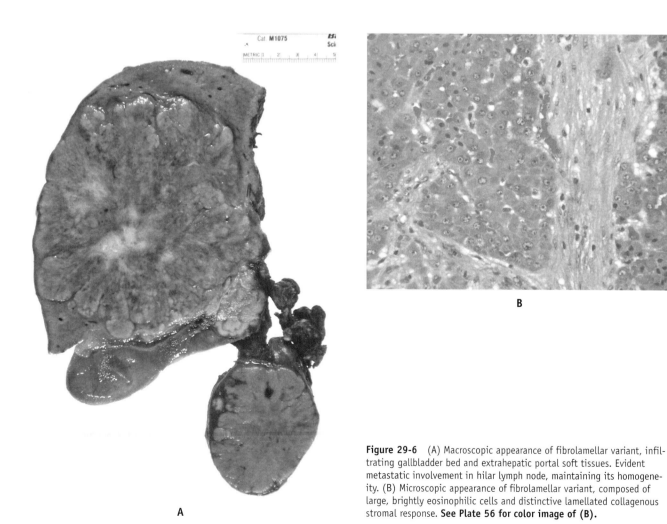

Figure 29-6 (A) Macroscopic appearance of fibrolamellar variant, infiltrating gallbladder bed and extrahepatic portal soft tissues. Evident metastatic involvement in hilar lymph node, maintaining its homogeneity. (B) Microscopic appearance of fibrolamellar variant, composed of large, brightly eosinophilic cells and distinctive lamellated collagenous stromal response. **See Plate 56 for color image of (B).**

very large, brightly eosinophilic cells growing as cords delimited by lamellated sclerotic collagenous tissue[12,131] and warrants distinction from conventional HCC, given its different biologic behavior[132] (Figure 29-6A,B).

5. *Transitional Liver Cell Tumors:* In older children and adolescents, some tumors show hybrid features of hepatoblastoma, with HCC making precise classification in either category unsatisfactory; some of these features may be found after chemotherapy. The use of β-catenin expression in different patterns by immunohistochemistry appears to support this concept. These tumors are highly aggressive.[133]

6. *Metastatic Tumors:* Metastatic epithelial or epithelioid tumors to the liver in the differential diagnosis include: rare adenocarcinomas of childhood, primary or metastatic endodermal sinus tumor (EST) characterized by mutlifocality, and a distinctive morphology with conspicuous AFP staining eosinophilic globules, Schiller-Duval bodies, and vesicular microcystic formations. Of note is that EST has a hepatoid variant that can be virtually indistinguishable from either hepatoblastoma or HCC, and thus exclusion of a gonadal primary is warranted; the use of HepPar1 antibody is useful in confirming the hepatocellular nature of a neoplasm[134,135]; metastatic mixed malignant germ cell tumor; primary choriocarcinoma of the liver, which is usually seen in infancy and may encompass the "infantile choriocarcinoma syndrome" characterized by presentation during infancy, anemia, bleeding, hepatomegaly, and elevated HCGβ;[136,137] metastatic placental and gonadal pure choriocarcinoma; and extremely rare metastatic transplacental maternal carcinomas. Metastatic nonepithelial tumors include epithelioid angiomyolipoma, which usually shows distinctive morphology and positivity for HMB45, myogenic markers, and CD117. Also included are gastrointestinal stromal tumors (GIST), which are usually positive for CD117 or C-Kit and CD34. Lymphoreticular large-cell tumors include Hodgkin lymphoma, identified by morphologic features and positivity of CD15 (LeuM1) and CD30 (Ki-1), usually accompanied by a mature cellular infiltrate forming portal-centered nodular aggregates, and large-cell non-Hodgkin lymphoma, usually positive for leukocytic lineage markers and histiocytic disorders, including Langerhans cell histiocytosis (CD1a and/or S100+) and true histiocytic lymphomas. Epithelioid hemangioendothelioma mimics carcinoma, composed of large epithelioid cells with occasional cytoplasmic lumen formation.[138] These cells grow in a fibroblastic stroma; by immunohistochemistry they are positive for factor VIII–related antigen, CD34, factor XIII, and occasionally keratin and epithelial membrane antigen (EMA). A very important differential consideration reflects the propensity of ocular and other melanomas to metastasize to the liver. Amelanotic melanoma pose a diagnostic difficulty, requiring confirmation with S100 protein, HMB45, and MelanA antibodies.

Small-Cell Tumors

1. *Undifferentiated Embryonal Sarcoma of the Liver:* Grossly, these tumors are large, circumscribed or diffusely infiltrative, and solid or solid/cystic with a propensity to invade the inferior vena cava and extend to the right atrium. There are reports of associated peripheral eosinophilia. These tumors usually show extensive necrosis, making their sampling for biopsy problematic. Although UESL tumors are predominantly composed of small, stellate and/or pleomorphic cells, diffusely growing in a myxoid or fibroblastic background, they frequently incorporate larger pleomorphic and anaplastic cells with small pink to orange eosinophilic globules[21] (Figure 29-7A). Immunochemistry shows that these tumors have variable expression of epithelial and mesenchymal markers, including alpha-1 antitrypsin, alpha-1 antichymotrypsin, lysozyme, CD68, desmin, HHF35, and rarely keratin. Unless distinct and widespread myogenesis is clearly documented by either morphology or immunochemistry, intrahepatic sarcomas with undifferentiated morphology should be considered UESL[139] with the caveat that skeletal muscle differentiation can be present in these tumors[140] but not to the degree shown in ERMS. Recently, there have been reports of UESL arising within mesenchymal hamartomas, showing a distinct cytogenetic alteration, involving t(11; 19) (q13, 13.4).

2. *Embryonal Rhabdomyosarcoma of the Liver or Biliary Tree:* This tumor may arise from the wall of the common bile duct, where it may grow into the lumen as the "botryoid" type (Figure 29-7B) or arise within the liver as a solid, fleshy, and homogeneous mass[141] and is rarely reported as arising in the gallbladder. Microscopically, it shows alternating myxoid and cellular areas imparted by growth of short, hyperchromatic spindle cells, many with brightly eosinophilic cytoplasm and evidence of cross-striations. When this tumor grows into an epithelium-lined cavity, the tumor cells condense in the subepithelial zone, creating a "cambium" layer of tumor cell condensation (Figure 29-7C). Less-differentiated examples are composed of small round cells, some with vacuolization and circular filamentous inclusions surrounding the nucleus. If no cross-striations are apparent, immunohistochemistry is warranted to confirm rhabdomyogenic phenotype by desmin, muscle specific actin, and myogenin. Poorly differentiated intrahepatic examples are sometimes impossible to separate from UESL (see above).

3. *Small-Cell Hepatoblastoma:* Usually a component of conventional hepatoblastoma, small-cell hepatoblastoma (SCHB) may constitute a significant portion of the hepatoblastoma or, rarely, can be the predominant pattern.[142] It is composed of small round cells or spindle cells with focal trabecular formations but little differentiation (Figure 29-8). It may show positivity for keratin. These small cells are considered pluripotent stem cells.[143]

4. *Neuroendocrine Tumors—Carcinoid:* These tumors are rare in childhood, arising as primary hepatic or metastatic tumors composed of uniform small round cells, growing in cords and trabecular formations. These tumors are usually positive for chromogranin-A and other endocrine markers. These tumors must be differentiated from desmoplastic small round cell tumors (DSRCTs).

5. *Metastatic Small Round-Cell Tumors:* Neuroblastoma and DSRCTs, as well as other primitive sarcomas that may originate within the abdominal cavity, may metastasize to the liver and be the most accessible site for biopsy.

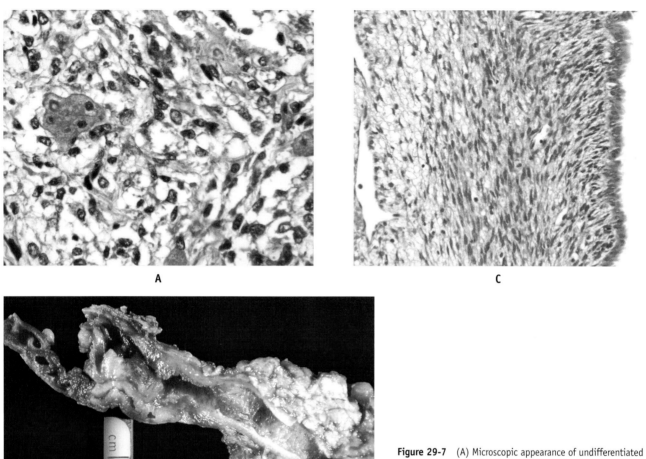

A

B

C

Figure 29-7 (A) Microscopic appearance of undifferentiated embryonal sarcoma showing a spectrum of cells; some appear primitive, other cells are large and pleomorphic. (B) Gross appearance of embryonal rhabdomyosarcoma arising from the common bile duct; note myxoid expansion of wall, narrowing the lumen. (C) Microscopic image of embryonal rhabdomyosarcoma showing condensation of mesenchymal cells under the epithelium. **See Plate 57 for color image of (A).**

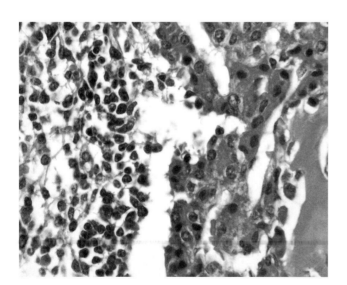

Figure 29-8 Microscopic image of small cell hepatoblastoma component (center) as part of mixed hepatoblastoma showing osteoid (upper right). **See Plate 58 for color image.**

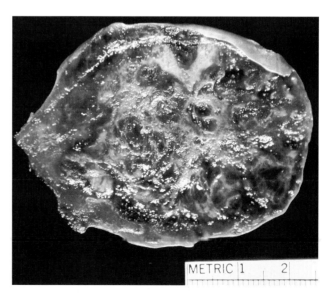

Figure 29-9 Resected, pedunculated hemangioma type I showing readily apparent cavernous spaces filled with blood and sclerotic changes.

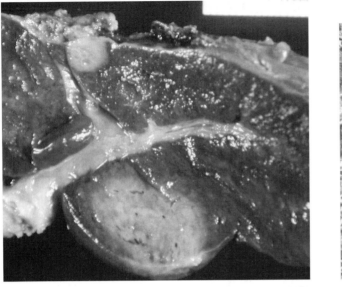
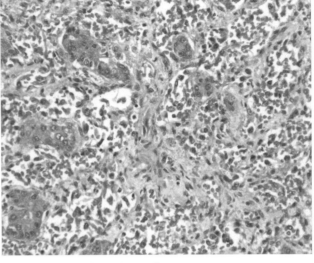

A   B

Figure 29-10 (A) Incidental autopsy findings of multicentric hemangioendothelioma type II, growing as solid, circumscribed, but infiltrative tumors. (B) Microscopic appearance of hemangioendothelioma composed of solid growth of spindle cells defining occasional inconspicuous vascular structures. There is mild pleomorphism of the endothelial cells but no malignant features. Note entrapped hepatocyte clusters. **See Plate 59 for color image of (B).**

Neuroblastoma shows some degree of neuropil formation, facilitating its diagnosis. Desmoplastic small round cell tumors usually show marked desmoplasia, the absence of which may suggest the morphologic diagnosis of endocrine tumors. Desmoplastic small round cell tumors co-express desmin, keratin, and MIC2 and WT1 (Wilms tumor 1 gene product) by immunochemistry.[144] Confirmation may require reverse transcriptase-polymerase chain reaction (RT-PCR) analysis for the EWS/WT1 gene fusion. Other tumors that may metastasize to the liver include Wilms tumor, lymphomas, and malignant germ cell tumors.

Spindle Cell Tumors

1. *Infantile Hemangioendothelioma and Angiosarcoma:* These tumors are small or very large single or multifocal tumors; they may be associated with similar tumors in other sites and may show spontaneous regression. They may be associated with congestive heart failure and the Kasabach-Merritt syndrome and intraabdominal bleeding. Two morphologic types I and II exist. Type I is identified by ectatic vascular spaces and conspicuous myxoid background infiltrating the liver, and type II is identified by solid proliferation of spindle and epithelioid cells defining vascular channels (Figure 29-9 and 29-10A,B)[145] and must be distinguished from angiosarcoma, which shows morphologic atypia of cells;[146] some, however, are indistinguishable. A recent review of these tumors separates them as arteriovenous malformations, infantile hemangioendotheliomas, and cavernous hemangioma.[147]

2. *Smooth Muscle Tumors in Immunosuppressed Patients and Metastatic Sarcomas to the Liver:* Leiomyomas and leiomyosarcomas may occur in the liver, presenting as single or multicentric lesions; their morphology and im-

munochemistry are identical to those occurring in the soft tissue and viscera. These tumors are associated with the Epstein-Barr virus (EBV). Other spindle-cell sarcomas, usually those arising within the abdominal cavity, include cellular mesoblastic nephroma, clear cell sarcoma of the kidney, and GISTs.

3. *Inflammatory Myofibroblastic Tumors:* When primary in the liver, these tumors are associated with sclerosis and conspicuous plasma and lymphocytic cell infiltration. Primary liver inflammatory myofibroblastic tumor (IMT) is frequently associated with EBV.[148,149] Metastatic inflammatory fibrosarcoma[150] shows morphologic atypia, pleomorphism, and mitotic activity and mimics pseudo-sarcomatous fibroblastic tumors.[151] Rarely, usually in adults, HCC may have sarcomatoid morphology.

Mixed, Teratoid, and Cystic Tumors

1. *Mixed and Teratoid Hepatoblastoma:* These tumors show similar gross morphology as conventional hepatoblastoma but with apparent variable mineralization, usually osteoid intermixed with cellular tumor. Extensive necrosis or osteoid matrix production may be apparent in hepatoblastoma after chemotherapy (Figure 29-10A,B). Morphologically, conventional epithelial hepatoblastoma elements are intermixed with conspicuous spindle cell myxoid proliferation, punctuated by cysts of intestinal type epithelium and/or squamous epithelium. The mesenchymal components may show skeletal muscle differentiation, chondroid, and osteoid matrix production (Figure 29-10C).

2. *Hepatic Teratoma and Metastatic Teratoma with Malignant Germ Cell Tumor:* Teratoma of the liver is highly unusual; primarily reported in infants and young children, it may be congenital. Grossly these tumors may be massive but are usually well circumscribed.[152] It is

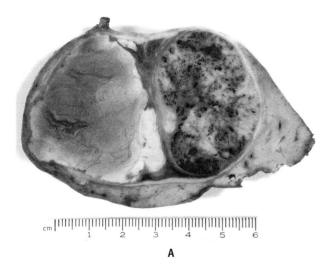

A

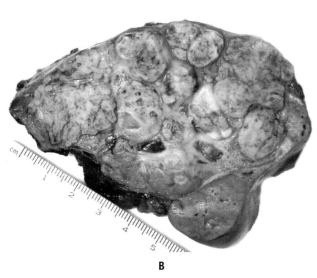

B

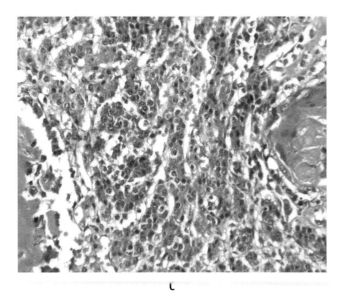

C

Figure 29-11 (A and B) Hepatoblastoma resected after chemotherapy; (A) shows partial necrosis and grossly viable appearing nodule; (B) shows extensive osteoid differentiation throughout this HBL. (C) Histology of mixed (epithelial / mesenchymal) HBL with primitive appearing mesenchyme and bone production. **See Plate 60 for color image of (C).**

important to differentiate teratoid hepatoblastoma from true teratoma of the liver or postchemotherapy maturation of malignant germ cell tumor (MGCT).

3. *Mesenchymal Hamartoma:* Mesenchymal hamartoma (MH) is grossly either a circumscribed or interdigitating solid and cystic tumor or a large multicystic unresectable tumor, with myxoid fluid- or mucin-filled cystic cavities, mimicking cystadenomata (Figure 29-12A). Microscopically, MH is characterized by biliary epithelium-lined cysts, disorganized bile ducts defined by a poorly defined myxoid and vascular proliferation permeating the liver and dissociating regional structures at its border.[153] No morphologic atypia or increased cellularity of the epithelium or stromal components should be seen (Figure 29-12B,C). There is a reported association with UESL.[154,155] Translocations involving chromosome 19 have been reported.[43,156]

4. *Desmoplastic Nested Spindle Cell Tumor of Liver/ Nested Stromal Epithelial Tumor of the Liver:* A tumor recently characterized by Hill et al, the reported experience consists of 10 cases in 2 series[157,158] showing a distinctive morphology occurring in children and adolescents.

These are well-circumscribed lobular tumors ranging in size from 2 cm to 30 cm. Spindle and epithelioid cohesive cell nests growing in a desmoplastic myofibroblastic stroma characterize them. Both series describe calcification and/or ossification. Most cases follow a benign course.

Treatment

Complete tumor resection is the cornerstone of therapy for liver tumors and offers the only realistic chance of long-term disease-free survival.[13,14,121,159] Chemotherapy has increasingly become an important part of the therapy for children with hepatoblastoma. It has been used as adjuvant therapy for patients who undergo complete tumor resection at the time of diagnosis, to induce tumor shrinkage preoperatively in those tumors considered unresectable or when primary resection is considered hazardous, and to control metastatic disease. Hepatocellular carcinomas have consistently been treated according to therapeutic trials for hepatoblastoma, despite the fact that the two malignancies are biologically different. Hepatocellular carcinomas most often present as multifocal tumors with vascular invasion and frequent metastases at diagnosis, making complete surgical excision almost impossible.[14,160]

Surgery

Biopsy

Pathological determination of the diagnosis remains the cornerstone of any therapeutic strategy. The combination of relevant clinical findings such as a hepatic mass in a young child associated with an elevated AFP level strongly suggests the diagnosis of hepatoblastoma, and outside of the context of a study, in certain cases it may allow for treatment without histological confirmation. Tissue diagnosis is strongly recommended in very young children (younger than 6 months) due to the large variety of hepatic tumors occurring in this age group and of the

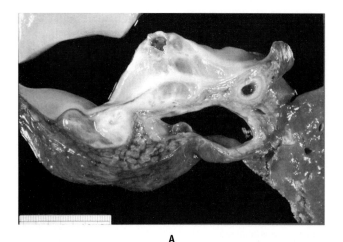

A

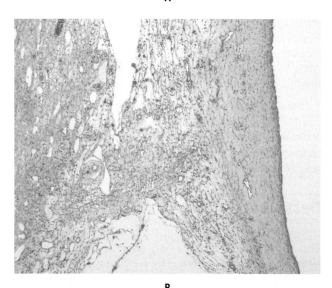

B

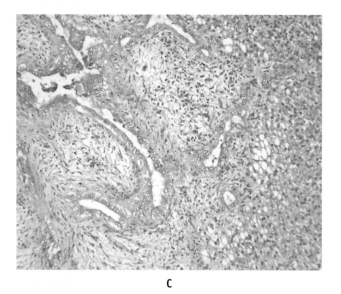

C

Figure 29-12 (A) Gross hamartomatous appearance of mesenchymal hamartoma showing interdigitation within liver structures. This was a pedunculated growth, circumscribed from underlying liver, but not encapsulated. (B and C) Large myxoid degenerative areas with cyst devoid of any lining; other areas show the multifocal, hamartomatous features of bile ducts formation, mesenchyme, and vascular structures amid liver tissue. **See Plates 61 and 62 for color images of (B) and (C).**

confounding effects of a physiologically elevated AFP level. Similarly, biopsy should be mandatory in all children presenting with a hepatic mass and older than 4 years; fewer than 5% of cases of hepatoblastoma have been diagnosed in children older than 4 years.[3]

The aim of biopsy in HCC is to obtain sufficient tissue to allow an accurate diagnosis while avoiding intraoperative complications, especially hemorrhage. There is also the possibility of seeding tumor cells into an uninvolved segment of the liver, the abdominal wall, or peritoneal cavity. These risks can be minimized by using a percutaneous coaxial technique or (in the case of a laparoscopic approach) using a protecting needle to guide Tru-cut biopsies.

Obviously, in a resectable tumor suspected most likely of being an HCC (ie, if the patient is an older child or young adult with a predisposing condition) primary resection should be undertaken without any attempt at biopsy alone. In clear cases of HCC arising within cirrhotic liver, the tumor diagnosis can be made on clinical grounds providing the tumor is more than 2 cm in diameter and is associated with unequivocal rise in AFP and imaging findings. However, one must keep in mind that in cirrhotic patients, AFP may be permanently elevated due to an ongoing liver regeneration process.

Tumor Resection

Irrespective of whether surgery is timed at initial diagnosis or upon subsequent second surgery following chemotherapy, complete resection of tumor represents the main goal of any treatment strategy. In fact, only gross tumor resection offers a realistic hope of cure. Hepatic surgery for tumor removal always implies a small, but significant, risk of fatal complications, mainly represented by uncontrolled blood loss. Actually, the loss of about one unit of blood in uncomplicated liver resections is quite a common event. Thus, it is strongly recommended to have tumor resection performed by surgical and anesthesiology teams experienced in hepatic surgery. Complete tumor resection is possible at diagnosis in 30% to 40% of cases, while it becomes possible at different time points following chemotherapy in 70% to 80% of cases overall.

In the case of tumors located in close proximity to the main liver vessels, in which circumstance resection would require peeling tumor off the vessels or even vascular reconstruction, such hazardous resections—which would in any event certainly leave microscopic residual tumor—should be avoided, due to the excellent survival rates of primary liver transplantation, if patients can be referred to a liver transplant center in a timely fashion.[161]

However, the prognostic relevance of leaving microscopic residual tumor is not clearly established. Unpublished SIOPEL 1 and SIOPEL 2 experience has shown that microscopic residual tumor does not necessarily carry an adverse prognosis. In the SIOPEL 1 trial of 11 patients with a positive resection margin, only 2 died, but neither of these patients experienced a local relapse. None of the 11 had a second resection, and all but 1 (who received local irradiation) were treated with postoperative chemotherapy alone. No relapse occurred and all survivors were in complete remission at their last follow-up (at a mean follow-up of 5.5 years). These favorable and quite unexpected results might possibly be explained by the use of the Cavitron ultrasound dissection and aspiration (CUSA) device during surgery. The resection margin is "vacuum cleaned" and therefore ablated. One could hypothesize that, despite the positive margin at the specimen site, there may have been a tumor-free margin at the patient's site. Alternatively or in addition, residual tumor may not be "viable" because of the lethal cell damage from preoperative chemotherapy. However, these data require further studies and should be interpreted with caution. At the present time, both the SIOPEL and the North American (Children's Cancer Group [CCG]) studies do not recommend any special therapeutic changes in patients with microscopic residual tumor.

Surgical resection is also advocated for those patients with isolated lung metastases remaining after chemotherapy. The role of aggressive thoracic surgery has been documented essentially in the case of salvage therapy; however, thoracotomy and resection also have an important role as the first line of therapy if feasible.

All recent studies have confirmed the importance of complete tumor resection in order to achieve cure in patients with HCC. However, fewer than 20% of patients are amenable to initial surgical resection. Nevertheless, the ultimate goal of treatment for HCC is to achieve complete tumor removal in either a primary or delayed setting. Standard hepatic resection techniques should be recommended, including segmentectomies, hemi-hepatectomies, and extended hemi-hepatectomies in advanced cases. However, limited hepatic reserve may be a problem in patients with liver cirrhosis, precluding any liver resection. As emphasized earlier, only a gross total resection offers realistic hope of cure for patients with HCC. Therefore, all options should be explored before declaring a tumor unresectable. In this regard, intraoperative ultrasound examination might be very useful, and it is essential when segmental hepatic resection is planned. Sampling of lymph nodes from the hepatoduodenal ligament should be performed in every patient with HCC, because their involvement has a significant impact on prognosis. In fact, even more extensive lymphadenectomy of the hepatic pedicle should be recommended.

In general, primary tumor excision of a biliary ERMS is rarely undertaken nowadays, although IRS I and II study data from the early 1980s demonstrated that 6 out of 10 tumors were primarily resected, and 4 patients became long-term survivors.[141] However, biliary ERMS may require very extensive operations, including pancreatico-duodenectomy, when operated primarily or following an inadequate response to initial chemotherapy. Embryonal rhabdomyosarcoma is generally a chemosensitive tumor, and in most cases it shrinks with chemotherapy, thus facilitating conservative surgery.[18,162] Porta hepatis lymph nodes should be biopsied during definitive surgery. In some cases associated with severe biliary obstruction, excessive toxicity due to cytostatic drugs excreted with bile, such as vincristine and doxo-

rubicin, must be avoided. In such patients, external drainage of the biliary tree needs to be established prior to starting chemotherapy by placement of an external biliary draining catheter (EBD) or by internal-external biliary drainage (IEBD).[18,163]

Chemotherapy

The introduction of effective chemotherapeutic regimens for the treatment of hepatoblastoma has significantly improved the survival of children diagnosed with this tumor. Agents with therapeutic efficacy in the treatment of hepatoblastoma include vincristine,[164,165] 5-fluorouracil,[165–168] doxorubicin,[169–171] cisplatin,[172] and carboplatin.[173] Cyclophosphamide, ifosfamide, and etoposide have been used as part of some chemotherapeutic regimens; however, their individual efficacy against liver tumors has not been determined.[174–177]

Adjuvant Versus Neoadjuvant Chemotherapy

Hepatoblastoma: With the advent of effective chemotherapy for the treatment of hepatoblastoma, two different schools of thought have emerged in regards to the utilization of chemotherapy. Investigators from the North American COG and the German and Japanese cooperative groups support the use of chemotherapy as adjuvant therapy following initial surgical resection whenever feasible. This recommendation is based on several different factors: gross total resection of the tumor continues to be the most important favorable factor predictive of cure; approximately one-third of hepatoblastoma patients can successfully achieve a gross total resection of tumor at diagnosis, and among them it is possible to identify some that require minimal or no chemotherapy; postsurgical complications are not less frequent—and may in fact be more frequent[178]—in patients submitted to surgery following initial chemotherapy.[179]

The SIOPEL proposes the use of delayed surgery following initial chemotherapy with the following objectives: to increase the number of patients for whom complete surgical resection of the tumor is feasible; to reduce the surgical morbidity; and to provide more time for making definitive surgical plans, including liver transplantation when indicated.[180] Due to the large numbers of countries participating in the SIOPEL studies, standardization of both sophisticated surgical approaches and supportive care measures has been difficult; therefore, the use of upfront chemotherapy prior to surgery has permitted patients from countries with limited resources to participate in these studies.

The benefit of adjuvant chemotherapy for patients with completely resected tumors was documented in early studies conducted jointly by the CCG and the POG.[119] In this study, stage I patients, achieving complete tumor resection, received chemotherapy with vincristine, cyclophosphamide, doxorubicin, and 5-fluorouracil, and had a tumor recurrence rate of only 6%. This rate is significantly lower than the 64% recurrence rate reported for patients who did not receive adjuvant chemotherapy. In the same study, the 2-year survival was only 26% for patients with unresectable tumors who received chemotherapy with cyclophosphamide, actinomycin D, vincristine, and 5-fluorouracil. The introduction of cisplatin in combination with other chemotherapeutic agents has resulted in a significant improvement in the outcome of patients with unresectable tumors at diagnosis. In 1991, CCG reported that the use of chemotherapy with cisplatin (90 mg/m^2 continuous infusion over 6 hours) followed by doxorubicin (80 mg/m^2 continued infusion over 96 hours) for patients with stage III and IV tumors improved their 3-year disease-free survival to 55% and 30%, respectively.[95] Douglass et al reported for the POG event-free survivals of 67% and 12.5% for patients with stage III and IV tumors, respectively, when treated with a combination of cisplatin (90 mg/m^2 continuous infusion over 6 hours on day 1), vincristine (1.5mg/m^2 on day 2), and 5-fluorouracil (600mg/m^2 on day 2).[181]

The following North American Intergroup study (INT-0098) was designed with the main objective of determining, in a randomized fashion, which of the above regimens was superior. The 5-year event-free survival for all patients (except stage I with pure fetal histology) was 57% for patients treated with Regimen A (cisplatin, vincristine, and 5-fluorouracil) and 69% for those treated with Regimen B (cisplatin and doxorubicin).[178] Although this difference was not statistically significant, the types of events associated with each regimen were notably different. Although tumor progression accounted for 86% of all reported events for patients treated with Regimen A, it represented only 56% of all events observed in those patients treated with Regimen B. However, Regimen B was associated with an increased number of treatment complications and toxic deaths. Based on these results, the COG adopted the regimen of cisplatin, vincristine, and 5-fluorouracil as the standard for the treatment of children with hepatoblastoma.

Patients with stage I favorable histology (pure fetal) treated on INT-0098 were not randomized and received 4 courses of doxorubicin (20 mg/m^2/bolus for 3 consecutive days). The event-free survival for the 9 patients entered in this group was 100%. Patients with stage I unfavorable histology (43 patients) were randomized between Regimens A and B as previously described. The 5-year event-free survival in this group was 91%.[178] Based on this experience, on the next COG study (P9645) stage I patients with pure fetal histology receive no further chemotherapy following the initial surgery, while those with stage I unfavorable histology receive 4 cycles of chemotherapy with cisplatin, vincristine, and 5-fluorouracil.[182] Preliminary analysis of this study has demonstrated that only 1 of 10 patients with pure fetal histology hepatoblastoma has developed disease progression, for an event-free survival of 95%. The survival rate for patients with favorable histology is 100%. This experience suggests that gross total resection of the tumor may be sufficient as treatment for those patients with favorable histology.

The German Cooperative Study HB89 used a combination of ifosfamide, cisplatin, and doxorubicin for the treatment of children with unresected hepatoblastoma at diagnosis. Their results were similar to those of the American Intergroup Hepatoblastoma Study and demonstrated that gross total resection of tumor was feasible in 78% of the patients after 2 to 4 courses of chemotherapy, and that the 3-year survival was 75%.[183] The German group recently reported upon the results obtained with their HB94 study. In this study, all patients received following diagnosis 2 cycles of chemotherapy with ifosfamide, cisplatin, and doxorubicin. Patients who did not demonstrate tumor response or who had metastatic or advanced disease went on to receive therapy with carboplatin and etoposide. The 3-year disease-free survival rate for stage III and IV patients was 76% and 21%, respectively.[184]

The Japanese study for pediatric liver tumors, JPLT-1, conducted between 1991 and 1999, used a modified TNM staging system to classify patients. For this study, 154 patients were entered, and of those, 145 were diagnosed with hepatoblastoma. According to this study, which emphasized initial tumor resection, stage I and II patients received chemotherapy courses of cisplatin (40 mg/m^2) and tetrahydropyranyl-adriamycin (30 mg/m^2). For stage IIIA, IIIB, and IV patients, the dose of cisplatin and adriamycin were increased to 80 mg/m^2 and 30 mg/m^2 for 2 days, respectively.[185] Survival and event-free survival rates for the 134 hepatoblastoma patients were 73% and 66%, respectively.

The SIOPEL-1 study was developed to expand and further confirm the results obtained in a pilot study using the PLADO regimen—that is, cisplatin 80 mg/m^2 followed by doxorubicin 60 mg/m^2 administered as a continuous infusion over 48 hours.[186] Patients entered on this study were staged according to the PRETEXT classification system, and all patients underwent preoperative chemotherapy with PLADO. Patients were evaluated following 4 courses of PLADO and followed by surgical resection if feasible. Of 154 patients entered in the study, 134 patients received preoperative chemotherapy and 106 patients (79%) subsequently achieved a gross total resection of the tumor (including 6 by liver transplantation). Thirteen patients received primary surgery for various reasons, 3 died early in the course of treatment, and data on 4 are missing. The 5-year event-free survival was 66%, comparable to the 69% obtained with a similar cisplatin and doxorubicin regimen in the North American Intergroup study.[180] However, the toxicity associated with the chemotherapy used in the SIOPEL-1 study was less than that reported in the North American study, most likely a result of the reduced length of doxorubicin infusion. It is however, important to notice that the surgical morbidity and mortality rates associated with this postchemotherapy surgical approach were 18% and 5%, respectively,[187] higher than those observed in the North American studies that used upfront surgical resection of the tumor followed by chemotherapy. However, this discrepancy can be explained by the large multicenter design of the SIOPEL study. The centers that participated in the study had different levels of experience in hepatobiliary surgery and were located in countries of varying economic status; these factors might have contributed to the observed differences between the SIOPEL and North American studies.

The main objectives of SIOPEL-2 were to determine the activity of 2 different regimens for patients identified as having standard- or high-risk hepatoblastoma. Standard-risk patients (with tumor limited to the liver, with no more than 3 sectors involved) received 4 courses of cisplatin (80 mg/m²) at 14-day intervals before surgery. High-risk patients (with tumor extension to all 4 liver sectors with or without pulmonary metastasis and/or intra-abdominal or vascular extension) received cisplatin alternating every 14 days with carboplatin (500 mg/m²) and doxorubicin (60 mg/m²). Of the 150 patients entered onto the study, 77 were considered standard risk and 58 high risk. The 3-year survival and event-free survival rates for standard-risk patients were 91% and 73%, respectively.[99] For high-risk patients, the 3-year survival and event-free survival rates were 52% and 47%, respectively.[188] Table 29-6 shows the results obtained in recent studies according to the approach (adjuvant vs neoadjuvant) and the chemotherapeutic regimen used.

Based on previous studies that suggested cisplatin to be the most effective chemotherapeutic agent for the treatment of hepatoblastoma, and considering the experience acquired with the intensification of cisplatin in pediatric germ cell tumors, COG developed a study to determine if the intensification of the platinum agent would improve the outcome for patients with stage III and IV hepatoblastoma. This study was also designed to determine if amifostine, a cytoprotective agent, is effective in reducing the toxicities associated with the administration of platinum-containing compounds in children with hepatoblastoma. Patients were randomized to receive either an intensified platinum regimen with carboplatin alternating with cisplatin with or without amifostine, or the standard regimen of cisplatin, vincristine, and 5-fluorouracil with or without amifostine. However, this randomization was discontinued in January 2002 when preliminary analysis demonstrated an event-free survival rate of 37% in the 56 patients randomized to the intensified platinum regimen, which was significantly inferior to the event-free survival rate of 57% observed in 53 patients treated with the standard regimen.[189] Despite the efforts to intensify therapy for patients with metastatic disease at diagnosis, outcome for these patients continues to be poor, with survival rates of less than 25%. Furthermore, the use of amifostine in the doses and schedule used in this study failed to reduce significantly the incidence of platinum-induced toxicities in patients with hepatoblastoma. The incidence of significant hearing loss, of greater than 40 dB, was similar for patients treated with or without amifostine: 38% (14 of 37) versus 38% (17 of 45) ($p = 0.68$), respectively.[190]

Table 29-6

Results of recent studies.

Adjuvant				
Group	Regimen	Patients	Patients	SOS/EFS
INT. 0098	A: CDDP/VCR/5FU	43	IUH	98%/91%
(CCG 8881/POG 8945)[108]	B: CDDP/DOXO	7	II	100%/100%
		83	III	69%/64%
		40	IV	37%/25%
GC PLTS	CDDP/IFOSF/DOXO		III	/76%
HB-94[153]			IV	/25%
JPLT[203]	91A2 CDDP/THT DOXO	48	IIIA	76.6%/67.5%
		25	IIIB	50.3%/47.5%
		20	IV	64%/40.6%
Neoadjuvant				
Group	Regimen	Patients	Patients	OS/EFS
SIOPEL 2[205,206]	SR: CDDP	77	I, II, III	91%/73%
	HR: CARBO/DOXO/CDDP	58	IV, Met.	52%/47%
FSPO/AmCA[154]	SR: CARBO/EPIRUB	18	I, II, III	/71%
	HR: CARBO/EPIRUB	11	IV, Met.	/30%

Abbreviations: CDDP, cisplatin; VCR, vincristine; 5FU, 5-fluorouracil; DOXO, doxorubicin; CARBO, carboplatin; EPIRUB, epirubricin; SR, standard risk; HR, high risk; OS, overall survival; EFS, event-free survival; CCG, Children's Cancer Group; POG, Pediatric Oncology Group; GCPLTS, German Cooperative Pediatric Liver Tumor Study; JPLT, Japanese Group for Pediatric Liver Tumors; SIOP, International Society of Pediatric Oncology; FSPO/ANCA, French Society of Pediatric Oncology/Academic Medical Center—Amsterdam.

Hepatocellular Carcinoma

Katzenstein and Czauderna have reported upon the results of children and adolescents with HCC treated on the recently completed North American Intergroup Hepatoma study (INT-0098) and the SIOPEL-1.[160,191] Both studies utilized preoperative chemotherapy in an attempt to increase surgical resectability, because this is the foundation for curative therapy of liver tumors.

Forty-six patients were entered onto the North American Intergroup Hepatoma study. After initial surgery or biopsy, all patients, 8 with stage I completely resected tumors, 25 with stage III unresectable tumor, and 13 with stage IV metastatic tumor were randomized to receive cisplatin with either doxorubicin or 5-fluorouracil and vincristine. There were no differences regarding response or survival rates between the 2 treatment regimens.

Seven of the 8 stage I patients (88%) with complete tumor excision at time of diagnosis followed by adjuvant cisplatin-based chemotherapy survived. This improvement is significant when compared with only 12 of 33 patients (36%) treated before the consistent use of adjuvant chemotherapy. This result suggests that adjuvant chemotherapy may be of benefit for patients with completely resected HCC. However, since one-third of these initially resected patients have fared well without any additional chemotherapy, the question of the necessity for adjuvant chemotherapy will be answered only in a randomized trial. In contrast, outcome was uniformly poor for patients with advanced-stage disease. The 5-year event-free survival rates for stage III and IV patients were 23% and 10%, respectively. Gross total resection of tumor after neoadjuvant chemotherapy was feasible in only 2 patients, and although these 2 patients did experience a prolonged survival, they eventually died of recurrent disease.

Thirty-nine patients were entered onto the SIOPEL-1 study. Of these, 2 underwent complete resection of the tumor at diagnosis followed by chemotherapy, and 37 had preoperative chemotherapy with cisplatin and doxorubicin. The determination of extent of tumor was based on radiological findings and classified according to the PRETEXT system. Disease was often advanced at the time of diagnosis, with 24 of 39 patients (62%) classified as PRETEXT III and IV. Metastases were identified in 31% of the patients, and extrahepatic tumor extension, vascular invasion, or both were identified in 39%. The tumor was multifocal in 56% of the patients. Although partial tumor response to chemotherapy was observed in 49% (18 of 37) of the patients, complete tumor resection was achieved in only 36% (14 of 39) of the patients. Outcome of patients on this study was also unsatisfactory, with a 5-year event-free survival of 17%. All long-term survivors had complete surgical excision of their tumor.

Twenty-one patients diagnosed with HCC were registered on the SIOPEL 2 study between March 1994 and May 1998, and data are available for 17 of these patients. Disease was advanced in most patients at diagnosis. Metastases occurred in 18% of the patients, extrahepatic tumor extension and/or vascular invasion were found in 35% of patients, and the tumor was multifocal in 53% of the patients. One

patient died 17 days after diagnosis from massive gastrointestinal bleeding and never received treatment. Thirteen of the 16 treated patients received preoperative chemotherapy ("SuperPLADO"—cisplatin, carboplatin, and doxorubicin). Partial response to preoperative chemotherapy was observed in 6 of 13 cases (46%). Gross total tumor resection was achieved in 8 patients (47%), 3 at the time of diagnosis and 1 through liver transplantation. Nine tumors (53%) never became operable. One patient was lost to follow up just before planned surgery. Four of the resected patients were alive at a median follow-up time of 53 months (range of 35 to 73 months). Twelve patients died due to progressive disease, and one from surgical complications. The 3-year overall survival for this study was 22%.

In the SIOPEL-2 study, treatment intensity was increased compared with the SIOPEL 1 study by rapidly alternating the administration of cisplatin (every 14 days) with carboplatin and doxorubicin. Despite this intensification of standard systemic chemotherapy, no improvement in event-free or overall survival has been achieved.

In the cooperative studies of the German Society for Pediatric Oncology and Hematology, childhood HCC was treated with the same regimen as hepatoblastoma, although throughout all three trials surgeons were obliged to attempt a primary complete resection in all cases with suspected HCC. In the first study, HB89 (conducted between 1989 and 1993), neoadjuvant and adjuvant chemotherapy consisted of conventionally dosed ifosfamide, cisplatin, and doxorubicin (IPA), which did not show any substantial benefit (D. von Schweinitz, personal communication, 2003). Thus, of the 12 registered patients, only 4 with resectable tumor survived. In the second study, HB94 (conducted between 1994 and 1998), patients with nonresectable HCC received conventionally dosed carboplatin and etoposide in addition to IPA, which seemed to produce at least short-term partial benefit (D. von Schweinitz, personal communication, 2003). Of the 25 registered patients, 9 had locally unresectable and 11 metastatic HCC. Three of the 9 and 1 of the 11 patients survived free of disease, in addition to 4 of 5 patients with resectable tumor (total 8 of 25 = 32%). In the current study, HB99, unresectable HCC is treated neoadjuvantly with conventionally dosed and high-dose carboplatin and etoposide, and some initial effect on tumor regression has been observed as well as some effect on microscopic residual tumor. Since 1999, 33 patients have been registered: all 7 patients with primary gross total resection are free of tumor, as well as 1 of 2 with primary microscopic residual tumor, and all 6 with presumed tumor spillage at primary operation. However, all 5 patients with unresectable tumor died of disease, as well as 8 of 11 with metastatic HCC. Of the latter, 2 are in remission and 1 still under therapy. Thus, there seems to be some response of HCC to carboplatin and etoposide, which, however, remains unsatisfactory.

In comparing the results of these studies with three North American studies conducted between 1973 and 1984,[192] the outcome for patients with HCC has shown no significant improvement despite the progress in surgical techniques, chemotherapy delivery, and patient support. It seems obvious that a completely new treatment approach is needed to increase the cure rate of childhood HCC.

First described in 1956 by Edmonson[193] as a distinct pathologic variant, the fibrolamellar type of hepatocellular carcinoma has been traditionally associated with a higher resection rate and better survival when compared with the typical pathological variant of HCC in both adolescents and young adults.[7,194–197]

The higher resection rate for patients with the fibrolamellar variant of HCC was not supported by the studies reported by Katzenstein[198] and Czauderna.[189] Ten of 46 patients (22%) entered onto the Intergroup Hepatoma study had a fibrolamellar HCC. Resectability at diagnosis and response to therapy were not different from those patients with typical HCC. Patients with the fibrolamellar variant did not have a better outcome when compared with those with typical HCC; the 5-year event-free survival was 30%, compared with 14%, respectively ($p = 0.18$), although the median survival was longer for patients with the fibrolamellar variant. The same results were seen in the SIOPEL-1 study; 4 of 6 patients with fibrolamellar variant of HCC died of disease. However, their survival was much longer (25 months vs 11 months) than that of the rest of the group.

Sorafenib, a new multikinase inhibitor with anti-angiogenic, pro-apoptotic, and Raf kinase inhibitory activity, was recently evaluated in a multicenter, randomized, placebo-controlled Phase III trial for patients with advanced HCC[199]. Sorafenib was well tolerated and demonstrated a statistically significant improvement in overall survival for patients with advanced HCC.

Liver Sarcomas

Adjuvant chemotherapy is indicated for all liver sarcomas, especially UESL and ERMS. In the era of surgical treatment alone, the survival was very poor and did not reach 30%.[22] Liver sarcomas were initially treated with chemotherapy regimens similar to those for hepatoblastoma, utilizing cisplatin, doxorubicin, 5-FU, and vincristine, but in recent years alkylator-based soft-tissue sarcoma protocols have more commonly been used. Tumors unresectable at diagnosis require preoperative, neoadjuvant chemotherapy. Typically, 3 or 4 chemotherapy courses are given. Webber et al reported that 7 children with unresectable UDS were treated with neoadjuvant chemotherapy. In 2 of these children, significant tumor shrinkage was observed; all 7 patients received postoperative chemotherapy, and 4 of them were cured, 2 experienced relapse and died, and 1 died from chemotherapy complications.[22] Bisogno et al reported 17 cases of UDS. Tumor resection at diagnosis was performed in 11 of these cases;[17] excision was complete in 4 cases. Six patients underwent biopsy only as an initial procedure, followed by neoadjuvant chemotherapy and delayed resection in all cases, which was complete in 4, while micro- or macroscopic residual tumor was left in 2; all 6 patients responded to preoperative chemotherapy, although response was minor in 2 of them. Pathologic examination showed that 3 of 4 completely resected tumors displayed greater than 90% necrosis of tumor. All patients received postoperative chemotherapy: 5 were treated with vincristine, actino-

mycin, and cyclophosphamide (VAC) alternating with cyclophosphamide and doxorubicin), 9 children received (VAC) plus adriamycin (VACA) or vincristine, actinomycin, ifosfamide, and doxorubicin (VAIA), one received cisplatin, etoposide, vincristine, doxorubicin, ifosfamide, actinomycin, and another one was treated initially with cisplatin and doxorubicin and then VAIA after recurrence. One patient died after surgery and did not receive any chemotherapy. Eleven of these 17 patients are alive in first remission, and one is alive in the third remission (4 years after the last recurrence), for a 70% overall survival rate with a follow-up ranging from 2.4 years to 20 years.

Other smaller series also noted a significant degree of response to preoperative chemotherapy in the range of 50% to 60%).[200–202] Most of these tumors became largely necrotic and could be successfully resected. In a recently published small series by Kim et al, the overall survival of patients with hepatic UDS treated by surgery and chemotherapy was 83%, with a follow-up time from 40 months to 122 months.[19]

The improved survival rate achieved in a recent series of patients with UESL in which chemotherapy has been uniformly used supports the strategy of using both pre- and postoperative chemotherapy in hepatic UESL. This result contrasts sharply with the poor cure rates in which surgical treatment alone was employed. It is difficult to determine which drugs in these chemotherapy regimens are the most effective, but it would appear that the use of alkylating agents is crucial, because soft-tissue sarcoma protocols were found to be more effective than hepatoblastoma (anthracycline, platinum, and/or 5-fluorouracil) regimens. Nevertheless, anthracyclines and platinum derivatives probably have some activity against UESL. According to the German and Italian Soft Tissues Sarcoma Groups, the VAIA regimen (VCR 1.5 mg/m² [maximum 2 mg] weekly for 4 weeks plus actinomycin 0.5 mg/m² [maximum 2 mg] on days 1-3 on weeks 1 and 7, plus ifosfamide 3 g/m² on days 1 and 2 of weeks 1, 4, and 7, plus doxorubicin 40 mg/m² on days 1 and 2 of week 4) is considered currently the first-line treatment, while a carboplatin and etoposide combination constitutes second-line chemotherapy.[17]

Biliary ERMS are treated with similar chemotherapy to UESL (VAC, VACA, VAIA, IVA protocols). Usually, modern preoperative chemotherapy produces very significant tumor shrinkage, in the range of 75% to 80%.[18]

New Chemotherapeutic Agents

The identification of new, effective chemotherapeutic agents for the treatment of malignant liver tumors is a challenge, because Phase I and II studies frequently include fewer than a handful of patients with these types of tumors.

Topotecan, a water-soluble analog of camptothecin, an inhibitor of topoisomerase I, has been shown to have antitumor activity against human hepatoblastoma subcutaneously implanted in immunodeficient mice.[203] In this animal model, the activity of topotecan was similar to that of doxorubicin. Recently, Palmer and Williams[204] have reported dramatic tumor response to irinotecan, also an inhibitor of topoisomerase I, similar to topotecan, in a single patient with a multiply recurrent hepatoblastoma. The current

COG study has been designed to determine the response rate following 2 cycles of novel regimens when administered as initial "window" chemotherapy for the treatment of children with metastatic (stage IV) hepatoblastoma; the first regimen consists of the combination of vincristine and irinotecan. The SIOPEL and German Hepatoblastoma Liver groups are currently investigating the activity of irinotecan in a Phase II study for patients with relapsing and chemotherapy refractory hepatoblastoma.

Radiation Therapy

The role of radiation therapy in the treatment of hepatoblastoma and HCC has not been established. A retrospective study conducted by SIOPEL investigators of patients with hepatoblastoma and HCC treated in different European institutions suggested that radiation therapy might be useful in some cases to control residual disease.[205] One of the objectives of the pilot study, CCG-829, reported in 1991 was to determine the activity of radiation therapy in patients with tumors that could not be surgically resected after 4 courses of cisplatin and doxorubicin. However, due to the limited number of patients that received irradiation, the activity of this therapeutic modality was never proven.[95] Radiation therapy doses ranged between 1200 cGy and 2000 cGy; however, higher doses to limited areas were also used. Radiation therapy has also been used as palliative treatment for patients with pulmonary metastases, but limited information on the efficacy of this approach is available.

Chemoembolization and Other Methods of Local Control

Hepatic arterial chemoembolization refers to the intra-arterial administration of chemotherapeutic and vascular occlusive agents (generally gelatin or Lipiodol) along with cytotoxic agents. The agents that have been most frequently used for chemoembolization are doxorubicin, mitomycin, and cisplatin.[206–208] Intra-arterial injection of cytotoxic agents results in higher local concentration of drugs with reduced systemic side effects, while the intra-arterial embolization causes ischemic necrosis of the tumor. This therapeutic strategy has been used in a small number of children and adolescents with recurrent HCC while awaiting the availability of a liver donor, or as adjuvant therapy in an attempt to facilitate tumor resection.[209–212] Recently, Malogolowkin et al[209] reported on the efficacy and toxicity of hepatic chemoembolization in 11 pediatric patients (6 hepatoblastoma, 3 HCC, and 2 hepatic UESL). All patients with the exception of one had previously received systemic chemotherapy. Complete resection or resection with microscopic residual disease was achieved in 5 patients, and 3 of them were alive and free of disease at the time of report. In conclusion, chemoembolization is a feasible therapeutic alternative for patients with hepatoblastoma whose tumor remains unresectable after initial systemic chemotherapy or for patients with nonmetastatic HCC.

Other methods of local control may be considered, especially in recurrent tumors. They include percutaneous radiofrequency ablation (RFA) and percutaneous ethanol injection (PEI). In most cases, these treatment approaches are of palliative capability and are suitable for smaller tumors only, generally below 3 cm to 4 cm maximum diameter. However, these techniques are of low risk, are repeatable, and do not damage nonneoplastic tissue, which is especially important in cirrhotic patients. Additionally, a combination of these techniques can be applied in the same patient. Neither PEI nor RFA can be used, at least percutaneously, if the lesion is not recognizable upon ultrasound examination.

Percutaneous ethanol injection is particularly suitable for HCC foci in a cirrhotic liver and can be performed under ultrasonic guidance. Hypervascularization and the difference in consistency between neoplastic and cirrhotic tissue favor the toxic action of ethanol. It can be repeated up to 15 times for larger and/or recurrent lesions. Percutaneous ethanol injection is also safe. The overall survival at 1, 3, and 5 years of Child's A, B, and C class patients with single HCC of less than 5 cm have been reported to be: 98%, 79%, and 47%; 93%, 63%, and 29%; and 64%, 12%, and 0, respectively.[213,214] The overall survival rates at 1, 3, and 5 years for Child's A class multifocal HCC are 94%, 68%, and 36%, respectively. Rate of tumor necrosis is usually 90% to 100%. Recently, ethanol has been substituted with other agents such as acetic acid.

Tumor thermo-ablation with radiofrequency (RFA) provides even better effect than PEI (90% vs 80% complete tumor necrosis) with less sessions (mean of 1.2 vs 4.8).[214] It is also associated with fewer side effects; thus, in many centers RFA is now preferred over PEI; however, RFA is contraindicated in lesions adjacent to the major biliary ducts or to bowel loops. The presence of immediately adjacent tumor satellite lesions is a relative contraindication to this technique. Complications of these percutaneous HCC treatment techniques occur in about 8% to 9% of cases, mainly in the form of bleeding, tumor seeding, and gastrointestinal perforation.[215] However, this therapeutic approach has not been well studied in children.

Liver Transplantation

The number of children with malignant liver tumors treated with total hepatectomy followed by orthotopic liver transplantation has increased significantly over the past 15 years.[216] Approximately 2% of the liver transplants performed in North America are in patients with liver tumors.[217] Initial results showed a better survival for patients with unifocal tumors when compared with patients with multifocal tumors.[216] Reyes et al[218] reported the results obtained in a series of 31 children with unresectable liver tumors treated with chemotherapy followed by total hepatectomy and liver transplantation. The 5-year survival rates post-transplantation were 83% and 68% for patients with hepatoblastoma and HCC, respectively.

In SIOPEL-1, 12 patients underwent liver transplantation (8% of all patients), as the initial surgical option in 7 children and as the second-line salvage procedure in 5 patients who had undergone a previous partial hepatectomy.[161] The median follow-up as of December 2001 was 127 (10 to 135) months since diagnosis and 117 (52 to 125) months since liver transplant for patients who were surviving. The overall patient survival was 75% after 5 years and 66% after 10 years following liver transplantation.

Recently, Otte et al[219] reviewed the world experience with the use of liver transplantation for children with hepatoblastoma. One hundred and forty-seven cases from 24 centers were collected with a medium age of 26 months (2 to 223 months). Of these 147 patients, 106 (72%) were submitted to liver transplantation as primary treatment, and in 41 patients (28%) transplantation was used as rescue therapy following tumor recurrence after partial hepatectomy. The 6-year survival for those that submitted to primary liver transplantation was 82% but only 30% in the group undergoing liver transplantation as rescue therapy. The impact of sex, age, presence of pulmonary metastasis, intravascular invasion at diagnosis, time to transplantation, type of transplantation, and chemotherapy post-transplantation on survival was analyzed. Of all these factors, only the presence of intravascular invasion at diagnosis was found to be an important factor affecting the survival of patients undergoing primary transplant. Of interest was the finding that 7 of 12 patients (58%) with pulmonary metastasis survived.

The scarcity of cadaveric organs of appropriate size for hepatic transplantation in children frequently leads to long delays, resulting at times in disease progression. This has promoted the use of living, related donor liver transplantations.[220] There are several advantages of using living, related donors: there are fewer delays in submitting the patient for transplantation, the transplanted liver is not impacted by transportation problems, the mortality associated with the use of living related donor is very low, and, finally, the procedure offers psychological advantage for the donor and other family members.[221] The benefits of using living, related livers were confirmed in a review of the world experience with liver transplantation for children with hepatoblastoma.[219] Of the 147 patients, the survival rate for the 28 patients who received a liver from a living, related donor was 82%. This result compares favorably with the 71% survival rate observed in 119 patients who received a cadaveric transplant.

Liver transplantation has added a new dimension for the treatment of hepatoblastoma and represents a feasible alternative for the treatment of patients with unresectable tumors. Also, patients who continue to have extensive unresectable tumors after systemic chemotherapy should be considered for liver transplantation. Data are available to support the use of liver transplantation in patients with metastatic disease responsive to chemotherapeutic treatment.[219,221]

The experience of liver transplantation in children with HCC is quite limited. There is only one pediatric series of transplanted HCCs (19 cases), from Pittsburgh, with promising 63% 5-year disease-free-survival, which confirms the negative influence of tumor size and vascular invasion on prognosis—very much like the case in adults.[218] Two other, earlier reports—one by Tagge[159] and one by Iwatsuki[222]—show low survival: in the range of 29% to 35% in patients with unresectable tumors. Nevertheless, liver transplantation in HCC can be curative in otherwise unresectable tumors, especially in patients with liver cirrhosis. Thus, expansion of its indications in children should be considered. Until now, however, no uniform criteria for liver transplantation in pediatric HCC exist. The value of this approach cannot be confirmed due to the small number of reported cases.[223]

New Therapeutic Modalities

There is a great need for the development of new therapeutic strategies for the treatment of liver tumors in children, especially for HCC. Angiogenesis is important for the growth of both primary and metastatic tumors, and for the growth of HCC.[224] Therefore, drugs that inhibit angiogenesis may be useful in the treatment of malignant tumors. Angiogenesis is dependent on the interaction of various factors, such as vascular endothelial growth factor (VEGF), platelet-derived endothelial growth factor (PDGF), interleukin-8 (IL-8), cyclooxygenase-2 (COX-2), tumor necrosis factor-α (TNFα), and others that lead to endothelial cell proliferation, migration, invasion, differentiation, and capillary tube formation.[225] Various factors have already been associated with the development and progression of hepatocellular carcinomas. Their expression has also been associated with histology grade, proliferative activity, invasion, and patient survival. Multiple studies have demonstrated that agents with antiangiogenic activity (TNP-470, thalidomide, ACE inhibitors, etc) may reduce the size and frequency of development of experimentally induced HCC in rats and inhibit tumor growth, invasion, and metastasis of human HCC in nude mouse models.[226–228] The role of sorafenib, a multikinase inhibitor, and other such inhibitors alone or in combination with other chemotherapy agents need to be further explored in the treatment of patients with advanced HCC.[199] The use of radiolabeled antibodies against AFP and ferritin has been used in many experimental studies; however, their role in the treatment of these diseases has yet to be established.[229,230]

Future Plans

Efforts directed toward the early detection of hepatoblastoma in high-risk populations would increase the possibility of complete tumor resection at diagnosis. Patients with predisposing conditions such as Beckwith-Wiedemann syndrome, hemihypertrophy, FAP, and possibly premature birth should be closely monitored during the first 4 years of life. Also, patients with viral hepatitis,[231–233] chronic cholestasis, and certain congenital metabolic conditions frequently associated with the development of cirrhosis are at higher risk of developing HCC and therefore should be monitored carefully.[234] Epidemiological studies may reveal important factors related to the cause of hepatic tumors in children and eventually allow for the eradication of these tumors. The role of liver transplantation and the use of living related donors require further evaluation.

The cooperative groups should carry out the development of a universal staging system that will allow comparison between different therapeutic studies in collaboration. Finally, due to the small number of children diagnosed with these tumors, international cooperation will be essential in the future design and implementation of biologic and therapeutic studies.

References

1. Bulterys N, Goodman M, Smith M, Buckley J. Hepatic tumors. In: Ries L, Smith M, Gurney JG, et al, eds. *Cancer Incidence and Survival Among Children and Adolescents. United States SEER Program 1975–1995.* Bethesda, MD: National Cancer Institute, SEER Program; 1999.
2. Young JL, Ries L, Silverberg E, et al. Cancer incidence, survival and mortality for children younger than 15 years. *Cancer.* 1986;58(Suppl 2):598–602.
3. Exelby PR, Filler RM, Grosfeld JL. Liver tumors in children in the particular reference to hepatoblastoma and hepatocellular carcinoma: American Academy of Pediatrics Surgical Section Survey—1974. *J Pediatr Surg.* 1975;10(3): 329–337.
4. Weinberg AG, Finegold MJ. Primary hepatic tumors of childhood [review]. *Hum Pathol.* 1983;14(6):512–537.
5. Harada T, Matsuo K, Kodama S, Higashihara H, Nakayama Y, Ikeda S. Adult hepatoblastoma: case report and review of the literature [review]. *Aust N Z J Surg.* 1995;65(9):686–688.
6. Bortolasi L, Marchiori L, Dal Dosso I, Colombari R, Nicoli N. Hepatoblastoma in adult age: a report of two cases [review]. *Hepatogastroenterology.* 1996;43(10):1073–1078.
7. Lack EE, Neave C, Vawter GF. Hepatocellular carcinoma: review of 32 cases in childhood and adolescents. *Cancer.* 1983;52:1510–1515.
8. Ross JA, Gurney JG. Hepatoblastoma incidence in the United States from 1973 to 1992. *Med Pediatr Oncol.* 1998;30(3):141–142.
9. Kenney L, Miller B, Ries L, et al. Increased incidence of cancer in infants in the U.S.: 1980–1990. *Cancer.* 1998;82:1396–1400.
10. Parkim D, Stiller C, Draper GJ, et al. *International Incidence of Childhood Cancer.* Vol 87. Lyon, France: Lyon International Agency for Research on Cancer Scientific Publications; 1988.
11. Ishak KG, Glunz PR. Hepatoblastoma and hepatocarcinoma in infancy and childhood: report of 47 cases. *Cancer.* 1967;20(3):396–422.
12. Craig JR, Peters RL, Edmonson HA, Omata M. Fibrolamellar carcinoma of the liver: a tumor of adolescents and young adults with distinctive clinicopathologic features. *Cancer.* 1980;46:372–379.
13. Chen JC, Chen CC, Chen WJ, et al. Hepatocellular carcinoma in children: clinical review and comparison with adult cases. *J Pediatr Surg.* 1998;33: 1350–1354.
14. Czauderna P. Adult type vs Childhood hepatocellular carcinoma—are they the same or different lesions? biology, natural history, prognosis, and treatment. *Med Pediatr Oncol.* 2002;39(5):519–523.
15. Di Bisceglie AM, Rustig VK, Hoofnagle JH, et al. NIH conference. Hepatocellular carcinoma. *Ann Intern Med.* 1988;108:390–401.
16. Chang M, Chen C, Lai M, et al. Universal hepatitis B vaccination in Taiwan and the incidence of hepatocellular carcinoma in children: Taiwan Childhood Hepatoma Study Group. *N Engl J Med.* 1997;336:1855–1859.
17. Bisogno G, Pilz T, Perilongo G, et al. Undifferentiated sarcoma of the liver in childhood: A curable disease. *Cancer.* 2002;94:252–257.
18. Pollono DG, Tomarchio S, Berghoff R, et al. Rhabdomyosarcoma of extrahepatic biliary tree initial treatment with chemotherapy and conservative surgery. *Med Pediatr Oncol.* 1998;30:290–293.
19. Kim DY, Kim KH, Jung SE, Lee SC, Park KW, Kim WK. Undifferentiated (embryonal) sarcoma of the liver: combination treatment by surgery and chemotherapy. *J Pediatr Surg.* 2002;37(10):1419–1423.
20. Siegel MJ. Pediatric liver imaging. *Semin Liver Dis.* 2001;21:251–269.
21. Stocker JT, Ishak KG. Undifferentiated embryonal sarcoma of the liver: report of 31 cases. *Cancer.* 1978;42:336–348.
22. Webber EM, Morrison KB, Pritchard SL, Sorensen PHB. Undifferentiated embryonal sarcoma of the liver: results of clinical management in one center. *J Pediatr Surg.* 1999;34:1641–1644.
23. Patil KK, Omojola MF, Khurana P, et al. Embryonal rhabdomyosarcoma within a choledochal cyst. *Can Assoc Radiol J.* 1992;43:145–148.
24. Koufos A, Hansen MF, Copeland NG, Jenkins NA, Lampkin BC, Cavenee WK. Loss of heterozygosity in three embryonal tumours suggests a common pathogenetic mechanism. *Nature.* 1985;316(6026):330–334.
25. De Baum M, Tucker M. Risk of cancer during the first four years of life in children from the Beckwith-Wiedemann Syndrome Registry. *J Pediatr.* 1998; 132:398–400.
26. Haas OA, Zoubek A, Grumayer ER, Gadner H. Constitutional interstitial deletion of 11p11 and pericentric inversion of chromosome 9 in a patient with Wiedemann-Beckwith syndrome and hepatoblastoma. *Cancer Genet Cytogenet.* 1986;23(2):95–104.
27. Little MH, Thomson DB, Hayward NK, Smith PJ. Loss of alleles on the short arm of chromosome 11 in a hepatoblastoma from a child with Beckwith-Wiedemann syndrome. *Hum Genetics.* 1988;79(2):186–189.
28. Hatada I, Ohashi H, Fukushima Y, et al. An imprinted gene p57K1P2 is mutated in Beckwith-Wiedemann syndrome. *Nat Genet.* 1996;14:171–173.
29. Hartmann W, Waha A, Koch A, et al. p57(KIP2) is not mutated in hepatoblastoma but shows increased transcriptional activity in a comparative analysis of the three imprinted genes p57(KIP2), IGF2, and H19. *Am J Pathol.* 2000;157(4):1393–1403.
30. Ross JA, Radloff GA, Davies SM. H19 and IGF-2 allele-specific expression in hepatoblastoma. *Br J Cancer.* 2000;82(4):753–756.
31. Rainier S, Dobry CJ, Feinberg AP. Loss of imprinting in hepatoblastoma. *Cancer Res.* 1995;55(9):1836–1838.
32. Kingston JE, Herbert A, Draper GJ, Mann JR. Association between hepatoblastoma and polyposis coli. *Arch Dis Child.* 1983;58(12):959–962.
33. Li FP, Thurber WA, Seddon J, Holmes GE. Hepatoblastoma in families with polyposis coli. *JAMA.* 1987;257(18):2475–2477.
34. Garber JE, Li FP, Kingston JE, et al. Hepatoblastoma and familial adenomatous polyposis [erratum appears in *J Natl Cancer Inst.* 1989;81(6):461]. *J Natl Cancer Inst.* 1988;80(20):1626–1628.
35. Broduer W, Bailey C, Bodmer N, et al. Localisation of the gene for familial adenomatous polyposis on chromosome 5. *Nature.* 1987;328:614–616.
36. Oda H, Imai Y, Nakatsuru Y, Hata J, Ishikawa T. Somatic mutations of the APC gene in sporadic hepatoblastomas. *Cancer Res.* 1996;56(14):3320–3323.
37. Jeng YM, Wu MZ, Mao TL, Chang MH, Hsu HC. Somatic mutations of beta-catenin play a crucial role in the tumorigenesis of sporadic hepatoblastoma. *Cancer Lett.* 2000;152(1):45–51.
38. Mann JR, Kasthuri N, Raafat F, et al. Malignant hepatic tumours in children: incidence, clinical features and aetiology. *Paediatr Perinat Epidemiol.* 1990; 4(3):276–289.
39. Mamlok V, Nichols M, Lockhart L, Mamlok R. Trisomy 18 and hepatoblastoma. *Am J Med Genet.* 1989;33(1):125–126.
40. Bove KE, Soukup S, Ballard ET, Ryckman F. Hepatoblastoma in a child with trisomy 18: cytoGenet, liver anomalies, and literature review [review]. *Pediatr Pathol Lab Med.* 1996;16(2):253–262.
41. Tanaka K, Uemoto S, Asonuma K, et al. Hepatoblastoma in a 2 year old girl with trisomy 18. *Eur J Pediatr Surg.* 1992;2:298–300.
42. Teraguchi M, Nogi S, Ikemoto Y, et al. Multiple hepatoblastomas associated with trisomy 18 in a 3-year-old girl. *Pediatr Hematol Oncol.* 1997;14(5):463–467.
43. Mascarello JT, Krous HF. Second report of a translocation involving 19q13.4 in a mesenchymal hamartoma of the liver. *Cancer Genet Cytogenet.* 1992;58: 141–142.
44. Bardi G, Johansson B, Pandis N, et al. Trisomy 2 as the sole chromosomal abnormality in a hepatoblastoma. *Genes Chromosomes Cancer.* 1992;4:78–80.
45. Ma SK, Cheung AN, Choy C, et al. Cytogenetic characterization of childhood hepatoblastoma. *Cancer Genet Cytogenet.* 2000;119(1):32–36.
46. Schneider NR, Cooley LD, Finegold MJ, Douglass EC, Tomlinson GE. The first recurring chromosome translocation in hepatoblastoma: der(4)t(1;4) (q12;q34). *Genes Chromosomes Cancer.* 1997;19(4):291–294.
47. Sainati L, Leszl A, Stella M, et al. Cytogenetic analysis of hepatoblastoma: hypothesis of cytogenetic evolution in such tumors and results of a multicentric study. *Cancer Genet Cytogenet.* 1998;104(1):39–44.
48. Parada LA, Limon J, Iliszko M, et al. CytoGenet of hepatoblastoma: further characterization of 1q rearrangements by fluorescence in situ hybridization: an international collaborative study. *Med Pediatr Oncol.* 2000;34(3):165–170.
49. Hashizume K, Nakajo T, Kawarasaki H, et al. Prader-Willi syndrome with del(15)(q11,q13) associated with hepatoblastoma. *Acta Paediatr Jpn.* 1991; 33(6):718–722.
50. Chen TC, Hsieh LL, Kuo TT. Absence of p53 gene mutation and infrequent overexpression of p53 protein in hepatoblastoma. *J Pathol.* 1995;176(3):243–247.
51. Feusner J, Plaschkes J. Hepatoblastoma and low birth weight: a trend or chance observation? *Med Pediatr Oncol.* 2002;39(5):508–509.
52. Maruyama K, Ikeda H, Koizumi T. Prenatal and postnatal histories of very low birth weight infants who develop hepatoblastoma. *Pediatr Intl.* 1999; 41(1):82–89.
53. Ross JA, Severson RK, Swenson AR, et al. Seasonal variations in the diagnosis of childhood cancer in the United States. *Br J Cancer.* 1999;8(3):549–553.
54. Ikeda H, Hachitanda Y, Tanimura M, Maruyama K, Koizumi T, Tsuchida Y. Development of unfavorable hepatoblastoma in children of very low birth weight: results of a surgical and pathologic review. *Cancer.* 1998;82(9):1789–1796.
55. Ikeda H, Matsuyama S, Tanimura H, et al. Association between hepatoblastoma in children with very low birth weight: a trend or a chance. *J Pediatr.* 1997;130:557–560.
56. Tanimura M, Matsui I, Abe J, et al. Increased risk of hepatoblastoma among immature children with a lower birth weight. *Cancer Res.* 1998;58(14):3032–3035.
57. Feusner J, Buckley J, Robison L, Ross J, Van Tornout J. Prematurity and hepatoblastoma: more than just an association? [comment]. *J Pediatr.* 1998; 133(4):585–586.
58. Ribons L, Slovis TL. Hepatoblastoma and birth weight. *J Pediatr.* 1998;132(4): 750.
59. Meyer P, LiVolsi V, Cornog JL. Letter: Hepatoblastoma associated with an oral contraceptive. *Lancet.* 1974;2(7893):1387.
60. Otten J, Smets R, De Jager R, Gerard A, Maurus R. Hepatoblastoma in an infant after contraceptive intake during pregnancy. *N Engl J Med.* 1977; 297(4):222.

61. Buckley JD, Sather H, Ruccione K, et al. A case-control study of risk factors for hepatoblastoma: a report from the Children's Cancer Study Group. *Cancer.* 1989;64(5):1169–1176.
62. Weinberg AG, Mize CE, Worthen HG. The occurrence of hepatoblastoma in the chronic form of hereditary tyrosenemia. *J Pediatr.* 1976;88:434–438.
63. Limmer J, Fleig WF, Leupold D, et al. Hepatocellular carcinoma in type I glycogen storage disease. *Hepatology.* 1988; 8:531–537.
64. Ugarte N, Gonzalez-Crussi F. Hepatoma in siblings with progressive familial cholestatic cirrhosis of childhood. *Am J Clin Pathol.* 1981;76:172–177.
65. Eriksson S, Carlson J, Velez R. Risk of cirrhosis and primary liver cancer in alpha 1-antitrypsin deficiency. *N Engl J Med.* 1986;296:1411–1412.
66. Morkrohisky ST, Ambruso DR, Hathaway WE. Fulminant hepatic neoplasia after androgen therapy. *N Engl J Med.* 1977; 296:1411–1412.
67. Buendia MA. Genetic alterations in hepatoblastoma and hepatocellular carcinoma: common and distinctive aspects [review]. *Med Pediatr Oncol.* 2002; 39(5):530–535.
68. Feitelson MA, Sun B, Satiroglu Tufan NL, et al. Genetic mechanisms of hepatocarcinogenesis. *Oncogene.* 2002;21:2593–2604.
69. Thorgeirsson SS, Grisham JW. Molecular pathogenesis of human hepatocellular carcinoma. *Nature Genet.* 2002;31:339–346.
70. Breslow NE, Tikashima JR, Whitton JA, et al. Second malignant neoplasm following treatment for Wilms' tumor: a report from the National Wilms' Tumor Study Group. *J Clin Oncol.* 1995;13(8):1855–1859.
71. Sage D, Sasco A, Little J. Antenatal drug exposure and fetal/neonatal tumours: review of 89 cases. *Paediatr Perinat Epidemiol.* 1998;12:84–117.
72. Delattre O, Zucman J, Ploustagel B, et al. Gene fusion with an ETS DNA binding domain caused by chromosome translocation in human cancers. *Nature.* 1992;359:162–165.
73. Sorensen PHB, Lessnick SL, Lopez-Terrada D, et al. A second Ewing sarcoma translocation, t21.22, fuses EWS gene to another ETS-family transcription factor. ERG. *Nature Genet.* 1994;6:146–151.
74. Iliszko M, Czauderna P, Babinska M, et al. Cytogenetic findings in an embryonal sarcoma of the liver. *Cancer Genet Cytogenet.* 1998;102:142–144.
75. Leuschner I, Schmidt D, Harms D. Undifferentiated sarcoma of the liver in childhood morphology: flow cytometry and literature review. *Hum Pathol.* 1990;21:68–76.
76. Arshad RR, Woo SY, Abbassi V, Hoy GR, Sinks LF. Virilizing hepatoblastoma: precocious sexual development and partial response of pulmonary metastases to cis-platinum. *CA Cancer J Clin.* 1982;32(5):293–300.
77. Behrle FC, Manta FA, Olson RL, et al. Virilisation accompanying hepatoblastoma. *Paediatrics.* 1963;63:895–903.
78. Braunstein GD, Bridson WE, Glass A, Hull EW, McIntire KR. In vivo and in vitro production of human chorionic gonadotropin and alpha-fetoprotein by a virilizing hepatoblastoma. *J Clin Endocrinol Metabol.* 1972;35(6):857–862.
79. Hung WT, Blizzard RM, Migeon CJ, et al. Precocious puberty in a boy with hepatoma and circulating gonadotrophin. *J Pediatr.* 1963;63:895–903.
80. Teng CT, Daeschner CW III, Singleton EB, et al. Liver diseases and osteoporosis in children: clinical observations. *J Pediatr.* 1961;59:684.
81. Chen CC, Au C. Spontaneous rupture of hepatocellular carcinoma in a child: a report of survival. *J Pediatr Surg.* 1989;24(4):404–405.
82. Gauthier F, Saliou C, Valayer J, Montupet P. [Surgery of hepatoblastoma and hepatocarcinoma in children in the era of preoperative chemotherapy: current progress and limitations] [in French]. *Chirurgie Pediatrique.* 1988;29(6):307–312.
83. Rao GN, Green AA. Hepatic tumors in children and adolescents. *Sci Pract Surg.* 1987;8:187–218.
84. Geary TR, Maclennan AC, Irwin GJ. Hypertrophic osteopathy in primary liver rhabdomyosarcoma. *Pediatr Radiol.* 2004;34:250–252.
85. Komura-Naito E, Matsumura T, Sawada T, et al. Thrombopoietin in patients with hepatoblastoma. *Blood.* 1997;90:2849–2850.
86. Nickerson HJ, Silberman TL, McDonald TP. Hepatoblastoma, thrombocytosis, and increased thrombopoietin. *Cancer.* 1980;45(2):315–317.
87. vonSchweinitz D, Schmiidt D, Fuchs J, et al. Extramedullary hematopoiesis and intratumoral production of cytokines in childhood hepatoblastoma. *Pediatr Res.* 1995;38:555–563.
88. Ikeda H, Kimua N, Suita S, et al. Pre and post operative changes of alpha-fetoprotein and human chorionic gonadotropin in hepatoma of children. *Z Kinderchir.* 1981;1:42–55.
89. Mann JR, Lakin GE, Leonard JC, et al. Clinical applications of serum carcinoembryonic antigen and alpha-fetoprotein levels in children with solid tumors. *Arch Dis Child.* 1978;53:366–374.
90. Gitlin D. Normal biology of alpha-fetoprotein. *Ann NY Acad Sci.* 1975;239:7.
91. Yachnin S. The clinical significance of human alpha-fetoprotein. *Ann Clin Lab Sci.* 1978;8:84–90.
92. Ortega JA, Siegel SE. Biological markers in pediatric solid tumors. In: Pizzo AP, Poplack DG, eds. *Principles and Practice of Pediatric Oncology.* Philadelphia: Lippincott; 1993:179–194.
93. Van Tornout JM, Buckley JD, Ortega JA. Timing and magnitude of decline in alpha-fetoprotein levels in treated children with unresectable or metastatic hepatoblastoma are predictors of outcome: a report from the Children's Cancer Group. *J Clin Oncol.* 1997;15:1190–1197.
94. Buamah PK, James OF, Skillen AW, et al. The value of tumor marker kinetics in the management of patients with primary hepatocellular carcinoma. *J Surg Oncol.* 1988;37:161–164.
95. Ortega JA, Krailo MD, Haas JE, et al. Effective treatment of unresectable or metastatic hepatoblastoma with cisplatin and continuous infusion doxoru-

bicin chemotherapy: a report from the Children's Cancer Study Group. *J Clin Oncol.* 1991;9:2167–2176.
96. Tsuchida Y, Kaneko M, Fukui M, Sakaguchi H, Ishiguro T. Three different types of alpha-fetoprotein in the diagnosis of malignant solid tumors: use of a sensitive lectin-affinity immunoelectrophoresis. *J Pediatr Surg.* 1989;24(4):350–355.
97. Walhof CM, Van Sonderen L, Voute PA, Delemarre JF. Half-life of alpha-fetoprotein in patients with a teratoma, endodermal sinus tumor, or hepatoblastoma. *Pediatr Hematol Oncol.* 1988;5(3):217–227.
98. von Schweinitz D, Hecker H, Schmidt-von-Arndt G, Harms D. Prognostic factors and staging systems in childhood hepatoblastoma. *Intl J Cancer.* 1997; 74(6):593–599.
99. Perilongo G, Shafford E, Maibach R, et al. Risk-adapted treatment for childhood hepatoblastoma: final report of the second study of the International Society of Paediatric Oncology—SIOPEL 2. *Eur J Cancer.* 2004;40(3):411–421.
100. Murthy AS, Vawter GF, Lee AB, Jockin H, Filler RM. Hormonal bioassay of gonadotropin-producing hepatoblastoma. *Arch Pathol Lab Med.* 1980; 104(10):513–517.
101. Watanabe I, Yamaguchi M, Kasai M. Histologic characteristics of gonadotropin-producing hepatoblastoma: a survey of seven cases from Japan. *J Pediatr Surg.* 1987;22(5):406–411.
102. Geiser CF, Shih VE. Cystathioninuria and its origin in children with hepatoblastoma. *J Pediatr.* 1980;96(1):72–75.
103. Liu HC, Chang MH, Wu MZ, Lin DT, Chen WJ. Pretreatment serum cholesterol level as a prognostic indicator in infants and children with hepatoblastoma [in Chinese]. *Chung-Hua Min Kuo Hsiao Erh Ko i Hsueh Hui Tsa Chih.* 1988;29(4):254–260.
104. Lee CL, Ko YC. Survival and distribution pattern of childhood liver cancer in Taiwan [review]. *Eur J Cancer.* 1998;34(13):2064–2067.
105. LeThai B. Prognostic factors in hepatocarcinoma. *J Chirurgie.* 1989;126(6):405–412.
106. Muraji T, Woolley MM, Sinatra F, Siegel SM, Isaacs H. The prognostic implication of hypercholesterolemia in infants and children with hepatoblastoma. *J Pediatr Surg.* 1985;20(3):228–230.
107. Paradinas FJ, Melia WM, Wilkinson ML, et al. High serum vitamin B12 binding capacity as a marker of fibrolamelar variant of hepatocellular carcinoma. *Br Med J.* 1982;25(285):840–842.
108. Miller JH, Gates GH, Stanley P. The radiologic investigation of hepatic tumors in childhood. *Radiology.* 1977;124:451–464.
109. Liu P, Daneman A, Stringer DA. Diagnostic imaging of liver masses in children. *J Can Assoc Radiol.* 1985;36:296–300.
110. de Campo M, de Campo JF. Ultrasound of primary hepatic tumours in childhood. *Pediatr Radiol.* 1988;19(1):19–24.
111. King S, Babyn P, Greenberg MA, et al. Value of CT in determining the resectability of hepatoblastoma before and after chemotherapy. *Am J Roentgenol.* 1993;160:793–799.
112. Korobkin M, Kirks DR, Sullivan DC, Mills SR, Bowie JD. Computed tomography of primary liver tumors in children. *Radiology.* 1981;139(2):431–438.
113. Boechat MI, Kangarloo H, Ortega J, et al. Primary liver tumors in children: comparison of CT and MR imaging. *Radiology.* 1988;169(3):727–732.
114. Wong KK, Lan LC, Lin SC, Tam PK. The use of positron emission tomography in detecting hepatoblastoma recurrence: a cautionary tale. *J Pediatr Surg.* 2004;39:1779–1781.
115. Sironi S, Messa C, Cistaro A, et al. Recurrent hepatoblastoma in orthotopic transplanted liver: detection with FDG positron emission tomography. *Am J Roentgenol.* 2004;182:1214–1216.
116. Ros PR, Olmsted WM, Dachman AH, et al. Undifferentiated embryonal sarcoma of the liver radiologic-pathologic correlation. *Radiology.* 1986;160:141–145.
117. Roebuck DJ, Yang WT, Lam WW, et al. Hepatobiliary rhabdomyosarcoma in children diagnostic radiology. *Pediatr Radiol.* 1998;28:101–108.
118. Reynolds M. Pediatric liver tumors. *Sem Surg Oncol.* 1999;16:159–172.
119. Evans AE, Land VJ, Newton WA Jr. Combination chemotherapy in the treatment of children with malignant hepatoma. *Cancer.* 1982;50:821–826.
120. MacKinlay G, Pritchard J. A common language for childhood liver tumours. *Pediatr Surg Intl.* 1992;7:325–326.
121. Brown J, Perilongo G, Shafford E, et al. Pretreatment prognostic factors for children with hepatoblastoma: results from the International Society of Paediatric Oncology (SIOP) study SIOPEL 1. *Eur J Cancer.* 2000;36(11):1418–1425.
122. Aronson DC, Schnater JM, Staalman CR, et al. Predictive value of the pretreatment extent of disease system in hepatoblastoma: results from the International Society of Pediatric Oncology Liver Tumor study group SIOPEL-1 study. *J Clin Oncol.* 2005;23:1245–1252.
123. Meyers RL, Katzenstein HM, Malogolowkin MH. Predictive value of staging systems in hepatoblastoma. *J Clin Oncol.* 2007;20:737.
124. Llovet JM, Bruix J. Systematic review of randomized trials for unresectable hepatocellular carcinoma chemoembolization improves survival. *Hepatology.* 2003;37:429–442.
125. Rowland JM. Hepatoblastoma: assessment of criteria for histologic classification. *Med Pediatr Oncol.* 2002;39:478–483.
126. Zimmermann A. Hepatoblastoma with cholangioblastic features ("cholangioblastic hepatoblastoma") and other liver tumors with bimodal differentiation in young patients. *Med Pediatr Oncol.* 2002;39:487–491.

127. O'Brien, WJ, Finlay JL, et al. (1989). "Patterns of antigen expression in hepatoblastoma and hepatocellular carcinoma in childhood." Pediatric Hematology & Oncology 6(4): 361–5.

128. Gupta A and Chou PM. C-Kit expression in hepatoblastoma—Evidence of stem-like cell in histogenesis? USCAP Annual Meeting, San Antonio, TX, 2005, Abstract: 1289.

129. Fiegel H, Gluer S, Roth B, Rischewski J, Schweinitz D, Ure B, Lambrecht W, and Kluth D. Stem-like Cells in Human Hepatoblastoma. J Histochem Cytochem, 2004;52(11):1495–1501.

130. Kondo Y. Histologic features of hepatocellular carcinoma and allied disorders. Pathol Annu. 1985;20(2):405–424.

131. Edmonson HA. Differential diagnosis of tumor and tumor-like lesions of liver in infancy and childhood. Am J Dis Child. 1956;97:168–186.

132. Epstein B, Pajak T, Haulk T, Herpst J, Order S, Abrams R. Metastatic nonresectable fibrolamellar hepatoma: prognostic features and natural history. Am J Clin Oncol. 1999;22(1):22–28.

133. Prokurat A, Kluge P, Kosciesza A, Perek D, Kappeler A, Zimmermann A. Transitional liver cell tumors (TLCT) in older children and adolescents: a novel groups of aggressive hepatic tumors expressing beta-catenin. Med Pediatr Oncol. 2002;39:510–518.

134. Chu PG, Ishizawa S, et al. (2002). "Hepatocyte antigen as a marker of hepatocellular carcinoma: an immunohistochemical comparison to carcinoembryonic antigen, CD10, and alpha-fetoprotein." American Journal of Surgical Pathology 26(8):978–88.

135. Fasano M, Theise ND, et al. (1998). "Immunohistochemical evaluation of hepatoblastomas with use of the hepatocyte-specific marker, hepatocyte paraffin 1, and the polyclonal anti-carcinoembryonic antigen." Modern Pathology 11(10):934–8.

136. Witzleben CL, Bruninga G. Infantile choriocarcinoma: a characteristic syndrome. J Pediatr. 1968;73:374–378.

137. Belchis DA, Mowry J, Davis JH. Infantile choriocarcinoma: re-examination of a potentially curable entity. Cancer. 1993;72:2028–2032.

138. Ishak KG, Sesterhenn I, Goodman Z, Rabin L, Stromeyer W. Epithelioid hemangiondothelioma of the liver: a clinicopathologic and follow-up study of 32 cases. Hum Pathol. 1984;15:839–852.

139. Parham D, Kelly DR, Donnelly WH, Douglass EC. Immunohistochemical and ultrastructural spectrum of hepatic sarcomas of childhood: evidence for a common histogenesis. Mod Pathol.1991;4(5):648–653.

140. Aoyama C, Hachitanda Y, Sato JK, Said JW, Shimada H. Undifferentiated (embryonal) sarcoma of the liver. Am J Surg Pathol. 1991;15:615–624.

141. Ruymann FB, Raney RB Jr, Crist WM, Lawrence W Jr, Lindberg RD, Soule EH. Rhabdomyosarcoma of the biliary tree in childhood: a report from the Intergroup Rhabdomyosarcoma Study. Cancer. 1985;56(3):575–581.

142. Hass JE, Feusner JH, Finegold MJ. Small cell undifferentiated histology in hepatoblastoma may be unfavorable. Cancer. 2001;92:3130–3134.

143. Ruck P, Xiao JC, Kaiserling E. Small epithelial cells and the histogenesis of hepatoblastoma. Am J Pathol. 1996;148:321–329.

144. Hill DA, Pfeifer JD, Marley EF, et al. WT1 staining reliably differentiates desmoplastic small round cell tumor from Ewing sarcoma/primitive neuroectodermal tumor: an immunohistochemical and molecular diagnostic study. Am J Clin Pathol. 2000;114(3):345–353.

145. Dehner LP, Ishak KG. Vascular tumors of the liver in infants and children. Arch Path. 1971;92:101–111.

146. Selby DM, Stocker JT, Ishak KG. Angiosarcoma of the liver in childhood. Pediatr Pathol. 1992;12:485–498.

147. Prokurat A, Prezemyslaw K, Chrupek M, Kosciesza A, Rajszys P. Hemangioma of the liver in children: proliferating vascular tumor or congenital vascular malformation? Med Pediatr Oncol. 2002;39:524–529.

148. Chan JK. Inflammatory pseudotumor: a family of lesions of diverse nature and etiologies. Adv Anat Pathol. 1996;3:156–171.

149. Arber DA, Weiss LM, Chang KL. Detection of Epstein-Barr virus in inflammatory pseudotumor. Sem Diagn Pathol. 1998;15(2):155–160.

150. Meis JM, Enzinger FM. Inflammatory fibrosarcoma of the mesentery and retroperitoneum: a tumor closely simulating inflammatory pseudotumor. Am J Surg Pathol. 1991;15(12):1146–1156.

151. Albores-Saavedra J, Manivel JC, Essenfeld H, et al. Pseudosarcomatous myofibroblastic proliferations in the urinary bladder of children. Cancer. 1990;66:1234–1241.

152. Todani T, Tabuchi K, Watanabe Y, Tsutsumi A. True hepatic teratoma with high alpha-fetoprotein in serum. J Pediatr Surg. 1977;12:591–592.

153. Stocker JT, Ishak KG. Mesenchymal hamartoma of the liver: report of 30 cases and review of the literature. Pediatr Pathol. 1983;1:245–267.

154. De Chadarevian JP, Pawel BR, Faerber EN, Wintraub WH. Undifferentiated (embryonal) sarcoma in conjunction with mesenchymal hamartoma of the liver. Mod Pathol. 1994;7(4):490–493.

155. Lauwers GY, Grant LD, Donnelly WH, et al. Hepatic undifferentiated (embryonal) sarcoma arising in a mesenchymal hamartoma. Am J Surg Pathol. 1997; 21(10):1248–1254.

156. Spelman F, De Tolder V, De Petter KR, et al. Cytogenetic analysis of a mesenchymal hamartoma of the liver. Cancer Genet Cytogenet. 1989;40:29–32.

157. Hill DA, Swanson PE, et al. (2005). "Desmoplastic nested spinal cell tumor of liver: report of four cases of a proposed new entity." American Journal of Surgical Pathology 29(1):1–9.

158. Heerema-McKenney A, Leuschner I, et al. (2005). "Nested stromal epithelial tumor of the liver: six cases of a distinctive pediatric neoplasm with frequent calcifications and association with cushing syndrome." American Journal of Surgical Pathology 29(1):10–20.

159. Tagge EP, Tagge DV, Reyes J, et al. Resection including transplantation for hepatoblastoma and hepatocellular carcinoma. J Pediatr Surg. 1992;21:292–297.

160. Katzenstein HM, Krailo MD, Malogolowkin MH, et al. Hepatocellular carcinoma in children and adolescents: results from the Pediatric Oncology Group and the Children's Cancer Group intergroup study. J Clin Oncol. 2002;20(12):2789–2797.

161. Otte JB, Aronson D, Vrasus H, et al. Preoperative chemotherapy, major liver resection and transplantation for primary malignancies in children. Transplant Proc. 1996;28:2393–2394.

162. Spunt SL, Lobe T, Pappo AS, et al. Aggressive surgery is unwarranted for biliary tract hepatoblastoma. J Pediatr Surg. 2000;35:309–316.

163. Roebuck DJ. Interventional radiology in children with hepatobiliary rhabdomyosarcoma [comment]. Med Pediatr Oncol. 1998;31(3):187–188.

164. Lascari AD. Vincristine therapy in an infant with probable hepatoblastoma. Pediatr. 1970;45(1):109–112.

165. Selawry OS, Holland JF, Wolman IJ. Effect of vincristine on malignant solid tumors in children. Cancer Chemother Rep. 1968;52:497.

166. Amsfield F, Schroeder J, Curreri A. Five year clinical experience with 5-fluorouracil. JAMA. 1962;181:295.

167. Ikeda K, Suita S, Nakagawara A, Takabayashi K. Preoperative chemotherapy for initially unresectable hepatoblastoma in children: survival in two cases. Arch Surg. 1979;114(2):203–207.

168. Jacobs EM, Luce JK, Wood DA. Treatment of cancer with weekly intravenous 5-fluorouracil. Cancer. 1968;22:1233.

169. Ragab AH, Sutow WW, Komp DM, et al. Adriamycin in the treatment of childhood solid tumors. Cancer. 1975;36:1567–1571.

170. Tan C, Rosen G, Ghavimi F, et al. Adriamycin (NSC 123127) in pediatric malignancies. Cancer Chemother Rep. 1975;6:259–266.

171. Wang JH, Holland JF, Sinks L. Phase II study of adriamycin (123127) in childhood solid tumors. Cancer Chemother Rep. 1975;6:267–270.

172. Champion J, Green AA, Pratt CB. Cisplatin (DDP) an effective therapy for unresectable or recurrent hepatoblastoma. Proc Am Assoc Clin Oncol. 1982; 671:173.

173. Katzenstein HM, London WB, Douglass EC, et al. Treatment of unresectable and metastatic hepatoblastoma: a Pediatric Oncology Group Phase II study. J Clin Oncol. 2002;20(16):3438–3444.

174. Cacciavillano WD BL, Childs M, Shafford E, et al. Phase II study of high-dose cyclophosphamide in relapsing and/or resistant hepatoblastoma in children: a study from the SIOPEL group. Eur J Cancer. 2004;40:2274–2279.

175. Fuchs J, Wenderoth M, von Schweinitz D, Haindl J, Leuschner I. Comparative activity of cisplatin, ifosfamide, doxorubicin, carboplatin, and etoposide in heterotransplanted hepatoblastoma. Cancer. 1998;83(11):2400–2407.

176. Pinkerton CR, Pritchard J. A phase II study of ifosfamide in paediatric solid tumours. Cancer Chemother Pharmacol. 1989;24(Suppl 1):S13–S15.

177. Schiavetti A, Varrasso G, Maurizi P, et al. Ten-day schedule oral etoposide therapy in advanced childhood malignancies. J Pediatr Hematol Oncol. 2000; 22:119–124.

178. Ortega JA, Douglass EC, Feusner JH, et al. Randomized comparison of cisplatin/vincristine/fluorouracil and cisplatin/continuous infusion doxorubicin for treatment of pediatric hepatoblastoma: a report from the Children's Cancer Group and the Pediatric Oncology Group. J Clin Oncol. 2000;18(14):2665–2675.

179. King DR, Ortega J, Campbell JR, et al. The surgical management of children with incompletely resected hepatic cancer is facilitated by intensive chemotherapy. J Pediatr Surg. 1991;26:1074–1080.

180. Pritchard J, Brown J, Shafford E, et al. Cisplatin, doxorubicin, and delayed surgery for childhood hepatoblastoma: a successful approach—results of the first prospective study of the International Society of Pediatric Oncology. J Clin Oncol. 2000;18(22):3819–3828.

181. Douglass EC, Reynolds M, Stalen JP. Effectiveness and toxicity of cisplatin, vincristine and fluorouracil therapy for hepatoblastoma: a Pediatric Oncology Group Study. J Clin Oncol. 1991;11:96–99.

182. Malogolowkin MH, Kazenstein H, Krailo M, Rowland J, Haas J, Meyers R, Finegold M. Complete surgical resection is curative children with pure fetal histology hepatoblastoma (PFH): A report of the Childrens Oncology Group (COG). ASCO Annual Meeting, Chicago, IL 2008.

183. von Schweinitz D, Byrd DJ, Hecker H, et al. Efficiency and toxicity of ifosfamide, cisplatin and doxorubicin in the treatment of childhood hepatoblastoma. Study Committee of the Cooperative Paediatric Liver Tumour Study HB89 of the German Society for Paediatric Oncology and Haematology. Eur J Cancer. 1997;33(8):1243–1249.

184. Fuchs J, Rydzynski J, Von Schweinitz D, et al. Pretreatment prognostic factors and treatment results in children with hepatoblastoma: a report from the German Cooperative Pediatric Liver Tumor Study HB 94. Cancer. 2002;95(1): 172–182.

185. Sasaki F, Matsunaga T, Iwafuchi M, et al. Outcome of hepatoblastoma treated with the JPLT-1 (Japanese Study Group for Pediatric Liver Tumor) Protocol-1: A report from the Japanese Study Group for Pediatric Liver Tumor. J Pediatr Surg. 2002;37(6):851–856.

186. Ninane J, Perilongo G, Stalen JP. Effectiveness and toxicity of cisplatin and doxorubicin (PLADO) in childhood hepatoblastoma and hepatocellular carcinoma: a SIOP pilot study. Med Pediatr Oncol. 1991(19):199–203.

187. Schnater JM, Aronson DC, Plaschkes J, et al. Surgical view of the treatment of patients with hepatoblastoma: results from the first prospective trial of the International Society of Pediatric Oncology Liver Tumor Study Group. *Cancer.* 2002;94(4):1111–1120.

188. Zsiros J, Brock P, Brugieres L, et al. High risk hepatoblastoma (HR-HB): Final treatment results of the SIOPEL-2 study. *Med Pediatr Oncol.* 2002; 39(4):264.

189. Malogolowkin MH. Intensive versus standard platinum therapy for the treatment of children with hepatoblastoma: a report of the Intergroup Hepatoblastoma Study P9645. Paper presented at: American Society of Clinical Oncology, 2004; New Orleans, LA.

190. Katzenstein HM, Chang K, Krailo M, et al. A randomized study of platinum based chemotherapy with or without amifostine for the treatment of children with hepatoblastoma (HB): a report of the Intergroup Hepatoblastoma Study P9645. *Proc ASCO.* 2004;23:799(8518).

191. Czauderna P, Mackinlay G, Perilongo G, et al. Hepatocellular carcinoma in children: results of the first prospective study of the International Society of Pediatric Oncology group. *J Clin Oncol.* 2002;20(12):2798–2804.

192. Haas JE, Muczynski KA, Krailo M, et al. Histopathology and prognosis in childhood hepatoblastoma and hepatocarcinoma. *Cancer.* 1989;64(5):1082–1095.

193. Edmonson H. Differential diagnosis of tumors and tumor-like lesions of liver in infancy and childhood. *Arch Dis Child.* 1956;1:168–186.

194. Farhi DC, Shikes RH, Murari PJ, et al. Hepatocellular carcinoma in young adults. *Cancer.* 1983;52:1516–1525.

195. Craig J, Peters R, Edmonson H, Omata M. Fibrolamellar carcinoma of the liver: a tumor of adolescents and young adults with distinctive clinico-pathologic features. *Cancer.* 1980;46:372–379.

196. Epstein BE, Pajak TF, Haulk TL, et al. Metastatic nonresectable fibrolamellar hepatocellular carcinoma: prognostic features and natural history. *Am J Clin Pathol.* 1999;22:22–28.

197. Saab S, Yao F. Fibrollamellar hepatocellular carcinoma: case reports and a review of the literature. *Dig Dis Sci.* 1996;41(10):1981–1985.

198. Katzenstein HM, Krailo MD, Malogolowkin MH, et al. Fibrolamellar hepatocellular carcinoma in children and adolescents [review]. *Cancer.* 2003;97(8):2006–2012.

199. Llovet J, Ricci S, Mazzaferro V, et al; for the SHARP Investigators Study Group. Randomized Phase III trial of sorafenib versus placebo in patients with advanced hepatocellular carcinoma. *Proc ASCO* (Post-Meeting edition). 25(18S, June 20 suppl); 2007:LBA1.

200. Horowitz ME, Etcubanas E, Webber BL, et al. Hepatic undifferentiated embryonal sarcoma and rhabdomyosarcoma in children. *Cancer.* 1987;59:396–402.

201. Moon WK, W.S. K, Choi BI, et al. Undifferentiated embryonal sarcoma of the liver treated with chemotherapy CT imaging in four patients. *Abdom Imaging.* 1995;20:133–137.

202. Urban CE, Mache CJ, Schwinger W, et al. Undifferentiated embryonal sarcoma of the liver in childhood: successful combined modality therapy in four patients. *Cancer.* 1993;72:2511–2516.

203. Warmann SW, Fuchs J, Wilkens L, Gratz KF, von Schweinitz D, Mildenberger H. Successful therapy of subcutaneously growing human hepatoblastoma xenografts with topotecan. *Med Pediatr Oncol.* 2001;37(5):449–454.

204. Palmer RD, Williams DM. Dramatic response of multiply relapsed hepatoblastoma to irinotecan (CPT-11). *Med Pediatr Oncol.* 2003;41(1):78–80.

205. Habrand JL, Pritchard J. Role of radiotherapy in hepatoblastoma and hepatocellular carcinoma in children and adolescents: results of a survey conducted by the SIOP Liver Tumor Study Group. *Med Pediatr Oncol.* 1991;19:208.

206. Golladay ES, Mollitt DL, Osteen PK, et al. Conversion to resectability by intra-arterial infusion chemotherapy after failure of systemic chemotherapy. *J Pediatr Surg.* 1985;20(6):715–717.

207. A comparison of lipiodol chemoembolization and conservative treatment for unresectable hepatocellular carcinoma. *N Engl J Med.* 1995;332:1256–1261.

208. Rose DM, Chapman WC, Brockenbrough AT, et al. Transcatheter arterial chemoembolization as primary treatment for hepatocellular carcinoma. *Am J Surg.* 1999;177:405–410.

209. Malogolowkin MH, Stanley P, Ortega JA, et al. Feasibility and toxicity of chemoembolization for children with liver tumors. *J Clin Oncol.* 2000;18:1279–1284.

210. Ogita S, Tokiwa K, Taniguchi H, Takahashi T. Intraarterial chemotherapy with lipid contrast medium for hepatic malignancies in infants. *Cancer.* 1987; 60(12):2886–2890.

211. Ogita S, Tokiwa K, Taniguchi H, Takahashi T. Intraarterial injection of anti-tumor drugs dispersed in lipid contrast medium: a choice for initially unresectable hepatoblastoma in infants. *J Pediatr Surg.* 1987;22(5):412–414.

212. Sue K, Ikeda K, Nakagawara A, et al. Intrahepatic arterial injections of cisplatin-phosphatidylcholine-Lipiodol suspension in two unresectable hepatoblastoma cases. *Med Pediatr Oncol.* 1989;17(6):496–500.

213. Whang-Peng J, Chao Y. Clinical trials of HCC in Taiwan. *Hepatogastroenterology.* 1998;45:1937–1943.

214. Venook AP. Treatment of hepatocellular carcinoma too many options? *J Clin Oncol.* 1994;12:1323–1334.

215. Llovet JM, Burroughs A, Bruix J. Hepatocellular carcinoma. *Lancet Oncol.* 2003;362:1907–1917.

216. Koneru B, Flye MW, Busuttil R, et al. Liver transplantation for hepatoblastoma: the American experience. *Ann Surg.* 1991;213:118–121.

217. Reyes J, Marariegos G. Pediatric transplantation. *Surg Clin North Am.* 1999; 79:163–189.

218. Reyes JD, Carr B, Dvorchik I, et al. Liver transplantation and chemotherapy for hepatoblastoma and hepatocellular cancer in childhood and adolescence. *J Pediatr.* 2000;136(6):795–804.

219. Otte JB, Pritchard J, Aronson DC, et al. Liver transplantation for hepatoblastoma: results from the International Society of Pediatric Oncology (SIOP) study SIOPEL-1 and review of the world experience [review]. *Pediatr Blood Cancer.* 2004;42(1):74–83.

220. Singer PA, Siegler M, Whittingin PF, et al. Ethics of liver transplantation with living donors. *N Engl J Med.* 1989;321:620–622.

221. Dower NA, Smith LV. Liver transplantation for malignant liver tumors in children. *Med Pediatr Oncol.* 2000;34:136–140.

222. Iwatsuki S, Starzl TE, Sheahan DG, et al. Hepatic resection vs. transplantation for hepatocellular carcinoma. *Ann Surg.* 1991;214:221–229.

223. Finlay JL, Kalayoglu M, Odell GB, Dinndorf PA, Frierdich S. Liver transplantation for primary hepatic cancer in childhood. *Lancet.* 1987;2(8567):1086–1087.

224. Zhao ZC, Zheng SS, Wan YL, Jia CK, Xie HY. The molecular mechanism underlying angiogenesis in hepatocellular carcinoma: the imbalance activation of signaling pathways. *Hepatobiliary Pancreat Dis Intl.* 2003;2:529–536.

225. Imura S, Miyake H, Izumi K, Tashiro S, Uehara H. Correlation of vascular endothelial cell proliferation with microvessel density and expression of vascular endothelial growth factor and basic fibroblast growth factor in hepatocellular carcinoma. *J Med Invest.* 2004:202–209.

226. Hsu C, Chen CN, Chen LT, et al. Low-dose thalidomide treatment for advanced hepatocellular carcinoma. *Oncol.* 2003(65):242–249.

227. Hsu C, Cheng JC, Cheng AL. Recent advances in non-surgical treatment for advanced hepatocellular carcinoma. *J Formos Med Assoc.* 2004;103(7):483–495.

228. Kinoshita S, Hirai R, Yamano T, Yuasa I, Tsukuda K, Shimizu N. Angiogenesis inhibitor TNP-470 can suppress hepatocellular carcinoma growth without retarding liver regeneration after partial hepatectomy. *Surg Today.* 2004;34:40–46.

229. Order SE, Leibel SA. Radiolabeled antibodies in the treatment of primary liver cancer. *Appl Radiol.* 1984;13:67–73.

230. Wharam MD, Klein JC, Leichner PK, et al. Preliminary experience with radioisotope labelled immunoglobulin for therapy of pediatric hepatoma. *Med Pediatr Oncol.* 1987;15:339–342.

231. Bruno S, et al. Hepatitis C virus genotypes and risk of hepatocellular carcinoma in cirrhosis: a prospective study. *Hepatology.* 1997(25):754–758.

232. Liaw YF, Tai DI, Chu CM, et al. Early detection of hepatocellular carcinoma in patients with chronic type B hepatitis: a prospective study. *Gastroenterology.* 1986;90(2):263–267.

233. Sun Z, Lu P, Gail MH. Increased risk of hepatocellular carcinoma in male hepatitis B surface antigen carriers with chronic hepatitis who have detectable aflatoxin metabolite M1. *Hepatology.* 1999;30:379–383.

234. Christopherson WM, Mays ET. *Risk factors, pathology, and pathogenesis of selected benign and malignant liver neoplasm.* New York: Marcel Decker; 1987.

Retinoblastoma

Carlos Rodriguez-Galindo and Anna T. Meadows

Incidence and Epidemiology

Retinoblastoma is the most frequent neoplasm of the eye in childhood, and the third most common intraocular malignancy in all ages, following malignant melanoma and metastatic carcinoma. Retinoblastoma represents 2.5% to 4% of all pediatric cancers, but 11% of cancers in the first year of life.[1] The average age-adjusted incidence rate of retinoblastoma in the United States and Europe is 2 to 5 per million children (approximately one in 14,000 to 18,000 live births).[2,3] Thus, an estimated 300 children develop retinoblastoma each year in the United States.[1]

The human retina is far from having completed its maturation by the end of gestation, and most retinoblasts are not terminally differentiated until three years of age. It is during this period of time, before these primitive photo-receptor cells differentiate into the mature retina that cells are at risk of sustaining oncogenic events that result in the development of a neoplasm. Retinoblastoma is therefore a cancer of the very young; two-thirds of all cases of retinoblastoma are diagnosed before two years of age, and 95% of cases are diagnosed before 5 years of age.[1] For these reasons, therapeutic approaches need to consider not only the cure of the disease, but also the need to preserve vision with minimal long-term side effects.

Retinoblastoma presents in two distinct clinical forms: (1) A bilateral or multifocal, heritable (40% of all cases) form, characterized by the presence of germline mutations of the *RB1* gene. Multifocal retinoblastoma may be inherited from an affected survivor (25%) or be the result of a new germline mutation (75%); and (2) a unilateral form in which about 90% of such unilateral or unifocal retinoblastomas are nonhereditary (60% of all cases). About 10% of germline cases are unilateral; in the absence of a positive family history, however, it is not possible without genetic screening to determine which unilateral cases are capable of being transmitted to the next generation.

The incidence of retinoblastoma is not distributed equally around the world. It appears to be higher (6 to 10 cases per million children) in Africa,[2,4] India,[5] and among children of native American descent in the North Ameri-

can continent.[6,7] The increased incidence in those groups occurs primarily in unilateral cases. Whether these geographical variations are due to ethnic or socio-economic factors is not well known. However, the fact that even in industrialized countries an increased incidence of retinoblastoma is associated with poverty and low levels of maternal education[8] suggests a role for the environment. Decreased dietary intake of vegetables and fruits during pregnancy, resulting in decreased intake of nutrients such as folate and carotenoids, which are necessary for DNA methylation and synthesis as well as for retinal formation, has also been associated with an increased risk of unilateral sporadic retinoblastoma.[9]

It is well known that exposure to certain toxic agents during gestation increases the frequency of germinal mutations in animals. The vast majority of germline mutations in sporadic heritable retinoblastoma are paternally derived,[10] and studies have suggested an association between paternal age[7,8,11] and occupation[12] with the occurrence of sporadic heritable retinoblastoma. Reports have also suggested an association between retinoblastoma and increased sunlight exposure[13,14] or *in vitro* fertilization.[15,16]

Retinoblastoma tumors arise from fetal retinal cells that have lost function of both allelic copies of the *RB1* gene, the first of the tumor suppressor genes to be cloned. The first event may be either a germline or a somatic mutation, but the second and perhaps subsequent events are always somatic. Molecular analyses have thus far been able to detect mutations in *RB1* in only 90% of cases, suggesting that there is either another gene or alternate mechanisms for inactivation of *RB1* function.[17] For example, the *RB1* gene can be epigenetically silenced through hypermethylation of the promoter.[18,19] In recent years, studies have suggested a role for human papilloma viruses (HPVs) in the pathogenesis of retinoblastoma. The viral oncoprotein E7 of high-risk HPV types has been shown to bind to and inactivate the *RB1* gene product (pRB). Therefore, it is plausible that HPV infection could be functionally equivalent to the biallelic loss of *RB1*.[20] Transgenic mice expressing HPV16 E6 and E7 proteins develop retinoblastoma.[21] Presumably, exposure to HPV would occur peripartum from genital infection of the mother. In this regard, the use of barrier methods of contraception is associated with a reduced incidence of both retinoblastoma and HPV infection.[8,22] Interestingly, there is an overlap between those countries in which the relative incidence of retinoblastoma is greatest and those in which the incidence of cervical carcinoma is highest.[22] High-risk HPV sequences have been detected in 28% to 36% of tumors.[22,23]

Biology

Retinoblastoma is among the best understood of human neoplasms and has served as an important model for understanding tumorigenesis. In 1971, based on the mathematical analysis of the age at presentation of bilateral (hereditary) and unilateral (mostly nonhereditary) cases of retinoblastoma, Knudson proposed the "two-hit hypothesis", in which two mutational events in a developing retinal cell lead to the development of retinoblastoma.[24] This hypothesis was subsequently extended to suggest that the two events could be mutations of both alleles of the *RB1* gene. *RB1*, located in chromosome 13q14, was identified and cloned in 1986.[25,26] Its product, pRb, is a 110 kilodalton nuclear phosphoprotein that acts by binding and inhibiting several proteins with growth-stimulatory activity. pRb is a key substrate for G1 cyclin-cdk complexes, which phosphorylate target gene products required for the transition of the cell through the G1 phase of the cell cycle. The active pRb is the unphosphorylated gene product, which binds to several cellular proteins, among which is the transcription factor E2F, which will activate the transcription of genes whose products are required for entry into the S phase of the cell cycle. During progression through the G1 phase, pRb undergoes additional phosphorylations resulting in a hyper-phosphorylated form that persists through S, G2, and M phases. pRb appears to function as a tumor suppressor at least in part by inhibiting cell-cycle progression past the G1-S restriction point. Once cells traverse the G1-S restriction point and enter S phase, they become irreversibly committed to cell division. Thus, pRb stands as the major gatekeeper to control this critical point in growth regulation. The lack of pRb or its inactivation will remove the pRb constraint on cell cycle control, with the consequence of deregulated cell proliferation.[27] Two other RB family members have been identified, p107 and p130. These proteins have functions in common with pRb, but they also have some unique features.[28] Tumor development occurs after silencing or loss of both alleles at the *RB1* locus, but other events must also occur.

The first hit: The *RB1* gene is a large gene, containing 27 exons over about 200 kilobases of DNA, and mutations have been described in almost every exon.[17,29] Nonsense and frame shift are the most common germ-line and somatic mutations, although deletions and duplications are also frequently encountered.[17,29,30] There are no mutational hot-spots, although new germline mutations have an overwhelming preference for the paternal allele, suggesting that deamination of methylated CpG pairs has an important role in mutagenesis.[10] These mutations are *bona*

fide deleterious mutations because they result in premature termination codons.[29] The type of mutation appears to have geographic variations, probably reflecting ethnic differences in DNA repair mechanisms.[30] As further understanding is gained of the mutation heterogeneity, genotype-phenotype correlations are becoming apparent.[17,30] The penetrance of the trait is greater than 90%, but pedigrees with reduced penetrance (that is, carriers without tumor) or reduced expressivity (unilateral disease or fewer tumors per patient) have been described. The molecular mechanisms of low-penetrance retinoblastoma are being elucidated, and can be grouped into two functional classes: (1) Mutations that reduce the level of expression of normal pRb; and (2) Mutations that result in a mutant pRb that is partially inactivated. The first class is comprised by those promoter mutations that interfere with the assembly of the transcriptional machinery reducing efficient gene expression, and by splice site mutations that result in transcribed messenger RNA from the mutant allele that encodes only 10% of the normal protein. In the second class, mutations affect the coding region of pRb and are thought to partially inactivate the protein.[31]

The second hit: In both hereditary and nonhereditary retinoblastoma, the second tumorigenic event is usually chromosomal in nature, often as a result of mitotic recombination errors.[31,32] This second hit occurs at a much higher frequency than the first hit, and it is more sensitive to environmental factors such as ionizing irradiation, perhaps explaining the increased risk of irradiation-induced malignancies in survivors of retinoblastoma.[33]

After the *second hit* has taken place, retinoblastoma cells rapidly accumulate additional genetic damage, and tumors develop. Tumorigenesis is a multi-stage process, and additional alterations may be necessary for the development of retinoblastoma.[27] Despite the knowledge accumulated since the discovery of the *RB1* gene two decades ago, the pathogenesis of retinoblastoma remains incompletely understood. Part of the problem is the lack of an animal model. Mice with hemizygous mutations of the retinoblastoma gene, generated to recapitulate the human condition, do not develop retinoblastoma—although some of them develop midbrain tumors[34]—and "knock-out" mice die at gestational day 14 due to hematopoietic and neuronal defects.[35] It is possible that other members of the retinoblastoma gene family, such as *p107*, play a role in the abrogation of tumor formation in mice (through a compensatory up-regulation, for example). In the mouse retina, *p107* is up-regulated in a compensatory manner when *Rb* is inactivated, thus preventing ectopic cell division. The same phenomenon occurs in mouse embryonic fibroblasts following *Rb* inactivation.[36] *The p107* gene is E2F-regulated, and when *Rb* repression of E2F at the *p107* promoter is relieved, *p107* expression is activated. However, this *p107* compensation does not occur in human retinal progenitor cells when *RB1* is inactivated. Both *Rb* and *p107*[37,38] or *Rb* and *p130*[39] must be inactivated in proliferating retinal progenitor cells in order for mice to develop retinoblastoma. Recently, the first knockout mouse models of retinoblastoma were generated by conditionally deleting *Rb* in retinal progenitor cells of *p107*-deficient mice.[37,38] When *p53* is simultaneously inactivated in *RB; p107*-deficient retinal progenitor cells, a more aggressive form of retinoblastoma, similar to the human disease, is observed.[37] Hemizygous mice do develop tumors if there is a simultaneous inactivation of *p53*.[40] However, *p53* does not appear to be mutated in human retinoblastoma,[27] suggesting that although the bilallelic loss of the *RB1* gene is a rate-limiting step for the development of retinoblastoma, additional mutations or gene amplifications are required. Tumorigenesis involves sequential genetic lesions in pathways that regulate cell proliferation and cell survival.[41] It has been proposed that both the *p16Ink4a-CycD/Cdk4-pRb* and *Arf-MDM2/MDMX-p53* pathways must be inactivated during tumorigenesis.[41] A key component of the *p53* tumor surveillance pathway is *p14^{ARF}*. When pRb activity is lost, the transcription factor E2F activates transcription of *p14^{ARF}*; *p14^{ARF}* then inactivates *MDM2*, leading to *p53*-mediated apoptosis and exit from the cell cycle. Therefore, loss of *RB1* in the developing human retina (or loss of *Rb* and *p107* in the mouse retina) should cause derepression of *Arf* and activation of the tumor surveillance mechanism. Because human retinoblastomas express wild-type *p53*, it was assumed that the p53 pathway was intact and the status of the other genes in the pathway (such as *p14^{ARF}*, *MDM2* and *MDMX*) was not considered. Furthermore, studies correlating apoptosis with retinal cell-type markers in these *Rb; p107*-deficient mouse retinas led to the proposal that retinoblastoma is a unique tumor that originates from intrinsically death-resistant cells.[42] A recent study has shown that inactivation of the Rb pathway in the developing mouse or human retina leads to ectopic proliferation and activation of the Arf-MDM2/MDMX-p53 tumor surveillance pathway. The ectopic proliferation caused by the loss of the Rb pathway is balanced by p53 mediated apoptosis. The defining event appears to be *MDMX/MDM2* amplification leading to inactivation of the *p53* pathway. In the animal model, expression of *MDMX* promoted proliferation and survival in developing retinal cells lacking *Rb* and *p107*. Furthermore, in human retinas, inactivation of *RB1* and over-expression of *MDMX* promoted retinoblastoma; *MDMX* blocked cell death in *Rb*-deficient human retinoblasts through its ability to bind and inactivate *p53*.[43] In the same study, *MDMX* and *MDM2* amplification was found in 65% and 10% of human retinoblastomas, respectively. Based on these studies, the most likely model of tumorigenesis of retinoblastoma proposes that following *RB1* inactivation, inactivation of the p53 pathway promotes the transition from differentiated retinoblastoma cells with amacrine, horizontal cell features to a more immature cell with retinal progenitor cell features. It is also possible, however, that there are two distinct tumor cell types (amacrine, horizontal and progenitor cell types) that originate from distinct cells of origin.[42,43] Finally, other genes and pathways are probably also involved; studies using comparative genomic hybridization have consistently shown chromosomal gains and amplifications at 6p and 1q, and losses at 16 q1.[44,45]

Genetic Counseling for Retinoblastoma Families

Retinoblastoma is a unique neoplasm, in that the genetic form imparts a predisposition to developing tumor in an autosomal dominant fashion with almost complete penetrance (85% to 95%).[46] The majority of such children acquire the first mutation as a new germline mutation, with only 15% to 25% having a positive family history. However, some families display an inheritance pattern characterized by reduced penetrance and expressivity.[17] As discussed above, these low-penetrance retinoblastoma mutations either cause a reduction in the amount of normal pRb produced, or result in a partially functional mutant pRb.[31] Also, the *RB1* gene mutation can occur at a late stage of embryogenesis, resulting in a variable expression depending on the tissue, causing mosaicisms in 10% to 15% of the patients or their progenitors.[47] In general, however, based on the inheritance pattern and considering the existence of mosaicisms, the following risk estimates can be made:[46]

1. *Risk for offspring of survivors of retinoblastoma:*
   a. The risk of retinoblastoma arising in the offspring of survivors of bilateral disease is 45%.
   b. In the case of patients with unilateral disease, investigators have estimated the risk of retinoblastoma overall to be 2.5%. However, this estimate includes offspring of survivors of unilateral retinoblastoma who have a positive family history and whose risk is similar to that of bilateral cases—45%. If the family history is negative and genetic screening has not been done, the actual risk is probably less than 2%.
2. *Risk for siblings of patients with retinoblastoma:* In the case of siblings of bilaterally affected children whose parents are also affected, the risk of developing retinoblastoma is 45%; if the sibling is unilaterally affected, the risk is 30%. For those cases without a family history, the empirically derived risk is 2% for siblings of bilateral cases, and 1% for siblings of unilateral cases.

Genetic counseling is of the utmost importance to assist parents in understanding the genetic consequences of each form of retinoblastoma and to estimate the risk in relatives. Counseling is relatively straightforward when a parent is affected, or when the child presents with bilateral disease; these patients all have the genetic form. For children without a parent involved who have only a single tumor, there is always a question about whether they carry the mutated gene or not. Children with unilateral disease who are over the age of two at the time of diagnosis are not likely to be gene carriers; we recommend that younger children be screened for mutations in *RB1*. Because the chromosomal location of the gene is known, it is theoretically possible to screen for mutations. However, because of the size of the *RB1* gene and the lack of mutational hot spots, exhaustive analysis of the *RB1* gene is required for clinical DNA testing. With the refinement in methods of mutational analysis over the last decade, detection rates have increased from 20 to 30%[48,49] to 70 to 80%,[29,30] to greater than 90% at present.[17] Given the heterogeneity in the site and type of gene defects, no single technology will be sensitive and effective, and a multi-step approach must be taken. More than 80% of the mutations can be detected with sequencing of the 27 exons of the *RB1* using a quantitative multiplex polymerase chain reaction (QMPCR).[17,29] However, 10% to 20% of the defects are due to large deletions,[29,49] and therefore deletion scanning and Southern blot is required for those cases with no detectable mutations by QMPCR. Finally, a small proportion of cases (probably fewer than 5%-10%) may result from gene inactivation by promoter methylation, and therefore screening for constitutional methylation should be considered if the other methods do not reveal a mutation.[17,29] With the recent improvements in the detection rates, genetic testing could be performed in the offspring of retinoblastoma survivors who are known to have the mutated gene (and detection of the mutation is relatively easily accomplished if the parental mutation is known). Even if genetic screening is negative for the mutation, newborn siblings of children with retinoblastoma should be examined periodically under anesthesia until they are about two years of age, because inherited retinoblastoma would be extremely rare beyond that age. In the future, if the false negative rate is negligible, one might expect that molecular diagnosis of mutations would lead to earlier treatment and better health outcomes for patients with retinoblastoma, with lower cost than conventional surveillance for those children at risk.[17]

Pathology

Retinoblastoma arises from the photoreceptor elements of the inner layer of the retina, usually extending into the vitreous cavity as a fleshy nodular mass (endophytic retinoblastoma).[50] Less frequently, it extends externally, causing a secondary retinal detachment, in which case there is no localized visible vitreous nodule (exophytic retinoblastoma). Macroscopically, retinoblastoma is soft and friable, and it tends to outgrow its blood supply, with resulting necrosis and calcification. Because of its friability, dissemination within the vitreous and retina in the form of small, white nodules (seeds) is common (Figure 30-1). In those cases, it may be difficult to distinguish a multi-centric primary from a disseminated tumor.[51]

Microscopically, the appearance of retinoblastoma depends on the degree of differentiation. Undifferentiated retinoblastoma is composed of small, round, densely packed cells with hypochromatic nuclei and scant cytoplasm. Several degrees of photoreceptor differentiation have been described and are characterized by distinctive arrangements of tumor cells. The Homer-Wright rosettes are composed of irregular circlets of tumor cells arranged around a tangle of fibrils with no lumen or internal limiting membrane. They are infrequently seen in retinoblastoma and are most often seen in other neuroblastic tumors

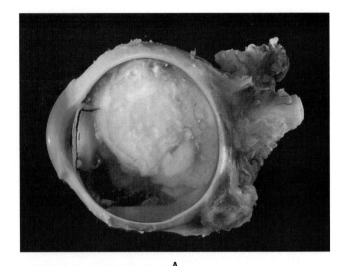

A

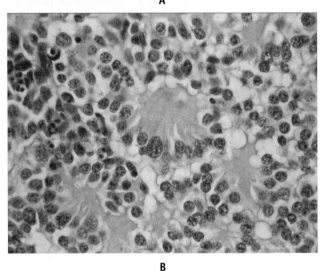

B

Figure 30-1 (A) Cross-section of an enucleation specimen showing retinoblastoma occupying most of the posterior chamber. The tumor is adherent to the retina, which is secondarily detached, and also adheres to the posterior aspect of the lens. (B) High-power microscopic image of retinoblastoma depicting multiple Homer-Wright rosettes composed of concentric arrangements of neoplastic cells around a tangle of cellular processes. More commonly, retinoblastomas contain Flexner-Wintersteiner rosettes, which are circular arrangements of neoplastic cells around a hollow central lumen. Rosette formation is an indication of differentiation in retinoblastoma.

such as neuroblastoma and medulloblastoma. The Flexner-Wintersteiner rosettes, on the other hand, are specific for retinoblastoma. These structures consist of a cluster of low columnar cells arranged around a central lumen that is bounded by an eosinophilic membrane analogous to the external membrane of the normal retina. The lumen contains an acid mucopolysaccharide similar to that found around normal rods and cones. These rosettes are seen in 70% of tumors. The fleurettes are less often seen. In this case, the cells exhibit even more ultrastructural characteristics of photoreceptor differentiation. They are composed of larger cells with abundant eosinophilic cytoplasm arranged in a distinctive *fleur de lis* pattern. Especially well-differentiated tumors composed almost entirely of fleurettes have been called retinomas or retinocytomas. Ultrastructurally, retinoblastoma cells also demonstrate photoreceptor differentiation with the presence of the 9-0 microtubule doublet pattern, abundant cytoplasmic microtubules, synaptic ribbons, and neurosecretory granules.[51,52]

Dissemination of retinoblastoma occurs via several routes. Choroidal invasion provides access to a rich vascular network that serves as a potential route for distant metastases. In advanced cases, direct extension occurs through the sclera into the orbit. Retinoblastoma can also invade the iris and the ciliary body, and metastasize to the regional lymph nodes. Finally, retinoblastoma can extend along the optic nerve, gaining access to the subarachnoid space and intracranial cavity.

Clinical Manifestations

Retinoblastoma is by definition a tumor of the young child, and the age at presentation correlates with laterality. Patients with bilateral retinoblastoma tend to present at a younger age (usually before one year of age) than patients with unilateral disease (often in the second or third year of life).[46,53] Half of the cases of retinoblastoma diagnosed during the first year are bilateral, compared with fewer than 10% of cases diagnosed after one year of age.[1] It is rare for retinoblastoma to be diagnosed during the first month of life, except in familial cases where examination has been recommended early; however, regardless of the family history, more than 90% of neonatal cases have either bilateral disease at presentation or will develop asynchronous bilateral retinoblastoma.[54]

In more than half of the cases, the presenting sign is leukocoria, which is occasionally first noticed after a flash photograph (Figure 30-2). Strabismus is the second most common presenting sign, and usually correlates with macular involvement. Very advanced intraocular tumors may become painful as a result of secondary glaucoma.[53] Differential diagnosis must be made from other childhood diseases that can present with leukocoria, such as persistent hyperplastic primary vitreous (PHPV), retrolental fibrodysplasia, Coats' disease, congenital cataracts, toxocariasis, and toxoplasmosis (Figure 30-3). In some series, these non-malignant conditions account for a significant proportion of enucleated eyes.[55,56] In familial cases, the diagnosis is usually made through screening, although almost 50% of familial cases are diagnosed later in life, when patients pre-

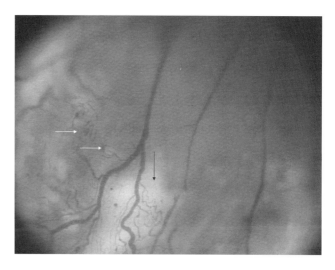

Figure 30-3 Coats' Disease: Exudative detachment, telangiectatic vessels (white arrows), and hyperplasia of the retinal pigment epithelium (black arrow).

sent with the typical signs of retinoblastoma, underscoring the importance of genetic counseling.[53]

The successful management of retinoblastoma depends on the ability to detect the disease while it is still intraocular. Disease stage correlates with delay in diagnosis.[57,58] In developing countries, late referrals are strongly associated with orbital and metastatic disease.[58–60] It is for this reason that eye assessment should be performed in all newborns and at all subsequent health supervision visits by the primary care provider.[61] Mass screening is also being considered, especially where the tumor is common, such as areas of South America and Asia. Photo-screening is a system by which a photograph is produced by a calibrated camera under prescribed lighting conditions, which shows a red reflex in both pupils. A trained observer can identify ocular abnormalities by recognizing characteristic changes in the photographed pupillary reflex. This technique is fast, efficient, and reproducible, but it is still evolving.[62]

Although most patients with bilateral retinoblastoma carry a germline mutation of the *RB1* gene, only a small proportion (5%-6%) carry a deletion involving the 13q14 locus, which is large enough to be detected by karyotype analysis, either as a deletion or as part of a balanced translocation, most typically t(X;13).[63] In those cases, retinoblastoma is part of a more complex syndrome resulting from the loss of

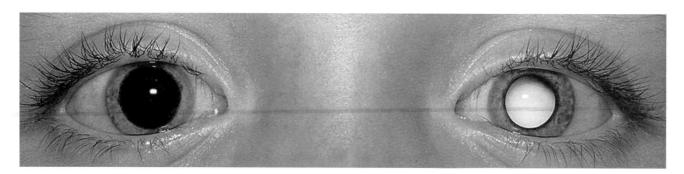

Figure 30-2 Leukocoria in a patient with unilateral retinoblastoma.

additional genetic material. Patients with the 13q-Syndrome are characterized by typical facial dysmorphic features, subtle skeletal abnormalities, and different degrees of mental retardation and motor impairment.[64–66] Dysmorphic features more consistently found include thick anteverted ear lobes, high and broad forehead, prominent philtrum, and short nose.[64,65] A proportion of patients also have overlapping fingers and toes, microcephaly, and delayed skeletal maturation.[65,66] The severity of the deficits correlate with the size of the deletion; normal psychomotor development may be seen in those patients in whom the deletion is restricted to the 13q14 band.[64]

Trilateral retinoblastoma refers to the association of bilateral retinoblastoma with an asynchronous intracranial tumor.[67–69] Tumors comprising trilateral retinoblastoma are primitive neuroectodermal tumors (PNETs) exhibiting varying degrees of neuronal or photoreceptor differentiation, suggesting an origin from the germinal layer of primitive cells.[70] This association can occur in 3% to 9% of patients with the genetic form and appears to be more common in familial cases. The prognosis has until recently been almost uniformly fatal. Trilateral retinoblastoma has been the principal cause of death from retinoblastoma during the first decade of life in the United States.[69] The majority of these tumors are pineal region PNETs (pineoblastomas), but in 20% to 25% of the cases, the tumors are suprasellar or parasellar. Rare cases of quadrilateral retinoblastoma have been reported in which bilateral retinoblastoma is associated with both pineal region and suprasellar intracranial primary PNETs. In most cases, the intracranial PNETs in association with retinoblastoma resemble undifferentiated retinoblastomas with the more frequent formation of Homer-Wright rosettes. The median age at diagnosis of trilateral retinoblastoma is 23 to 48 months,[67–69,71] and the interval between the diagnosis of bilateral retinoblastoma and the diagnosis of the brain tumor is usually more than 20 months.[67,72] Suprasellar tumors are usually diagnosed earlier[72] and in 15% to 20% of cases, the intracranial tumor antecedes the diagnosis of retinoblastoma.[68] In recent years, with the more widespread use of chemo-reduction treatments for patients with bilateral retinoblastoma, the incidence of trilateral retinoblastoma has decreased dramatically, almost to the point that patients with the genetic form of retinoblastoma are now considered to be protected against this commonly fatal complication.[73] However, approximately 5% of patients with bilateral disease develop pineal cysts; these appear to be a *forme fruste* of trilateral retinoblastoma.[74,75]

Diagnosis and Extent of Disease Evaluations

The diagnosis of intraocular retinoblastoma is usually made without pathologic confirmation. An examination under anesthesia with a maximally dilated pupil and scleral indentation is required to examine the entire retina. A

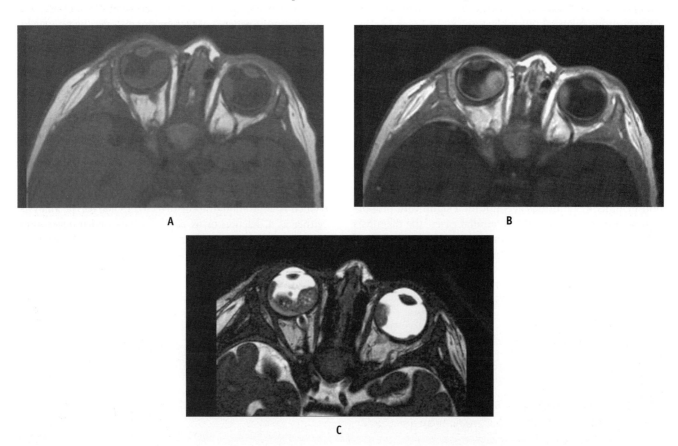

Figure 30-4 Axial T1 weighted pre (A) and post (B), and axial CISS 3-D images (C) through the orbits demonstrate multiple bilateral hypercellular enhancing retinal masses consistent with retinoblastoma, with a small right posterolateral retinal detachment.

careful examination of the iris and the anterior chamber is first performed, and the intraocular pressure is measured. Retinoblastoma usually appears as a mass projecting into the vitreous, although the presence of retinal detachment or vitreous hemorrhage may make its visualization difficult. Endophytic tumors are those that grow inward to the vitreous cavity. Because of its friability, endophytic retinoblastoma may seed the vitreous cavity. Exophytic retinoblastoma grows into the subretinal space, thus causing progressive retinal detachment and subretinal seeding. Exophytic tumors frequently resemble Coats' disease. Less frequently, retinoblastoma can adopt an infiltrative pattern, without an obvious mass. This infiltrative pattern appears to be more frequent among older children.

A very detailed documentation of the number, location, and size of tumors, the presence of retinal detachment and subretinal fluid, and the presence of vitreous and subretinal seeds must be performed. Wide-angle real-time retinal imaging systems such as RetCam® provide a 130 degree field of view and digital recording, facilitating diagnosis and monitoring.

Additional imaging studies that aid in the diagnosis include bi-dimensional ultrasound, computerized tomography, and magnetic resonance imaging (MRI). These imaging studies are particularly important to evaluate extraocular extension and to differentiate retinoblastoma from other causes of leukocoria. Computerized tomography is very helpful to detect calcifications, and MRI is very helpful in the differential diagnosis from Coats' disease and other inflammatory conditions, and with PHPV[76] (Figures 30-4 and 30-5). Evaluation for the presence of metastatic disease also needs to be considered in a subgroup of patients. Metastatic disease occurs in approximately 10% to 15% of patients, and it usually occurs in association with distinct intraocular histological features, such as deep choroidal and scleral invasion, or with involvement of the iris or ciliary body and optic nerve beyond the lamina cribrosa.[77] In these cases, additional staging procedures, including bone scintig-

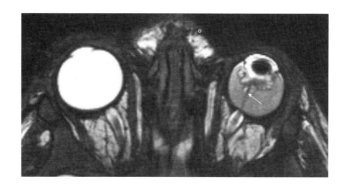

Figure 30-5 Persistent hyperplastic primary vitreous–Axial CISS 3-D image of the orbits. Normal right globe. Small left globe demonstrating persistent hyaloid artery (arrow) and hypointense primary vitreous of the posterior chamber, and an abnormally large lens.

raphy, bone marrow aspirates and biopsies, and lumbar puncture, must be performed.

Staging

The Reese-Ellsworth (R-E) grouping system has been generally accepted as the standard for intraocular disease. This grouping system was initially designed to predict the outcome after external beam radiation therapy. It divides eyes into five groups on the basis of the size, location, and number of lesions, and on the presence of vitreous seeding (Table 30-1).[78] However, developments in the conservative management of intraocular retinoblastoma have made the R-E grouping system less predictable of eye salvage, and less helpful in guiding treatment.[79] A new staging system (International Classification of Retinoblastoma) has been developed, with the goal of providing a simpler, more user-friendly classification more applicable to current therapies. This new system is based on extent of tumor seeding within the vitreous cavity and subretinal space, rather than on tumor size and location, and seems to be a better predictor of treatment success[80] (Table 30-2) (Figure 30-6).

Table 30-1

Reese-Ellsworth grouping for suitability for treatment of retinoblastoma by radiation therapy.[78]

GROUP I. VERY FAVORABLE

Ia Solitary tumor smaller than 4 dd at or behind the equator

Ib Multiple tumors, none larger than 4 dd, all at or behind equator

GROUP II. FAVORABLE

IIa Solitary tumor 4-10 dd, at or behind equator

IIb Multiple tumors 4-10 dd, at or behind equator

GROUP III. DOUBTFUL

IIIa Any lesion anterior to equator

IIIb Solitary tumor larger than 10 dd behind equator

GROUP IV. UNFAVORABLE

IVa Multiple tumors, some larger than 10 dd

IVb Any lesion extending anteriorly to the ora serrata

GROUP V. VERY UNFAVORABLE

Va Massive tumors involving more than half the retina

Vb Vitreous seeding

Abbreviation: dd, disk diameter (1.5 mm).

Table 30-2

International classification for intraocular retinoblastoma.

Group A

Small tumors away from foveola and disc

- Tumors ≤ 3 mm in greatest dimension confined to the retina, *and*
- Located at least 3 mm from the foveola and 1.5 mm from the optic disc

Group B

All remaining tumors confined to the retina

- All other tumors confined to the retina not in Group A
- Subretinal fluid (without subretinal seeding) ≤ 3 mm from the base of the tumor

Group C

Local subretinal fluid or seeding

- Local subretinal fluid alone > 3 to ≤ 6 mm from the tumor
- Vitreous seeding or subretinal seeding ≤ 3 mm from the tumor

Group D

Diffuse subretinal fluid or seeding

- Subretinal fluid alone > 6 mm from the tumor
- Vitreous seeding or subretinal seeding > 3 mm from tumor

Group E

Presence of any or more of these poor prognosis features

- More than 2/3 globe filled with tumor
- Tumor in anterior segment
- Tumor in or on the ciliary body
- Iris neovascularization
- Neovascular glaucoma
- Opaque media from hemorrhage
- Tumor necrosis with aseptic orbital cellulitis
- Phthisis bulbi

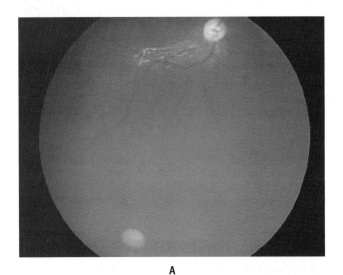

A

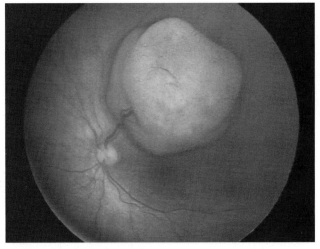

B1

Figure 30-6 International Classification of Retinoblastoma. (A) Small tumor (≤ 3 mm) confined to the retina, distant from the foveola and optic nerve. (B1) **Case 1:** Tumor > 3 mm, confined to the retina.

For patients undergoing enucleation, pathologic staging that incorporates other features known to influence the modality of treatment and the prognosis, such as choroidal and scleral involvement, optic nerve extension, and presence of metastatic disease are used.[81–83] A newly proposed staging system developed by an international consortium of ophthalmologists and pediatric oncologists incorporates the most important elements of the older systems[84] (Table 30-3). Growth and invasion occur as a sequence of events, and extra-retinal extension occurs only once the tumor has reached large intraocular dimensions (R-E Groups IV and V).[85] As part of this process, retinoblastoma extends into the ocular coats (choroids and sclera), the optic nerve, and the anterior segment. Extraocular disease is the next step in this progression; loco-regional dissemination occurs by direct extension through the sclera into the orbital contents and pre-auricular lymph nodes, and extraorbital disease manifests as intracranial dissemination and hematogenous metastases.

While the clinical significance of extraocular extension is obvious, there is no uniform agreement on the prognostic implications of the different histological characteristics; thus the different staging systems used. Even in the absence of extraocular disease, a variable risk of develop-

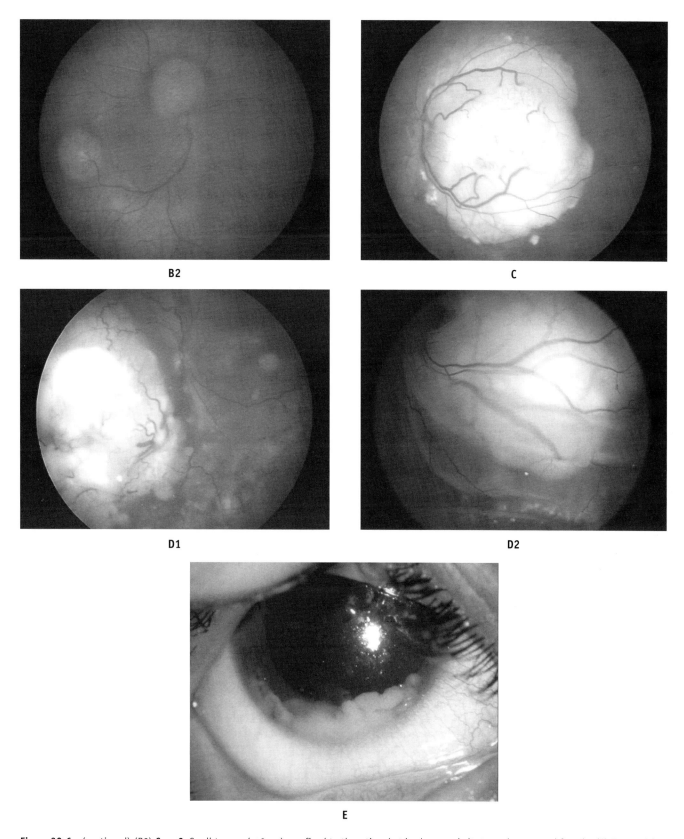

B2

C

D1

D2

E

Figure 30-6 (continued) **(B2) Case 2:** Small tumors (≤ 3mm), confined to the retina, but in close proximity to optic nerve and foveola. **(C)** Tumor with localized subretinal fluid and local seeding. **(D1) Case 1:** Tumor with diffuse seeding **(D2) Case 2:** Tumor with diffuse subretinal fluid and subretinal seeding. **(E)** Tumor in anterior segment.

Table 30-3

International retinoblastoma staging system.[84]

Stage 0. Patients treated conservatively

Stage I. Eye enucleated, completely resected histologically

Stage II. Eye enucleated, microscopic residual tumor

Stage III. Regional extension
  a. Overt orbital disease
  b. Preauricular or cervical lymph node extension

Stage IV. Metastatic disease
  a. **Hematogenous metastasis** (without CNS involvement)
    1. Single lesion
    2. Multiple lesions
  b. **CNS extension** (with or without any other site of regional or metastatic disease)
    1. Prechiasmatic lesion
    2. CNS mass
    3. Leptomeningeal and CSF disease

ing metastatic disease exists.[86–90] Many studies have attempted to evaluate the risk associated with the different histological variables. Two-thirds of patients have exclusive retinal disease, and invasion of the anterior segment, choroid, and optic nerve occur in variable proportions and combinations in the remaining patients (Table 30-4). The metastatic risk and mortality rate appear to be proportional to the extent of invasion of the ocular coats and the optic nerve. Extension of tumor into the sclera and across the line of transection of the optic nerve are associated with elevated mortality and by definition are considered to represent extraocular disease. The question arises when interpreting the other variables, because the risk associated with each variable is confounded by the lack of standardized grading methods and biased by the use of adjuvant therapy.[86,87,91]

Optic nerve involvement is common (in 25%-45% of all cases), but its impact on outcome appears to be limited to the involvement beyond the *lamina cribrosa* (where the meninges insert), and to the extension up to the transection line.[86,87,91–93] The mortality rates for the rare, untreated patients with those features are 40% to 60%, and greater than 80%, respectively.[87–90]

Choroidal involvement is found in up to 40% of patients, although massive invasion occurs in less than 10% of cases.[90,91,94] This is an important distinction, because although choroidal invasion might have prognostic implications,[77,86,92,95] its impact appears to be limited to those cases with massive replacement by tumor.[91] However, contrary to optic nerve evaluation, criteria for determining the extent of choroidal disease are more subjective and the grading of invasion is seldom reported.[91]

Evaluating the risk for each histological variable individually is insufficient; different combinations of simultaneously occurring factors are very frequent.[85] When choroidal invasion is present, half the cases will also show optic nerve involvement, whereas optic nerve invasion is uncommon (20%) if the choroid is intact.[86,89,96] Conversely, when the optic nerve is invaded, 30% to 40% of cases will have choroidal replacement (> 80% if the tumor has spread to the transection line), but choroidal invasion is quite rare (< 20%) if the optic nerve is free of tumor.[86,88,89,96] Therefore, the risk associated with each histological variable can be estimated only in the light of its association with others. Most available data support the notion that choroidal invasion alone is not associated with increased risk of extraocular spread, although massive choroidal replacement by tumor may be an exception.[91] Similarly, retro-laminar optic nerve invasion is of prognostic significance only when there is concomitant choroidal invasion,[89,94,96,97] but this represents fewer than 10% of cases.[86,89] The significance of other histological features, such as invasion of the anterior segment or grade of differentiation remains unclear.[91,92] The presence of extensive tumor necrosis appears to correlate with high-risk histological features, such as post-laminar optic nerve involvement and choroidal invasion.[98]

Principles of Treatment

Treatment of retinoblastoma aims to save life and preserve useful vision, and thus needs to be individualized. Factors that need to be considered include unilaterality or bilaterality of the disease, potential for preserving vision, and intraocular and extraocular staging.

Surgery

Enucleation is indicated for large tumors filling the vitreous for which there is little or no likelihood of restoring vision, and in cases of tumor present in the anterior chamber or in the presence of neovascular glaucoma. Enucleation should be performed by an experienced ophthalmologist; the eye must be removed intact, without seeding the malignancy into the orbit and avoiding globe perforation.[99] For optimal staging, a long section (10 mm-15 mm) of the optic nerve needs to be removed with the globe. An orbital implant is usually fitted during the same procedure, and the extraocular muscles are attached to it. In the past, orbital implants were avoided because it was felt that they would interfere with the palpation of the socket and clinical detection of orbital recurrence. However, with improved understanding of the histological risk factors, and the availability of better imaging techniques to detect orbital disease, implants should be placed at the time of the enucleation. Different orbital implants are available, including polymethylmethacrylate, polyethylene, and coralline and bovine hydroxyapatite spheres. A tissue wrap to the implant is placed, which will allow the four rectus muscles to be anatomically re-attached, thus providing implant motility with little resistance in the orbit.[99] The size and type of implant are important to stimulate orbital growth.[100] A ceramic false eye is later fitted in the orbital socket. Orbital

Table 30-4

Histologic findings in enucleated eyes.

Histologic Variables	Messner[86]	Kopelman[87]	Magramm[88]	Shields[89]	Khelfaoui[91]	Chantada[94]	Uusitalo[90]
Retinal only	56%	57%		58%		21%	
Anterior segment	6.9%				13%		7.7%
Optic nerve	24%	39%	29.4%	29%	43%	31.2%	63.5%
Prelaminar	14.8%	12.8%*	14.7%	22%	15%	7.6%	52%
Retrolaminar	5.6%		8%	6%	19%	17.7%	8.5%
+ transection	3.8%	26%	6%	1%	9.8%	5.9%	3%
Choroid (massive)	12.4%	22%		23.5%	42%	31.9%	33%
					(11.6%)	(7.6%)	(9%)
Sclera	1.2%	7.8%			8%	3%	2.3%
Combinations							
Choroid only	6%			12.8%			
Optic nerve only	10%			18%			
Choroid + optic nerve (all)	7%			10.7%			
Choroid + optic nerve (RL only)	1.4%						

*Prelaminar and retrolaminar; RL, retrolaminar.

exenteration is very seldom indicated. For patients presenting with orbital disease, a judicious use of chemotherapy, surgery, and radiation therapy will result in good tumor control, avoiding the need for orbital exenteration.

Focal Therapies

Focal treatments are used for small tumors (<3 mm-6 mm), usually in patients with bilateral disease, and in combination with chemotherapy. *Photocoagulation* with Argon laser is used for the treatment of tumors situated at or posterior to the equator of the eye, and for the treatment of retinal neo-vascularization due to radiation therapy.[101] This technique is limited to tumors measuring no greater than 4.5 mm in base, and no greater than 2.5 mm in thickness. The treatment is directed to de-limit the tumor and coagulate all blood supply to the tumor, and two or three monthly sessions are usually required. Tumor control rates approach 70%.[99] *Cryotherapy* is used for the treatment of small equatorial and peripheral lesions, measuring no more than 3.5 mm in base and no more than 2 mm thickness.[99,102] One or two monthly sessions of triple freeze and thaw are performed, and tumor control rates are usually excellent. Finally, an important focal method is *transpupillary thermotherapy*, which applies focused heat at sub-photocoagulation levels, usually with diode laser.[103] In thermotherapy, the goal is to deliver a temperature of 42°C to 60°C for 5 to 20 minutes to the tumor, sparing retinal vessels from photocoagulation.

The use of focal treatments is especially important in conjunction with chemotherapy, and both treatment modalities appear to have a synergistic effect. The sequential administration of thermotherapy with carboplatin enhances the anti-tumor effect by increasing the platinum-DNA adducts, for which reason *thermochemotherapy* is becoming a very important component in the treatment of intraocular retinoblastoma.[104,105] Also, in addition to its effect on tumor control, cryotherapy contributes to increase the intraocular penetration of chemotherapy agents, presumably through disruption of the blood-vitreous barrier.[106,107] In general, local control rates of 70% to 80% can be achieved.[101,102,104] Complications of focal treatments include transient serous retinal detachment, retinal traction and tears, and localized fibrosis.[99]

Chemotherapy

Chemotherapy is indicated in patients with extraocular disease, in the subgroup of patients with intraocular disease with high-risk histological features, and in patients with bilateral disease in conjunction with aggressive focal therapies. Agents effective in the treatment of retinoblastoma include platinum compounds, etoposide, cyclophosphamide, doxorubicin, vincristine, and ifosfamide.[108]

Radiotherapy

Retinoblastoma is a very radiosensitive tumor. Radiotherapy in combination with focal treatments can provide excellent tumor control.[109–111] However, since radiation therapy increases the risk of second malignancies, contemporary management of intraocular retinoblastoma is designed to avoid or delay its use, and the role of irradiation is mainly as salvage management for eyes that have failed chemotherapy and focal treatments, usually due to progression of vitreous and sub-retinal seeding. Radiation therapy continues to have a major role in the treatment of patients with extraocular disease (see below).

Since most patients with intraocular retinoblastoma undergoing radiotherapy have multi-focal disease, the entire retinal surface needs to be irradiated to a uniform dose. Several techniques can be used, usually through lateral or anterior fields.[109–111] Recommended total doses are 4,000 cGy to 4,500 cGy, in 180 cGy to 200 cGy fractions, although doses of 3,600 cGy may be effective in conjunction with other techniques.[112,113] *Radioactive plaque technique* is useful when treating localized tumors, both because the procedure time is short, and because a high dose of irradiation is delivered to the areas of interest while minimizing irradiation effects to extraocular structures. Indications for plaque therapy include solitary tumors with a diameter ranging between 6 mm and 15 mm, tumor thickness of 10 mm or less, and location of the lesion more than 3 mm from the optic disc or *fovea*. The radioactive implant is placed on the sclera over the base of the tumor, and is kept for 2 to 4 days, the time needed to deliver approximately 4,000 cGy to the apex of the tumor. Different radioactive epi-scleral plaques can be used, although radio-iodine I[124] is the most widely used. Control rates of 85% to 90% can be achieved.[114]

Treatment of Intraocular Retinoblastoma
Unilateral Retinoblastoma

In the absence of extraocular disease, enucleation alone is curative for 85% to 90% of children with unilateral retinoblastoma.[55,91,94,115] The outcome for patients with unilateral disease that has been enucleated is excellent, with good functional results and minimal long-term effects.[116] In view of the apparent success in treating bilateral intraocular disease with chemo-reduction, some clinicians are salvaging single eyes with chemotherapy and focal measures, especially in very young children who may develop metachronous bilateral disease. In these cases, the combination of chemo-reduction with aggressive focal consolidation techniques, usually thermochemotherapy and brachytherapy, is necessary.[99]

Adjuvant treatment is indicated in those cases with scleral invasion and in patients with positive tumor at the transection line of the optic nerve (see below, under treatment of extraocular retinoblastoma). Adjuvant treatment for the remaining patients with intraocular disease is debatable. In the absence of randomized studies, available information would suggest that the use of adjuvant chemotherapy is beneficial for the selected group of patients with higher risk of extraocular dissemination (patients with concurrent retro-laminar and choroidal involvement, and possibly patients with massive choroidal involvement).[85,90,91,94] Adjuvant chemotherapy is not indicated for patients with pre-laminar involvement[90,117] or isolated focal choroidal involvement.[90,94,115,117] The value of adjuvant chemotherapy in the setting of isolated retro-laminar involvement is controversial.[74,94] Different chemotherapy regimens have been proposed. Six-month treatment with vincristine, cyclophosphamide, and doxorubicin; vincristine, carboplatin, and etoposide; or a hybrid with alternating courses of both regimens, appears to be effective.[55,85,94] Radiation therapy is not indicated in these cases.

Bilateral Retinoblastoma

Patients with germ line mutation of the *RB1* gene develop multiple, bilateral retinoblastomas at an earlier age, and they are at risk of developing new tumors until the completion of retinal differentiation.[118,119] In the past, the treatment for patients with bilateral retinoblastoma has been enucleation of those eyes with advanced intraocular disease and no visual potential, and the use of external beam radiation therapy for the remaining eyes. However, there are several complications associated with radiation therapy. Irradiation of the orbit during a period of rapid growth results in a major decrease in orbital volume, resulting in mid-facial deformities.[120,121] More importantly, however, is the greatly increased risk for the development of a sarcoma within the radiation therapy field, compared to the underlying increased risk of secondary neoplasms in these predisposed individuals. This risk may be age-related and decreases as irradiation is delayed.[122] These concerns have resulted in the development of new and more conservative approaches. The treatment of patients with bilateral retinoblastoma now incorporates up-front chemotherapy, which is intended to achieve maximum chemo-reduction of the intraocular tumor burden early in the treatment, followed by aggressive focal therapies (Figure 30-7). Chemo-reduction coupled with intensive use of sequential focal therapies (cryotherapy, laser photocoagulation, thermotherapy, and brachytherapy) has resulted in an increase in the eye salvage rates and in a decrease (and delay) in the use of radiation therapy. Different chemotherapy combinations are used, although the best results are achieved with a combination of vincristine, carboplatin and etoposide (or teniposide).[104,113,123–126] An alternative chemotherapy regimen includes the addition of cyclosporin to the three-drug regimen.[127] The rationale for the use of cyclosporin originates from the documentation of the presence of the P-glycoprotein efflux pump in a significant proportion of retinoblastomas, an expression that appears to correlate with treatment failure.[128] The concurrent administration of cyclosporin could potentially abrogate the efflux of drugs from the cancer cell.[127,129] However, the expression of P-glycoprotein does not always seem to predict response,[130] and cyclosporin adds additional toxicity.[115] For patients with early intraocular stages (R-E Groups I-III, International Group B), a less intensive regimen with vincristine and carboplatin alone appears to be effective.[74,125,126] (Tables 30-5 and 30-6).

Salvage rates for R-E Groups I-III eyes approach 100% using these techniques. For patients with advanced intraocular tumors (R-E Groups IV-V), ocular salvage rates are not better than 50% to 70%, and external beam radiation therapy is usually required.[113] However, the use of radiation therapy is usually delayed for several months, which allows for better orbital growth and a decrease in the risk of second malignancies. A major proportion of failures occur because of progression of tumor in the vitreous, or as sub-retinal implants, two areas of difficult access for anti-neoplastic agents.[132] Carboplatin diffuses well into the vitreous.[133] Intraocular concentrations are 7 to 10 times higher when carboplatin is administered sub-conjunctivally,[133] and animal studies have shown a dose-dependent inhibition of intraocular tumor growth by sub-conjuctival carboplatin.[107,134] These encouraging pre-clinical data, however, have not been effectively translated into an improvement in the outcome of advanced eyes;[134] prospective studies are planned in the Children's Oncology Group to evaluate the role of this modality of carboplatin administration. Great caution should be exerted if peri-ocular carboplatin is administered; there is a risk of

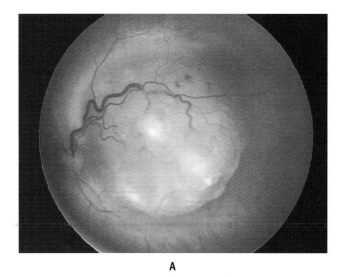

A

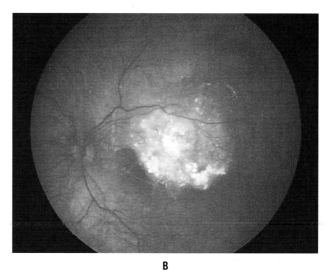

B

Figure 30-7 Response of intraocular retinoblastoma to chemotherapy. (A) Group B tumor before therapy. (B) Same tumor, after two courses of vincristine and carboplatin.

Table 30-5

Treatment of intraocular retinoblastoma.

Author	N pts (eyes)	Upfront Enucleation	Evaluable Eyes	Reese-Ellsworth Group	Cytoreduction Regimen	Required EBRT	Ocular Salvage	Overall Ocular Salvage*
Levy[131]	23 (43)	5 (12%)	38	I-III: 15 (39%) IV-V: 23 (60%)	ETO 150 mg/m² d 1-3 CBP 200 mg/m² d 1-3 × 2 courses	20 (53%)	82% RE I-III: 100% RE IV-V: 60%	72% RE I-III: 100% RE IV-V: 57%
Friedman[132]	47 (85)	10 (12%)	75	I-III: 39 (52%) IV-V: 36 (48%)	VCR 1.5 mg/m² d 1 ETO 150 mg/m² d 1-2 CBP 560 mg/m² d 1 × 6 courses	11 (17%)	85% RE I-III: 100% RE IV-V: 70%	75% RE I-III: 100% RE IV-V: 54%
Gallie[127]	21 (42)	14 (33%)	28	I-III: 15 (54%) IV-V: 13 (46%)	VCR 0.05 mg/kg d 1 TEN 239 mg/m² d 1 CBP 560 mg/m² d 1 CsA: 33 mg/kg d 1 × 3-12 courses	1 (4%)	93% RE I-III: 100% RE IV-V: 85%	62% RE I-III: 100% RE IV-V: 48%
Beck[123]	24 (42)	9 (21%)	33	I-III: 18 (56%) IV-V: 15 (44%)	ETO 150 mg/m² d 1-3 CBP 200 mg/m² d 1-3 × 2-5 courses	4 (12%)	85% RE I-III 100% RE IV-V: 66%	67% RE I-III: 100% RE IV-V: 56%
Rodriguez-Galindo[74]	25 (43)	0	43	I-III: 24 (56%) IV-V: 19 (44%)	VCR 0.05 mg/kg d 1 CBP 560 mg/m² d 1 × 8 courses	19 (44%)	70% RE I-III: 83% RE IV-V: 53%	70% RE I-III: 83% RE IV-V: 53%
Chantada[125]	58 (97)	19 (20%)	78	I-III: 24 (31%) IV-V: 54 (69%)	VCR 0.05 /kg d 1 CBP 560 mg/m² d 1 ETO# 100 mg/m² d 1-2 × 2-8 courses	28 (48%)	64% RE I-III: 96% RE IV-V: 50%	52% RE I-III: 96% RE IV-V: 37%
Wilson[126]	16 (27)	0	27	I-III: 7 (26%) IV-V: 20 (64%)	VCR 0.05 mg/kg d 1 CBP 560 mg/m² d 1 × 8 courses	8 (30%)	82% RE I-III: 100% RE IV-V: 75%	82% RE I-III: 100% RE IV-V: 75%

*Overall ocular salvage includes upfront enucleation

#Only to patients with RE group IV-V eyes

Abbreviations: ETO, etoposide; CBP, carboplatin; VCR, vincristine; TEN, teniposide; CsA, cyclosporin A; RE, Reese-Ellsworth group.

Table 30-6

Recommended approach to the treatment of intraocular retinoblastoma.

RE Group	ABC Group	Treatment		
		Focal Tx	Chemotherapy	Radiation
I-II	A	+	−	If PD
I-III	B	+	VCR 0.05 mg/kg d 1 CBP 18.6 mg/kg d 1 × 2 – 6 courses	If PD
IV-V	C-D	+ +/− subtenon carboplatin × 3	VCR 0.05 mg/kg d 1 CBP 14 mg/kg d 1, 2 ETO 6 mg/kg d 1, 2 × 6 courses + G-CSF	If PD Consider early EBRT if massive vitreous seeding at completion of chemotherapy
V b	E	Enucleation		

ischemic necrosis and atrophy of the optic nerve, and sub-tenon administration is preferred.[136]

Thus the treatment of patients with advanced intraocular disease (R-E Groups IV and V, International Groups C and D) remains a major challenge. Although randomized studies have not been performed, compared to radiation therapy and focal treatments alone, chemo-reduction does not seem to improve overall ocular salvage significantly for patients with very advanced intraocular disease.[109–111] Chemotherapy intensification appears to correlate with outcome, and better results are obtained with protocols that include at least six courses of vincristine, etoposide, and carboplatin.[113,137,138] Central retinal tumors usually respond better to chemotherapy than do tumors in the peripheral retina,[139] but large central tumors may be associated with sub-retinal seeds, which ultimately may cause treatment failure.[140] Despite the addition of aggressive sequential focal therapies, globe retention is still no better than 50% for R-E Group V eyes (International Group D), and most patients eventually require irradiation.[113,123,126] A major proportion of failures occur because of progression of tumor in the vitreous or as sub-retinal implants, two areas of difficult access for anti-neoplastic agents.[132] In contrast to the highly protein-bound etoposide, which remains in the plasma and lacks intraocular penetration, carboplatin diffuses well into the vitreous.[133] The intraocular penetration of carboplatin is enhanced by disruption of the blood-vitreous barrier by the tumor[140] and it is enhanced after cryotherapy.[106,107]

Radiation therapy appears to be the only valid alternative for these patients, and with the incorporation of irradiation early in the treatment, in a situation of minimal disease, before disease progression occurs, ocular salvage rates for International Group D eyes may improve.[124]

New agents with better intraocular penetration are being investigated. Topotecan, a topoisomerase-I inhibitor with well documented efficacy against pediatric tumors, is a promising alternative. Studies performed in the animal model have shown that topotecan has excellent intraocu-

lar penetration and is among the most effective agents for treating retinoblastoma.[142] Suicide gene therapy using an adenoviral vector to locally deliver (by intraocular injection) the herpes simplex tyrosine kinase gene, followed by systemic administration of ganciclovir, has been shown to be safe and to induce responses of the vitreous lesions in a recently reported phase I study.[143] This is a promising treatment for patients with vitreous disease, and phase II studies are being developed. Finally, the recent description of *MDMX* amplification as the mechanism of inactivation of the p53 pathway in retinoblastoma has opened the door to the use of specific targeted molecular therapies. Nutlin-3 is a small-molecule inhibitor of the MDM2-p53 interaction.[144] MDMX and MDM2 bind p53 with similar affinities, and studies have shown that nutlin-3 prevents the MDMX-p53 interaction in retinoblastoma cells, inducing p53-mediated apoptosis *in vitro* and *in vivo*. Importantly, sub-conjunctival injection of nutlin-3 to mice with intraocular retinoblastoma resulted in significant tumor responses. Importantly, the combination of nutlin-3 with a DNA damaging agent such as topotecan resulted in a synergistic effect.[43]

Treatment of Extraocular Retinoblastoma

Extraocular dissemination of retinoblastoma bears a close relationship with the socio-economic conditions that result in delayed diagnosis and treatment. In Europe and the United States, fewer than 5% of patients present with extraocular disease,[86,145,146] in contrast to 12% to 20% in South America,[115,147] 25% to 40% in Mexico and India[60,148,149] and greater than 50% in less developed countries.[150]

Four patterns of extraocular disease have been recognized: (1) Loco-regional dissemination, including orbital disease, tumor extending to the cut end of the optic nerve, and lymphatic spread to the pre-auricular lymph nodes; (2) Central nervous system (CNS) dissemination;

(3) Metastatic retinoblastoma, and (4) Trilateral retino-blastoma.

Orbital and Loco-regional Retinoblastoma

Orbital retinoblastoma occurs as a result of progression of the tumor through the emissary vessels and sclera. For this reason, scleral disease is considered to be extraocular, and should be treated as such. Orbital retinoblastoma is isolated in 60% to 70% of cases; lymphatic, hematogenous, and CNS metastases occur in the remaining patients.[150] Treatment should include systemic chemotherapy and radiation therapy; with this approach, 60% to 85% of patients can be cured. Since most recurrences occur in the CNS, regimens using drugs with well documented CNS penetration are recommended. Different chemotherapy regimens have proven to be effective, including vincristine, cyclophosphamide, and doxorubicin, platinum- and epipodophyllotoxin-based regimens, or a combination of both.[55,93,115,147,152–155] For patients with macroscopic orbital disease, it is recommended that surgery is delayed until response to chemotherapy has been obtained (usually two or three courses of treatment). Enucleation should then be performed, and an additional four to six courses of chemotherapy administered. Local control should then be consolidated with orbital irradiation (4,000 cGy to 4,500 cGy). Using this approach, orbital exenteration is not indicated.[153,154] Similar management should be followed for patients with scleral disease, including radiation therapy, although good outcomes without irradiation have also been reported.[147] Patients with isolated involvement of the optic nerve at the transection level should also receive similar systemic treatment, and irradiation should include the entire orbit (3,600 cGy) with 1,000 cGy boost to the chiasm (total 4,600 cGy). Also, because metastases in parameningeal bones have been associated with intracranial dissemination,[156] irradiation fields should be adjusted carefully. The pre-auricular and cervical lymph nodes should be explored carefully, because 20% of patients with orbital retinoblastoma have lymphatic metastases.[151] Lymphatic dissemination does not carry a worse prognosis, provided that the involved lymph nodes are also irradiated.[94,115,145,154,157] Patients with spontaneous or accidental ocular perforation and patients with intraocular surgery for unsuspected retinoblastoma should be considered to have orbital disease by definition, and treated accordingly.

Central Nervous System Disease

Intracranial dissemination occurs by direct extension through the optic nerve, and its prognosis is dismal.[94,145,147,153–158] Treatment for these patients should include platinum-based intensive systemic chemotherapy and CNS directed therapy. Although intrathecal methotrexate (with or without cytosine arabinoside) has traditionally been used, there is no preclinical or clinical evidence to support its use.[159] Other intrathecal

agents with documented effect against retinoblastoma include topotecan[160,161] and thiotepa.[157,162] However, there is no evidence that their use can impact outcome. Although the use of irradiation in these patients is controversial, responses have been observed with craniospinal irradiation, using 2,500 cGy to 3,500 cGy to the entire craniospinal axis, and a boost (1,000 cGy) to sites of measurable disease.[147,154,156,157,163] Therapeutic intensification with high-dose, marrow ablative chemotherapy and autologous hematopoietic progenitor cell rescue has been explored[156] but its role is not yet clear. Despite the intensity of the treatment and the documented responses of the intracranial disease,[152] patients succumb to their disease, and survivors are anecdotal.[153,156]

Trilateral Retinoblastoma

The prognosis for patients with trilateral retinoblastoma is very poor; most patients die of disseminated neuroaxis disease in less than nine months.[67,71,72] The rare survivors are usually those diagnosed with screening imaging and treated with intensive chemotherapy with or without craniospinal irradiation.[67] Pineal PNETs (pineoblastoma) occurring in non-retinoblastoma patients are also associated with a poor prognosis in younger patients. However, with an appropriately aggressive multimodal approach, these patients can be cured. Primitive neuroectodermal tumors are chemo-sensitive tumors, and they appear to have a steep dose-response curve for alkylating agents. Studies in older patients with pineoblastoma have recently shown that a treatment with complete resection and intensive alkylator- and cisplatin-based therapy, followed by craniospinal irradiation (3,600 cGy with boost to the pineal gland to 5,900 cGy), and consolidation with high-dose, myeloablative chemotherapy and autologous hematopoietic progenitor cell rescue, may produce survival rates in more than two-thirds of patients.[164] It is therefore possible that similar treatment guidelines could be used for trilateral retinoblastoma. One must, however, consider the serious long term toxicities of such doses of irradiation in the very young child. Therefore, current strategies are directed toward avoiding irradiation using intensive chemotherapy followed by consolidation with myeloablative chemotherapy and autologous hematopoietic progenitor cell rescue, an approach similar to those being used in the treatment of brain tumors in infants. Using the Head Start regimen, which uses this approach, improved outcomes have been reported in young children with supratentorial PNETs, including pineoblastomas.[165]

Because of the poor prognosis of trilateral retinoblastoma, screening neuro-imaging is a common practice. One-fourth of the cases in the literature correspond to cases found during screening.[67] Given the short interval between the diagnosis of retinoblastoma and the occurrence of trilateral retinoblastoma, routine screening might detect the majority of cases within two years.[67] While it is not clear whether early diagnosis can impact survival,[166] it is usually recommended to perform neuro-imaging every six months until five years of age.[67,72,167]

(Extracranial) Metastatic Retinoblastoma

Hematogenous metastases may develop in the bones, bone marrow and, less frequently, in the liver.[147,154,155,158,163] Although long-term survivors have been reported with conventional chemotherapy,[155] these cures should be considered anecdotal; metastatic retinoblastoma is not curable with conventional chemotherapy.[147,154] In recent years, however, small series of patients have shown that metastatic retinoblastoma can be cured using high-dose, marrow-ablative chemotherapy and autologous hematopoietic progenitor cell rescue (Table 30-7).[156,158,163,168–170] The approach is similar to metastatic neuroblastoma; patients receive short and intensive induction regimens, usually containing alkylating agents, anthracyclines, etoposide, and platinum compounds and are then consolidated with marrow-ablative chemotherapy and autologous hematopoietic cell rescue.

Using this approach, the outcome appears to be excellent. As for any 'megatherapy' consolidation, the agents selected may be important. In general, recurrences are intracranial, and for this reason, agents with proven efficacy in intracranial retinoblastoma should be used. In this regard, the combination of carboplatin and etoposide has been shown to be effective against CNS disease,[152] and for this reason it should be part of the regimen. In the largest published series, seven patients received consolidation with the CARBOPEC combination (carboplatin 1250-1750 mg/m^2, etoposide 1750 mg/m^2, and cyclophosphamide 6.4 g/m^2), five of them were cured, and two patients failed due to CNS relapse. Two other series have used a thiotepa-based consolidation (thiotepa 900 mg/m^2, etoposide 750–1200 mg/m^2, and carboplatin 1500 mg/m^2). There is a strong rationale for using thiotepa: retinoblastoma is responsive to alkylating agents such as thiotepa, a group of agents for which dose escalation is shown to overcome resistance. Furthermore, thiotepa has excellent CNS penetration.[163,171] An interesting observation

Table 30-7

Treatment of metastatic retinoblastoma.

Author	N	Sites of Disease	Induction	Radiation	Megatherapy	Outcome	Site of Failures
Dunkel[163]	4	BM (4) Bone (2) Liver (2) Orbit/ skull (3)	[VCR-DOX-CYC] [CP-ETO]	Skull (21 Gy) Orbit (40 Gy) Liver (19.5 Gy) Bone (30 Gy)	TT-CBP±ETO	4/4 Alive	—
Namouni[156]	7	Bone (6) BM (1)	[VCR-DOX-CYC] [CBP-ETO] [CP-ETO]	None	CBP-ETO-CYC	5/7 Alive	CNS (2)
Kremens[168]	4	BM (4) Bone (1) Orbit (1)	[CP-ETO-VD] [VCR-DTIC-IFO-DOX] [CBP-ETO] [CBP-CYC] [CYC-ETO]	None	TT-CBP-ETO	4/4 Alive	—
Rodriguez-Galindo[169]	4	BM (4) Bone (1) Orbit/ skull (4) LN (1)	[CYC/DOX/CP] [CBP/ETO] [CYC/DOX/CBP]	Orbit/skull (36.5 – 46 Gy) LN (18 Gy)	CBP-ETO (1) BUS-CYC-MEL (1) MEL-CYC-ETO (1) CYC-TOP (1)	2/4	CNS (2) BM (1)
Matsubara[158]	3	BM (3) Bone (1) Orbit (1)	[VCR-DOX-CYC] [CP-ETO] [CBP-ETO]	Bone (45 Gy)	MEL-ETO-CBP MEL-CYC-TT	3/3	

Abbreviations: BM, bone marrow; LN, lymph nodes; VCR, vincristine; DOX, doxorubicin; CYC, cyclophosphamide; CP, cisplatin; ETO, etoposide; CBP, carboplatin; VD, vindesine; IFO, ifosfamide; TT, thiotepa; BUS, busulfan; MEL, melphalan; TOP, topotecan; CNS, central nervous system.

is that patients with distant (outside orbit and skull) bone metastases that show good response to induction chemotherapy may not require radiation therapy when treated with marrow-ablative chemotherapy.[156,168]

Long Term Effects of Retinoblastoma and Its Treatment

The cumulative incidence of second cancers in patients with germ-line mutations of the *RB1* gene is greatly increased with the use and dose of radiation therapy, and this incidence is reported to increase steadily with age, to up to 40% to 60% at 40 to 50 years of age, although a more recent study estimates a considerably lower risk.[118,119,172,173] Patients with non-hereditary retinoblastoma are not inherently at an increased risk.[118,173] The risk of second cancer appears to correlate as well with timing of radiation therapy; children receiving radiation therapy during their first year may have a higher risk of developing a second cancer within the field of irradiation.[122] However, the need for earlier irradiation may also be an indication of a biologically and clinically more aggressive disease.

Almost any neoplasm has been described in survivors of retinoblastoma[173] and 60% to 70% of the tumors occur in the head and neck areas.[122,172,173] The most common second tumor is osteogenic sarcoma, arising both inside and outside the irradiation field, which accounts for approximately one-third of all cases of second cancers.[172,173] Osteogenic sarcomas usually develop during the growth spurt years (even those arising within irradiation fields), not significantly different from the normal population.[174] Soft tissue sarcomas and melanomas are second in frequency, accounting for 20% to 25% of cases.[172,175] In recent years, it has become apparent that patients with hereditary retinoblastoma are also at risk of developing epithelial cancers late in adulthood.[176] Of those, lung cancer appears to be the most common.[176,177] This is not surprising because somatic mutations of the *RB1* gene are known to contribute to the development of lung cancer.[177,178] Finally, an interesting observation is the increased incidence of lipomas in survivors of hereditary retinoblastoma. The incidence of a second neoplasm appears to be higher in those patients with lipomas, suggesting that the presence of lipomas could be a clinical marker of susceptibility to second neoplasms.[179]

Because their orbital growth is still in progress, children treated for retinoblastoma are at risk of functionally and cosmetically significant bony orbital abnormalities. These sequelae become evident by early adolescence, when orbital growth is largely complete, and result in the "hour-glass facial deformity."[120] Both enucleation, which causes orbital contraction, and radiotherapy, which induces arrest of bone growth, adversely affect orbital growth. In children treated for bilateral retinoblastoma, the impact of enucleation in orbital development is not different from that of irradiation. However, final orbital volumes after enucleation correlate with the size of the prosthetic implant.[121]

Delay of radiation therapy should therefore be a goal when designing treatment for children with bilateral retinoblastoma. Studies show that the therapeutic strategy of chemo-reduction and aggressive focal treatments can successfully delay the use of radiation therapy for at least six or seven months, (median age 21 months).[74,113] In addition to theoretically decreasing the risk of second cancers, delaying radiation therapy may also allow more complete facial and orbital growth, thus reducing the degree of mid-facial deformities.[120,121] However, with the use of a multi-disciplinary approach, the dose of irradiation needed for disease control may also be reduced.[112]

References

1. Young JL, Smith MA, Roffers SD, Liff JM, Bunin GR. Retinoblastoma. In: Ries LAG, Smith MA, Gurney JG, et al. (eds). *Cancer Incidence and Survival Among Children and Adolescents: United States SEER Program, 1975–1995*, National Cancer Institute, SEER Program. NIH Pub. No. 99–4649. Bethesda, MD; 1999.
2. Parkin DM, Stiller CA, Draper GJ, Bieber CA. The international incidence of childhood cancer. *Int J Cancer.* 1988;42:511–520.
3. Stiller CA, McKinney PA, Bunch KJ, Bailey CC, Lewis IJ. Childhood cancer and ethnic group in Britain: a United Kingdom Children's Cancer Study Group (UKCCSG) study. *Br J Cancer.* 1991;64:543–548.
4. Koulibaly M, Kabba IS, Cisse A, et al. Cancer incidence in Conakry, Guinea: first results from the cancer registry 1992–1995. *Int J Cancer.* 1997;70:39–45.
5. Schultz KR, Ranade S, Negllia JP, Ravindranath Y. An increased relative frequency of retinoblastoma at a rural regional referral hospital in Miraj, Maharashtra, India. *Cancer.* 1993;72:282–286.
6. Duncan MH, Wiggins CL, Samet JM, Key CR. Childhood cancer epidemiology in New Mexico's American Indians, Hispanic Whites, and Non-Hispanic Whites, 1970–82. *J Natl Cancer Inst.* 1986;76:1013–1018.
7. Lanier AP, Holck P, Day GE, Key C. Childhood cancer among Alaska natives. *Pediatrics.* 2003;112:396–403.
8. Bunin GR, Meadows AT, Emanuel BS, et al. Pre- and postconception factors associated with sporadic heritable and nonheritable retinoblastoma. *Cancer Res.* 1989;49:5730–5735.
9. Orjuela MA, Titievsky L, Liu X, et al. Fruit and vegetable intake during pregnancy and risk for development of sporadic retinoblastoma. *Cancer Epidemiol Biomarkers Prev.* 2005;14:1433–1440.
10. Dryja TP, Mukai S, Petersen R, Rapaport JM, Walton D, Yandell DW. Parental origin of mutations of the retinoblastoma gene. *Nature.* 1989;339:556–558.
11. Moll AC, Imhof SM, Kuik J, et al. High parental age is associated with sporadic hereditary retinoblastoma: the Dutch Retinoblastoma Register 1862–1994. *Hum Genet.* 1996;98:109–112.
12. Bunin GR, Petrakova A, Meadows AT, et al. Occupations of parents of children with retinoblastoma: a report from the Children's Cancer Study Group. *Cancer Res.* 1990;50:7129–7133.
13. Jemal A, Devesa SS, Fears TR, Fraumeni JF. Retinoblastoma incidence and sunlight exposure. *Br J Cancer.* 2000;82:1875–1878.
14. Hooper ML. Is sunlight an aetiological agent in the genesis of retinoblastoma? *Br J Cancer.* 1999;79:1273–1276.
15. Niemitz EL, Feinberg, AP. Epigenetics and assisted reproductive technology: a call for investigation. *Am J Hum Genet.* 2004;74:599–609
16. Moll A, Imhof S, Cruysberg JRM, Schouten-van Meeteren AYN, Boers M, van Leeuwen FE. Incidence of retinoblastoma in children born after in-vitro fertilisation. *Lancet.* 2003;361:309–310.
17. Richter S, Vandezande K, Chen N, et al. Sensitive and efficient detection of *RB1* gene mutations enhances care for families with retinoblastoma. *Am J Hum Genet.* 2003;72:253–269.
18. Greger V, Passarge E, Hopping W, Messmer E, Horsthemke B. Epigenetic changes may contribute to the formation and spontaneous regression of retinoblastoma. *Hum Genet.* 1989;83:155–158.
19. Ohtani-Fujita N, Fujita T, Aoike A, Osifchin NE, Robbins PD, Sakai T. CpG methylation inactivates the promoter activity of the human retinoblastoma tumor-suppressor gene. *Oncogene.* 2003;8:1063–1067.
20. Gillison ML, Shah KV. Role of mucosal human papillomavirus in nongenital cancers. *J Natl Cancer Inst Monogr.* 2003;31:57–65.
21. Griep A, Krawcek J, Lee D, et al. Multiple genetic loci modify risk for retinoblastoma in transgenic mice. *Invest Ophthalmol Vis Sci.* 1998;39:2723–2732.
22. Orjuela M, Ponce Castaneda V, Ridaura C, et al. Presence of human papilloma virus in tumor tissue from children with retinoblastoma: an alternative mechanism for tumor development. *Clin Cancer Res.* 2000;6:4010–4016.
23. Palazzi MA, Yunes JA, Cardinalli IA, et al. Detection of oncogenic human papillomavirus in sporadic retinoblastoma. *Acta Ophthalmol Scand.* 2003;81: 396–398.
24. Knudson AG. Mutation and cancer: statistical study of retinoblastoma. *Proc Natl Acad Sci USA.* 1971;68:820–823

25. Lee WH, Bookstein R, Hong F, Young LJ, Shew JY, Lee EY. Human retinoblastoma susceptibility gene: cloning, identification, and sequence. *Science.* 1987; 235:1394–1399.

26. Friend SH, Bernards R, Rogelj S, et al. A human DNA segment with properties of the gene that predisposes to retinoblastoma and osteosarcoma. *Nature.* 1986;323:643–646.

27. Brantley MA, Harbour JW. The molecular biology of retinoblastoma. *Ocul Immunol Inflamm.* 2001;9:1–8.

28. Classon M, Dyson N. p107 and p130: versatile proteins with interesting pockets. *Exp Cell Res.* 2001;264:135–147.

29. Houdayer C, Gauthier-Villars M, Laugé A, et al. Comprehensive screening for constitutional *RB1* mutations by DHPLC and QMPSF. *Hum Mutat.* 2004;23: 193–202.

30. Alonso J, Garcia-Miguel P, Abelairas J, et al. Spectrum of germline *RB1* gene mutations in Spanish retinoblastoma patients: phenotypic and molecular epidemiological implications. *Hum Mutat.* 2001;17:412–422.

31. Harbour JW. Molecular basis of low-penetrance retinoblastoma. *Arch Ophthalmol.* 2001;119:1699–1704.

32. Zhu X, Dunn JM, Goddard AD, et al. Mechanisms of loss of heterozygosity in retinoblastoma. *Cytogenet Cell Genet.* 1992;59:248–252.

33. Weinberg RA. The tumor suppressor genes. *Science.* 1991;254:1138–1146.

34. Jacks T, Fazeli A, Schmitt EM, Bronson RT, Goodell MA, Weinberg RA. Effects of an Rb mutation in the mouse. *Nature.* 1992;359:295–300.

35. Lee EY, Chang CY, Hu N, et al. Mice deficient for Rb are nonviable and show defects in neurogenesis and haematopoiesis. *Nature.* 1992;359:288–294.

36. Sage J, Miller AL, Perez-Mancera PA, Wysocki JM, Jacks T. Acute mutation of retinoblastoma gene function is sufficient for cell cycle re-entry. *Nature.* 2003; 424:223–228.

37. Zhang J, Schweers B, Dyer MA. The first knockout mouse model of retinoblastoma. *Cell Cycle.* 2004;3:952–959.

38. Chen D, Livne-bar I, Vanderluit JL, Slack RS, Agochiya M, Bremner R. Cell-specific effects of RB or RB/p107 loss on retinal development implicate an intrinsically death-resistant cell-of-origin in retinoblastoma. *Cancer Cell.* 2004;5:539–551.

39. MacPherson D, Sage J, Kim T, Ho D, McLaughlin ME, Jacks T. Cell type-specific effects of Rb deletion in the murine retina. *Genes Dev.* 2004;18:1681–1694.

40. Windle JJ, Albert DM, O'Brien NM, et al. Retinoblastoma in transgenic mice. *Nature.* 1990;343:665–669.

41. Vogelstein B, Kinzler KW. Cancer genes and the pathways they control. *Nat Med.* 2004;10:789–799.

42. Dyer MA, Bremner R. The search for the retinoblastoma cell of origin. *Nat Rev Cancer.* 2005;5:91–101.

43. Laurie NA, Donovan SL, Shih C-S, et al. Inactivation of the p53 pathway in retinoblastoma. *Nature.* 2006;444:61–66.

44. van der Wal JE, Hermsen MAJA, Gille HJP, et al. Comparative genomic hybridisation divides retinoblastomas into a high and a low level chromosomal instability group. *J Clin Pathol.* 2003;56:26–30.

45. Lillington DM, Kingston JE, Coen PG, et al. Comparative genomic hybridization of 49 primary retinoblastoma tumors identifies chromosomal regions associated with histopathology, progression, and patient outcome. *Genes Chromosomes Cancer.* 2003;36:121–128.

46. Draper GJ, Sanders BM, Brownhill PA, Hawkins MM. Patterns of risk of hereditary retinoblastoma and applications to genetic counselling. *Br J Cancer.* 1992;66:211–219.

47. Sippel KC, Fraioli RE, Smith GD, et al. Frequency of somatic and germ-line mosaicism in retinoblastoma: implications for genetic counseling. *Am J Hum Genet.* 1998;62:610–619.

48. Lohmann DR, Brandt B, Höpping W, Passarge E, Horsthemke B. The spectrum of RB1 germ-line mutations in hereditary retinoblastoma. *Am J Hum Genet.* 1996;58:940–949.

49. Blanquet V, Turleau C, Gross-Morand MS, Sénamaud-Beaufort C, Doz F, Besmond C. Spectrum of germline mutations in the RB1 gene: a study of 232 patients with hereditary and nonhereditary retinoblastoma. *Hum Mol Genet.* 1995;4:383–388.

50. Perentes E, Herbort CP, Rubinstein LJ, et al. Immunohistochemical characterization of human retinoblastomas in situ with multiple markers. *Am J Ophthalmol.* 1987;103:647–658.

51. Sang DN, Albert DM. Retinoblastoma: clinical and histopathologic features. *Hum Pathol.* 1982;13:133–147.

52. Wang MX, Jenkins JJ, Cu-Unjieng AB, Meyer D, Donoso LA. Eye tumors. In: Parham DM, ed. *Pediatric Neoplasia: Morphology and Biology.* Philadelphia: Lippincott-Raven; 1996:405–422.

53. Abramson DH, Frank CM, Susman M, Whalen MP, Dunkel IJ, Boyd NW. Presenting signs of retinoblastoma. *J Pediatr.* 1998;132:505–508.

54. Abramson DH, Du TT, Beaverson KL. (Neonatal) retinoblastoma in the first month of life. *Arch Ophthalmol.* 2002;120:738–742.

55. Zelter M, Damel A, Gonzalez G, Schwartz L. A prospective study on the treatment of retinoblastoma in 72 patients. *Cancer.* 1991;68:1685–1690.

56. Shields CL, Shields JA. Differential diagnosis of retinoblastoma. *Retina.* 1991; 11:232–243.

57. Goddard AG, Kingston JE, Hungerford JL. Delay in diagnosis of retinoblastoma: risk factors and treatment outcome. *Br J Ophthalmol.* 1999;83:1320–1323.

58. Chantada G, Fandiño A, Manzitti J, Urrutia L, Schvartzman E. Late diagnosis of retinoblastoma in a developing country. *Arch Dis Child.* 1999;80:171–174.

59. Erwenne C, Franco E. Age and lateness of referral as determinants of extraocular retinoblastoma. *Ophthalmic Paediatr Genet.* 1989;10:179–184.

60. Leal-Leal C, Rivera-Luna R, Tovar-Guzman V, Hernandez-Giron C, Lazcano-Ponce E. Risk of dying of retinoblastoma in Mexican children. *Med Pediatr Oncol.* 2002;38:211–213.

61. American Academy of Pediatrics, Committee on Practice and Ambulatory Medicine and Section of Ophthalmology. Eye examination in infants, children, and young adults by pediatricians. *Pediatrics.* 2003;111:902–907.

62. American Academy of Pediatrics, Committee on Practice and Ambulatory medicine and Section on Ophthalmology. Use of photoscreening for children's vision screening. *Pediatrics.* 2002;109:524–525.

63. Bunin GR, Emanuel BS, Meadows AT, Buckley JD, Woods WG, Hammond GD. Frequency of 13q abnormalities among 203 patients with retinoblastoma. *J Natl Cancer Inst.* 1989;81:370–374.

64. Baud O, Cormier-Daire V, Lyonnet S, Desjardins L, Turleau C, Doz F. Dysmorphic phenotype and neurological impairment in 22 retinoblastoma patients with constitutional cytogenetic 13q deletion. *Clin Genet.* 1999;55:478–482.

65. Pratt CB, Raimondi SC, Kaste SC, et al. Outcome for patients with constitutional 13q chromosomal abnormalities and retinoblastoma. *Pediatr Hematol Oncol.* 1994;11:541–547.

66. Kaste SC, Pratt CB. Radiographic findings in 13q- syndrome. *Pediatr Radiol.* 1993;23:545–548.

67. Kivelä T. Trilateral retinoblastoma: a meta-analysis of hereditary retinoblastoma associated with primary ectopic intracranial retinoblastoma. *J Clin Oncol.* 1999;17:1829–1837.

68. Amoaku WMK, Willshaw HE, Parkes SE, Shah KJ, Mann JR. Trilateral retinoblastoma: a report of five patients. *Cancer.* 1996;78:858–863.

69. Blach LE, McCormick B, Abramson DH, Ellsworth RM. Trilateral retinoblastoma—incidence and outcome: decade of experience. *Int J Radiat Oncol Biol Phys.* 1994;29:729–733.

70. Marcus DM, Brooks SE, Leff G, et al. Trilateral retinoblastoma: insights into histogenesis and management. *Surv Ophthalmol.* 1998;43:59–70.

71. Holladay DA, Holladay A, Montebello JF, Redmond KP. Clinical presentation, treatment, and outcome of trilateral retinoblastoma. *Cancer.* 1991;67:710–715.

72. Paulino AC. Trilateral retinoblastoma: is the location of the intracranial tumor important? *Cancer.* 1999;86:135–141.

73. Shields CL, Meadows AT, Shields JA, Carvalho C, Smith AF. Chemoreduction for retinoblastoma may prevent intracranial neuroblastic malignancy (trilateral retinoblastoma). *Arch Ophthalmol.* 2001;119:1269–1272.

74. Rodriguez-Galindo C, Wilson MW, Haik BG, et al. Treatment of intraocular retinoblastoma with vincristine and carboplatin. *J Clin Oncol.* 2003;21:2019–2025.

75. Beck-Popovic M, Balmer A, Maeder P, Braganca T, Munier FL. Benign pineal cysts in children with bilateral retinoblastoma: A new varian of trilateral retinoblastoma? *Pediatr Blood Cancer.* 2006;46:755–761.

76. Beets-Tan RG, Hendriks MJ, Ramos LM, Tan KE. Retinoblastoma: CT and MRI. *Neuroradiology.* 1994;36:59–62.

77. Karcioglu ZA, al-Mesfer SA, Abboud E, Jabak MH, Mullaney PB. Workup for metastatic retinoblastoma: a review of 261 patients. *Ophthalmology.* 1997; 104:307–312.

78. Reese AB, Ellsworth RM. The evaluation and current concept of retinoblastoma therapy. *Trans Am Acad Ophthalmol Otolaryngol.* 1963;67:164–172.

79. Shields CL, Mashayekhi A, Demirci H, Meadows AT, Shields JA. Practical approach to management of retinoblastoma. *Arch Ophthalmol.* 2004;122:729–735.

80. Shields CL, Mashayekhi A, Au AK, et al. The international classification of retinoblastoma predicts chemoreduction success. *Ophthalmology.* 2006;113: 2276–2280.

81. Pratt CB, Fontanesi J, Lu X, Parham DM, Elfervig J, Meyer D. Proposal for a new staging scheme for intraocular and extraocular retinoblastoma based on an analysis of 103 globes. *Oncologist.* 1997;2:1–5.

82. Grabowski EF, Abramson DH. Intraocular and extraocular retinoblastoma. *Hematol Oncol Clin North Am.* 1987;1:721–735.

83. Retinoblastoma. In: *AJCC Cancer Staging Manual,* 6th ed. New York: Springer-Verlag; 2002:371–376.

84. Chantada G, Doz F, Antonelli CBG, et al. A proposal for an international retinoblastoma staging system. *Pediatr Blood Cancer.* 2008;50(3):733.

85. Honavar SG, Singh AD, Shields CL, et al. Postenucleation adjuvant therapy in high-risk retinoblastoma. *Arch Ophthalmol.* 2002;120:923–931.

86. Messmer EP, Heinrich T, Höpping W, de Sutter E, Havers W, Sauerwein W. Risk factors for metastases in patients with retinoblastoma. *Ophthalmology.* 1991;98:136–141.

87. Kopelman JE, McLean IW, Rosenberg SH. Multivariate analysis of risk factors for metastsis in retinoblastoma treated by enucleation. *Ophthalmology.* 1987; 94:371–377.

88. Magramm I, Abramson DH, Ellsworth RM. Optic nerve involvement in retinoblastoma. *Ophthalmology* 1989;96:217–222.

89. Shields CL, Shields JA, Baez K, Cater JR, De Potter P. Optic nerve invasion of retinoblastoma: metastatic potential and clinical risk factors. *Cancer.* 1994;73: 692–698.

90. Uusitalo MS, Van Quill KR, Scott IU, Matthay KK, Murray TG, O'Brien JM. Evaluation of chemoprophylaxis in patients with unilateral retinoblastoma with high-risk features on histopathologic examination. *Arch Ophthalmol.* 2001;119:41–48.

91. Khelfaoui F, Validire P, Auperin A, et al. Histopathologic risk factors in retinoblastoma: a retrospective study of 172 patients treated in a single institution. *Cancer.* 1996;77:1206–1213.

92. Rubin CM, Robison LL, Cameron JD, et al. Intraocular retinoblastoma group V: an analysis of prognostic factors. *J Clin Oncol.* 1985;3:680–685.

93. Mustafa MM, Jamshed A, Khafaga Y, et al. Adjuvant chemotherapy with vincristine, doxorubicin, and cyclophosphamide in the treatment of postenucleation high risk retinoblastoma. *J Pediatr Hematol Oncol.* 1999;21:364–369.

94. Chantada G, Fandiño A, Dávila MTG, et al. Results of a prospective study for the treatment of retinoblastoma. *Cancer.* 2004;100:834–842.

95. Wang A-G, Hsu W-M, Hsia W-W, Liu J-H, Yen M-Y. Clinicopathologic factors related to metastasis in retinoblastoma. *J Pediatr Ophthalmol Strabismus.* 2001;38:166–171.

96. Shields CL, Shields JA, Baez KA, Cater J, De Potter PV. Choroidal invasion of retinoblastoma: metastatic potential and clinical risk factors. *Br J Ophthalmol.* 1993;77:544–548.

97. Stannard C, Lipper S, Sealy R, Sevel D. Retinoblastoma: correlation of invasion of the optic nerve and choroid with prognosis and metastases. *Br J Ophthalmol.* 1979;63:560–570.

98. Chong E-M, Coffee RE, Chintagumpala M, Hurwitz RL, Hurwitz MY, Chevez-Barrios P. Extensively necrotic retinoblastoma is associated with high-risk prognostic factors. *Arch Pathol Lab Med.* 2006;130:1669–1672.

99. Shields CL, Shields JA. Recent developments in the management of retinoblastoma. *J Pediatr Ophthalmol Strabismus.* 1999;36:8–18.

100. Shields JA, Shields CL, DePotter P. Enucleation technique for children with retinoblastoma. *J Pediatr Ophthalmol Strabismus.* 1992;29:213–215.

101. Shields JA, Shields CL, DePotter, P. Photocoagulation of retinoblastoma. *Int Ophthalmol Clin.* 1993;33:95–99.

102. Shields JA, Parsons H, Shields CL, Giblin ME. The role of cryotherapy in the management of retinoblastoma. *Am J Ophthalmol.* 1989;106:260–264.

103. Shields CL, Santos MCM, Diniz W, et al. Thermotherapy for retinoblastoma. *Arch Ophthalmol.* 1999;117:885–893.

104. Murphree AL, Villablanca JG, Deegan WF, et al. Chemotherapy plus local treatment in the management of intraocular retinoblastoma. *Arch Ophthalmol.* 1996;114:1348–1356.

105. Lumbroso L, Doz F, Urbieta M, et al. Chemothermotherapy in the management of retinoblastoma. *Ophthalmology.* 2002;109:1130–1136.

106. Wilson TW, Chan HSL, Moselhy GM, Heydt DD, Frey CM, Gallie BL. Penetration of chemotherapy into vitreous is increased by cryotherapy and cyclosporine in rabbits. *Arch Ophthalmol.* 1996;114:1390–1395.

107. Murray TG, Cicciarelli N, O'Brien JM, et al. Subconjunctival carboplatin therapy and cryotherapy in the treatment of transgenic murine retinoblastoma. *Arch Ophthalmol.* 1997;115:1286–1290.

108. Schouten-van Meeteren AYN, Moll AC, Imhof SM, Veerman AJP. Chemotherapy for retinoblastoma: an expanding area of clinical research. *Med Pediatr Oncol.* 2002;38:428–438.

109. Scott IU, Murray TG, Feuer WJ, et al. External beam radiotherapy in retinoblastoma: tumor control and comparison of 2 techniques. *Arch Ophthalmol.* 1999;117:766–770.

110. Hungerford JL, Toma NMG, Plowman PN, Kingston, JE. External beam radiotherapy for retinoblastoma: I. whole eye technique. *Br J Ophthalmol.* 1995;79:109–111

111. Toma NMG, Hungerford JL, Plowman PN, Kingston JE, Doughty D. External beam radiotherapy for retinoblastoma: II. lens sparing technique. *Br J Ophthalmol.* 1995;79:112–117.

112. Merchant TE, Gould CJ, Hilton NE, et al. Ocular preservation after 36 Gy external beam radiation therapy for retinoblastoma. *J Pediatr Hematol Oncol.* 2002;24:246–249.

113. Shields CL, Honavar SG, Meadows AT, et al. Chemoreduction plus focal therapy for retinoblastoma: factors predictive of need for treatment with external beam radiotherapy or enucleation. *Am J Ophthalmol.* 2002;133:657–664.

114. Shields CL, Shields JA, Cater J, et al. Plaque radiotherapy for retinoblastoma: long-term control and treatment complications in 208 tumors. *Ophthalmology.* 2001;108:2116–2121.

115. Schvartzman E, Chantada G, Fandiño A, de Dávila MT, Raslawski E, Manzitti J. Results of a stage-based protocol for the treatment of retinoblastoma. *J Clin Oncol.* 1996;14:1532–1536.

116. Ross G, Lipper EG, Abramson D, Preiser L. The development of young children with retinoblastoma. *Arch Pediatr Adolesc Med.* 2001;155:80–83.

117. Chantada GL, Davila MTG, Fandiño A, et al. Retinoblastoma with low risk for extraocular relapse. *Ophthalmic Genet.* 1999;20:133–140.

118. Eng C, Li FP, Abramson DH, et al. Mortality from second tumors among long-term survivors of retinoblastoma. *J Natl Cancer Inst.* 1993;85:1121–1128.

119. Mohney BG, Robertson DM, Schomberg PJ, Hodge DO. Second nonocular tumors in survivors of heritable retinoblastoma and prior radiation therapy. *Am J Ophthalmol.* 1998;126:269–277.

120. Yue NC, Benson ML. The hourglass deformity as a consequence of orbital irradiation for bilateral retinoblastoma. *Pediatr Radiol.* 1996;26:421–423.

121. Kaste SC, Chen G, Fontanesi J, Crom DB, Pratt CB. Orbital development in long-term survivors of retinoblastoma. *J Clin Oncol.* 1997;15:1183–1189.

122. Abramson DH, Frank CM. Second nonocular tumors in survivors of bilateral retinoblastoma: a possible age effect on radiation-related risk. *Ophthalmology.* 1998;105:573–580.

123. Nenadov Beck M, Balmer A, Dessing C, Pica A, Munier F. First-line chemotherapy with local treatment can prevent external-beam irradiation and enucleation in low-stage intraocular retinoblastoma. *J Clin Oncol.* 2000;18:2881–2887.

124. Kingston JE, Hungerford JL, Madreperla SA, Plowman PN. Results of combined chemotherapy and radiotherapy for advanced intraocular retinoblastoma. *Arch Ophthalmol.* 1996;114:1339–1343.

125. Chantada GL, Fandiño A, Raslawski EC, et al. Experience with chemoreduction and focal therapy for intraocular retinoblastoma in a developing country. *Pediatr Blood Cancer.* 2005;44:455–460.

126. Wilson MW, Haik BG, Liu T, Merchant TE, Rodriguez-Galindo C. Effect on ocular survivalo of adding early intensive focal treatments to a two-drug chemotherapy regimen in patients with retinoblastoma. *Am J Ophthalmol.* 2005;140:397–406.

127. Gallie BL, Budning A, DeBoer G, et al. Chemotherapy with focal therapy can cure intraocular retinoblastoma without radiotherapy. *Arch Ophthalmol.* 1996;114:1321–1328.

128. Chan HSL, Lu Y, Grogan TM, et al. Multidrug resistance protein (MRP) expression in retinoblastoma correlates with the rare failure of chemotherapy despite cyclosporine for reversal of P-glycoprotein. *Cancer Res.* 1997;57:2325–2330.

129. Chan HSL, DeBoer G, Thiessen JJ, et al. Combining cyclosporin with chemotherapy controls intraocular retinoblastoma without requiring radiation. *Clin Cancer Res.* 1996;2:1499–1508.

130. Krishnakumar S, Mallikarjuna K, Desai N, et al. Multidrug resistance proteins: P-glycoprotein and lung resistance protein expression in retinoblastoma. *Br J Ophthalmol.* 2004;88:1521–1526.

131. Levy C, Doz F, Quintana E, et al. Role of chemotherapy alone or in combination with hyperthermia in the primary treatment of intraocular retinoblastoma: preliminary results. *Br J Ophthalmol.* 1998;82:1154–1158.

132. Friedman DL, Himelstein B, Shields CL, et al. Chemoreduction and local ophthalmic therapy for intraocular retinoblastoma. *J Clin Oncol.* 2000;18:12–17.

133. Mendelsohn ME, Abramson DH, Madden T, Tong W, Tran HT, Dunkel IJ. Intraocular concentrations of chemotherapeutic agents after systemic or local administration. *Arch Ophthalmol.* 1998;116:1209–1212.

134. Hayden BH, Murray TG, Scott IU, et al. Subconjunctival carboplatin in retinoblastoma. Impact of tumor burden and dose schedule. *Arch Ophthalmol.* 2000;118:1549–1554.

135. Abramson D, Frank CM, Dunkel IJ. A phase I/II study of subconjunctival carboplatin for intraocular retinoblastoma. *Ophthalmology.* 1999;106:1947–1950.

136. Schmack I, Hubbard B, Kang SJ, Aaberg TM, Grossniklaus HE. Ischemic necrosis and atrophy of the optic nerve after periocular carboplatin injection for intraocular retinoblastoma. *Am J Ophthalmol.* 2006;142:310–315.

137. Gündüz K, Shields CL, Shields JA, et al. The outcome of chemoreduction treatment in patients with Reese-Ellsworth group V retinoblastoma. *Arch Ophthalmol.* 1998;116:1613–1617.

138. Shields CL, Shields JA, Needle M, et al. Combined chemoreduction and adjuvant treatment for intraocular retinoblastoma. *Ophthalmology.* 1997;104:2101–2111.

139. Gombos DS, Kelly A, Coen PG, Kingston JE, Hungerford JL. Retinoblastoma treated with primary chemotherapy alone: the significance of tumor size, location, and age. *Br J Ophthalmol.* 2002;86:80–83.

140. Shields CL, Honavar SG, Shields JA, Demirci H, Meadows AT, Naduvilath TJ. Factors predictive of recurrence of retinal tumors, vitreous seeds, and subretinal seeds following chemoreduction for retinoblastoma. *Arch Ophthalmol.* 2002;120:460–464.

141. Abramson DH, Frank CM, Chantada GL, et al. Intraocular carboplatin concentrations following intravenous administration for human intraocular retinoblastoma. *Ophthalmic Genet.* 1999;20:31–36.

142. Laurie NA, Gray JK, Zhang J, et al. Topotecan combination chemotherapy in two new rodent models of retinoblastoma. *Clin Cancer Res.* 2005;11:7569–7578.

143. Chevez-Barrios P, Chintagumpala M, Mieler W, et al. Response of retinoblastoma with vitreous tumor seeding to adenovirus-mediated delivery of thymidine kinase followed by gancyclovir. *J Clin Oncol.* 2005;23:7927–7935.

144. Vassilev LT, Vu BT, Graves B, et al. In vivo activation of the p53 pathway by small-molecule antagonists of MDM2. *Science.* 2004;303:844–888.

145. Jubran RF, Erdreich-Epstein A, Butturini A, Murphree AL, Villablanca JG. Approaches to treatment for extraocular retinoblastoma: Children's Hospital Los Angeles experience. *J Pediatr Hematol Oncol.* 2004;26:31–34.

146. Kingston JE, Hungerford JL, Plowman PN. Chemotherapy in metastatic retinoblastoma. *Ophthalmic Paediatr Genet.* 1986;8:69–72.

147. Antonelli CBG, Steinhorst F, Ribeiro KCB, et al. Extraocular retinoblastoma: a 13–year experience. *Cancer.* 2003;98:1292–1298.

148. Amozorrutia-Alegria V, Bravo-Ortiz JC, Vazquez-Viveros J, et al. Epidemiological characteristics of retinoblastoma in children attending the Mexican Social Security Institute in Mexico City, 1990–94. *Paediatr Perinat Epidemiol.* 2002;16:370–374.

149. Sahu S, Banavali SD, Pai SK, et al. Retinoblastoma: problems and perspectives from India. *Pediatr Hematol Oncol.* 1998;15:501–508.

150. Menon BS, Reddy SC, Maziah W, Ham A, Rosline H. Extraocular retinoblastoma. *Med Pediatr Oncol.* 2000;35:75–76.

151. Doz F, Khelfaoui F, Mosseri V, et al. The role of chemotherapy in orbital involvement of retinoblastoma. *Cancer.* 1994;74:722–732.

152. Doz F, Neuenschwander S, Plantaz D, et al. Etoposide and carboplatin in extraocular retinoblastoma: a study by the Société Française d'Oncologie Pédiatrique. *J Clin Oncol.* 1995;13:902–909.

153. Kiratli H, Bilgiç S, Özerdem U. Management of massive orbital involvement of intraocular retinoblastoma. *Ophthalmology.* 1998;105:322–326. .

154. Chantada G, Fandiño A, Casak S, Manzitti J, Raslawski E, Schvartzman E. Treatment of overt extraocular retinoblastoma. *Med Pediatr Oncol.* 2003;40: 158–161.

155. Gündüz K, Muftuoglu O, Gunalp I, Unal E, Tacyildiz N. Metastatic retinoblastoma: Clinical features, treatment, and prognosis. *Ophthalmology.* 2006; 113:1558–1566.

156. Namouni F, Doz F, Tanguy ML, et al. High-dose chemotherapy with carboplatin, etoposide and cyclophosphamide followed by a haematopoietic stem cell rescue in patients with high-risk retinoblastoma: a SFOP and SFGM study. *Eur J Cancer.* 1997;33:2368–2375.

157. Pratt CB, Fontanesi J, Chenaille P, et al. Chemotherapy for extraocular retinoblastoma. *Pediatr Hematol Oncol.* 1994;11:301–309.

158. Marsubara H, Makimoto A, Higa T, et al. A multidisciplinary treatment strategy that includes high-dose chemotherapy for metastatic retinoblastoma without CNS involvement. *Bone Marrow Transplantation.* 2005;35:763–766.

159. Chan HS, Canton MD, Gallie BL. Chemosensitivity and multidrug resistance to antineoplastic drugs in retinoblastoma cell lines. *Anticancer Res.* 1989;9: 469–474.

160. Blaney SM, Heideman R, Berg S, et al. Phase I clinical trial of intrathecal topotecan in patients with neoplastic meningitis. *J Clin Oncol.* 2003;21:143–147.

161. Chantada G, Fandino A, Casak S, Mato G, Manzitti J. A phase II study of topotecan in children with retinoblastoma. *Med Pediatr Oncol.* 2001;37:236.

162. Fisher PG, Kadan-Lottick NS, Koroner DN. Intrathecal thiotepa: reapprisal of an established therapy. *J Pediatr Hematol Oncol.* 2002;24:274–278.

163. Dunkel IJ, Aledo A, Kernan NA, et al. Successful treatment of metastatic retinoblastoma. *Cancer.* 2000;89:2117–2121.

164. Gururangan S, McLaughlin C, Quinn J, et al. High-dose chemotherapy with autologous stem-cell rescue in children and adults with newly diagnosed pineoblastomas. *J Clin Oncol.* 2003;21:2187–2191.

165. Dhall G, Grodman H, Ji L, Sands S, Gardner S, Dunkel IJ, McCowage GB, Diez B, Allen JC, Gopalan A, et al. Outcome of children less than three years old at diagnosis with non-metastatic medulloblastoma treated with chemotherapy on the "Head Start" I and II protocols. *Pediatr Blood Cancer.* 2008;50: 1169–1175.

166. Moll AC, Imhof SM, Schouten-van Meeteren AYN, Boers M. Trilateral retinoblastoma: is the location of the intracranial tumor important? [letter to the editor]. *Cancer.* 2000;88:965–966.

167. Singh AD, Shields CL, Shields JA. New insights into trilateral retinoblastoma. *Cancer.* 1999;86:3–5.

168. Kremens B, Wieland R, Reinhard H, et al. High-dose chemotherapy with autologous stem cell rescue in children with retinoblastoma. *Bone Marrow Transplant.* 2003;31:281–284.

169. Rodriguez-Galindo C, Wilson MW, Haik BG, et al. Treatment of metastatic retinoblastoma. *Ophthalmology.* 2003;110:1237–1240.

170. Saarinen UM, Sariola H, Hovi L. Recurrent disseminated retinoblastoma treated with high-dose chemotherapy, total body irradiation, and autologous bone marrow rescue. *Am J Pediatr Hematol Oncol.* 1991;13:315–319.

171. Heideman RL, Cole DE, Balis F, et al. Phase I and pharmacokinetic evaluation of thiotepa in the cerebrospinal fluid and plasma of pediatric patients: evidence for dose-dependent plasma clearance of thiotepa. *Cancer Res.* 1989;49: 736–741.

172. Kleinerman RA, Tucker MA, Tarone RE, et al. Risk of new cancers after radiotherapy in long-term survivors of retinoblastoma: an extended follow-up. *J Clin Oncol.* 2005;23:2272–2279.

173. Wong FL, Boice JD, Abramson DH, et al. Cancer incidence after retinoblastoma: radiation dose and sarcoma risk. *JAMA.* 1997;278:1262–1267.

174. Chauveinc L, Mosseri V, Quintana E, et al. Osteosarcoma following retinoblastoma: age at onset and latency period. *Ophthalmic Genet.* 2001;22:77–88.

175. Kleinerman RA, Tucker MA, Abramson DH, Seddon JM, Tarone RE, Fraumeni JF. Risk of soft tissue sarcomas by individual subtype in survivors of hereditary retinoblastoma. *J Natl Cancer Inst.* 2007;99:24–31.

176. Fletcher O, Easton D, Anderson K, Gilham C, Jay M, Peto J. Lifetime risks of common cancers among retinoblastoma survivors. *J Natl Cancer Inst.* 2004; 96:357–363.

177. Kleinerman RA, Tarone RE, Abramson DH, Seddon JM, Li FP, Tucker MA. Hereditary retinoblastoma and risk of lung cancer. *J Natl Cancer Inst.* 2000; 92:2037–2039.

178. Harbour JW, Lai SL, Whang-Peng J, Gazdar AF, Minna JD, Kaye FJ. Abnormalities in structure and expression of the human retinoblastoma gene in SCLC. *Science.* 1988;241:353–357.

179. Li FP, Abramson DH, Tarone RE, Kleinerman RA, Fraumeni JF Jr, Boice JD. Hereditary retinoblastoma, lipoma, and second primary cancers. *J Natl Cancer Inst.* 1997;89:83–84.

Thyroid Cancer in Childhood

Chintan Parekh and Hollie A. Jackson

Thyroid malignancies are rare in children and include papillary, follicular, and medullary carcinomas. Anaplastic and poorly differentiated carcinomas are almost unheard of in children,[1] and metastatic lesions to the thyroid from breast and colon carcinomas that are seen in adults have not been reported in children. Other rare thyroid neoplasms include teratomas[2] and non-Hodgkin lymphoma.[3] Because most childhood thyroid malignancies are of the papillary type, the discussion in this chapter mainly pertains to papillary carcinomas, but the management recommendations are applicable to most cases of follicular carcinoma as well.

Epidemiology

The incidence of thyroid carcinomas is roughly 4.9 per 10^6 in children. From 2000 to 2004, 2.1% of all thyroid carcinomas were diagnosed in children. These carcinomas constitute the most common carcinoma during childhood.[1] The peak incidence is in the 15- to 19-year-old age group (1.8 per 10^6).[1] The female-to-male ratio is 1.6 in the 5- to 9-year age group, 3.3 in the 10- to 14-year age group, and 5.2 in the 15- to 19-year age group.[4] Ninety percent of the carcinomas are papillary carcinomas or follicular variants of papillary carcinomas.[5] Thyroid carcinomas constitute 7% of all head and neck cancers and 1.4% of all newly diagnosed childhood malignancies.[1]

Etiology

Exposure to head and neck irradiation is associated with an increased risk for the development of thyroid carcinoma. Several studies have shown a high rate of previous irradiation for treatment of benign conditions in children with thyroid cancers.[6] Latent periods to thyroid cancer onset of 8 to 11 years have been reported.[7] Thyroid cancers developing after therapeutic irradiation for children treated for initial cancers at Memorial Sloan-Kettering Cancer Center were reported by Acharya et al to occur at a median latency of 13 years.[8] Thirty-nine percent (of 33 thyroid tumors) in this series were malignant (11 papillary and 2 follicular), all malignant tumors were confined to the neck, and after a median follow-up of 6.5 years, no

patients had developed recurrent or progressive disease. The median dose of irradiation to the thyroid was lower in patients developing malignant thyroid tumors compared with those developing benign lesions (2000 cGy vs 2950 cGy; $p = 0.03$).

An increased incidence of thyroid malignancies was observed in children in Belarus and other areas of the former Soviet Union following the Chernobyl nuclear accident.[9] The age-standardized incidence of thyroid carcinoma in children in Belarus from 1989 to 1997 was 23.6 per million, in contrast to the incidence of 0.5 to 1.2 per million for the rest of Europe during the same time period.[10] A latent period as short as 4 years was noted, and most of the carcinomas were solid variants of the papillary type. The tumors tended to have a high rate of metastasis (this may be due to the relatively young age of the patients), despite which these children had a high survival rate.[11] In comparison with adults, young children are more sensitive to the carcinogenic effect of irradiation, perhaps because of the higher proliferative index of thyroid cells in children.[12]

The increased incidence of thyroid malignancies following the Chernobyl incident has been linked to exposure to large amounts of radioiodine.[11,13] In a retrospective review of 740 cases of pediatric thyroid carcinomas, 681 of which had a history of irradiation exposure from the Chernobyl incident, 94.9% were papillary carcinomas, 4.7% were follicular carcinomas, and 0.4% were medullary carcinomas.[14]

In a retrospective European study, no correlation was found between iodine deficiency and the incidence of childhood thyroid carcinoma.[10]

Pathogenesis

A positive family history is seen in medullary carcinoma[15] and in 3% of papillary carcinomas (chromosome 19p13.2).[16] A high incidence of papillary thyroid carcinomas is seen in familial adenomatosis polyposis coli[17] and Cowden disease.[18] Inherited medullary carcinoma is seen in multiple endocrine neoplasia type 2a and 2b (MEN 2a and 2b) or as part of familial medullary carcinoma.[19] Multiple endocrine neoplasia type 2a and 2b syndromes are caused by germline point mutations in the *RET* (rearranged during transfection) proto-oncogene. The *RET* proto-oncogene located on chromosome 10q11.2 is a tumor-suppressor gene that encodes a transmembrane receptor with a tyrosine kinase domain. Patients with MEN type 2a develop medullary thyroid carcinoma, pheochromocytoma, and parathyroid neoplasms. MEN type 2b is characterized by pheochromocytoma, medullary thyroid carcinoma, and Marfanoid body habitus with mucosal neuromas and ganglioneuromatosis. Patients with MEN 2a develop medullary thyroid carcinoma, pheochromocytoma, and parathyroid neoplasms. Medullary carcinoma in these syndromes develops in childhood, and there is a correlation between the type of *RET* mutation and the age of development of medullary carcinoma.[19]

Rearrangements resulting in juxtaposition of the *RET* kinase and COOH terminus encoding domains to unrelated genes result in dominantly transforming oncogenes called *RET/PTC*. They cause activation of the MAPK (mitogen-activated protein kinase) pathway, and this signaling cascade has been shown to play a role in thyroid cell transformation.[20] These rearrangements are seen in both sporadic and irradiation-induced childhood papillary thyroid carcinoma. Three types—*PTC* 1, *PTC* 2, and *PTC* 3—have been described, of which *PTC* 1 is seen commonly in sporadic cases[21] and *PTC* 3 is most commonly seen in post-Chernobyl irradiation-induced cases with short latency periods.[20] A study undertaken on 33 cases of papillary carcinoma in patients ranging from 6 to 21 years of age showed the presence of *RET/PTC* rearrangements in 45% of the cases. There was no correlation between the type of *RET/PTC* rearrangement and age of presentation, tumor size, focality of tumor, extent of disease at diagnosis, or recurrence rate.[21] In contrast, adult papillary thyroid carcinomas show a high incidence of the *BRAF* (V raf murine sarcoma viral oncogene homolog B1) mutation.[22]

Clinical Features

Childhood thyroid carcinoma is biologically and clinically different from that seen in adults. The most common clinical presentation is a solitary thyroid nodule, which was noted in 73% of cases reported by Harness.[23] Palpable cervical adenopathy was seen in 37% of the cases. Other presenting manifestations such as dysphonia or dysphagia due to local invasion of surrounding structures are rare in children.

Children present with cervical node involvement (60%) [Figure 31-2] and pulmonary metastases (13%)[24] [Figures 31-3 and 31-4] more often than adults.[25] They have more advanced disease and a higher rate of recurrence.[25] The pulmonary metastases are almost always

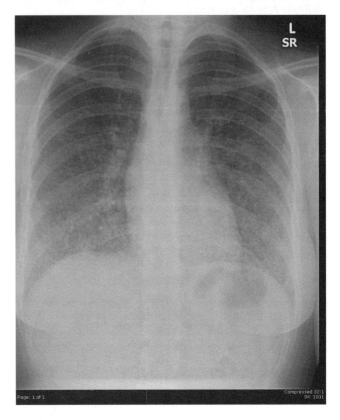

Figure 31-2 Chest X-ray showing military pulmonary metastases in the same patient.

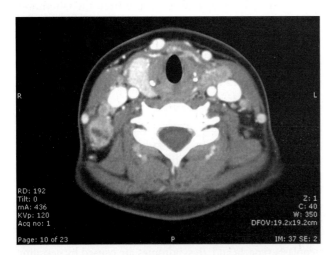

Figure 31-1 CT scan showing cervical lymph node metastases in a 14-year-old girl with papillary thyroid carcinoma.

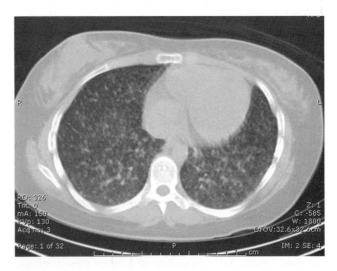

Figure 31-3 Chest CT scan showing military pulmonary metastases in the same patient.

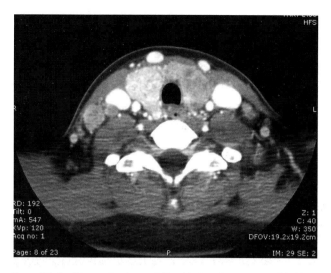

Figure 31-4 CT scan showing multifocal lesions in a 14-year-old girl with papillary thyroid carcinoma.

functional and tend to be miliary.[26] However, children with thyroid carcinoma have an excellent 5-year survival rate of 95%[4] and a 20-year survival rate greater than 90%.[10] These results may be due to differences in tumor biology[27] as well as an enhanced immune response to the tumor in children.[28] Even children with pulmonary metastases have an excellent outcome. Brink et al, in a retrospective review of 14 children with papillary carcinoma with pulmonary metastases, found no deaths during a mean follow-up period of 19.3 years.[29]

Lymph nodes are the most common site of dissemination, followed by the lungs. Bone metastases are rare.[26]

Pathology

Papillary carcinomas consist of a firm, partially encapsulated, or nonencapsulated mass that may show calcifications and cystic changes. Histologically, there is a papillary growth pattern with "ground glass" or "Orphan Annie" nuclei. Peripheral or central sclerosis are typical features. There is intralymphatic invasion resulting in a high incidence of intraglandular multifocal lesions (Figure 31-4) and lymph node metastases. The diffuse sclerosing variant, which causes diffuse replacement of both lobes with hard calcified tumor, tends to affect children and young adults. The tall cell, columnar cell, and solid variants are rare in children. The follicular variant shows a follicular growth pattern, but the nuclear features are those of papillary carcinoma.

Pure follicular cancers with a follicular growth pattern and no nuclear features of papillary carcinomas are rare in children and are usually of the minimally invasive variety with low recurrence and mortality rates.[27]

Staging

The American Joint Committee on Cancer (AJCC) recommends a TNM staging system that includes age (Table 31-1). This system is not useful for children because under 45 years of age, only the presence of distant metastases raises the stage from I to a higher stage. Children have a high recurrence risk. The metastases, age, completeness of resection, extrathyroid invasion, and size staging system may have a higher prognostic value and may be more useful for planning treatment for children, most of whom have stage I AJCC disease.[27]

A younger age at diagnosis has been found to be associated with a higher risk for recurrence in univariate analyses, but not in multivariate analyses that included treatment-related factors. Total thyroidectomy, radioiodine, and thyroid-stimulating hormone (TSH) suppressive therapy have been shown to be predictive of recurrence in some studies but not in others.[26]

Management

The reported occurrence of thyroid nodules in children is 1% to 1.5%.[31] Previous studies reported a higher rate of malignancy (30%-50%) in thyroid nodules in children when compared with adults.[32] However, a recent study showed a 19.9% prevalence of malignancy in thyroid nodules in children.[33] Factors that increase the probability of a thyroid nodule being malignant include young age,[31] past history of irradiation,[34] and possibly autoimmune thyroiditis.[35]

The initial workup of a thyroid nodule generally includes measurement of thyroxine and TSH levels, but these are rarely helpful in differentiating between malignant and benign nodules. Nuclear medicine thyroid scintigraphy is often used in the evaluation of a thyroid nodule. Increased uptake in a nodule almost always indicates that the nodule is benign. Some very rare thyroid carcinomas can demonstrate increased radioisotope uptake on thyroid scintigraphy.[36] There are also rare cases of a benign adenoma or carcinoma that have the ability to trap the radioisotope but do not organify the iodide; this situation results in a discordant nodule that is hot on $^{99m}TcO4$ studies but cold on radioiodine (I^{123}) studies.[37]

Although lack of uptake in a thyroid nodule on scintigraphy may indicate malignancy, the majority of "cold" nodules are benign, with follicular adenomas being the most common cause of a cold nodule (68.9%) in one series.[32] Therefore, other imaging modalities, such as ultrasound, are often used to evaluate a thyroid nodule. The presence of indistinct margins, hypo-echogenicity, predominantly solid composition, vascularity, absence of an echo-lucent halo surrounding the nodule, and calcifications on ultrasound are more suggestive of malignancy.[38] The ultrasound can also help guide the clinician while performing a fine needle aspiration (FNAC). FNAC is recommended for all thyroid nodules.[39] Gharib et al undertook a retrospective study of 47 FNACs in children and found one false negative result and no false positive results.[40] In cases of an inconclusive result, surgical removal should be performed for high-risk patients such as those who are younger than 10 years, have suspicious features on ultrasound, have a past history of irradiation exposure, or have a positive family history. In low-risk adolescent patients, an inconclusive result can be followed with a repeat FNAC.[39]

Table 31-1

TNM AJCC (sixth edition) for differentiated thyroid carcinoma.[30]

Tx	Primary tumor cannot be assessed
T0	No evidence of primary tumor
T1	Tumor size ≤2 cm
T2	Tumor size >2 and ≤4 cm, intrathyroidal
T3	Tumor size >4 cm intrathyroidal or any tumor with minimal extrathyroidal extension (eg, extension to sternothyroid muscle or perithyroid soft tissues)
T4	T4a: any tumor invaded to subcutaneous soft tissues, larynx, trachea, esophagus, or recurrent laryngeal nerve. T4b: any tumor invaded to prevertebral fascia or encasing carotid artery or mediastinal vessels
Nx	Regional lymph nodes cannot be assessed
N0	No regional lymph node metastasis
N1a	Metastasis to level VI (pretracheal, paratracheal, and prelaryngeal/delphian lymph nodes)
N1b	Metastasis to unilateral, bilateral, or contralateral cervical or superior mediastinal lymph nodes
Mx	Distant metastases cannot be assessed
M0	No distant metastasis
M1	Distant metastasis
Stage I	M0 <45 years or T1 only ≥45 years
Stage II	M1 <45 years or T2 only ≥45 years
Stage III	T1-3 N1a M0 or T3 N0 M0 ≥5 years
Stage Iva	T1-3 N1b M0 or T4a N0–1 M0 ≥45 years
Stage IVb	T4b N0-1 M0 ≥45 years
Stage IVc	M1 ≥45 years

When histological evidence of thyroid malignancy is documented, a neck ultrasound or magnetic resonance imaging (MRI) scan should be performed to look for metastatic lymph nodes, and a chest radiograph or computed tomography (CT) scan should be performed to assess for pulmonary metastases. A chest CT scan is more sensitive and can detect micronodular and interstitial patterns of metastases[41] much better than conventional chest radiographs. An MRI may also be helpful to evaluate and delineate the extent of local invasion.

Treatment

Because of the rarity of thyroid malignancies, and the low death rate from thyroid malignancies in children, there are no randomized prospective studies regarding management strategies, and recommendations are based on retrospective multicenter reviews, small cohort studies, and extrapolations from adult studies and guidelines.

Surgery

Surgery is the mainstay of treatment for all stages of thyroid carcinoma. A total or near total thyroidectomy is recommended by most experts in the United States.[5,27] and is believed to decrease the incidence of locoregional recurrence.[42] It also enables the use of thyroglobulin levels and whole-body radioiodine scans for monitoring for disease recurrence and persistence. Massimino et al have suggested removal of the involved thyroid lobe and selective neck node dissection followed by TSH suppressive therapy for papillary carcinoma that is grossly limited to one lobe without radiographic evidence of distant metastases.[43] Children tend to have a higher incidence of multifocal disease and local recurrence, however, making this a less attractive option. Because of the high incidence of lymph node metastases, routine central compartment lymph node dissection is recommended in adults by the American Thyroid Association, but there are no specific recommendations for children. Modified lateral neck dissection is recommended when there is lateral node involvement on clinical examination, preoperative ultrasound, or intraoperative biopsy.[26,34] This dissection reduces the recurrence rate when compared with "berry picking."[44]

Adjuvant Therapy

Radioiodine

Routine postoperative radioiodine ablation is recommended in children. Remnant thyroid tissue (greater than 0.3% uptake on radioiodine scan) is seen in most cases even after total thyroidectomy.[5] The thyroid remnant can interfere with the detection of residual or recurrent disease on whole-body scans or by thyroglobulin measurements. As a result, routine radioablation is performed in most centers. The use of radioiodine ablation has been shown to decrease the incidence of locoregional recurrence in retrospective studies.[45] Prior to radioablation, a diagnostic whole-body scan with I[123] or 0.5 to 2 mci of I[131] is obtained.[46] Images are obtained 24 to 48 hours after administration of the radioisotope. Some experts also recommend a noncontrast spiral chest CT at this point in order to detect interstitial pulmonary metastases.[5] A spiral CT scan, together with the whole-body scan, helps rule out pulmonary metastases. The pre-ablation scan also shows the extent of thyroid remnant as well as disease burden post-thyroidectomy. Because this scan involves significant irradiation exposure, some experts recommend against obtaining a pre-ablation whole-body scan or chest CT scan and relying on a post-ablation scan instead.[47] Neither approach has been shown to have superiority over the other. One of the concerns about I[131] diagnostic scans is that they might cause sublethal damage to the thyroid cells and carcinoma cells, causing a decrease in radioiodine uptake at the time of ablation. This phenomenon is called "stunning."[48] Whether stunning actually occurs is controversial.[49] There is no unequivocal evidence showing that there is significant stunning when a low dose (less than 2 mci) of radioiodine is used. An I[123] scan can be obtained to avoid stunning.[50] However, I[123] is more expensive and less easily available than I[131]. Dosimetry calculations cannot be deduced from I,[123] because it is a different isotope from I[131].

The uptake of radioiodine is dependent on TSH stimulation of thyroid tissue as well as carcinoma tissue. The TSH level should be greater than 30 µU/ml for optimum uptake. The diagnostic scan followed by ablation is performed 6 weeks after thyroidectomy. Thyroid hormone medications must be withheld for a sufficient time to permit an adequate rise in the TSH level needed for optimum uptake. Additionally, the patient is administered a low iodine diet for 2 weeks prior to the scan to increase the avidity of the thyroid remnant for iodine.[26] Triiodothyronine (T3) can be given until 2 weeks before the scan,[5] because T3 has a short half-life and thus needs less time for reversal of effect.

The normal thyroid remnant tissue is more efficient than the carcinoma tissue at concentrating radioiodine. As a result, the first diagnostic whole-body scan done after thyroidectomy might not detect residual tumor or metastases. These may show up on the scan obtained following radioablation, because much higher doses of radioiodine are used for ablation.

In children, the maximally safe radioiodine dose can be calculated based on quantitative blood and whole-body dosimetry, and the minimally effective dose can be calculated based on lesional dosimetry.[51] Because this calculation is complicated, most centers use a fixed dose of 30 mci.[52] Rarely, a second treatment may be needed to completely ablate the remnant. A much higher dose of up to 175 to 200 mci is required to ablate pulmonary metastases.[53] It is customary to obtain a scan 5 to 7 days after radioablation, which will demonstrate avid uptake in the thyroid remnant and may show metastases not apparent on the previous diagnostic scan.[5]

Thyroid-Stimulating Hormone Suppressive Treatment

Based on the belief that thyroid carcinoma cells are dependent on TSH stimulation for growth, TSH suppressive therapy with thyroxine is used to suppress tumor growth. Adult studies suggest the value of thyroid hormone suppression.[54] Most pulmonary metastases are sensitive to TSH suppression.[26] The optimum TSH level that needs to be maintained is not known. Initially, TSH levels of less than 0.1 µU/ml are recommended, but once remission has been achieved levels of less than 0.5 µU/ml may be acceptable.[27]

Treatment of Metastases

Radioiodine is the treatment of choice for metastases once adequate thyroid ablation has been achieved. Papillary carcinoma cells in children show more sodium iodide symporters (transport proteins that simultaneously move two substances across the membrane in the same direction) than adult papillary carcinoma cells[26] and are hence more sensitive to radioiodine. Treatment is given every 6 months until negative whole-body scans are achieved. This may take several treatments. Doses of 175 to 200 mci for pulmonary metastases and 200 mci for bone metastases are recommended.[53] These doses may be reduced based on body weight and surface area.[28]

Follow-Up

Because the recurrence rate in children with thyroid carcinoma is high, periodic follow-up is recommended. Follow-up should initially be every 6 months, and the interval between follow-ups can be increased once remission has been achieved. The first whole-body scan is obtained 6 months after radioablation, and successful ablation is defined as less than 0.1% uptake in the thyroid bed. Thyroxine, TSH and thyroglobulin levels, neck ultrasound (the most sensitive method to detect recurrence), and whole-body diagnostic radioiodine scans are obtained during follow-up.[5] A detectable thyroglobulin level in the presence of TSH suppression is suggestive of recurrent or residual disease. Since tumor cells may not secrete thyroglobulin in the presence of TSH suppression, an undetectable level in the presence of TSH suppression should prompt one to obtain a level of thyroxine for 6 weeks. Because thyroid deprivation needs to be carried out for the whole-body scan, a thyroglobulin level can be obtained at the same time. Another approach to obtaining a scan in a non-thyroid-suppressed state is to give thyroxine replacement and give recombinant TSH (rTSH) just prior to the scan. This approach has been validated with studies showing equivalent disease detection rates when rTSH-stimulated whole-body scans are used in combination with rTSH-stimulated thyroglobulin levels (compared with thyroid deprivation scans) in adults.[55] The accuracy of rTSH-stimulated scans was studied in 8 children.[56] The images are obtained earlier (6-24 hours) when rTSH is used, because radioiodine is cleared faster in the euthyroid state.

Antithyroglobulin autoantibodies that interfere with thyroglobulin assays have been detected in 20% of cases of thyroid cancer.[57] Therefore, these antibodies should be assayed, and if they are detected, determination of thyroglobulin levels is of no value. Also, thyroglobulin assays vary from one laboratory to another in terms of sensitivity; therefore, all measurements should be obtained in the same laboratory. A trend in values is more important than a single value.

Sometimes an elevated thyroglobulin level can be seen in the absence of any uptake on a whole-body scan. Since children in remission on the basis of negative scans with unknown thyroglobulin levels have done well,[39] some authors recommend observation in such cases. Also, in many of these instances, the persistent disease turns out to be locoregional foci that need surgery rather than radioiodine.[26] Other researchers recommend empiric treatment with radioiodine ablation, because some of these cases show uptake on the post-treatment scan.[5] Adult studies suggest that fluorodeoxyglucose positron emission tomography (PET) scans may be useful in detecting and localizing disease in such patients.[58]

The goal of treatment is to achieve a negative whole-body scan, a negative neck ultrasound, and a thyroid hormone withdrawal thyroglobulin level of less than 8 ng/ml.[5,59]

Treatment of Recurrence

The majority of recurrences are cervical lymph node recurrences. Macroscopic recurrence, including excisable pulmonary and bone metastases, is treated surgically. If surgery is not possible, radioiodine is the treatment of choice.[27] A dose of 175 to 200 mci for pulmonary metastases and 200 mci for bone metastases is used.

Side Effects of Treatment

The major side effects of surgery are permanent hypoparathyroidism and permanent recurrent laryngeal nerve palsy. In a retrospective review of 744 cases of surgery for thyroid carcinoma by Demdichik, 12.9% developed permanent hypoparathyroidism, and 6.2% developed permanent recurrent laryngeal injury. Other complications reported in this review included transient recurrent laryngeal nerve injury, transient hypoparathyroidism, wound bleeding, lymph leakage, Horner syndrome, glossopharyngeal nerve injury, and wound infection.[14]

Radioiodine can cause painful swelling of remnant tissue or metastases, nausea, vomiting, transient anosmia or aguesia, and sialadenitis.[52] If the sialadenitis is permanent, it may result in dental problems. Transient bone marrow suppression with a nadir in platelet and white blood cell counts at 6 to 8 weeks can be seen. Pulmonary fibrosis may be seen when treating extensive pulmonary metastases. A retained dose of greater than 80 mci in the lungs increases the risk of pulmonary fibrosis.[5] A European study found an increased risk of leukemias and solid tumors with increasing cumulative doses of administered I[131].[60] Total cumulative doses of I[131] should be kept below

500 mci in children and 800 mci in adolescents. The rate of miscarriages is increased during the first year after treatment, but subsequent pregnancies are not affected. Cumulative doses of greater than 300 mci have been reported to cause azoospermia in adults.[5]

Concerns with thyroid-suppressive therapy include the possibilities of osteoporosis and ventricular hypertrophy[26] as well as unmasking of attention deficit disorders.

Other Treatment Modalities

External radiotherapy has been used in cases of locally invasive disease that could not be completely resected, in cases of metastases refractory to radioiodine and metastases that do not concentrate radioiodine. In adults with locally invasive nonresectable disease, radiotherapy has been shown to decrease recurrence rates.[61] It can be used to palliate painful oligo-osseous metastases.

Chemotherapy is ineffective. A doxorubicin- and cisplatin-based regimen may have partial or temporary efficacy in rapidly growing refractory metastatic disease, but the experience in children is limited and this approach is more relevant in adult cases of aggressive disease. In adults efficacy is short lived and partial.[62]

Newer Therapeutic Agents

Newer therapeutic agents include molecularly targeted treatments, which are being tested in adult patients with thyroid carcinomas that are refractory to conventional therapies. A potential target is the MAPK pathway. An abnormality in one of the encoding genes is seen in 80% of papillary carcinomas. Another strategy is to increase the expression of sodium iodide symporters in radioiodine-refractory dedifferentiated cells and then using radioiodine. BAY 43-9006 is a compound in Phase II trials that is antiangiogenic and also inhibits *BRAF* kinase (*BRAF* mutations activate the MAPK pathway). *BRAF* kinase inhibitors block the growth of thyroid cancer cells that have the *PET/RET* rearrangement or the *BRAF* mutation.[63]

Medullary Thyroid Carcinoma

Medullary thyroid carcinomas (MTCs) account for 5% of childhood thyroid carcinomas. They arise from the neuroendocrine parafollicular C cells. The development of MTC is preceded by multifocal C cell hyperplasia. These carcinomas may be sporadic, but in children they are generally inherited (see pathogenesis section). Medullary thyroid carcinoma is the first endocrine malignancy to develop in most patients with MEN 2 and shows almost complete penetrance. Multiple endocrine neoplasia type 2b is less common than MEN 2a; however, in MEN 2b, MTC develops at an earlier age, is more aggressive, and may present with metastatic disease in patients as young as one year of age. Prophylactic thyroidectomy before the onset of MTC is recommended in individuals that carry the *RET* mutation. There is a genotype/phenotype correlation, and the age at which thyroidectomy is recommended depends on the type of *RET* mutation. Children with MEN should be screened for other endocrine complications.

Medullary thyroid carcinoma tends to metastasize to the cervical and mediastinal lymph nodes, liver, lungs, and bones. Serum calcitonin levels and imaging of the neck, chest, and abdomen should be undertaken. Nuclear medicine scans with octeotride, dimercaptosuccinate or technetium 99m, and FDG PET scans are useful imaging modalities. The treatment for medullary carcinoma is total thyroidectomy with at least bilateral dissection of the central compartment lymph nodes. There is no role for radioiodine. Thyroid hormone replacement but not suppression is needed because C cells are TSH nonresponsive. The survival rate for patients with lymph node metastases is poor. Serum calcitonin levels are followed postoperatively to identify persistent or recurrent disease.[19,39]

Conclusion

Thyroid malignancies are rare in children and represent a disease that is biologically and clinically distinct from that in adults. Children with papillary thyroid carcinoma, including those who have metastases at presentation, have an excellent overall survival of greater than 90% at 20 years. The standard treatment includes total thyroidectomy, radioiodine ablation, and TSH suppression, along with periodic follow-up.

References

1. Bernstein L, Gurney JC. Carcinomas and other malignant epithelial neoplasms ICCCC xi. Cancer Incidence and Survival Among Children and Adolescents: United States SEER Program, 1975–1995. Bethesda, MD: National Cancer Institute; 1999.
2. Thompson LD, Rosai J, Heffess CS. Primary thyroid teratomas: a clinicopathologic study of 30 cases. *Cancer.* 2000;88(5):1149–1158.
3. Hart S, Horsman JM, Radstone CR, et al. Localised extranodal lymphoma of the head and neck: the Sheffield Lymphoma Group experience (1971–2000). *Clin Oncol (R Coll Radiol).* 2004;16(3):186–192.
4. SEER Cancer Statistics Review, 1975–2004. Bethesda, MD: National Cancer Institute; 2007.
5. Hung W, Sarlis NJ. Current controversies in the management of pediatric patients with well-differentiated non-medullary thyroid cancer: a review. *Thyroid.* 2002;12(8):683–702.
6. Winship T, Rosvoll R. Thyroid carcinoma in children: final report of a 20-year study. *Clin Proc Child Hosp DC.* 1970;26:11.
7. Viswanathan K, Gierlowski TC, Schneider AB. Childhood thyroid cancer: characteristics and long-term outcome in children irradiated for benign conditions of the head and neck. *Arch Pediatr Adolesc Med.* 1994;148(3):260–265.
8. Acharya S, Sarafoglou K, LaQuaglia M, et al. Thyroid neoplasms after therapeutic radiation for malignancies during childhood or adolescence. *Cancer.* 2003;97(10):2397–2403.
9. Bennett B, Repacholi M, Carr Z. Health effects of the Chernobyl accident and special health care programmes: report of the UN Chernobyl Forum Expert Group "Health." Geneva: World Health Organization; 2006.
10. Steliarova-Foucher E, Stiller CA, Pukkala E, et al. Thyroid cancer incidence and survival among European children and adolescents (1978–1997): report from the Automated Childhood Cancer Information System project. *Eur J Cancer.* 2006;42(13):2150–2169.
11. Ron E. Thyroid cancer incidence among people living in areas contaminated by radiation from the Chernobyl accident. *Health Phys.* 2007;93(5):502–511.
12. Williams ED. Biological mechanisms underlying radiation induction of thyroid carcinoma. In: Thomas G, Karaoglou A, Williams ED, eds. *Radiation and Thyroid Cancer.* Singapore: World Scientific; 1999:177–188.
13. Cardis E, Kesminiene A, Ivanov V, et al. Risk of thyroid cancer after exposure to 131-I in childhood. *J Natl Cancer Inst.* 2005;97(10):724–732.
14. Demidchik YE, Demidchik EP, Reiners C, et al. Comprehensive clinical assessment of 740 cases of surgically treated thyroid cancer in children of Belarus. *Ann Surg.* 2006;243(4):525–532.
15. Chi DD, Moley JF. Medullary thyroid carcinoma: genetic advances, treatment recommendations, and the approach to the patient with persistent hypercalcitoninemia. *Surg Oncol Clin N Am.* 1998;7(4):681–706.
16. Canzian F, Amati P, Harach HR, et al. A gene predisposing to familial thyroid tumors with cell oxyphilia maps to chromosome 19p13.2. *Am J Hum Genet.* 1998;63(6):1743–1748.
17. Herraiz M, Barbesino G, Faquin W, et al. Prevalence of thyroid cancer in familial adenomatous polyposis syndrome and the role of screening ultrasound examinations. *Clin Gastroenterol Hepatol.* 2007;5(3):367–373.
18. Haggitt RC, Reid BJ. Hereditary gastrointestinal polyposis syndromes. *Am J Surg Pathol.* 1986;10(12):871–887.
19. Marini F, Falchetti A, Del Monte F, et al. Multiple endocrine neoplasia type 2. *Orphanet J Rare Dis.* 2006;1:45.
20. Santoro M, Melillo RM, Fusco A. RET/PTC activation in papillary thyroid carcinoma: European Journal of Endocrinology Prize Lecture. *Eur J Endocrinol.* 2006;155(5):645–653.
21. Fenton CL, Lukes Y, Nicholson D, et al. The RET/PTC mutations are common in sporadic papillary thyroid carcinoma of children and young adults. *J Clin Endocrinol Metab.* 2000;85(3):1170–1175.
22. Penko K, Livezey J, Fenton C, et al. BRAF mutations are uncommon in papillary thyroid cancer of young patients. *Thyroid.* 2005;15(4):320–325.
23. Harness JK. Childhood thyroid carcinoma. In: Clark OH, Duh Q-Y, eds. *Textbook of Endocrine Surgery.* Philadelphia: Saunders; 1997:75–81.
24. Grigsby PW, Gal-or A, Michalski JM, Doherty GM. Childhood and adolescent thyroid carcinoma. *Cancer.* 2002;95(4):724–729.
25. Zimmerman D, Hay ID, Gough IR, et al. Papillary thyroid carcinoma in children and adults: long-term follow-up of 1039 patients conservatively treated at one institution during three decades. *Surgery.* 1988;104(6):1157–1166.
26. Jarzab B, Handkiewicz-Junak D, Wloch J. Juvenile differentiated thyroid carcinoma and the role of radioiodine in its treatment: a qualitative review. *Endocr Relat Cancer.* 2005;12(4):773–803.
27. Thompson GB, Hay ID. Current strategies for surgical management and adjuvant treatment of childhood papillary thyroid carcinoma. *World J Surg.* 2004; 28(12):1187–1198.
28. Gupta S, Patel A, Folstad A, et al. Infiltration of differentiated thyroid carcinoma by proliferating lymphocytes is associated with improved disease-free survival for children and young adults. *J Clin Endocrinol Metab.* 2001;86(3): 1346–1354.
29. Brink JS, van Heerden JA, McIver B, et al. Papillary thyroid cancer with pulmonary metastases in children: long-term prognosis. *Surgery.* 2000;128(6): 881–6; discussion 886–887.
30. Patel SG, Shah JP. TNM staging of cancers of the head and neck: striving for uniformity among diversity. *CA Cancer J Clin.* 2005;55(4):242–258; quiz 261–262, 264.
31. Wartofsky L. The thyroid nodule. In: Wartofsky L, ed. *Thyroid Cancer: A Comprehensive Guide to Clinical Management.* Totowa, NJ: Humana Press; 2000:3–7.
32. Hung W. Nodular thyroid disease and thyroid carcinoma. *Pediatr Ann.* 1992; 21(1):50–57.
33. Hung W. Solitary thyroid nodules in 93 children and adolescents: a 35-year experience. *Horm Res.* 1999;52(1):15–18.
34. La Quaglia MP, Black T, Holcomb GW 3rd, et al. Differentiated thyroid cancer: clinical characteristics, treatment, and outcome in patients under 21 years of age who present with distant metastases: a report from the Surgical Discipline Committee of the Children's Cancer Group. *J Pediatr Surg.* 2000; 35(6):955–959.
35. Tamimi DM. The association between chronic lymphocytic thyroiditis and thyroid tumors. *Int J Surg Pathol.* 2002;10(2):141–146.
36. Nagai GR, Pitts WC, Basso L, et al. Scintigraphic hot nodules and thyroid carcinoma. *Clin Nucl Med.* 1987;12:123–127.
37. Dekeyser LFM, Van Herle A. Differentiated thyroid cancer in children. *Head Neck Surg.* 1985;8:100–114.
38. Frates MC, Benson CB, Charboneau JW, et al. Management of thyroid nodules detected at US: Society of Radiologists in Ultrasound consensus conference statement. *Ultrasound Q.* 2006;22(4):231–238; discussion 239–240.
39. Dinauer C, Francis GL. Thyroid cancer in children. *Endocrinol Metab Clin North Am.* 2007;36(3):779–806, vii.
40. Gharib H, Zimmerman D, Goellner JR, Bridley SM, Le Blanc SM. Fine-needle aspiration biopsy: use in diagnosis and management of pediatric thyroid diseases. *Endocr Pract.* 1995;1(1):9–13.
41. Piekarski JD, Schlumberger M, Leclere J, et al. Chest computed tomography (CT) in patients with micronodular lung metastases of differentiated thyroid carcinoma. *Int J Radiat Oncol Biol Phys.* 1985;11(5):1023–1027.
42. Harness JK, Thompson NW, McLeod MK, Pasieka JL, Fukuuchi A. Differentiated thyroid carcinoma in children and adolescents. *World J Surg.* 1992;16(4): 547–553; discussion 553–554.
43. Massimino M, Collini P, Leite SF, et al. Conservative surgical approach for thyroid and lymph-node involvement in papillary thyroid carcinoma of childhood and adolescence. *Pediatr Blood Cancer.* 2006;46(3):307–313.
44. Musacchio MJ, Kim AW, Vijungco JD, et al. Greater local recurrence occurs with "berry picking" than neck dissection in thyroid cancer. *Am Surg.* 2003; 69(3):191–196; discussion 196–197.
45. Handkiewicz-Junak D, Wloch J, Roskosz J, et al. Total thyroidectomy and adjuvant radioiodine treatment independently decrease locoregional recurrence risk in childhood and adolescent differentiated thyroid cancer. *J Nucl Med.* 2007;48(6):879–888.
46. Sisson JC. Selection of the optimal scanning agent for thyroid cancer. *Thyroid.* 1997;7(2):295–302.
47. Reynolds JC. Percent 131-I uptake and post-therapy 131-I scans: their role in the management of thyroid cancer. *Thyroid.* 1997;7(2):281–284.

48. Muratet JP, Daver A, Minier J-F, Larra F. Influence of scanning doses of iodine-131 on subsequent first ablative treatment outcome in patients operated on for differentiated thyroid carcinoma. *J Nucl Med.* 1998;39(9):1546–1550.

49. Silberstein EB. Comparison of outcomes after (123) I *versus* (131) I pre-ablation imaging before radioiodine ablation in differentiated thyroid carcinoma. *J Nucl Med.* 2007;48(7):1043–1046.

50. Yaakob W, Gordon L, Spicer KM, Nitke SJ. The usefulness of iodine-123 whole-body scans in evaluating thyroid carcinoma and metastases. *J Nucl Med Technol.* 1999;27(4):279–281.

51. Maxon HR. Quantitative radioiodine therapy in the treatment of differentiated thyroid cancer. *Q J Nucl Med.* 1999;43(4):313–323.

52. Yeh SD, La Quaglia MP. 131-I therapy for pediatric thyroid cancer. *Semin Pediatr Surg.* 1997;6(3):128–133.

53. Beierwaltes WH, Nishiyama RH, Thompson NW, Copp JE, Kubo A. Survival time and "cure" in papillary and follicular thyroid carcinoma with distant metastases: statistics following University of Michigan therapy. *J Nucl Med.* 1982;23(7):561–568.

54. Wang PW, Wang ST, Liu R-T, et al. Levothyroxine suppression of thyroglobulin in patients with differentiated thyroid carcinoma. *J Clin Endocrinol Metab.* 1999;84(12):4549–4553.

55. Haugen BR, Pacini F, Reiners C, et al. A comparison of recombinant human thyrotropin and thyroid hormone withdrawal for the detection of thyroid remnant or cancer. *J Clin Endocrinol Metab.* 1999;84(11):3877–3885.

56. Lau WF, Zacharin MR, Waters K, et al. Management of paediatric thyroid carcinoma: recent experience with recombinant human thyroid stimulating hormone in preparation for radioiodine therapy. *Intern Med J.* 2006;36(9):564–570.

57. Spencer CA, Takeuchi M, Kazarosyan M, et al. Serum thyroglobulin autoantibodies: prevalence, influence on serum thyroglobulin measurement, and prognostic significance in patients with differentiated thyroid carcinoma. *J Clin Endocrinol Metab.* 1998;83(4):1121–1127.

58. Roberts M, Maghami E, Kandeel F, et al. The role of positron emission tomography scanning in patients with radioactive iodine scan-negative, recurrent differentiated thyroid cancer. *Am Surg.* 2007;73(10):1052–1056.

59. Pineda JD, Lee T, Ain K, Reynolds JC, Robbins J, et al. Iodine-131 therapy for thyroid cancer patients with elevated thyroglobulin and negative diagnostic scan. *J Clin Endocrinol Metab.* 1995;80(5):1488–1492.

60. Roldan Schilling V, Fernandez Abellan P, Dominguez E, et al. Acute leukemias after treatment with radioiodine for thyroid cancer. *Haematologica.* 1998;83(8):767–768.

61. Mazzarotto R, Cesaro MG, Lora O, et al (2000). The role of external beam radiotherapy in the management of differentiated thyroid cancer. *Biomed Pharmacother.* 2000;54(6):345–349.

62. Williams SD, Birch R, Einhorn LH. Phase II evaluation of doxorubicin plus cisplatin in advanced thyroid cancer: a Southeastern Cancer Study Group Trial. *Cancer Treat Rep.* 1986;70(3):405–407.

63. Baudin E, Schlumberger M. New therapeutic approaches for metastatic thyroid carcinoma. *Lancet Oncol.* 2007;8(2):148–156.

Rare Cancers of Childhood and Adolescence

Geoffrey B. McCowage and Leo Mascarenhas

Introduction

This chapter deals with some of the cancers that are rare in childhood and adolescence. Some of these cancers arise predominantly in adults while others are unique to children. For those tumors that are more common in adults, we must rely on the experience of our colleagues who treat adults but apply the information judiciously in the management of children while continuing to report on our experiences. Special tumor registries that can compile useful information for the management of these rare conditions best serve unique pediatric cancers. This chapter is meant not to be an exhaustive resource but rather to provide a framework to approach and manage these cancers. The cancers are discussed below in alphabetical order.

Adrenocortical Carcinoma

Adrenocortical carcinoma (ACC) is a rare malignancy in children and adolescents; about 14 cases per year in individuals younger than 20 years have been reported by the Surveillance, Epidemiology, and End Results (SEER) registry in the United States.[1] Adrenocortical carcinoma occurs mainly in adults and is characterized by a poor prognosis, with fewer than 38% of patients surviving for 5 years following diagnosis.[2,3] The incidence of ACC peaks in both the first and fourth decades of life, with a frequency of 0.4 per 10^6 during the first 4 years of life.[4,5] The incidence of ACC varies worldwide and is particularly high in the south of Brazil.[6–8] Patients with Beckwith-Weidemann syndrome and hemihypertrophy have an increased incidence of ACC.[9,10] Adrenocortical carcinoma has also been reported in association with congenital adrenal hyperplasia and multiple endocrine neoplasia I syndrome.[11,12] The incidence of ACC in Li-Fraumeni syndrome is well described, and germline mutations in the p53 tumor suppressor gene may contribute to the etiology of the majority of pediatric cases in the United States and Brazil.[13–15] In the United States, germline mutations frequently occur in the DNA-binding domains of the p53 gene, while in Brazilian patients a single mutation in exon 10 is consistently observed with low penetrance.[13,16,17] The molecular mechanisms contributing to the development of ACC remain unclear at this time. One recent review

describes the signaling pathways that have been postulated in the development of ACC.[18] Alterations that have frequently been observed in ACC include upregulation of the IGF-II system, as well as mutations in p53 and RAS.

The International Pediatric Adrenocortical Tumor Registry (IPACTR) recently reported on 255 patients younger than 20 years, providing some valuable insight on this rare neoplasm.[19] It occurs more frequently in females. Adrenocortical carcinoma may be functionally inactive or active, secreting hormones that include cortisol, androgens, estrogens, aldosterone, and other intermediates encountered in steroid synthesis.[4,19–22] Functional tumors are more common in children and are discovered usually on investigation for clinical symptoms of steroid hormone production.[4,19,21–24] Patients usually have signs and symptoms of hypercortisolism (Cushing syndrome) and/or hyperandrogenism (virilization) (Figure 32-1). Sometimes, patients present with clinical features of hyperaldosteronism or hyperestrogenism. Other presenting features include abdominal pain and rarely weight loss.

The diagnosis of ACC is usually made based on an endocrine syndrome and the presence of a suprarenal

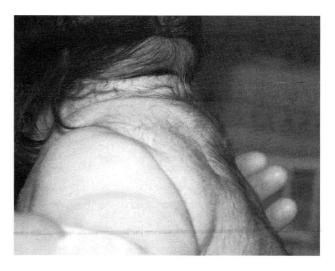

Figure 32-1 Photograph of an infant with adrenocortical carcinoma depicting the "buffalo hump" associated with hypercortisolism and hirsutism associated with hyperandrogenism.

tumor with elevated concentrations of adrenocortical hormones and their bio-intermediates in the serum or urine. Primary tumors are frequently large, and patients present with advanced regional or metastatic disease.[25] Visceral metastases usually involve the liver, lungs, kidneys, and bones. Radiographic studies are necessary for both staging and planning surgical resection. Computed tomography (CT) scan or magnetic resonance imaging (MRI) of the abdomen in addition to CT scan of the chest and bone scan is recommended at the time of diagnosis. The disease staging system used by the IPACTR is depicted in Table 32-1.[19] This staging system is highly predictive of outcome: more than 90% of patients with stage I disease survive long term, while only 10% of those with stage IV disease survive overall.

Adrenocortical carcinoma is locally aggressive and has a thin pseudo-capsule. Numerous mitoses are noted in pleomorphic cells with scant cytoplasm. Hemorrhage and necrosis are usually notable features within these tumors.[26,27] Tumor size (greater than 200 gm) and high mitotic activity correlate with aggressive behavior in these tumors and help distinguish ACC from the more favorable adrenocortical adenoma.[28]

Surgery is the only proven effective therapy for ACC, and curative surgical excision should be considered in every child.[21,22,29,30] Surgery is usually performed transabdominally. Adrenocortical carcinoma is a very friable tumor because of the thin pseudo-capsule, extensive hemorrhage, and necrosis. Spontaneous rupture has been observed after needle biopsy.[31,32] Even though laparoscopic excisions have been performed successfully, laparoscopy is not recommended as the procedure of choice for the primary resection of ACC because it is associated with a high incidence of peritoneal carcinomatosis.[33] Surgery is also indicated in the management of metastatic and recurrent disease, because it can prolong survival. Mitotane, a synthetic derivative of the insecticide dichlorodiphenyltrichloroethane, is an adrenocorticolytic agent and has been used to treat ACC in both adults and children.[22,34,35] It has been studied more extensively in adults and has not been evaluated systematically in children.[4,19,21,23,29] At lower doses, mitotane decreases clinical symptomatology by suppressing adrenal steroids. However, higher doses are necessary to have an adrenolytic effect. A third of adults with advanced-stage disease have objective responses to mitotane alone, with complete responses possible.[20,21,36,37] Mitotane is therefore indicated in those patients with advanced-stage disease and those who have a high risk of recurrence. Adjuvant mitotane has also recently been shown to benefit patients who have undergone complete surgical excision of ACC, though these results need to be validated.[29] The side effects of mitotane are significant and include gastrointestinal and neurologic toxicity. Patients can experience severe nausea, vomiting, diarrhea, and abdominal pain, as well as lethargy, somnolence, ataxia, vertigo, and depression. Mitotane can also cause hypothyroidism. Close monitoring is therefore necessary, and dose adjustment is indicated to decrease toxicity. Since mitotane is adrenolytic, patients who receive this drug should be considered to be adrenal insufficient. Therefore they should be supplemented with hydrocortisone and fludrocortisone to prevent glucocorticoid and mineralocorticoid deficiencies. Other chemotherapeutic agents including cisplatin, etoposide, 5-fluorouracil (5-FU), doxorubicin, and cyclophosphamide have been used as single agents or in combination, with or without mitotane.[38-44] Adrenocortical carcinoma is generally considered to be a radioresistant tumor.[20] Because many children with ACC also carry the *p53* gene mutation, radiation therapy may increase the incidence of second tumors in these patients.[45]

The Children's Oncology Group (COG) is conducting a study in children with ACC. COG ARAR0332 will evaluate the role of surgery, retroperitoneal lymph node (RPLN) dissection, and chemotherapy with mitotane in combination with cisplatin, etoposide, and doxorubicin. Patients with stage I or II disease are treated with radical surgery with or without RPLN dissection, respectively, while patients with stage III or IV undergo surgery, RPLN dissection, and chemotherapy. This study will also evaluate the incidence of germline *p53* mutations and characterize cooperating molecular alterations and the presence of embryonal markers associated with ACC in children.

Chordoma

Chordomas are epithelial tumors that arise from notochordal rests along the spinal axis. The most common sites are the skull base, particularly the clivus, and the sacrococcygeal region, though tumors may occur anywhere along the spinal column.[46-49] Skull-base tumors predominate in children, whereas sacrococcygeal tumors predominate in adults. Classic cases in adults exhibit benign or locally invasive behavior; pediatric cases appear to have a higher incidence of more aggressive tumor behavior and metastasis.[46,48-51]

Classic chordoma comprises large epithelioid cells with vacuolated cytoplasm, described as phyliferous, in a background of myxoid cytoplasm. Atypical variant forms are described, with varying levels of malignancy. Immunohistochemical stains may be required to distinguish chordoma

Table 32-1	
International Pediatric Adrenocortical Tumor Registry (IPACTR) staging system.	
Stage	**Description**
I	Tumor completely excised with negative margins, tumor weight ≤ 200 g, and absence of metastases
II	Tumor completely excised with negative margins, tumor weight > 200 g, and absence of metastases
III	Residual* or inoperable tumor
IV	Hematogenous metastases at presentation

*Residual tumor is defined as the presence of microscopic or gross tumor after surgical resection.

from other sarcomas of childhood. Patients with base-of-skull lesions may present with a mass, neurologic deficits, or nasopharyngeal symptoms. Computed tomography and MRI imaging reveal a destructive intraosseous lesion with variable enhancement (Figure 32-2). Extension into the nasopharynx may be seen with clival lesions, and distinction from nasopharyngeal carcinoma or rhabdomyosarcoma may be difficult.

Common sites of metastatic disease are lungs, lymph nodes, skin, and bone. Surgery is the most effective therapy, but because radical resection of clival lesions is frequently not possible, radiotherapy is generally required. Proton therapy offers the advantage of decreasing the irradiation dose to surrounding tissues and is preferred, if available, for treatment of these base-of-skull lesions.[52–54] Chemotherapy has been employed in patients with metastatic disease with mixed results.[50] Occasional tumor responses have been observed, but long-term disease control is infrequent. Sarcoma protocols of chemotherapy have been used in general, including ifosfamide and doxorubicin and other agents. Intrathecal chemotherapy has been effective in the management of meningeal disease.[50]

Colon Carcinoma in Children

Colorectal carcinoma is common in adults in Western societies, affecting some 130 000 people each year in the United States alone.[55] The disease is the second leading cause of adult cancer-related deaths, and the cumulative lifetime risk is around 6%. Approximately 1% of cases of colorectal carcinoma cases occur in patients younger than 30 years, and about 0.1% in patients younger than 20 years.[56] The incidence in individuals younger than 20 years is 0.1 case per 10^6, rising to 0.7 case per 10^6 in individuals aged 10 to

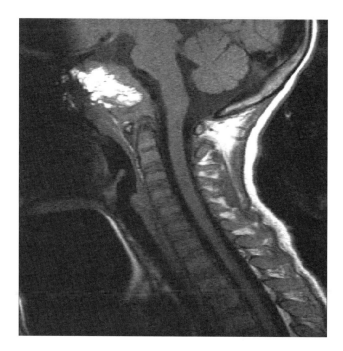

Figure 32-2 T2-weighted magnetic resonance imaging sagittal sections of the brain in a 6-year-old boy diagnosed with a clival chordoma.

19 years. Approximately 1% of malignant tumors in children are colonic in origin.

A number of conditions are associated with an increased risk of colon carcinoma. In particular, the gastrointestinal polyposis syndromes have a high risk of colon carcinoma.[57] In discussing these syndromes, distinction needs to be made between those associated with adenomatous polyps and those with inflammatory or hamartomatous polyps. The risk of colon carcinoma is increased in both settings, but this risk is highest in patients with syndromes of adenomatous polyposis. Syndromes of adenomatous polyposis include familial polyposis coli (FPC), Gardener syndrome, and Turcot syndrome. Juvenile polyposis is a distinct entity from familial polyposis coli: there are familial and sporadic forms of the disease, and the condition is characterized by multiple inflammatory polyps in the colon. The malignant potential of these lesions is much less than that of the adenomatous polyps of FPC, but malignant change may occur, and gastrointestinal surveillance is advised. Generalized juvenile polyposis is a closely related condition in which the polyps are found throughout the gastrointestinal tract rather than being limited to the colon. Peutz-Jeghers syndrome is characterized by hamartomatous gastrointestinal polyps and brown pigmentation of lips, oral mucosa, and skin. There is an increased risk of gastrointestinal and extraintestinal cancers in this syndrome. Inflammatory bowel disease is associated with an increased risk of colon carcinoma. The risk increases according to the anatomic extent and the duration of ulcerative colitis.[58–61] Crohn's disease is also associated with an increased risk of gastrointestinal neoplasia.

A large group of adult patients with a heritable tendency to colon carcinoma are those with hereditary nonpolyposis colorectal cancer (HNPCC). These include the Lynch syndromes I and II, with risk of colon cancer only, and colonic and extracolonic cancers, respectively.[62] The mean age of onset of carcinoma in these patients is 45 years, and the lifetime risk approaches 80%. The condition is associated with DNA microsatellite instability and autosomal dominant inheritance of germline mutations, the most common being in the DNA mismatch repair genes *MSH2*, *MSH6*, and *MLH1*. In a series of 16 patients younger than 24 years with colon carcinoma,[63] 8 of 11 had DNA microsatellite instability, 6 of 12 had germline mutations in mismatch repair genes, and 10 of 16 met the Amsterdam criteria[64] for the diagnosis of HNPCC. Other pediatric cases have been described.[65,66]

Symptoms of colon carcinoma include abdominal pain, rectal bleeding, vomiting, constipation, and weight loss. Pediatric patients have a higher rate of right-sided lesions than adults: between 40% and 50% of young patients have right-sided tumors, compared with 20% to 30% of older subjects.[67,68] A further difference from adult patients is the finding that young patients more often present with advanced disease. Over 80% of one series of young patients had tumors that had penetrated the bowel wall, involved lymph nodes, or spread to distant sites.[69] Another analysis of adult patients younger and older than

40 years showed that the younger cohort presented with more advanced disease and more aggressive histology than the older patients.[70]

The principal modality of therapy for carcinoma of the colon is surgery. Advice from an adult colorectal surgeon should be sought whenever possible before undertaking resection of the lesion. In addition to the usual surgical techniques utilized for bowel resection in other settings, a number of well-described surgical maneuvers are critical to accurate staging of colorectal tumors and can reduce the risk of local recurrence. Lymph node sampling needs to be systematically performed: studies have showed that a minimum of 12 to 15 lymph nodes must be examined to accurately determine regional node involvement.[71–73] Furthermore, there are well-described regional lymph node groups draining the colorectum, which can be considered regional, while others are considered sites of distant metastasis in the TNM staging system. Adequate margins both proximal and distal to the tumor need to be obtained: if 5-cm margins can be obtained, anastomotic recurrences are very rare. With rectal tumors, such margins may be difficult to achieve: a margin of 2 cm is usually adequate to prevent local recurrence, and distal margins of 1 cm may also prove sufficient.[74,75] Other margins to be considered include the mesenteric margin and the circumferential radial margin (CRM). The CRM is the retroperitoneal or perineal adventitial soft tissue margin closest to the deepest penetration of a rectal tumor.[76–78]

Other surgical strategies include the technique of total mesorectal excision (TME). Large studies have demonstrated significantly improved local control when TME is performed compared with historic controls.[75] Laparoscopic resection of tumors has been performed, but the benefits as far as surgical morbidity and disease control are not yet well defined. Finally, functional issues of sexual function and bowel function following tumor resection need also to be considered.

The pediatric pathologist should likewise work closely with a pathologist who is experienced in the evaluation of colorectal cancer. Various subtypes of colon carcinoma exist including unfavorable forms such as signet ring cell carcinoma and small cell carcinoma and the more favorable medullary carcinoma. Mucinous adenocarcinoma is found more commonly in younger patients than in older subjects.[68] Histologic grade has also been shown to be a stage-independent prognostic factor in colorectal cancer.[79] The subtleties of involvement of the lamina propria, the muscularis mucosa, the submucosa, and proximal, distal, and circumferential margins are all best evaluated in collaboration with the colorectal pathologist.

Chemotherapy is not routinely recommended in patients with stage I tumors. Tumors in these patients are limited to the mucosa and submucosa, may involve but do not penetrate the full thickness of the muscularis, and have not spread to local regional lymph nodes. Where there is full-thickness penetration of the bowel wall (stage II) and/or local/regional lymph node involvement (stage III), adjuvant chemotherapy should be considered. There is consensus that adjuvant chemotherapy is appropriate in adult patients with node-positive colon cancer. Until recently, standard therapy was with regimens that combined 5-FU with leucovorin.[80] More recently, oxaliplatin, irinotecan, and capecitabine have emerged as active agents.[81–88] Oxaliplatin and irinotecan have been combined with 5-FU and leucovorin in the FOLFOX[81] and IFL[82,87] regimens, respectively; capecitabine is a pro-drug of fluorouracil that is administered orally as a single agent and is active in this disease.[85,88]

More controversial is the role of chemotherapy in adult patients with stage II disease.[80,89,90] Some large series have demonstrated statistically significantly improved outcomes when chemotherapy is administered, but the magnitude of this benefit is modest and must be balanced against the toxicities. The American Society of Clinical Oncology recommended in 2004 that some patients with stage II disease could be considered for adjuvant therapy, including patients with inadequately sampled nodes, T4 lesions, perforation, or poorly differentiated histology.[91] The European Society of Medical Oncology similarly recommended against routine use of chemotherapy in this setting, though it did state that chemotherapy may be considered in selected node-negative patients.[91] The role of chemotherapy in stage II disease remains a subject of investigation and is developing further as newer agents such as oxaliplatin are evaluated.[81] Chemotherapy is recommended for patients with metastatic disease. Of regimens employing conventional cytotoxic chemotherapy, the FOLFOX regimen appears most effective[83]; alternatives include the IFL regimen.[82,87] Bevacizumab is a monoclonal antibody against vascular endothelial growth factor, a critical regulator of angiogenesis. Improved outcomes were seen in adult patients with metastatic colorectal cancer when combined with fluorouracil/leucovorin, with[92,93] or without irinotecan.[94] Cetuximab is a monoclonal antibody that specifically blocks the epidermal growth factor receptor. It was active against chemotherapy-resistant metastatic colorectal cancer, when given alone or in combination with irinotecan.[95]

Patients with carcinoma of the rectum may be candidates for adjuvant or neoadjuvant radiation therapy. In adult practice it has been standard to use irradiation as an adjuvant for patients with T3 or node-positive disease. Other studies have demonstrated an improvement in local control, disease-free survival, and overall survival with the use of preoperative radiation therapy. Such radiotherapy is often combined with chemotherapy. Radiotherapy may also be useful for disease palliation at metastatic sites such as the lung or brain.

The prognosis for children and adolescents with colon carcinoma is poor. Rao reported 30 patients younger than 30 years, of whom 3 survived[68]; these 3 were patients who were able to have a complete tumor resection. Minardi described 37 patients younger than 40 years, with a 26% 5-year survival.[96] Many pediatric patients present with advanced disease, and in these situations the prognosis for long-term survival is dismal.

Gastrointestinal Stromal Tumor

Gastrointestinal stromal tumor (GIST) is a mesenchymal neoplasm of the gastrointestinal tract. Many tumors previously labeled leiomyoma, leiomyosarcoma, or leiomyoblastoma are now considered to be GISTs.[97] Most cases occur in adults, with a peak incidence in the sixth and seventh decades. Gastrointestinal stromal tumors are characterized by cell-surface expression of CD117 in the great majority of cases and typical molecular abnormalities; the majority of adult cases have gain-of-function mutations in the receptor tyrosine kinases, Kit, or platelet-derived growth factor receptor-α (PDGFR-A),[98] and these mutations are of great importance in predicting response to therapy using tyrosine kinase inhibitors.[99] Gastrointestinal stromal tumors in adults may be associated with neurofibromatosis type 1 or Carney triad, which typically affects young females and includes GIST, paraganglioma, and pulmonary chondroma[100,101]; more recently, the occurrence of benign adrenocortical tumors has also been described in Carney triad.[102] A separate familial syndrome of GIST and paraganglioma has also been described.[103,104] While Carney triad is rarely present in pediatric patients with GIST,[97,102,105] there are similarities in the pathology and course of non–Carney-associated GISTs in children to those adult patients with Carney triad, particularly the histologic subtype and indolent nature of the disease.[100–102] A further group of patients with familial GISTs have germline mutations in Kit or PDGFR-A.[106,107] These kindreds have not included pediatric cases, and the molecular features differ from childhood GISTs.[105]

Fewer than 100 cases of GISTs in patients younger than 16 years have been described in the literature.[97,104,105,105,108–121] These cases occurred predominantly in the second decade, though patients as young as 4 years are described.[110] The overwhelming majority of patients are females, 25 of 28 in the largest series.[105] While adult cases occur in the stomach in only two-thirds of cases, the great majority of pediatric cases are gastric in origin, with only case reports of lesions in the duodenum, rectum, and elsewhere.[105,122,123] Gastrointestinal bleeding is the most common presentation, including hematemesis, melena, or anemia. An abdominal mass may be present. Metastasis occurred in 5 of 5 patients[97] and 11 of 32 patients[105]: the liver is the most common site of metastasis; abdominal lymph nodes and lung may also be involved.[97,121,124] There is a suggestion that early-stage primary tumors, which have a low rate of metastasis in adult patients, may be more likely to metastasize in the pediatric age group.[105]

Pathologic findings in pediatric patients differ in important ways from the adult experience: first, many pediatric patients have multifocal disease affecting the stomach, with normal tissue between tumor nodules.[97,124] Adult cases with multiple tumors are described, but with proliferation of the interstitial cells of Cajal in the intervening areas.[125] Second, the epithelioid form of GIST is most common, rather than the spindle variant that predominates in adults.[97,105] Third, most childhood cases are

notable for the absence of any mutation of Kit or PDGFR-A: the largest series described such abnormalities in none of 11, none of 5, and 1 of 3 cases[105,97,120]; 3 case reports[116–118] also found no mutations. Interestingly, this same germline configuration of Kit and PDGFR-A has been found in GISTs from adult patients with neurofibromatosis[126] and 1 patient with Carney triad.[127]

Surgical resection of the gastric primary is indicated; the possibility of multifocal disease needs to be considered in determining resection margins. The primary tumor can be assigned a prognostic group based on adult parameters combining tumor size and the frequency of mitotic figures.[98,105] Analysis for mutations in Kit and PDGFR-A is imperative.

Imatinib mesylate, an inhibitor of Kit, is active against adult GISTs and is prescribed for patients with high-risk primary disease or metastases.[128] The majority of adults with metastatic GIST benefit from such therapy, but the late emergence of imatinib resistance is problematic. Adult patients who do not have mutations in Kit or PDGFR-A have suboptimal results or primary resistance to imatinib: GISTs with Kit mutations in exon 11, exon 9, and with no mutations in Kit or PDGFR-A had partial response rates to imatinib of 84%, 48%, and 0%, respectively.[99] Since most pediatric GISTs lack Kit or PDGFR-A mutations, a similar lack of imatinib efficacy may be encountered. Prakash described 2 children with wild-type Kit and PDGFR-A who were treated with imatinib: one failed to respond and one experienced stable disease.[97] Kuroiwa described a single patient who remained disease free during 25 months of imatinib therapy; a PDGFR-A mutation was present in the tumor.[116] Janeway described 3 patients selected for treatment with sunitinib because of imatinib resistance[121]; the first had wild-type Kit and PDGFR-A and exhibited primary resistance to imatinib. The second patient had wild-type Kit and PDGFR-A, and developed local recurrence while on imatinib 14 months from diagnosis. The third patient remained disease free for 18 months while on imatinib and then developed a recurrence 6 months later, the genotype of which was not reported.

In contrast to imatinib, which is selective in targeting specific tyrosine kinases, newer agents such as sunitinib target multiple tyrosine kinases including Kit, PDGFR, VEGFR, RET, and FLT3. Sunitinib has demonstrated efficacy in adult patients with imatinib-resistant GIST, including patients with wild-type Kit and PDGFR-A. The 3 children (above) described by Janeway were treated with sunitinib: all GIST lesions stabilized or decreased in size.[121] Such agents remain investigational but may be shown to be effective in pediatric patients with GISTs and wild-type Kit and PDGFR-A, or in those who develop imatinib resistance.

The prognosis for children with GIST is variable. Most tumors exhibit indolent behavior, even after recurrence.[97,105,108,120,124] There may be late recurrences, and further surgery and/or drug treatment is appropriate, since prolonged periods of stable disease may be observed. Miettinen's series,[122,123] which was confined to children and young adults with gastric tumors, described 11 of 32 patients with follow-up developing liver metastases, and 6 dying from disease. Of the 5 children described by Prakash,[97] all developed recurrent disease in liver, peritoneum, or both sites, at 3 to 136 months from diagnosis. One died at 138 months from diagnosis; the other 4 were alive with disease at 24 to 148 months from diagnosis, and 4 to 33 months from the time of recurrence. Kerr described 4 patients with the gastrointestinal autonomic nerve tumor subtype of GIST[124]: one developed metastases, and all 4 were alive at 8 to 108 months from diagnosis.

Melanoma

Data from the U.S.' SEER program indicate that malignant melanoma accounts for 0.9% of cases of cancer in children younger than 15 years.[1] The incidence rises after puberty to account for 7% of all cancers in the 15- to 19-year age group. In recent decades, the incidence of adolescent melanoma has increased at an annual rate of 2.6% and 4.1% in the United States and Europe, respectively.[1,129] Compared with adult cases, the SEER data indicate a slightly higher proportion of females (61%) and of non-Caucasians (6.5%).

The most important risk factor numerically for the development of melanoma is the interaction between fair skin type, family history, and sun exposure. Other risk factors are implicated in a minority of cases of melanoma. These include congenital cases, including cases of transplacental spread from an affected mother, lesions arising within large congenital melanocytic nevi,[130] and patients with xeroderma pigmentosum, immune deficiency, or those undergoing radiation therapy.[131-134] Known predisposing melanoma genetic markers, such as mutations within the CDKN2A and CDK4 genes, have been found in only 1.6% of cases.[135-137]

The most common presenting features relate to change in a pigmented nevus, such as change in color, bleeding, itching, enlargement, or ulceration. In a review of 8 series, totaling 322 children with melanoma, primary tumors most commonly affected the extremities, followed by the trunk and head and neck regions.[138] Eighty-five percent of children had localized disease at presentation, and in 61% the primary lesion was less than 1.5 mm in thickness. Metastatic disease at presentation was unusual; the most common sites of metastasis when such did occur were the regional lymph nodes.

The approach to management of melanoma can be considered under 3 headings:

- Evaluation and treatment of the primary lesion
- Detection and management of regional lymph node involvement
- Detection and management of distant metastasis

The primary lesion is evaluated for thickness, as described by Breslow,[139] and microanatomic invasion as described by the Clark level.[140] Wide local excision is required for the primary tumor, with resection margins depending largely on the thickness of the lesion. The proper resection margin has been determined in adult randomized studies,[141] and there are no data to support deviations from these guidelines in younger patients, subject to anatomic considerations. For melanoma in situ, margins of 0.5 to 1.0 cm are recommended. For lesions in which the thickness is 1 mm or less, a 1-cm margin is accepted. For lesions that are 1 to 2 mm thick, most recommend a margin of 2 cm if this can be achieved. For lesions over 2 mm in thickness, a 2- to 3-cm margin is recommended.[142,143] Lesions that are thicker than 4 mm have a high risk of spread to lymph nodes and distant sites. A 2- to 3-cm margin is probably adequate for these patients, because more radical removal may not significantly affect the rate of metastatic failure insofar as such spread is likely to have occurred before resection was undertaken.[143]

The 2002 American Joint Committee on Cancer (AJCC) recommends staging melanoma on the basis of the thickness of the lesion, the presence or absence of ulceration, the number of lymph nodes involved, the size of the nodes, and the presence or absence of distant metastases.[144] Historically, the pediatric melanoma literature has described many cases using more arbitrary staging systems such as "localized," "nodal spread," and "metastatic." Such systems should be avoided; because pediatric units should seek advice from colleagues in adult oncology when evaluating such patients, the use of the same staging system that adult units use will facilitate such a discussion and allow the application of "adult" principles to the child with melanoma.

In patients with lesions less than 1.0 mm without ulceration or advanced Clark level and who have no clinically detectable disease, plain chest radiographs, blood count, and serum biochemistries are adequate. Where there is more advanced disease at the primary site, sentinel lymph node biopsy should be considered. If nodal disease is detected, complete lymph node dissection is recommended and more comprehensive staging studies are indicated; these typically include CT scan of the chest, MRI scan of the brain, and whole-body positron emission tomography (PET) scan if available.

Nodal disease is best evaluated using sentinel lymph node biopsy. The first draining lymph node is defined using radionuclide and a vital dye, then excised for histopathologic analysis, which must include immunohistochemical stains[145-147] (Figure 32-3). The sentinel node can be identified more than 95% of the time with less than 5% false negative results.[141] The rate of sentinel node positivity varies according to the thickness of the primary lesion, from 1% in tumors less than 0.8 mm to 23% if 1.5 mm to 4.0 mm and 36% if thicker than 4 mm.[147,148] Because the rates of nodal involvement are low in lesions less than 1.0 mm thick, the test is not routinely performed in such cases, though it may be considered if there are more invasive features clinically or histologically. With thicker tumors, the procedure is useful to refine prognosis and determine the need for adjuvant therapy. There is a strong negative correlation between the presence of melanoma in the sentinel node and survival.[147,149] Where the sentinel node is positive for melanoma, complete lymph node dissection should be

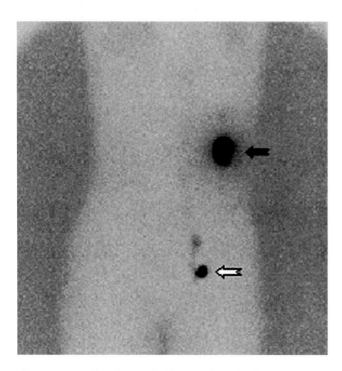

Figure 32-3 Radionuclide sentinel lymph node study of a 7-year-old girl with melanoma in the skin of the left flank. Intradermal injection of technetium-99-antimony sulphide colloid into the primary site was performed (black arrow). Lymphoscintigraphy demonstrated that the draining lymph node was in the left inguinal region (white arrow). The sentinel node was then biopsied to determine whether nodal spread of disease had occurred.

performed because it leads to improved survival compared with delayed lymphadenectomy performed at the time of overt nodal recurrence.[147]

In adult studies, adjuvant medical therapies have been evaluated in patients with high-risk primary disease and/or nodal disease. Only interferon *alpha*-2b has been shown to provide reproducible benefit.[150–152] Candidate patients would typically have disease stage IIB, IIC, or III. Tumor vaccines remain under experimental evaluation in this subset of patients.

Curative therapies for disseminated melanoma remain elusive. Patients with hematogenous spread of their disease are unlikely to survive 2 years. Surgery may be useful in selected cases—for instance, with solitary metastasis to lung or brain. Dacarbazine chemotherapy has been the most widely used agent, but responses are seen in fewer than 20% of patients, and durable responses are rare. High-dose interleukin-2 was approved for use in the United States for adult patients with stage IV disease, but experience in children is limited and toxicity is significant.[153] Temozolomide is an analogue of dacarbazine with a more favorable toxicity profile and greater penetration into the central nervous system, but efficacy was equal to that of dacarbazine in one randomized Phase III trial.[154] Various chemo-immunotherapy combinations of temozolomide or dacarbazine with interferon, interleukin, thalidomide, cisplatin, and other agents have been reported in adult studies; despite some improvements in response rates and duration of disease control, no survival advantage has been seen compared with treatment with chemotherapy or immunotherapy alone.[155,156] Earlier reports described activity with vincristine, actinomycin-D, and cyclophosphamide (VAC), then with cisplatin/etoposide, VAC, and interferon.[157,158] Radiotherapy may be useful for palliation.

Outcome for children with melanoma is similar to that seen in adult patients. Five-year survival in the SEER database was 91% from 1985 to 1994.[1,138] The prognosis in pediatric patients with nodal or distant metastasis is approximately 60% and 25% 10-year survival, respectively.

Nasopharyngeal Carcinoma

Nasopharyngeal carcinoma (NPC) is a distinct head and neck malignancy that arises in the lining of the nasal cavity and pharynx.[159,160] It is a rare disease with an incidence of 0.5 to 2 cases per 100 000 persons per year.[161] It is even more rare in the pediatric age group, with approximately 3% of all NPC occurring in those younger than 19 years.[162] Nasopharyngeal carcinoma occurs endemically in certain groups such as Southeast Asians and Alaskan Eskimos, where the incidence is between 15 and 80 cases per 100 000 persons per year,[163,164] and sporadically in the Western hemisphere, where it is associated with tobacco and alcohol use.[159,164] Nasopharyngeal carcinoma constitutes less than 3% of pediatric malignancies and 20% to 50% of all nasopharyngeal malignancies in children.[1] The highest prevalence is in the southern United States and in African American children.[165]

The World Health Organization classifies NPC into 3 distinct histologic subtypes: type 1, squamous cell carcinoma; type 2, nonkeratinizing carcinoma with or without lymphoid stroma; and type 3, undifferentiated carcinoma with or without lymphoid stroma.[160] The sporadic form is typically type 1.[166] Type 2 and type 3 subtypes are usually observed with endemic NPC and are associated with infectious, environmental, and genetic factors.[161,163,164,166] Almost all pediatric NPC is type 3 (also referred to as lymphoepithelioma).[160] There is a strong association between the Epstein-Barr virus (EBV) and NPC. High antibody titers against EBV have been observed in patients with NPC.[167] Epstein-Barr virus DNA is also present in almost all NPC cancer cells and is present as a monoclonal episome, suggesting that EBV may be responsible for the transformation of nasopharyngeal cells.[160,164,168–174] Several EBV genes, including EBV nuclear antigen 1 (*EBNA 1*), latent membrane protein 1 (*LMP1*), and EBV-encoded RNA 1 and 2 (*EBER 1* and *EBER 2*), are also expressed on NPC cells.[159,160,164,173,175–178] Circulating EBV DNA is readily detected in the plasma of NPC patients and has been shown to correlate with tumor response and clinical outcome.[179–187] Serologic measurement of antibodies to EBV immunoglobulin A/viral capsid antigen (IgA/VCA) and early antigen (IgA/EA) has been used to screen for NPC in China. However, plasma EBV DNA is a more sensitive and specific marker than IgA/VCA for the diagnosis, monitoring, and prognosis of NPC.[188,189] The incidence of NPC is increased in individuals with certain human leukocyte antigen (HLA) haplotypes. Increased incidence has been reported with HLA A2 sin2 and AW19, BW46, and B17 haplotypes.[160,164,190] Cytogenetic analysis has revealed several abnormalities in NPC, the most consistent of which are deletions in 3p and 16q.[191] p53 overexpression has also been reported in a considerable subset of NPC biopsies tested by immunochemistry.[192] An association with ingestion of Cantonese-style salted fish and NPC has been reported from China.[193]

Nasopharyngeal carcinoma can occur in all age groups. The peak incidence is in the fifth to sixth decades with median duration of symptoms of 8 months.[194] In children, the median age at diagnosis is 13 years with a median duration of symptoms of 5 months. Nasopharyngeal carcinoma is more common in males. It usually presents as a painless mass in the upper neck. Local effects of the tumor include epistaxis, nasal congestion, otitis and otorrhea, hearing loss, tinnitus, dysphasia, dysphonia, and diplopia. Rarely, there can be loss of vision, dysphagia, and taste disorders. These symptoms are secondary to cranial nerve involvement, intraorbital, intratemporal, and intracranial extension of the tumor. Up to 80% of patients can have cervical lymph node metastases at the time of diagnosis.[166] The next most common site of metastasis is the lungs. Bone, bone marrow, mediastinal, and visceral metastases have also been reported. Paraneoplastic syndromes such as hypertrophic pulmonary osteoarthropathy, syndrome of inappropriate antidiuretic hormone secretion, and dermatomyositis have all been reported in patients with widespread metastatic disease or at the time of recurrence.[160,195,196] The differential diagnoses to be considered in a child or adolescent with NPC include malignancies such as Hodgkin and non-Hodgkin lymphoma, rhabdomyosarcoma, and thyroid cancer. Benign angiofibroma and certain infectious conditions can also present with similar clinical features. Diagnosis is confirmed by incision biopsy. Epstein-Barr virus–associated NPC should be distinguished from NUT-rearranged carcinomas. These poorly differentiated carcinomas are characterized by the t(15;19) translocation resulting in the BRD4-NUT fusion oncogene and are usually fatal despite intensive therapies.[197,198]

The AJCC system is used to stage NPC based on primary tumor, regional lymph nodes, and distant metastases (TNM) definitions (Table 32-2).[199] The majority of children present with advanced (stage III or IV) disease.[160,200] The accurate extent of the primary tumor can be assessed with MRI (Figure 32-4), while metastatic disease can be evaluated with CT scan, technetium bone scan, and bone marrow aspiration/biopsy. In patients who have intracranial extension or bony erosion of the skull base, analysis of the cerebrospinal fluid for malignant cells is appropriate.[160,192,201]

Due to its anatomical location and local invasiveness, the role of surgery in the management of NPC is limited to the diagnostic biopsy. High-dose radiation therapy (doses of 6500-7000 cGy) is the main component in the treatment of NPC and may be sufficient in the management of low-stage disease.[160,202–204] The radiation field should include the nares, nasopharyngeal cavity, pharynx, posterior ethmoid and maxillary sinuses, base of skull, and cer-

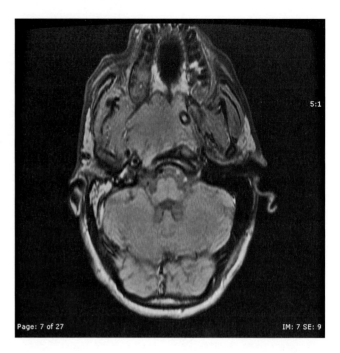

Figure 32-4 T2-weighted magnetic resonance imaging axial section of the brain in a 15-year-old African American male with undifferentiated nasopharyngeal carcinoma.

vical lymph nodes including supraclavicular lymph nodes. Undifferentiated NPC (Type 3) is more sensitive to irradiation and is associated with a better outcome.[205] Survival for patients with T1 and T2 lesions is excellent with radiation therapy alone, with local control rates of approximately 80%.[160,203] However, patients with T3 and T4 tumors fare less well, with survival rates in the 30% range.[160,203] Nasopharyngeal carcinoma is a chemosensitive tumor, and chemotherapy may be beneficial for patients with locally advanced or metastatic disease. Several chemotherapy agents such as cisplatin, carboplatin, methotrexate, bleomycin, and 5-FU have activity as single agents and in combination against NPC.[206,207] Cisplatin-containing regimens are superior to non–cisplatin-containing regimens.[208,209] Several randomized studies have been conducted to define the role of chemotherapy in the treatment of NPC.[210–214] None of these studies have demonstrated a significant benefit for patients receiving chemotherapy. Therefore, the role of chemotherapy in the treatment of NPC remains unclear at this time. The role of concurrent chemoradiotherapy with cisplatin-containing regimens has also been investigated in nonrandomized and randomized clinical trials.[215–220] These trials have resulted in progression-free survival rates of 66% to 81% and overall survival rates of 78% to 90%.

Several pediatric studies have used cisplatin- or doxorubicin-based therapies in the neoadjuvant or adjuvant setting.[221–231] These studies report survival rates of 60% to 70% in patients with advanced-stage disease. St Jude Children's Research Hospital conducted a collaborative study utilizing neoadjuvant chemotherapy. Patients received 4 courses of chemotherapy with methotrexate, leucovorin, 5-FU, and cisplatin followed by radiation therapy. All 21

Table 32-2

TNM definitions.[199]

Primary tumor (T)

- TX: Primary tumor cannot be assessed
- T0: No evidence of primary tumor
- Tis: Carcinoma in situ
- T1: Tumor confined to the nasopharynx
- T2: Tumor extends to soft tissues
  - T2a: Tumor extends to the oropharynx and/or nasal cavity without parapharyngeal extension*
  - T2b: Any tumor with parapharyngeal extension*
- T3: Tumor invades bony structures and/or paranasal sinuses
- T4: Tumor with intracranial extension and/or involvement of cranial nerves, infratemporal fossa, hypopharynx, orbit, or masticator space

Regional lymph nodes (N)

- NX: Regional lymph nodes cannot be assessed
- N0: No regional lymph node metastasis
- N1: Unilateral metastasis in lymph node(s), not more than 6 cm in greatest dimension, above the supraclavicular fossa*
- N2: Bilateral metastasis in lymph node(s), not more than 6 cm in greatest dimension, above the supraclavicular fossa*
- N3: Metastasis in a lymph node(s)* larger than 6 cm and/or to supraclavicular fossa
  - N3a: larger than 6 cm
  - N3b: Extension to the supraclavicular fossa**

Distant metastasis (M)

- MX: Distant metastasis cannot be assessed
- M0: No distant metastasis
- M1: Distant metastasis

---

patients achieved a complete remission and 20 of them were survivors.[232] The preliminary results of a multicenter study using combined chemotherapy, radiotherapy, and postirradiation interferon-β in children and adolescents was recently reported from Germany.[233] Fifty-four of 58 high-risk patients remain in first remission with a median follow-up of 4 years. The dose of irradiation used on this trial was lower than that traditionally used in the treatment of NPC (5940 cGy to the primary site and 4500 cGy to the neck). A recent pediatric study from France suggests that the irradiation dose to the nasopharynx and neck may be decreased to lower than traditional doses in those children who have a good clinical response to chemotherapy.[234] High-dose-rate brachytherapy has also been used in conjunction with multidisciplinary treatment of childhood NPC.[235]

Several side effects are associated with the treatment of NPC related to irradiation and chemotherapy. The most common side effects include mucositis, xerostomia, and hearing loss. Late effects include decreased salivation, dental complications and sinusitis, trismus, endocrine effects such as thyroid dysfunction and hypopituitarism, carotid artery disease, neck fibrosis, second malignancies, and encephalopathy.[164,236] Amifostine has been used effectively to decrease the incidence of xerostomia and mucositis in patients irradiated for head and neck carcinomas.[237,238] A recent randomized trial concluded that intensity-modulated radiation therapy was superior to 2-dimensional radiation therapy in preserving parotid function in patients with early-stage NPC resulting in less-severe delayed xerostomia.[239]

The COG is currently conducting a clinical trial in children and adolescents with NPC (ARAR0331). This trial will evaluate the efficacy of neoadjuvant chemotherapy with cisplatin and 5-FU followed by chemo-radiotherapy (using cisplatin) for those with AJCC stage IIB-IV. Amifostine, administered daily prior to irradiation, is also being investigated in this trial. Patients with lower-stage disease will receive irradiation alone together with amifostine. This trial will also seek to characterize the role of EBV in the pathogenesis of NPC in children, investigate the predictive value of *EBV-DNA* in the peripheral blood of children with NPC, and determine the incidence of *NUT* rearrangements in childhood NPC.

Pleuropulmonary Blastoma

Pleuropulmonary blastoma (PPB) is a rare primary intrathoracic malignancy that occurs almost always in early childhood.[240] Pleuropulmonary blastoma was first described in 1988 as a distinct neoplasm in 11 children with pulmonary, mediastinal, or pleural-based masses that had the common histologic feature of small, primitive cells resembling blastema separated by an uncommitted stroma.[241] It is considered a true dysembryonic neoplasm of the pulmonary/pleural mesenchyme in childhood and is classified with the group of tumors that are almost exclusively observed in childhood Wilms tumor, neuroblastoma, rhabdomyosarcoma, and hepatoblastoma. This tumor used to be referred to as the "pulmonary blastoma" of childhood but differs by the absence of malignant biphasic epithelial stromal morphology that is seen in classic adult pulmonary blastoma.[240–242]

Approximately 25% of PPB cases have a constitutional or familial association with other dysplasias and neoplastic diseases.[243] Associated conditions included other cases of PPB, sarcomas, medulloblastomas, malignant germ cell tumors, Hodgkin lymphoma, leukemia, Langerhans cell histiocytosis, thyroid cancer and dysplasia, pulmonary cysts, and cystic nephromas. The reasons for these associations are unclear at this time. Several cytogenetic and molecular studies have been performed in PPB, but no specific abnormality has been defined. Trisomy 8 and trisomy 2 have been most consistently seen, while double minutes, p53 mutations, and MYCN amplification have been reported.[244–248] The Wilms tumor (WT)-1 and WT-2 gene loci have also been preliminarily investigated in PPB with no abnormalities detected thus far.[243]

Three morphologic subtypes have been described based on gross and microscopic appearance and may have prognostic implications.[240] Type I PPB is always cystic and is seen at an earlier age (usually younger than 2 years) than type II and III PPB. Type II is characterized by both cystic and solid components, while type III is a purely solid neoplasm. These morphologic subtypes also define the clinical symptomatology with this disease.[240,249] Children younger than 2 years often present with a pneumothorax or recurrent pneumothoraces, and chest radiographs reveal simple or multiloculated cysts. Older children usually present with respiratory distress, fever, and chest pain. Based on these symptoms and a chest radiograph, a clinical diagnosis of pneumonia is often made. However, when these "pneumonias" do not respond to antibiotics, further investigation reveals a mass that is usually a type II or III PPB. Pleural effusions are common but usually do not contain malignant cells. The tumors are locally aggressive and have a propensity for vascular invasion and hematogenous metastases.[240,249,250] Various metastatic sites have been noted, but the 3 most common sites are the brain, bone, and liver. Therefore, it is essential that the staging workup include a CT scan of the head, chest, abdomen, and pelvis and a bone scan. A large pleural-based mass with an associated cyst in a young child is highly suggestive of a diagnosis of PPB (Figure 32-5).

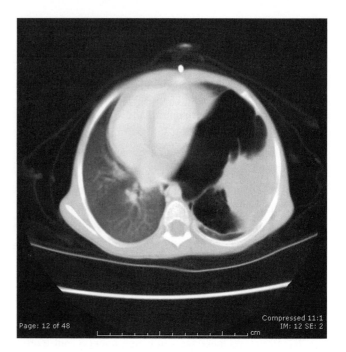

Figure 32-5 Computed tomography of the lungs in a 3-year-old girl with left thoracic pleuropulmonary blastoma demonstrating large mass with associated cyst.

Diagnosis is confirmed on histology usually after a thoracoscopic or open-wedge biopsy. Needle biopsies are rarely diagnostic. Complete surgical excision is rarely accomplished at diagnosis except in type I disease. In type II and III disease, the tumor may be grossly necrotic and hemorrhagic with extensive spillage.[240] In type I PPB, the pathologist must extensively examine cysts because they can be mistaken for congenital cystic adenomatoid malformation (CCAM) if the malignant component is missed. Multiloculated cysts separated by thin fibrous septa and lined by ciliated columnar epithelium are pathologically characteristic of type I PPB. Beneath this epithelium, primitive mesenchymal tumor cells are noted interspersed with larger cells that have features of rhabdomyoblasts.[240] Embryonal rhabdomyosarcoma is the exclusive malignant component in type I PPB. In fact, many type I PPBs may have been reported in the past as rhabdomyosarcomas arising in a CCAM, congenital pulmonary cyst, or mesenchymal hamartoma.[251–254] In type II and III PPB the solid components have mixed blastematous and sarcomatous features. The rhabdomyosarcomatous component is also a prominent feature of type II and III PPB. However, cartilaginous, blastemal, fibrosarcoma-like, and anaplastic foci can also be noted.[240–242,255]

Treatment for PPB includes surgery, chemotherapy, and radiotherapy.[240,256–258] Complete surgical excision at any time during the course of treatment improves the prognosis of PPB.[259] Surgery as a single modality may be sufficient in type I PPB when combined with careful postoperative monitoring for recurrence.[255] There are several reports of the successful role of multiagent chemotherapy in patients with PPB, especially those with type II or III disease.[240,249,255–260] Chemotherapy used is similar to various sarcoma regimens and includes vincristine, dactinomycin, cyclophosphamide, doxorubicin, cisplatin, ifosfamide, carboplatin, and etoposide. There are also reports of the use of high-dose chemotherapy followed by autologous hematopoietic progenitor cell rescue in PPB patients.[261,262] Whether this modality adds anything to standard multimodal therapy has yet to be determined. The role of radiation therapy in the treatment of PPB is also unclear. There are several reports of successful treatment of PPBs without the use of irradiation.[240,249,260] Radiation therapy dose used is similar to that for rhabdomyosarcoma and is reserved mainly for patients with type II or III PPBs when there is residual disease after definitive surgery. Significant acute and late effects of irradiation can be expected because of the young age of and location of tumors in patients with PPB and therefore should be used judiciously.

A PPB registry has been set up between the Children's Hospitals of St Paul and Minneapolis, Minnesota, and Barnes Jewish and St Louis Children's Hospitals, Missouri, in the United States. This registry is a valuable resource for both health care workers and patients and their families and can be accessed at www.ppbregistry.org. Active participation in this registry can further our understanding of this rare and unique childhood malignancy.

References

1. Ries LAG, Smith MA, Gurney JG, et al., eds. *Cancer Incidence and Survival Among Children and Adolescents: United States SEER Program 1975–1999;* National Cancer Institute, SEER Program. NIH Pub. No. 99–4649. Bethesda, MD; 1999.
2. Allolio B, Fassnacht M. Clinical review: adrenocortical carcinoma: clinical update. *J Clin Endocrinol Metab.* 2006;91(6):2027–2037.
3. Dackiw AP, Lee JE, Gagel RF, Evans DB. Adrenal cortical carcinoma. *World J Surg.* 2001;25(7):914–926.
4. Wooten MD, King DK. Adrenal cortical carcinoma: epidemiology and treatment with mitotane and a review of the literature. *Cancer.* 1993;72(11):3145–3155.
5. Rodgers SE, Evans DB, Lee JE, Perrier ND. Adrenocortical carcinoma. *Surg Oncol Clin N Am.* 2006;15(3):535–553.
6. Parkin DM, Stiller CA, Draper GJ, Bieber CA. The international incidence of childhood cancer. *Int J Cancer.* 1988;42(4):511–520.
7. Sandrini R, Ribeiro RC, DeLacerda L. Childhood adrenocortical tumors. *J Clin Endocrinol Metab.* 1997;82(7):2027–2031.
8. Stiller CA. International variations in the incidence of childhood carcinomas. *Cancer Epidemiol Biomarkers Prev.* 1994;3(4):305–310.
9. Steenman M, Westerveld A, Mannens M. Genetics of Beckwith-Wiedemann syndrome-associated tumors: common genetic pathways. *Genes Chromosomes Cancer.* 2000;28(1):1–13.
10. Hoyme HE, Seaver LH, Jones KL, Procopio F, Crooks W, Feingold M. Isolated hemihyperplasia (hemihypertrophy): report of a prospective multicenter study of the incidence of neoplasia and review. *Am J Med Genet.* 1998;59(4):274–278.
11. Brandi ML, Gagel RF, Angeli A, et al. Guidelines for diagnosis and therapy of MEN type 1 and type 2. *J Clin Endocrinol Metab.* 2001;86(12):5658–5671.
12. Varan A, Unal S, Ruacan S, Vidinlisan S. Adrenocortical carcinoma associated with adrenogenital syndrome in a child. *Med Pediatr Oncol.* 2000; 35(1):88–90.
13. Wagner J, Portwine C, Rabin K, Leclerc JM, Narod SA, Malkin D. High frequency of germline p53 mutations in childhood adrenocortical cancer. *J Natl Cancer Inst.* 1994;86(22):1707–1710.
14. Kleihues P, Schauble B, zur HA, Esteve J, Ohgaki H. Tumors associated with p53 germline mutations: a synopsis of 91 families. *Am J Pathol.* 1997;150(1):1–13.
15. Birch JM, Alston RD, McNally RJ, et al. Relative frequency and morphology of cancers in carriers of germline *TP53* mutations. *Oncogene.* 2001;20(34):4621–4628.
16. Ribeiro RC, Sandrini F, Figueiredo B, et al. An inherited *p53* mutation that contributes in a tissue-specific manner to pediatric adrenal cortical carcinoma. *Proc Natl Acad Sci USA.* 2001;98(16):9330–9335.
17. Figueiredo BC, Sandrini R, Zambetti GP, et al. Penetrance of adrenocortical tumours associated with the germline *TP53 R337H* mutation. *J Med Genet.* 2006;43(1):91–96.
18. Kirschner LS. Signaling pathways in adrenocortical cancer. *Ann N Y Acad Sci.* 2002;222–239.
19. Michalkiewicz E, Sandrini R, Figueiredo B, et al. Clinical and outcome characteristics of children with adrenocortical tumors: a report from the International Pediatric Adrenocortical Tumor Registry. *J Clin Oncol.* 2004;22(5):838–845.
20. Wajchenberg BL, Albergaria Pereira MA, Medonca BB, et al. Adrenocortical carcinoma: clinical and laboratory observations. *Cancer.* 2000;88(4):711–736.
21. Luton JP, Cerdas S, Billaud L, et al. Clinical features of adrenocortical carcinoma, prognostic factors, and the effect of mitotane therapy. *N Engl J Med.* 1990;322(17):1195–1201.
22. Ribeiro RC, Figueiredo B. Childhood adrenocortical tumours. *Eur J Cancer.* 2004;40(8):1117–1126.
23. Ribeiro RC, Sandrini Neto RS, Schell MJ, Lacerda L, Sambaio GA, Cat I. Adrenocortical carcinoma in children: a study of 40 cases. *J Clin Oncol.* 1990;8(1):67–74.
24. Mishra A, Agarwal G, Misra AK, Agarwal A, Mishra SK. Functioning adrenal tumours in children and adolescents: an institutional experience. *ANZ J Surg.* 2001;71(2):103–107.
25. van Slooten H, Schaberg A, Smeenk D, Moolenaar AJ. Morphologic characteristics of benign and malignant adrenocortical tumors. *Cancer.* 1985;55(4):766–773.
26. Koch CA, Pacak K, Chrousos GP. The molecular pathogenesis of hereditary and sporadic adrenocortical and adrenomedullary tumors. *J Clin Endocrinol Metab.* 2002;87(12):5367–5384.
27. Weiss LM. Comparative histologic study of 43 metastasizing and nonmetastasizing adrenocortical tumors. *Am J Surg Pathol.* 1984;8(3):163–169.
28. Weiss LM, Medeiros LJ, Vickery AL Jr. Pathologic features of prognostic significance in adrenocortical carcinoma. *Am J Surg Pathol.* 1989;8(3):202–206.
29. Terzolo M, Angeli A, Fassnacht M, et al. Adjuvant mitotane treatment for adrenocortical carcinoma. *N Engl J Med.* 2007;356(23):2372–2380.
30. Rodriguez-Galindo C, Figueiredo BC, Zambetti GP, Ribeiro RC. Biology, clinical characteristics, and management of adrenocortical tumors in children. *Pediatr Blood Cancer.* 2005;45(3):265–273.
31. O'Kane HF, Duggan B, Lennon G, Russell C. Spontaneous rupture of adrenocortical carcinoma. *J Urol.* 2002;168(6):2530.
32. Kardar AH. Rupture of adrenal carcinoma after biopsy. *J Urol.* 2001;166(3):984.
33. Gonzalez RJ, Shapiro S, Sarlis N, et al. Laparoscopic resection of adrenal cortical carcinoma: a cautionary note. *Surgery.* 2005;138(6):1078–1085;discussion 1085–1086.
34. Schteingart DE. Conventional and novel strategies in the treatment of adrenocortical cancer. *Braz J Med Biol Res.* 2000;33(10):1197–1200.
35. Schteingart DE. Current perspective in the diagnosis and treatment of adrenocortical cancer. *Rev Endocr Metab Disord.* 2001;2(3):323–333.
36. Becker D, Schumacher OP. o,p'DDD therapy in invasive adrenocortical carcinoma. *Ann Intern Med.* 1975;82(5):677–679.
37. Ilias I, Alevizaki M, Philippou G, Anastasiou E, Souvatzoglou A. Sustained remission of metastatic adrenal carcinoma during long-term administration of low-dose mitotane. *J Endocrinol Invest.* 2001;24(7):532–535.
38. Ishikawa S, Kazama T, Akiyama T, Nakada T, Katayama T. [Cis-platinum used for the prevention of the recurrence of adrenal cortical carcinoma: report of a case] [in Japanese]. *Hinyokika Kiyo.* 1985;(5):801–805.
39. Berruti A, Terzolo M, Pia A, Angeli A, Dogliotti L. Mitotane associated with etoposide, doxorubicin, and cisplatin in the treatment of advanced adrenocortical carcinoma. Italian Group for the Study of Adrenal Cancer. *Cancer.* 1998;83(10):2194–2200.
40. Williamson SK, Lew D, Miller GJ, Balcerzak SP, Baker LH, Crawford ED. Phase II evaluation of cisplatin and etoposide followed by mitotane at disease progression in patients with locally advanced or metastatic adrenocortical carcinoma: a Southwest Oncology Group Study. *Cancer.* 2000;88(5):1159–1165.
41. Abraham J, Bakke S, Rutt A, et al. A phase II trial of combination chemotherapy and surgical resection for the treatment of metastatic adrenocortical carcinoma: continuous infusion doxorubicin, vincristine, and etoposide with daily mitotane as a P-glycoprotein antagonist. *Cancer.* 2002;94(9):2333–2343.
42. Hovi L, Wikstrom S, Vettenranta K, Heikkila P, Saarinen-Pihkala UM. Adrenocortical carcinoma in children: a role for etoposide and cisplatin adjuvant therapy? preliminary report. *Med Pediatr Oncol.* 2003;40(5):324–326.
43. Berruti A, Terzolo M, Sperone P, et al. Etoposide, doxorubicin and cisplatin plus mitotane in the treatment of advanced adrenocortical carcinoma: a large prospective phase II trial. *Endocr Relat Cancer.* 2005;12(3):657–666.
44. Zancanella P, Pianovski MA, Oliveira BH, et al. Mitotane associated with cisplatin, etoposide, and doxorubicin in advanced childhood adrenocortical carcinoma: mitotane monitoring and tumor regression. *J Pediatr Hematol Oncol.* 2006;28(8):513–524.
45. Driver CP, Birch J, Gough DC, Bruce J. Adrenal cortical tumors in childhood. *Pediatr Hematol Oncol.* 1998;15(6):527–532.
46. Coffin CM, Swanson PE, Wick MR, Dehner LP. Chordoma in childhood and adolescence: a clinicopathologic analysis of 12 cases [see comment]. *Arch Pathol Lab Med.* 1993;117(9):927–933.
47. Azzarelli A, Quagliuolo V, Cerasoli S, et al. Chordoma: natural history and treatment results in 33 cases. *J Surg Oncol.* 1988;37(3):185–191.

48. Borba LA, Al-Mefty O, Mrak RE, Suen J. Cranial chordomas in children and adolescents.[see comment] [review]. *J Neurosurg.* 1996;84(4):584–591.

49. Hoch BL, Nielsen GP, Liebsch NJ, Rosenberg AE. Base of skull chordomas in children and adolescents: a clinicopathologic study of 73 cases. *Am J Surg Pathol.* 2006;30(7):811–818.

50 Scimeca PG, James-Herry AG, Black KS, Kahn E, Weinblatt ME. Chemotherapeutic treatment of malignant chordoma in children [review]. *J Pediatr Hematol/Oncol.* 1996;18(2):237–240.

51 Iwasa Y, Nakashima Y, Okajima H, Morishita S. Sacral chordoma in early childhood: clinicopathological and immunohistochemical study. *Pediatr Dev Pathol.* 1998;1(5):420–426.

52. Habrand JL, Mammar H, Ferrand R, et al. [Proton beam therapy (PT) in the management of CNS tumors in childhood] [in German]. *Strahlentherapie und Onkologie.* 1999;175(Suppl 2):91–94.

53. Hug EB, Loredo LN, Slater JD, et al. Proton radiation therapy for chordomas and chondrosarcomas of the skull base [see comment]. *J Neurosurg.* 1999; 91(3):432–439.

54. Noel G, Feuvret L, Calugaru V, et al. Chordomas of the base of the skull and upper cervical spine: one hundred patients irradiated by a 3D conformal technique combining photon and proton beams. *Acta Oncologica.* 2005; 44(7):700–708.

55. Greenlee RT, Murray T, Bolden S, Wingo PA. Cancer statistics, 2000. *CA Cancer J Clin.* 2000;50(1):7–33.

56. Steele GD Jr. The National Cancer Data Base report on colorectal cancer [see comment]. *Cancer.* 1994;74(7):1979–1989.

57. Haggitt RC, Reid BJ. Hereditary gastrointestinal polyposis syndromes [review]. *Am J Surg Pathol.* 1986;10(12):871–887.

58. Devroede GJ, Taylor WF, Sauer WG, Jackman RJ, Stickler GB. Cancer risk and life expectancy of children with ulcerative colitis. *N Engl J Med.* 1971; 285(1):17–21.

59. Ekbom A, Helmick C, Zack M, Adami HO. Ulcerative colitis and colorectal cancer: a population-based study. *N Engl J Med.* 1990;323(18):1228–1233.

60. Gillen CD, Walmsley RS, Prior P, Andrews HA, Allan RN. Ulcerative colitis and Crohn's disease: a comparison of the colorectal cancer risk in extensive colitis [see comment]. *Gut.* 1994;35(11):1590–1592.

61. Greenstein AJ, Sachar DB, Smith H, Janowitz HD, Aufses AH Jr. A comparison of cancer risk in Crohn's disease and ulcerative colitis. *Cancer.* 1981; 48(12):2742–2745.

62. Lynch HT, de la Chapelle A. Hereditary colorectal cancer. *N Engl J Med.* 2003; 48(10):919–932.

63. Durno C, Aronson M, Bapat B, Cohen Z, Gallinger S. Family history and molecular features of children, adolescents, and young adults with colorectal carcinoma [see comment]. *Gut.* 2005;54(8):1146–1150.

64. Vasen HF, Watson P, Mecklin JP, Lynch HT. New clinical criteria for hereditary nonpolyposis colorectal cancer (HNPCC, Lynch syndrome) proposed by the International Collaborative group on HNPCC. *Gastroenterology.* 1999;16(6): 1453–1456.

65. Marcos I, Borrego S, Urioste M, Garcia-Valles C, Antinolo G. Mutations in the DNA mismatch repair gene *MLH1* associated with early-onset colon cancer. *J Pediatr.* 2006;148(6):837–839.

66. Aiges HW, Kahn E, Silverberg M, Daum F. Adenocarcinoma of the colon in an adolescent with the family cancer syndrome. *J Pediatr.* 1979;94(4):632–633.

67. Angel CA, Pratt CB, Rao BN, et al. Carcinoembryonic antigen and carbohydrate 19-9 antigen as markers for colorectal carcinoma in children and adolescents. *Cancer.* 1992;69(6):1487–1491.

68. Rao BN, Pratt CB, Fleming ID, Dilawari RA, Green AA, Austin BA. Colon carcinoma in children and adolescents: a review of 30 cases. *Cancer.* 1985;55(6): 1322–1326.

69. Enker WE, Palovan E, Kirsner JB. Carcinoma of the colon in the adolescent: a report of survival and an analysis of the literature. *Am J Surg.* 1977;133(6): 737–741.

70. O'Connell JB, Maggard MA, Livingston EH, Yo CK. Colorectal cancer in the young [see comment] [review]. *Am J Surg.* 2004;187(3):343–348.

71. Tepper JE, O'Connell MJ, Niedzwiecki D, et al. Impact of number of nodes retrieved on outcome in patients with rectal cancer. *J Clin Oncol.* 2001;19(1): 157–163.

72. Blenkinsopp WK, Stewart-Brown S, Blesovsky L, Kearney G, Fielding LP. Histopathology reporting in large bowel cancer. *J Clin Pathol.* 1981;34(5):509–513.

73. Swanson RS, Compton CC, Stewart AK, Bland KI. The prognosis of T3N0 colon cancer is dependent on the number of lymph nodes examined. *Ann Surg Oncol.* 2003;10(1):65–71.

74. Quirke P, Durdey P, Dixon MF, Williams NS. Local recurrence of rectal adenocarcinoma due to inadequate surgical resection: histopathological study of lateral tumour spread and surgical excision. *Lancet.* 1986;2(8514):996–999.

75. Stocchi L, Nelson H, Sargent DJ, et al. Impact of surgical and pathologic variables in rectal cancer: a United States community and cooperative group report. *J Clin Oncol.* 2001;19(18):3895–3902.

76. Adam IJ, Mohamdee MO, Martin IG, et al. Role of circumferential margin involvement in the local recurrence of rectal cancer [see comment]. *Lancet.* 1994;344(8924):707–711.

77. Birbeck KF, Macklin CP, Tiffin NJ, et al. Rates of circumferential resection margin involvement vary between surgeons and predict outcomes in rectal cancer surgery. *Ann Surg.* 2002;235(4):449–457.

78. Chan KW, Boey J, Wong SK. A method of reporting radial invasion and surgical clearance of rectal carcinoma. *Histopathology.* 1985;9(12):1319–1327.

79. Compton CC, Fielding LP, Burgart LJ, et al. Prognostic factors in colorectal cancer. College of American Pathologists Consensus Statement 1999 [review]. *Arch Pathol Lab Med.* 2000;124(7):979–994.

80. Gill S, Loprinzi CL, Sargent DJ, et al. Pooled analysis of fluorouracil-based adjuvant therapy for stage II and III colon cancer: who benefits and by how much? [see comment]. *J Clin Oncol.* 2004;22(10):1797–1806.

81. Andre T, Boni C, Mounedji-Boudiaf L, et al. Oxaliplatin, Fluorouracil, and Leucovorin as adjuvant treatment for colon cancer. *N Engl J Med.* 2004; 50(23):2343–2351.

82. Douillard JY, Cunningham D, Roth AD, et al. Irinotecan combined with fluorouracil compared with fluorouracil alone as first-line treatment for metastatic colorectal cancer: a multicentre randomised trial [erratum appears in *Lancet.* 2000;355(9212):1372]. *Lancet.* 2000;355(9209):1041–1047.

83. Goldberg RM, Sargent DJ, Morton RF, et al. Randomized controlled trial of reduced-dose bolus fluorouracil plus leucovorin and irinotecan or infused fluorouracil plus leucovorin and oxaliplatin in patients with previously untreated metastatic colorectal cancer: a North American Intergroup Trial [see comment]. *J Clin Oncol.* 2006;24(21):3347–3353.

84. Goldberg RM, Sargent DJ, Morton RF, et al. A randomized controlled trial of fluorouracil plus leucovorin, irinotecan, and oxaliplatin combinations in patients with previously untreated metastatic colorectal cancer [see comment]. *J Clin Oncol.* 2004;22(1):23–30.

85. Hoff PM, Ansari R, Batist G, et al. Comparison of oral capecitabine versus intravenous fluorouracil plus leucovorin as first-line treatment in 605 patients with metastatic colorectal cancer: results of a randomized phase III study. *J Clin Oncol.* 2001;19(8):2282–2292.

86. Saltz LB, Douillard JY, Pirotta N, et al. Irinotecan plus fluorouracil/leucovorin for metastatic colorectal cancer: a new survival standard [see comment]. *Oncologist.* 2001;6(1):81–91.

87. Saltz LB, Cox JV, Blanke C, et al. Irinotecan plus fluorouracil and leucovorin for metastatic colorectal cancer. *N Engl J Med.* 2000;343(13):905–914.

88. Van Cutsem E, Twelves C, Cassidy J, et al. Oral capecitabine compared with intravenous fluorouracil plus leucovorin in patients with metastatic colorectal cancer: results of a large phase III study. *J Clin Oncol.* 2001;19(21):4097–4106.

89. Efficacy of adjuvant fluorouracil and folinic acid in B2 colon cancer. International Multicentre Pooled Analysis of B2 Colon Cancer Trials (IMPACT B2) Investigators [see comment]. *J Clin Oncol.* 1999;17(5):1356–1363.

90. Mamounas E, Wieand S, Wolmark N, et al. Comparative efficacy of adjuvant chemotherapy in patients with Dukes' B versus Dukes' C colon cancer: results from four National Surgical Adjuvant Breast and Bowel Project adjuvant studies (C-01, C-02, C-03, and C-04) [see comment]. *J Clin Oncol.* 1999; 17(5):1349–1355.

91. Sobrero A. Should adjuvant chemotherapy become standard treatment for patients with stage II colon cancer? for the proposal [see comment] [erratum appears in *Lancet Oncol.* 2006;7(7):533]. *Lancet Oncology.* 2006;7(6):515–516.

92. Kabbinavar F, Hurwitz HI, Fehrenbacher L, et al. Phase II, randomized trial comparing bevacizumab plus fluorouracil (FU)/leucovorin (LV) with FU/LV alone in patients with metastatic colorectal cancer. *J Clin Oncol.* 2003;21(1): 60–65.

93. Kabbinavar FF, Hambleton J, Mass RD, Hurwitz HI, Bergsland E, Sarkar S. Combined analysis of efficacy: the addition of bevacizumab to fluorouracil/leucovorin improves survival for patients with metastatic colorectal cancer. *J Clin Oncol.* 2005;23(16):3706–3712.

94. Hurwitz H, Fehrenbacher L, Novotny W, et al. Bevacizumab plus irinotecan, fluorouracil, and leucovorin for metastatic colorectal cancer. *N Engl J Med.* 2004;350(23):2335–2342.

95. Cunningham D, Humblet Y, Siena S, et al. Cetuximab monotherapy and cetuximab plus irinotecan in irinotecan-refractory metastatic colorectal cancer. *N Engl J Med.* 2004;351(4):337–345.

96. Minardi AJ Jr, Sittig KM, Zibari GB, McDonald JC. Colorectal cancer in the young patient. *Am Surg.* 1998;64(9):849–853.

97. Prakash S, Sarran L, Socci N, et al. Gastrointestinal stromal tumors in children and young adults: a clinicopathologic, molecular, and genomic study of 15 cases and review of the literature [review]. *J Pediatr Hematol Oncol.* 2005; 27(4):179–187.

98. Miettinen M, Sobin LH, Lasota J. Gastrointestinal stromal tumors of the stomach: a clinicopathologic, immunohistochemical, and molecular genetic study of 1765 cases with long-term follow-up. *Am J Surg Pathol.* 2005;29(1): 52–68.

99. Heinrich MC, Corless CL, Demetri GD, et al. Kinase mutations and imatinib response in patients with metastatic gastrointestinal stromal tumor. *J Clin Oncol.* 2003;21(23):4342–4349.

100. Carney JA. The triad of gastric epithelioid leiomyosarcoma, pulmonary chondroma, and functioning extra-adrenal paraganglioma: a five-year review. *Medicine.* 1983;62(3):159–169.

101. Carney JA, Sheps SG, Go VL, Gordon H. The triad of gastric leiomyosarcoma, functioning extra-adrenal paraganglioma and pulmonary chondroma. *N Engl J Med.* 1977;296(26):1517–1518.

102. Carney JA. Gastric stromal sarcoma, pulmonary chondroma, and extra-adrenal paraganglioma (Carney Triad): natural history, adrenocortical component, and possible familial occurrence [see comment]. *Mayo Clin Proc.* 1999;74(6):543–552.

103. Carney JA, Stratakis CA. Familial paraganglioma and gastric stromal sarcoma: a new syndrome distinct from the Carney triad. *Am J Med Genet.* 2002;108(2):132–139.

104. Boccon-Gibod L, Boman F, Boudjemaa S, Fabre M, Leverger G, Carney AJ. Separate occurrence of extra-adrenal paraganglioma and gastrointestinal stromal tumor in monozygotic twins: probable familial Carney syndrome. *Pediatr Dev Pathol.* 2004;7(4):380–384.

105. Miettinen M, Lasota J, Sobin LH. Gastrointestinal stromal tumors of the stomach in children and young adults: a clinicopathologic, immunohistochemical, and molecular genetic study of 44 cases with long-term follow-up and review of the literature. *Am J Surg Pathol.* 2005;29(10):1373–1381.

106. Hirota S, Okazaki T, Kitamura Y, O'Brien P, Kapusta L, Dardick I. Cause of familial and multiple gastrointestinal autonomic nerve tumors with hyperplasia of interstitial cells of Cajal is germline mutation of the c-kit gene. *Am J Surg Pathol.* 2000;24(2):326–327.

107. Chompret A, Kannengiesser C, Barrois M, et al. PDGFRA germline mutation in a family with multiple cases of gastrointestinal stromal tumor. *Gastroenterology.* 2004;126(1):318–321.

108. Budzynski A, Stachura T, Ostrowska M, Zasada J, Grochowska E. [Stromal tumor of the stomach in a 14 year old girl] [in Polish]. *Przeglad Lekarski.* 2003;60(Suppl 7):81–85.

109. Dijoud F, Frachon S, Basset T, Bertrand Y, Bergeron C. [Stromal gastrointestinal tumors in children: about a case] [in French]. *Ann Pathol.* 2004;24(6):628–631.

110. Durham MM, Gow KW, Shehata BM, Katzenstein HM, Lorenzo RL, Ricketts RR. Gastrointestinal stromal tumors arising from the stomach: a report of three children. *J Pediatr Surg.* 2004;39(10):1495–1499.

111. Haider N, Kader M, Mc Dermott DM, Devaney D, Corbally MT, Fitzgerald RJ. Gastric stromal tumors in children. *Pediatr Blood Cancer.* 2004;42(2):186–189.

112. Hayashi Y, Okazaki T, Yamataka A, et al. Gastrointestinal stromal tumor in a child and review of the literature [review]. *Pediatr Surg Int.* 2005;21(11):914–917.

113. Hughes JA, Cook JV, Said A, Chong SK, Towu E, Reidy J. Gastrointestinal stromal tumour of the duodenum in a 7-year-old boy. *Pediatr Radiol.* 2004;34(12):1024–1027.

114. Iwasaki M, Morimoto T, Sano K, et al. A case of pediatric gastrointestinal stromal tumor of the stomach [review]. *Pediatr Int.* 2005;47(1):102–104.

115. Kau W, Stessel U, Schoellnast H. [Gastric stromal tumor in childhood—a rare diagnosis with an initial consideration of Hodgkin's disease] [in German]. *Rofo.* 2006;178(1):112–114.

116. Kuroiwa M, Hiwatari M, Hirato J, et al. Advanced-stage gastrointestinal stromal tumor treated with imatinib in a 12-year-old girl with a unique mutation of PDGFRA. *J Pediatr Surg.* 2005;40(11):1798–1801.

117. Li P, Wei J, West AB, Perle M, Greco MA, Yang GC. Epithelioid gastrointestinal stromal tumor of the stomach with liver metastases in a 12-year-old girl: aspiration cytology and molecular study [see comment]. *Pediatr Dev Pathol.* 2002;5(4):386–394.

118. O'Sullivan MJ, McCabe A, Gillett P, Penman ID, MacKinlay GA, Pritchard J. Multiple gastric stromal tumors in a child without syndromic association lacks common KIT or PDGFRalpha mutations. *Pediatr Dev Pathol.* 2005;8(6):685–689.

119. Oguzkurt P, Akcoren Z, Senocak ME, Caglar M, Buyukpamukcu N. A huge gastric stromal tumor in a 13-year-old girl. *Turkish J Pediatr.* 2002;44(1):65–68.

120. Price VE, Zielenska M, Chilton-MacNeill S, Smith CR, Pappo AS. Clinical and molecular characteristics of pediatric gastrointestinal stromal tumors (GISTs). *Pediatr Blood Cancer.* 2005;45(1):20–24.

121. Janeway K, Matthews D, Butrynski J, et al. Sunitinib treatment of pediatric metastatic GIST after failure of imatinib. 2006 ASCO Annual Meeting Proceedings. *J Clin Oncol.* 2006;24(18S):9519.

122. Miettinen M, Kopczynski J, Makhlouf HR, et al. Gastrointestinal stromal tumors, intramural leiomyomas, and leiomyosarcomas in the duodenum: a clinicopathologic, immunohistochemical, and molecular genetic study of 167 cases. *Am J Surg Pathol.* 2003;27(5):625–641.

123. Miettinen M, Furlong M, Sarlomo-Rikala M, Burke A, Sobin LH, Lasota J. Gastrointestinal stromal tumors, intramural leiomyomas, and leiomyosarcomas in the rectum and anus: a clinicopathologic, immunohistochemical, and molecular genetic study of 144 cases. *Am J Surg Pathol.* 2001;25(9):1121–1133.

124. Kerr JZ, Hicks MJ, Nuchtern JG, et al. Gastrointestinal autonomic nerve tumors in the pediatric population: a report of four cases and a review of the literature [review]. *Cancer.* 1999;85(1):220–230.

125. Chen H, Hirota S, Isozaki K, et al. Polyclonal nature of diffuse proliferation of interstitial cells of Cajal in patients with familial and multiple gastrointestinal stromal tumours. *Gut.* 2002;51(6):793–796.

126. Kinoshita K, Hirota S, Isozaki K, et al. Absence of c-kit gene mutations in gastrointestinal stromal tumours from neurofibromatosis type 1 patients. *J Pathol.* 2004;202(1):80–85.

127. Diment J, Tamborini E, Casali P, Gronchi A, Carney JA, Colecchia M. Carney triad: case report and molecular analysis of gastric tumor. *Human Pathol.* 2005;36(1):112–116.

128. Demetri GD, von Oosterom MM, Blanke CD, et al. Efficacy and safety of imatinib mesylate in advanced gastrointestinal stromal tumors [see comment]. *N Engl J Med.* 2002;347(7):472–480.

129. de Vries VE, Steliarova-Foucher E, Spatz A, Ardanaz E, Eggermont AM, Coebergh JW. Skin cancer incidence and survival in European children and adolescents (1978–1997): report from the Automated Childhood Cancer Information System project. *Eur J Cancer.* 2006;42(13):2170–2182.

130. Krengel S, Hauschild A, Schafer T. Melanoma risk in congenital melanocytic naevi: a systematic review [review]. *Br J Dermatol.* 2006;155(1):1–8.

131. Buyukpamukcu M, Varan A, Yazici N, et al. Second malignant neoplasms following the treatment of brain tumors in children. *J Child Neurol.* 2006;21(5):433–436.

132. Cohen RJ, Curtis RE, Inskip PD, Fraumeni JF Jr. The risk of developing second cancers among survivors of childhood soft tissue sarcoma. *Cancer.* 2005;103(11):2391–2396.

133. Guerin S, Dupuy A, Anderson H, et al. Radiation dose as a risk factor for malignant melanoma following childhood cancer. *Eur J Cancer.* 2003;39(16):2379–2386.

134. Curtis RE, Rowlings PA, Deeg HJ, et al. Solid cancers after bone marrow transplantation [see comment]. *N Engl J Med.* 1997;336(13):897–904.

135. Berg P, Wennberg AM, Tuominen R, et al. Germline CDKN2A mutations are rare in child and adolescent cutaneous melanoma. *Melanoma Res.* 2004;14(4):251–255.

136. Tsao H, Zhang X, Kwitkiwski K, Finkelstein DM, Sober AJ, Haluska FG. Low prevalence of germline CDKN2A and CDK4 mutations in patients with early-onset melanoma. *Arch Dermatol.* 2000;136(9):1118–1122.

137. Whiteman DC, Milligan A, Welch J, Green AC, Hayward NK. Germline CDKN2A mutations in childhood melanoma. *J Natl Cancer Inst.* 1997;89(19):1460.

138. Pappo AS. Melanoma in children and adolescents [review]. *Eur J Cancer.* 2003;39(18):2651–2661.

139. Breslow A. Thickness, cross-sectional areas and depth of invasion in the prognosis of cutaneous melanoma. *Ann Surg.* 1970;172(5):902–908.

140. Clark WH, Jr., From L, Bernardino EA, Mihm MC. The histogenesis and biologic behavior of primary human malignant melanomas of the skin. *Cancer Res.* 1969;29(3):705–727.

141. Tsao H, Atkins MB, Sober AJ. Management of cutaneous melanoma [see comment] [erratum appears in *N Engl J Med.* 2004;351(23):2461] [review]. *N Engl J Med.* 2004;351(10):998–1012.

142. Thomas JM, Newton-Bishop J, A'Hern R, et al. Excision margins in high-risk malignant melanoma.[see comment]. *N Engl J Med.* 2004;350(8):757–766.

143. Balch CM, Soong SJ, Smith T, et al. Long-term results of a prospective surgical trial comparing 2 cm vs. 4 cm excision margins for 740 patients with 1-4 mm melanomas [see comment]. *Ann Surg Oncol.* 2001;8(2):101–108.

144. Balch CM, Buzaid AC, Soong SJ, et al. Final version of the American Joint Committee on Cancer Staging System for cutaneous melanoma. *J Clin Oncol.* 2001;19(16):3635–3648.

145. Shah NC, Gerstle JT, Stuart M, Winter C, Pappo A. Use of sentinel lymph node biopsy and high-dose interferon in pediatric patients with high-risk melanoma: the Hospital for Sick Children experience. *J Pediatr Hematol Oncol.* 2006;8(8):496–500.

146. Uren RF, Howman-Giles R, Thompson JF. Patterns of lymphatic drainage from the skin in patients with melanoma [see comment] [review]. *J Nucl Med.* 2003;44(4):570–582.

147. Morton DL, Thompson JF, Cochran AJ, et al. Sentinel-node biopsy or nodal observation in melanoma. *N Engl J Med.* 2006;355(13):1307–1317.

148. Bleicher RJ, Essner R, Foshag LJ, Wanek LA, Morton DL. Role of sentinel lymphadenectomy in thin invasive cutaneous melanomas. *J Clin Oncol.* 2003;21(7):1326–1331.

149. Vuylsteke RJCL, van Leeuwen PAM, Muller MGS, Gietema HA, Kragt DR, Meijer S. Clinical outcome of stage I/II melanoma patients after selective sentinel lymph node dissection: long-term follow-up results. *J Clin Oncol.* 2003;21(6):1057–1065.

150. Kirkwood JM, Ibrahim JG, Sosman JA, et al. High-dose interferon alfa-2b significantly prolongs relapse-free and overall survival compared with the GM2-KLH/QS-21 vaccine in patients with resected stage IIB-III melanoma: results of intergroup trial E1694/S9512/C509801 [see comment]. *J Clin Oncol.* 2001;19(9):2370–2380.

151. Kirkwood JM, Ibrahim JG, Sondak VK, et al. High- and low-dose interferon alfa-2b in high-risk melanoma: first analysis of intergroup trial E1690/S9111/C9190 [see comment]. *J Clin Oncol.* 2000;18(12):2444–2458.

152. Kirkwood JM, Strawderman MH, Ernstoff MS, Smith TJ, Borden EC, Blum RH. Interferon alfa-2b adjuvant therapy of high-risk resected cutaneous melanoma: the Eastern Cooperative Oncology Group Trial EST 1684 [see comment]. *J Clin Oncol.* 1996;14(1):7–17.

153. Bauer M, Reaman GH, Hank JA, et al. A phase II trial of human recombinant interleukin-2 administered as a 4-day continuous infusion for children with refractory neuroblastoma, non-Hodgkin's lymphoma, sarcoma, renal cell carcinoma, and malignant melanoma: a Children's Cancer Group study. *Cancer.* 1995;75(12):2959–2965.

154. Middleton MR, Grob JJ, Aaronson N, et al. Randomized phase III study of temozolomide versus dacarbazine in the treatment of patients with advanced metastatic malignant melanoma [see comment] [erratum appears in *J Clin Oncol.* 2000;18(11):2351]. *J Clin Oncol.* 2000;18(1):158–166.

155. Keilholz U, Punt CJA, Gore M, et al. Dacarbazine, cisplatin, and interferon-alfa-2b with or without interleukin-2 in metastatic melanoma: a randomized phase III trial (18951) of the European Organisation for Research and Treatment of Cancer Melanoma Group. *J Clin Oncol.* 2005;23(27):6747–6755.

156. Atkins MB LSFLSJSVKJ[correct?]. A prospective randomised phase III trial of concurrent biochemotherapy (BCT) with cisplatin, vinblastine, dacarbazine (CVD), IL-2 and interferon alpha 2b (IFN) versus CVD alone in patients with

metastatic melanoma (E3695): an ECOG-coordinated intergroup trial [abstract]. *Proc Am Soc Clin Oncol.* 2003:22.

157. Hayes FA, Green AA. Malignant melanoma in childhood: clinical course and response to chemotherapy. *J Clin Oncol.* 1984;2(11):1229–1234.

158. Boddie AW Jr., Cangir A. Adjuvant and neoadjuvant chemotherapy with dacarbazine in high-risk childhood melanoma. *Cancer.* 1987;60(8):1720–1723.

159. Vasef MA, Ferlito A, Weiss LM. Nasopharyngeal carcinoma, with emphasis on its relationship to Epstein-Barr virus. *Ann Otol Rhinol Laryngol.* 1997;106(4):348–356.

160. Ayan I, Kaytan E, Ayan N. Childhood nasopharyngeal carcinoma: from biology to treatment. *Lancet Oncol.* 2003;4(1):13–21.

161. Fandi A, Altun M, Azli N, Armand JP, Cvitkovic E. Nasopharyngeal cancer: epidemiology, staging, and treatment. *Semin Oncol.* 1994;21(3):382–397.

162. Marks JE, Phillips JL, Menck HR. The National Cancer Data Base report on the relationship of race and national origin to the histology of nasopharyngeal carcinoma. *Cancer.* 1998;83(3):582–588.

163. Fandi A, Cvitkovic E. Biology and treatment of nasopharyngeal cancer. *Curr Opin Oncol.* 1995;7(3):255–263.

164. Spano JP, Busson P, Atlan D, et al. Nasopharyngeal carcinomas: an update. *Eur J Cancer.* 2003;39(15):2121–2135.

165. Greene MH, Fraumeni JF, Hoover R. Nasopharyngeal cancer among young people in the United States: racial variations by cell type. *J Natl Cancer Inst.* 1977;58(5):1267–1270.

166. Vokes EE, Liebowitz DN, Weichselbaum RR. Nasopharyngeal carcinoma. *Lancet.* 1997;350(9084):1087–1091.

167. Chien YC, Chen JY, Liu MY, et al. Serologic markers of Epstein-Barr virus infection and nasopharyngeal carcinoma in Taiwanese men. *N Engl J Med.* 2001;346(26):1877–1882.

168. Chang YS, Tyan YS, Liu ST, Tsai MS, Pao CC. Detection of Epstein-Barr virus DNA sequences in nasopharyngeal carcinoma cells by enzymatic DNA amplification. *J Clin Microbiol.* 1990;28(11):2398–2402.

169. Pathmanathan R, Prasad U, Sadler R, Flynn K, Raab-Traub N. Clonal proliferations of cells infected with Epstein-Barr virus in preinvasive lesions related to nasopharyngeal carcinoma. *N Engl J Med.* 1995;333(11):693–698.

170. Pathmanathan R, Prasad U, Chandrika G, Sadler R, Flynn K, Raab-Traub N. Undifferentiated, nonkeratinizing, and squamous cell carcinoma of the nasopharynx: variants of Epstein-Barr virus-infected neoplasia. *Am J Pathol.* 1995;146(6):1355–1367.

171. Raab-Traub N, Flynn K. The structure of the termini of the Epstein-Barr virus as a marker of clonal cellular proliferation. *Cell.* 1986;47(6):883–889.

172. Niedobitek G, Agathanggelou A, Nicholls JM. Epstein-Barr virus infection and the pathogenesis of nasopharyngeal carcinoma: viral gene expression, tumour cell phenotype, and the role of the lymphoid stroma. *Semin Cancer Biol.* 1996;7(4):165–174.

173. Wu TC, Mann RB, Epstein JI, et al. Abundant expression of EBER1 small nuclear RNA in nasopharyngeal carcinoma: a morphologically distinctive target for detection of Epstein-Barr virus in formalin-fixed paraffin-embedded carcinoma specimens. *Am J Pathol.* 1991;138(6):1461–1469.

174. Chen CL, Wen WN, Chen JY, Hsu MM, Hsu HC. Detection of Epstein-Barr virus genome in nasopharyngeal carcinoma by in situ DNA hybridization. *Intervirology.* 1993;36(2):91–98.

175. Huang DP, Ho HC, Henle W, Henle G, Saw D, Lui M. Presence of EBNA in nasopharyngeal carcinoma and control patient tissues related to EBV serology. *Int J Cancer.* 1978;22(3):266–274.

176. Pagano JS. Epstein-Barr virus: the first human tumor virus and its role in cancer. *Proc Assoc Am Phys.* 1999;111(6):573–580.

177. Young LS, Dawson CW, Clark D, et al. Epstein-Barr virus gene expression in nasopharyngeal carcinoma. *J Gen Virol.* 1988;69(Pt 5):1051–1065.

178. Murray PG, Niedobitek G, Kremmer E, et al. In situ detection of the Epstein-Barr virus-encoded nuclear antigen 1 in oral hairy leukoplakia and virus-associated carcinomas. *J Pathol.* 1996;178(1):44–47.

179. Lo YM, Chan AT, Chan LY, et al. Molecular prognostication of nasopharyngeal carcinoma by quantitative analysis of circulating Epstein-Barr virus DNA. *Cancer Res.* 2000;60(24):6878–6881.

180. Lo YM, Chan LY, Chan AT, et al. Quantitative and temporal correlation between circulating cell-free Epstein-Barr virus DNA and tumor recurrence in nasopharyngeal carcinoma. *Cancer Res.* 1999;59(21):5452–5455.

181. Lo YM, Chan LY, Lo KW, et al. Quantitative analysis of cell-free Epstein-Barr virus DNA in plasma of patients with nasopharyngeal carcinoma. *Cancer Res.* 1999;59(6):1188–1191.

182. Lo YM, Leung SF, Chan LY, et al. Kinetics of plasma Epstein-Barr virus DNA during radiation therapy for nasopharyngeal carcinoma. *Cancer Res.* 2000;60(9):2351–2355.

183. Chan AT, Lo YM, Zee B, et al. Plasma Epstein-Barr virus DNA and residual disease after radiotherapy for undifferentiated nasopharyngeal carcinoma. *J Natl Cancer Inst.* 2002;94(21):1614–1619.

184. Leung SF, Zee B, Ma BB, et al. Plasma Epstein-Barr viral deoxyribonucleic acid quantitation complements tumor-node-metastasis staging prognostication in nasopharyngeal carcinoma. *J Clin Oncol.* 2006;24(34):5414–5418.

185. Ma BB, King A, Lo YM, et al. Relationship between pretreatment level of plasma Epstein-Barr virus DNA, tumor burden, and metabolic activity in advanced nasopharyngeal carcinoma. *Int J Radiat Oncol Biol Phys.* 2006;66(3):714–720.

186. Chan AT, Ma BB, Lo YM, et al. Phase II study of neoadjuvant carboplatin and paclitaxel followed by radiotherapy and concurrent cisplatin in patients with locoregionally advanced nasopharyngeal carcinoma: therapeutic monitoring with plasma Epstein-Barr virus DNA. *J Clin Oncol.* 2004;22(15):3053–3060.

187. Leung SF, Chan AT, Zee B, et al. Pretherapy quantitative measurement of circulating Epstein-Barr virus DNA is predictive of posttherapy distant failure in patients with early-stage nasopharyngeal carcinoma of undifferentiated type. *Cancer.* 2003;98(2):288–291.

188. Twu CW, Wang WY, Liang WM, et al. Comparison of the prognostic impact of serum anti-EBV antibody and plasma EBV DNA assays in nasopharyngeal carcinoma. *Int J Radiat Oncol Biol Phys.* 2007;67(1):130–137.

189. Shao JY, Li YH, Gao HY, et al. Comparison of plasma Epstein-Barr virus (EBV) DNA levels and serum EBV immunoglobulin A/virus capsid antigen antibody titers in patients with nasopharyngeal carcinoma. *Cancer.* 2004;100(6):1162–1170.

190. Simons MJ, Wee GB, Goh EH, et al. Immunogenetic aspects of nasopharyngeal carcinoma: IV. increased risk in Chinese of nasopharyngeal carcinoma associated with a Chinese-related HLA profile (A2, Singapore 2). *J Natl Cancer Inst.* 1976;57(5):977–980.

191. Chien G, Yuen PW, Kwong D, Kwong YL. Comparative genomic hybridization analysis of nasopharyngeal carcinoma: consistent patterns of genetic aberrations and clinicopathological correlations. *Cancer Genet Cytogenet.* 2001;126(1):63–67.

192. Agaoglu FY, Dizdar Y, Dogan O, et al. P53 overexpression in nasopharyngeal carcinoma. *In Vivo.* 2004;18(5):555–560.

193. Yu MC, Mo CC, Chong WX, Yeh FS, Henderson BE. Preserved foods and nasopharyngeal carcinoma: a case-control study in Guangxi, China. *Cancer Res.* 1988;48(7):1954–1959.

194. Lee AW, Foo W, Law SC, et al. Nasopharyngeal carcinoma: presenting symptoms and duration before diagnosis. *Hong Kong Med J.* 1997;3(4):355–361.

195. Roebuck DJ. Skeletal complications in pediatric oncology patients. *Radiographics.* 1999;19(4):873–885.

196. Bass IS, Haller JO, Berdon WE, Barlow B, Carsen G, Khakoo Y. Nasopharyngeal carcinoma: clinical and radiographic findings in children. *Radiology.* 1985;156(3):651–654.

197. French CA, Kutok JL, Faquin WC, et al. Midline carcinoma of children and young adults with *NUT* rearrangement. *J Clin Oncol.* 2004;22(20):4135–4139.

198. French CA, Miyoshi I, Kubonishi I, Grier HE, Perez-Atayde AR, Fletcher JA. *BRD4-NUT* fusion oncogene: a novel mechanism in aggressive carcinoma. *Cancer Res.* 2003;63(2):304–307.

199. American Joint Committee on Cancer. *AJCC Cancer Staging Manual,* 6th ed. New York: Springer-Verlag, 2002.

200. Ayan I, Altun M. Nasopharyngeal carcinoma in children: retrospective review of 50 patients. *Int J Radiat Oncol Biol Phys.* 1996;35(3):485–492.

201. Stambuk HE, Patel SG, Mosier KM, Wolden SL, Holodny AI. Nasopharyngeal carcinoma: recognizing the radiographic features in children. *Am J Neuroradiol.* 2005;26(6):1575–1579.

202. Lee AW, Poon YF, Foo W, et al. Retrospective analysis of 5037 patients with nasopharyngeal carcinoma treated during 1976–1985: overall survival and patterns of failure. *Int J Radiat Oncol Biol Phys.* 1992;23(2):261–270.

203. Perez CA, Devineni VR, Marcial-Vega V, Marks JE, Simpson JR, Kucik N. Carcinoma of the nasopharynx: factors affecting prognosis. *Int J Radiat Oncol Biol Phys.* 1992;23(2):271–280.

204. Mendenhall WM, Morris CG, Hinerman RW, Malyapa RS, Amdur RJ. Definitive radiotherapy for nasopharyngeal carcinoma. *Am J Clin Oncol.* 2006;29(6):622–627.

205. Sanguineti G, Geara FB, Garden AS, et al. Carcinoma of the nasopharynx treated by radiotherapy alone: determinants of local and regional control. *Int J Radiat Oncol Biol Phys.* 1997;35(5):985–996.

206. Decker DA, Drelichman A, Al Sarraf M, Crissman J, Reed ML. Chemotherapy for nasopharyngeal carcinoma: a ten-year experience. *Cancer.* 1983;52(4):602–605.

207. Chan AT, Teo PM, Leung TW, Johnson PJ. The role of chemotherapy in the management of nasopharyngeal carcinoma. *Cancer.* 1998;82(6):1003–1012.

208. Huang SC, Lui LT, Lynn TC. Nasopharyngeal cancer: study III: a review of 1206 patients treated with combined modalities. *Int J Radiat Oncol Biol Phys.* 1985;11(10):1789–1793.

209. Chi KH, Chan WK, Cooper DL, Yen SH, Lin CZ, Chen KY. A phase II study of outpatient chemotherapy with cisplatin, 5-fluorouracil, and leucovorin in nasopharyngeal carcinoma. *Cancer.* 1994;73(2):247–252.

210. Preliminary results of a randomized trial comparing neoadjuvant chemotherapy (cisplatin, epirubicin, bleomycin) plus radiotherapy vs. radiotherapy alone in stage IV(+AD4- or +AD0- N2, M0) undifferentiated nasopharyngeal carcinoma: a positive effect on progression-free survival. International Nasopharynx Cancer Study Group. VUMCA I trial. *Int J Radiat Oncol Biol Phys.* 1996;35(3):463–469.

211. Hong S, Wu HG, Chie EK, et al. Neoadjuvant chemotherapy and radiation therapy compared with radiation therapy alone in advanced nasopharyngeal carcinoma. *Int J Radiat Oncol Biol Phys.* 1999;45(4):901–905.

212. Ma J, Mai HQ, Hong MH, et al. Results of a prospective randomized trial comparing neoadjuvant chemotherapy plus radiotherapy with radiotherapy alone in patients with locoregionally advanced nasopharyngeal carcinoma. *J Clin Oncol.* 2001;19(5):1350–1357.

213. Chan AT, Teo PM, Leung TW, et al. A prospective randomized study of chemotherapy adjunctive to definitive radiotherapy in advanced nasopharyngeal carcinoma. *Int J Radiat Oncol Biol Phys.* 1995;33(3):569–577.

214. Chua DT, Sham JS, Choy D, et al. Preliminary report of the Asian-Oceanian Clinical Oncology Association randomized trial comparing cisplatin and epirubicin followed by radiotherapy versus radiotherapy alone in the treatment of patients with locoregionally advanced nasopharyngeal carcinoma. Asian-Oceanian Clinical Oncology Association Nasopharynx Cancer Study Group. *Cancer.* 1998;83(11):2270–2283.

215. Chan AT, Teo PM, Ngan RK, et al. Concurrent chemotherapy-radiotherapy compared with radiotherapy alone in locoregionally advanced nasopharyngeal carcinoma: progression-free survival analysis of a phase III randomized trial. *J Clin Oncol.* 2002;20(8):2038–2044.

216. Chan AT, Leung SF, Ngan RK, et al. Overall survival after concurrent cisplatin-radiotherapy compared with radiotherapy alone in locoregionally advanced nasopharyngeal carcinoma. *J Natl Cancer Inst.* 2005;97(7):536–539.

217. Cheng SH, Jian JJ, Tsai SY, et al. Long-term survival of nasopharyngeal carcinoma following concomitant radiotherapy and chemotherapy. *Int J Radiat Oncol Biol Phys.* 2000;48(5):1323–1330.

218. Wolden SL, Zelefsky MJ, Kraus DH, et al. Accelerated concomitant boost radiotherapy and chemotherapy for advanced nasopharyngeal carcinoma. *J Clin Oncol.* 2001;19(4):1105–1110.

219. Rischin D, Corry J, Smith J, Stewart J, Hughes P, Peters L. Excellent disease control and survival in patients with advanced nasopharyngeal cancer treated with chemoradiation. *J Clin Oncol.* 2002;20(7):1845–1852.

220. Al Sarraf M, LeBlanc M, Giri PG, et al. Chemoradiotherapy versus radiotherapy in patients with advanced nasopharyngeal cancer: phase III randomized Intergroup study 0099. *J Clin Oncol.* 1998;16(4):1310–1317.

221. Lobo-Sanahuja F, Garcia I, Carranza A, Camacho A. Treatment and outcome of undifferentiated carcinoma of the nasopharynx in childhood: a 13-year experience. *Med Pediatr Oncol.* 1986;14(1):6–11.

222. Roper HP, Essex-Cater A, Marsden HB, Dixon PF, Campbell RH. Nasopharyngeal carcinoma in children. *Pediatr Hematol Oncol.* 1986;3(2):143–152.

223. Gasparini M, Lombardi F, Rottoli L, Ballerini E, Morandi F. Combined radiotherapy and chemotherapy in stage T3 and T4 nasopharyngeal carcinoma in children. *J Clin Oncol.* 1988;6(3):491–494.

224. Pao WJ, Hustu HO, Douglass EC, Beckford NS, Kun LE. Pediatric nasopharyngeal carcinoma: long term follow-up of 29 patients. *Int J Radiat Oncol Biol Phys.* 1989;17(2):299–305.

225. Arush MW, Stein ME, Rosenblatt E, Lavie R, Kuten A. Advanced nasopharyngeal carcinoma in the young: the Northern Israel Oncology Center experience, 1973–1991. *Pediatr Hematol Oncol.* 1995;12(3):271–276.

226. Werner-Wasik M, Winkler P, Uri A, Goldwein J. Nasopharyngeal carcinoma in children. *Med Pediatr Oncol.* 1996;26(5):352–358.

227. Strojan P, Benedik MD, Kragelj B, Jereb B. Combined radiation and chemotherapy for advanced undifferentiated nasopharyngeal carcinoma in children. *Med Pediatr Oncol.* 1997;28(5):366–369.

228. Ghim TT, Briones M, Mason P, et al. Effective adjuvant chemotherapy for advanced nasopharyngeal carcinoma in children: a final update of a long-term prospective study in a single institution. *J Pediatr Hematol Oncol.* 1998; 20(2):131–135.

229. Ozyar E, Selek U, Laskar S, et al. Treatment results of 165 pediatric patients with non-metastatic nasopharyngeal carcinoma: a Rare Cancer Network study. *Radiother Oncol.* 2006;81(1):39–46.

230. Bakkal BH, Kaya B, Berberoglu S, et al. The efficiency of different chemoradiotherapy regimens in patients with paediatric nasopharynx cancer: review of 46 cases. *Int J Clin Pract.* 2007;61(1):52–61.

231. Kupeli S, Varan A, Ozyar E, et al. Treatment results of 84 patients with nasopharyngeal carcinoma in childhood. *Pediatr Blood Cancer.* 2006;46(4): 454–458.

232. Douglass EC, Fontanesi J, Ribeiro RC, Hawkins E. Improved long-term disease-free survival in nasopharyngeal carcinoma (NPC) in childhood and adolescence: a multi-institution treatment protocol. *Proc Am Soc Clin Oncol.* 1996;15(Abstract 1470): 2007.

233. Mertens R, Granzen B, Lassay L, et al. Treatment of nasopharyngeal carcinoma in children and adolescents: definitive results of a multicenter study (NPC-91-GPOH). *Cancer.* 2005;104(5):1083–1089.

234. Orbach D, Brisse H, Helfre S, et al. Radiation and chemotherapy combination for nasopharyngeal carcinoma in children: radiotherapy dose adaptation after chemotherapy response to minimize late effects. *Pediatr Blood Cancer.* 2008; 50(4):849–853.

235. Nakamura RA, Novaes PE, Antoneli CB, et al. High-dose-rate brachytherapy as part of a multidisciplinary treatment of nasopharyngeal lymphoepithelioma in childhood. *Cancer.* 2005;104(3):525–531.

236. Louis CU, Paulino AC, Gottschalk S, et al. A single institution experience with pediatric nasopharyngeal carcinoma: high incidence of toxicity associated with platinum-based chemotherapy plus IMRT. *J Pediatr Hematol Oncol.* 2007;29(7):500–505.

237. Brizel DM, Wasserman TH, Henke M, et al. Phase III randomized trial of amifostine as a radioprotector in head and neck cancer. *J Clin Oncol.* 2000; 18(19):3339–3345.

238. Bourhis J, Rosine D. Radioprotective effect of amifostine in patients with head and neck squamous cell carcinoma. *Semin Oncol.* 2002;29(6 Suppl 19): 61–62.

239. Kam MK, Leung SF, Zee B, et al. Prospective randomized study of intensity-modulated radiotherapy on salivary gland function in early-stage nasopharyngeal carcinoma patients. *J Clin Oncol.* 2007;25(31):4873–4879.

240. Priest JR, McDermott MB, Bhatia S, Watterson J, Manivel JC, Dehner LP. Pleuropulmonary blastoma: a clinicopathologic study of 50 cases. *Cancer.* 1997;80(1):147–161.

241. Manivel JC, Priest JR, Watterson J, et al. Pleuropulmonary blastoma: the so-called pulmonary blastoma of childhood. *Cancer.* 1988;62(8):1516–1526.

242. Dehner LP. Pleuropulmonary blastoma is THE pulmonary blastoma of childhood. *Semin Diagn Pathol.* 1994;11(2):144–151.

243. Priest JR, Watterson J, Strong L, et al. Pleuropulmonary blastoma: a marker for familial disease. *J Pediatr.* 1996;128(2):220–224.

244. Taube JM, Griffin CA, Yonescu R, et al. Pleuropulmonary blastoma: cytogenetic and spectral karyotype analysis. *Pediatr Dev Pathol.* 2006;9(6):453–461.

245. Hong B, Chen Z, Coffin CM, et al. Molecular cytogenetic analysis of a pleuropulmonary blastoma. *Cancer Genet Cytogenet.* 2003;142(1):65–69.

246. Kusafuka T, Kuroda S, Inoue M, et al. *P53* gene mutations in pleuropulmonary blastomas. *Pediatr Hematol Oncol.* 2002;19(2):117–128.

247. Yang P, Hasegawa T, Hirose T, et al. Pleuropulmonary blastoma: fluorescence in situ hybridization analysis indicating trisomy 2. *Am J Surg Pathol.* 1997; 21(7):854–859.

248. Novak R, Dasu S, Agamanolis D, Herold W, Malone J, Waterson J. Trisomy 8 is a characteristic finding in pleuropulmonary blastoma. *Pediatr Pathol Lab Med.* 1997;17(1):99–103.

249. Indolfi P, Casale F, Carli M, et al. Pleuropulmonary blastoma: management and prognosis of 11 cases. *Cancer.* 2000;89(6):1396–1401.

250. Priest JR, Magnuson J, Williams GM, et al. Cerebral metastasis and other central nervous system complications of pleuropulmonary blastoma. *Pediatr Blood Cancer.* 2007;49(3):266–273.

251. Pai S, Eng HL, Lee SY, Hsiao CC, Huang WT, Huang SC. Rhabdomyosarcoma arising within congenital cystic adenomatoid malformation. *Pediatr Blood Cancer.* 2005;45(6):841–845.

252. Allan BT, Day DL, Dehner LP. Primary pulmonary rhabdomyosarcoma of the lung in children: report of two cases presenting with spontaneous pneumothorax. *Cancer.* 1987;59(5):1005–1011.

253. Krous HF, Sexauer CL. Embryonal rhabdomyosarcoma arising within a congenital bronchogenic cyst in a child. *J Pediatr Surg.* 1981;16(4):506–508.

254. Ueda K, Gruppo R, Unger F, Martin L, Bove K. Rhabdomyosarcoma of lung arising in congenital cystic adenomatoid malformation. *Cancer.* 1977;40(1): 383–388.

255. Priest JR, Hill DA, Williams GM, et al. Type I pleuropulmonary blastoma: a report from the International Pleuropulmonary Blastoma Registry. *J Clin Oncol.* 2006;24(27):4492–4498.

256. Romeo C, Impellizzeri P, Grosso M, Vitarelli E, Gentile C. Pleuropulmonary blastoma: long-term survival and literature review. *Med Pediatr Oncol.* 1999; 33(4):372–376.

257. Parsons SK, Fishman SJ, Hoorntje LE, et al. Aggressive multimodal treatment of pleuropulmonary blastoma. *Ann Thorac Surg.* 2001;72(3):939–942.

258. Yusuf U, Dufour D, Jenrette JM, III, Abboud MR, Laver J, Barredo JC. Survival with combined modality therapy after intracerebral recurrence of pleuropulmonary blastoma. *Med Pediatr Oncol.* 1998;30(1):63–66.

259. Indolfi P, Bisogno G, Casale F, et al. Prognostic factors in pleuro-pulmonary blastoma. *Pediatr Blood Cancer.* 2007;48(3):318–323.

260. Ozkaynak MF, Ortega JA, Laug W, Gilsanz V, Isaacs H Jr. Role of chemotherapy in pediatric pulmonary blastoma. *Med Pediatr Oncol.* 1990;18(1):53–56.

261. Kaneko K, Isogai K, Kondo M, et al. Autologous peripheral blood stem cell transplantation in a patient with relapsed pleuropulmonary blastoma. *J Pediatr Hematol Oncol.* 2006;28(6):383–385.

262. de Castro CG Jr., de Almeida SG, Gregianin LJ, et al. High-dose chemotherapy and autologous peripheral blood stem cell rescue in a patient with pleuropulmonary blastoma. *J Pediatr Hematol Oncol.* 2003;25(1):78–81.

Supportive Care

Oncologic Emergencies

Kara M. Kelly

Introduction

Over the past several decades, the prognosis for childhood cancer has improved dramatically. With these advances comes the increased need for proper recognition and treatment of complications arising in children with cancer. Initial attention must be directed toward those problems that threaten vital organs or compromise the long-term quality of life of the child. Even before definitive therapy for the malignancy can begin, stabilization of the patient, often by the primary care physician, is required. Recognition of some common emergencies arising in a previously well child, which are the first sign of cancer, is essential. These conditions are reversible if recognized and treated promptly but have serious consequences if proper emergent care is not delivered.

Superior Vena Cava Syndrome

Superior vena cava syndrome (SVCS) is a clinical syndrome of superior vena cava compression or obstruction, frequently caused by mediastinal tumors.[1] Signs and symptoms are related to decreased venous return to the heart and increased venous pressure in the head, neck, and upper chest. These include orthopnea, headache, facial swelling, dizziness, or fainting, with symptoms often exacerbated by the Valsalva maneuver. Physical examination may reveal plethora and edema of the face and neck, jugular venous distension, papilledema, pulsus paradoxus, pallor, and possibly cardiorespiratory arrest with postural changes. In children, compression of the trachea, bronchi, and pulmonary vessels may coexist, and subsequent respiratory insufficiency may predominate. Symptoms may include cough, dyspnea, and air hunger with uncontrollable anxiety. Physical examination may reveal decreased air entry, wheezing, stridor, or cyanosis.

Malignant tumors are the most common primary cause of SVCS,[2] especially non-Hodgkin lymphoma (NHL) (primarily lymphoblastic or large cell), Hodgkin disease (HD), or T-cell acute lymphoblastic leukemia (ALL). Rarely, malignant teratoma, thymoma, thyroid cancer, neuroblastoma (NBL), rhabdomyosarcoma (RMS), or Ewing sarcoma (ES) may lead to obstruction. Thrombosis of central venous catheters is a secondary cause of SVCS.[1]

Initial investigations must be carefully planned because severe cardiovascular and/or respiratory collapse may occur following induction of general anesthesia, even in children without symptoms.[3] Laboratory studies should be used to determine the severity of the obstruction. Pulse oximetry and arterial blood gas measurement may be used to assess tissue oxygenation. Posteroanterior and lateral chest radiographs will reveal superior mediastinal widening, with tracheal compression or deviation if airway compromise coexists. Computed tomography (CT) imaging of the chest is used to assess the airway and the extent of thrombosis and collateral circulation, if the patient can tolerate recumbency (Figure 33-1). Imaging in the prone or lateral position may be better tolerated. Sedation should be avoided.

The diagnosis should be established by the least invasive measures.[1] Anemia, thrombocytopenia, leukopenia, or leukocytosis, as well as elevations of serum uric acid (UA) and lactate dehydrogenase, may be observed in patients with leukemia or lymphoma. Lymph node or bone marrow aspiration and biopsy, pleurocentesis, or periocardiocentesis may obviate the need for mediastinal

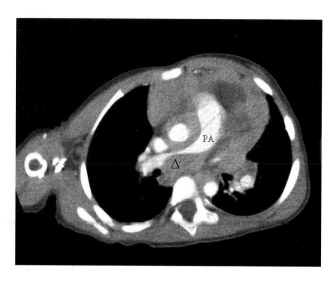

Figure 33-1 Compression of the pulmonary artery by a large anterior mediastinal mass in a child with a lymphoblastic lymphoma. Arrow demonstrates area of narrowing. Abbreviation: PA, pulmonary artery.

biopsy. Measurement of the serum markers α-fetoprotein and β-human chorionic gonadotropin may help diagnose a malignant germ cell tumor. If these studies are nondiagnostic, the patient must be carefully assessed prior to induction of general anesthesia. When tracheal area measured by CT of the chest is at least 50% of the area predicted for normal and pulmonary function tests show peak expiratory flow rates to be greater than 50% of predicted, general anesthesia should be tolerated.[4,5] Echocardiogram is necessary to evaluate cardiac motility and the degree of venous return impairment with suspected SVC obstruction. The anesthesiologist should consider the need for induction of anesthesia in the sitting position, avoidance of neuromuscular blocking agents, turning the patient to the semiprone position, and the availability of direct laryngoscopy, rigid bronchoscopy, and cardiopulmonary bypass. Factors associated with development of acute airway compromise include anterior location of the mediastinal mass, histologic diagnosis of lymphoma, symptoms and signs of SVCS, radiologic evidence of vessel compression or displacement, and presence of a pericardial effusion or pleural effusion.[6]

If a tissue diagnosis cannot be obtained, empiric therapy is necessary. The patient should be followed closely for improvement so that a biopsy may be performed as soon as possible. Chemotherapy including corticosteroids is recommended for children when HD, NHL, ALL, and chemosensitive solid tumors are suspected. Radiation therapy has historically been used, but its use may lead to tracheal swelling and further respiratory deterioration. Radiation therapy and chemotherapy, even when administered at low doses, may render the histologic diagnosis uninterpretable within 48 hours.[7,8] In patients with tumors less sensitive to chemotherapy or radiation, endovascular stent placement within the superior vena cava is associated with rapid and persistent symptom resolution.[9]

Spinal Cord Compression

Spinal cord compression occurs in approximately 2.7% to 5% of children with cancer[10,11] and 4% of children at diagnosis of cancer.[12] Although infrequent, prompt investigation and management are necessary to minimize irreversible neurologic damage with paralysis, sensory loss, and sphincter incompetence. Most often epidural compression of the cord results from extension of tumor through the intervertebral foramina (eg, "dumbbell tumor"), and less often from extension of tumor in the vertebral column. At the time of diagnosis, most cases in children are secondary to ES, NBL, NHL, and HD.[11,12] Cord compression is most often seen in the setting of disseminated disease. In patients with RMS or osteosarcoma, cord compression is associated with tumor recurrence. Rarely, primary astrocytoma and ependymoma present as intramedullary lesions. Compression of the vertebral venous plexus by tumor leads to vasogenic cord edema, venous hemorrhage, demyelination, and ischemia.[13,14]

Back pain in children should be investigated promptly, especially if a neurologic deficit is detected. Once a neurologic deficit appears, paraplegia may evolve within hours or days.[15] Back pain, localized or radicular, occurs in 80% to 94% of children with cord compression[12,16] and may be aggravated by movement, straight leg raising, neck flexion, recumbency, or the Valsalva maneuver.[15] Nighttime or constant pain and symptoms of less than 3 months' duration are more often associated with a diagnosis of tumor.[17] Weakness, sensory loss, and incontinence secondary to sphincter disturbance usually develop later. Sensory deficits are difficult to ascertain, especially in young children.

Imaging studies are necessary for further investigation. Although spine radiographs show abnormalities in up to 85% of adults,[18] in children, where cord compression typically occurs via extension through the intervertebral foramina, radiographs are abnormal in only 30% to 35% of patients.[12] Magnetic resonance imaging (MRI) is the imaging modality of choice.[19] Magnetic resonance imaging is noninvasive and provides the best images of the spinal cord, epidural space, and paravertebral areas (Figure 33-2). If MRI is unavailable, CT scan with contrast can be informative.[16]

History and neurologic examination determine the need and time course for radiologic investigations and institution of therapy. The patient with a history of rapidly progressing spinal cord dysfunction or the finding of neurologic deficits needs immediate attention. Dexamethasone, 1 mg/kg intravenously, should be administered, followed by emergent MRI study. A patient with a history of back pain but no abnormalities on neurologic exam may receive a lower dose of dexamethasone, 0.25 to 0.5 mg/kg orally every 6 hours, followed by MRI examination within the next 24 hours.[1] Although the doses are empiric, there is laboratory evidence for a dose-related benefit.[20,21]

In the patient where a tumor is demonstrated, the spinal cord must be relieved of the effects of compression promptly. Options include surgery, chemotherapy, and radiotherapy. The decision is based on the availability of a histologic diagnosis, the anticipated response to chemotherapy or radiotherapy, the extent of neurologic deficit, and the rate of progression of symptoms.[22] Surgery should

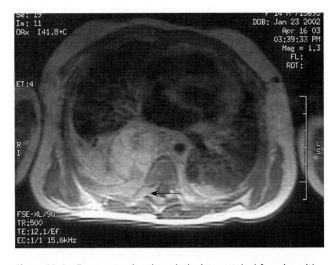

Figure 33-2 Tumor extension through the intervertebral foramina with subsequent spinal cord compression in a child with neuroblastoma. Arrow demonstrates tumor impingement on the cord.

be considered for the patient in whom the etiology of the tumor is not known to decompress the cord and to obtain tissue for diagnosis. Posterior laminectomy is usually sufficient in decompressing tumors that have reached the epidural space via the intervertebral foramina but may result in subluxation, scoliosis, and kyphosis in long-term survivors.[23,24] Chemotherapy is effective for certain tumor types, particularly NBL, NHL, HD, and ES,[10,25–27] and treats tumor at other sites too. Radiotherapy is effective for radiosensitive tumors in which the diagnosis is already known but is also associated with long-term scoliosis and kyphosis.[24,28] The full extent of disease must be delineated by MRI studies so that all sites of tumor can be included in the radiation field. If initially unrecognized, later radiotherapy may be compromised because of the need for overlapping portals.

The prognosis for neurologic recovery is most related to degree of disability at diagnosis, which in turn is associated with the duration of symptoms and time to diagnosis.[12,15] Patients who are ambulatory at diagnosis usually remain ambulatory. Children who are nonambulatory at diagnosis fare better than nonambulatory adults. Most adults will not regain function, but 50% of children regain the ability to ambulate.[12]

Hyperleukocytosis

Hyperleukocytosis, defined as a white blood cell count greater than $100\,000/\mu l$, is seen in 5% to 20% of children diagnosed with leukemia.[29] Clinically significant leukostasis is more often observed in patients with acute myeloid leukemia (AML). The presence of high numbers of circulating leukemic blast cells is associated with early morbidity and mortality from metabolic complications of rapid cell lysis, especially in children with ALL (see section on tumor lysis syndrome) or leukostasis in the pulmonary or cerebral vasculature, more commonly observed in children with AML.

The excessive leukocytes have been proposed to obstruct circulation in the lung, brain, or other organs by forming aggregates and white thrombi in small veins.[29] Viscosity is related to the deformability of cells

and the packed erythrocyte and packed leukocyte volumes.[30] Subsets of leukemia at greater risk for complications of hyperleukocytosis are listed in Table 33-1.[31] Myeloblasts and monoblasts, which tend to be larger than lymphoblasts and more rigid, are associated with a greater risk for vascular obstruction. Leukemic blast-endothelial cell interactions leading to microvascular disruption and bleeding may be related to upregulation and downregulation of adhesion molecules by leukemic blasts.[32-34]

The intracerebral and pulmonary circulations are more often affected by hyperleukocytosis. Patients may have no symptoms or present with mental status changes, seizures, papilledema or retinal venous distention, or frontal headache. Pulmonary leukostasis may lead to dyspnea, hypoxemia, and right ventricular failure. Chest radiographs may be normal or reveal diffuse interstitial infiltrates. Other signs include renal failure, bowel infarction, priapism, or dactylitis. Risk factors for early death include increasing leukocyte count, especially greater than $300\,000/\mu l$ in patients with myelomonocytic and monocytic subtypes of AML, and a cytocrit (hematocrit + leukocrit) greater than 30%.[35] Older age and the presence of respiratory distress, renal failure, neurologic symptoms, or coagulopathy are also poor prognostic factors.[36]

Specific antileukemic therapy should be initiated as soon as the patient is stabilized. Hydration should be started promptly. Platelet transfusions should be given to reduce the risk of intracranial hemorrhage in patients with thrombocytopenia. Coagulopathy, more prevalent with AML, should be corrected with fresh frozen plasma and vitamin K. Packed red blood cell transfusions will increase blood viscosity; the hemoglobin should not be raised above 10 g/dl. Similarly, diuretic use should be avoided until the white blood cell count is lowered.

The therapies for hyperleukocytosis have not been subject to a controlled study. Exchange transfusion and leukapheresis may rapidly lower the white blood cell count and metabolic load. Both are effective, with mean reductions in leukocyte count of 66% for exchange transfusion and 48% for leukapheresis.[37] In uncontrolled series, leukapheresis reduced the risk of tumor lysis syndrome in patients with

Table 33-1

Leukemic subsets associated with elevated risk for development of complications from hyperleukocytosis.

Type of Leukemia	Subset
Acute myeloid leukemia	Myelomonocytic
	Monocytic
	Microgranular variant of acute promyelocytic leukemia
	Presence of chromosome 11q23 rearrangements
	Presence of internal tandem duplications of the *FLT3* gene
Acute lymphoblastic leukemia	Presence of chromosome 11q23 rearrangements
	T cell

ALL,[35,38] but there are scant data for evaluating the effects of these procedures on the outcome of intracerebral hemorrhage or pulmonary leukostasis. Problems include a rapid rebound in leukocyte count, difficulty with intravascular access, and need for anticoagulation. In general, leukapheresis should be avoided in acute promyelocytic leukemia, because the procedure may further exacerbate the coagulopathic risk.[31]

Cranial radiation to a dose of 400 cGy has been used to decrease the risk of intracranial hemorrhage in patients with ALL[39,40] but is rarely used in current practice. Drugs targeting the leukocyte-endothelium interface, such as dexamethasone, require investigation.[34]

Tumor Lysis Syndrome

Tumor lysis syndrome (TLS) is a pattern of metabolic abnormalities resulting from rapid cell lysis. This syndrome results in the rapid release of potassium, phosphates, and nucleic acids into the circulation, leading to hyperkalemia, hyperphosphatemia, and hyperuricemia. It may progress to multiple organ failure and death.

Tumor lysis syndrome typically occurs at diagnosis or up to 5 days after the start of cytotoxic therapy. Tumor types associated with TLS are listed in Table 33-2. Highest risk for TLS is seen with a large tumor burden and high sensitivity to chemotherapy, as seen with Burkitt lymphoma or T-cell ALL.[41] Risk factors include bulky abdominal disease, elevated pretreatment serum UA and lactate dehydrogenase levels, and poor urine output.[42] Renal parenchymal tumor infiltration or ureteral or venous obstruction from tumor compression further increases the risk for renal failure.

Symptoms of hyperkalemia include gastrointestinal symptoms, weakness, or paralysis. At serum potassium levels of 7.0 to 7.5 mEq/L, an electrocardiogram will reveal QRS widening and peaked T waves. Without intervention, ventricular arrhythmias and death may occur. The risk of calcium phosphate precipitation is increased when the in vivo solubility of calcium-phosphorus (Ca × P) is greater than 58.[43] Tissue damage may present as renal failure, pruritic or gangrenous changes in the skin, or inflammation of the eyes or joints. Signs and symptoms of hypocalcemia include anorexia, vomiting, cramps, carpopedal spasms, tetany, seizures, alterations in consciousness, or cardiac arrest. Patients with UA levels of 10 to 15 mg/dl may present with nonspecific symptoms of lethargy, nausea, or vomiting.[44] Frank renal failure is usually not seen until the level reaches 20 mg/dl, but it may occur at lower levels in association with other metabolic derangements.[44]

The treatment of TLS is ideally preventative.[1] Metabolic stability should be achieved prior to initiation of chemotherapy but not delayed too long, because there will be a continued increase in tumor burden until definitive tumor-directed therapy is started. A risk assessment based on laboratory findings has been developed (Table 33-3).[45] Patients with laboratory TLS are at higher risk for progression to cardiac arrhythmias, seizures, and death. General preventative measures include aggressive intravenous hydration (3 L/m2/day) with appropriate use of diuretics to promote urine output and close monitoring of laboratory values to correct electrolyte imbalances promptly. Urine alkalinization through the use of intravenous sodium bicarbonate has been recommended for prevention and treatment of hyperuricemia. Its use is generally not required with the use of newer hypouricemic agents such as recombinant urate oxidase.[46] Historically, allopurinol has been widely used to decrease UA production, and its use has led to a reduction in the incidence of UA-associated obstructive uropathy in patients with hematologic malignancies.[47,48] Allopurinol is a competitive inhibitor of xanthine oxidase, the enzyme that catalyzes the conversion of the purine degradation products, xanthine, and hypoxanthine to UA. Its effectiveness may be limited in some patients with exceptionally high serum UA levels. Xanthine precipitation may contribute to renal failure.[49] Also, allopurinol does not reduce preformed UA; thus, significant decrements in serum UA levels may take

Table 33-2

Tumor types associated with risk for development of tumor lysis syndrome.

Risk Group	Tumor Type
High	Burkitt lymphoma
	Lymphoblastic lymphoma
	T-cell acute lymphoblastic leukemia
Moderate	Large cell lymphoma
	B-precursor acute lymphoblastic leukemia
	Acute myeloid leukemia
Low (case reports only)	Neuroblastoma
	Medulloblastoma
	Hepatoblastoma
	Germ cell tumor

Table 33-3

Laboratory results associated with increased risk for development of complications of TLS. The risk is increased with an abnormality in 2 or more of the following and occurs within the period from 3 days before or 7 days after chemotherapy.[45]

Laboratory Test	Value
Uric acid	>8 mg/dL, or 25% increase
Potassium	>6 meq/L, or 25% increase
Phosphate	>4.5 mg/dL or 25% increase
Calcium	<7 mg/dL, or 25% decrease

2 to 3 days, assuming normal renal function.[46] Allopurinol is primarily excreted in the urine and not readily removed during hemodialysis, so significant dose reductions may be needed with renal failure.[50] Allopurinol may be safely used in patients with a low risk for development of TLS.[46]

Urate oxidase, an enzyme that occurs in all mammals other than primates, converts UA to allantoin, 5 to 10 times more soluble than UA, thereby promoting UA excretion.[51,52] Recombinant urate oxidase more rapidly and significantly lowers UA levels in patients with hematologic malignancies compared with allopurinol.[53] Its use should be considered in patients at moderate to high risk for development of TLS.[46] Hemolysis may occur in patients with G-6PD deficiency or methemoglobinemia.[46]

Prevention and treatment of electrolyte imbalances is critical.[1] Oral potassium intake should be stopped. The potassium-binding resin Kayexalate may be given. Rectal administration should be avoided. Calcium gluconate may be given to augment myocardial conduction and shift potassium intracellularly. Sodium bicarbonate will also lead to potassium influx by inducing efflux of hydrogen ions. Similarly, regular insulin with dextrose will promote intracellular flow of potassium. Phosphate excretion may be aided with the addition of aluminum hydroxide, although its utility in lowering phosphorus levels may be slow and unpredictable. Treatment of hypocalcemia must take into account the level of serum phosphorus, because administration of calcium may increase calcium phosphate precipitation. Calcium gluconate is given if severe symptoms of hypocalcemia are present. Severe alkalosis may further reduce ionized calcium and therefore should be avoided.

When conservative measures are ineffective in correcting electrolyte disturbances and improving urinary flow, dialysis may be necessary. Hemodialysis is preferred over peritoneal dialysis because it is more rapid and effective at removing UA and phosphorus.[54] Although conventional hemodialysis is most efficient at correcting the metabolic abnormalities, continuous hemofiltration may play a role in the management of those critically ill patients who cannot tolerate the osmotic shifts associated with hemodialysis.[55]

References

1. Kelly KM, Lange B. Oncologic emergencies. *Pediatr Clin North Am.* 1997;44(4):809–830.
2. King RM, Telander RL, Smithson WA, Banks PM, Han MT. Primary mediastinal tumors in children. *J Pediatr Surg.* 1982;17(5):512–520.
3. Hammer GB. Anaesthetic management for the child with a mediastinal mass. *Paediatr Anaesth.* 2004;14(1):95–97.
4. Shamberger RC. Preanesthetic evaluation of children with anterior mediastinal masses. *Sem Pediatr Surg.* 1999;8(2):61–68.
5. Shamberger RC, Holzman RS, Griscom NT, Tarbell NJ, Weinstein HJ, Wohl ME. Prospective evaluation by computed tomography and pulmonary function tests of children with mediastinal masses. *Surgery.* 1995;118(3):468–471.
6. Lam JCM, Chui CH, Jacobsen AS, Tan AM, Joseph VT. When is a mediastinal mass critical in a child? an analysis of 29 patients. *Pediatr Surg Int.* 2004;20(3):180–184.
7. Halpern S, Chatten J, Meadows AT, Byrd R, Lange B. Anterior mediastinal masses: anesthesia hazards and other problems. *J Pediatr.* 1983;102(3):407–410.
8. Loeffler JS, Leopold KA, Recht A, Weinstein HJ, Tarbell NJ. Emergency prebiopsy radiation for mediastinal masses: impact on subsequent pathologic diagnosis and outcome. *J Clin Oncol.* 1986;4(5):716–721.
9. Rowell NP, Gleeson FV. 2002. Steroids, radiotherapy, chemotherapy and stents for superior vena caval obstruction in carcinoma of the bronchus: a systematic review. *Clin Oncol (R Coll Radiol).* 2002;14(5):338–351.
10. Ch'ien LT, Kalwinsky DK, Peterson G, et al. Metastatic epidural tumors in children. *Med Pediatr Oncol.* 1982;10(5):455–462.
11. Klein SL, Sanford RA, Muhlbauer MS. Pediatric spinal epidural metastases. *J Neurosurg.* 1991;74(1):70–75.
12. Lewis DW, Packer RJ, Raney B, Rak IW, Belasco J, Lange B. Incidence, presentation, and outcome of spinal cord disease in children with systemic cancer. *Pediatrics.* 1986;78(3):438–443.
13. Kato A, Ushio Y, Hayakawa T, Yamadak K, Ikeda H, Mogami H. Circulatory disturbance of the spinal cord with epidural neoplasm in rats. *J Neurosurg.* 1985;63(2):260–265.
14. Manabe S, Tanaka H, Higo Y, Park P, Ohno T, Tateishi A. Experimental analysis of the spinal cord compressed by spinal metastasis. *Spine.* 1989;14(12):1308–1315.
15. Byrne TN. Spinal cord compression from epidural metastases. *N Engl J Med.* 1992;327(9):614–619.
16. Pollono D, Tomarchia S, Drut R, Ibanez O, Ferreyra M, Cedola J. Spinal cord compression: a review of 70 pediatric patients. *Pediatr Hematol Oncol.* 2003;20(6):457–466.
17. Feldman DS, Hedden DM, Wright JG. The use of bone scan to investigate back pain in children and adolescents. *J Pediatr Orthoped.* 2000;20(6):790–795.
18. Stark RJ, Henson RA, Evans SJW. Spinal metastases: a retrospective survey from a general hospital. *Brain.* 1982;105(Pt 1):189–213.
19. Zimmerman RA, Bilaniuk LT. Imaging of tumors in the spinal canal and cord. *Radiol Clin North Am.* 1988;26(5):965–1007.
20. Delattre JY, Arbit E, Thaler HT, Rosenblum MK, Posner JB. A dose-response study of dexamethasone in a model of spinal cord compression caused by epidural tumor. *J Neurosurg.* 1989;70(6):920–925.
21. Ushio Y, Posner R, Posner JB, Shapiro WR. Experimental spinal cord compression by epidural neoplasm. *Neurology.* 1977;27(5):422–429.
22. Nicolin G. Emergencies and their management. *Eur J Cancer.* 2002;38(10):1365–1377.
23. Raimondi AJ, Gutierrez FA, Di Rocco C. Laminotomy and total reconstruction of the posterior spinal arch for spinal canal surgery in childhood. *J Neurosurg.* 1976;45(5):555–560.
24. Mayfield JK, Riseborough EJ, Jaffe N, Nehme ME. Spinal deformity in children treated for neuroblastoma. *J Bone Joint Surg.* 1981;63(2):183–193.
25. Posner JB, Howieson J, Cvitkovic E. "Disappearing" spinal cord compression: oncolytic effect of glucocorticoids (and other chemotherapeutic agents) on epidural metastases. *Ann Neurol.* 1977;2(5):409–413.
26. Sanderson IR, Pritchard J, Marsh HT. Chemotherapy as the initial treatment of spinal neuroblastoma. *J Neurosurg.* 1989;70(5):688–690.
27. Plantaz D, Rubie H, Michon J, et al. The treatment of neuroblastoma with intraspinal extension with chemotherapy followed by surgical removal of residual disease. *Cancer.* 1996;78(2):311–319.
28. Riseborough EJ, Grabias SL, Burton RI, Jaffe N. Skeletal alterations following irradiation for Wilms' tumor: with particular reference to scoliosis and kyphosis. *J Bone Joint Surg.* 1976;58(4):526–536.
29. Lichtman MA, Rowe JM. Hyperleukocytic leukemias: rheological, clinical, and therapeutic considerations. *Blood.* 1982;60(2):279–283.
30. Field M, Block JB, Levin R, Rall DP. Significance of blood lactate elevations among patients with acute leukemia and other neoplastic proliferative disorders. *Am J Med.* 1966;40:528–547.
31. Blum W, Porcu P. Therapeutic apheresis in hyperleukocytosis and hyperviscosity syndrome. *Sem Thromb Hemost.* 2007;33(4):350–354.
32. Opdenakker G, Fibbe WE, Van Damme J. The molecular basis of leukocytosis. *Immunol Today.* 1998;19(4):182–189.
33. Stucki A, Rivier AS, Gikic M, Monai N, Shapira M, Spertini O. Endothelial cell activation by myeloblasts: molecular mechanisms of leukostasis and leukemic cell dissemination. *Blood.* 2001;97(7):2121–2129.
34. Porcu P, Farag S, Marcucci G, Cataland SR, Kennedy MS, Bissell M. Leukocytoreduction for acute leukemia. *Ther Apher.* 2002;6(1):15–23.
35. Bunin NJ, Pui CH. Differing complications of hyperleukocytosis in children with acute lymphoblastic or acute nonlymphoblastic leukemia. *J Clin Oncol.* 1985;3(12):1590–1595.
36. Porcu P, Danielson CF, Orazi A, Heerema NA, Gabig TG, McCarthy LJ. Therapeutic leukapheresis in hyperleukocytic leukemias: lack of correlation between degree of cytoreduction and early mortality rate. *Br J Haematol.* 1997;98:433–436.
37. Nelson SC, Bruggers CS, Kurtzberg J, Friedman HS. Management of leukemic hyperleukocytosis with hydration, urinary alkalinization, and allopurinol: are cranial irradiation and invasive cytoreduction necessary? *Am J Pediatr Hematol/Oncol.* 1993;15(3):351–355.
38. Maurer HS, Steinherz PG, Gaynon PS, et al. The effect of initial management of hyperleukocytosis on early complications and outcome of children with acute lymphoblastic leukemia. *J Clin Oncol.* 1988;6(9):1425–1432.
39. Gilchrist GS, Fountain KS, Dearth JC, Smithson WA, Burget EO Jr. Cranial irradiation in the management of extreme leukemic leukocytosis complicating childhood acute lymphocytic leukemia. *J Pediatr.* 1981;98(2):257–259.
40. Wald BR, Heisel MA, Ortega JA. Frequency of early death in children with acute leukemia presenting with hyperleukocytosis. *Cancer.* 1982;50(1):150–153.
41. Stapleton FB, Strother DR, Roy S III, Wyatt RJ, McKay CP, Murphy SB. Acute renal failure at onset of therapy for advanced stage Burkitt lymphoma and B cell acute lymphoblastic lymphoma. *Pediatrics.* 1988;82(6):863–869.

42. Cohen LF, Balow JE, Magrath IT, Poplack DG, Ziegler JL. Acute tumor lysis syndrome: a review of 37 patients with Burkitt's lymphoma. *Am J Med.* 1980; 68(4):486–491.

43. Herbert LA, Lemann J Jr, Petersen JR, Lennon EJ. Studies of the mechanism by which phosphate infusion lowers serum calcium concentration. *J Clin Invest.* 1966;45(2):1886–1894.

44. Allegretta GJ, Weisman SJ, Altman AJ. Oncologic emergencies. I. metabolic and space-occupying consequences of cancer and cancer treatment. *Pediatr Clin North Am.* 1985;32(3):601–611.

45. Cairo MS, Bishop M. Tumour lysis syndrome: new therapeutic strategies and classification. *Br J Haematol.* 2004;127(1):3–11.

46. Cairo MS. Prevention and treatment of hyperuricemia in hematological malignancies. *Clin Lymphoma.* 2002;3:S26–S31.

47. Spector T. Inhibition of urate production by allopurinol. *Biochemical Pharmacology.* 1977;26(5):355–358.

48. DeConti RC, Calabresi P. Use of allopurinol for prevention and control of hyperuricemia in patients with neoplastic disease. *N Engl J Med.* 1966;274(9): 481–486.

49. Andreoli SP, Clark JH, McGuire WA, Bergstein JM. Purine excretion during tumor lysis in children with acute lymphocytic leukemia receiving allopurinol: relationship to acute renal failure. *J Pediatr.* 1986;109(2):292–298.

50. Elion GB, Benezra FM, Beardmore TD, Kelley WN. Studies with allopurinol in patients with impaired renal function. *Adv Exp Med Biol.* 1980;122A:263–267.

51. Masera G, Jankovic M, Zurlo MG, et al. Urate-oxidase prophylaxis of uric acid-induced renal damage in childhood leukemia. *J Pediatr.* 1982;100(1): 152–155.

52. Brogard JM, Coumaros D, Franckhauser J, Stahl A, Stahl J. Enzymatic uricolysis: a study of the effect of a fungal urate-oxydase. *Eur J Clin Biol Res.* 1972; 17(9):890–895.

53. Goldman SC, Holcenberg JS, Finklestein JZ, et al. A randomized comparison between rasburicase and allopurinol in children with lymphoma and leukemia at high risk for tumor lysis. *Blood.* 2001;97(10):2998–3003.

54. Jeha S. Tumor lysis syndrome. *Sem Hematol.* 2001;38(4 Suppl 10):4–8.

55. Bishof NA, Welch TR, Strife CF, Ryckman FC. Continuous hemodiafiltration in children. *Pediatrics.* 1990;85(5):819–823.

Prevention, Diagnosis, and Treatment of Infectious Complications

Thomas W. McLean and Sarah W. Alexander

Introduction

Infection in pediatric oncology patients is a common cause of morbidity and mortality. Patients may have immune suppression from both the underlying malignancy and, often to an even greater degree, the therapy. This chapter reviews the current practices for the prevention, diagnosis, and treatment of infectious complications in pediatric oncology patients.

Prevention

General Preventive Measures

Education of the patient and family is crucial in helping to prevent infection in the immunocompromised host. Although a simple concept, hand washing remains the single best intervention for lowering infection risks in the hospital.[1,2] Alcohol-based hand antiseptics are equally efficacious and may promote better compliance with hand cleansing.[3,4] In general, patients should avoid sick contacts, dirty or crowded environments, and construction sites.[5] Good nutrition is an important preventative measure, although there is little evidence of the benefits of the "neutropenic diet."[6] Good oral hygiene is also important for preventing infection and minimizing mucositis pain.[7,8] The hospital and clinic environment should be clean, and there should be appropriate respiratory isolation rooms, laminar airflow rooms, high-efficiency particulate air filters, and (ideally) separate clinic waiting areas apart from the general pediatric waiting areas.

Central venous lines (CVLs) have well-documented benefits as well as risks, including infection. Strategies to minimize CVL-associated infection include avoiding insertion with neutropenia and the use of perioperative antibiotics.[9–11] Blood products should be routinely screened for infectious agents and filtered (and irradiated, to prevent graft-versus-host disease) for all immunosuppressed patients. Although clear data are lacking, severely immunocompromised patients (eg, undergoing stem cell transplant or acute myeloid leukemia [AML] induction) should probably avoid plants and flowers (dried or fresh).[5]

The pediatric oncology patient should have minimal to no manipulation of the anus and rectum because of the area's potential to seed the bloodstream with bacteria should the rectal mucosa become breached.[12] On a practical level, this means that neutropenic patients should not have enemas or suppositories given, rectal temperatures taken, or digital rectal exams performed. Educating the patient and family of this risk is crucial for preventing such infections.

Immunizations

The schedule of routine childhood immunizations needs to be significantly modified for children undergoing cancer chemotherapy. In general, vaccines are not given while a child is receiving chemotherapy or for the 3 to 6 months following, a time period to allow for T-cell reconstitution.[13]

Inactivated vaccines (DTaP, Hep B, IPV, Hib, pneumococcal, and HPV) are usually not administered during this period because the response to the vaccine may be inadequate. An exception is the influenza vaccine, which is recommended yearly for children with cancer.[14] Most live vaccines (MMR, OPV, BCG, *Salmonella typhi*) are contraindicated during this period.[15] The exception to this is the use of varicella vaccine in children with acute lymphoblastic leukemia (ALL) who have been in remission for more than 1 year, for whom it has been shown to be safe and effective.[16] It should be noted, however, that at least 1 death has been attributed to the varicella vaccine given to a child on therapy for ALL.[17] Household contacts (siblings) should receive immunizations per the regularly recommended schedule (including the live vaccines MMR and varicella); however, they should receive IPV instead of OPV. In addition, family members should be encouraged to receive yearly influenza vaccines.[15]

Prophylaxis

Antimicrobial prophylaxis is widely used in the care of children and adults with cancer. As with any pharmacologic prophylaxis, there is always a concern for the regimen leading to the emergence of resistant pathogens.

Prophylaxis for pneumonia caused by *Pneumocystis jiroveci* (formerly known as *P. carinii*) is indicated in almost all children undergoing cancer chemotherapy. In addition, children receiving high-dose steroids need *Pneumocystis* prophylaxis. The drug of choice is trimethoprim-sulfamethoxazole (TMP-SMX). The dose should be approximately 150 mg TMP/m^2/day divided twice a day, for 3 consecutive days a week. A recent study shows that 2 days a week is also efficacious.[18] Alternative prophylactic agents include aerosolized or intravenous pentamidine, dapsone, and atovaquone.[19–22]

The use of prophylactic antibacterial agents during periods of neutropenia is generally not recommended.[23] Studies of both TMP-SMX and ciprofloxacin in both pediatric and adult patients have shown decreased rates of infection but have not decreased overall mortality.[24–26] The use of quinolone antibiotics (such as ciprofloxacin) in children is limited somewhat by concern of toxicity to cartilage and other connective tissue. The primary concern with either regimen is the emergence of resistant pathogens.

Fluconazole is recommended for prophylaxis against invasive *Candida albicans* infections in patients undergoing stem cell transplantation.[27–29] Concern for broader application of fluconazole prophylaxis is the finding of colonization with more resistant Candidal species, specifically *C. krusei* and *C. glabrata*.[30] The use of amphotericin or its lipid formulations for prophylaxis is not generally recommended.[31–33] Newer agents such as voriconazole, caspofungin, and posaconazole may prove to be effective preventative agents in the future.

Common viruses can cause severe disease in children receiving chemotherapy. Any child who is at risk for varicella and has an exposure should receive varicella-zoster virus (VZV) immune globulin with 96 hours, and steroid therapy should be held.[15,34] In stem cell transplant patients, acyclovir decreases VZV infection during the first year after transplant.[35] Respiratory syncytial virus (RSV) can cause fatal pneumonias in children with cancer, especially those being treated for AML and those undergoing stem cell transplantation.[36] Respiratory syncytial virus–immune globulin and palivizumab have been extensively studied in premature infants,[37] and palivizumab is now recommended (15 mg/kg IM every month during RSV season) for infants being treated for ALL. Prophylaxis against herpes simplex virus (HSV) and cytomegalovirus (CMV) (with acyclovir and ganciclovir, respectively) has become an important component of the care of stem cell transplant patients but usually is not required for those receiving standard chemotherapy.

Intravenous immunoglobulin is not generally recommended for children undergoing cancer chemotherapy; however, there may be a subset of children (such as infants with ALL and patients of any age following a stem cell transplant) who develop hypogammaglobulinemia who may benefit from monthly prophylaxis.[38]

Lastly, similar to children with congenital heart disease at risk of endocarditis,[39] patients with cancer are widely presumed to be at risk of CVL infection during episodes of transient bacteremia. Despite a lack of clear data, pediatric oncology patients with CVLs are generally treated with amoxicillin (or clindamycin for those who are penicillin allergic) 1 hour prior to invasive procedures such as dental manipulations or procedures involving the gastrointestinal or genitourinary tract.

Hematopoietic Colony-Stimulating Factors

Filgrastim (granulocyte colony-stimulating factor [G-CSF]) and sargramostim (granulocyte-macrophage colony-stimulating factor [GM-CSF]) increase the number and phagocytic function of polymorphonuclear cells in the blood. The use of these agents in patients receiving chemotherapy has been shown to cause a modest reduction in number of days of neutropenia, days of fever, and length of hospitalization. No clear evidence for decreasing overall infection-related mortality has been demonstrated.[40,41]

The American Society of Clinical Oncology has created guidelines for the use of CSFs. In general, primary prophylaxis is recommended when the expected frequency of febrile neutropenia is ≥ 40%. In addition, special circumstances (such as extensive prior chemotherapy or a history of fever and neutropenia) may warrant CSF use. Colony-stimulating factors are also warranted following autologous and allogeneic stem cell therapy.[42] The initiation of growth factors at the time of presentation with febrile neutropenia (secondary prophylaxis) has shown little clinical benefit.[43,44]

Diagnosis

History

Obtaining a history is obviously important in establishing a diagnosis of infection in the pediatric oncology patient, and the chief complaint is usually the most important part of the history. For any symptom it is important to explore quality, duration, location, severity, and precipitating events. Fever (typically defined as an oral temperature > 38° C or 100.4° F) is often the only symptom, but chills, pain (eg, throat, chest, or abdominal), cough, rhinorrhea, nausea, vomiting, diarrhea, or rash may all result from infection. The presence of localizing symptoms should be explored. The patient's type and location of malignancy, most recent therapy, and past infection history should be obtained from both the patient and medical records, if available, because these factors may influence management.

Physical Exam

A thorough physical exam should be done on all patients suspected of having infection, with a focus on the sites of concern. Vital signs should be done on all patients, avoiding rectal temperatures. The anus and perirectal site should be inspected and gently palpated, however, because abscesses may arise there. Of note is that neutropenic patients may not produce pus due to lack of neutrophils. Upon count recovery, abscesses may become more evident. Purplish discoloration around otherwise minor skin lesions may represent cellulitis. In herpes-zoster infections, pain may precede the skin eruption.

Laboratory and Radiologic Assessment

All febrile patients should have a blood culture and complete blood count obtained. The presence and degree of neutropenia will usually have direct management implications. If a CVL is present, all lumens should be cultured. It is unclear whether a peripheral blood culture is needed in addition. Other cultures (urine, stool, throat, sputum, skin/wound, cerebrospinal fluid) should be obtained as clinically indicated. Nasopharyngeal swabs may be indicated to test for viral infections such as RSV, influenza, parainfluenza, and adenovirus. Electrolytes, renal, and liver function tests should be assessed if clinically indicated. Routine chest radiographs are not necessary unless the patient has respiratory signs or symptoms.[45] Ultrasound, computed tomography (CT) and/or magnetic resonance imaging scanning may be useful if deep-seeded infection is suspected. In addition, if fever and neutropenia persist for 5 days or more, CT scans (typically of the sinuses, chest, abdomen, and pelvis) are often obtained prior to starting antifungal therapy.

Treatment

Antibiotics

The most appropriate treatment for febrile oncology patients needs to be assessed on an individual basis; however, evidence-based guidelines for empiric antimicrobial choices are broadly employed.[23] Factors that affect decision making often include the history and physical exam as well as laboratory parameters, most importantly the absolute neutrophil count (ANC). Figure 34-1 summarizes the evaluation and management of the child with fever and neutropenia.

Patients who are febrile and neutropenic (ANC < 500 per mm^3) should be treated with broad-spectrum intravenous antibiotics as inpatients. There are multiple well-studied empiric regimens, some of which utilize

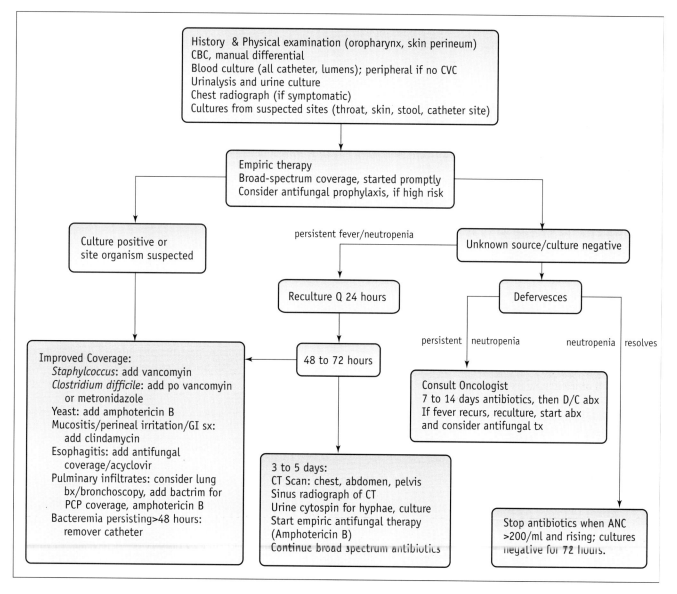

Figure 34-1 Evaluation and management of the child with fever and neutropenia. Abbreviations: CBC, complete blood count; CVC, central venous catheter; PCP, *Pneumocystis carinii* pneumonia; CT, computed tomography; ANC, absolute neutrophil count.

monotherapy where others employ a combination of antimicrobial agents (Table 34-1). Regimens are designed to provide early coverage for pathogens that are potentially lethal if not treated expeditiously. There is no single best regimen. Choice of antibiotics depends on awareness of the resistance patterns of bacteria in one's own institution, as well as side effects, ease of administration, and costs.

Modifications of empiric therapy at the time of the patient's presentation with fever and neutropenia are often required based on specific clinical and laboratory findings (see Figure 34-1). A history of penicillin or cephalosporin allergy often complicates antibiotic choice.

The use of empiric vancomycin has received considerable attention with studies providing mixed results.[46–48] There are some clinical situations in which the empiric use of vancomycin is indicated,[23] as for patients presenting with signs of overt or impending sepsis, those with obvious CVL infections, and those whose therapy is associated with a higher risk of invasive streptococcal infections—for example, patients undergoing AML induction.[49,50] If started empirically, vancomycin should be stopped as soon as it is deemed unnecessary. In general, however, the routine empiric use of vancomycin is discouraged because of concerns of evolving resistance in staphylococcal and enterococcal pathogens.

Not all patients with fever and neutropenia are at the same level of risk for invasive bacterial infections. Investigators have suggested that factors contributing to lower risk of infection include being clinically well, having a nonfocal physical exam, having cancer that is in remission, and becoming afebrile shortly after presentation with evidence of bone marrow recovery. Several studies have been done to assess whether patients with "low risk" febrile neutropenia can be safely treated with modified therapy, including the use of oral antibiotics in the outpatient setting.[51] In general, results have been encouraging; however, no consensus exists regarding the definition of "low risk," and this practice should be used with caution.

Individuals with an ANC greater than 500 per mm³ (with or without a CVL) who are clinically well without focal infection and who have reliable care providers are often treated with empiric intravenous antibiotics (eg, ceftriaxone) in the outpatient setting; however, evaluation and management of these patients varies considerably.[52]

Antifungal Agents

Patients with persistent fevers and neutropenia (5 days or more) are at significant risk for invasive fungal infections (most commonly *Candida* and *Aspergillus*) and require empiric antifungal therapy, the standard of which is amphotericin B. In some institutions, liposomal amphotericin has largely replaced standard amphotericin because several large studies have shown equal efficacy and less renal toxicity; however, the cost is significantly higher.[53,54] For patients with documented fungal infections the drug of choice may be modified. For example, a patient with fungemia due to a sensitive *Candida* species may be treated successfully with fluconazole. Voriconazole is more effective and less toxic than amphotericin B for patients with invasive aspergillosis.[55] New antifungal agents such as caspofungin, posaconazole are increasingly being used in pediatric oncology patients, and studies to date suggest they are safe and effective.[56]

Antiviral Agents

Viral infections may be life threatening in the immuno-compromised host. Acyclovir is indicated for the treatment of infections caused by VZV and HSV types 1 and 2. Ganciclovir is indicated for the treatment of CMV infection. Aerosolized ribavirin may be considered in the treatment of RSV pneumonia. Amantadine is effective in the treatment of influenza A; oseltamivir and zanamivir are active against both influenza A and B, although their roles have yet to be defined in pediatric oncology patients.[57]

Conclusions and Future Directions

In summary, pediatric oncology patients are at serious risk of infection. With patient and family education, prophylactic strategies, and prompt evaluation and treatment, most infections can be prevented and successfully treated. As we move into the era of targeted cancer therapies, the degree of immunosuppression and infection risk should lessen. Improved disease risk stratification will allow less toxic therapy to some patients and identification of other patients at high risk for infection. Faster and more accurate diagnostic tests will lead to improved management.

Table 34-1		
Empiric antibiotic regimens for pediatric oncology patients with fever and neutropenia.		
Monotherapy	Cefepime	
	Ceftazidime	
	Carbapenum (imipenum-cilastin or meropenum)	
	Pipericillin-tazobactam	
Two-drug therapy	Cefepime	
	Ceftazidime	+ aminoglycoside
	Carbapenum	(gentamicin, tobramycin,
	Antipseudomonal penicillin	or amikacin)

Finally, the development and assessment of new antimicrobial agents will aid clinicians caring for pediatric oncology patients.

References

1. Rowin ME, Patel VV, Christenson JC. Pediatric intensive care unit nosocomial infections: epidemiology, sources and solutions. *Crit Care Clin.* 2003;19:473–487.
2. Saloojee H, Steenhoff A. The health professional's role in preventing nosocomial infections. *Postgrad Med J.* 2001;77:16–19.
3. Barrau K, Rovery C, Drancourt M, Brouqui P. Hand antisepsis: evaluation of a sprayer system for alcohol distribution. *Infect Control Hosp Epidemiol.* 2003;24:180–183.
4. Maury E, Alzieu M, Baudel JL, et al. Alcohol-based handwashing agent improves hand washing. *Infect Control Hosp Epidemiol.* 2000;21:617–618.
5. Dykewicz CA, Kaplan JE. *Guidelines for Preventing Opportunistic Infections Among Hematopoietic Stem Cell Transplant Recipients: Recommendations of CDC, the Infectious Disease Society of America, and the American Society of Blood and Marrow Transplantation.* MMWR. 2000;49(RR10):1–128. http://www.cdc.gov/mmwr//preview/mmwrhtml/rr4910a1.htm. Accessed July 30, 2007.
6. Moody K, Charlson ME, Finlay J. The neutropenic diet: what's the evidence? *J Pediatr Hematol Oncol.* 2002;24:717–721.
7. Cheng KK, Molassiotis A, Chang AM, Wai WC, Cheung SS. Evaluation of an oral care protocol intervention in the prevention of chemotherapy-induced oral mucositis in paediatric cancer patients. *Eur J Cancer.* 2001;37:2056–2063.
8. Scully C, Epstein J, Sonis S. Oral mucositis: a challenging complication of radiotherapy, chemotherapy, and radiochemotherapy. Part 2: diagnosis and management of mucositis. *Head Neck.* 2004;26:77–84.
9. Rackoff WR, Ge J, Sather HN, Cooper HA, Hutchinson RJ, Lange BJ. Central venous catheter use and the risk of infection in children with acute lymphoblastic leukemia: a report from the Children's Cancer Group. *J Pediatr Hematol Oncol.* 1999;21:260–267.
10. Shaul DB, Scheer B, Rokhsar S, et al. Risk factors for early infection of central venous catheters in pediatric patients. *J Am Coll Surg.* 1998;186:654–658.
11. De Gaudio AR, Di Filippo A. Device-related infections in critically ill patients: part I: prevention of catheter-related bloodstream infections. *J Chemother.* 2003;15:419–427.
12. North JH Jr, Weber TK, Rodriguez-Bigas MA, Meropol NJ, Petrelli NJ. The management of infectious and noninfectious anorectal complications in patients with leukemia. *J Am Coll Surg.* 1996;183:322–328.
13. Alexander SW, Walsh TJ, Freifeld AG, Pizzo PA. Infectious complications in pediatric cancer patients. In: Pizzo PA, Poplack DG, eds. *Principles and Practice of Pediatric Oncology.* Philadelphia: Lippincott Williams & Wilkins, 2002:1239–1284.
14. Brydak LB, Rokicka-Milewska R, Machala M, Jackowska T, Sikorska-Fic B. Immunogenicity of subunit trivalent influenza vaccine in children with acute lymphoblastic leukemia. *Pediatr Infect Dis J.* 1998;17:125–129.
15. American Academy of Pediatrics. Immunizations in special clinical circumstances. *Red Book: 2003 Report of the Committee on Infectious Diseases.* Elk Grove Village, IL: American Academy of Pediatrics; 2003:66–98.
16. LaRussa P, Steinberg S, Gershon AA. Varicella vaccine for immunocompromised children: results of collaborative studies in the United States and Canada. *J Infect Dis.* 1996;174(Suppl 3):S320–323.
17. Schrauder A, Henke-Gendo C, Seidemann K, et al. Varicella vaccination in a child with acute lymphoblastic leukaemia. *Lancet.* 2007;369:1232.
18. Lindemulder S, Albano E. Successful intermittent prophylaxis with trimethoprim/sulfamethoxazole 2 days per week for Pneumocystis carinii (jiroveci) pneumonia in pediatric oncology patients. *Pediatrics.* 2007;120:e47–51.
19. Ioannidis JP, Cappelleri JC, Skolnik PR, Lau J, Sacks HS. A meta-analysis of the relative efficacy and toxicity of Pneumocystis carinii prophylactic regimens. *Arch Intern Med.* 1996;156:177–188.
20. Hughes WT. Use of dapsone in the prevention and treatment of *Pneumocystis carinii* pneumonia: a review. *Clin Infect Dis.* 1998;27:191–204.
21. Madden RM, Pui CH, Hughes WT, Flynn PM, Leung W. Prophylaxis of Pneumocystis carinii pneumonia with atovaquone in children with leukemia. *Cancer.* 2007;109:1654–1658.
22. Kim SY, Dabb AA, Glenn DJ, Snyder KM, Chuk MK, Loeb DM. Intravenous pentamidine is effective as second line Pneumocystis pneumonia prophylaxis in pediatric oncology patients. *Pediatr Blood Cancer.* 2007.
23. Hughes WT, Armstrong D, Bodey GP, et al. 2002 guidelines for the use of antimicrobial agents in neutropenic patients with cancer. *Clin Infect Dis.* 2002;34:730–751.
24. Gualtieri RJ, Donowitz GR, Kaiser DL, Hess CE, Sande MA. Double-blind randomized study of prophylactic trimethoprim/sulfamethoxazole in granulocytopenic patients with hematologic malignancies. *Am J Med.* 1983;74:934–940.
25. Wilson JM, Guiney DG. Failure of oral trimethoprim-sulfamethoxazole prophylaxis in acute leukemia: isolation of resistant plasmids from strains of Enterobacteriaceae causing bacteremia. *N Engl J Med.* 1982;306:16–20.
26. Dekker AW, Rozenberg-Arska M, Verhoef J. Infection prophylaxis in acute leukemia: a comparison of ciprofloxacin with trimethoprim-sulfamethoxazole and colistin. *Ann Intern Med.* 1987;106:7–11.
27. Winston DJ, Chandrasekar PH, Lazarus HM, et al. Fluconazole prophylaxis of fungal infections in patients with acute leukemia: results of a randomized placebo-controlled, double-blind, multicenter trial. *Ann Intern Med.* 1993;118:495–503.
28. Marr KA. The changing spectrum of candidemia in oncology patients: therapeutic implications. *Curr Opin Infect Dis.* 2000;13:615–620.
29. Goodman JL, Winston DJ, Greenfield RA, et al. A controlled trial of fluconazole to prevent fungal infections in patients undergoing bone marrow transplantation. *N Engl J Med.* 1992;326:845–851.
30. Wingard JR, Merz WG, Rinaldi MG, Johnson TR, Karp JE, Saral R. Increase in Candida krusei infection among patients with bone marrow transplantation and neutropenia treated prophylactically with fluconazole. *N Engl J Med.* 1991;325:1274–1277.
31. Wolff SN, Fay J, Stevens D, et al. Fluconazole vs low-dose amphotericin B for the prevention of fungal infections in patients undergoing bone marrow transplantation: a study of the North American Marrow Transplant Group. *Bone Marrow Transplant.* 2000;25:853–859.
32. Timmers GJ, Zweegman S, Simoons-Smit AM, van Loenen AC, Touw D, Huijgens PC. Amphotericin B colloidal dispersion (Amphocil) vs fluconazole for the prevention of fungal infections in neutropenic patients: data of a prematurely stopped clinical trial. *Bone Marrow Transplant.* 2000;25:879–884.
33. Kelsey SM, Goldman JM, McCann S, et al. Liposomal amphotericin (AmBisome) in the prophylaxis of fungal infections in neutropenic patients: a randomised, double-blind, placebo-controlled study. *Bone Marrow Transplant.* 1999;23:163–168.
34. Hill G, Chauvenet AR, Lovato J, McLean TW. Recent steroid therapy increases severity of varicella infections in children with acute lymphoblastic leukemia. *Pediatrics.* 2005;116:e525–529.
35. Boeckh M, Kim HW, Flowers ME, Meyers JD, Bowden RA. Long-term acyclovir for prevention of varicella zoster virus disease after allogeneic hematopoietic cell transplantation—a randomized double-blind placebo-controlled study. *Blood.* 2006;107:1800–1805.
36. Whimbey E, Englund JA, Couch RB. Community respiratory virus infections in immunocompromised patients with cancer. *Am J Med.* 1997;102:10–18; discussion 25–26.
37. Group TI-RS. Palivizumab, a humanized respiratory syncytial virus monoclonal antibody, reduces hospitalization from respiratory syncytial virus infection in high-risk infants. *Pediatrics.* 1998;102:531–537.
38. Yap PL. Prevention of infection in patients with B cell defects: focus on intravenous immunoglobulin. *Clin Infect Dis.* 1993;17(Suppl 2):S372–S375.
39. Dajani AS, Taubert KA, Wilson W, et al. Prevention of bacterial endocarditis: recommendations by the American Heart Association. *J Am Dent Assoc.* 1997;128:1142–1151.
40. Holdsworth MT, Mathew P. Efficacy of colony-stimulating factors in acute leukemia. *Ann Pharmacother.* 2001;35:92–108.
41. Lehrnbecher T, Zimmermann M, Reinhardt D, Dworzak M, Stary J, Creutzig U. Prophylactic human granulocyte colony-stimulating factor after induction therapy in pediatric acute myeloid leukemia. *Blood.* 2007;109:936–943.
42. Ozer H, Armitage JO, Bennett CL, et al. 2000 update of recommendations for the use of hematopoietic colony-stimulating factors: evidence-based, clinical practice guidelines. American Society of Clinical Oncology Growth Factors Expert Panel. *J Clin Oncol.* 2000;18:3558–3585.
43. Riikonen P, Saarinen UM, Makipernaa A, et al. Recombinant human granulocyte-macrophage colony-stimulating factor in the treatment of febrile neutropenia: a double blind placebo-controlled study in children. *Pediatr Infect Dis J.* 1994;13:197–202.
44. Mitchell PL, Morland B, Stevens MC, et al. Granulocyte colony-stimulating factor in established febrile neutropenia: a randomized study of pediatric patients. *J Clin Oncol.* 1997;15:1163–1170.
45. Korones DN, Hussong MR, Gullace MA. Routine chest radiography of children with cancer hospitalized for fever and neutropenia: is it really necessary? *Cancer.* 1997;80:1160–1164.
46. Vancomycin added to empirical combination antibiotic therapy for fever in granulocytopenic cancer patients. European Organization for Research and Treatment of Cancer (EORTC) International Antimicrobial Therapy Cooperative Group and the National Cancer Institute of Canada-Clinical Trials Group. *J Infect Dis.* 1991;163:951–958.
47. Feld R. Vancomycin as part of initial empirical antibiotic therapy for febrile neutropenia in patients with cancer: pros and cons. *Clin Infect Dis.* 1999;29:503–507.
48. Shenep JL, Hughes WT, Roberson PK, et al. Vancomycin, ticarcillin, and amikacin compared with ticarcillin-clavulanate and amikacin in the empirical treatment of febrile, neutropenic children with cancer. *N Engl J Med.* 1988;319:1053–1058.
49. Gamis AS, Howells WB, DeSwarte-Wallace J, Feusner JH, Buckley JD, Woods WG. Alpha hemolytic streptococcal infection during intensive treatment for acute myeloid leukemia: a report from the Children's cancer group study CCG-2891. *J Clin Oncol.* 2000;18:1845–1855.
50. Reilly AF, Lange BJ. Infections with viridans group streptococci in children with cancer. *Pediatr Blood Cancer.* 2007;49(6):774–780.
51. Orudjev E, Lange BJ. Evolving concepts of management of febrile neutropenia in children with cancer. *Med Pediatr Oncol.* 2002;39:77–85.
52. Salzer W, Steinberg SM, Liewehr DJ, Freifeld A, Balis FM, Widemann BC. Evaluation and treatment of fever in the non-neutropenic child with cancer. *J Pediatr Hematol Oncol.* 2003;25:606–612.

53. Walsh TJ, Finberg RW, Arndt C, et al. Liposomal amphotericin B for empirical therapy in patients with persistent fever and neutropenia. National Institute of Allergy and Infectious Diseases Mycoses Study Group. *N Engl J Med.* 1999; 340:764–771.

54. Wingard JR, White MH, Anaissie E, Raffalli J, Goodman J, Arrieta A. A randomized, double-blind comparative trial evaluating the safety of liposomal amphotericin B versus amphotericin B lipid complex in the empirical treatment of febrile neutropenia. L Amph/ABLC Collaborative Study Group. *Clin Infect Dis.* 2000;31:1155–1163.

55. Herbrecht R, Denning DW, Patterson TF, et al. Voriconazole versus amphotericin B for primary therapy of invasive aspergillosis. *N Engl J Med.* 2002; 347:408–415.

56. Sable CA, Strohmaier KM, and Chodakewitz JA. Advances in antifungal therapy. *Annu Rev Med.* 2008;59:361–379.

57. Whitley RJ, Monto AS. Prevention and treatment of influenza in high-risk groups: children, pregnant women, immunocompromised hosts, and nursing home residents. *J Infect Dis.* 2006;194(Suppl 2):S133–S138.

Transfusion Therapy in Pediatric Patients with Cancer

Thomas C. Hofstra and John J. Quinn

Introduction

The remarkable advances that have occurred in the treatment of pediatric patients with cancer would not have been possible without the ability to aggressively support the patients at initial diagnosis and throughout the various phases of therapy. Management of the consequences of deficiency of one or more formed blood elements and of coagulopathies is crucial to the successful outcome of treatment. Infectious complications due to a paucity of phagocytic cells will be dealt with in another chapter. This chapter will focus on transfusion therapy and its role in the management of deficiencies of red cells, platelets, and granulocytes and in the therapy of hemostatic abnormalities. It is important to recognize the invaluable contributions of specialists in transfusion medicine whose investigations and vigilant protection of the blood supply have contributed so much to the safety and efficacy of blood product support.

General Transfusion Guidelines

Consent

Written consent must be obtained for transfusion of blood products. If the patient is a minor, a parent or legal guardian gives consent, and once majority is reached, the patient consents. Children old enough to assent should be requested to do so. The consent process should include discussion of the risks and benefits of transfusion, alternatives to transfusion, and sources of blood products, including the option for directed donation. However, directed donor blood products are not safer than those from the general inventory.[1] When directed donation is chosen, blood relatives are best avoided if the patient has a disease for which related donor hematopoietic progenitor cell transplantation may be an option. The potential recipient could be sensitized to minor histocompatibility antigens present in the donor but absent in the recipient, which could increase the risk of graft rejection.

Irradiation

All blood products containing cellular elements should be irradiated to avoid the rare but often lethal complication of post-transfusion graft-versus-host disease (GVHD). This form of GVHD develops because the patient, immunosuppressed as a consequence of the underlying malignancy or its therapy, cannot reject donor T lymphocytes. Affected patients develop a fulminant disease with skin rash, diarrhea, hepatitis, and marrow failure. Irradiation of the product to 25 Gy completely avoids this complication and does not decrease the function of transfused platelets or granulocytes but their is a decrease in red cell viability. Therefore, red blood cells should be transfused within 28 days of irradiation.[2]

Leukoreduction

Blood products, with the exception of granulocytes, should be leukocyte reduced. This process usually occurs prior to storage rather than prior to administration. Effective filtration removes greater than 99.99% of leukocytes so that less than 5×10^6 leukocytes remain per unit of blood. Leukocytes express both class I and class II human leukocyte antigens (HLAs), while platelets express class I HLA but not class II HLA. Sensitization to class I HLA on platelets can result in refractoriness, but it occurs only when the antigens are presented by cells such as leukocytes, which also express class II HLA. Leukocyte depletion not only decreases sensitization but also greatly decreases the risk of transmission of cytomegalovirus (CMV). Prevention of CMV transmission by leukoreduction appears to be almost as effective as the use of blood products from CMV seronegative donors. However, for patients at highest risk of serious CMV infection, such as CMV seronegative hematopoietic progenitor cell transplant recipients, leukocyte-reduced blood products from CMV seronegative donors provide the least risk of infection.[3,4]

Leukocyte reduction decreases the number of febrile nonhemolytic transfusion reactions, the most common adverse complication of transfusion. Transfusion of allogeneic leukocytes may be immunosuppressive and may increase the risk of cancer recurrence, and it may also increase the risk for bacterial infections, including sepsis.[5] Recent studies have demonstrated reduced sepsis rates in patients with indwelling venous access devices who receive leukoreduced blood products. Studies have also shown reduction in infectious complications in children with acute lymphoblastic leukemia (ALL) who undergo induction chemotherapy while receiving leukoreduced products.[6,7] In aggregate, these concerns about complications have prompted the shift in policy toward leukoreduction at the times of blood collection and storage.

Red Blood Cells

Anemia in the Oncology Patient

Anemia develops in most pediatric patients with cancer.[8] In some, it is present at the time of initial diagnosis. This is especially so with acute leukemia, the anemia of which is due to extensive replacement of the normal hematopoietic elements by leukemic blasts. Severe thrombocytopenia is often present as well and may cause additional red cell loss from bleeding. Disseminated intravascular coagulation (DIC) may occur with certain types of acute leukemia and can produce a severe hemorrhagic diathesis. Disseminated intravascular coagulation is most frequently encountered in patients with acute promyelocytic leukemia (FAB M3) but may also be seen with acute monocytic leukemia (FAB M5) and T-cell ALL.[9] Patients with solid tumors are less likely to be anemic at initial diagnosis. Patients with advanced Hodgkin disease, osteosarcoma, and Ewing sarcoma may present with anemia of chronic inflammation, while patients with large, vascular, and/or necrotic Wilms tumors, liver tumors, germ cell tumors, or neuroblastomas may have hemorrhage into the tumor. Additionally, patients with neuroblastoma, Ewing sarcoma, and alveolar rhabdomyosarcoma may have decreased erythrocyte production from widespread marrow metastases.[10] Pediatric cancer patients produce erythropoietin (EPO) normally in response to their anemia. Their decreased erythrocyte production is due to a paucity of erythroid precursors, due either to excessive marrow infiltration by malignant cells or, in the absence of this, inhibition of erythropoiesis by inflammatory cytokines.[11]

Anemia is most commonly encountered as a consequence of myelosuppressive chemotherapy. The more intense the therapy administered, the greater the degree of anemia. Radiation therapy may also cause anemia, especially if the field of irradiation encompasses a significant amount of bone marrow. Infection with parvovirus B19 and with CMV may suppress erythropoiesis. Trimethoprim and sulfamethoxazole, used for pneumocystis carinii prophylaxis, may also cause anemia. For some patients, additional factors that contribute to anemia development include blood loss from frequent blood draws for laboratory tests and poor nutrition.

Anemia can produce distressing symptoms in children with terminal cancer. Fatigue is one of the most bothersome issues for these children and their parents.[12] Red cell transfusions can ameliorate this fatigue, and a plan should be developed for their use when the patient can most benefit from this intervention.[13]

Erythrocytes carry oxygen to the tissues. If their numbers decline, compensatory mechanisms develop to maintain tissue oxygenation. These include shift in the oxyhemoglobin dissociation curve to the right, which favors increased extraction of oxygen from hemoglobin, preferential redistribution of blood flow away from the splanchnic bed and to critical organs such as heart and brain, and increase in cardiac output due to increase in heart rate and stroke volume.[14] With slowly developing anemia, the increase in cardiac output results in increased venous return, increased end diastolic pressure, and stretching of cardiac muscle fibers, which increases force of contraction and maintenance of the high output state and preservation of oxygen delivery to tissue.[15] However, the heart is working at the peak of the Frank-Starling curve (Figure 35-1), and any further increase in blood volume and stretching of cardiac muscle fibers will cause a shift to the descending portion of the curve with a fall in cardiac output and heart failure. Therefore, severely anemic patients should receive only small volumes of red cells initially during transfusion (see below).

Signs and symptoms of anemia depend on its severity and the rapidity with which it develops. Rapidly developing anemia from acute blood loss can cause hypovolemic shock with tachycardia, hypotension, and poor perfusion. Frequently, anemia develops more insidiously as red cell production declines and cardiovascular adaptations limit symptomatology. As signs and symptoms do develop, they include pallor, fatigue, irritability, anorexia, and decreased activity. More severely anemic patients can have headaches, syncope, dyspnea, and altered mental status. Life-threatening respiratory distress and congestive heart failure occur in those with the most severe anemia.[16]

Red Cell Transfusion Practices

For patients with active bleeding, the goal is to replace the ongoing loss. With brisk bleeding, rapid transfusion of multiple units may be indicated. For unstable patients in whom it may be difficult to judge whether they have received too little or too much volume, central venous pressure monitoring is very helpful.

For preoperative oncology patients, transfusion requirements must be anticipated. Surgeries to resect large and vascular tumors are likely to require red cell transfusion. For musculoskeletal tumors, transfusion support is most often needed for malignant bone tumors undergoing wide resection.[17]

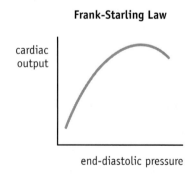

Figure 35-1 The Frank-Starling Law of the heart indicates that stretch of myocardial muscle fibers will, up to a point, increase force of contraction. On the ascending limb of the curve, increased end diastolic volume and pressure from increased venous return result in increased systolic force of contraction and cardiac output. However, the descending limb of the curve demonstrates that stretch of myocardial fibers beyond a certain point will decrease force of contraction and cardiac output. This can occur with too rapid transfusion of severely anemic individuals.

For patients who are not actively bleeding, there is no consensus on the degree of anemia that requires transfusion support. The 2004 transfusion guidelines for neonates and older children of the British Committee for Standards in Haematology acknowledge the lack of controlled trials and indicate that the decision to transfuse depends on clinical judgment, the child's general condition, presence or absence of bleeding, and imminence of marrow recovery.[18] Recently published guidelines from the Children's Oncology Group suggest transfusion with red cells for symptomatic children with hemoglobin less than 6 to 7 g/dL, for hemoglobin less than 9 g/dL if an invasive procedure is planned, and for less than 10 g/dL in concomitantly thrombocytopenic patients.[2] A recent survey of pediatric hematology/oncology specialists from North America indicated wide variations in practice.[19,20] Many would not transfuse for a hemoglobin greater than 7 g/dL unless the patient was unstable (having febrile neutropenia with tachypnea) or lived far (more than 3 hours away) from the treating facility.[19] The transfusion threshold was often somewhat higher for patients receiving radiation therapy. The effectiveness of irradiation requires generation of free radicals, which may be compromised by hypoxia.[21] There are no pediatric studies that address this issue, and adult studies that show a positive effect for maintaining a higher hemoglobin have been undertaken primarily in cervical and head and neck cancer patients.[22,23] There also remains concern that transfusions may be harmful due to their potentially immunosuppressive effect, especially when leukocytes have not been removed.

The use of red cell transfusions depends on therapeutic intensity. Studies indicate that only 12.5% of patients receiving less-intense regimens for brain tumors, Wilms tumor, or Hodgkin disease required red cells as compared with 59.5% receiving more-intense regimens for leukemia, bone and soft tissue sarcomas, and germ cell tumors.[24] A risk model for solid-tumor patients receiving intermittent pulse chemotherapy has been proposed that stratifies on the basis of decreased performance status; hemoglobin less than 12 g/dL and absolute lymphocyte count of less than 700 μL. Children with 2 or 3 risk factors had a 59% and 96% probability of red cell transfusion for severe anemia, respectively.[25] Patients who are severely thrombocytopenic are more likely to bleed if anemic, and therefore it would seem prudent to maintain a higher hemoglobin level through transfusion than would otherwise be necessary.[20] There is no consensus about what hemoglobin level should prompt transfusion in critically ill children cared for in the pediatric intensive care unit. A hemoglobin level less than 9 g/dL is often the trigger, but the patient population is quite heterogeneous and generally includes fewer than 10% with oncologic diseases.[26] Although many patients have cardiac or pulmonary compromise or both and would seem to benefit from increase in oxygen-carrying capacity from correction of anemia, there are no data to support this contention. Indeed, patients requiring transfusion have increased resource utilization (increase in days of oxygen use, mechanical ventilation, vasoactive agent infusions, and hospital stay) and poorer outcome.[27] Oncology patients are more likely to fall into this category,

but it is not clear that they would benefit from a more restrictive transfusion policy.[28]

In the absence of acute hemorrhage or severe anemia, patients generally receive a transfusion of 10 cc/kg of packed red blood cells. The preservative used for erythrocyte storage determines shelf life and hematocrit of the product. If CPDA (citrate, phosphate buffer, dextrose, adenine) is used, the product has a hematocrit between 50% and 80% and can be stored for 35 days; if AS (adenine, dextrose, saline, mannitol) is used, the product has a hematocrit between 50% and 60% and can be stored for 42 days.

Transfusion of 10 cc/kg of the CPDA product will increase hemoglobin by 2.5 g/dL and hematocrit by 8% to 9%; transfusion of 10 cc/kg of the AS product will increase hemoglobin by 2 g/dL and hematocrit by 6% to 7%.[2]

The total volume of red blood cells (RBCs) transfused can be calculated from the following formula:

Volume of packed RBCs transfused = total blood volume × (target hgb − current hgb)/hgb of donor unit

An estimated blood volume of 80 cc/kg for infants and children can be used with this formula.

A simplified formula for pediatric patients has recently been published and is as follows:

Volume of packed RBCs transfused = 1.6 × weight in kg × desired % increase in hct[29]

For severely anemic patients with hemoglobin of 5 g/dL or less, transfusion should consist of no more than 5 cc/kg of tightly packed red cells administered over 3 to 4 hours. To avoid volume overload that could precipitate heart failure (Figure 35-1), it may be necessary to administer a small dose (0.5-1 mg/kg) of furosemide. After a 1- to 2-hour interval, the transfusion can be repeated using a volume of approximately 5 to 7 ml/kg, and if necessary this procedure can be repeated a third time after another short equilibration period. For infants and small children, the blood bank should be instructed to split the unit into 2 to 3 aliquots, which can be used in this stepwise approach to correcting severe anemia. This technique minimizes exposure to blood products. For patients already in congestive heart failure from severe anemia, it may be necessary to perform an isovolemic exchange transfusion.

Hyperleukocytosis

Leukemic patients with hyperleukocytosis (white blood cell [WBC] count greater than 100 000/μL) have increased blood viscosity as a consequence of their high WBC count. This may lead to sludging and capillary obstruction by leukocyte thrombi, especially in the lungs and brain. This complication is more likely in acute myeloid leukemia (AML) than in ALL or chronic myelogenous leukemia (CML) because immature myeloid cells are larger in size, are relatively more rigid, and are more prone to adhere to each other and to vascular endothelium and form aggregates. Aggregates in the pulmonary vasculature produce hypoxemia that manifests as dyspnea and tachypnea, and pulmonary hemorrhage may subsequently develop; aggregates in the central nervous system may produce visual disturbance, confusion, somnolence, or coma. For these patients, until the leukocyte count has declined, red cell transfusions should be given with caution if at all. It is better to maintain the patient's hemoglobin at 8 g/dL or less than to increase viscosity by red cell transfusions. However, the platelet count should be kept greater than 20000/μL due to a propensity for these patients to bleed. In addition, measures should be undertaken as rapidly as possible to lower the WBC count. The principal components of treatment for ALL patients with hyperleukocytosis are hydration, management of tumor lysis, and initiation of chemotherapy. Cytoreduction by leukapheresis or exchange transfusion is generally not needed and can be reserved for symptomatic patients or those with a WBC count greater than 400000/μL.[30] For AML patients the same principles would apply, but these children often need management of an associated coagulopathy because a high WBC count is especially common with FAB M5 AML. These patients may be more likely to benefit from cytoreduction by leukapheresis or exchange transfusion, provided the technical obstacles can be overcome and it can be accomplished expeditiously.[31]

Erythropoietin

Erythropoietin is widely used as an alternative to transfusion to correct or prevent anemia in adult cancer patients. Practice guidelines exist for its administration, and in many adults it has resulted in improved quality of life.[32] The fully published studies of its use for pediatric cancer patients are few and consist of small numbers of patients.[33] In children undergoing intensive chemotherapy, such as induction therapy for high-risk neuroblastoma, it offers no benefit.[34] However, with less aggressive regimens, especially if cisplatin is not used, it does appear to decrease transfusion requirements.[35–37] Two larger pediatric studies have been conducted, and both employed a once-weekly intravenous administration schedule. In the European trial, which compared transfusion rates for ALL and non-ALL patients either receiving or not receiving 20 weeks of weekly intravenous EPO, benefit was limited to patients with ALL who had a 66% rate of transfusion with EPO and an 89% transfusion rate without it. For non-ALL patients, the transfusion rates were similar in both groups and approximately 60%.[38] The American study was limited to patients 5 years or older treated in a similar manner for 16 weeks and demonstrated that 35% of patients receiving EPO were transfusion free as compared with 22% who did not receive it. Patients who responded to EPO had improved quality of life, but this could be conclusively demonstrated only for children 5 to 7 years old and not for older children. Furthermore, there was an increased incidence of serious thrombotic events in the EPO recipients.[39] These modest benefits from decrease in transfusion requirements must also be counterbalanced by ongoing concerns that some tumors may have erythropoietin receptors and in them its administration could promote tumor growth. Indeed, there are reports of increased recurrence rates in adults treated with EPO.[40,41] Erythropoietin receptors have also been demonstrated on a wide variety of pediatric solid tumors and from cells lines derived from them.[42] This issue is of extreme importance in pediatrics, where successful outcome of therapy cannot simply be measured in increased comfort for a number of years but must be a cure with long-term survival. Currently, less than 15% of pediatric hematologist/oncologists from North America favor use of EPO in children with cancer.[19] However, it might be considered in patients whose religious beliefs forbid the use of blood products, such as Jehovah's Witnesses (see below).

Platelets

Thrombocytopenia occurs for a variety of reasons in children with cancer. At diagnosis, it is due to extensive marrow infiltration by malignant cells, a frequent occurrence in acute leukemia and more rarely in metastatic solid tumors such as neuroblastoma and alveolar rhabdomyosarcoma. Intensive chemotherapy, radiation therapy, prophylactic sulfamethoxazole and trimethoprim, or complications of therapy such as sepsis, veno-occlusive disease (VOD), or DIC, may also lead to thrombocytopenia. Paraneoplastic syndromes or immune thrombocytopenia may also lead to thrombocytopenia in the child with cancer.

Platelet transfusions have improved the survival of children with cancer. Currently, hemorrhage accounts for less than 1% of deaths in patients being treated for hematologic malignancies.[43] The ability to transfuse platelets safely has significantly contributed to this improved survival. While utilization of RBC transfusions has plateaued, platelet transfusions have continued to increase at a rate of approximately 5% per year for the past several years.[44] Although the increase in utilization of platelets for transfusion has improved outcomes for children with cancer, concerns remain regarding the ongoing availability of platelets, appropriate dosing of platelets, a platelet threshold, and refractoriness to platelet transfusions.

Platelet Triggers and Platelet Dosing

Establishing a platelet count above which there would be minimal risk of bleeding and below which there is a significant risk of serious bleeding remains is an as yet unrealized goal. Several studies comparing different platelet thresholds or comparing prophylactic platelet transfusions to on-demand therapy (transfusion only for significant bleeding) failed to establish a definitive platelet count at which transfusions offer an obvious benefit.[43]

The first study attempting to show a relationship between platelet count and risk of bleeding was performed by Gaydos et al.[45] Although this study was unable to establish a relationship between platelet count and the risk of significant bleeding, a platelet threshold of 20000/μL became the accepted threshold for platelet transfusions. It is important to note that when this study was performed, aspirin therapy, which interferes with platelet function, was common, and the ability to measure accurately platelet counts at low levels was limited.

Subsequent studies attempted to lower the trigger threshold by comparing various platelet thresholds, usually 10000/μL to 20000/μL, or a threshold of 10000/μL, to treatment for bleeding only.[46–53] These studies used various inclusion criteria, rarely blinded investigators, and did not have the power to establish one threshold as superior.[43] Despite these limitations, most institutions and consensus opinions consider the platelet count trigger of 10000/µL as the standard.[19,54,55] By using this lower threshold, fewer platelet products are transfused, offering a cost savings, reducing exposure to multiple donors, and preserving this limited resource, all without an increased risk of morbidity.[46,56,57]

Certain children with an increased risk for bleeding may require a higher platelet threshold than 10000/µL. They include patients with fever, sepsis, hyperleukocytosis, mucositis, DIC or other coagulation abnormalities, rapidly falling platelet counts and recipients of amphotericin B or imatinib therapy.[48,55,58,59] Children with cancer undergoing surgical procedures generally need platelet counts greater than 50000/µL to ensure hemostasis at the time of the operation. These levels are also needed for insertion of indwelling catheters. For surgeries in which excessive bleeding would result in significant morbidity, such as extensive tumor resection or neurosurgical or ophthalmologic procedures, the preoperative platelet count may need to be as high as 100000/µL. Platelet counts should be maintained above these target levels for at least 3 days following surgery. For patients with coagulation abnormalities, higher platelet counts may be necessary as well as attempts to improve the coagulopathy.

Platelets are often administered to thrombocytopenic patients prior to lumbar puncture. However, investigators at St Jude Children's Research Hospital (SJCRH) reported in 2000 that children with acute leukemia who had platelet counts of 10000/µL or greater could safely undergo lumbar puncture (LP). There were not enough children with lower counts to determine if there was an adverse outcome for them.[60] Lowering of the trigger for transfusion to 10000/µL for all such patients may not always be safe and must be viewed in the broader context of risk of relapse from introduction of blasts into the cerebrospinal fluid (CSF) if the LP is traumatic. Indeed, investigators from SJCRH subsequently reported, as did others from Germany and the Netherlands, that traumatic LP at initial diagnosis may increase the risk of relapse.[61–63] Current recommendations from SJCRH are that the initial LP be done under deep sedation or general anesthesia by experienced clinicians, intrathecal chemotherapy should be given once CSF is collected and, for thrombocytopenic patients, platelets be transfused prior to the procedure.[64] A platelet count of less than 100000/µL was their suggested trigger for transfusion.[65] It would be prudent to continue this practice for additional LPs as long as blasts persist in the peripheral blood.[64]

Platelet transfusions are not needed prior to bone marrow aspiration and biopsy.[55] Guidelines for use of platelet transfusions with various procedures are provided in Table 35-1.

Once the decision has been made to transfuse the thrombocytopenic patient with platelets, optimal dosing becomes a key issue. Platelet dosing is usually based on patient size, either weight or body surface area (BSA). Var-

Table 35-1

Platelet levels needed for invasive procedures.

Procedure	Minimal Platelet Count
Acute leukemia initial LP	$100 \times 10^3/\mu L$
Acute leukemia subsequent LP	$10 \times 10^3/\mu L$
Surgery	$50 \times 10^3/\mu L$
Extensive tumor resection	$100 \times 10^3/\mu L$
Neuro/ophthal surgery	$100 \times 10^3/\mu L$
Central line insertion	$50 \times 10^3/\mu L$
Marrow aspiration/biopsy	no minimum

ious formulas can be used to determine platelet dose. One random donor unit per square meter should increase the platelet count by 10000/µL. When calculations are based on BSA, one random donor unit should increase the platelet count by 10000/L per square meter. For the infant with cancer and thrombocytopenia, 10 cc/kg of platelets will increase the platelet count by approximately 30000/µL. In order to optimize utilization of this limited resource, these formulas generally translate to transfusing one half of an apheresis unit or 3 random donor units for children weighing less than 30 kg, and one apheresis unit for children weighing greater than 30 kg. Larger platelet doses may reduce the total number of transfusions, thus reducing donor exposure and the risk of alloimmunization.[66,67] Coordination with the blood bank will allow splitting units so that each apheresis unit can be used for more than one transfusion. If platelets are filtered at the bedside, the equivalent of one random donor unit is lost through the leukocyte filter.

Platelet Preparations

Platelet transfusions in children with cancer can be prepared either from random donor platelets obtained from whole blood donations or from platelet apheresis procedures. Random donor platelets are processed from whole blood donations through centrifugation and storage of the platelets in a closed system. Each unit of random donor platelets contains 0.5 to 0.75×10^{11} platelets in 50 ml of plasma.[68] Random donor platelets offer the benefit of cost savings, although with the requirement of testing each unit for bacterial contamination and time spent pooling units, cost benefits are not as great as previously described. A significant disadvantage of random donor platelets is the exposure of the oncology patient to multiple donors, increasing the potential for alloimmunization or of receiving a product contaminated by bacteria.[69,70] Because of these risks, random donor platelets are less commonly used than in the past.

Apheresis units are obtained from a single donor in a procedure lasting 90 to 120 minutes, during which platelet-rich plasma is extracted from donor blood within a closed system while returning red blood cells to the donor. An apheresis unit contains the equivalent of 4 to 10 random donor units of platelets (3-8 × 10[11] platelets) in 200 to 300 ml of plasma but may be split into smaller aliquots for transfusion.[70] Apheresis platelets reduce the child's risk of exposure to multiple donors. Leukocyte reduction at the time of donation reduces cytokine release from leukocytes during storage and decreases the likelihood of developing refractoriness to platelet transfusions (see below). Both apheresis and random donor platelets are now routinely leukocyte reduced prior to storage, improving the platelet yield at the time of transfusion.

Regardless of the method of acquisition, platelets are stored at 20°C to 24°C on a horizontal agitator to prevent platelet clumping. Units are collected and stored in polyurethane bags that allow carbon dioxide and oxygen exchange, improving the viability of the platelets. Platelets can be stored under these conditions for up to 7 days.[71] However, the increased risk of bacterial contamination and cytokine-related reactions with longer storage times limits storage time to 5 days.[70]

Children with cancer may develop fluid overload from causes such as renal insufficiency, VOD, congestive heart failure, or the syndrome of inappropriate antidiuretic hormone secretion. For children requiring restriction of fluid intake, the clinician may request that the blood bank reduce the volume of platelets for transfusion by recentrifugation. Although this manipulation will reduce volume, it will also reduce the platelet transfusion yield by as much as 50%.[55,72] Because of this poorer yield, volume-reduced platelet transfusions should be limited to patients for whom increased intravascular volume will result in adverse clinical consequences.

Platelet Refractoriness

Platelet refractoriness, the failure to increase or sustain platelet counts after repeated transfusions, may be due to a variety of mechanisms, both immune and nonimmune. Alloimmunization results from antibody-mediated clearance of transfused platelets and is a significant complication in multiply transfused patients. Host factors and platelet product factors also influence responses to platelet transfusions. In alloimmunized patients, antibodies are frequently directed against class I HLA antigens and less frequently against various platelet glycoproteins.[73] Risk factors for development of alloimmunization include prior platelet transfusions and a history of pregnancy.[74]

Refractoriness is measured using the corrected platelet count index (CCI).[73] The formula for determining the CCI is as follows:

$$\frac{(\text{post-transfusion platelet count} - \text{pre-transfusion count}) - \text{body surface area}}{\text{number of platelets transfused} \times 10^{11}}$$

This calculation requires that the blood bank measure the quantity of platelets being transfused and requires a 1- and 24-hour platelet count. A CCI less than 5000 to 7500 indicates platelet refractoriness. If the l-hour CCI is less than 7500, the most likely mechanism of platelet destruction is alloimmunization to HLA or other platelet antigens. A CCI above 7500 at 1 hour and less than 7500 at 24 hours indicates a probable nonimmune mechanism. Another and simpler means of assessing refractoriness is the post-transfusion platelet increment. A rise in the platelet count of less than 11 000/μL one hour post transfusion on two successive occasions correlates with a CCI of 5000 if a standard platelet transfusion is given.[75]

Strategies for preventing alloimmunization include limiting the number of donors to which the patient is exposed and modifying the platelet product to decrease its ability to induce an immune response. As discussed above, leukocyte reduction decreases the risk of sensitization to class I HLA antigens. Ultraviolet (UV) irradiation of platelets or other blood products inactivates WBCs and makes them less immunogenic but does not greatly decrease platelet survival. However, it is not generally available.[73]

In the Trial to Prevent Alloimmunization to Platelets, adults with AML were randomized to receive pooled random donor platelets (control), UV-irradiated pooled platelets, or leukocyte-filtered pooled or apheresis platelets. The results of this study demonstrated the effectiveness of leukocyte reduction and UV irradiation in reducing alloimmunization. Patients in the control arm had a 13% incidence of HLA antibodies compared with 3% in the pooled filtered arm, 5% in the apheresis arm, and 4% in the UV-irradiated arm. Interestingly, there was no difference in development of antibodies directed against platelet glycoproteins in any of the 4 groups.[73] Although the subjects of this study subjects were adults with AML, extrapolation of its conclusions to the pediatric population can be made and are supported by smaller, nonrandomized studies involving children with cancer.[76-78]

Given the intensity of treatment for children with cancer and the likelihood of need for repeated platelet transfusions, the standard of care is to use leukocyte-depleted platelets. Leukocyte reduction usually occurs at the time of donation but may occur at the bedside depending on the policy of the institutional blood bank. Bedside leukoreduction reduces platelet yield by 25% to 35%.[55] Leukocyte reduction at the time of apheresis or whole blood collection will not result in transfused platelet loss at the time of transfusion and has the added advantage of reducing cytokine release from the residual WBC in the stored product.[79,80] Thus pre-storage leukocyte reduction is the preferable method.

Nonimmune platelet refractoriness may be secondary to platelet product factors or to host factors. Although alloimmunization is the most significant long-term complication in the multiply transfused patient, nonimmune causes are more common.[75,81] Host factors predisposing to nonimmune refractoriness include presence of fever, infection, DIC, bleeding, splenomegaly, vascular endothelial damage from chemotherapy and from hemolytic uremic syndrome or VOD, and GVHD.[82] The presence of fever with or without evidence of infection reduces platelet transfusion yield by as much as 40%.[82] The spleen holds approximately 30% of circulating platelets. Thus, hypersplenism will result in a larger percentage of transfused platelet being sequestered in the spleen, resulting in a lower than expected yield from any platelet transfusion.[83] Concomitant use of multiple antibiotics, administration of amphotericin-B, or exposure to heparin are additional host factors that can decrease transfused platelet survival.[75] Furthermore, as the number of platelet transfusions increases, there may be a decrease in the post-transfusion increment and in the interval to next transfusion.[75]

Platelet product variables may also contribute to transfusion refractoriness. Platelet counts may vary by unit resulting in a less than expected rise in platelet count. Age of the transfused unit also will affect platelet yield. Older platelets produce a smaller incremental rise due to increasing acidosis over time and activation of platelets from constant agitation during storage. Slower transfusion rates result in lower transfusion yields by allowing platelets to adhere to the surface of tubing. Use of ABO-matched platelets improves the survival of transfused platelets.[75,84]

Management of the Refractory Patient

When a patient demonstrates refractoriness to platelet transfusions, various techniques can be utilized to attempt to improve transfusion yield. Strategies depend on whether the cause is immune or nonimmune. For patients with nonimmune refractoriness, management of the underlying cause should improve the transfused platelet yield. Additional strategies include using fresh platelets or platelet transfusions for symptomatic bleeding only.

Patients with immune-mediated platelet refractoriness present a greater challenge. For them, HLA typing or cross matching should be considered. Children refractory to platelets due to antibodies directed against class I HLA antigens should benefit from HLA-matched platelets, which will increase the transfusion yield in as many as 90% of cases.[68] HLA-matched platelets are expensive due to costs incurred for HLA typing. They are not always available and are not beneficial if alloimmunization is due to antibodies against antigens other than class I HLA proteins. Cross matching platelets when HLA compatible platelets are unavailable or if alloimmunization is due to other antigens may improve platelet yield.[75,84] Additional strategies include using platelets from a blood relative or transfusing only for symptomatic bleeding.[19,81,85]

Wong et al[19] surveyed pediatric oncologists about their use of platelet transfusions for patients with suspected or confirmed refractoriness. For suspected refractoriness, practitioners elected to use ABO-compatible apheresis platelets, HLA-matched apheresis platelets, cross-matched apheresis platelets, platelets less than 3 days old, and apheresis platelets from a blood relative, in descending order of preference. If refractoriness was confirmed, they chose HLA-matched apheresis platelets, ABO-compatible apheresis platelets, cross-matched apheresis platelets,

apheresis platelets from a blood relative, and platelets less than 3 days old, in descending order of preference. Because HLA-matched platelets increase the cost of transfusions, recognizing the need for this product is of utmost importance. Understanding the mechanisms of platelet refractoriness affords the pediatric oncologist strategies to improve platelet yield in a cost-effective manner.

Fresh Frozen Plasma and Cryoprecipitate

Fresh frozen plasma (FFP) is prepared from whole blood donations and is stored at $-30°C$ until used. Bags of FFP range in volume from 180 to 400 ml. Each milliliter of FFP contains approximately one international unit of each coagulation factor. Cryoprecipitate is prepared by thawing FFP at 4°C. Cryoprecipitate contains high levels of Factor VIII, Factor XIII, von Willebrand factor, and fibrinogen. The volume of each bag of cryoprecipitate is 20 to 40 ml.

The use of FFP or cryoprecipitate in the pediatric oncology patient is limited. The most common reasons to transfuse these plasma products include DIC, symptomatic l-asparaginase (L-ASP) induced coagulopathy, massive blood transfusions, or liver synthetic dysfunction. Disseminated intravascular coagulation may occur with acute leukemia, sepsis, disseminated malignancy, or acute hemolytic transfusion reactions.[86–88] Therapy with L-ASP may result in coagulopathy secondary to depletion of natural anticoagulants and coagulation factors, especially anti-thrombin III and fibrinogen, resulting in both hypercoaguable and hypocoaguable states.

Management of DIC requires treatment of the underlying cause. The use of plasma products is supportive until the underlying cause is controlled. The use of FFP in DIC should be limited to symptomatic bleeding, because prophylactic plasma transfusions have not been shown to prevent bleeding or thrombotic complications.[89] Prophylactic FFP has not been shown to prevent thrombosis associated with L-ASP.[90–92]

When FFP is indicated, the dose is 10 to 20 ml/kg as often as every 6 hours. Monitoring response to FFP requires serial measurements of coagulation studies including prothrombin time, partial thromboplastin time, fibrinogen, and fibrin degradation products as well as cessation of bleeding.[89]

For the child with cancer, cryoprecipitate is usually limited to treatment of hypofibrinogenemia due to DIC or L-ASP therapy. For patients with DIC, transfusion of cryoprecipitate is indicated when the fibrinogen is less than 100 mg/dl, although no absolute threshold has been established.[89] In the absence of bleeding, cryoprecipitate is generally not used for patients being treated with L-ASP. Institution of cryoprecipitate infusions in the absence of bleeding after L-ASP may result in thrombotic complications.[93,94] The dose of cryoprecipitate for hypofibrinogenemia due to DIC or L-ASP therapy is one bag for each 5 to 10 kg of body weight to raise the fibrinogen level by 50 to 100 mg/dl.[95] As with FFP, sequential monitoring of coagulation studies to assess response is indicated.

Pharmacologic Interventions in Thromocytopenic Patients

In addition to platelet transfusions, pharmacologic interventions may reduce bleeding complications in thrombocytopenic patients. Medications can be used to improve platelet function, enhance thrombus formation, or interfere with clot breakdown.

Desmopressin acetate (DDAVP) activates platelets and may reduce bleeding in selected thrombocytopenic patients.[96,97] In the severely thrombocytopenic patient, DDAVP is unlikely to offer benefit. The dose of DDAVP depends on the route of administration: 150 μg intranasally for children who weigh less than 30 kg or 300 μg for children who weigh more than 30 kg, 0.3 μg/kg intravenously or 0.3 to 0.4 μg/kg subcutaneously. Side effects of DDAVP include hypertension, facial flushing, and hyponatremia from fluid retention, usually after repeated doses.

Recombinant VIIa (rVIIa) is licensed for the management of hemophilia A or B when inhibitors are present, as well as for Glanzmann thrombocytopenia and congenital Factor VII deficiency. Recombinant VIIa may improve primary hemostasis in patients with thrombocytopenia by generating additional thrombin on the platelet surface, signaling activation of surrounding platelets and improving platelet function.[98] There is anecdotal evidence that rVIIa improves hemostasis in refractory thrombocytopenic patients in whom other therapies have failed.[99–101] However, there are probably many patients whom it does not benefit. In bone marrow transplant patients with alveolar hemorrhage or hemorrhagic cystitis, rVIIa may be useful provided a platelet count of at least 75 000/μL can be maintained.[102] The dose of rVIIa is unknown for control of bleeding in patients with thrombocytopenia. It has ranged from 40 to 270 μg/kg administered as often as every 2 to 3 hours. The use of rVIIa in these patients should be considered an off-label use and be considered only after other therapies fail to stop bleeding.[103]

Antifibrinolytic agents may play a role in hemostasis for thrombocytopenic children. Aminocaproic acid and tranexamic acid, lysine analog antifibrinolytics, interfere with plasminogen and plasmin binding to fibrin and are indicated for management of bleeding associated with fibrinolysis. Some authors have observed variable improvement in hemostasis in thrombocytopenic cancer and bone marrow transplant patients.[104,105] However, use of aminocaproic acid should be considered only an adjunct to other therapies to control bleeding. The use of local measures such as topical thrombin or fibrin glues may help with bleeding in the oral cavity.

Granulocytes

When granulocytes were first used in neutropenic cancer patients with progressive infection uncontrolled by antibiotics, the only individuals with sufficient numbers of granulocytes for donation were CML patients in chronic phase with high white cell counts. Their numbers were clearly limited, but they were the only ones who could supply 40 to 60 × 10^9 cells/day needed to achieve a therapeutic effect. As methods of collection improved from normal donors, and corticosteroid stimulation to mobilize their granulocytes became an option, enthusiasm for this form of therapy increased, but studies from the 1970s through the 1980s failed to show that these transfusions were clearly beneficial. However, this method of donor stimulation produced only 50% of the dose needed for a therapeutic effect. Furthermore, during this time period, major improvements in supportive care of the infected neutropenic patient occurred, including introduction of colony-stimulating factors and improvements in antibiotic and antifungal therapies. These advances in management of febrile neutropenia decreased the number of potential beneficiaries of granulocyte transfusions. With the advent of granulocyte colony-stimulating factor (G-CSF) mobilization from normal donors and the subsequent collection of the cells by continuous-flow centrifugation leukapheresis, therapeutic doses of granulocytes could be collected. These mobilized cells retained their function.[106,107] As a consequence of being able to transfuse sufficient numbers of granulocytes to achieve a therapeutic effect, the issue of granulocyte transfusions has been readdressed.[108] Case reports with both small and large numbers of patients suggest efficacy in otherwise unresponsive progressive bacterial and fungal infections.[109–112] However, none of these studies are large, prospective, and well controlled.[107] All prior randomized controlled trials were performed in the era prior to G-CSF and dexamethasone mobilization, and they are inconclusive as to efficacy.[113] New studies are needed, and until they are undertaken, granulocyte transfusion must be considered experimental.[114]

Current recommendations are that the donor, either related or unrelated to the recipient, be primed with both G-CSF (5 μg/kg subcutaneously) and dexamethasone (8 mg orally) 12 hours prior to collection. ABO compatibility between donor and recipient is required because the product contains large numbers of red cells as well as large numbers of platelets. HLA compatibility is also desirable but not always possible to achieve. The product must be irradiated to 25 Gy to prevent post-transfusion GVHD. If the recipient is CMV seronegative, the donor should be as well. Granulocyte transfusion should be administered for at least 4 treatments, preferably on a daily basis. In children, the volume administered with each infusion is generally 10 to 15 cc/kg, and premedication with hydrocortisone and antihistamines is recommended.[115] Granulocytes should be administered as soon after collection as possible to prevent loss of function. However, it appears they can be stored for up to 24 hours at 10°C without loss of function.[116]

Candidates for granulocyte transfusion should generally meet the following criteria: (1) severe neutropenia with absolute neutrophil count less than 200/μL, (2) bacterial sepsis or progressive fungal infection uncontrolled by appropriate antibacterial or antifungal therapy, (3) progressive local bacterial infection such as typhlitis or necrotizing fasciitis unresponsive to appropriate antimicrobial therapy, and (4) bone marrow recovery expected to be delayed by 7 days or more.[106,115]

Granulocyte transfusions are not without risk to both donor and recipient. Granulocyte colony-stimulating factor administration to donors may be associated with mild and reversible side effects as myalgias, bone pain, headaches, and fatigue. Recipients may have reactions to the infused products and require treatment with antipyretics, antihistamines, meperidine, and corticosteroids. Granulocytes can transmit CMV, and CMV-seronegative patients should receive them from CMV-seronegative donors to avoid transmission of CMV. Transfusion-related acute lung injury (TRALI) may develop shortly after their administration. This is a serious and sometimes fatal complication (see below). Pulmonary infiltrates may develop when they are administered in close proximity to infusion of amphotericin B. This drug may cause neutrophil aggregation, and therefore, infusions of amphotericin B and granulocytes should be separated by at least 2 hours and often as many as 12 hours.[106,107] However, neutrophil aggregation is less likely to occur with use of liposomal preparations of amphotericin B.[117]

Complications of Transfusions

The past two decades have seen a remarkable (greater than 4 log) reduction in the risk of acquisition of human immunodeficiency virus (HIV) and hepatitis C from transfusion. These two viral infections no longer remain the principal causes of fatality from blood product administration. The three leading causes of fatality are now mismatched blood product administration resulting in an acute hemolytic transfusion reaction, TRALI, and bacterial sepsis from transfusion of a contaminated product, generally platelets (Figure 35-2).[118] These complications and others are discussed below.

Acute Hemolytic Transfusion Reaction

Acute hemolytic transfusion reaction is due to transfusion of incompatible RBCs and is due to a clerical error that results in the wrong product going to the wrong patient. Somewhere along the pathway from submitting a specimen for cross match, preparing the product in the blood bank, and administration of the product, mislabeling or misreading labels causes this potentially life-threatening complication. The error is at least as likely to occur at the bedside as in the blood bank. The most common error that occurs at the bedside is failure to check that the right blood product is being given to the right patient.[119] ABO incompatibility between donor and recipient results in immune-mediated intravascular hemolysis. The antibodies binding to the red cells cause complement activation with production of the C5b-9 complex that fixes to the red cell membrane and causes pores to form in it. This leads to red cell destruction by lysis in the vasculature with resultant hemoglobinemia and hemoglobinuria. A systemic inflammatory response and DIC often accompany the hemolysis.[120]

Soon after the infusion starts, the patient experiences fever, chills, nausea, vomiting, abdominal pain or flank pain, dyspnea, and hypotension. Younger patients may appear very anxious and uncomfortable. The first clue to its occurrence in the anesthetized patient may be bleeding from DIC. The transfusion must be immediately stopped and the product returned to the blood bank. Specimens must be obtained from the recipient for repeat cross match, direct Coombs test, repeat typing, and detection of hemoglobinemia and hemoglobinuria. The differential diagnosis includes those acute nonimmune hemolytic reactions due to bacterial contamination of the product, mechanical or thermal damage to the red cells, or infusion

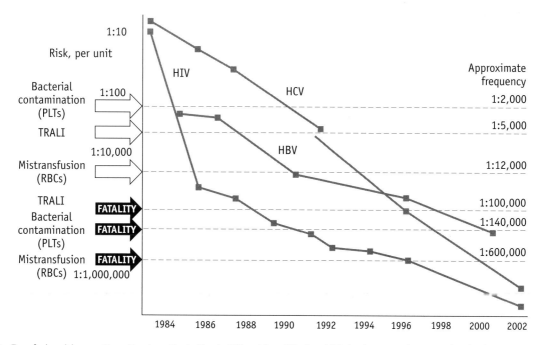

Figure 35-2 Transfusion risks over time. The dramatic decline in HIV and hepatitis B and C infections over the past 2 decades is contrasted with the nonvirologic hazards of transfusion: bacterial contamination of platelets, TRALI, and mismatched transfusion. The open arrows indicate frequency of these 3 complications, and the black arrows frequency of fatalities from these events.

with a hypotonic solution. Intravenous fluids should be administered with the goal of maintaining a good urine output. Sometimes, diuretics, mannitol, or low-dose dopamine may be needed as well. Patients should be evaluated for DIC and may need platelets, cryoprecipitate, and FFP if they are actively bleeding.[2,120,121] Some patients who survive the acute episode are left with permanent renal damage.

Less frequently, acute extravascular hemolytic transfusion reactions occur. IgG or complement in the form of C3b attaches to the red cell membrane, and these cells are then removed by the reticuloendothelial system. The acute systemic inflammatory reaction does not occur because there is no intravascular lysis or generation of complement components beyond C3b. There may be low-grade fever, and there will be a more rapid decline in hemoglobin than anticipated, hyperbilirubinemia that is predominantly due to indirect reacting (unconjugated) bilirubin, and development of a positive direct Coombs test.

Delayed Hemolytic Transfusion Reaction

This often unrecognized complication is much less dramatic than the acute reaction and is due to destruction of the transfused red cells by alloantibody. Alloantibody develops because of prior exposure to red blood cells through transfusion sometime in the past that was not detected at the time of cross match because the antibody titer in the recipient had become very low. However, the recipient develops an anamnestic response on repeat challenge with the alloantigen and produces higher titers of alloantibody, resulting in destruction of the transfused erythrocytes over the ensuing days. This extravascular immune-mediated hemolysis can cause low-grade fever, hyperbilirubinemia, and a more rapid fall in hemoglobin than would have been anticipated.[121]

Febrile Nonhemolytic Reactions

Febrile nonhemolytic reactions are characterized by a 1°C or greater increase in temperature, often accompanied by shaking chills, during or shortly after transfusion for which no other etiology can be ascertained. The symptoms are caused by cytokines generated by leukocytes in the donated blood or by cytokines produced by antibodies interacting with antigens on either platelets or leukocytes. Pre-storage leukoreduction has greatly diminished those reactions caused by donor leukocytes. When this reaction develops, the transfusion should be stopped and acetaminophen administered. If there are rigors, meperidine may be given to alleviate them. It is also critically important to rule out other causes of fever with transfusion, including a hemolytic transfusion reaction and sepsis. If these conditions are suspected, the unit should be returned to the blood bank for further study. If infection is a possibility, the returned unit should be cultured, and the patient should have blood cultures obtained and broad-spectrum intravenous antibiotic therapy initiated pending the results of cultures. Premedication with acetaminophen

may prevent febrile reactions with subsequent transfusions; more severely affected patients may require hydrocortisone as well.[121]

Allergic Reactions

Allergic reactions are usually IgE mediated reactions to plasma proteins. Histamine release can cause pruritis, cutaneous erythema, and urticaria. The transfusion should be stopped and diphenhydramine administered. If the symptoms resolve, the transfusion should resume. For future transfusions, premedication with diphenhydramine is commonly employed. Particularly severe anaphylactic reactions can develop in IgA-deficient individuals who develop antibodies to IgA in the transfusion product. Fortunately, these events are uncommon, even in IgA-deficient individuals. Should a severe allergic reaction develop, however, the recipient should be evaluated for IgA deficiency.[121] Not every allergic reaction that develops in close proximity to transfusion is due to the blood product. In many cases, the patient is on medications that could cause allergy. All drugs administered within 4 hours of the reaction should be reviewed for this possibility. It is also prudent not to administer drugs to which allergy could develop during a transfusion. This approach should help reduce uncertainty as to the cause of an allergic reaction. For instance, L-ASP should not be given in close temporal relation to blood product administration.

Premedication

As indicated above, acetaminophen and diphenhydramine are often used to treat febrile and allergic reactions, respectively, and for patients who develop these reactions, as premedication to prevent their recurrence. This prophylactic intervention may not be necessary if products are leukoreduced prior to storage and irradiated, and if platelet transfusions are limited to single-donor apheresis units stored for 5 days or less. Investigators at SJCRH found a remarkably low 1% incidence of either type reaction when using these products and, if anything, a greater incidence of reactions in premedicated patients. They do not recommend premedication as standard practice for patients transfused with the types of products they used, except for the small group of patients with multiple or severe reactions.[122]

Transfusion-Related Acute Lung Injury

Transfusion-related acute lung injury is an uncommon event, and yet it has become one of the leading causes of death from transfusion.[123,124] It can be seen following infusion of any type of plasma-containing blood product and typically develops within 6 hours of the start of the transfusion. Patients develop noncardiogenic pulmonary edema with bilateral pulmonary infiltrates and hypoxemia. They may also have hypotension or hypertension, fever, and chills. Patients who are not neutropenic may have a transient decline in neutrophil count.[125] Differential diagnosis includes allergic reactions, volume overload, and transfusion-related sepsis. The clinical findings are those of acute respiratory distress syndrome (ARDS). However, in contrast to other forms of ARDS, patients typically recover within hours to days and there is no permanent lung injury.[124,126–128]

Transfusion-related acute lung injury is almost certainly underdiagnosed and complicates at least 1 out of every 5000 transfusions. Most cases are misdiagnosed as fluid overload or as acute lung injury from other etiologies.[123] In the cancer population, TRALI is most commonly encountered in patients with hematologic malignancies undergoing induction chemotherapy, and in pediatrics, these are usually children with ALL.[124,128] Two mechanisms have been proposed for its occurrence. The first postulates an immune-mediated reaction whereby antigranulocyte antibodies, some with specificity for HLA class I or class II antigens, mediate the reaction. Usually the antibodies are from the donor and activate recipient granulocytes that damage pulmonary endothelial cells. Acute lung injury ensues with capillary leak syndrome and hypoxemia. This type of TRALI often follows transfusion of frozen plasma or platelet concentrates. Donors of these products are usually multiparous women. Less commonly, the recipient may have antibodies to donor granulocytes. This reaction is likely to develop when a product that has not been leukocyte reduced is infused and may be a reason for TRALI occurring in granulocyte transfusion recipients. With these forms of TRALI, antibody should be identified in donor or in recipient. However, there are cases of TRALI that are not immune mediated, and they more commonly occur after transfusion of stored blood products such as red cells or platelets. Patients who develop this nonimmune form of TRALI are generally sick, either infected or recovering from major surgery, and are thought to have primed neutrophils. The stored product is thought to have biologically active lipids and cytokines that activate these neutrophils in the lungs.[128–130] In neutropenic patients, another mechanism is postulated whereby substances in the product have a direct effect on pulmonary vascular endothelium and cause the capillary leak syndrome. These substances may be high levels of vascular endothelial growth factor or antibodies against HLA class II antigens on pulmonary vascular endothelial cells.[124]

Treatment is primarily with supportive care that can range from administration of supplemental oxygen to mechanical ventilation. Severe cases can be fatal.[126–128] Immune-mediated TRALI is more severe than non-immune-mediated TRALI, and it is more likely to require mechanical ventilation or be fatal.[129] If any type of TRALI is suspected, the transfusion should be immediately stopped and any remaining product returned to the blood bank. Workup of donor and recipient for antineutrophil and anti-HLA antibodies should be undertaken. Donors of products causing TRALI should be deferred from future donations.[126]

Transfusion-Transmitted Diseases

The contamination of the blood supply with HIV in the 1970s, the slow initial recognition of and response to this catastrophe, and the tragic consequences have been elo-

quently documented.[131] Subsequent corrective actions have dramatically altered the practice of transfusion medicine. The lessons learned from the HIV tragedy have resulted in the virtual elimination from the blood supply of this virus and the viruses for hepatitis B and C and human T-cell lymphotrophic virus (HTLV) I and II. The heightened awareness that blood products can be the source of serious and fatal disease transmission has generated a set of standards that will hopefully preclude future tragedies. Deferral of donors at risk of transmitting disease by transfusion is an important aspect of this process. These include individuals at risk for certain diseases such as HIV and those who are acutely ill at the time of donation. However, increasingly sensitive methods for detection of transfusion-transmitted diseases are the mainstays for prevention of infectious complications in recipients of blood products.

Screening that employs serologic testing and nucleic acid testing (NAT) of blood products is so effective that individuals rarely acquire via transfusion the viral diseases for which testing is available. Using these technologies the risk for transfusion-transmitted hepatitis C and HIV has been drastically reduced to the point where an individual is more likely to die from a lightning strike than from acquiring these diseases from a blood product (Figure 35-2).[132] Currently, the principal infectious complication from blood transfusion is sepsis resulting from bacterial contamination of the product, and this particular complication is the second leading cause of death from transfusion.

Viral Diseases

All units must be screened for HIV, HTLV I and II, and hepatitis B and C. Combining serologic testing for HIV 1 and 2 with NAT has resulted in risk of acquisition of these infections to less than 1 in 10^6 units transfused. The window period during which all these tests will be negative in an infected individual has been reduced to 10 days. Similar tests are used to screen for hepatitis C virus and have resulted in an equally low risk of transmission via blood products. The window period has also decreased to 10 to 30 days.[133] Hepatitis B screening employs both HBsAg and anti-HBc and decreases risk of transmission to 1 in 200 000 units transfused. The 60-day window period for hepatitis B is greater than for the other diseases.[134] HTLV I and II screening is serologic and so effective that risk of transmission is less than 1 in 2×10^6 units transfused.

Screening for other viral diseases is not mandatory. There have been at least 23 cases of transmission of West Nile virus by blood transfusions. Since the incidence of this infection varies with geographic location and season, the need for screening all donors for this virus has been questioned, and it has been suggested that screening be limited to donors from locations where there is an outbreak.[135] Provision of CMV-safe blood products can be accomplished by either selection of CMV-seronegative donors or by leukoreduction. As indicated above, for the highest risk patients, use of CMV-seronegative donors appears to be the safest option. Parvovirus B19 can cause persistent hypoproliferative anemia in immunocompromised hosts, including patients on chemotherapy. Most infections with this virus occur in childhood, producing erythema infectiousum or Fifth disease, and once humoral immunity develops, the virus is cleared and infection ceases. However, approximately, 1% of normal or immunocompetent individuals do not clear their infection, even after development of antibody. They may serve as a reservoir for its transmission by transfusion to immunocompromised recipients.[136]

Bacterial Contamination of Blood Products

Bacterial contamination is now the greatest infectious risk of blood transfusion and is much more common with platelets than with red blood cells. Bacterial contamination may be decreased by improved methods of donor skin disinfection, by diversion of the first 30 ml of blood collected into a separate system used for testing rather than infusion, and by leukoreduction. However, bacterial contamination still occurs in 1 out of every 1000 to 2000 platelet products and 1 out of 10^6 red cell products.[137] When the product is transfused, the inoculum of bacteria can cause fever and chills, rigors, hypotension, and hypoxemia. With gram-negative organisms, endotoxic shock and DIC may occur. Pediatric oncology patients are frequently neutropenic when receiving transfusions and already have decreased capacity to fight infection. It may be difficult to discern if a fever spike during transfusion is due to an acute hemolytic reaction, a febrile nonhemolytic transfusion reaction, infection unrelated to the blood product administration, or sepsis from a contaminated product. Patients experiencing nonhemolytic reactions are generally less sick than those with sepsis or an acute hemolytic reaction. Once bacterial infection is suspected, the transfusion should be stopped, the product and the patient's blood cultured, and broad-spectrum intravenous antibiotics administered promptly.

Platelets are a much more likely source for bacterial contamination because they are stored for a number of days at room temperature.[138] Current policy dictates they be screened for bacterial contamination before they can be transfused. Nonspecific methods such as pH and glucose alterations are less precise than culture techniques, which are the preferred method for detection of bacterial contamination.[70,139] Platelets are tested after 24 hours of storage, a time usually sufficient to allow enough bacterial growth for detection by culture; the culture is usually positive within 12 to 24 hours. Therefore, 2 days must elapse before the platelets are administered.[139] Apheresis units are less likely to be contaminated than pooled platelet units because they are from a single donor rather than multiple donors. When bacteria are present in platelet concentrates, they are predominantly gram-positive organisms, especially *Staphylococci*, with coagulase-negative organisms more common than *Staphylococcus aureus*. Red blood cells are much less likely to be contaminated because they are stored in the cold. *Yersinia enterocolitica* is the most frequent pathogen recovered from stored red cells and can produce severe sepsis of rapid onset with a high fatality rate.[133,137]

Pathogen Reduction Methods

For acelluar products, solvent detergent methods are effective in removing lipid-enveloped viruses such as HIV and hepatitis C but are much less effective for viruses such as parvovirus B19 and hepatitis A that lack a lipid envelope. Other processes must be used with cellular products so that the cells remain functional. For platelets, photosensitive compounds such as psoralens are added and activated by subsequent exposure to UV light. The photoactivated psoralens bind to RNA or DNA, or both, in pathogens. Nucleic acids are modified in such a manner to prevent pathogen replication.[140] Use of this technology for platelets has demonstrated that they retain their function but that there is an increase in the number of units needed and decrease in the time interval for transfusions.[141] A number of nucleic acid-modifying compounds have been added to red cells to inactivate pathogens.[142] Pathogen reduction methods for cellular products have not been universally embraced or adopted. There remain concerns about alteration in the function of the cells by this treatment, as well as concerns that infusion of these nucleic acid-altering substances could mutate recipient DNA and promote oncogenesis or alter nucleic acids in donor or recipient cells and make them immunogenic.[143] Indeed, this has already occurred for red cells. Antibodies have developed to erythrocytes subjected to pathogen reduction technology, and this has led to suspension of their use for individuals requiring repeated transfusions.[118] However, this technology offers great promise because it is not specific for any given pathogen. If it is proved safe and effective, it may protect against as yet unknown pathogens when they enter the blood supply.[140]

Prion-Transmitted Disease

The only documented type of prion-associated disease transmitted by blood products is variant Creutzfeldt-Jakob disease (vCJd). The agent that causes vCJd also causes bovine spongiform encephalopathy, and it develops in humans who ingest meat from cows with this disease. There was an outbreak of the cattle disease in the 1980s and 1990s in the United Kingdom and subsequent infection of individuals who ate meat from diseased cattle. Variant Creutzfeldt-Jakob disease initially presents with neuropsychiatric symptoms such as anxiety, depression, dysaesthesia, and ataxia, and it progresses to dementia, myoclonus, and choreoathetosis, with death occurring within 6 to 24 months of onset of symptoms. Approximately one-third of the population of the United Kingdom is particularly susceptible to CId. They are individuals homozygous for the methionine coding polymorphism at codon 129 of prion protein, and they are genetically predisposed to develop vCJd when exposed to the causative prion. The abnormal prions in individuals with vCJd are felt to reside in the lymphoid tissue, including circulating B-lymphocytes, during early preclinical stages of the disease and are therefore transmissible in blood products. Transmission through blood products has been documented to have occurred only twice, but it is of sufficient concern in the United Kingdom that major alterations in transfusion practices have been instituted as a consequence. There are no serologic tests to detect prion-transmitted disease. Therefore, donors who received blood transfusions from 1980 onward (the period of risk for acquiring vCJd) are deferred. For children born after 1995 and therefore not exposed to the causative prion from contaminated meat, the only plasma products given to them are from the United States rather than the United Kingdom.[134,144]

Patients and Families Who Refuse Transfusion

Patients and families may refuse transfusions for a variety of reasons. They may have concerns about blood safety or may object to transfusions on religious grounds. If a family objects to blood based on safety issues, education regarding blood product safety and the possibility for directed donor blood usually alleviates their concerns.

Families that object to blood products on a religious basis present a unique challenge to the pediatric hematologist/oncologist. Jehovah's Witnesses represent the most common religious group refusing blood. Jehovah's Witnesses decline any nonprocessed blood products, including packed RBCs, platelets, WBCs, FFP, and cryoprecipitate. The use of albumin, plasma-derived factor concentrates, or other fractionated plasma proteins is considered a matter of individual conscience.

Managing the patient who refuses blood products requires creativity and compassion. Practitioners must assure families that they will attempt to avoid blood product transfusions if at all possible but also must state realistically that transfusions may be necessary. Preparation is key to the management of these special patients. This preparation starts prior to initiation of therapy and continues during and after institution of treatment for the child's cancer.

Prior to initiating treatment for a patient who refuses transfusion therapy, hemoglobin and platelet counts should be optimized. This can be attempted by using hematopoietic growth factors. Clinicians have the most experience with EPO, a red cell growth factor. In patients with preoperative/pretherapy anemia, EPO at doses of 100 to 300 μ/kg, 3 times a week, given in conjunction with exogenous iron, will improve the hemoglobin and hematocrit.[145,146] Erythropoietin should be considered if time permits prior to surgery or chemotherapy.

Other pretreatment interventions include preparing the family for the possibility of transfusions and obtaining court consent for transfusion. This requires a multidisciplinary approach including nursing, social work, and a medical liaison from the Jehovah's Witness community. Parents with religious objections should not be pressured to consent for transfusion for their child. Instead, the court should be petitioned to supersede the parental right to refuse therapies.

Although regulations vary from state to state, court orders can usually be obtained quickly. In emergency situations, agreement of two physicians confirming the necessity of transfusion is usually sufficient. However, an understanding of individual state law is essential to protect the clinician. Even if a court order is obtained, attempts to prevent transfusions should persist. The perception of the family that their religious beliefs are respected will improve the physician–patient relationship.

If surgeries are planned, the following strategies will decrease need for transfusions: staging procedures to reduce blood loss with each procedure and delaying surgery to allow improvement in hemoglobin level by utilizing EPO and exogenous iron. Intraoperatively, hemodilution and cell-saver techniques can reduce blood loss. Cell saver during a cancer surgery may be contraindicated due to the concern of reinfusing cancer cells. Chemotherapy regimens also must be considered. Therapies that are less myelosuppressive but have similar outcomes should be offered to families. Clinical trials where one arm increases the probability of transfusion should not be offered.

Once therapy has been determined, strategies to avoid potential transfusions should persist. Minimizing blood tests, withdrawing minimal amounts of blood by batching studies and employing micro-container draws, and returning discard (as permitted by hospital policy) will reduce iatrogenic contributions toward anemia. Utilization of EPO after doses of chemotherapy will improve the hemoglobin level and possibly cause the platelet count to rise more rapidly, thereby reducing the likelihood of transfusion.[147–149] Finally, the decision to transfuse in this patient population should be based on symptoms and not on any specific cell count number.

If a transfusion is deemed necessary for a patient opposed to transfusion, the patient and family should be prepared as soon as possible and reassured that no alternatives exist. For patients and families that refuse transfusion, it is the transfusion itself, not the amount transfused, that is the problem. Patients describe transfusions as equivalent to assault (personal communication, medical liaison). Thus, if a transfusion is required, a sufficient volume should be infused to decrease the likelihood of another transfusion being necessary.

Summary

Transfusion therapy is one of the major aspects of supportive care of pediatric oncology patients. Appropriate and judicious use of blood components enables patients to progress through the various phases of therapy for their malignancy. Cure for many patients would not be possible without blood product support. Recommendations made for use of specific components are offered as good clinical practice guidelines. Clinicians must also be aware of the potential complications associated with transfusion of blood products, both infectious and noninfectious, and strive to minimize these complications whenever possible. Vigilance must be maintained to provide pathogen-free products and to detect any new pathogens that enter the blood supply. Research must continue with the goal of providing better and safer products for transfusion, more precise guidelines for the use of these products, and for alternatives to transfusion.

References

1. Wales PW, Lau W, Kim PC. Directed blood donation in pediatric general surgery: is it worth it? *J Pediatr Surg.* 2001;36:722–725.
2. Barnard D, Rogers C. Blood component therapy. In: Altman A, ed. *Supportive Care of Children with Cancer: Current Therapy and Guidelines from the Children's Oncology Group,* 3rd ed. Baltimore: Johns Hopkins University Press; 2004:39–57.
3. Bowden RA, Slichter SJ, Sayers M, et al. A comparison of filtered leukocyte-reduced and cytomegalovirus (CMV) seronegative blood products for the prevention of transfusion-associated CMV infection after marrow transplant. *Blood.* 1995;86:3598–3603.
4. Nichols WG, Price TH, Gooley T, Corey L, Boeckh M. Transfusion-transmitted cytomegalovirus infection after receipt of leukoreduced blood products. *Blood.* 2003;101:4195–4200.
5. Goodnough LT, Brecher ME, Kanter MH, AuBuchon JP. Transfusion medicine: first of two parts—blood transfusion. *N Engl J Med.* 1999;340:438–447.
6. Blumberg N, Fine L, Gettings KF, Heal JM. Decreased sepsis related to indwelling venous access devices coincident with implementation of universal leukoreduction of blood transfusions. *Transfusion.* 2005;45:1632–1639.
7. Rios JA, Korones DN, Heal JM, Blumberg N. WBC-reduced blood transfusions and clinical outcome in children with acute lymphoid leukemia. *Transfusion.* 2001;41:873–877.
8. Michon J. Incidence of anemia in pediatric cancer patients in Europe: results of a large, international survey. *Med Pediatr Oncol.* 2002;39:448–450.
9. Sanz MA, Tallman MS, Lo-Coco F. Tricks of the trade for the appropriate management of newly diagnosed acute promyelocytic leukemia. *Blood.* 2005; 105:3019–3025.
10. Hockenberry MJ, Hinds PS, Barrera P, et al. Incidence of anemia in children with solid tumors or Hodgkin disease. *J Pediatr Hematol Oncol.* 2002;24:35–37.
11. Corazza F, Beguin Y, Bergmann P, et al. Anemia in children with cancer is associated with decreased erythropoietic activity and not with inadequate erythropoietin production. *Blood.* 1998;92:1793–1798.
12. Wolfe J, Grier HE, Klar N, et al. Symptoms and suffering at the end of life in children with cancer. *N Engl J Med.* 2000;342:326–333.
13. Beardsmore S, Fitzmaurice N. Palliative care in paediatric oncology. *Eur J Cancer.* 2002;38:1900–1907.
14. Desmet L, Lacroix J. Transfusion in pediatrics. *Crit Care Clin.* 2004;20:299–311.
15. Hebert PC, Van der Linden P, Biro G, Hu LQ. Physiologic aspects of anemia. *Crit Care Clin.* 2004;20:187–212.
16. Hetzel TM, Losek JD. Unrecognized severe anemia in children presenting with respiratory distress. *Am J Emerg Med.* 1998;16:386–389.
17. Kawai A, Kadota H, Yamaguchi U, Morimoto Y, Ozaki T, Beppu Y. Blood loss and transfusion associated with musculoskeletal tumor surgery. *J Surg Oncol.* 2005;92:52–58.
18. Gibson BE, Todd A, Roberts I, et al. Transfusion guidelines for neonates and older children. *Br J Haematol.* 2004;124:433–453.
19. Wong EC, Perez-Albuerne E, Moscow JA, Luban NL. Transfusion management strategies: a survey of practicing pediatric hematology/oncology specialists. *Pediatr Blood Cancer.* 2005;44:119–127.
20. Buchanan GR. Blood transfusions in children with cancer and hematologic disorders: why, when, and how? *Pediatr Blood Cancer.* 2005;44:114–116.
21. Varlotto J, Stevenson MA. Anemia, tumor hypoxemia, and the cancer patient. *Int J Radiat Oncol Biol Phys.* 2005;63:25–36.
22. Dische S, Anderson PJ, Sealy R, Watson ER. Carcinoma of the cervix: anaemia, radiotherapy and hyperbaric oxygen. *Br J Radiol.* 1983;56:251–255.
23. Knight K, Wade S, Balducci L. Prevalence and outcomes of anemia in cancer: a systematic review of the literature. *Am J Med.* 2004;116(Suppl 7A):11S-26S.
24. Ruggiero A, Riccardi R. Interventions for anemia in pediatric cancer patients. *Med Pediatr Oncol.* 2002;39:451–454.
25. Marec-Berard P, Blay JY, Schell M, Buclon M, Demaret C, Ray-Coquard I. Risk model predictive of severe anemia requiring RBC transfusion after chemotherapy in pediatric solid tumor patients. *J Clin Oncol.* 2003;21:4235–4238.
26. Armano R, Gauvin F, Ducruet T, Lacroix J. Determinants of red blood cell transfusions in a pediatric critical care unit: a prospective, descriptive epidemiological study. *Critical Care Med.* 2005;33:2637–2644.
27. Goodman AM, Pollack MM, Patel KM, Luban NL. Pediatric red blood cell transfusions increase resource use. *J Pediatr.* 2003;142:123–127.
28. Bratton SL, Annich GM. Packed red blood cell transfusions for critically ill pediatric patients: when and for what conditions? *J Pediatr.* 2003;142:95–97.
29. Morris KP, Naqvi N, Davies P, Smith M, Lee PW. A new formula for blood transfusion volume in the critically ill. *Arch Dis Child.* 2005;90:724–728.
30. Lowe EJ, Pui CH, Hancock ML, Geiger TL, Khan RB, Sandlund JT. Early complications in children with acute lymphoblastic leukemia presenting with hyperleukocytosis. *Pediatr Blood Cancer* 2005;45:10–15.
31. Creutzig U, Zimmermann M, Reinhardt D, Dworzak M, Stary J, Lehrnbecher T. Early deaths and treatment-related mortality in children undergoing therapy for acute myeloid leukemia: analysis of the multicenter clinical trials AML-BFM 93 and AML-BFM 98. *J Clin Oncol.* 2004;22:4384–4393.
32. Rizzo JD, Lichtin AE, Woolf SH, et al. Use of epoetin in patients with cancer: evidence-based clinical practice guidelines of the American Society of Clinical Oncology and the American Society of Hematology. *Blood.* 2002;100: 2303–2320.
33. Feusner J, Hastings C. Recombinant human erythropoietin in pediatric oncology: a review. *Med Pediatr Oncol.* 2002;39:463–468.
34. Wagner LM, Billups CA, Furman WL, Rao BN, Santana VM. Combined use of erythropoietin and granulocyte colony-stimulating factor does not decrease blood transfusion requirements during induction therapy for high-risk neuroblastoma: a randomized controlled trial. *J Clin Oncol.* 2004; 22:1886–1893.
35. Varan A, Buyukpamukcu M, Kutluk T, Akyuz C. Recombinant human erythropoietin treatment for chemotherapy-related anemia in children. *Pediatrics.* 1999;103:E16.
36. Yilmaz D, Cetingul N, Kantar M, Oniz H, Kansoy S, Kavakli K. A single institutional experience: is epoetin alpha effective in anemic children with cancer? *Pediatr Hematol Oncol.* 2004;21:1–8.
37. Kronberger M, Fischmeister G, Poetschger U, Gadner H, Zoubek A. Reduction in transfusion requirements with early epoetin alfa treatment in pediatric patients with solid tumors: a case-control study. *Pediatr Hematol Oncol.* 2002; 19:95–105.
38. Henze G, Michon J, Morland B, et al. Phase III randomized study: efficacy of epoetin alpha in reducing blood transfusions in newly diagnosed pediatric cancer patients receiving chemotherapy. *Proc Am Soc Clin Oncol.* 2002;21:387a.
39. Razzouk BI, Hord JD, Hockenberry M, et al. Double-blind, placebo-controlled study of quality of life, hematologic end points, and safety of weekly epoetin alfa in children with cancer receiving myelosuppressive chemotherapy. *J Clin Oncol.* 2006;24:3583–3589.
40. Henke M, Laszig R, Rube C, et al. Erythropoietin to treat head and neck cancer patients with anaemia undergoing radiotherapy: randomised, double-blind, placebo-controlled trial. *Lancet.* 2003;362:1255–1260.
41. Leyland-Jones B. Breast cancer trial with erythropoietin terminated unexpectedly. *Lancet Oncol.* 2003;4:459–460.
42. Batra S, Perelman N, Luck LR, Shimada H, Malik P. Pediatric tumor cells express erythropoietin and a functional erythropoietin receptor that promotes angiogenesis and tumor cell survival. *Lab Invest.* 2003;83:1477–1487.
43. Stanworth SJ, Hyde C, Heddle N, Rebulla P, Brunskill S, Murphy MF. Prophylactic platelet transfusion for haemorrhage after chemotherapy and stem cell transplantation. *Cochrane Database Syst Rev.* 2004;CD004269.
44. Kruskall MS. The perils of platelet transfusions. *N Engl J Med.* 1997;337: 1914–1915.
45. Gaydos LA, Freireich EJ, Mantel N. The quantitative relation between platelet count and hemorrhage in patients with acute leukemia. *N Engl J Med.* 1962; 266:905–909.
46. Wandt H, Frank M, Ehninger G, et al. Safety and cost effectiveness of a 10 × 10(9)/L trigger for prophylactic platelet transfusions compared with the traditional 20 x 10(9)/L trigger: a prospective comparative trial in 105 patients with acute myeloid leukemia. *Blood.* 1998;91:3601–3606.
47. Callow CR, Swindell R, Randall W, Chopra R. The frequency of bleeding complications in patients with haematological malignancy following the introduction of a stringent prophylactic platelet transfusion policy. *Br J Haematol.* 2002;118:677–682.
48. Friedmann AM, Sengul H, Lehmann H, Schwartz C, Goodman S. Do basic laboratory tests or clinical observations predict bleeding in thrombocytopenic oncology patients? a reevaluation of prophylactic platelet transfusions. *Transfus Med Rev.* 2002;16:34–45.
49. Rebulla P. Trigger for platelet transfusion. *Vox Sang.* 2000;78(Suppl 2):179–182.
50. Heckman KD, Weiner GJ, Davis CS, Strauss RG, Jones MP, Burns CP. Randomized study of prophylactic platelet transfusion threshold during induction therapy for adult acute leukemia: 10 000/microL versus 20 000/microL. *J Clin Oncol.* 1997;15:1143–1149.
51. Zumberg MS, del Rosario ML, Nejame CF, et al. A prospective randomized trial of prophylactic platelet transfusion and bleeding incidence in hematopoietic stem cell transplant recipients: 10 000/L versus 20 000/microL trigger. *Biol Blood Marrow Transplant.* 2002;8:569–576.
52. Higby DJ, Cohen E, Holland JF, Sinks L. The prophylactic treatment of thrombocytopenic leukemic patients with platelets: a double blind study. *Transfusion.* 1974;14:440–446.
53. Slichter SJ. Relationship between platelet count and bleeding risk in thrombocytopenic patients. *Transfus Med Rev.* 2004;18:153–167.
54. Stanworth SJ, Hyde C, Brunskill S, Murphy MF. Platelet transfusion prophylaxis for patients with haematological malignancies: where to now? *Br J Haematol.* 2005;131:588–595.
55. Schiffer CA, Anderson KC, Bennett CL, et al. Platelet transfusion for patients with cancer: clinical practice guidelines of the American Society of Clinical Oncology. *J Clin Oncol.* 2001;19:1519–1538.
56. Lawrence JB, Yomtovian RA, Hammons T, et al. Lowering the prophylactic platelet transfusion threshold: a prospective analysis. *Leuk Lymphoma.* 2001; 41:67–76.

57. Murphy S, Snyder E, Cable R, et al. Platelet dose consistency and its effect on the number of platelet transfusions for support of thrombocytopenia: an analysis of the SPRINT trial of platelets photochemically treated with amotosalen HCl and ultraviolet A light. *Transfusion.* 2006;46:24–33.

58. Benjamin RJ, Anderson KC. What is the proper threshold for platelet transfusion in patients with chemotherapy-induced thrombocytopenia? *Crit Rev Oncol Hematol.* 2002;42:163–171.

59. Kulpa J, Zaroulis CG, Good RA, Kutti J. Altered platelet function and circulation induced by amphotericin B in leukemic patients after platelet transfusion. *Transfusion.* 1981;21:74–76.

60. Howard SC, Gajjar A, Ribeiro RC, et al. Safety of lumbar puncture for children with acute lymphoblastic leukemia and thrombocytopenia. *JAMA.* 2000; 284:2222–2224.

61. Gajjar A, Harrison PL, Sandlund JT, et al. Traumatic lumbar puncture at diagnosis adversely affects outcome in childhood acute lymphoblastic leukemia. *Blood.* 2000;96:3381–3384.

62. Burger B, Zimmermann M, Mann G, et al. Diagnostic cerebrospinal fluid examination in children with acute lymphoblastic leukemia: significance of low leukocyte counts with blasts or traumatic lumbar puncture. *J Clin Oncol.* 2003;21:184–188.

63. Te Loo DMWM, Kamps WA, van der Does-van den Berg A, de Graaf SSN. Prognostic significance of blasts in the cerebrospinal fluid without pleiocytosis or a traumatic lumbar puncture in children with acute lymphoblastic leukemia: experience of the Dutch Childhood Oncology Group. *J Clin Oncol.* 2006;24:2332–2336.

64. Pui CH. Toward optimal central nervous system-directed treatment in childhood acute lymphoblastic leukemia. *J Clin Oncol.* 2003;21:179–181.

65. Howard SC, Gajjar AJ, Cheng C, et al. Risk factors for traumatic and bloody lumbar puncture in children with acute lymphoblastic leukemia. *JAMA.* 2002;288:2001–2007.

66. Tinmouth AT, Freedman J. Prophylactic platelet transfusions: which dose is the best dose? a review of the literature. *Transfus Med Rev.* 2003;17:181–193.

67. Klumpp TR, Herman JH, Gaughan JP, et al. Clinical consequences of alterations in platelet transfusion dose: a prospective, randomized, double-blind trial. *Transfusion.* 1999;39:674–681.

68. Saxonhouse M, Slayton W, Sola M. Platelet transfusions in the infant and child. In: Hillyer C, Strauss R, Luban N, eds. *Handbook of Pediatric Transfusion Medicine.* San Diego, CA: Academic Press; 2004:253–269.

69. Klein HG. Pathogen inactivation technology: cleansing the blood supply. *J Intern Med.* 2005;257:224–237.

70. Brecher ME, Hay SN. Bacterial contamination of blood components. *Clin Microbiol Rev.* 2005;18:195–204.

71. Simon TL, Nelson EJ, Carmen R, Murphy S. Extension of platelet concentrate storage. *Transfusion.* 1983;23:207–212.

72. Simon TL, Sierra ER. Concentration of platelet units into small volumes. *Transfusion.* 1984;24:173–175.

73. McFarland J, Menitove J, Kagen L, et al. Leukocyte reduction and ultraviolet B irradiation of platelets to prevent alloimmunization and refractoriness to platelet transfusions. *New Engl J Med.* 1997;337:1861–1869.

74. Sintnicolaas K, Vriesendorp HM, Sizoo W, et al. Delayed alloimmunisation by random single donor platelet transfusions: a randomised study to compare single donor and multiple donor platelet transfusions in cancer patients with severe thrombocytopenia. *Lancet.* 1981;1:750–754.

75. Slichter SJ, Davis K, Enright H, et al. Factors affecting posttransfusion platelet increments, platelet refractoriness, and platelet transfusion intervals in thrombocytopenic patients. *Blood.* 2005;105:4106–4114.

76. Saarinen UM, Kekomaki R, Siimes MA, Myllyla G. Effective prophylaxis against platelet refractoriness in multitransfused patients by use of leukocyte-free blood components. *Blood.* 1990;75:512–517.

77. Saarinen UM, Koskimies S, Myllyla G. Systematic use of leukocyte-free blood components to prevent alloimmunization and platelet refractoriness in multi-transfused children with cancer. *Vox Sang.* 1993;65:286–292.

78. Hogge DE, McConnell M, Jacobson C, Sutherland HJ, Benny WB, Massing BG. Platelet refractoriness and alloimmunization in pediatric oncology and bone marrow transplant patients. *Transfusion.* 1995;35:645–652.

79. Chalandon Y, Mermillod B, Beris P, et al. Benefit of prestorage leukocyte depletion of single-donor platelet concentrates. *Vox Sang.* 1999;76:27–37.

80. Couban S, Carruthers J, Andreou P, et al. Platelet transfusions in children: results of a randomized, prospective, crossover trial of plasma removal and a prospective audit of WBC reduction. *Transfusion.* 2002;42:753–758.

81. Schiffer CA. Prevention of alloimmunization against platelets. *Blood.* 1991; 77:1–4.

82. McFarland JG, Anderson AJ, Slichter SJ. Factors influencing the transfusion response to HLA-selected apheresis donor platelets in patients refractory to random platelet concentrates. *Br J Haematol.* 1989;73:380–386.

83. Berman RS, Feig BW, Hunt KK, Mansfield PF, Pollock RE. Platelet kinetics and decreased transfusion requirements after splenectomy for hematologic malignancy. *Ann Surg.* 2004;240:852–857.

84. Heal JM, Blumberg N. Optimizing platelet transfusion therapy. *Blood Rev.* 2004;18:149–165.

85. Jimenez TM, Patel SB, Pineda AA, Tefferi A, Owen WG. Factors that influence platelet recovery after transfusion: resolving donor quality from ABO compatibility. *Transfusion.* 2003;43:328–334.

86. Zeerleder S, Hack CE, Wuillemin WA. Disseminated intravascular coagulation in sepsis. *Chest.* 2005;128:2864–2875.

87. Higuchi T, Toyama D, Hirota Y, et al. Disseminated intravascular coagulation complicating acute lymphoblastic leukemia: a study of childhood and adult cases. *Leuk Lymphoma.* 2005;46:1169–1176.

88. Contreras M, Ala FA, Greaves M, et al. Guidelines for the use of fresh frozen plasma. British Committee for Standards in Haematology, Working Party of the Blood Transfusion Task Force. *Transfus Med.* 1992;2:57–63.

89. O'Shaughnessy DF, Atterbury C, Bolton MP, et al. Guidelines for the use of fresh-frozen plasma, cryoprecipitate and cryosupernatant. *Br J Haematol.* 2004;126:11–28.

90. Halton JM, Mitchell LG, Vegh P, Eves M, Andrew ME. Fresh frozen plasma has no beneficial effect on the hemostatic system in children receiving L-asparaginase. *Am J Hematol.* 1994;47:157–161.

91. Nowak-Gottl U, Rath B, Binder M, et al. Inefficacy of fresh frozen plasma in the treatment of L-asparaginase-induced coagulation factor deficiencies during ALL induction therapy. *Haematologica.* 1995;80:451–453.

92. Hongo T, Okada S, Ohzeki T, et al. Low plasma levels of hemostatic proteins during the induction phase in children with acute lymphoblastic leukemia: a retrospective study by the JACLS. Japan Association of Childhood Leukemia Study. *Pediatr Int.* 2002;44:293–299.

93. Musa MO, Al Fair F, Al Mohareb F, Al Saeed H, Aljurf M. Cryoprecipitate-induced mesenteric venous thrombosis during L-asparaginase therapy for acute lymphoblastic leukaemia. *Leuk Lymphoma.* 2001;40:429–431.

94. Imamura T, Morimoto A, Kato R, et al. Cerebral thrombotic complications in adolescent leukemia/lymphoma patients treated with L-asparaginase-containing chemotherapy. *Leuk Lymphoma.* 2005;46:729–735.

95. Hattersley PG, Kunkel M. Cryoprecipitates as a source of fibrinogen in treatment of disseminated introvascular coagulation (DIC). *Transfusion.* 1976;16:641–645.

96. Castaman G, Bona ED, Schiavotto C, Trentin L, D'Emilio A, Rodeghiero F. Pilot study on the safety and efficacy of desmopressin for the treatment or prevention of bleeding in patients with hematologic malignancies. *Haematologica.* 1997;82:584–587.

97. Kobrinsky NL, Tulloch H. Treatment of refractory thrombocytopenic bleeding with 1-desamino-8-D-arginine vasopressin (desmopressin). *J Pediatr.* 1988;112:993–996.

98. Monroe DM, Hoffman M, Allen GA, Roberts HR. The factor VII-platelet interplay: effectiveness of recombinant factor VIIa in the treatment of bleeding in severe thrombocytopathia. *Semin Thromb Hemost.* 2000;26:373–377.

99. Heuer L, Blumenberg D. Management of bleeding in a multi-transfused patient with positive HLA class I alloantibodies and thrombocytopenia associated with platelet dysfunction refractory to transfusion of cross-matched platelets. *Blood Coagul Fibrinolysis.* 2005;16:287–290.

100. Vidarsson B, Onundarson PT. Recombinant factor VIIa for bleeding in refractory thrombocytopenia. *Thromb Haemost.* 2000;83:634–635.

101. Gerotziafas GT, Zervas C, Gavrielidis G, et al. Effective hemostasis with rFVIIa treatment in two patients with severe thrombocytopenia and life-threatening hemorrhage. *Am J Hematol.* 2002;69:219–222.

102. Blatt J, Gold SH, Wiley JM, Monahan PE, Cooper HC, Harvey D. Off-label use of recombinant factor VIIa in patients following bone marrow transplantation. *Bone Marrow Transplant.* 2001;28:405–407.

103. Mittal S, Watson HG. A critical appraisal of the use of recombinant factor VIIa in acquired bleeding conditions. *Br J Haematology.* 2006;133:355–363.

104. Benson K, Fields K, Hiemenz J, et al. The platelet-refractory bone marrow transplant patient: prophylaxis and treatment of bleeding. *Semin Oncol.* 1993; 20:102–109.

105. Garewal HS, Durie BG. Anti-fibrinolytic therapy with aminocaproic acid for the control of bleeding in thrombocytopenic patients. *Scand J Haematol.* 1985;35:497–500.

106. Bishton M, Chopra R. The role of granulocyte transfusions in neutropenic patients. *Br J Haematol.* 2004;127:501–508.

107. Robinson SP, Marks DI. Granulocyte transfusions in the G-CSF era: where do we stand? *Bone Marrow Transplant.* 2004;34:839–846.

108. Dale DC, Liles WC, Price TH. Renewed interest in granulocyte transfusion therapy. *Br J Haematol.* 1997;98:497–501.

109. Cesaro S, Chinello P, De Silvestro G, et al. Granulocyte transfusions from G-CSF-stimulated donors for the treatment of severe infections in neutropenic pediatric patients with onco-hematological diseases. *Support Care Cancer.* 2003;11:101–106.

110. Johnston DL, Waldhausen JH, Park JR. Deep soft tissue infections in the neutropenic pediatric oncology patient. *J Pediatr Hematol Oncol.* 2001;23:443–447.

111. Mousset S, Hermann S, Klein SA, et al. Prophylactic and interventional granulocyte transfusions in patients with haematological malignancies and life-threatening infections during neutropenia. *Ann Hematol.* 2005;84:734–741.

112. Safdar A, Hanna HA, Boktour M, et al. Impact of high-dose granulocyte transfusions in patients with cancer with candidemia: retrospective case-control analysis of 491 episodes of Candida species bloodstream infections. *Cancer.* 2004;101:2859–2865.

113. Stanworth SJ, Massey E, Hyde C, et al. Granulocyte transfusions for treating infections in patients with neutropenia or neutrophil dysfunction. *Cochrane Database Syst Rev.* 2005;CD005339.

114. Bohme A, Ruhnke M, Buchheidt D, et al. Treatment of fungal infections in hematology and oncology: guidelines of the Infectious Diseases Working Party (AGIHO) of the German Society of Hematology and Oncology (DGHO). *Ann Hematol.* 2003;82(Suppl 2):S133–S140.

115. Sulis M, Harrison L, Cairo M. Granulocyte transfusion in the neonate and child. In: Hillyer C, Strauss R, Luban N, eds. *Handbook of Pediatric Transfusion Medicine.* San Diego, CA: Academic Press; 2006:167–180.
116. Hubel K, Rodger E, Gaviria JM, Price TH, Dale DC, Liles WC. Effective storage of granulocytes collected by centrifugation leukapheresis from donors stimulated with granulocyte-colony-stimulating factor. *Transfusion.* 2005;45: 1876–1889.
117. Sulis ML, van de Ven C, Henderson T, Anderson L, Cairo MS. Liposomal amphotericin B (AmBisome) compared with amphotericin B +/− FMLP induces significantly less in vitro neutrophil aggregation with granulocyte-colony-stimulating factor/dexamethasone-mobilized allogeneic donor neutrophils. *Blood.* 2002;99:384–386.
118. AuBuchon JP. Pathogen reduction technologies: what are the concerns? *Vox Sang.* 2004;87(Suppl 2):84–89.
119. Stainsby D, Russell J, Cohen H, Lilleyman J. Reducing adverse events in blood transfusion. *Br J Haematol.* 2005;131:8–12.
120. Wu Y, Snyder E. Transfusion reactions. In: Hoffman R, Benz E, Shattil S, eds. *Hematology: Basic Principles and Practice,* 4th ed. Philadelphia: Elsevier; 2005:2515–2526.
121. Eder A. Transfusion reactions. In: Hillyer C, Strauss R, Luban N, eds. *Handbook of Pediatric Transfusion Medicine.* San Diego, CA: Academic Press; 2004: 301–316.
122. Sanders RP, Maddirala SD, Geiger TL, et al. Premedication with acetaminophen or diphenhydramine for transfusion with leucoreduced blood products in children. *Br J Haematol.* 2005;130:781–787.
123. Gajic O, Moore SB. Transfusion-related acute lung injury. *Mayo Clin Proc.* 2005;80:766–770.
124. Silliman CC, Ambruso DR, Boshkov LK. Transfusion-related acute lung injury. *Blood.* 2005;105:2266–2273.
125. Marques MB, Tuncer HH, Divers SG, Baker AC, Harrison DK. Acute transient leukopenia as a sign of TRALI. *Am J Hematol.* 2005;80:90–91.
126. Sanchez R, Toy P. Transfusion related acute lung injury: a pediatric perspective. *Pediatr Blood Cancer.* 2005;45:248–255.
127. Shander A, Popovsky MA. Understanding the consequences of transfusion-related acute lung injury. *Chest.* 2005;128:598S-604S.
128. Silliman CC, Boshkov LK, Mehdizadehkashi Z, et al. Transfusion-related acute lung injury: epidemiology and a prospective analysis of etiologic factors. *Blood.* 2003;101:454–462.
129. Bux J. Transfusion-related acute lung injury (TRALI): a serious adverse event of blood transfusion. *Vox Sang.* 2005;89:1–10.
130. Toy P, Popovsky MA, Abraham E, et al. Transfusion-related acute lung injury: definition and review. *Crit Care Med.* 2005;33:721–726.
131. Shilts R. *And the Band Played On: Politics, People and the AIDS Epidemic.* New York: St. Martin's Press; 1987.
132. Bolton-Maggs PH, Murphy MF. Blood transfusion. *Arch Dis Child.* 2004;89: 4–7.
133. Jamali F, Ness P. Infectious complications. In: Hillyer C, Strauss R, Luban N, eds. *Handbook of Pediatric Transfusion Medicine.* San Diego, CA: Academic Press; 2004:329–342.
134. Fiebig E, Busch M, Menitove J. Transfusion-transmitted disease. In: Hoffman R, Benz E, Shattil S, eds. *Hematology: Basic Principles and Practice,* 4th ed. Philadelphia: Elsevier; 2005:2527–2540.
135. Custer B, Busch MP, Marfin AA, Petersen LR. The cost-effectiveness of screening the US blood supply for West Nile virus. *Ann Intern Med.* 2005;143: 486–492.
136. Lefrere JJ, Servant-Delmas A, Candotti D, et al. Persistent B19 infection in immunocompetent individuals: implications for transfusion safety. *Blood.* 2005;106:2890–2895.
137. Goodnough LT. Risks of blood transfusion. *Anesthesiol Clin North Am.* 2005; 23:241–252,v.
138. Kickler T. Principles of platelet transfusion therapy. In: Hoffman R, Benz E, Shattil S, eds. *Hematology: Basic Principles and Practice,* 4th ed. Philadelphia: Elsevier, 2005;2433–2440.
139. Fang CT, Chambers LA, Kennedy J, et al. Detection of bacterial contamination in apheresis platelet products: American Red Cross experience, 2004. *Transfusion.* 2005;45:1845–1852.
140. Wu YY, Snyder EL. Safety of the blood supply: role of pathogen reduction. *Blood Rev.* 2003;17:111–122.
141. McCullough J. Progress toward a pathogen-free blood supply. *Clin Infect Dis.* 2003;37:88–95.
142. McCullough J, Vesole DH, Benjamin RJ, et al. Therapeutic efficacy and safety of platelets treated with a photochemical process for pathogen inactivation: the SPRINT Trial. *Blood.* 2004;104:1534–1541.
143. AuBuchon JP. Managing change to improve transfusion safety. *Transfusion.* 2004;44:1377–1383.
144. Ludlam CA, Turner ML. Managing the risk of transmission of variant Creutzfeldt Jakob disease by blood products. *Br J Haematol.* 2006;132:13–24.
145. Tamir L, Fradin Z, Fridlander M, et al. Recombinant human erythropoietin reduces allogeneic blood transfusion requirements in patients undergoing major orthopedic surgery. *Haematologia (Budap).* 2000;30:193–201.
146. Braga M, Gianotti L, Gentilini O, Vignali A, Di Carlo V. Erythropoietic response induced by recombinant human erythropoietin in anemic cancer patients candidate to major abdominal surgery. *Hepatogastroenterology.* 1997; 44:685–690.
147. Beguin Y. Erythropoietin and platelet production. *Haematologica.* 1999;84: 541–547.
148. Pronzato P, Jassem J, Mayordomo J. Epoetin beta therapy in patients with solid tumours. *Crit Rev Oncol Hematol.* 2006;58:46–52.
149. Boogaerts M, Coiffier B, Kainz C. Impact of epoetin beta on quality of life in patients with malignant disease. *Br J Cancer.* 2003;88:988–995.

Palliative Care

Sarah Friebert

Introduction

The impact of scientific and technological advances in pediatric oncology is best showcased by a dramatic decline in childhood mortality rates from cancer. Practitioners in pediatric oncology now have the luxury of enjoying long-term relationships with children and their families, largely because so many children with cancer are cured. Despite the tremendous progress in the treatment of pediatric malignancy, approximately 20% to 25% of children with cancer continue to die of their disease or its complications, and cancer remains the top disease-related cause of death in children.[1,2]

Pediatric oncology providers have long recognized that care of the child with advanced cancer has been inadequate; improvement is already occurring, largely due to growing interest in pediatric palliative care training and availability of specialized programs. Until recently, lack of evidence-based models for delivery of quality pediatric end-of-life care has resulted in inadequate attention to physical, psychological, practical, social, educational, and spiritual needs of dying children, causing needless suffering.[3,4] The burgeoning evidence base in pediatric end-of-life care research is demonstrating what practitioners have known anecdotally for decades: terminal symptoms and the accompanying suffering often remain unaddressed and untreated;[4-6] palliative care and hospice programs can improve the illness experience for families, but multiple barriers prevent successful integration and utilization;[6-11] children themselves want and need to participate as much as they are able in their own illness and death experience;[12,13] and parents and providers alike need extensive anticipatory guidance as well as bereavement support when experiencing the death of a child.[11,14,15]

Despite many other barriers, availability of quality palliative care services is rapidly becoming the standard of care for hospitals, including pediatric institutions.[12,16-18] Palliative care is comprehensive, interdisciplinary care that "seeks to prevent or relieve the physical and emotional distress produced by a life-threatening medical condition or its treatment, to help patients with such conditions and their families live as normally as possible, and to provide them with timely and accurate information and support in decision-making." Such care and assistance "can be provided concurrently with curative or life-prolonging treatments."[11] Palliative care does not exclude chemotherapy, surgery, radiation, or other therapies that focus on relieving symptoms; in fact, no disease-modifying treatment is excluded.

A primary focus of this chapter will be on the integration of palliative care into the care of many pediatric oncology patients, not just for those who will not survive. Additionally, this chapter will not focus on specific algorithms of symptom management because numerous recent publications detail developmental stages in the understanding of death, common symptoms experienced, and pharmacologic/nonpharmacologic interventions. Instead, the focus will be to present a conceptual framework in which to understand and actualize the natural integration and transdisciplinary potential of oncology and palliative care teams working together to improve quality of life for patients and families challenged with childhood cancer.

Palliative Care Is NOT Terminal Care

The American Academy of Pediatrics Policy Statement on Palliative Care for Children reiterates the concept that such care is not limited to the end of life and can be provided simultaneously with curative treatment.[17] An integrated model of palliative care, one in which the components of palliative care are offered at diagnosis and continued throughout the course of illness, includes all children living with a life-threatening illness. Such an inclusive approach allows all children who need palliative care to benefit.[19] In addition to focusing on assessment and treatment of symptoms interfering with quality of life, palliative care teams also work with patients and families to promote understanding of medical information; to facilitate informed decision making; to coordinate the services of different subspecialties; to restore or maintain functional capacity; to create opportunities for growth, memory-making, and closure; and to provide continued bereavement support for families and communities.[20-22] In a conceptual framework, palliative care can be understood to encompass five essential "practice spheres," each with its own areas of assessment and subsequent plans to be implemented; these spheres include physical, psycho-social, spiritual, and practical concerns along with advance care planning.[23]

Integration of Palliative Therapy with Antineoplastic Therapy

The receipt of palliative care is not and should not be mutually exclusive with cure-directed therapy—parents and children should not need to choose between palliative care and continued treatment of the cancer. In fact, treatment options for cancer are often appropriate for palliating symptoms of progressive malignancy. Similarly, improved symptom control (especially sleep, nutrition, and pain control) affects a patient's ability to tolerate therapy. The meanings of such treatments in this context, however, need to be made clear to patients and families.

When physicians and parents are able to recognize that a child has no realistic chance for cure, palliative care is more easily integrated into the treatment plan. However, research indicates that on average there is a 3-month delay between when the primary oncologist recognizes that cure is unlikely and when the parents come to terms with this.[24] Discrepancies may exist because of denial on the part of the family (or refusal to hear anything but positive information); an alternative explanation is that the family has been presented with confusing, conflicting, or unrealistic information regarding the likely outcome of their child's illness course.[25,26] It is well described that families need to leave no stone unturned in the battle against their child's malignancy; rather than labeling this fighting attitude as an unrealistic expectation for cure or as denial, families would be better served if physicians recognized this attitude as reality.[4,14,15,21]

One solution to the problem is to introduce palliative care early in the trajectory of illness for those children whose prognoses are less favorable or whose treatments, whatever the outcome, are likely to be burdensome. Specifically, "the same moral obligation to alleviate the suffering of a terminally ill child is also a valid standard in the care of children suffering from other serious diseases, many of which do not have a fatal outcome, but may significantly affect growth and development."[27] Understood in this way, it could be argued that the provision of palliative care to any child with cancer (as the prototype of a life-threatening illness) not only represents medical standard-of-care practice but is also a moral standard of care.

Advantages to this approach are numerous. By helping to establish open and ongoing communication among all care team members with the child and family, the palliative care team can be instrumental in helping to bridge the gap and allow hope for comfort to exist in parallel with hope for life extension.[21,24] Introducing the palliative care team early as part of the oncology treatment team can also alleviate many of the barriers that have heretofore restricted the number of children receiving these services. Such a collaborative approach lessens the chance that a jarring transition will occur between care teams at the most difficult time in the child's life.[28] By working together and complementing each other's strengths and

time limitations, palliative care and oncology teams can improve access to palliative care services, broaden the array of supports available to the family, and lessen the burden on any one provider. Benefits of early integration of palliative care and pediatric oncology are shown in Table 36-1.

Pediatric oncology services have an opportunity to model team integration with pediatric palliative care.[29] Pediatric oncologists have demonstrated a long-standing interest in collaborative approaches with a focus on family-centered care as well as in research in the context of cooperative group clinical trials. Clearly, oncology teams have the benefit and privilege of working intimately with families struggling with life-threatening illness and death. Even while oncologists continue to strive to improve cure rates in pediatric oncology, prototypes can be developed for integration of palliative care into other pediatric subspecialty teams and services.

How might this integration be accomplished? Every pediatric oncology service is different, as is every program's access to palliative care expertise and services. Within institutions, models need to be individualized to meet child/family, clinician, and community needs efficiently, thoroughly, and compassionately. Some general suggestions to improve integration of palliative care and oncology teams are presented in Table 36-2.

Communication and Decision Making

Introducing Palliative Care to Families

Pediatric oncology patients and their families need to maintain hope for cure and choose aggressive curative therapy. As mentioned earlier, systems of care must accommodate this reality rather than trying to change families. Palliative care may be introduced to families without indicating a terminal prognosis as part of the dialogue; in fact, such language may be inappropriate for many families who would benefit from palliative care but whose child is not, in fact, terminally ill.[30,31] When intro-

Table 36-1
Benefits of early integration.
1. Prevents disruptive transition to new care team at worst possible time for the family
2. Decreases feelings of abandonment
3. Minimizes fragmentation of care and lack of coordination among providers
4. Provides umbrella of support through entire draining process
5. Allows patient and family self-determination about treatment options
6. Empowers parents to maintain dual goals of care concurrently
7. Provides additional support for the oncology team (time, resources, self-care, prevention of compassion fatigue)

Table 36-2

Strategies to accomplish early integration of palliative care and oncology teams.

1. Consider palliative care as an adjunct medical specialty that comes as part of a package with oncology services, not as an optional service

2. Find a symptom or reason to introduce the team to the family early on (eg, pain control, spiritual care needs)

3. Remove idea of prognosis altogether: the difficulty of the journey merits involvement of additional support people (this approach avoids having to decide who is appropriate and who is not)

4. If access to full palliative care team is limited, educate care team members to practice palliative care principles

5. Structure the collaboration so that families do not have to have a whole other team if only certain services are needed

6. Think about list of diagnoses or conditions appropriate for palliative care at or soon after diagnosis:
   a. Acknowledge likelihood of cure
   b. Acknowledge burdensome treatment course
   c. Perform honest appraisal of "doing to" vs "doing for"

7. Evaluate various time points on illness trajectory to think of incorporating palliative care
   a. Overwhelmed at diagnosis
   b. Phase I enrollment
   c. Relapse/recurrence
   d. Serious complications (multiorgan failure with sepsis, superior vena cava syndrome, spinal cord compression)
   e. Intensive care unit admissions/transfers

ducing the concept of palliative care to families, open-ended questions, such as "What concerns you most about your child's illness?" or "What are your hopes for your child's future?" provide a means to explore the possibilities that palliative care can offer.[32,33]

Communication with Child and Adolescent Patients

Though a growing literature supports open and compassionate communication with families of seriously ill children, little is known regarding communication about palliative care issues directly with children who have cancer. Many investigators have shown that children living with life-limiting illness are well aware when they are dying.[34–41] This awareness may arise either directly, through provision of information, or indirectly, through awareness of physiologic changes or of feelings and actions of others around them.[42,43] Studies have similarly

indicated that children with cancer want to know about their prognosis.[44,45] In a survey of 50 children with cancer aged 8 to 17, 95% of patients wanted to be told if they were dying. Although most of the children felt that treatment decisions were up to the physician, 63% of the adolescents and 28% of the younger children wanted to make their own decisions about palliative therapy.[43] Direct communication with the ill child is usually also preferred by parents. Recent studies indicate that parents of children who die of cancer rated the quality of care provided by oncologists more highly when the physicians communicated directly with their child.[46] Rarely, families forbid communication directly with their children about palliative or end-of-life issues, or even the cancer diagnosis itself; here, too, a palliative care team can be a useful "objective" third party to explore the meaning of these proscriptions and facilitate honest information exchange.

General guidelines surrounding children's developmental understanding of death and dying are widely available and often useful to provide starting points for discussion.[11,19,23,34,47–49] In clinical practice, however, knowledge of how an individual patient conceptualizes death is an essential part of the communication process with that child and family. As uncomfortable as starting the discussion can be, children must actively participate in the process to the extent that they are able, making decisions in their care and accomplishing grief work, in order to achieve control over their own dying.

When a Child or Adolescent Is Dying

Just as principles of informed consent mandate the provision of information regarding possibilities of side effects of anticancer treatments, it is equally incumbent upon the health care team to communicate the possibility or increasing probability of a child's death. Certainly, this information needs to be delivered in a time- and context-sensitive fashion, and many resources exist to help health care professionals present devastating information in ways that it can be heard and understood by families.[50–53] Nevertheless, when the outcome is likely to be death, it is not sufficient to assume that once the words have been spoken, a family generates a clear understanding of that reality. Additionally, when treatment goals shift from primarily cure-driven to comfort-driven care, it is particularly important to listen to the child and other family members and to understand a family's concerns and priorities. Goals and priorities are not static—they need to be reassessed frequently.

Care of children with life-threatening illness involves a great deal of uncertainty, especially related to prognosis. Predicating a palliative care referral on the determination of the actual moment that a child has transitioned from active treatment to dying necessarily shortchanges the family and the care team. Missed opportunities may be created on many levels, including memory-making, improved symptom control, establishment of rapport with home-based care agencies if these are to be utilized, or even choice of location of care and/or death. Here again, if palliative care is conceptualized as an integral part of the services provided for a child with cancer, the transition to comfort care as a predominant approach can occur seamlessly. If uncertainty about prognosis is not acknowledged, the care team and family may prioritize interventions that favor quantity over quality of life, perhaps resulting in adverse effects on a child's remaining time.[27,33] Surveys of parents of children who died of cancer have demonstrated that parents are capable of maintaining dual goals of cancer-directed therapy and comfort care concurrently.[4,21,54] Introducing palliative care early to the child with cancer will allow patients and their families to view palliative care as an integral part of the services provided rather than as an indicator of loss of hope.

Ethical Issues

A full treatment of the complex and numerous ethical issues in pediatric palliative care is beyond the scope of this chapter. Suffice it to say that ethical issues differ substantially from the ethics of caring for adults with life-threatening illness. Principles do exist with regard to guidance of care of children with life-threatening conditions. In a recent study examining caregiver agreement with widely published pediatric ethical guidelines, national recommendations in end-of-life decision making were grouped into the following categories: withholding versus withdrawing life support; medically supplied food and fluids; use of opioids; use of paralytic agents; brain death criteria; and the dead-donor rule.[55] This survey of 781 clinicians in the field revealed that attending physicians, house officers, and nurses who rated their knowledge of medical ethics as quite high in fact demonstrated significant lack of knowledge regarding basic ethical guidelines for pediatric end-of-life decision making.

The above list of what might be considered *primary* ethical issues in pediatrics is incomplete. It should include resuscitation decisions, palliative sedation, euthanasia/physician-assisted suicide, informed consent, quality of life determination, resource allocation, and genetic testing issues. Ethical issues in pediatrics have numerous secondary considerations, which are particularly heightened in palliative or end-of-life situations. Children, by virtue of age alone, are not considered to be competent, except in the rare circumstance of emancipated minors. Thus, decisions are made on the basis of the best interest standard in which a surrogate decision maker (usually a parent) weighs burdens and benefits, and makes decisions on behalf of the child. Many factors influence the relative weights of burdens and benefits in every situation. Unless their rights are removed, parents are given decision-making rights for their minor children and are presumed to keep their children's best interests front and center. However, children with life-threatening illness are often able to demonstrate decisional capacity beyond their chronological years. Even children who are not chronically or seriously ill should have the opportunity, if willing and able, to participate in treatment decisions.[56,57] If a child can understand the situation, appreciate the consequences of different available courses of action, communicate a clear preference among alternatives, and demonstrate consistency between a stated preference and his or her own value system—thus demonstrating decisional capacity—the child should be invited to participate in medical decision making and his or her preferences should be strongly considered, if not respected outright.[58] While many individual circumstances and dynamics influence the extent to which children are able to act as agents in their own health care decision making, every effort should be made to include them in these important discussions.

Resuscitation Status

At a certain time in a child's illness, planning for what will and will not occur at the time of a cardiac or respiratory arrest may become a priority. Without question, parents are better able to consider these decisions when they are not in the midst of a crisis. However, it is often a crisis that precipitates discussion of this emotionally-charged topic. Generally, acceptance of DNR (do-not-resuscitate) status is a process that should occur over a prolonged period of time and involve multiple discussions. Children and adolescents should be part of these discussions to the extent to which they are willing and able. In clinical practice, families usually want treatable problems or illnesses addressed until the ultimate outcome cannot be prolonged any further or until such prolongation is clearly causing more suffering for the child.

Parents often think that agreeing not to resuscitate is choosing death over life for their children. It is helpful to explain that death results from progressive cancer and not from failure to intervene. Presenting the idea as part of a "hope for the best, plan for the worst" strategy also eases the transition into the conversation. Recent initiatives across the country support the use of more positive terminology in resuscitation documents and policies; examples include "aggressive comfort treatment" and "allow natural death." Reframing communication around resuscitation to reinforce what will be done rather than what will not be done helps families realize they are allowing a natural death for their child rather than opting to remove or not to provide aggressive medical treatment.

Research shows that patients and their families prefer to be guided in these decisions by practitioners they know and trust[14,59] and is another reason to involve the palliative care team earlier in the child's illness course, giving the family and clinicians time to forge a collaborative relationship prior to discussing sensitive and overwhelming issues. Often, full understanding of resuscitation status represents a turning point for the family at which acceptance of the inevitability of the child's death is achieved.[60]

Home or Hospital?

It is important to discuss preferences regarding location of terminal care as early as possible and to revisit the discussion with significant changes in the child's condition. Options include inpatient hospitalization, home care with or without support of a home care or hospice team (wherever the patient calls home), or admission to an inpatient hospice facility, if available to the pediatric patient. Studies have found that slightly more than half of children with advanced cancer die at home. Some families choose to remain primarily at home, while other parents prefer their child to die in the hospital for multiple reasons. Death at home is not always better; the important outcome is that the child and family are supported wherever they feel most comfortable. Child preferences should be honored whenever possible, and families should be reassured that they may change from one primary location of care to another as the situation changes. Wherever the child is, families consistently cite continued involvement of the primary care team as a crucial factor in their ability to cope, both as the child is dying and afterward.[3,30,59,61]

Particularly for children who die at home, assistance from hospice is invaluable. Availability of hospice programs with pediatric expertise and flexibility in working with pediatric patients presents the biggest barrier to utilization of these important services.[11,20] Support from the hospice team does not replace the primary team. Rather, the role of the additional personnel is to extend holistic care of the family into the home and community, through the dying process and beyond. Hospice programs also provide bereavement services for family members, including siblings, who can potentially be underserved when a child is dying of cancer. For parents who decide to use home-based hospice care, the anxieties associated with taking a terminally ill child home may be great. Proactive attention to the fears of families caring for a dying child—the unknown, abandonment by care providers, not being able to control symptoms, and the like—will greatly assist the transition to home-based care.[59,61]

Comfort and Disease Therapy and Interventions

Cancer-Directed Therapy

Chemotherapy: Several agents have been well tolerated in children and have some antitumor effect. Common choices with low side-effect profiles include: VP16, topotecan, hydroxyurea, and cytarabine; newer agents such as temozolomide, imatinib, and rituximab may also improve quality of life without adding significant toxicity. The decision whether or not to continue cancer-directed therapy must rest on goals of care and must carefully balance considerations of efficacy, potential treatment-related complications with their attendant supportive care needs, and psychological impact.[62,63]

Phase I Clinical Trials: It is important to state clearly to families that the goal of Phase I research is to determine the toxicities and the maximum tolerated dose of an investigational agent. Despite high hopes of therapeutic benefit on the part of patients as well as treating physicians, actual tumor response in Phase I studies has historically ranged from only 4% to 6% among adults as well as children; fortunately, chances of fatal toxicity were also low at approximately 0.5%.[6,15,63,64] A recent meta-analysis indicates that toxic death rates in Phase I studies have decreased substantially over 3 time periods from 1991 to 2002 and now average 0.06%; objective response rates, however, have also decreased from 6.2% to 2.5%.[65] Risk-benefit analysis is very individualized in this setting, which is also fraught with ethical complexity. It is strongly recommended that children give their assent to participation and that palliative care be part and parcel of the treatment plan for any child enrolled

on a Phase I clinical trial.[56,65–68] Again, the approaches are not mutually exclusive.

Radiation Therapy: Short courses of radiation can often provide dramatic relief of troubling symptoms and should be incorporated into a palliative care plan whenever appropriate. Since late effects of therapy are not the major concern and complete elimination of the tumor is not necessary, higher fractions or treatment volumes can usually be delivered over shorter time frames. Possible palliative indications for radiation include: pain relief for bone or pulmonary metastases, control of bleeding, control of ulcerating or fungating masses, and tumor shrinkage for symptoms related to mass effect, including oncologic emergency situations.[69] Risks and benefits are particularly important to discuss with the family, as even abbreviated courses of radiation may cause undesired side effects, including the burdens of lost time, painful travel back and forth, or increased need for transfusion or supportive care.

Surgery: Surgical intervention may also be part of the palliative care plan. Partial surgical resection of recurrent or progressive tumor to provide pain or other symptomatic relief may be possible even when complete resection is not feasible or safe. Other surgical interventions, for such problems as bowel obstruction or spinal cord compression, may in fact be less morbid than medical management. As always, open discussion regarding risks and benefits in the context of a particular child's goals of care is of paramount importance. For patients who have advance directives or resuscitation orders in place, it is important to discuss resuscitation status when an operative procedure is planned. Institutional policies vary regarding suspension of DNR orders during surgery. The American College of Surgeons and the American Society of Anesthesiologists recommend implementing a process of "required reconsideration" in which a pre-op discussion occurs among the patient (when appropriate), parents or legal decision makers, managing physician, surgeon, and anesthesiologist to determine whether resuscitation will occur for a surgical or anesthetic issue; if DNR orders are suspended, the amount of time the suspension is in effect should also be specified.[70,71] Either suspension or activation of orders may be appropriate in any given situation; the important concept is that there must be explicit consideration of the wishes of the patient and family prior to surgery.

Symptom Management

Although pain is the most obvious cause of suffering, pediatric oncology patients experience many other distressing symptoms at the end of life. These include: infection, bleeding, dyspnea, cough, nausea and/or vomiting, diarrhea, pruritis, fatigue or lack of energy, depression, and anorexia, to name a few. Numerous excellent resources detail specific management of many of these symptoms.[4,9,20,21,49,60,72–75] A key concept to remember is that the symptom itself is relevant only when considered along with the burden it presents to the child or family. What a provider or parent may perceive as causing suffering may not, in fact, be troubling to the child; similarly, seemingly minor issues may detract significantly from a child's quality of life. As described by

Hinds and colleagues, this concept is perhaps best conceptualized as *symptom distress*: "an individual's report of his or her awareness of one or more changes in normal function, sensation, or appearance that cause him or her some degree of physical discomfort, mental anguish, or suffering."[76] Palliative care providers, as experts in symptom control, offer an additional resource to the oncology team in managing symptom distress.

When a child is dying, symptoms need to be described clearly to families. Most parents will want to be present at the time of their child's death, but uncertainty about what will happen at that time is a major cause of distress and fear. Children may also have questions about their own dying process, which should be answered as simply and honestly as possible, using familiar terminology. Most people have not experienced the death of a child firsthand and do not know what to expect or even what to ask. Gentle but clear descriptions of the dying process can go a long way in allaying anxiety.[14]

Occasionally, symptom management poses an ethical dilemma when symptom distress is perceived or reported by the family more (or less) than by the ill child. Education and holistic approaches to family-centered care can resolve many of these issues, with attention to open communication and/or use of time trials for interventions. For example, if a family member believes a child is not in pain but the care team feels the child is exhibiting pain behavior, a short trial of appropriate analgesia may be helpful in demonstrating whether a change in behavior occurs. When disagreements occur, it must be emphasized that the provider's primary obligation is toward the patient. Involvement of a palliative care team is often quite helpful in navigating conflict; ethics consultation can also be useful in extreme cases. These and other important general considerations regarding symptom management are listed in Table 36-3.

Quality of Life at the End of Life

Integration of palliative care into cancer treatment from the outset allows more consistent attention to addressing concerns of quality of life.[77] The impact of selected interventions on various dimensions of quality of life, such as pain and symptom management, is the focus of more and more research in pediatric oncology, particularly as quality of life measures have begun to be included in a greater percentage of cooperative group trials.[78,79] However, the particular domains that constitute quality of life for children at the end of life have not yet been fully elucidated.

One of the basic tenets of pediatric palliative care is that care is goal-directed and is defined in a way that is consistent with the beliefs and values of each family.[33,49] Despite methodologic obstacles in assessing care at the end of life, what constitutes quality of life for an individual patient and family can perhaps best be ascertained through the assessment and frequent reassessment of *goals of care*. While goals of care often shift many times in the course of the cancer journey, two clear priorities are to allow dying children to achieve optimal symptom relief and to solidify relationships with loved ones. In particular, school and friendships serve a very important social func-

tion for children. Roles for the care team during this period can include: encouraging the child's continued participation in school and social activities at whatever level is possible; helping families explore and carry out religious or cultural traditions of significance;[80] and facilitating memory-building for the child and family. Here again, open-ended questions with the child and family can be used to establish (rather than assume) what may be important for a child to complete to feel as if his or her life has had meaning.

Spiritual Care

Patients and their families undoubtedly think about spiritual issues when confronted with serious illness, suffering, and the possibility of dying.[81,82] In fact, the role of spirituality in health care is generating rising attention, largely due to consumer-driven interest. No consensus exists on a precise definition of spirituality or what domains such a construct might encompass. However, spirituality can be generally understood to offer a sense of hope and self-worth, meaning and purpose, and interconnectedness with others. Studies of hospitalized and chronically ill children reveal that the significance of spiritual and religious issues increases directly with seriousness of illness.[83–85]

Assessing and addressing spiritual needs should be viewed as part of a complete history, physical, and treatment plan of any oncology patient and family;[86] such a holistic approach presents more opportunities for healing and offers increased satisfaction for caregivers as well.[87,88] Pediatric-specific spirituality assessment tools have not yet been developed and validated for use with pediatric cancer patients, particularly those at the end of life. However, guidelines do exist, such as those put forth by the Children's International Project on Palliative/Hospice Services for addressing spirituality in ill children, parents, siblings, grandparents, and nonreligious or nontraditional families.[19,87] Through a few targeted yet open-ended questions, a baseline spirituality assessment can be initiated by anyone on the care team who enjoys a close relationship with a child. A family or palliative care/hospice spiritual care provider can then pursue further exploration, particularly of troubling or confusing issues.

Bereavement Care

Care for oncology patients and families does not end with the death of the child. Bereavement support for the patient's parents and siblings should be considered part and parcel of quality palliative and oncology team care. The death of a child is one of the most significant psychological stressors a person may ever face.[89–92] There are several concrete ways in which the care team can be helpful.

First, parents often have unanswered medical questions that need to be addressed before the psychological work of mourning may begin, or they may simply have little memory of the events leading up to the child's death. Siblings may harbor anxiety about their own health, and their parents may likewise be worried about them. At some time after the child's death, the family should be invited to review the medical events surrounding the illness and death. If an autopsy has been performed, this is an ideal time to discuss the findings; it may be helpful to include the examining pathologist or other subspecialists involved in the child's care. Siblings can be included in this discussion to the extent that they are interested and/or developmentally capable. If a sibling's health is in question, a relatively simple exam or even a blood test may go a long way in allaying a family's fears; simply brushing off the worry with an answer based in statistics may not allow the family significant comfort to move on.

Second, families should be offered educational materials about the process of grief and mourning. The health care team should provide information—such as reading materials, specialized grief counseling resources, support groups, and bereavement camps for siblings—so that family members may continue to receive the help that they will need for as long as needed after the death of their child. Traditional models of grief support timelines (such as the standard 13 months of bereavement follow-up provided by most hospice programs) need to be suspended, because mourning periods often extend beyond standard expectations.[93] Often, though, the care team is in the best position to recognize what might be considered pathologic grief and to make referrals to appropriate community resources.

Third, families often need and appreciate continued contact with their treatment team long after their child has died. This contact can occur in the context of formalized remembrance services, anniversary/birthday/holiday cards, or individual phone calls. While maintenance of professional boundaries is, of course, appropriate, ongoing relationships with families of children who have died can be beneficial to families and providers alike. In addition, siblings may need to revisit the death of a brother or sister at a later developmental time; input from the treatment team can be extremely valuable in correcting misconceptions and answering lingering questions.

In addition to family bereavement care, attention to staff and caregiver needs is also paramount after a child has died. Studies show that medical providers who care for dying children need approximately twice as long to recover from a child's death as do professionals caring for adults who die. The repeated losses experienced by health care professionals may constitute a significant source of personal stress.[94] Some staff find attendance at patient calling hours and funerals to be beneficial, while others benefit from team retreats or shared activities; division or hospital policies should be amended to allow attendance at these important rituals if desired. Importantly, staff stress may be substantially influenced by lack of palliative care training. A self-perceived lack of competence in symptom management and communication skills appears to influence post-death coping in providers who care for dying children.[3,95] Health care providers should be given the opportunity to improve their competency in pediatric palliative care, to share emotions and concerns with fellow staff, and to participate in formal or informal memorial services to grieve their losses. Caregivers should also be encouraged in their means of self-care, such as journaling or exercising, so that they may be able to continue to appreciate the honor and privilege it is to care for dying children.

Summary

In summary, the field of pediatric oncology offers many satisfying opportunities to forge meaningful and sustaining bonds with patients and families. Most of the time, our patients survive their diseases and go on to lead productive lives. For those who do not, and even for those who will but for whom the journey will prove arduous, palliative care offers additional support and resources. Palliative care should not be offered as an either/or option, nor should it be relegated to second-best status by reserving it until all other options for cure have been exhausted. In fact, palliative care is fast becoming the standard of care for pediatric patients. Early integration of palliative treatment with disease-directed oncology treatment improves care coordination, enables achievement of goals, and facilitates holistic healing of children and families by incorporating spiritual, emotional/psychological, physical, social, and practical dimensions of care. Rather than removing hope or detracting from the illness experience, pediatric palliative care enhances the cancer journey for patients, families, and care providers, regardless of whether the disease itself is cured, when provided in an integrated model.

Simply put, "The need to give care and attempt the relief of suffering is just as great as the need to cure and should be no less an ultimate goal of medicine."[98]

References

1. Jemal A, Tiwari RC, Murray T, et al. Cancer statistics, 2004. *CA J Clinicians.* 2004,54(1).8–28.
2. Martin JA, Kochanek KD, Strobino DM, et al. Annual summary of vital statistics – 2003. *Pediatrics.* 2005;115(3):619–634.
3. Contro NA, Larson J, Scofield S, et al. Hospital staff and family perspectives regarding quality of pediatric palliative care. *Pediatrics.* 2004;114(5):1248–1252.
4. Wolfe J, Grier HE, Klar N, et al. Symptoms and suffering at the end of life in children with cancer. *N Engl J Med.* 2000;342:326–333.
5. Collins JJ, Grier HE, Kinney HC, et al. Control of severe pain in children with terminal malignancy. *J Pediatr.* 1995;126(4):653–657.
6. Frager G. Pediatric palliative care: building the model, bridging the gaps. *J Palliat Care.* 1996;12(3):9–12.
7. Hilden JM, Emanuel EJ, Fairclough DL, et al. Attitudes and practices among pediatric oncologists regarding end-of-life care: results of the 1998 American Society of Clinical Oncology survey. *J Clin Oncol.* 2001;19(1):205–212.
8. Liben S. Pediatric palliative medicine: obstacles to overcome. *J Palliat Care.* 1996;12(3):24–28.
9. Collins JJ. Palliative care and the child with cancer. *Hematol Oncol Clin North Am.* 2002;16(3):657–670.
10. Hilden JM, Himelstein BP, Freyer DR, et al. End-of-life care: special issues in pediatric oncology. In: Foley KM, Gellband H, eds. *Improving Palliative Care for Cancer.* Washington, DC: National Academy Press; 2001:161–198.
11. Field MJ, Behrman R, eds. *When Children Die: Improving Palliative and End-of-Life Care for Children and Their Families.* Washington, DC: National Academy Press; 2003.
12. Bradshaw G, Hinds PS, Lensing S, et al. Cancer-related deaths in children and adolescents. *J Palliat Med.* 2005;8(1):86–95.
13. McAliley L, Hudson-Barr DC. The use of advance directives with adolescents. *Pediatr Nurs.* 2000;26(5):471–480.
14. Martinson IM. Improving care of dying children. *West J Med.* 1995;163(3):258–262.
15. Vickers JL, Carlisle C. Choices and control: parental experiences in pediatric terminal home care. *J Pediatr Oncol Nurs.* 2000;17(1):12–21.
16. Wolfe J, Grier HE. Care of the dying child. In: Pizzo PA, Poplack DG, eds. *Principles and Practice of Pediatric Oncology,* 4th ed. Philadelphia: Lippincott, Williams & Wilkins, 2002;1477–1493.
17. American Academy of Pediatrics Committees on Bioethics and Hospital Care. Palliative care for children. *Pediatrics.* 2000;106:351–357.
18. Council on Scientific Affairs, American Medical Association. Good care of the dying patient. *JAMA.* 1996;275(6):474–478.
19. Levetown M, ed. *Compendium of Pediatric Palliative Care.* Alexandria, VA: Children's International Project on Palliative/Hospice Services (ChIPPS), National Hospice and Palliative Care Organization; 2000.
20. Hilden JM, Friebert S, Himelstein BP, et al. Children and adolescents with cancer. In: Carter BS, Levetown M, eds. *Palliative Care for Infants, Children, and Adolescents: A Practical Handbook.* Baltimore: Johns Hopkins University Press; 2004:348–373.
21. Wolfe J, Friebert S, Hilden J. Caring for children with advanced cancer: integrating palliative care. *Pediatr Clin North Am.* 2002;49(5):1043–1062.
22. Chaffee S. Pediatric palliative care. *Prim Care.* 2001;28(2):365–390.
23. Himelstein BP, Hilden JM, Boldt AM, et al. Pediatric palliative care. *N Engl J Med.* 2004;350:1752–1762.
24. Wolfe J, Klar N, Grier HE, et al. Understanding of prognosis among parents of children who died of cancer: impact on treatment goals and integration of palliative care. *JAMA.* 2000;284:2469–2475.
25. Whittam EH. Terminal care of the dying child. Psychosocial implications of care. *Cancer.* 1993;71(10 Suppl):3450–3462.
26. Martinson IM, Cohen MH. Themes from a longitudinal study of family reactions to childhood cancer. *J Psychosoc Oncol.* 1988;(6):81–98.
27. Kane JR, Garrison BR, Jordan M, et al. Supportive/palliative care of children suffering from life-threatening and terminal illness. *Am J Hosp Palliat Care.* 2000;17(3):165–172.
28. Stevens MM, Jones P, O'Riordan E. Family responses when a child with cancer is in palliative care. *J Palliat Care.* 1996;12:51–55.
29. Postovsky S, Ben Arush M. Care of a child dying of cancer: the role of the palliative care team in pediatric oncology. *Pediatr Hematol Oncol.* 2004;21(1):67–76.
30. Harris MB. Palliative care in children with cancer: which child and when? *J Natl Cancer Inst Monogr.* 2004;32:144–149.
31. Billings JA. What is palliative care? *JAMA.* 1997;277(8):678–682.
32. Lo B, Quill T, Tulsky J. Discussing palliative care with patients: ACP-ASIM End-of-Life Care Consensus Panel. *Ann Intern Med.* 1999;130(9):744–749.
33. Kane JR, Primomo M. Alleviating the suffering of seriously ill children. *Am J Hosp Palliat Care.* 2001;18(3):161–169.
34. Bluebond-Langner M. *The Private Worlds of Dying Children.* Princeton, NJ: Princeton University Press; 1980.
35. Bluebond-Langner M. Worlds of dying children and their well siblings. *Death Stud.* 1989;13:465–483.
36. Sourkes BM. *Armfuls of Time: The Psychological Experience of the Child with a Life-Threatening Illness.* Pittsburgh: University of Pittsburgh Press; 1995.
37. Sourkes BM. The broken heart: anticipatory grief in the child facing death. *J Palliat Care.* 1996;12:56–59.
38. Hinds PS, Oakes L, Furman W, et al. End-of-life decision making by adolescents, parents, and healthcare providers in pediatric oncology: research to evidence-based practice guidelines. *Cancer Nurs.* 2001;24:122–134.
39. Freyer DR. Care of the dying adolescent: special considerations. *Pediatrics.* 2001;113(2):381–388.
40. Nitschke R, Meyer WH, Huszti HC. When the tumor is not the target, tell the children. *J Clin Oncol.* 2001;19:595–596.
41. Faulkner KW. Talking about death with a dying child. *Am J Nurs.* 1997;97:64–69.
42. Waechter EH. Children's awareness of fatal illness. *Am J Nurs.* 1971;7:1168–1170.
43. Spinetta JJ, Maloney J. Death anxiety in the outpatient leukemia child. *Pediatrics.* 1975;56:1035–1037.
44. Ellis K, Leventhal B. Information needs and decision-making preferences of children with cancer. *Psychooncology.* 1993;2:277–284.
45. Orr DP, Hoffmans MA, Bennets G. Adolescents with cancer report their psychosocial needs. *J Psychosocial Oncol.* 1984;2(2):47–59.
46. Mack JW, Hilden JM, Watterson J, et al. Parent and physician perspectives on quality of care at the end of life in children with cancer. *J Clin Oncol.* 2005;23(36):1–7.
47. American Academy of Pediatrics Committee on Psychosocial Aspects of Child and Family Health: the pediatrician and childhood bereavement. *Pediatrics.* 2000;105(2):445–447.
48. Faulkner K. Children's understanding of death. In: Armstrong-Dailey A, Zarbock S, eds. *Hospice Care for Children.* 2nd ed. New York: Oxford University Press; 2001:9–22.
49. Kane JR, Himelstein BP. Palliative care in pediatrics. In: Berger AM, Portenoy RK, Weissman DE, eds. *Principles and Practice of Palliative Care and Supportive Oncology.* Philadelphia: Lippincott, Williams & Wilkins; 2002:1044–1061.
50. Mack JW, Grier HE. The day one talk. *J Clin Oncol.* 2004;22(3):563–566.
51. Buckman R. *How to Break Bad News.* Baltimore: Johns Hopkins University Press; 1992.
52. Ptacek JT, Eberhardt TL. Breaking bad news: a review of the literature. *JAMA.* 1996;276(6):496–502.
53. Baile WF, Buckman R, Lenzi R, et al. SPIKES—a six-step protocol for delivering bad news: application to the patient with cancer. *Oncologist.* 2000;5(4):302–311.
54. Hurwitz CA, Duncan J, Wolfe J. Caring for the child with cancer at the close of life. *JAMA.* 2004;292(17):2141–2149.
55. Solomon MZ, Sellers DE, Heller KS, et al. New and lingering controversies in pediatric end-of-life care. *Pediatrics.* 2005;116(4):872–883.
56. American Academy of Pediatrics Committee on Bioethics. Informed consent, parental permission, and assent in pediatric practice. *Pediatrics.* 1995;95:314–317.
57. Weir RF, Peters C. Affirming the decisions adolescents make about life and death. *Hastings Center Report.* 1997(Nov-Dec):29–40.
58. Brock DW. Children's competence for health care decisionmaking. In: Kopelman LM, Moskop JC, eds. *Children and Health Care: Moral and Social Issues.* Boston: Kluwer Academic; 1989:181–212.
59. James L, Johnson B. The needs of parents of pediatric oncology patients during the palliative care phase. *J Pediatr Oncol Nurs.* 1997;14:83–95.
60. Hilden JM, Tobin DR, Lindsey K. *Shelter from the Storm: Caring for a Child with a Life-Threatening Condition.* Cambridge, MA: Perseus; 2003.
61. Contro N, Larson J, Scofield S, et al. Family perspectives on the quality of pediatric palliative care. *Arch Pediatr Adolesc Med.* 2002;156:14–19.
62. Goold SD, Williams B, Arnold RM. Conflicts regarding decisions to limit treatment: a differential diagnosis. *JAMA.* 2000;283(7):909–914.
63. Decoster G, Stein G, Holdener EE. Responses and toxic deaths in phase I clinical trials. *Ann Oncol.* 1990;1:175–181.
64. Estlin EJ, Cotterill S, Pratt CB, et al. Phase I trials in pediatric oncology. *J Clin Oncol.* 2000;18(9):1900–1905.
65. Roberts TG, Goulart BH, Squitieri L, et al. Trends in the risks and benefits to patients with cancer participating in phase I clinical trials. *JAMA.* 2004;292(17):2130–2140.
66. National Commission for Protection of Human Subjects of Biomedical and Behavioral Research. *Research Involving Children.* Washington, DC: US Government Printing Office; 1977.
67. Friebert SE, Kodish ED. Kids and cancer: ethical issues in treating the pediatric oncology patient. In: Angelos P, ed. *Ethical Issues in Cancer Patient Care.* Norwell, MA: Kluwer Academic; 1999:99–135.
68. Ulrich CM, Grady C, Wendler D. Palliative care: a supportive adjunct to pediatric phase I clinical trials for anticancer agents? *Pediatrics.* 2004;114:852–855.
69. Kirkbride P. The role of radiation therapy in palliative care. *J Palliat Care.* 1995;11(1):19–26.
70. American College of Surgeons. Statement on advance directives by patients: "do not resuscitate" in the operating room. *Bull Am Coll Surgeons.* 1994;79(9):29.
71. American Society of Anesthesiologists. Ethical guidelines for the anesthesia care of patients with do-not-resuscitate orders. House of Delegates, American Society of Anesthesiologists 1993, Amended 2001.

72. Friebert SE, Hilden JM. Palliative care for children with cancer. In: Altman A, ed. *Supportive Care of Children with Cancer*. Baltimore: Johns Hopkins University Press; 2004:379–396.

73. Drake R, Frost J, DipEd MN, et al. The symptoms of dying children. *J Pain Symptom Manage*. 2003;26;1:594–603.

74. Collins JJ, Devine TD, Dick GS, et al. The measurement of symptoms in young children with cancer: the validation of the Memorial Symptom Assessment Scale in children aged 7-12. *J Pain Symptom Manage*. 2002;23(1):10–16.

75. Collins JJ, Byrnes ME, Dunkel IJ, et al. The measurement of symptoms in children with cancer. *J Pain Symptom Manage*. 2000;19(5):363–377.

76. Hinds PS, Quargnenti AG, Wentz TJ. Measuring symptom distress in adolescents with cancer. *J Pediatr Oncol Nurs*. 1992;9(2):84–86.

77. MacDonald N. The interface between oncology and palliative medicine. In: Doyle D, Hanks GWC, MacDonald N, eds. *Oxford Textbook of Palliative Medicine*, 2nd ed. Oxford: Oxford University Press; 1998:11–17.

78. Bradlyn AS, Pollock BH. Quality-of-life research in the Pediatric Oncology Group: 1991–1995. *J Natl Cancer Inst*. 1996;20:49–53.

79. Bradlyn AS, Harris CV, Spieth LE. Quality of life assessment in pediatric oncology: a retrospective review of phase III reports. *Soc Sci Med*. 1995;41:1463–1465.

80. Mazanec P, Tyler MK. Cultural considerations in end-of-life care: how ethnicity, age, and spirituality affect decisions when death is imminent. *Am J Nurs*. 2003;103:50–58.

81. Barnes LL, Plotnikoff GA, Fox K, et al. Spirituality, religion, and pediatrics: intersecting worlds of healing. *Pediatrics*. 2000;106:S899–908.

82. Stuber ML, Houskamp BM. Spirituality in children confronting death. *Child Adolesc Psychiatr Clin N Am*. 2004;13:127–136.

83. Desai PP, Ng JB, Bryant SG. Care of children and families in the CICU: a focus on their developmental, psychosocial, and spiritual needs. *Crit Care Nurs Q*. 2002;25(3):88–97.

84. Pendleton SM, Cavalli KS, Pargament KI, et al. Religious/spiritual coping in childhood cystic fibrosis: a qualitative study. *Pediatrics*. 2002;109(1):E8.

85. Fulton RB, Moore CM. Spiritual care of the school-age child with a chronic condition. *J Pediatr Nurs*. 1995;10:224–231.

86. Brady MJ, Peterman AH, Fitchett G, et al. A case for including spirituality in quality of life measurement in oncology. *Psychooncology*. 1999;8(5):417–428.

87. Davies B, Brenner P, Orloff S, et al. Addressing spirituality in pediatric hospice and palliative care. *J Palliat Care*. 2002;18(1):59–67.

88. Puchalski CM, Romer AL. Taking a spiritual history allows clinicians to understand patients more fully. *J Palliat Med*. 2000;3(1):129–137.

89. Martinson IM, McClowry SG, Davies B, et al. Changes over time: a study of family bereavement following childhood cancer. *J Palliat Care*. 1994;10;1:19–25.

90. Rando T. An investigation of grief and adaptation in parents whose children have died from cancer. *J Pediatr Psychol*. 1983;8(1):3–20.

91. Lauer ME, Mulhern RK, Wallskog JM, et al. A comparison study of parental adaptation following a child's death at home or in the hospital. *Pediatrics*. 1983;71(1):107–112.

92. Meert KL, Thurston CS, Briller SH. The spiritual needs of parents at the time of their child's death in the pediatric intensive care unit and during bereavement: a qualitative study. *Pediatr Crit Care Med*. 2005;6(4):420–427.

93. Saunders CM. A comparison of adult bereavement in the death of a spouse, child, and parent. *Omega*. 1979;10:302–322.

94. Mount BM. Dealing with our losses. *J Clin Oncol*. 1986;47:1127–1134.

95. Andresen EM, Seecharan GA, Toce SS. Provider perceptions of child deaths. *Arch Pediatr Adolesc Med*. 2004;158:430–435.

Nutritional Supportive Care

Paul C. Rogers

Introduction

The prevalence of malnutrition (undernutrition) in children with malignancy ranges from 6% to 50% depending on primary diagnosis, stage, treatment, and socioeconomic status.[1–5] In developed countries, the degree of undernutrition is related to the pathological type of the malignancy and the degree of tumor involvement. It is most frequently seen in patients with advanced solid tumors such as neuroblastoma, Wilms tumor, rhabdomyosarcoma, and bone sarcomas, and it is less often observed in patients who present with leukemias or lymphomas. In developing countries, undernutrition is more frequently due to socioeconomic conditions associated with inadequate intake of calories and protein (protein calorie malnutrition, PCM; protein energy malnutrition, PEM) and probably is present in more than 50% of all children.[1,6,7] Complications during therapy can also exacerbate undernutrition.

Nutritional status and its relationship to overall survival and disease-free outcome is controversial.[4,7] Reports have shown that undernutrition correlates with decreased survival, especially in countries where overall undernutrition is prevalent. In developed countries it does not always appear to be a significant prognostic factor. The study reported by Donaldson[3] in 1981 shows a significant correlation of poor nutritional status with decrease in overall survival, most notably for patients with solid tumors. Protein energy malnutrition appears to be associated with impaired tolerance to chemotherapy, altered treatment schedules, and impaired immunity with increased risk of complications of therapy such as infections. Conversely, nutritional support improves the feeling of well-being and performance status while maintaining or improving immune competence.[1,7,8–12] Pharmocokinetics of drugs are also affected by PEM, which decreases clearance and alters distribution and metabolism of drugs.[13–16] These effects have been well described for methotrexate.[17,18]

Enhanced supportive care has played an important role in the overall improved prognosis for pediatric malignancies. However, nutritional support has been inconsistently applied. A recent review by the Children's Oncology Group (COG) Nutrition Committee reported a wide disparity in the practice of nutritional assessment and intervention.[19] This report showed that assessment of nutritional status does not occur on a consistent basis, and when it does, it usually looks at weight change alone. The study found that different indices were employed to indicate nutritional status; different guidelines were used to categorize malnutrition; and, when nutritional intervention appeared to be clinically indicated, a variety of approaches were employed. This current status of nutritional practice is due to the dearth of well-conducted nutritional trials in pediatric oncology that would allow for evidence-based recommendations. A great need exists for a consistent and rational approach to the supportive nutritional care of the pediatric oncology patient.

Guidelines for assessment of nutritional status, categorization, and algorithms for intervention are available and should be utilized[16,20,21] (see Figure 37-1). Evaluation of different interventions is required to ascertain whether they improve the well-being of children, decrease morbidities both on and off therapy, maintain normal growth and development, and impact on overall outcome. While the true impact of nutritional intervention in children with cancer is uncertain,[4] pediatricians accept as fundamental that appropriate nutrition is essential for growth, development, and well-being for children without disease. Thus, adequate nutrition should be ensured in cancer patients while investigators conduct specific interventional trials to clarify what is the most practical and effective way to assess and nutritionally supplement patients.

Pathogenesis of Cancer Malnutrition

Cancer cachexia is multifactorial[7,12,22,23] both at the time of diagnosis and during treatment, as shown in Table 37-1. It is critical to identify the factors contributing to malnutrition so appropriate interventions can be employed that may ameliorate some of those factors. While some of the contributing factors are recognized for cancer cachexia, many of the mechanisms are poorly understood and may well be different in the growing and developing pediatric patient compared with adult patients.[7,24,25] Animal studies and the adult literature indicate that pro-inflammatory

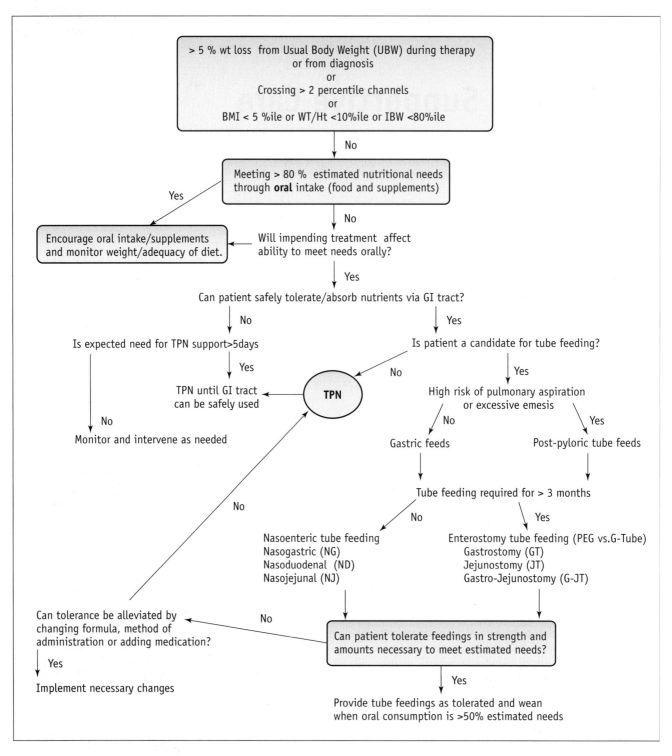

Figure 37-1 Algorithm for nutritional intervention in the pediatric oncology patient.

processes are implicated in the hypermetabolism and weight loss associated with cancer-associated cachexia.[22,23]

Nutritional Assessment

Nutritional assessment of the pediatric cancer patient is fundamentally no different from that of any other pediatric patient.[7,12,16,26–28] Assessments should ideally com-

mence at diagnosis of the malignancy and be carried out longitudinally during treatment as well as in the post-treatment period. As in most aspects of clinical medicine, the importance of history and physical assessment cannot be underestimated. Baseline evaluation should include dietary history to ascertain calorie protein intake and known food aversions, allergies, or intolerance. Clinical evaluation includes appropriate anthropometric and bio-

Table 37-1

Cancer cachexia/malnutrition.

Tumor- and Patient-Related Factors

- Socioeconomic conditions
- Inadequate supply of nutrients
- Anorexia
- Bowel obstruction
- Malabsorption of nutrients
- Pain
- Metastatic disease
- Metabolic effects (paraneoplastic)
- Altered metabolism of protein, fat, and carbohydrates
- Increased resting energy expenditure (REE)

Therapy-Related Effects

- Reaction to multimodal treatments (chemotherapy, radiation, and surgery)
- Gastrointestinal disorders: nausea and vomiting, mucositis, impaired digestion, diarrhea, ileus, morphological changes to gut mucosa, decreased appetite

- Infection from and reactions to antibiotics
- Reactions to other drugs
- Toxic effects in other organs

Psychological/Central Nervous System Factors

- Anorexia
- Food aversion
- Anticipatory vomiting
- Depression/anxiety
- Body image
- Loss of control by the patient over his or her environment
- Parental influence and perceptions
- Changes in taste and smell

---

chemical measurements (see Table 37-2). The extent of assessment can range from baseline routine assessment to the use of sophisticated biochemical parameters and newer technologies of body mass assessment. One such technology, the Dexa (dual-energy x-ray absorptiometry) scan, distinguishes adipose tissue from lean body mass as well as assesses bone density.

In practical terms, weight is used as the baseline measurement. Assessments based on weight alone can be misleading, especially in an acutely ill patient whose fluid balance may be disturbed or in a patient who has edema or mass disease. Additionally, weight may be maintained, but lean body mass can be diminished, as can be the case in a patient who is obese at the onset of treatment. Most physicians will assess the appropriate weight for a patient's height.[29] Body mass index (BMI)[30] is considered a more reasonable parameter for assessment for children over the age of 2, and ideal body weight (IBW) is measured for children under age 2. Body mass index has to be interpreted relative to population reference data, as it changes with age and differs for males and females. It is considered a better indication of body fat and lean body mass. It is the most appropriate index in assessing obesity that may be a long-term side effect of treatment.[31,32] Health care providers should measure and plot on the appropriate population charts a patient's weight for age, height for age, weight for height, BMI, head circumference (under age 3), and mid-arm circumference to better assess muscle wasting and use triceps skinfolds to estimate adipose tissue.[7,33] The latter two measurements should preferably be undertaken by the same observer to avoid inter-observer variability. Measurements should commence at the time of diagnosis, with consistent longitudinal observations in order to detect any changes that may require intervention. Also important is the continuous assessment of calorie protein intake. If the patient is hospitalized, dietitians and nutritionists can be asked to carry out this assessment. When possible this assessment should be done on a regular basis for patients known to be at high risk for nutritional depletion. Software is available to calculate protein and calories of daily intake. For outpatients, a dietician will still need to assess if the patient is nutritionally replete. Data can be gathered in several ways, including a 24-hour dietary recall, a 3- to 5-day food record, and a food frequency questionnaire.[26,27]

Biochemical assessments need to be interpreted carefully, as some proteins can also be acute phase reactants and give spurious values. Any condition that can alter the rate of synthesis, degradation, or excretion of proteins may alter the serum concentration of proteins. Albumin and prealbumin are the most frequent biochemical parameters used, of which the latter is a better indicator of the acute state due to its shorter half-life. Immune status is impaired by malnutrition,[34] but evaluation and interpretation of lymphocyte counts, lymphocyte subsets, and function are problematic in the patient receiving chemotherapy. Immune status can be followed sequentially to assess response to nutritional intervention, but this practice is not routine.

The pediatric cancer patient on treatment is at risk for episodes of sepsis with the associated catabolic state and depletion of nutrients. Ongoing cytotoxic therapy may also deplete the body of micronutrients. Decreased antioxidant

Table 37-2

Anthropometric, biochemical, and body mass evaluations.

Anthropometric Measurements and Assessments

- Weight
- Height/length
- Head circumference (for patients < 3 yrs)
- Weight for height/length
- Ideal body weight (IBW = patient's actual weight divided by the ideal weight for height × 100)
- Body mass index (BMI = weight in Kg divided by height in meters squared)
- Height and weight Z score
- Triceps skin fold (to measure fat stores)
- Arm circumference (to measure muscle stores)
- Waist circumference
- Height velocity
- Body composition assessment
  - ∼ Isotope dilution methods
    - –fat-free mass, fat mass, and % body fat
  - ∼ Bioelectrical methods
    - –TOBEC fat-free mass, fat mass, and % body fat
  - ∼ Absorptiometry methods
    - –Dual photon absorptiometry (DPA) and dual-energy x-Ray absorptiometry (DEXA)
    - –Measure bone mass, lean body mass, and fat mass

Biochemical Assessments

- Complete blood count, hepatic biochemistry, renal and fluid biochemistry, sugar
  - ∼ Albumin (half-life 14-21 days)
  - ∼ Transferrin (half-life 8-9 days)
  - ∼ Prealbumin (half-life 2-3 days)
  - ∼ Retinol binding protein (half-life 12 hours)
- Fat status
  - ∼ Cholesterol
  - ∼ Lipoproteins
- Trace elements: Zn, Cu, Se, Mg
- Vitamins: A, C, E, thiamine, riboflavin
- Global biochemical assessment of antioxidants

levels have been reported following chemotherapy.[35,36] Trace elements may also be depleted.[37] Zinc is important to both immune function and mucosal integrity. The patient who is not thriving; has persistent infections, delayed wound healing, or skin changes; and has unexplained impaired cognition should have vitamin and trace elements evaluated.

Nutritional Intervention

Nutritional support should be an active and continuous aspect of supportive care to sustain growth and development, plus improve well-being and quality of life (Figure 37-1).[1,38] Dietary intervention is most commonly undertaken if there is weight loss, despite the limitations of weight being the sole criteria.[39] A proactive approach to monitoring dietary intake should be considered in patients who are known to be at high risk for becoming malnourished[1,12] (Table 37-3). This monitoring will help the clinician ascertain if protein or calorie intake is falling below 80% of the required intake. If diminished intake persists, there should be an intervention before substantial weight loss occurs. Some criteria for intervention for both underweight and overweight patients are listed in Table 37-4.

Increasing oral intake of nutrients should be the first approach. A wide variety of oral supplements are available

to increase calorie and/or protein intake.[20,27] Children should be allowed to have a choice, as taste and tolerance varies. Enteral tube feeding may well be required to sustain adequate intake. Enteral feeding has numerous advantages over the parenteral route, such as the maintenance of gastrointestinal mucosal function. Moreover, it is cheaper and avoids the known complications of parenteral feeding.[40–43] Many physicians and nurses, however, are reluctant to use nasogastric (NG) tube feeding, as it is often misinterpreted as a punishment for not eating. They may be concerned for the child due to the inconvenience, discomfort, and poor body image associated with the placement of the NG tube. Feeding should be presented as a positive supportive care measure that will aid the patient's well-being. For patients in whom nasal tube placement is difficult or not well tolerated, the alternatives are gastrostomy, duodenostomy, or enterostomy tubes.[44–47] These are becoming increasingly acceptable for cosmetic reasons as well as the ability to place the tube percutaneously.

Many myths abound about NG tube feeding, such as that it is not to be used in the neutropenic or thrombocytopenic patient; it is not to be inserted if there is mucositis; and it may cause aspiration and sinusitis. Currently, there is insufficient evidence to either support or refute these perceptions. The importance of maintaining gut integrity is well established, however, and adequate enteral feeding avoids

Table 37-3

Patients at high risk of protein energy malnutrition.

- Patients who are undernourished or cachectic at diagnosis
- Patients with relapsed disease
- Patients younger than 2 months
- Patients who are under 90% of their ideal body weight
- Patients who have had irradiation of oropharynx/esophagus or abdomen
- Patients undergoing a chemotherapy treatment protocol associated with a high occurrence of GI or appetite-depressing side effects—eg, for Burkitt lymphoma, osteogenic sarcoma, CNS tumors
- Patients with postsurgical complications
- Stem cell transplant patients

Table 37-4

Criteria for intervention.

Anthropometric

- >5% weight loss
- <10th percentile or >90th percentile weight-for-height
- <90% or >120% IBW-for-height
- <5th percentile or >85th percentile BMI-for-age
- <10th percentile height-for-age
- <10th percentile weight-for-age
- Subcutaneous fat (triceps skinfolds) and muscle mass (upper mid-arm circumference) values under- or overweight
- Current percentile weight or height that has fallen 2 percentile channels

Nutrient intake

- <80% of estimated needs of calories and protein

Supportive Care of Children with Cancer. Current Therapy and Guidelines
From the Children's Oncology Group, 3rd ed., 2004.

the risks of parenteral nutrition.[48,49] The practical clinical approach should be to place a tube prior to the development of mucositis, neutropenia, or thrombocytopenia in a high-risk patient who is unlikely to maintain adequate voluntary oral intake. The early use of NG or other tube feeding is gaining acceptance.[43,50–52] Depending on the voluntary oral intake of the patient, tube feeding can commence as bolus feeds and progress to nocturnal continuous feeds with bolus feeds during the day or continuous drip-

feeding by pump. The aim is to supply the calculated required intake of proteins and calories enterally, as long as the method of feeding is tolerated. Diarrhea can be caused by hyperosmolar formulas, lactose intolerance, or refeeding syndrome. Refeeding syndrome can occur in a malnourished patient due to the rapid administration of calorically dense enteral or parenteral formulas. It may cause hyperglycemia, which in turn can lead to large shifts in phosphorus, magnesium, and potassium from the extracellular space to the intracellular space with associated nausea, vomiting, diarrhea, and metabolic disturbances.[53,54]

Many nutritionally complete formulas are now available.[20,27] The assistance of a registered dietician is often required to help choose which is most appropriate in a given clinical situation. Specialized elemental or simple peptide feeds should be used when malabsorption is a concern or when there has been prolonged damage to the gut. Formulas and supplements are available to improve immune status (eg, Immunocal™). There is now great interest in immunonutrition and nutriceuticals by the public and, to a lesser extent, clinicians. The Children's Oncology Group (COG) studied patients on chemotherapy using an undernatured whey protein–based formula (Immunocal™) to improve cysteine delivery, which is a precursor for glutathione production. The study did show preliminary results of an increase of glutathione over the baseline level.[55] Weight gain was documented in the majority of patients. A randomized trial is now proposed to assess if side effects of chemotherapy will be reduced. Specific enteral and parenteral formulae for organ toxicities such as hepatic and renal toxicity are available.[27] Glutamine has been advocated to improve mucosal turnover, especially in stem cell transplant patients. Reports give variable results in a heterogeneous group of patients.[38] A Cochrane review indicates there is evidence to support glutamine supplementation in stem cell transplant patients.[56] A neutropenic diet has been utilized for patients at high risk for infection, but there is little evidence to support its use.[57] A low-bacterial diet is probably appropriate for stem cell transplant patients.

Appetite stimulants are used but remain controversial.[58] Megace (megestrol acetate) may have endocrinological side effects (antiandrogen or progestational agonist, adrenal suppression), while Periactin (cyproheptadine hydrochloride) may have mild central depressant properties. The Children's Oncology Group (COG) is conducting a randomized trial in patients with sustained weight loss to assess these drugs' efficacy and toxicity.

Parenteral nutrition (PN) should be considered when all attempts for sufficient enteral feeding have failed or are contraindicated, as in the presence of neutropenic enterocolitis/typhlitis or a gut that is nonfunctional. Parenteral nutrition is associated with a significant increased risk of infection, hepatic toxicity, a variety of metabolic abnormalities, fluid/electrolyte imbalance, and increased risk of thrombosis of the central venous line.[59–62] The potential interaction of parenteral nutrition with many drugs remains unclear. The role and utility of PN has been best defined in stem cell transplant patients who have had prolonged gut damage due to the preparative regimen, graft-versus-host disease, and/or infections.[63,64] Short-term parenteral therapy is rarely of benefit.

A central venous device is required for prolonged parenteral nutrition to avoid damage of the peripheral veins by high-solute PN solution. To determine PN requirements, calculate the required fluids, calories, protein, fat, carbohydrates, vitamins, and trace elements.[65,66] Most hospitals have specific PN guidelines. Close monitoring, both clinically and biochemically, is necessary to prevent complications.[62] If PN is required there should still be an effort to maintain some enteral feeding, unless contraindicated, to preserve gut integrity and function.

Obesity

Malnutrition refers not only to those with inadequate intake or other reasons of cachexia but also to those with excessive intake or metabolic (thyroid, pituitary, hypothalamus) abnormalities causing significant weight gain and obesity. The pandemic of obesity in North America has been well documented, with at least 30% of children over age 6 having a BMI greater than the 85th percentile.[67] Pediatric oncology patients have not been spared.[68–72] Significant medical and psychosocial consequences accompany excessive weight gain. Obesity in adults frequently commences during childhood. Obese adults may have impaired glucose tolerance, diabetes mellitus, insulin resistance, hypercholesterolemia, hypertension, and cardiovascular disease. These individuals have higher rates of some forms of cancer, and inferior survival when they develop cancer.[73] This metabolic syndrome is now being seen in the pediatric population.[74] Obesity may be a prognostic factor in both acute myeloblastic leukemia (AML)[75] and lymphoblastic leukemia (ALL).[76] In AML, the inferior mortality of the obese patients was related to treatment-related mortality in the first months of therapy. Acute lymphoblastic leukemia patients who are obese have lower event-free survival rates due to excess relapse rather than treatment-related mortality. There also appear to be some ethnic differences related to obesity and outcome in patients with ALL, with Hispanic females at greatest risk.[77] Genetic variation in the leptin receptor gene may be a contributing factor.[78]

The pharmacodynamics and pharmacokinetics of cytotoxic agents may be altered in an obese patient. Several authors have reviewed pharmacokinetics of drugs in obese patients.[79–83] Appropriate dosing for overweight pediatric patients is unknown. Underdosing could be an issue for some drugs, and increased toxicity may be of concern for others. As yet no clear guidelines exist as to which drugs should have their dose altered due to a patient's obesity.[84] There is a need to retrospectively review completed studies to analyze for survival and toxicity of overweight and obese patients and correlate with the method of calculating dosage and dose received. At this time the consensus is initially to administer the appropriate calculated dose for surface area unless upper dose limits are given for a specific drug.

Patients may present at diagnosis with obesity, become obese during therapy, or become obese off therapy. Cranial radiation is a documented therapy-related risk factor for obesity.[85–88] High-risk groups are brain tumor patients, especially craniopharyngioma survivors. Obese patients should be assessed for metabolic syndrome since it raises the risks of treatment complications both on and off therapy. The long-term effects of obesity are likely to increase long-term morbidity and decrease quality of life for cancer survivors. These patients also have the added risk of a second malignancy associated with obesity.[73] Obesity and risk of cardiovascular disease is well documented. It is not certain whether obesity also increases the risk of late-onset cardiac failure documented up to 15 years after anthracycline exposure.[89,90] As cancer cure rates increase, ongoing surveillance is required to evaluate cancer survivors for the risk of long-term sequelae associated with obesity.

Interventions for obese patients, both preventive and therapeutic, need to be considered. These measures should include nutritional, physical, lifestyle, psychological, endocrinological, and pharmacological modifications.[91,92] Possible interventions can be introduced only by documenting all risk factors and by continuously assessing nutritional and anthropometrical status. Providing nutritional education and encouraging increased physical activity are rational preventative measures, as for the non-oncology population. The utility and effectiveness of any intervention need to be evaluated, as well as potential impact on the underlying disease.

Summary

Nutritional supportive care for pediatric oncology patients should be undertaken with the same diligence as for other supportive care issues, such as those related to infections and blood product support. Interventions should be aimed at maintaining the optimum intake required for growth, improving quality of life, and possibly overall survival. Vigilance by the whole multidisciplinary team of the patient is required. Assistance of those with expertise in nutrition should be sought with the same frequency as other consultants. The pandemic of obesity and its added morbidity necessitates long-term nutritional and anthropometric surveillance.

References

1. UICC International Workshop. Nutritional morbidity in children with cancer: mechanisms, measures and management. *Int J Cancer.* 1998;11 [page nos.?].
2. van Eys J. Malnutrition in children with cancer: incidence and consequence. *Cancer.* 1979;43(5 Suppl):2030–2035.
3. Donaldson SS, Wesley MN, Dewys WD, Suskind RM, Jaffe N, Van Eys J. A study of the nutritional status of pediatric-cancer patients. *Am J Dis Child.* 1981;135:1107–1112.
4. Barr RD, Gibson B. Nutritional status and cancer in childhood. *J Pediatr Hematol Oncol.* 2000;22:491–494.
5. Elhasid R, Laor A, Lischinsky S, Weyl Ben Arush M. Nutritional status of children with solid tumors. *Cancer.* 1999;86:119–125.
6. Barr RD, Ribeiro RC, Agarwal BR, Masera G, Hesseling PB, Magrath IT. Pediatric oncology in countries of limited resources. In: Pizzo PA, Poplack DG, eds. *Principles and Practice of Pediatric Oncology,* 4th ed. Philadelphia: Lippincott, Williams and Wilkins; 2002:1541–1552.
7. Sala A, Pencharz P, Barr RD. Children, cancer, and nutrition: a dynamic triangle in review. *Cancer.* 2004;100:677–687.
8. Pickard KA, Detamore CM, Coates TD, et al. Effect of nutrition staging on treatment delays and outcome in stage-IV neuroblastoma. *Cancer.* 1983;52: 587–598.

9. Gomez-Almaguer D, Montemayor J, Gonzalez-Llano O, Ruiz-Arguelles GJ, Betz NL, Marfil-Rivera J. Leukemia and nutrition. IV: improvement in the nutritional status of children with standard-risk acute lymphoblastic leukemia is associated with better tolerance to continuation chemotherapy. *Int J Pediatr Hematol Oncol.* 1995;2:53–56.

10. Rickard KA, Coates TD, Grosfeld JL, Weetman RM, Baehner RL. The value of nutrition support in children with cancer. *Cancer.* 1986;58(8 Suppl):1904–1910.

11. Delbecque-Boussard L, Gottrand F, Ategbo S, et al. Nutritional status of children with acute lymphoblastic leukemia: a longitudinal study. *Am J Clin Nutr.* 1997;65(1):95–100.

12. Mauer AM, Burgess JB, Donaldson SS, et al. Special nutritional needs of children with malignancies: a review. *JPEN J Parenter Enteral Nutr.* 1990;14(3):315–324.

13. Krishnaswamy K. Drug metabolism and pharmacokinetics in malnourished children. *Clin Pharmacokinet.* 1989;17(Suppl 1):68–88.

14. Murry DJ, Riva L, Poplack DG. Impact of nutrition on pharmacokinetics of anti-neoplastic agents. *Int J Cancer Suppl.* 1998;11:48–51.

15. Lee JH, Suh OK, Lee MG. Pharmacokinetic changes in drugs during protein-calorie malnutrition: correlation between drug metabolism and hepatic microsomal cytochrome P450 isoenzymes. *Arch Pharm Res.* 2004;27(7):693–712.

16. Ladas EJ, Sacks N, Meacham L, et al. A multidisciplinary review of nutrition considerations in the pediatric oncology population: a perspective from Children's Oncology Group. *Nutr Clin Pract.* 2005;20:377–393.

17. Mihranian MH, Wang YM, Daly JM. Effects of nutritional depletion and repletion on plasma methotrexate pharmacokinetics. *Cancer.* 1984;54(10):2268–2271.

18. Charland SL, Bartlett D, Torosian MH. Effect of protein-calorie malnutrition on methotrexate pharmacokinetics. *JPEN J Parenter Enteral Nutr.* 1994;18(1):45–49.

19. Ladas E, Sacks N, Brophy P, Rogers PC. Standards of nutritional care in pediatric oncology: results from a nationwide survey on the standards of practice in pediatric oncology. *Pediatr Blood Cancer.* 2006;46(3):339–344.

20. Sacks N, Ringwald-Smith K, Hale G. Nutritional Support. In: Altman A, ed. *Supportive Care of Children with Cancer.* Baltimore: Johns Hopkins University Press; 2004:243–261.

21. Bowman IC, Williams R, Sanders M, Ringwald-Smith K, Baker D, Gajjar A. Algorithm for nutritional support: experience of the metabolic and infusion support service of St Jude Children's Research Hospital. *Int J Cancer.* 1998;11(Suppl):76–80.

22. Deans C, Wigmore SJ. Systemic inflammation, cachexia and prognosis in patients with cancer. *Curr Opin Clin Nutr Metabol Care.* 2005;8(3):265–269.

23. Argiles JM, Moore-Carrasco R, Fuster G, Busquets S, Lopez-Soriano FJ. Cancer cachexia: the molecular mechanisms. *Int J Biochem Cell Biol.* 2003;35(4):405–409.

24. Saarinen UM, Koskelo EK, Teppo AM, Siimes MA. Tumor necrosis factor in children with malignancies. *Cancer Res.* 1990;50(3):592–595.

25. Van Eys J. Nutrition and cancer: physiological interrelationships. *Annu Rev Nutr.* 1985;5:435–461.

26. Bessler S. Nutritional assessment. In: Samour PQ, King K, eds. *Handbook of Pediatric Nutrition.* Sudbury, MA: Jones & Bartlett; 2005:11–33.

27. Kleinman RE, ed. *Pediatric Nutrition Handbook.* Elk Grove Village, IL: American Academy of Pediatrics; 2004.

28. Pietsch JB, Ford C. Children with cancer: measurements of nutritional status at diagnosis. *Nutr Clin Prac.* 2000;15:185–188.

29. Waterlow JC. Classification and definition of protein-calorie malnutrition. *Br Med J.* 1972;3:566–569.

30. Hammer LD, Kraemer HC, Wilson DM, Ritter PL, Dornbusch SM. Standardized percentile curves of body-mass index for children and adolescents. *Am J Dis Child.* 1991;145:259–263.

31. Pietrobelli A, Faith MS, Allison DB, Gallagher D, Chiumello G, Heymsfield SM. Body mass index as a measure of adiposity among children and adolescents: a validation study. *J Pediatr.* 1998;132:204–210.

32. Warner JT, Cowan FJ, Dunstan FD, Gregory JW. The validity of body mass index for the assessment of adiposity in children with disease states. *Ann Hum Biol.* 1997;24:209–215.

33. Motil KJ. Sensitive measures of nutritional status in children in hospital and in the field. *Int J Cancer Suppl.* 1998;11:2–9.

34. Stallings VA, Vaisman N, Chan HS, et al. Immune responses in malnutrition. In: Stiehm R, Ocks HD, Winkelstein JA, eds. *Immunological Disorders in Infants and Children.* [city]: Elsevier Sanders; 2004:761–784.

35. Ladas EJ, Jacobson JS, Kennedy DD, Teel K, Fleischauer A, Kelly KM. Antioxidants and cancer therapy: a systemic review. *J Clin Oncol.* 2004;22:517–552.

36. Kennedy DD, Ladas EJ, Rheingold SR, Blumberg J, Kelly KM. Antioxidant status decreases in children with acute lymphoblastic leukemia during the first six months of chemotherapy treatment. *Pediatr Blood Cancer.* 2005;44(4):378–385.

37. [author?]Trace elements. In: Kleinman RE, ed. *Pediatric Nutrition Handbook.* Elk Grove, IL: American Academy of Pediatrics; 2004.

38. Berchard L, Adiv O, Jaksic T, Duggan C. Nutritional supportive care. In: Pizzo PA, Poplack DG, eds. *Principles and Practice of Pediatric Oncology.* Philadelphia: Lippincott Williams & Wilkins; 2002:1285–1300.

39. Rickard K, Lopez A, Godshall BJ, Wetman R, Grosfeld J. Nutritional strategies for children with cancer. *Nutr Focus.* 1991;6(5):1–10.

40. den Broeder E, Lippens RJJ, van't Hof MA, et al. Association between the change in nutritional status in response to tube feeding and the occurrence of infections in children with a solid tumor. *Pediatr Hematol Oncol.* 2000;17:567–575.

41. Nevin-Folino N, Miller M. Enteral Nutrition. In: Samour PQ, King K, eds. *Handbook of Pediatric Nutrition.* Sudbury, MA: Jones & Bartlett; 2005:499–524.

42. Schattner M. Enteral nutrition support of the patient with cancer: route and role. *J Clin Gastroenterol.* 2003;36:297–3023.

43. den Broeder E, Lippens RJ, van't Hof MA, et al. Effects of naso-gastric tube feeding on the nutritional status of children with cancer. *Eur J Clin Nutr.* 1998;52(7):494–500.

44. Aquino VM, Smyrl CB, Hagg R, et al. Enteral nutritional support by gastrostomy tube in children with cancer. *J Pediatr.* 1995;127:58–62.

45. Mathew P, Bowman L, Williams R, et al. Complications and effectiveness of gastrostomy feedings in pediatric cancer patients. *J Pediatr Hematol Oncol.* 1996;18:81.

46. Mathew P, Bowman L, Williams R, et al. Complications and effectiveness of gastrostomy feedings in pediatric cancer patients. *J Pediatr Hematol Oncol.* 1996;18(1):81–85.

47. Aquino VM, Smyrl CB, Hagg R, McHard KM, Prestridge L, Sandler ES. Enteral nutritional support by gastrostomy tube in children with cancer. *J Pediatr.* 1995;127(1):58–62.

48. Heubi JE. Whenever possible, use the gut! *J Pediatr Hematol Oncol.* 1999;21:88–90.

49. Rees Parrish C. Enteral feeding: the art and the science. *Nutr Clin Prac.* 2003;18:76–85.

50. DeSwarte-Wallace J, Firouzbakhsh S, Finklestein JZ. Using research to change practice: enteral feedings for pediatric oncology patients. *J Pediatr Oncol Nurs.* 2001;18:217–223.

51. Pietsch JB, Ford C, Whitlock JA. Nasogastric tube feedings in children with high-risk cancer: a pilot study. *J Pediatr Hematol Oncol.* 1999;21:111–114.

52. Langdana A, Tully N, Molloy E, et al. Intensive enteral nutrition support in paediatric bone marrow transplantation. *Bone Marrow Transplant.* 2001;27:741–746.

53. Dunn R, Stettler N, Mascarenhas M. Refeeding syndrome in hospitalized pediatric patients. *Nutr Clin Pract.* 2003;18:327–332.

54. Solomon SM, Kirby DF. The refeeding syndrome: a review. *JPEN J Parenter Enteral Nutr.* 1990;14(1):90–97.

55. Melnick SJ, Rogers PC, Sacks N, et al. A pilot limited institutional study to evaluate the safety and tolerability of immunocal a nutriceutical cysteine delivery agent in the management of wasting in high risk childhood cancer patients [abstract]. Chicago Supportive Oncology Conference, September 2005.

56. Murray SM, Pindoria S. Nutrition support for bone marrow transplant patients. *Cochrane Database Syst Rev.* 2002;(2):CD002920.

57. Moody K, Charlson ME, Finlay J. The neutropenic diet: what's the evidence? *J Pediatr Hematol Oncol.* 2002;24(9):717–721.

58. Yavuzsen T, Davis MP, Walsh D, LeGrand S, Lagman R. Systematic review of the treatment of cancer-associated anorexia and weight loss. *J Clin Oncol.* 2005;23(33):8500–8511.

59. Christensen ML, Hancock ML, Gattuso J, et al. Parenteral nutrition associated with increased infection rate in children with cancer. *Cancer.* 1993;72(9):2732–2738.

60. Quigley EM, Marsh MN, Shaffer JL, Markin RS. Hepatobiliary complications of total parenteral nutrition. *Gastroenterology.* 1993;104(1):286–301.

61. Lenssen P, Bruemmer BA, Bowden RA, Gooley T, Aker SN, Mattson D. Intravenous lipid dose and incidence of bacteremia and fungemia in patients undergoing bone marrow transplantation. *Am J Clin Nutr.* 1998;67(5):927–933.

62. Mirtallo J, Canada T, Johnson D, et al. Safe practices for parenteral nutrition. *JPEN J Parenter Enteral Nutr.* 2004;28(6):S39–S70.

63. Barale K, Charuhas P. Oncology and hematopoietic cell transplantation. In: Samour P, King K, eds. *Handbook of Pediatric Nutrition.* Sudbury, MA: Jones & Bartlett; 2005:459–482.

64. Muscaritoli M, Grieco G, Capria S, Iori AP, Fanelli FR. Nutritional support in patients undergoing bone marrow transplantation. *Am J Clin Nutr.* 2002;75:183–190.

65. ASPEN Board of Directors and The Clinical Guidelines Task Force. Guidelines for the use of parenteral and enteral nutrition in adult and pediatric patients. *JPEN J Parenter Enteral Nutr.* 2002;26(1 Suppl):1SA–138SA.

66. National Academy of Sciences, Institute of Medicine. *Dietary Reference Intakes for Energy, Carbohydrate, Fiber, Fat, Fatty Acids, Cholesterol, Protein, and Amino Acids (Macronutrients).* Washington, DC: National Academy Press; 2002.

67. Lobstein T, Baur L, Uauy R. Obesity in children and young people: a crisis in public health. *Obesity Rev.* 2004;5(Suppl 1):4–85.

68. Rogers PC, Meacham LR, Oeffinger KC, Henry DW, Lange BJ. Review: obesity in pediatric oncology. *Pediatr Blood Cancer.* 2005;45:881–891.

69. Oeffinger KC, Mertens AC, Sklar CA, et al. Obesity in adult survivors of childhood acute lymphoblastic leukemia: a report from the Childhood Cancer Survivor Study. *J Clin Oncol.* 2003;21(7):1359–1365.

70. Zee P, Chen CH. Prevalence of obesity in children after therapy for acute lymphoblastic leukemia. *Am J Pediatr Hematol Oncol.* 1986;8(4):294–299.

71. Nysom K, Holm K, Michaelsen KF, Hertz H, Muller J, Molgaard C. Degree of fatness after treatment for acute lymphoblastic leukemia in childhood. *J Clin Endocrinol Metab.* 1999;84(12):4591–4596.

72. Didi M, Didcock E, Davies HA, Ogilvy-Stuart AL, Wales JK, Shalet SM. High incidence of obesity in young adults after treatment of acute lymphoblast leukemia in childhood. *J Pediatr.* 1995;127(1):63–67.

73. Calle EE, Kaaks R. Overweight, obesity and cancer: epidemiological evidence and proposed mechanisms. *Nature Rev Cancer.* 2004;4:579–591.

74. Kourti M, Tragiannidis A, Makedou A, Papageorgiou T, Rousso I, Athanassiadou F. Metabolic syndrome in children and adolescents with acute lymphoblastic leukemia after the completion of chemotherapy. *J Pediatr Hematol Oncol.* 2005;27(9):499–501.

75. Lange BJ, Gerbing R, Feusner J, et al. Mortality in overweight and underweight children with acute myeloid leukemia. *JAMA.* 2005;293(2):203–211.

76. Butturini AM, Dorey FJ, Gaynon PS, et al. Obesity and outcome in pediatric acute lymphoblastic leukemia: a report from the Children's Oncology Group. Submitted *Lancet.*

77. Baillargeon J, Langevin AM, Lewis M, et al. Therapy related changes in body size in Hispanic children with acute lymphoblastic leukemia. *Cancer.* 2005; 103(8):1725–1729.

78. Ross JA, Oeffinger KC, Davies SM, et al. Genetic variation in the leptin receptor gene and obesity in survivors of childhood acute lymphoblastic leukemia: a report from the Childhood Cancer Survivor Study. *J Clin Oncol.* 2004; 22(17):3558–3562.

79. Cheymol G. Effects of obesity on pharmacokinetics implications for drug therapy. *Clin Pharmacokinet.* 2000;39(3):215–231.

80. Blouin RA, Warren GW. Pharmacokinetic considerations in obesity. *J Pharm Sci.* 1999;88(1):1–7.

81. Rodvold KA, Rushing DA, Tewksbury DA. Doxorubicin clearance in the obese. *J Clin Oncol.* 1988;6(8):1321–1327.

82. Dunn TE, Ludwig EA, Slaughter RL, Camara DS, Jusko WJ. Pharmacokinetics and pharmacodynamics of methylprednisolone in obesity. *Clin Pharmacol Ther.* 1991;49(5):536–549.

83. Zuccaro P, Guandalini S, Pacifici R, et al. Fat body mass and pharmacokinetics of oral 6-mercaptopurine in children with acute lymphoblastic leukemia. *Ther Drug Monit.* 1991;13(1):37–41.

84. Baker SD, Grochow LB, Donehower RC. Should anticancer drug doses be adjusted in the obese patient? *J Natl Cancer Inst.* 1995;87(5):333–334.

85. Dalton VK, Rue M, Silverman LB, et al. Height and weight in children treated for acute lymphoblastic leukemia: relationship to CNS treatment. *J Clin Oncol.* 2003;21(15):2953–2960.

86. Sklar CA, Mertens AC, Walter A, et al. Changes in body mass index and prevalence of overweight in survivors of childhood acute lymphoblastic leukemia: role of cranial irradiation. *Med Pediatr Oncol.* 2000;35(2):91–95.

87. Lustig RH, Post SR, Srivannaboon K, et al. Risk factors for the development of obesity in children surviving brain tumors. *J Clin Endocrinol Metab.* 2003; 88(2):611–616.

88. Bakish J, Hargrave D, Tariq N, Laperriere N, Rutka JT, Bouffet E. Evaluation of dietetic intervention in children with medulloblastoma or supratentorial primitive neuroectodermal tumors. *Cancer.* 2003;98(5):1014–1020.

89. Gurney JG, Kadan-Lottick NS, Packer RJ, et al. Endocrine and cardiovascular late effects among adult survivors of childhood brain tumors: Childhood Cancer Survivor Study. *Cancer.* 2003;97(3):663–673.

90. Heikens J, Ubbink MC, van der Pal HP, et al. Long term survivors of childhood brain cancer have an increased risk for cardiovascular disease. *Cancer.* 2000;88(9):2116–2121.

91. Committee on Nutrition. American Academy of Pediatrics. Policy statement. Prevention of pediatric overweight and obesity. *Pediatrics.* 2003;112:424–430.

92. Dietz WH, Gortmaker SL. Preventing obesity in children and adolescents. *Annu Rev Public Health.* 2001;22:337–353.

Nausea

Ria G. Hawks

Introduction

Nausea and vomiting are among the most common and distressing side effects of cancer treatment.[1] Dealing with chemotherapy-induced nausea and vomiting (CINV) is a challenging problem in children being treated for malignancy. Despite the introduction in the 1990s of a highly effective new class of antiemetics, the 5-HT$_3$ receptor antagonists, a substantial number of chemotherapy patients still experience nausea and vomiting.[2] Certain highly emetogenic chemotherapy agents and combination regimens predictably induce severe nausea and vomiting. Poorly controlled nausea and vomiting may result in anticipatory nausea with subsequent treatment cycles[3,4] and generally impact negatively on treatment compliance and quality of life.

From the patient's perspective, nausea is a distinctly unpleasant state with decreased gastric motility, increased small intestine tone, and psychic distress. Nausea is a subjective, unobservable phenomenon that cannot be quantified. Nausea may progress to emesis, in which gastric and occasionally small intestinal contents are propelled up to and out of the mouth. Uncontrolled vomiting may progress to retching, a spasmodic respiratory movement against a closed glottis, with simultaneous contraction of the gastric antrum and relaxation of the fundus and cardia.

Important progress has been made in the control of CINV, with the rational use of antiemetic combinations and adjunctive modalities. Also, newer "targeted" cancer therapies appear to have less associated nausea and vomiting than standard cytotoxic chemotherapy agents. This chapter will review the pathophysiology and types of nausea and vomiting, the commonly used antiemetics, and newer agents, as well as nonpharmacologic approaches, particularly as they relate to the management of children with cancer.

Physiologic Control of Nausea and Vomiting

Nausea and vomiting are distinct physiologic processes. Nausea is mediated through the autonomic nervous system. Cytotoxic drugs cause damage to gastrointestinal (GI) cells, resulting in sudden release of the neurotransmitter serotonin (5-hydroxytryptamine) from enterochromaffin cells. Other neurotransmitters that have been associated with the pathogenesis of vomiting include dopamine, histamine, and substance P.[5]

Vomiting is controlled by a putative center in the lateral reticular formation of the fourth ventricle and medulla. The vomiting center appears to be stimulated by afferent signals from 4 sources. The primary source is the chemoreceptor trigger zone (CTZ), a neural network in the nucleus tractus solitarius that senses chemical abnormalities in the body (eg, emetic drugs, uremia, hypoxia, diabetic ketoacidosis). The CTZ is located in the area postrema on the dorsal surface of the medulla and floor of the fourth ventricle. Because it is located outside of the blood-brain barrier, the CTZ responds to stimuli in the blood as well as in the cerebrospinal fluid.

The vomiting center is also stimulated by visceral afferents from the GI tract, via the vagus or sympathetic nerves, signaling GI distension and mucosal irritation. Additional visceral afferents may emanate from the bile ducts and peritoneum as well as other organs. Afferents from the cerebral cortex and limbic system respond to sensory stimuli (particularly smell and taste) and report pain and psychological stress. Finally, afferents from the vestibular-labyrinthine apparatus of the inner ear respond to body motion, mainly causing motion sickness.

Once activated, the vomiting center induces vomiting by stimulating salivary and respiratory centers and the pharyngeal, GI, and abdominal musculature. To be effective, antiemetic agents must block activation of the vomiting center. Successful management of nausea and vomiting in cancer patients requires consideration of all potential causes, in addition to the direct effect of chemotherapy. This chapter addresses primarily CINV, but other factors that contribute to nausea and vomiting in pediatric patients should not be overlooked when developing a treatment plan for the child with nausea and vomiting (Table 38-1).

Table 38-1

Causes of nausea and vomiting in pediatric cancer patients.

- Chemotherapy
- Radiation therapy
- Cancer itself, including CNS disease or GI tract involvement
- Delayed gastric emptying
- Gastritis, gastroesophageal reflux, ulcer
- Pancreatitis, cholecystitis
- Gastric distension (eg, constipation, ileus)
- Hypercalcemia, hyperglycemia
- Dehydration, hypokalemia
- Renal insufficiency, uremia
- Infection (eg, *H. pylori* or *C. difficile*)
- Other medications, such as antibiotics and opioid analgesics
- Anxiety and anticipation

Chemotherapy-Induced Nausea and Vomiting

The pathogenesis of CINV involves multiple neurotransmitters and receptors. *Dopamine*, which is synthesized in the central nervous system (CNS), was the first neurotransmitter to be targeted in the development of antiemetics. Dopamine D_2 receptors predominate in the area postrema and are also found on enterochromaffin cells in the intestinal mucosa. Dopaminergic antagonists such as phenothiazines and metoclopramide appear to exert their antiemetic activity by blocking dopamine receptors in the CTZ. Other neurotransmitters involved in the vomiting reflex include histamine H_1 and muscarinic receptors, which are located in the nucleus tractus solitarius. Antagonists of these receptors are effective in treating motion sickness and potentially CINV as well.[5]

Serotonin (5-hydroxytryptamine, 5-HT) is widely distributed throughout the GI tract, especially in the enterochromaffin cells of the gut mucosa. Intestinal mucosal damage caused by chemotherapy agents results in a massive release of 5-HT primarily from enterochromaffin cells, sending a vomiting message to the brain. Of the 7 classes of 5-HT receptors, it is the $5-HT_3$ receptors (widely distributed both centrally and peripherally) that appear to be the main cause of chemotherapy-induced vomiting. In the GI tract, $5-HT_3$ receptors are found exclusively on enteric neurons such as the vagus and sympathetic nerves. In the brain they are located in areas that mediate emesis—namely, the area postrema, nucleus tractus solitarius, and presynaptically on vagal afferent terminals in the medulla.

Selective $5-HT_3$ receptor antagonists are highly effective in antagonizing the serotonin that is released from enterochromaffin cells in the gut, thereby preventing CINV.

Substance P is a regulatory peptide found in the nucleus tractus solitarii, the area postrema of the brain, as well as in the vagal afferents of the GI tract.[6] Substance P's involvement in the emetic reflex is mediated through the neurokinin-1 (NK1) receptor, coupled to the inositol phosphate signal transduction pathway. Neurokinin-1 receptor antagonists bind to the receptor sites of the neurotransmitter, substance P, within the nucleus tractus solitarii to effectively block the emetic response to central, peripheral, and combined stimuli.[7]

Factors Affecting Nausea and Vomiting

The degree of clinical nausea and vomiting associated with chemotherapy depends on a number of factors. The specific emetic potential of the chemotherapy must first be considered. The emetogenicity of the agent administered is the single most important determinant of nausea and vomiting in adults,[8] and this is likely true in pediatric patients as well. Dose, schedule, route, and duration of administration of the medication also contribute to the emetogenic potential of the therapy. Onset of emesis is more rapid with parenteral compared with oral administration, and emesis is more likely with short intravenous infusion than with protracted infusion.[5] Emesis is more severe with single high doses of chemotherapy agents such as cisplatin, compared with divided-dose multiple-day administration.

Combination therapy and/or frequent interval administration will also impact CINV. The effect can be additive in regimens combining multiple emetogenic agents.[9] Daily or weekly scheduling can lead to incomplete recovery from nausea and vomiting between treatments.[4]

Certain patient characteristics are associated with an increased risk of CINV. In pediatrics, these characteristics include female gender, age above 3 years, history of motion sickness, poor control of emesis with prior chemotherapy treatments, and treatment-associated anxiety.[10]

Types of Nausea and Vomiting

Chemotherapy-induced nausea and vomiting can be acute, delayed, or anticipatory. Breakthrough and refractory vomiting may also occur. Acute-onset nausea and vomiting occurs within minutes to hours, peaking after 5 to 6 hours, and ends within 24 hours. The $5-HT_3$ serotonin receptors have made their biggest impact in controlling acute nausea and vomiting.[3]

Delayed-onset nausea and vomiting develops more than 24 hours after administration of chemotherapy (eg, cisplatin-related vomiting peaks at 48 to 72 hours and may last up to 7 days). Delayed emesis can also occur in patients treated with a combination of moderately emetogenic chemotherapy. Until recently, delayed nausea and vomiting did not attract the attention of investigators interested in minimizing CINV. The vomiting is less severe and the nausea hard to quantify. Risk factors for delayed CINV in children include occurrence of acute nausea and vomiting with the accompanying cycle of chemotherapy; cycles that contain cisplatin, carboplatin, or cyclophosphamide; or cycles extending over 2 or more days.[11] A history of motion sickness and development of taste aversions have also been reported as risk factors for delayed CINV in children.[12]

Anticipatory nausea and vomiting (ANV) is a learned behavior associated with previous experience of poorly controlled CINV and develops in up to 25% of patients. The literature is rich in the exploration of ANV as a classic conditioned response.[13–15] Standard antiemetics may be ineffective against ANV.

Breakthrough vomiting occurs despite previously effective control of vomiting—ie, there is a secondary failure of the antiemetic regimen. Refractory vomiting refers to the situation in which the patient no longer responds to treatment directed at preventing or controlling vomiting. Chronic nausea and vomiting may occur in patients with advanced cancer (eg, from medications, constipation, dehydration, or brain metastases).

Emetogenic Potential of Chemotherapy and Radiotherapy

Commonly used chemotherapeutic agents can be ranked according to emetogenic potential.[8] Emetogenic potential may vary with dose. Chemotherapy combinations will be more emetogenic than single agents. Table 38-2 lists the relative emetogenic potential of commonly used agents based on a series of studies.[3,16,17]

Omitted from Table 38-2, as well as the reviews mentioned, is the emetogenic potential of intrathecal chemotherapy, which is integral to the management of childhood leukemia. Most published reports are based on the adult experience, but Holdsworth et al[18] demonstrated that the administration of ondansetron significantly reduced the emetogenic potential of the combination of intrathecal methotrexate, hydrocortisone, and cytarabine. Anecdotal experience suggests that emesis with this combination is attributable to cytarabine. Knowing the emetogenic potential of the chemotherapy agent(s) can guide the pediatric oncologist in the selection of an antiemetic regimen.[13]

Radiation therapy (RT) for solid tumors, including brain tumors, and cranial spinal irradiation for the treatment of CNS leukemia may be accompanied by nausea and vomiting. Risk assessment for the child receiving RT is based primarily on the treatment field. However, dose and fractionation of radiotherapy also contribute to the emetic potential. The American Society for Clinical Oncology (ASCO) Guidelines for Antiemetics in Oncology Update[19] describe 4 emetic risk categories and drug recommendations for adult patients receiving RT. The patients who receive total-body irradiation are in the highest risk group, and the recommendation is prophylaxis with a 5-HT_3 receptor antagonist with each fraction and for 24 hours after the last fraction. The moderate-risk group, of which 60% to 90% of patients are at risk of vomiting, includes patients receiving standard fractionated doses of 180 to 200 cGy to the abdomen who may experience nausea and vomiting, typically 1 to 2 hours after treatment. The ASCO recommendation is again a

Table 38-2
Emetogenetic risk of chemotherapeutic agents.

Level	Frequency of N/V[a]	Agents
5	>90%	Carmustine (>250 mg/m²), cisplatin (>50 mg/m²), cyclophosphamide (>1500 mg/m²), dacarbazine, lomustine (>60 mg/m²), d'actinomycin mechlorethamine, streptozocin
4	60%–90%	Busulfan (high dose), carboplatin, carmustine (<250 mg/m²), cisplatin (<50 mg/m²), cyclophosphamide (750-1500 mg/m²), cytarabine (>1000 mg/m²), doxorubicin (>v60 mg/m²), methotrexate (>1000 mg/m²), procarbazine
3	30%–60%	Cyclophosphamide (<750 mg/m²), doxorubicin (<60 mg/m²), epirubicin (<90 mg/m²), hexamethylmelamine, idarubicin, ifosfamide, methotrexate (250-1000 mg/m²), mitoxantrone (<15 mg/m²)
2	10%–30%	Capecitabine, cytarabine (low dose), docetaxel, etoposide, 5-fluorouracil (<1000 mg/m²), gemcitabine, irinotecan, methotrexate (50-250 mg/m²), mitomycin, paclitaxel, rituximab, temozolamide, topotecan
1	<10%	Asparaginase, bleomycin, busulfan (low dose), chlorambucil, 2-chlorodeoxyadenosine, fludarabine, hydroxyurea, methotrexate (<50 mg/m²), L-phenylalanine mustard, mercaptopurine, tamoxifen, thioguanine, vinblastine, vincristine, vinorelbine

[a]Percentage of patients experiencing N/V if no antiemetics are administered.

5-HT$_3$ receptor antagonist but does not require an additional dose to cover the 24 hours after the fraction has been administered. The third category is for low-risk patients (30%–60%), including patients who receive craniospinal, pelvic, or lower-thorax RT. The recommendation is that these patients also receive a 5-HT$_3$ receptor antagonist prior to each fraction.[20] Although these recommendations are for adults, they are applicable to the child receiving RT.

Results of Clinical Trials of Antiemetic Therapy

Most studies of antiemetics for chemotherapy-induced nausea and vomiting have been conducted in adults. In addition, most studies have evaluated the response in the setting of acute, and not chronic, nausea and vomiting. As with many other medications, antiemetics may have different metabolism and side effects in children, so there is a clear need for more pediatric studies. Table 38-3 summarizes the wide range of antiemetic agents by category and target receptors that will be discussed and referenced in this section.

In children as in adults, the 5-HT$_3$ receptor antagonists are generally superior to other antiemetics. The toxicity profile is minimal and the drugs are well tolerated. The most commonly reported toxicity is headache (10%–15% of patients) and constipation (10%–15% of patients). If a patient exhibits one of these side effects, switching to another agent often eliminates the toxicity, while continuing to provide equivalent prophylaxis. Rare adverse reactions include anxiety, dizziness, diarrhea, and fatigue.[21] An early study showed that ondansetron is superior to metoclopramide against highly emetic chemotherapy and has a better toxicity profile.[22] In children as in adults, a single daily dose is as effective as 3 divided doses.[23] In this prospective, double-blind, randomized trial, 31 chemotherapy-naive patients receiving either moderately or highly emetogenic chemotherapy were given either a single high dose of ondansetron (0.6 mg/kg, maximum 32 mg) or multiple

Table 38-3

Antiemetic agents in clinical use.

Category	Generic Name	Brand Name	Target Receptor
NK$_1$ receptor antagonist	Aprepitant[c]	Emend	Neurokinin
5-HT$_3$ receptor antagonists[a]	Ondansetron[a]	Zofran	Serotonin
	Granisetron[a]	Kytril	
	Dolasetron	Anzemet	
	Palestron: 2nd-generation 5-HT$_3$, Phase III clinical trials	Aloxi	
Benzamides	Metoclopramide	Reglan	Dopamine and serotonin
Butyrophenones	Haloperidol	Haldol	Dopamine
	Droperidol	Inapsine	
Phenothiazines	Prochlorperazine	Compazine	Dopamine
	Chlorpromazine	Thorazine	
	Thiethylperazine	Torecan	
	Promethazine	Phenergan	
Benzodiazepines	Lorazepam[b]	Ativan	
	Alprazolam	Xanax	
Cannabinoids	Dronabinol	Marinol	Cannabinoid
Antihistamines	Diphenhydramine	Benadryl	Histamine
Corticosteroids[a]	Dexamethasone	Decadron	Unknown
	Methylprednisolone	SoluMedrol	

[a]Standard of care for highly emetic chemotherapy.

[b]For anticipatory N/V related to CINV.

[c]Phase III clinical trials in combination with *5-HT$_3$ receptor antagonists and corticosteroid for acute and delayed CINV.

standard doses (0.15 mg/kg, maximum 8 mg, given every 4 hours for 4 doses). Efficacy was rated according to an emesis scale: (1) no nausea or emesis, (2) nauseous but able to eat, (3) nauseous and unable to eat, and (4) emesis. The proportion of patients rating 1 or 2 was 81% in the high-dose group and 80% in the standard-dose group ($p = 0.93$). No patient experienced any clinical or laboratory toxicity.

Another study addressed route of administration of ondansetron.[24] In this double-blind multicenter trial, 439 children receiving moderately or highly emetogenic chemotherapy were administered ondansetron 5 mg/m² intravenously and placebo syrup orally, or ondansetron syrup 8 mg orally and placebo intravenously, with each group receiving dexamethasone 2 to 4 mg orally. Ondansetron syrup 4 mg was given orally twice daily for 2 days after completion of chemotherapy. Complete or major control of emesis on the worst chemotherapy treatment day was achieved in 89% of patients in the intravenous group and in 88% of patients in the oral syrup group.

Granisetron and dolasetron are pharmacologically distinct from ondansetron but appear equally efficacious and safe. In a study of 294 pediatric patients receiving moderately or highly emetogenic chemotherapy, oral granisetron at 20 or 40 micrograms per kg twice daily (before and 6 to 12 hours after chemotherapy) resulted in a complete response (no vomiting, only mild nausea, and no need for rescue therapy) in 51% and 53% of children, respectively.[25] There was also no difference between these 2 doses in children with leukemia receiving high-dose methotrexate or cytarabine.[26] Single doses of granisetron have also been studied in children. Dolasetron has not been compared with other 5-HT₃ antagonists in children.

The 5-HT₃ receptor antagonists, as single agents, have demonstrated superior efficacy as a class of antiemetics, with acute response rates ranging from 50% to 70%.[27] To improve on this outcome, the second-generation 5-HT₃ receptor antagonists, with distinct pharmacologic differences from the current 5-HT₃ receptor antagonists, are now in development. Of these, palonosetron has been studied the most extensively. Palonosetron is a potent and selective 5-HT₃ antagonist with a 100-fold enhanced binding affinity for the 5-HT₃ receptor compared with first-generation 5-HT₃ antagonists. The plasma elimination half-life is extended to 40 hours, significantly longer than the others in this class.[28] Palonosetron is well tolerated. In 3 well-conducted double-blind studies, palonosetron demonstrated similar efficacy to ondansetron in cisplatin-treated patients and was superior to ondansetron and doleasetron in patients receiving moderately emetogenic chemotherapy.[28–30] Palonosetron has recently been evaluated with respect to the other 5-HT₃ antagonists when combined with dexamethasone and aprepitant, demonstrating promising results.[31] Again, these are adult studies; future studies are needed to confirm dosing in children.

The 5-HT₃ receptor antagonists are most effective when given with corticosteroids, usually as single intravenous doses of dexamethasone 12 mg/m² or methylprednisolone 100 mg/m². The exact mechanism of action corticosteroids is unknown. Animal studies suggest that corticosteroids exert a direct effect on the solitary tract in the medulla in the CNS, as well as a mode of action that is additive to that of a 5HT₃ receptor antagonist.[32] Despite the lack of understanding of how corticosteroids work, their efficacy has been well established in clinical trials. Corticosteroids are more potent antiemetics than metoclopramide or chlorpromazine.[33,34] The combination of a corticosteroid and metoclopramide is more effective than chlorpromazine alone.[35]

In a meta-analysis of 32 adult studies involving 5500 patients, addition of dexamethasone improved control of acute vomiting from 55% to 69% and delayed vomiting from 45% to 61%.[36] In children as well, the combination of a 5-HT₃ receptor antagonist and dexamethasone was superior to the 5-HT₃ antagonist alone.[37] In this randomized, double-blind, crossover placebo-controlled trial, 61% of pediatric cancer patients receiving ondansetron and dexamethasone had complete control of emesis, compared with 21% receiving ondansetron alone. Two or fewer vomiting episodes occurred in 86% of patients receiving both agents, compared with 67% with ondansetron alone. Minimal or no nausea occurred in 74% of courses with both drugs, compared with 52% of courses with ondansetron alone.

The combination of ondansetron and dexamethasone affords some control of delayed nausea and vomiting. In one double-blind, prospective, randomized multicenter trial, the combination of ondansetron and dexamethasone was effective in protecting 90% of patients from vomiting during the first 24 hours after chemotherapy.[38] In these patients, dexamethasone with or without ondansetron was superior to placebo in preventing delayed emesis. In patients who had vomiting on day 1, dexamethasone with ondansetron was superior to dexamethasone alone in controlling delayed emesis.

Although antiemetic clinical trials support the use of corticosteroids in controlling nausea and vomiting, the question of corticosteroids interfering with antitumor effects of chemotherapy has been of theoretical concern. This issue is specifically raised in the treatment of children with brain tumors. Corticosteroids may influence the blood-brain barrier, and, as a result, may limit access of the drugs to CNS tumors.[39] Glaser et al[39] suggest that children being treated for CNS malignancies receive steroids only if other therapies have failed to control the CINV. Another area where corticosteroids are discouraged is in their nonprotocol mandated use in clinical trials in which they may function therapeutically. In spite of these concerns, corticosteroids continue to be incorporated into treatment guidelines and play an important role in preventing CINV.[32]

The newest and most promising class of agents in clinical trials is the NK1 (substance P) antagonists. Substance P belongs to a family of neuropeptides known as tachykinins. Substance P is found primarily in the GI tract and in the CNS and functions through specific cell-surface receptors for NK1 receptors. Neurokinin-1 receptors are found in brain regions critical for regulation of the vomiting reflex. The NK1 receptor antagonists inhibit the action of substance P, and as a result, nausea and vomiting stimulated by chemotherapy are suppressed. Substance P has a role in both acute and delayed CINV. One agent, aprepitant, is currently marketed for use in combination with standard antiemetic agents for acute and delayed nausea and vomiting with highly emetogenic chemotherapy. Aprepitant is approved for use in children aged 12 years and older.

Review of the literature indicates that these agents have similar efficacy to that of 5-HT$_3$ antagonists in acute nausea and vomiting and superior efficacy in delayed nausea and vomiting.[40,41] The addition of aprepitant to standard ondansetron and dexamethasone also resulted in improved effectiveness against moderately emetogenic chemotherapy.[16] A Phase III study indicates that addition of a substance P antagonist, aprepitant, to a 5-HT$_3$ antagonist and a corticosteroid affords better prevention of CINV than that achieved with the 5-HT$_3$ antagonist and corticosteroid alone.[42] Aprepitant is available in oral formulation only. The regimen of 125 mg on day 1 and 80 mg on days 2 to 5 was found to be optimal.[43]

Dopamine blockers include metoclopramide, domperidone, and haloperidol. Metoclopramide is a relatively weak 5-HT$_3$ antagonist except at higher doses, but it also enhances gastric emptying, which may contribute to its antiemetic effect. Metoclopramide was widely used prior to the availability of newer 5-HT$_3$ antagonists and is clearly effective in children. Its use is limited by the occurrence of dystonic extrapyramidal reactions, however, particularly in younger patients.[44] However, given at lower doses to promote gastric emptying, metroclopramide is generally tolerated and has been used in the treatment of delayed nausea and vomiting.

Butyrophenones have potent antiemetic activity but may produce extrapyramidal reactions, hypotension, and sedation. Domperidone does not cross the blood-brain barrier, so there is less risk of dystonic reactions. Haloperidol is not used routinely for acute CINV, but it may have a place in refractory or chronic nausea and vomiting.

The phenothiazines also target dopamine receptors and are effective antiemetics in adults and children, but their use in younger patients is limited by concern about extrapyramidal reactions. Chlorpromazine appears to be more effective than metoclopramide in children.[45] Prochlorperazine is perhaps the most frequently used dopamine antagonist prescribed as an antiemetic in adults and may be useful for delayed nausea and vomiting with cisplatin. Common side effects of prochlorperazine are extrapyramidal reactions and sedation, limiting its use in pediatric patients.[46] Levomepromazine, although not widely studied in children and not available in the United States, is a relatively nonsedating phenothiazine that targets dopamine, histamine, acetylcholine, and some serotonin receptors and could be useful in refractory nausea and vomiting.

Benzodiazepines are valuable adjuncts in combination with acute antiemetic regimens, especially in teenagers, because they moderate anxiety. Benzodiazepines have no intrinsic antiemetic activity but produce anxiolytic, sedative, and anterograde amnesic effects and are thus useful in preventing and treating anticipatory nausea and vomiting.[13] Clinical trials have not evaluated the use of benzodiazepines in pediatric patients. Formulations with rapid onset and short duration of action (such as lorazepam or midazolam) are preferred.

Cannabinoids have a low therapeutic index but may be accepted and useful in selected patients. Most studies have evaluated their effect on pain. Synthetic cannabinoids may be more effective than metoclopramide or prochlorperazine.[47,48] Chemotherapy-induced nausea and vomiting is a proven indication for Dronabinol.[49] Nabilone, a derivative of marijuana, can help dissociate anxiety and nausea. Tolerance to effects on mood may occur within days to weeks. Side effects, including euphoria, sedation, dysphoria, depression, and hallucinations, limit the patient population who will tolerate this drug.[50] Adolescents have been the most tolerant group in the pediatric population to utilize this class of agents in the adjuvant setting to treat delayed nausea and decreased appetite.

Antihistamines such as diphenhydramine are frequently used because of their known effectiveness against motion sickness and the involvement of histamine receptors in mediation of CINV. Cyclizine is both an antihistamine and an anticholinergic that could be more effective but is poorly tolerated in children due to excessive dizziness and drowsiness.[46] There are no clinical trials supporting the use of diphenhydramine, although it has been utilized in clinical practice. Hydroxyzine hydrochloride has been used as an adjuvant antiemetic based primarily on anecdotal efficacy. However, one published study[51] suggests that hydroxyzine hydrochloride adds to the antiemetic control provided by granisetron.

Evidence-Based Recommendations for the Treatment of Chemotherapy-Induced Nausea and Vomiting in the Pediatric Patient

Chemotherapy-induced nausea and vomiting should be considered a single process that can occur throughout a treatment cycle, and patient management should be comprehensive over a 4 to 5 day period rather than dealing only with the chemotherapy treatment day(s). Most of the studies are conducted in the adult oncology setting.

For patients receiving highly emetogenic chemotherapy, the combination of a 5-HT$_3$ antagonist and dexamethasone results in complete control of acute nausea and vomiting in 70% of patients. Thus, the Antiemetic Subcommittee of the Multinational Association of Supportive Care in Cancer recommends that all pediatric cancer patients receiving highly or moderately emetogenic chemotherapy should receive antiemetic prophylaxis with this combination.[52] The ASCO antiemetic guidelines' recommendation for children receiving highly emetogenic chemotherapy includes the addition of an NK1 receptor antagonist.[20]

Highly emetogenic chemotherapy may also cause delayed nausea and vomiting, although this effect may be less common in children than adults.[53] Other risk factors include multi-day regimens and secondary failure of antiemetic prophylaxis.[11] Strategies for prevention of delayed nausea and vomiting in adults include extending the 5-HT$_3$ antagonist for 48 hours after chemotherapy or addition of corticosteroids or metoclopramide. The newer agent aprepitant, an NK1 antagonist, appears promising for prevention of delayed nausea and vomiting. In adults, the addition of aprepitant to standard ondansetron and dexamethasone resulted in improved effectiveness against moderately emetogenic chemotherapy.[16] Clinical trials in children have yet to be completed. Smith et al[54] reported on 2 case studies for CINV in adolescents, demonstrating safety and efficacy in treating pediatric patients for both acute and delayed emesis after chemotherapy. It is hoped that the results of ongoing clinical trials will define the evidence to incorporate this class of agents into the recommendations for standard of care to treat delayed nausea and vomiting.

For patients receiving moderately emetogenic chemotherapy, prophylaxis should include a 5-HT$_3$ antagonist with dexamethasone. Orally administered medications should be sufficient. This therapy should provide complete control of acute CINV in 75% to 80% of patients, and fewer than half will have delayed CINV, which may be reduced with dexamethasone with or without metoclopramide.[20]

Anticipatory nausea and vomiting may occur in up to 25% of children, typically 1 to 4 hours before chemotherapy but sometimes days in advance.[13] The recommended treatment approach is the best possible control of acute and delayed emesis, up front. Benzodiazepines and/or behavioral therapies involving relaxation, particularly systemic sensitization, have proven efficacy.[13,20,52]

The ASCO guidelines have the following recommendations for patients receiving RT. Patients receiving total-body irradiation are in the highest risk group, and the recommendation is prophylaxis with a 5-HT$_3$ receptor antagonist with each fraction and for 24 hours after the last fraction. Radiation therapy to the upper abdomen places patients in the moderate risk group, of which 60% to 90% of patients are at risk of vomiting. The ASCO recommendation is the same as for the high-risk group but does not require an additional dose to cover the 24 hours after the fraction has been administered. The third category, for patients at low risk (30%–60%) for vomiting, includes patients who receive cranial, spinal, pelvic, or lower-thorax RT. For these patients, the recommendation is to either receive rescue antiemetics with a dopamine or 5-HT$_3$ as prophylaxis or rescue. Patients at minimal risk (30%) should receive rescue antiemetics with a dopamine or 5-HT$_3$ receptor antagonist.[20]

Antiemetics in Development

With the recent introduction of the NK1 (substance P) antagonists, ongoing research continues to develop more effective agents as well as to address the optimal use of available agents.

Newer 5-HT$_3$ receptor antagonists under evaluation include batanopride and tropisetron. There is also evidence that the 5-HT$_3$ receptors in the CNS are associated with control of mood and may be the site of action of selective serotonin reuptake inhibitor medications in their antidepressive effect. Casopitant is a potent and selective oral NK1 receptor antagonist that has shown activity in preventing CINV in preclinical studies. Preliminary results of a Phase II study evaluating casopitant in combination with 5-HT$_3$ receptor antagonists and dexemethasone showed promising results.[19] Other CNS-acting agents in development include newer cannabinoid receptor agonists, which may have antiemetic activity superior to dronabinol. Olanazapine is an antipsychotic drug that blocks multiple neurotransmitters. A retrospective chart review of 28 patients, who received olanzapine on an as-needed basis following moderately to highly emetogenic chemotherapy, suggests that olanzapine may decrease delayed emesis.[55] A recent Phase II trial administered the antiemetic regime of olanzapine, dexamethasone, and palonosetron to 41 chemotherapy-naive patients who received moderately or highly emetic chemotherapy. This study concluded that this combination of antiemetics was very effective in controlling both delayed and CINV in these patients.[56]

It is hoped that new insights into the pathophysiology of nausea and vomiting will result in improved management. A representative area of research is the measurement of gastric motility by electrogastrogram, a noninvasive methodology. This technique can be used to quantify the effect of various chemotherapy agents and antiemetic medications on gastric emptying.

Nonpharmacologic Treatment for Anticipatory and Chemotherapy-Induced Nausea and Vomiting

Behavioral interventions and complementary and alternative medicine (CAM) are also effective in reducing ANV and CINV. Behavioral interventions evolve around a variety of adaptive behavioral skills designed to prevent or interrupt the conditioning cycle of nausea and vomiting. These methods are most successful in the management of ANV. Integrating the research that focuses on the biological understanding with behavioral interventions may help to advance the field.[57] Specific interventions including hypnosis, progressive muscle relaxation, biofeedback, guided imagery, music therapy, and distraction/videogames are known to have efficacy in ameliorating nausea and vomiting.

This is an area that welcomes more vigorous scientific research, particularly in the area of pediatrics. Complementary and alternative medicine offers a number of primary or adjuvant options to alleviate the discomfort and consequences of the progressive triad of nausea, retching, and emesis. Examples of CAM modalities that are currently being offered include acupuncture, acustimulation, acupressure, aromatherapy, and the use of herbs, such as ginger.

Acupuncture is the insertion and manual rotation of a very fine needle. Acustimulation, or electrical stimulation, is the use of an electrical current passed through an inserted needle. This type of stimulation can also be applied by noninvasive electrostimulation or acupressure. Evidence is emerging that the stimulation of acupuncture points, particularly the Neiguan (P6) acupuncture point (located on the inside of the wrist), is helpful in controlling nausea and vomiting. The safety of acupuncture-point stimulation, by any method, has been demonstrated by several large prospective trials.[58] A study published by Reindl, Geilen, and Hartmann[59] demonstrates the feasibility, effectiveness, and acceptance of acupuncture as a supportive therapy for pediatric oncology patients receiving emetic chemotherapy. The 1997 National Institutes of Health consensus statement conference concurred that acupuncture has been found to be effective in reducing CINV and encouraged further studies.[60]

In 2005 the Children's Oncology Group opened a randomized clinical trial in selected institutions to investigate the efficacy of electroacupuncture treatment to reduce delayed CINV in pediatric and young adult patients with solid tumors. The blinded design addressed the potential placebo effects by offering a sham arm. Accrual to this study is not yet complete, and results are, to date, not known. Alternative medicine practitioners also recommend the use of elastic bands designed to apply pressure to the P6 acupuncture point to control CINV. Several trials have demonstrated their effectiveness, primarily in decreasing the severity of nausea and vomiting.[58,61,62] Traditional acupuncture is also offered by licensed acupuncture practitioners at pediatric oncology CAM programs in centers that are fortunate enough to have an acupuncturist on staff.

Aromatherapy is the use of essential oils for therapeutic or medical purposes.

Research is ongoing to evaluate the use of aromatherapy as an adjunctive therapy to reduce CINV. Current literature suggests that aromatherapy massage has a mild transient anxiolytic effect.[63]

Complementary and alternative medicine modalities, such as herbs, are widely used in the pediatric oncology population.[64] Ginger (*Zingiber officinale*) has been advocated as a promising antiemetic herbal preparation. A monograph for ginger has been approved by the US pharmacopeia and is included in the National Formulary. Nausea and vomiting are listed as indications. The exact mechanism of action remains unknown. One area of research has suggested that the composition of ginger may stimulate serotonin receptors.[65] Clinical evidence supports the use of ginger for pregnancy-related nausea and vomiting.[66] Further research in needed on the use of ginger as an adjunctive therapy for CINV.

Summary

Dealing with CINV remains a challenging problem in pediatric oncology. The introduction of 5-HT$_3$ receptor antagonists either alone or in combination with corticosteroids has reduced the incidence and severity of CINV. Challenges remain in the optimization of established adult regimens for pediatric use, in the control of delayed nausea and vomiting, and in reducing nausea and vomiting associated with dose-intensive chemotherapy regimens.

Complete control of CINV should be the goal, to enhance the family and child's quality of life. Care should be convenient for the family and child, and treatment should reduce hospitalization and time spent in the ambulatory setting. The NK1 (substance P) antagonists appear to offer improved control of nausea and vomiting. Adjunctive methods such as acupuncture, aromatherapy, and behavior modification are increasingly used. Areas for further research included targeted therapy for CINV and CAM and related nonpharmacologic interventions.

References

1. de Boer-Dennert M, de Wit R, Schmitz PI, et al. Patient perspectives of the side-effects of chemotherapy: the influence of 5HT3 antagonists. *Br J Cancer*. 1997;76(8):1055–1061.
2. Hesketh PJ. New treatment options for chemotherapy-induced nausea and vomiting. *Support Care Cancer*. 2004;12(8):550–554.
3. Jordan K, Kasper C, Schmoll HJ. Chemotherapy-induced nausea and vomiting: current and new standards in the antiemetic prophylaxis and treatment. *Eur J Cancer*. 2005;41(2):199–205.
4. Oo TH, Hesketh PJ. Drug insight: new antiemetics in the management of chemotherapy-induced nausea and vomiting. *Nat Clin Pract Oncol*. 2005; 2(4):196–201.
5. Antonarakis ES, Hain RD. Nausea and vomiting associated with cancer chemotherapy: drug management in theory and in practice. *Arch Dis Child*. 2004;89(9):877–880.
6. Amin AH, Crawford TB, Gaddum JH. The distribution of substance P and 5-hydroxytryptamine in the central nervous system of the dog. *J Physiol*. 1954; 126(3):596–618.
7. Tattersall FD, Rycroft W, Francis B, et al. Tachykinin NK1 receptor antagonists act centrally to inhibit emesis induced by the chemotherapeutic agent cisplatin in ferrets. *Neuropharmacology*. 1996;35(8):1121–1129.
8. Hesketh PJ, Kris MG, Grunberg SM, et al. Proposal for classifying the acute emetogenicity of cancer chemotherapy. *J Clin Oncol*. 1997;15(1):103–109.
9. Kris MG, Hesketh PJ, Herrstedt J, et al. Consensus proposals for the prevention of acute and delayed vomiting and nausea following high-emetic chemotherapy. *Support Care Cancer*. 2005;13(2):85–96.
10. LeBaron S, Zeltzer LK, LeBaron C, et al. Chemotherapy side effects in pediatric oncology patients: drugs, age, and sex as risk factors. *Med Pediatr Oncol*. 1988;16(4):263–268.
11. Depuis LL, Lau R, Greenberg ML. Delayed nausea and vomiting in children receiving antineoplastics. *Med Pediatr Oncol*. 2001;37(2):115–121.
12. Tyc VL, Mulhern RK, Barclay DR, et al. Variables associated with anticipatory nausea and vomiting in pediatric cancer patients receiving ondansetron antiemetic therapy. *J Pediatr Psychol*. 1997;22(1):45–58.
13. Aapro MS, Molassiotis A, Oliver I. Anticipatory nausea and vomiting. *Support Care Cancer*. 2005;13(2):117–121.
14. Morrow GR. Clinical characteristics associated with the development of anticipatory nausea and vomiting in cancer patients undergoing chemotherapy. *J Clin Oncol*. 1984;2(10):1170–1176.
15. Stockhorst U, Spennes-Saleh S, Körholz D. Anticipatory symptoms and anticipatory immune response in pediatric cancer patients receiving chemotherapy: features of a classically conditioned response? *Brain Behav Immun*. 2000; 14(3):198–218.
16. Herrstedt J, Muss HB, Warr DG, et al. Efficacy and tolerability of aprepitant for the prevention of chemotherapy-induced nausea and emesis over multiple cycles of moderately emetogenic chemotherapy. *Cancer*. 2005;104(7):1548–1555.
17. Koeller JM, Aapro MS, Gralla RJ, et al. Antiemetic guidelines: creating a more practical approach. *Support Care Cancer*. 2002;10(7):519–522.
18. Holdsworth MT, Raisch DW, Winter SS, Chavez CM. Assessment of the emetogenic potential of intrathecal chemotherapy and response to prophylactic treatment with ondansetron. *Support Care Cancer*. 1998;6(2):132–138.
19. Rolski J, Ramlau R, Dediu M, et al. Randomized phase II trial of neurokinin-1 receptor antagonist (NK-1 RA) casopitant mesylate with ondansetron (ond)/dexamethasone (dex) for chemotherapy induced nausea/vomiting (CINV) in patients (pts) receiving highly emetorgenic chemotherapy (HEC). *J Clin Oncology*, 2006 ASCO Annual Meeting Proceedings Part 1; 2006; 24(June 20 Suppl):8513.
20. Kris MG, Hesketh PJ, Herrstedt J, et al. American Society of Clinical Oncology guidelines for antiemetics in oncology: update 2006. *J Clin Oncol*. 2006; 24:18:2932–2947.
21. Schwartzberg LS. Chemotherapy-induced nausea and vomiting: which antiemetic for which therapy. *Oncology*. 2007;21(8):946–953.
22. Koseoglu V, Kurekci, AE, Sarici U, et al. Comparison of the efficacy and side-effects of ondansetron and metoclopramide-diphenhydramine administered to control nausea and vomiting in children treated with antineoplastic chemotherapy: a prospective randomized study. *Eur J Pediatr*. 1998;157:806–810.

23. Sandoval C, Corbi D, Strobino B, et al. Randomized double-blind comparison of single high-dose ondansetron and multiple standard-dose ondansetron in chemotherapy-naïve pediatric oncology patients. *Cancer Invest.* 1999;17: 309–313.

24. White L, Daly SA, McKenna CJ, et al. A comparison of oral ondansetron syrup or intravenous ondansetron loading dose regimens given in combination with dexamethasone for the prevention of nausea and emesis in pediatric and adolescent patients receiving moderately/highly emetogenic chemotherapy. *Pediatr Hematol Oncol.* 2000;17:445–455.

25. Mabro M, Cohn R, Zanesco L, et al. Oral granisetron solution as prophylaxis for chemotherapy-induced emesis in children: double-blind study of two doses. *Bull Cancer.* 2000;87:259–264.

26. Komada Y, Matsuyama T, Takao A, et al. A randomized dose-comparison trial of granisetron in preventing emesis in children with leukaemia receiving emetogenic chemotherapy. *Eur J Cancer.* 1999;35:1095–1101.

27. Hesketh PJ. Comparative review of 5-HT3 receptor antagonists in the treatment of acute chemotherapy-induced nausea and vomiting. *Cancer Investigat.* 2000;18:422–426.

28. Gralla R, Lichinister M, Van Der Begt S, et al. Palonosetron improves prevention of chemotherapy-induced nausea and vomiting following moderately emetogenic chemotherapy: results of a double-blind randomized phase III trial comparing single dose palonosetron with ondansetron. *Ann Oncol.* 2003; 14:1570–1577.

29. Eisenberg P, MacKintosh FR, Ritch P, Cornett PA, Macciocchii A. Efficacy, safety and pharmacokinetics of palonosetron in patients receiving highly emetogenic cisplatic-based chemotherapy: a dose-ranging clinical study. *Ann Oncol.* 2004;2:330–337.

30. Aapro MS, Grunberg SM, Manikhas GM, et al. A phase III, double-blind, randomized trial of palonosetron compared with ondansetron in preventing chemotherapy induced nausea and vomiting following highly emetogenic chemotherapy. *Ann Oncol.* 2006;17:1441–1449.

31. Grote T, Hajdenberg J, Cartmell A, Ferguson S, Ginkel A, Charu V. Combination therapy for chemotherapy-induced nausea and vomiting in patients receiving moderately emetogenic chemotherapy: palonosetron, dexamethasone, and aprepitant. *J Support Oncol.* 2006;4(8):403–409.

32. Grunberg SM. Antiemetic activity of corticosteroids in patients receiving cancer chemotherapy: dosing, efficacy, and tolerability analysis. *Ann Oncol.* 2007;18(2):233–240.33. Mehta P, Gross S, Graham-Pole J, et al. Methylprednisolone for chemotherapy-induced emesis: a double-blind randomized trial in children. *J Pediatr.* 1986;108:774–776.

34. Basade M, Kulkarni SS, Dhor AK, et al. Comparison of dexamethasone and metoclopramide as antiemetics in children receiving cancer chemotherapy. *Indian Pediatr.* 1996;33:321–323.

35. Marshall G, Kerr S, Vowels M, et al. Antiemetic therapy for chemotherapy-induced vomiting: metoclopramide, benztropine, dexamethasone, and lorazepam regimen compared with chlorpromazine alone. *J Pediatr.* 1989; 115:156–160.

36. Ioannidis JA, Hesketh JP, Lau J. Contribution of dexamethasone to control of chemotherapy-Induced nausea and vomiting: a meta-analysis of randomized evidence. *J Clin Oncol.* 2000;18:3409–3422.

37. Alvarez O, Freeman A, Bedros A. (1995). Randomized double-blind crossover ondansetron-dexamethasone versus ondansetron-placebo study for the treatment of chemotherapy-induced nausea and vomiting in pediatric patients with malignancies. *J Pediatr Hematol Oncol.* 1995;17(2):145–150.

38. Italian Group for Antiemetic Research. Dexamethasone alone or in combination with ondansetron for the prevention of delayed nausea and vomiting induced by chemotherapy. *New Eng J Med.* 2000;342:1554–1559.

39. Glaser AW, Buxton N, Walker D. Corticosteroids in the management of central nervous system tumors. *Arch Dis Child.* 1997;76:76–78.

40. Campos D, Pereira JR, Reinhardt RR, et al. Prevention of cisplatin-induced emesis by the oral neurokinin-1 antagonist, MK-869, in combination with granisetron and dexamethasone or with dexamethasone alone. *J Clin Oncol.* 2001;19:1759–1767.

41. Hesketh PJ, Grunberg SM, Gralla RJ, et al. The oral neurokinin-1 antagonist aprepitant for the prevention of chemotherapy-induced nausea and vomiting: a multinational, randomized, double-blind, placebo-controlled trial in patients receiving high-dose cisplatin-the aprepitant protocol 052 study group. *J Clin Oncol.* 2003;21:4112–4119.

42. Massaro AM, Lenz KL. Aprepitant: a novel antiemetic for chemotherapy-induced nausea and vomiting. *Ann Pharmacother.* 2005;39(1):77–85.

43. Chawla SP, Grunberg SM, Gralla RJ, et al. Establishing the dose of the oral NK1 antagonist aprepitant for the prevention of chemotherapy-induced nausea and vomiting. *Cancer.* 2003;97:2290–2300.

44. Allen JC, Gralla R, Reilly L, et al. Metoclopramide: dose-related toxicity and preliminary antiemetic studies in children receiving cancer chemotherapy. *J Clin Oncol.* 1985;3(8):1136–1141.

45. Graham-Pole J, Weare J, Engel S, et al. Antiemetics in children receiving cancer chemotherapy: a double-blind prospective randomized study comparing metoclopramide with chlorpromazine. *J Clin Oncol.* 1986;4:1110–1113.

46. Freedman SB, Fuchs S. Antiemetic therapy in pediatric emergency departments. *Pediatr Emerg Care.* 2004;20(9):625–635.

47. Ekert H, Waters KD, Jurk IH, et al. Amelioration of cancer chemotherapy-induced nausea and vomiting by delta-9-tetrahydrocannabinol. *Med J Aust.* 1979;2:657–659.

48. Chan HS, Correia JA, MacLeod SM. Nabilone versus prochlorperazine for control of cancer chemotherapy-induced emesis in children: a double-blind, crossover trial. *Pediatrics.* 1987;79:946–952.

49. Walsh D, Nelson KA, Mahmoud FA. Established and potential therapeutic applications of cannabinoids in oncology. *Support Care Cancer.* 2003;1(3):137–143.50. Sharma R, Tobin T, Clarke SJ. Management of chemotherapy-induced nausea, vomiting orla mucositis and diarrhoea. *Lancet Oncol.* 2005;6:93–102.

51. Tsukuda M, Furukawa S, Kokatsu S, et al. Comparison of granisetron alone and granisetron plus hydroxyzine hydrochloride for prophylactic treatment of emesis induced by cisplatin chemotherapy. *Eur J Cancer.* 1995;31A(10): 1647–1649.

52. Roila F, Hesketh PJ, Herrstedt J; Antiemetic Subcommittee of the Multinational Association of Supportive Care in Cancer. Prevention of chemotherapy- and radiotherapy-induced emesis: results of the Perugia Consensus Conference. *Ann Oncol.* 1998;9:811–819.

53. Kris MG, Roila F, DeMulder PH, et al. Delayed emesis following anticancer chemotherapy. *Support Care Cancer.* 1998;6:228–232.

54. Smith AR, Repla TL, Weigel BJ. Aprepitant for the control of chemotherapy induced nausea and vomiting in adolescents. *Pediatr Blood Cancer.* 2005;45: 857–860.

55. Passik SD, Kirsh KL, Theobald DE, et al. A retrospective chart review of the use of olanzapine for prevention of delayed emesis in cancer patients. *J Pain Symptom Manage.* 2003;25(5):485–488.

56. Navari RM, Einhorn LH, Lochrer PJ, Passik SD, Vinson J, McLean J, Chowhan N, Hanna NH, & Johnson CS, (2007). A phase II trialofolanzapine, dexamethasone, and palonosetron for the prevention of chemotherapy-induced nausea and vomiting: a Hoosier oncology group study. *Supportive Care Cancer* 15:1285–1291.

57. Morrow GR, Roscoe JA, Hickok JT, Andrews PR, Matteson S. Nausea and emesis: evidence for a biobehavioral perspective. *Support Care Cancer.* 2002; 10(2):96–105.

58. Ezzo J, Vickers A, Richardson MA, et al. Acupuncture-point stimulation for chemotherapy-induced nausea and vomiting. *J Clin Oncol.* 2005;23(28): 7188–7198.

59. Reindl TK, Geilen W, Hartmann R, et al. Acupuncture against chemotherapy-induced nausea and vomiting in pediatric oncology: interim results of a multicenter crossover study. *Support Care Cancer.* 2006;14:172–176.

60. National Institutes of Health Consensus Development Statement. *Acupuncture.* 1997.

61. Treish I, Shord S, Valgus J, et al. Randomized double-blind study of Reliefband as an adjunct to standard antiemetics in patients receiving moderately-high to highly emetic chemotherapy. *Support Care Cancer.* 2003;11(8):516–521.

62. Collins KB, Thomas DJ. Acupuncture and acupressure for the management of chemotherapy-induced nausea and vomiting. *J Am Acad Nurse Pract.* 2004; 16(2):76–80.

63. Cooke B, Ernst E. Aromatherapy: a systematic review. *Brit J Gen Pract.* 2000; 50(455):493–496.

64. Sencer SF, Kelly KM, (2007). Complementary and alternative therapies in pediatric oncology. *Pediatric Clinics of North America* 12 54(6):xiii.

65. Quimby EL. The use of herbal therapies in pediatric oncology patients: treating symptoms of cancer and side effects of standard therapies. *J Pediatr Oncol Nurs.* 2007;24(1):35–40.

66. Betz O, Kranke P, Geldner G, Wulf H, Eberhart LH. [Is ginger a clinically relevant antiemetic? A systematic review of randomized controlled trials.] *Forsch Komplementarmed Klass Naturheilkd.* 2005;12(1):14–23.

Management of Symptoms Associated with Cancer: Pain Management

John J. Collins

Introduction

Pain is one of the most common and one of the most feared symptoms of children and their families in their experience of illness related to cancer or its treatment. Despite data suggesting there is much room for improvement in pain management for children with cancer,[1] the majority of children can achieve adequate analgesia if contemporary pain management techniques are utilized. Intractable pain in children with cancer is relatively rare.[2] The World Health Organization (WHO) has established guidelines for pain management and palliative care as a universal standard of care for all children with cancer.[3]

The Epidemiology of Cancer Pain in Children

Pain is a common symptom experienced by children with cancer. It potentially occurs commonly at diagnosis,[4] as a result of treatment (eg, postoperative pain, mucositis, phantom limb pain, infection, antineoplastic therapy-related pain, and procedure-related pain),[5] at the time of tumor recurrence, and during the terminal phase of the illness.[1,6] Severe pain in terminal pediatric malignancy occurs more commonly in patients with solid tumors metastatic to the central nervous system (CNS) or peripheral nervous system.[6] It is uncommon for children who are cured of their cancer to have chronic nonmalignant pain as a consequence of their cancer.

An Approach to Pain Management in the Child with Cancer

Assessment

A complaint of pain in child with cancer warrants a thorough history, physical examination, and investigations, if appropriate, to make a diagnosis, because children rarely fabricate a complaint of pain. Treatments directed at the primary causes will often be more effective in providing longer-term analgesia. Assessment of pain includes some form of pain severity measurement. A cognitively normal child above the age of 4 can usually self-report pain severity

experience, and numerous tools have been created to determine such.[7] Behavioral scales and physiologic measures are usually reserved for the preverbal child. New scales have recently been formulated for the cognitively impaired.[8]

Integrating Nonpharmacologic Methods of Pain Control in Children with Cancer

The decision to use a psychological or pharmacologic approach or both as methods of pain control depends on the knowledge of the procedure, the skill of the practitioner, the understanding of the child, and the expectations of pain and anxiety for the particular child.[9] The choice of which nonpharmacologic method to use is based on the child's age, behavioral factors, coping ability, fear and anxiety, and the type of pain experienced.[10]

Nonpharmacologic methods of pain control include techniques categorized as physical (eg, heat, cold stimulation, electrical nerve stimulation, acupuncture, massage), behavioral (eg, relaxation, biofeedback, modeling, desensitization, art and play therapy), or cognitive (eg, distraction, imagery, thought stopping, hypnosis, music therapy), according to whether the intervention is focused on modifying an individual's sensory perception, behaviors, or thoughts and coping abilities.[10]

Performing a painful procedure in a quiet, calm environment conducive to reducing stress and anxiety, in a location separate from the child's room, is recommended. Providing a description of the steps of a given procedure and of the sensations that may be experienced are common interventions for the preparation of a child about to undergo a painful procedure. Unexpected stress is more anxiety provoking to children than anticipated or predictable stress.[9,11]

Analgesic Prescription for Cancer-Related Pain

The prescription of analgesics for children with cancer pain is based on the WHO analgesic ladder.[3] This tool emphasizes pain intensity as the guide to the choice of analgesic. In other words, the prescription of analgesics should be according to pain severity, ranging from acetaminophen and nonsteroidal anti-inflammatory drugs (NSAIDs) for mild pain to opioids for moderate to severe pain. The choice of analgesic is individualized to achieve an optimum balance between analgesia and side effects.[3]

Although the pharmacokinetic and the major pharmacodynamic properties (analgesia and sedation) of most opioids have been studied in pediatric populations and previously documented, little information is available about oral bioavailability, potency ratios, and other pharmacodynamic properties in children. In addition, there have been no controlled clinical trials of adjuvant analgesic agents in pediatrics.

Non-opioid Analgesics

Acetaminophen inhibits prostaglandin synthesis primarily in the CNS. It is one of the most commonly used non-opioid analgesics in children and does not have the side effects of gastritis and inhibition of platelet function found with aspirin and NSAIDs. Although acetaminophen has a potential for hepatic and renal injury,[12] this is uncommon in therapeutic doses. Acetaminophen does not have an association with Reye syndrome.

The antipyretic action of acetaminophen may be contraindicated in neutropenic patients in whom it is important to monitor fever. Pediatric dosing of acetaminophen is based on the dose response for fever control. Oral dosing of 15 mg/kg every 4 hours is recommended, with a maximum daily dose of 90 mg/kg/day in children and 60 mg/kg/day in younger children. There are no data on the safety of chronic administration of acetaminophen in children.

In selected children with adequate platelet number and function, NSAIDs may be helpful analgesics, both alone and in combination with opioids. However, aspirin and NSAIDs are often contraindicated in pediatric oncology patients who are at risk of bleeding if thrombocytopenic. There are no data on the safety, efficacy, and tolerability of Cox-2 inhibitors in children with cancer.

Opioid Analgesics

The starting doses of commonly used opioids are outlined in Table 39-1.[13]

Codeine

Codeine is a phenanthrene alkaloid derived from morphine. It is usually prescribed for moderate pain. Codeine is commonly administered orally in children and is often administered in combination with acetaminophen. In equipotent doses, codeine has a similar analgesic and side effect profile to that of morphine. Pharmacogenetic studies have demonstrated that 4% to 14% of the population lack the hepatic enzyme responsible for the conversion of codeine to morphine. A pediatric study has shown that 35% of children showed inadequate conversion of codeine to morphine.[14] For this reason the prescription of codeine as an analgesic in pediatrics is declining.

Oxycodone

Oxycodone is a semi-synthetic opioid and is used for moderate to severe pain in children with cancer. Oxycodone is available as a long-acting preparation and as an oral preparation in combination with acetaminophen in some countries. Oxycodone has a higher clearance value and a shorter elimination half-life ($t_{1/2}$) in children aged 2 to 20 years than in adults.[15,16]

Morphine

Morphine is perhaps the most widely used opioid for moderate to severe cancer pain in children. The major hepatic metabolite of morphine, morphine-6-glucuronide, produces analgesia and side effects comparable to those of morphine with chronic dosing. Morphine-6-glucuronide may accumulate and result in opioid side effects in patients with renal insufficiency.

Morphine clearance is delayed in the first 1 to 3 months of life. The half-life of morphine ($t_{1/2}$) changes from 10 to

Table 39-1

Starting drug doses of commonly used opioids in pediatrics.[13]

Drug	Usual IV Starting Dose (< 50 kg)	Usual IV Starting Dose (> 50 kg)	Usual Oral Starting Dose (< 50 kg)	Usual Oral Starting Dose (> 50 kg)
Morphine	0.1 mg/kg every 3-4 h	5-10 mg every 3-4 h	0.3 mg/kg every 3-4 h	30 mg every 3-4 h
Hydromorphone	0.015 mg/kg every 3-4 h	1-1.5 mg every 3-4 h	0.06 mg/kg every 3-4 h	6 mg every 3-4 h
Oxycodone	N/A	N/A	0.3 mg/kg every 3-4 h[b]	10 mg every 3-4 h
Meperidine[a]	0.75mg/kg every 2-3 h	75-100 mg every 3 h	N/R	N/R
Fentanyl	0.5-1.5 μ/kg every 1-2 h	25-75 μ/kg every 1-2 h	N/A	N/A

Abbreviations: IV, intravenous; h, hours; N/A, not available; N/R, not recommended.
[a]Meperidine is not recommended for chronic use because of the accumulation of the toxic metabolite normeperidine.
[b]Smallest tablet size is 5 mg.

20 hours in preterm infants to 1 to 2 hours in young children.[17,18] Starting doses in very young infants should be reduced by approximately 25% to 30% on a per kg basis relative to the dosing recommended for older children. During the neonatal period for term infants, the volume of distribution is linearly related to age and body surface area.[19–21] One study[22] suggests that when given an equivalent dose for weight, younger children are likely to have significantly lower plasma morphine and metabolite concentrations. A starting dose for oral morphine of 1.5 to 2 mg/kg/day is recommended for children with pain unrelieved by mild or moderate-strength analgesics.[23]

Oral morphine has a significant first-pass metabolism in the liver. An oral to parenteral potency ratio of approximately 3 to 1 is commonly employed during chronic administration. Typical starting intravenous morphine infusion rates are 0.02 to 0.03 mg/kg per hour beyond the first 3 months of life, and 0.015 mg/kg per hour in younger infants. Sustained release oral preparations of morphine are available for children and are usually administered at twice daily intervals. Dosing at 8-hour intervals may be appropriate in children.[22] Crushing sustained released tablets produces immediate release of morphine. Thus, their use is limited in children who must chew tablets.

Hydromorphone

Hydromorphone is an alternative opioid used when the dose escalation of morphine is limited by side effects. Hydromorphone is available for oral, intravenous (IV), subcutaneous, epidural, and intrathecal administration. A double-blinded randomized crossover comparison of morphine and hydromorphone using patient-controlled analgesia (PCA) in children and adolescents with mucositis following bone marrow transplantation showed that hydromorphone was well tolerated and had a potency ratio of approximately 6 to 1 relative to morphine in this setting.[24] Adult studies indicate that IV hydromorphone is 5 to 8 times as potent as morphine. Hydromorphone is convenient for subcutaneous infusion because of its high potency and aqueous solubility. Little is known about the pharmacokinetics of hydromorphone in infants.

Fentanyl

Fentanyl is a synthetic opioid approximately 50 to 100 times more potent than morphine during acute IV administration. Fentanyl has a very rapid onset following IV administration, due to its high lipid solubility. Fentanyl is eliminated almost entirely by hepatic metabolism. The half-life of fentanyl is prolonged in preterm infants undergoing cardiac surgery,[25] but values comparable to those of adults are reached within the first months of life.[25–28] The clearance of fentanyl is higher in infants and young children than in adults.[27,28]

The duration of action of fentanyl following single IV bolus administration is much shorter than that for morphine. These features make fentanyl useful for procedures in which rapid onset and short duration are important. Fentanyl may also be used for continuous infusion for selected patients with dose-limiting side effects from morphine. Rapid administration of high doses of IV fentanyl may result in chest wall rigidity and severe ventilatory difficulty.

Schechter[29] described the use of oral transmucosal fentanyl for sedation/analgesia during bone marrow biopsy/aspiration and lumbar puncture in children with cancer. This formulation was safe and effective, although the frequency of vomiting may be a limiting factor in its tolerability. In a small study utilizing a clinical protocol, the utility, feasibility, and tolerability of transdermal fentanyl were demonstrated in children with cancer pain.[30] The mean clearance and volume of distribution of transdermal fentanyl were the same for both adults and children, but the variability was higher for adults.[30] A larger study is required to confirm these findings.

Meperidine

Meperidine is a short-half-life synthetic opioid and has been used for procedural and postoperative pain in children. Neonates have a slower elimination of meperidine than children and young infants.[14,31–34] Normeperidine, a major metabolite of meperidine, can cause CNS excitatory effects, including tremors and convulsions.[35] These effects occur particularly in patients with renal impairment. Meperidine is not generally recommended for children with chronic pain but may be an acceptable alternative opioid for short, painful procedures. Meperidine in low doses (0.25-0.5 mg/kg IV) may be used for the prophylaxis and treatment of rigors following the infusion of amphotericin.

Methadone

Methadone is a synthetic opioid that has a long and variable half-life. The oral to parenteral potency ratio is approximately 2 to 1. In children receiving postoperative analgesia, methadone produced equivalent but more prolonged analgesia than morphine.[36,37] Due to its prolonged half-life, methadone has a risk of delayed sedation and overdosage occurring several days after the initiation of treatment.

Frequent patient assessment is the key to safe and effective use of methadone. If a patient becomes oversedated, it is recommended to stop dosing, not just reduce the dose, and to observe the patient until alertness is improved. Although "as needed" dosing is discouraged for most patients with cancer pain, some clinicians find this approach a useful way to establish a dosing schedule for methadone.[36,37] Methadone remains a long-acting agent when administered either as an elixir or as crushed tablets.

Routes and Methods of Analgesic Administration

Analgesics should be administered to children by the simplest, safest, most effective, and least painful route. The oral route of administration of analgesics is therefore the first choice for the majority of patients. The intramuscular administration of an opioid is painful and may lead to the underreporting of pain. This route of administration does not permit easy dose titration or infusion and should be avoided. Rectal administration is also discouraged in children with cancer because of concern regarding infection and the great variability of rectal absorption of drugs.[38]

The eutectic mixture of local anesthetics (EMLA) is a topical preparation that provides local anesthesia to the skin, dermis, and subcutaneous tissues. It must be applied under an occlusive dressing for at least 1 hour, but depth of penetration is greater with a longer application time (90–120 minutes). EMLA has been shown to be useful for providing topical local anesthesia for procedural pain, including lumbar puncture[38] and central venous port access,[39] in children with cancer. Preliminary studies of topical amethocaine for percutaneous analgesia prior to venous cannulation in children have demonstrated promising safety and efficacy data.[40]

Intravenous administration of opioids has the advantage of rapid onset of analgesia, easier opioid dose titration, bioavailability, and continuous effect when infusions are used. The subcutaneous route is an alternative route of administration for children with no IV access.[41] Subcutaneous infusion rates generally do not exceed 1 to 3 ml per hour.[42] A small catheter or butterfly needle (27 gauge) may be placed under the skin of the thorax, abdomen, or thigh. Subcutaneous infusion sites are changed approximately every 3 days.

Patient-controlled analgesia has been used successfully for the management of prolonged oropharyngeal mucositis pain following bone marrow transplantation in children and adolescents.[24,43,44] Patient-controlled analgesia is a method of opioid administration that permits the patient to self-administer a small bolus dose of opioid within set time limits. In postoperative use, PCA is widely used successfully by children aged 6 and above. Patient-controlled analgesia caters to an individual's variation in pharmacokinetics, pharmacodynamics, and pain intensity. Patient-controlled analgesia allows children to have control over their analgesia when appropriate and to choose a balance between the benefits of analgesia and the side effects of opioids.

Breakthrough Pain in Children

A prospective study to determine the prevalence, characteristics, and impact of breakthrough pain in children with cancer was conducted in a major children's hospital. Twenty-seven pediatric in- and outpatients with cancer (aged 7–18 years) who had severe pain requiring treatment with opioids participated in this study. The children responded to a structured interview (Breakthrough Pain Questionnaire for Children) designed to characterize breakthrough pain in children. Measures of pain, anxiety, and depressed mood were completed.

Fifty-seven percent of the children had experienced one or more episodes of breakthrough pain during the preceding 24 hours, each episode lasting seconds to minutes, occurring 3 to 4 times daily, most commonly characterized as "sharp" and "shooting" by the children. Younger children (7–12 years) had a significantly higher risk of experiencing breakthrough pain compared with teenagers. Although no statistical difference could be shown between children with and without breakthrough pain in regard to anxiety and depression, children with breakthrough pain reported significantly more interpersonal problems on a Child Depression Inventory subtest. The most effective treatment of an episode of breakthrough pain was a PCA opioid bolus dose.[45]

Opioid Dose Schedules

Unless painful episodes are truly incidental and unpredictable, analgesics should generally be administered at regular times to provide continuous pain relief. Should breakthrough pain occur, "rescues" are supplemental "as-needed" doses of opioid incorporated into the analgesic regimen to allow a patient to have additional analgesia should breakthrough pain occur. Rescue doses of opioid may be calculated as approximately 5% to 10% of the total daily opioid requirement and may be administered every hour.[46]

Opioid dose escalation may be required after opioid administration begins and periodically thereafter. The size of an opioid dose increment may be calculated as follows:

1. If greater than approximately 6 rescue doses of opioid are given in a 24-hour period, then the total daily opioid dose should be increased by the total of opioid given as "rescue" medication. For example, the hourly average of the total daily rescue opioid should be added to the baseline opioid infusion. An alternative to this method would be to increase the baseline infusion by 50%.[46]
2. Rescue doses are kept as a proportion of the baseline opioid dose. A rescue dose can be 5% to 10% of the total daily dose.[46] An alternative guideline for opioid infusions is between 50% to 200% of the hourly basal infusion rate.[46]

Opioid Switching

The usual indication for an opioid switch to an alternative opioid is dose-limiting toxicity. In other words, the dose of opioid required to achieve adequate analgesia is limited by opioid side effects. A favorable change in opioid analgesia to side effect profile will be experienced if there is less cross-tolerance at the opioid receptors mediating analgesia than at those mediating adverse effects.[47]

Following long-term opioid dosing, equivalent analgesia may be attained with a dose of a second opioid that is smaller than that calculated from an equianalgesic table,[47] approximately 50% for short-half-life opioids. In contrast to short-half-life opioids, the doses of methadone required for equivalent analgesia after switching may be on the order of 10% to 20% of the equianalgesic dose of the previously used short-half-life opioid. A protocol for methadone dose conversion and titration has been reported.[48]

A retrospective study was conducted to determine the therapeutic value of opioid rotation in a large pediatric oncology center. The study looked at the details of opioid prescriptions over the course of a year, obtained from the medical records of children with cancer who had a rotation of opioid therapy during their admission. Twenty-two children, or 14% of children, on opioid therapy underwent 30 opioid rotations. Mucositis was the cause of pain in 19 (70%) children, bone pain in 3 (11%) children, and postoperative, visceral, or neuropathic pain in the remainder.

The opioid was rotated either for excessive side effects with adequate analgesia (70%), excessive side effects with inadequate analgesia (16.7%), or tolerance (6.7%). Five (23%) children required 2 rotations, 3 during the same admission. The favored rotations were morphine to fentanyl in 20 (67%) children and fentanyl to hydromorphone in 6 (20%). Adverse opioid effects were resolved in 90% of cases; all failures occurred when morphine was rotated to fentanyl. There was no significant loss of pain control or increase in mean morphine equivalent dose requirements. Opioid rotation had a positive impact on managing dose-limiting side effects of, or tolerance to, opioid therapy during cancer pain treatment in children. This rotation was accomplished without loss of pain control or having to significantly increase the dose of opioid therapy.[49]

Opioid Side Effects

Children do not necessarily report opioid side effects voluntarily (eg, constipation, pruritus, dreams) and should be asked specifically about these problems. An assessment of opioid side effects is included in an assessment of analgesic effectiveness. All opioids can potentially cause the same constellation of side effects. If opioid side effects limit opioid dose escalation, then consideration should be given to an opioid switch. Tolerance to some opioid side effects (eg, sedation, nausea and vomiting, pruritus) often develops within the first week of starting opioids. Children do not develop tolerance to constipation, and concurrent treatment with laxatives should be considered.

Adjuvant Analgesics in Children with Cancer

Adjuvant analgesics are a heterogeneous group of medications that are analgesic in some painful conditions but have a primary indication other than pain.[50] These drugs are commonly prescribed with primary analgesics. Common classes of these adjuvant agents include antidepressants, anticonvulsants, neuroleptics, psychostimulants, antihistamines, corticosteroids, and centrally acting skeletal muscle relaxants.

References

1. Wolfe J, Grier HE, Klar N, et al. Symptoms and suffering at the end of life in children with cancer. *N Engl J Med.* 2000;342(5):326–333.
2. Collins JJ, Grier HE, Kinney HC, Berde CB. Control of severe pain in terminal pediatric malignancy. *J Pediatr.* 1995;126(4):653–657.
3. *Cancer Pain Relief and Palliative Care in Children.* Geneva: World Health Organization; 1998.
4. Miser AW, McCalla J, Dothage P, Wesley M, Miser JS. Pain as a presenting symptom in children and young adults with newly diagnosed malignancy. *Pain.* 1987;29:363–377.
5. Miser AW, Dothage P, Wesley RA, et al. The prevalence of pain in a pediatric and young adult population. *Pain.* 1987;29:265–266.
6. Collins JJ, Grier HE, Kinney HC, Berde CB. Control of severe pain in terminal pediatric malignancy. *J Pediatr.* 1995;126(4):653–657.
7. Champion GD, Goodenough B, von Baeyer CL, Thomas W. Measurement of pain by self-report. In: Finlay GA, McGrath PJ, eds. *Measurement of Pain in Infants and Children.* Seattle: IASP Press, 1998:123–160.
8. Breau LM, Finley GA, McGrath PJ, Camfield CS. Validation of the Non-communicating Children's Pain Checklist-Postoperative Version. *Anesthesiology.* 2002;96(3):523–526.
9. Zeltzer L, Jay S, Fisher D. The management of pain associated with pediatric procedures. *Pediatr Clin North Am.* 1989;36(4):914–964.
10. McGrath PA. Intervention and management. In: Bush JP, Harkins SW, eds. *Children in Pain.* New York: Springer-Verlag; 1991:83–115.
11. Siegal LJ. Preparation of children for hospitalization: a selected review of the research literature. *J Pediatr Psychol.* 1976;1(26):36.
12. Sandler DP, Smit JC, Weinberg CR, et al. Analgesic use and chronic renal disease. *N Engl J Med.* 1989;320:1238–1243.
13. Berde CB, Billett AL, Collins JJ. Symptom management in supportive care. In: Pizzo PA, Poplack DG, eds. *Principles and Practice of Pediatric Oncology.* Baltimore: Lippincott Williams & Wilkins; 2006:1358.
14. Mather LE, Tucker GT, Pflug AE, et al. Meperidine kinetics in man: intravenous injection in surgical patients and volunteers. *Clin Pharmacol Ther.* 1975;17:21–30.
15. Poyhia R, Seppala T. Lipid solubility and protein binding of oxycodone in vitro. *Pharmacol Toxicol.* 1994;74:23–27.
16. Pelkonen O, Kaltiala EH, Larmi TKL. Comparison of activities of drug metabolizing enzymes in human fetal and adult liver. *Clin Pharmacol Ther.* 1973;14:840–846.
17. Stanski DR, Greenblatt DJ, Lowenstein E. Kinetics of intravenous and intramuscular morphine. *Clin Pharmacol Ther.* 1978;24:52–59.
18. Olkkola KT, Maunuksela EL, Korpela R, Rosenberg PH. Kinetics and dynamics of postoperative intravenous morphine in children. *Clin Pharmacol Ther.* 1988;44(2):128–136.
19. McRorie TI, Lynn A, Nespeca MK. The maturation of morphine clearance and metabolism. *Amer J Dis Child.* 1992;146:972–976.
20. Bhat R, Chari G, Gulati A, et al. Pharmacokinetics of a single dose of morphine in pre-term infants during the first week of life. *J Pediatr.* 1990;117:477–481.
21. Pokela ML, Olkkala KT, Seppala T. Age-related morphine kinetics in infants. *Dev Pharm Ther.* 1993;20:26–34.
22. Hunt AM, Joel S, Dick G, Goldman A. Population pharmacokinetics of oral morphine and its glucuronides in children receiving morphine as immediate-release liquid or sustained-release tablets. *J Pediatr.* 1999;135(1):47–55.
23. Hunt AM. A survey of signs, symptoms and symptom control in 30 terminally ill children. *Dev Med Child Neurol.* 1990;32:347–355.
24. Collins JJ, Geake J, Grier HE, et al. Patient-controlled analgesia for mucositis pain in children: a three-period crossover study comparing morphine and hydromorphone. *J Pediatr.* 1996;129(5):722–728.
25. Collins C, Koren G, Crean P, et al. Fentanyl pharmacokinetics and hemodynamic effects in preterm infants during ligation of patent ductus arteriosus. *Anesth Analg.* 1985;64:1078–1080.
26. Koren G, Goresky G, Crean P, et al. Unexpected alterations in fentanyl pharmacokinetics in children undergoing cardiac surgery: age related or disease related? *Dev Pharm Ther.* 1986;9:183–191.
27. Johnson K, Erickson J, Holley F, Scott J. Fentanyl pharmacokinetics in the pediatric population. *Anesthesiology.* 1984;61(3A):A441.
28. Gauntlett IS, Fisher DM, Hertzka RE, et al. Pharmacokinetics of fentanyl in neonatal humans and lambs: effects of age. *Anesthesiology.* 1988;69:683–687.
29. Schechter NL, Weisman SJ, Rosenblum M, et al. The use of oral transmucosal fentanyl citrate for painful procedures in children. *Pediatrics.* 1995;95:335–339.
30. Collins JJ, Dunkel I, Gupta SK, et al. Transdermal fentanyl in children with cancer: feasibility, tolerability, and pharmacokinetic correlates. *J Pediatr.* 1999;134:319–323.
31. Tamsen A, Hartvig P, Fagerlund C, et al. Patient-controlled analgesic therapy, part 1: pharmacokinetics of pethidine in the pre- and postoperative periods. *Clin Pharmacokinetics.* 1982;7:149–163.
32. Hamunen K, Maunuksela EL, Seppala T, et al. Pharmacokinetics of iv and rectal pethidine in children undergoing ophthalmic surgery. *Br J Anaesth.* 1993;71:823–826.
33. Koska AJ, Kramer WG, Romagnoli A, et al. Pharmacokinetics of high dose meperidine in surgical patients. *Anesth Analg.* 1981;60:8–11.
34. Pokela ML, Olkkala KT, Kovisto M, et al. Pharmacokinetics and pharmacodynamics of intravenous meperidine in neonates and infants. *Clin Pharmacol Ther.* 1992;52:342–349.
35. Kaiko RF, Foley KM, Grabinsky PY, et al. Central nervous system excitatory effects of meperidine in cancer patients. *Ann Neurol.* 1983;13:180–185.
36. Berde CB, Beyer JE, Bournaki MC, Levin CR, Sethna NF. Comparison of morphine and methadone for prevention of postoperative pain in 3- to 7-year-old children. *J Pediatr.* 1991;136:141.

37. Berde CB, Sethna NF, Holzman RS, Reidy P, Gondek EJ. Pharmacokinetics of methadone in children and adolescents in the perioperative period. *Anesthesiology.* 1987;67:A519.

38. Kapelushnik J, Koren G, Solh H, et al. Evaluating the efficacy of EMLA in alleviating pain associated with lumbar puncture: comparison of open and double-blinded protocols in children. *Pain.* 1990;42:31–34.

39. Miser AW, Goh TS, Dose AM, et al. Trial of a topically administered local anesthetic (EMLA cream) for pain relief during central venous port accesses in children with cancer. *J Pain Symptom Manage.* 1994;9(4):259–264.

40. Van Kan HJM, Egberts ACG, Rijnvos WPM, Ter Pelkwijk NJ, Lenderink AW. Tetracaine versus lidocaine-prilocaine for preventing venipuncture-induced pain in children. *Am J Obstet Gynecol.* 1997;54:388–392.

41. Miser AW, Davis DM, Hughes CS, Mulne AF, Miser JS. Continuous subcutaneous infusion of morphine in children with cancer. *Am J Dis Child.* 1983; 137(4):383–385.

42. Bruera E, Brenneis C, Michaud M, et al. Use of the subcutaneous route for the administration of narcotics in patients with cancer pain. *Cancer.* 1988;62: 407–411.

43. Mackie AM, Coda BC, Hill HF. Adolescents use patient controlled analgesia effectively for relief for relief from prolonged oropharyngeal mucositis pain. *Pain.* 1991;46:265–269.

44. Dunbar PJ, Buckley P, Gavrin JR, Sanders JE, Chapman CR. Use of patient-controlled analgesia for pain control for children receiving bone marrow transplants. *J Pain Symptom Manage.* 1995;10:604–611.

45. Friedrichsdorf SJ, Finney D, Bergin M, Stevens M, Collins JJ. Breakthrough pain in children with cancer. *J Pain Symptom Manage.* 2007;34(2):209:216.

46. Cherny NI, Foley KM. Nonopioid and opioid analgesic pharmacotherapy of cancer pain. *Hematol Oncol Clin North Am.* 1996:79–102.

47. Portenoy RK. Opioid tolerance and responsiveness: research findings and clinical observations. In: Gebhart GF, Hammond DI, Jensen TS, eds. *Progress in Pain Research and Management.* Seattle: IASP Press; 1994:615–619.

48. Inturrisi CE, Portenoy RK, Max M, Colburn WA, Foley KM. Pharmacokinetic-pharmacodynamic relationships of methadone infusions in patients with cancer pain. *Clin Pharmacol Ther.* 1990;47:565–577.

49. Drake R, Longworth J, Collins JJ. Opioid rotation in children with cancer. *J Palliat Med.* 2004;7(3):419–422.

50. Portenoy RK. Adjuvant analgesics in pain management. In: Doyle D, Hanks GWC, MacDonald N, eds. *Oxford Textbook of Palliative Medicine.* Oxford: Oxford University Press; 1993:187–203.

CHAPTER 40

Psychological Support of the Child with Cancer and the Family: Neurobehavioral Outcomes

Thomas A. Kaleita

Introduction

Psychological support of the child with cancer and the family begins at the time of diagnosis and includes a broad range of health care providers. Pediatric oncologists and nurses are the first caregivers to encounter the child and his or her family. Some time later, psychologists, social workers, and other pediatric specialists, most often radiotherapists and surgeons, will join the health care team. The pattern of psychological support varies according to the staffing at an individual treatment center as well as to the natural course of developing interpersonal relationships. However, psychological support, in various forms, is an essential part of an effective treatment plan for the child diagnosed with cancer. At some centers, the psychology staff becomes active early in treatment and continues to provide a broad range of services even after completion of cancer therapy in long-term follow-up. At many other institutions, psychologists serve in a more limited role, acting as consultants who address specific, predetermined issues, such as school-related problems. Psychological support may focus primarily on family functioning, simultaneously with the psychological well-being and the neurobehavioral functioning of the pediatric patient in the context of treatment. The focus of this chapter is on the neurobehavioral outcome of the pediatric cancer patient and the support provided to the child and the family.

Neurobehavioral Sequelae of Childhood Cancer and Treatment

Improvements in the treatments for childhood cancer have been achieved in large part by increased aggressiveness of therapy. This approach presents a biological challenge to normal tissue and organs at risk of injury. The developing central nervous system (CNS) is particularly vulnerable to various types of treatment, especially when treatments are used in combination. Among long-term survivors of childhood cancer, neurobehavioral examinations have been used increasingly in clinical service and in research to characterize patterns and severity of disease- and therapy-associated sequelae as measurable treatment endpoints (ie, outcomes). Most research efforts have concerned children diagnosed with acute lymphoblastic leukemia (ALL) or brain tumor,[1,2] the most frequently occurring neoplasms in childhood. Both conditions can involve irradiation treatment to the entire brain (and sometimes to the complete neuraxis) and multiagent systemic chemotherapy. Some types of lymphoma are also treated with schedules of chemotherapeutic agents and with intrathecal therapy very similar to those used for ALL. There have not been systematic neurobehavioral outcome studies of patients with other forms of cancer, however. Neurobehavioral outcomes of pediatric cancer patients treated for lymphoma or rarer forms of cancer have been reported in the context of large studies containing subjects with heterogeneous diagnoses, most of which are ALL.[3] Thus, existing research on ALL and brain tumor patients serves as a basis for understanding neurobehavioral outcomes of children and adolescents treated for all types of cancer.

Much has been learned in the past 20 years about the long-term effects of CNS-directed irradiation and chemotherapy on the developing brain, but new questions are emerging due to the increasing systemic chemotherapeutic intensity in modern therapeutic trials. Treatment regimens with specified CNS-directed therapy components may lead to permanent neurocognitive sequelae, primarily involving deficits in attention/concentration, memory, visual-motor skills, and psychomotor processing speed.[4,5] These sequelae compose a foundation for poor academic achievement, and often, poor social and behavioral adaptation. Clinically relevant neurocognitive impairments are estimated in approximately 32% of all childhood cancer survivors, most frequently in survivors diagnosed with CNS tumors (47%), acute leukemia (34%), retinoblastoma (31%), and bone tumors (29%).[6] Younger age at diagnosis of ALL and lower socioeconomic status of the family are also well-known risk factors for neurocognitive disabilities.[1] A recently completed Children's Cancer Group study of neurocognitive, motor, and academic outcomes in children treated for ALL concluded that age younger than 6 years was a particular risk factor for neurobehavioral abnormalities and was independent of CNS treatment with or without whole-brain radiotherapy and intensified chemotherapy.[7] This finding has potential implications for children with other types of cancer; psychological support and family interventions should be particularly focused on very young cancer patients, regardless of cancer diagnosis and treatment strategy.

The long-term neurobehavioral effects and the risk factors for these sequelae from regional brain irradiation used to treat many pediatric brain tumor patients are far less well established.[2] Risk of late neurobehavioral sequelae in these patients depends on age at diagnosis and tumor location, especially when the affected brain region involves language or motor skills. Younger children treated with craniospinal irradiation for brain tumors (>75%) are at highest risk for disabilities in addition to a number of other medical complications.[6] In recent times, conformal radiotherapy has been used increasingly at pediatric cancer treatment centers, with the justification that it produces less injury and allows for better repair of normal tissues. Some initial reports of comparatively less severe impairments after regional brain treatments with the modern conformal approaches have recently been published.[8,9] Systematic comparisons of outcomes with children treated with conventional regional radiotherapy have not yet been performed. Because optimal treatment for brain tumors often includes regional brain irradiation, more outcomes research is greatly needed to determine the comparative impact of conventional versus conformal treatment approaches on long-term neurocognitive and social/behavioral functioning. Irradiation dose distribution to specific brain regions can now be calculated with great precision using modern radiotherapy planning technology.[10] Thus, very refined studies of the relationships between conformal radiotherapy and neurobehavioral outcomes are now feasible.

Neurobehavioral Assessment and Clinical Psychological Management

Neurobehavioral examination of a pediatric cancer patient can range from a brief screening during a medical clinic appointment to a comprehensive evaluation involving multiple appointments and several hours of time. In the clinic setting, in which health care providers usually spend only one hour or less with the family, basic screening of neurocognitive functions and emotional/behavioral status can be efficiently accomplished. Based on the information obtained from a screening exam, the child or adolescent may return for a more comprehensive assessment or perhaps for serial brief assessments. An initial screening examination combined with brief follow-up assessments can document trends in neurocognitive functioning in the context of the overall multidisciplinary management of the pediatric cancer patient and generate longitudinal data in a repeated measures design for clinical research. All children and adolescents whose treatment requires either regional or whole-brain irradiation, and infants and preschool-age patients diagnosed with malignant disease, should have neurobehavioral screening as part of the initial workup at presentation.

The screening examination should include brief assessment of neurocognitive status and behavioral adaptation

in children of all ages. This assessment can most efficiently be accomplished by administration of selected standardized tests with the patient and/or completion of structured interview/questionnaires administered to parents or caretakers. Many of these instruments are now published in Spanish and in an increasing number of other languages. For infant patients, a standardized screening test of development requiring less than 30 minutes of observation and parent query may be administered depending on a number of practical factors in the clinic. Neurocognitive tests administered to preschool- and school-age children should emphasize measures of attention, visual motor skills, psychomotor speed and, if requested, selected academic skills (see Tables 40-1 and 40-2 for suggested screening exam tests and measures). Results obtained from the individual measures indicate the status of specific neurocognitive functions. These data can then be combined to form an aggregate outcome measure, reflecting the dynamic balance among the neurocognitive functions tested. This aggregate measure can be used efficiently to provide a statistically powerful marker of the global neurocognitive status of the patient in clinical research paradigms.[11]

The purposes of the neurobehavioral examination are:

- *Determination of neurocognitive, motor, and social/behavioral functioning in children at an initial point in time after diagnosis of disease*, with estimations of developmental levels that existed prior to disease/treatment.
- *Determination of strengths and areas of deficit at the time of the neurobehavioral examination*, with consideration of the impact of disease and treatment factors on the various neurocognitive and motor abilities and the behaviors that are being measured.
- *Documentation of the improvement, stability, or decline in various neurocognitive, motor, and social/behavioral functions measured.* Serial examinations are needed to determine whether or not abilities that normally develop over time are affected by disease or treatment. It is especially important to make these determinations for children younger than 6 years. Studies indicate consistently that young children have an increased vulnerability to disruptions in cognitive and motor development, regardless of whether or not irradiation was a part of treatment. Because brain maturation continues into early adulthood, longitudinal examinations should be performed on a regular basis for older children and adolescents.
- *Differential diagnosis of biologic versus psychogenic components in expression of emotional and social/behavioral difficulties.* The emotional and behavioral effects of a tumor and the various treatments (especially irradiation and chemotherapy) may depend on the nature of the treatments themselves. One notable example of dramatic changes in behavior during cancer treatment is a part of somnolence syndrome, a transient encephalopathy characterized by excessive daytime drowsiness and increased night sleep in addition to EEG slowing and reduced white blood cell count.[12] Combinations of these behaviors are symptoms caused by regional or whole-brain irradiation which may be interpreted as laziness or

depression. Some pediatric patients, especially long term survivors, may have episodic or chronic yet vague complaints that do not fit criteria for a psychopathological diagnosis in the *Diagnostic and Statistical Manual of Mental Disorders,* fourth edition. Symptoms may include headache, anorexia, decreased activity, fatigue, irritability, low stamina, sleep problems, and social indifference. Any one or some combination of these complaints could be the behavioral expressions of hormonal depletion requiring endocrinology workup and treatment or, in previously identified patients, hormone imbalance requiring adjustment in hormone replacement medication doses.

- *Assistance in the development and implementation of rehabilitation and educational remediation plans.* Adjustments, particularly in the latter setting, may be necessary throughout a patient's educational experiences, which can continue through 21 years of age in the public schools. Though few systematic studies exist, numerous case reports of children and adolescents, who received educational accommodations specifically addressing their individual needs, indicate that academic achievement and social/behavior adaptation can be substantially improved. Review and modifications at least on a yearly basis should address changing expectations at various developmental and educational levels as well as any new areas of concern involving social adaptation. In recent times, cognitive remediation principles have been applied to rehabilitation efforts for some childhood cancer survivors.[13] This innovative approach is promising but is not yet generalizable to a broad range of patients.

- *Assistance to parents and families by increasing understanding and knowledge of an individual child's needs.* With increased knowledge of the goals and findings from neurobehavioral examinations, parents and caretakers become better equipped to provide insightful behavior management and proactive participation in educational planning meetings at school. Most importantly, a better understanding of the child's neurobehavioral assets and deficits may reduce the impact on all family members. Individual parent counseling and/or family psychotherapy can often address neurobehavioral issues as a springboard to a more expansive intervention involving individuals or the family as a unit.

Methods for Neurobehavioral Examination of the Child with Cancer

Neurobehavioral outcomes in long-term survivors of childhood cancer have been an increasing area of concern since the first reports of CNS abnormalities in ALL patients after therapy were published more than 20 years ago. Among pediatric patients treated for ALL and brain tumors, survivors with neurocognitive impairments by age at diagnosis range from 76% of infants to 38% of adolescents 15 to 19 years old when brain irradiation was part of treatment, and 27% to 29% across the entire pediatric age range when CNS-directed treatment involved chemotherapy only.[6] A myriad of retrospective and prospective studies have documented cognitive, motor, and behavioral functioning in patients mostly diagnosed with ALL or brain tumor.[1,2] Findings from these studies are typically presented in arrays of standardized test data that are challenging to integrate in the context of disease and complex treatment protocols. With the enormous progress made in the treatment of childhood cancers, a focus on *outcomes* has emerged in current clinical management. It has become imperative both to restore the child to complete health and to facilitate the child's potential to the greatest extent possible. Neurobehavioral examinations of patients during and after completion of treatment are being used increasingly in therapeutic trials to evaluate outcomes of disease and therapies and to establish these procedures as components of standard care for children and adolescents with cancer.

Over the same time period, many new approaches and techniques for the neurobehavioral examination have evolved, especially for the pediatric patient. These approaches offer different ways to conceptualize the process and include traditional test batteries as well as very specialized techniques. In general, there is considerable redundancy among the various standardized tests available. There are few tests which inspire consensus among psychologists for use in the neurobehavioral examination of the pediatric patient.

The common element of a neurobehavioral examination for a pediatric cancer patient of any age begins with a thorough review of medical history prior to the initial appointment. Documentation of neurologic, oncologic, and endocrine abnormalities and treatments should be emphasized. An understanding of clinical trials and the specific protocol used for treatment of the patient is recommended. A statement of parental concerns and a detailed perinatal history and developmental and educational history are essential. The specific neurocognitive tests and parent-completed questionnaires chosen for the neurobehavioral examination that follows will depend on the chronological age of the patient.

Following is an outline of recommended measures for a basic neurobehavioral examination of the school-age child with ALL. A more extensive examination may be indicated if, for example, language abnormalities are present or a more detailed assessment of academic skills is required for special education services. This test battery was derived from a previous study of children treated for ALL[14] and is currently being used in a large multicenter neurobehavioral outcomes study of children treated on 1 of 2 standard-risk ALL randomized therapeutic trials.[15] Many components of this approach may also be applied to children with other forms of cancer. (see Table 40-1.)

For a school-age child, tests of intelligence and academic achievement should be included in the examination of a broad range of neurocognitive abilities, or specific subtests from each category can be selected for serial examinations without significant practice effects. Administration of an entire standardized intelligence test should be repeated no less than once every 2 years, so as to minimize practice effects and therefore produce valid test results. Computerized tests are being used increasingly across a broad age

Table 40-1

Neurobehavioral test battery: school-age children.

1. **Intelligence**
   a. Wechsler Intelligence Scale for Children, 4th edition[16]
      - Digit Span, Letter-Number Sequencing, Coding, and Symbol Search subtests.*

2. **Academic Achievement**
   a. Wechsler Individual Achievement Test, 2nd edition, Abbreviated[17]
      - Word Reading subtest*

3. **Attention-Concentration**
   a. Conners' Continuous Performance Test II[18]
   b. Conners' Parent Rating Scale—Revised: Short Form (completed by parent)[19]*
   c. Conners' Teacher Rating Scale—Revised: Short Form (completed by teacher)[19]

4. **Visuoconstructive/Fine Motor Coordination**
   a. Beery Developmental Test of Visual Motor Integration, 5th edition[20]*
   b. Grooved Pegboard[21]

5. **Executive Functioning**
   a. FAS Word Fluency[22]*
   b. Behavior Rating Inventory of Executive Function (completed by parent and teacher)[23]

6. **Verbal and Nonverbal Memory**
   a. Children's Memory Scale[24]

7. **Social and Behavioral Adaptation**
   a. Child Behavior Checklist for Ages 6-18 (completed by parent)[25]*
   b. Teacher's Report Form (completed by teacher)[25]

*Potential screening measures.

range to measure attention/concentration in many dimensions. Other measures involve manual or oral responses to verbal, numerical, or nonverbal stimuli. Parent- and teacher-completed questionnaires are often used as secondary data sources and then combined with findings from the direct examination of the patient to reach a definitive conclusion about this essential building block of cognition. Visuoconstructive and visual motor tests include having the patient copy geometric designs with a pencil and form abstract designs with blocks. Fine motor tests involve the child or adolescent inserting pegs in a peg board or having very young children thread beads, build towers with blocks, or place geometric forms in form boards. Executive functioning is examined with tests requiring sorting of stimuli by category and producing words either beginning with specific letters of the alphabet or included within categories such as animals and foods. Tests of this kind are highly recommended, because they are sensitive to changes in the developing brain due to malignant diseases and treatments. In recent times, standardized parent- and teacher-completed questionnaires allow for measuring of executive behaviors in both preschool and school age patients. A more expansive neurobehavioral examination can involve detailed assessment of expressive and receptive language skills, especially if language areas have been affected by brain or head and neck tumors requiring surgery and/or irradiation. Comprehensive assessment of language adds considerable time to the examination of the school-age patient and may require audio recording of some test performances that are subsequently analysed in depth. Language assessment should always be performed with preschool-age children, as developmental arrests or even regressions are common. Memory tests are usually classified in terms of verbal and nonverbal stimuli and immediate and delayed recall. Stimuli typically include brief stories, word pairs, sentences, lists of unrelated words, faces, and round tokens placed on a grid. Simple and complex geometric figures are queried in a multiple-choice format or, more often, reproduced with paper and pencil.

Infants and preschool-age children should be given special considerations when scheduling a neurobehavioral examination due to the day-to-day variability in neurocognitive test performances and behavior. For these patients, it is often advisable to schedule 2 or more separate appointments in order to obtain an accurate assessment of neurocognitive and motor skills and social behaviors in addition to providing didactic information and much needed support and guidance to parents and caretakers. Infant testing may involve screening for developmental delays in language, motor skills, and adaptive behavior.[26] These tests, combined with parent-completed questionnaires on development, require one hour or less to obtain valid results. Depending on the findings, a more comprehensive, time-intensive examination of receptive and expressive language, gross and

Table 40-2

Neurodevelopmental tests: infants and preschool-age children.

1. **Infants: Screening and Basic Examination**
   a. Bayley III-Screening Test[26]*
   b. Bayley Scales of Infant and Toddler Development, 3rd edition[27]

2. **Preschool Age: Basic Examination of Neurocognitive Abilities and Social Behavior**
   a. Stanford-Binet Intelligence Scales, 5th edition[28]†
      • Object Series/Matrices and Vocabulary routing subtests*
   b. Child Behavior Checklist 1-1/2 to 5 and Language Development Survey (completed by parent)[29]*

3. **Birth Through Preschool Age: Assessment of Social Competence and Adaptive Behavior**
   a. Vineland Adaptive Behavior Scales, 2nd edition (completed by parent interview and observation of the patient)[30]*†

*Potential screening measures.

†This measure may be used with patients across the entire pediatric age range.

fine motor coordination, social/emotional functioning, and adaptive behavior may be indicated to provide specific recommendations for developmental stimulation and remediation.[27] Standardized tests for preschoolers measuring neurocognitive abilities and social/behavioral adaptation generally resemble the respective versions designed for school-age children, adolescents, and adults.[28,29] However, discrete domains and subdomains of neurocognitive functioning and adaptive behavior are less well delineated due to the comparatively immature brain development in this age range. (see Table 40-2.)

Emotional status and social/behavioral adaptation of the pediatric cancer patient can be examined using various approaches. An initial screening of social and behavioral adaptation can take place during the many reciprocal interactions involved in cognitive, motor, and academic testing or by administering an interview/rating scale of social competence to parents or caretakers.[30] Parent- and teacher-completed questionnaires are commonly used to obtain information that may be queried by additional interview to clarify and elaborate emotional and behavioral issues of concern. Another more comprehensive approach to understanding emotional status and social/behavioral adaptation of the pediatric cancer patient often addresses a specific referral question and provides the opportunity to identify and define difficulties with greater breadth. This examination may take place in the office, a playroom, or the hospital and extend over several appointments. This approach may later transition into a psychotherapeutic intervention. Parents and siblings become directly involved in the process to varying extents. Siblings often develop emotional or behavioral problems characteristic of their developmental stage. For example, a toddler reacting to the sudden attention now given to his or her acutely ill sibling may begin losing bladder or bowel control during the day or when asleep. Or, an adolescent sibling may react to the medical crisis by becoming more isolated socially or not completing school assignments and preparing for tests, resulting in declining

grades. In these situations psychotherapeutic interventions can be developed and implemented to involve the pediatric cancer patient, an individual family member, subsets of family members (e.g., with one or both parents), or the family as a unit. A presentation of specific psychosocial issues and adaptation of child and adolescent patients and family members has been elaborated and is recommended for additional reading.[31]

Summary

Psychological support of the child with cancer and the family is elaborated in terms of the neurobehavioral outcomes of malignant disease and subsequent clinical management. The most common sequelae of childhood cancer and the intensive treatments required to eradicate these diseases include deficits in attention/concentration, memory, visual-motor skills, and psychomotor processing speed. The primary risk factors for these sequelae are age at diagnosis; diagnosis of acute leukemia or CNS, eye, and bone tumors; and socioeconomic status. The purposes of the neurobehavioral examination are elaborated, with a summary of the key issues involved. Methods for the neurobehavioral examination are specified and discussed for patients in terms of chronological age range, including infancy, preschool age, childhood, and adolescence. Specific tests and a matrix of brain abilities to be measured in these age subgroups are included to guide screening and more comprehensive examinations of neurocognitive, motor, and social/behavioral functioning. Findings from these examinations can generate recommendations for school interventions and developmental stimulation and remediation programs, as well as serve as a springboard for individual psychotherapy and family counseling.

References

1. Stehbens JA, Kaleita TA, Noll RB, et al. CNS prophylaxis of pediatric leukemia: what are the long-term neurological, neuropsychological, and behavioral effects? *Neuropsych Rev.* 1991;2:147–177.

2. Ris MD, Noll RB. Long-term neurobehavioral outcome in pediatric brain tumor patients: review and methodological critique. *J Clin Exp Neuropsychol.* 1994;16:21–42.

3. Copeland DR, Moore BD, Francis DF, et al. Neuropsychologic effects of chemotherapy on children with cancer: a longitudinal study. *J Clin Oncol.* 1996;14:2826–2835.

4. Rodgers J, Horrocks J, Britton PG, et al. Attentional ability among survivors of leukemia. *Arch Dis Child.* 1999;80:318–323.

5. Cousens P, Ungerer JA, Crawford JA, et al. Cognitive effects of childhood leukemia therapy: a case for four specific deficits. *J Pediatr Psychol.* 1991;16: 475–488.

6. Pogany L, Barr RD, Shaw A, et al. Health status in survivors of cancer in childhood and adolescence. *Qual Life Res.* 2006;15:143–157.

7. Kaleita TA, Noll RB, Stehbens JA, et al. Age at diagnosis of acute lymphoblastic leukemia is associated with neurobehavioral outcomes independent of CNS-directed treatment with or without cranial irradiation and intensive chemotherapy: a Children's Cancer Group report. *J Pediatr Hematol Oncol.* 2002;24(3):A8.

8. Kiehna EN, Mulhern RK, Li C, et al. Changes in attentional performance of children and young adults with localized primary brain tumors after conformal radiation therapy. *J Clin Oncol.* 2006;24:5283–5290.

9. Jalali R, Goswami S, Sarin R, et al. Neuropsychological status in children and young adults with benign and low grade tumors treated prospectively with focal stereotactic radiotherapy. *Int J Radiat Oncol Biol Phys.* 2006;66(4 Suppl): S14–19.

10. Ding M, Newman F, Kavanagh BD, et al. Comparative dosimetric study of three-dimensional conformal, dynamic conformal arc, and intensity-modulated radiotherapy for brain tumor treatment using the Novalis system. *Int J Radiat Oncol Biol Phys.* 2006;66(4 Suppl):S82–86.

11. Kaleita TA, Wellisch DK, Cloughesy TF, et al. Prediction of neurocognitive outcome in adult brain tumor patients. *J Neurooncol.* 2004;67:245–253.

12. Uzal D, Ozyar E, Hayran M, et al. Reduced incidence of the somnolence syndrome after prophylactic cranial irradiation in children with acute lymphoblastic leukemia. *Radiother Oncol.* 1998;48:29–32.

13. Butler RW, Copeland DR. Attentional processes and their remediation in children treated for cancer: a literature review and the development of a theoretical approach. *J Int Neuropsych Soc.* 2002;8:113–124.

14. Kaleita TA, Tubergen DG, Stehbens JA, et al. Longitudinal study of cognitive, motor, and behavioral functioning in children diagnosed with acute lymphoblastic leukemia: a report from the Children's Cancer Group. *Haematol Blut Transfus.* 1997;38:680–673.

15. Kadan-Lottick N, Neglia J, Kaleita T, et al. Neurobehavioral outcomes in childhood acute lymphoblastic leukemia: ALTE02C2. Children's Oncology Group unpublished manuscript. 2004.

16. Wechsler D. *Manual for the Wechsler Intelligence Scale for Children—Fourth Edition.* San Antonio, TX: The Psychological Corporation; 2003.

17. Wechsler D. *Wechsler Individual Achievement Test—Second Edition—Abbreviated.* San Antonio, TX: The Psychological Corporation; 2001.

18. Conners CK. *Conners' Continuous Performance Test II Version 5 for Windows.* Toronto, ON: Multi-Health Systems; 2005.

19. Conners CK. *Conners' Rating Scales—Revised Technical Manual.* North Tonawanda, NY: Multi-Health Systems; 1997.

20. Beery K. *The Beery-Buktenica Developmental Test of Visual-Motor Integration: Administration, Scoring and Teaching Manual,* 5th ed. Minneapolis: NC Pearson; 2004.

21. Trites RL. *Neuropsychological Test Manual.* Ottawa, ON: Royal Ottawa Hospital; 1977.

22. Delis D, Kaplan E, Kramer J. *Delis-Kaplan Executive Function System.* San Antonio, TX: The Psychological Corporation; 2004.

23. Gioia GA, Isquith PK, Guy SC, et al. *Behavioral Rating Inventory of Executive Function.* Odessa, FL: Psychological Assessment Resources; 2000.

24. Cohen MJ. *Children's Memory Scale Manual.* San Antonio: The Psychological Corporation; 1997.

25. Achenbach TM, Rescorla LA. *Manual for the ASEBA School-Age Forms and Profiles.* Burlington: University of Vermont, Research Center for Children, Youth, and Families; 2001.

26. Bayley N. *Bayley-III Screening Test.* San Antonio, TX: Harcourt Assessment; 2005.

27. Bayley N. *Bayley Scales of Infant and Toddler Development,* 3rd ed. San Antonio, TX: Harcourt Assessment; 2005.

28. Roid GH. *Stanford-Binet Intelligence Scales,* 5th ed. Itasca, IL: Riverside Publishing; 2003.

29. Achenbach TM, Rescorla LA. *Manual for the ASEBA Preschool Forms and Profiles.* Burlington: University of Vermont Research Center for Children, Youth, and Families; 2000.

30. Sparrow SS, Cicchetti DV, Balla DA. *Vineland Adaptive Behavior Scales.* 2nd ed. Circle Pines, MN: AGS Publishing; 2005.

31. Noll RB, Kazak A. Psychosocial care. In: Ablin A, ed. *Supportive Care of Children with Cancer: Current Therapy and Guidelines from the Children's Cancer Group,* 2nd ed. Baltimore: Johns Hopkins University Press; 1997:263–227.

Complementary and Alternative Medicine

Elena J. Ladas and Janice Post-White

Introduction

The diagnosis of cancer in a child leaves parents and families devastated and vulnerable. In an effort to do everything possible, families often choose complementary and alternative medicine (CAM) to support their child through treatment. Surveys have found that 31% to 84% of children with cancer use CAM.[1] Practices and modalities that fall outside of the mainstream of conventional medicine are considered to be CAM. These treatments are either complementary (used in combination with conventional therapy) or alternative (used as a replacement to mainstream treatment). The National Center for Complementary and Alternative Medicine of the National Institutes of Health (NCCAM, NIH) has identified 4 domains of CAM therapies: mind-body, touch, energy, and biological therapies (www.nccam.nih .gov). Children with cancer most commonly use prayer and spiritual healing, mind-body therapies, biological therapies, and massage. Hypnosis, guided imagery, and biofeedback are considered standard approaches in pediatric pain centers.

This chapter will introduce the pediatric oncology caregiver to popular agents and methods currently used by families, and resources to evaluate evidence of safety and efficacy of CAM practices.

Evidence for Effectiveness

Despite the prevalent use of CAM in both adults and children with cancer, there are few scientifically rigorous studies determining whether CAM therapies in children are safe and effective and whether they lead to improved quality of life and positive clinical outcomes. Some therapies have more evidence for effectiveness (eg, hypnosis and acupuncture) than others (eg, herbal therapies and homeopathy). And some therapies require more caution prior to evidence of safety and efficacy because of known or potential toxicities (Table 41-1), while others carry less risk (massage therapy, energy therapies). The combination of the increased use of CAM therapies and the awareness of potential interactions has led to the need for reliable evidence of their safety and efficacy.[2]

Although CAM therapies are often criticized for being used despite a lack of evidence, hundreds of systematic reviews have evaluated specific therapies.[3] Over 900 reports of randomized clinical trials using a CAM intervention for children were found in 4 databases.[4] Table 41-2 summarizes select clinical CAM studies specific to children with cancer. Additional trials are ongoing. Information on active trials may be found at the Children's Oncology Group Web site (www.childrensoncologygroup.org) or the National Cancer Institute's clinical trials resource (www.cancer.gov). Until there is evidence for safety and efficacy, CAM therapies should not replace standard medical care.[5]

Nonbiological Agents
Acupuncture/Acupressure

Although the precise mechanism of acupuncture is unknown, its roots lie in the Traditional Chinese Medicine (TCM) theory of energy, or *chi*, flowing through meridians in the body. These meridians can be accessed through points located on the surface of the body. Integrating the concepts of yin and yang, practitioners identify imbalances in an individual's *chi* (or *qi*), which if left alone will manifest as disease. Acupuncture corrects the energy imbalances in the patient's body so as to prevent or treat disease.

In 1997 a National Institute of Health Consensus Development Panel concluded that there is clear evidence that acupuncture is effective for the treatment of adult postoperative and chemotherapy-induced nausea and vomiting.[6] Acupuncture has been found to be beneficial in alleviating chemotherapy-induced nausea and vomiting, pain management, alleviation of migraines, and fertility.[6] A thorough review of the literature suggests that acupuncture is safe in the pediatric population. The risk of an adverse event of acupuncture provided by a licensed acupuncturist is low. The incidence is reported to be between 1 in 10 000 to 1 in 100 000.[7]

Two small pilot studies found that acupuncture is feasible and accepted by children with cancer.[8,9] A retrospective study of 32 children with various cancer diagnoses found that acupuncture is also feasible in children with cancer with thrombocytopenia.[10] Larger trials in children with cancer are currently under way.

Table 41-1

Common classes of herbal or nutritional therapies to avoid during cancer therapy

Class of Herbal or Nutritional Therapies	Examples	Contraindications
Salicylate-containing	Meadowsweet, red clover, bilberry, White Willow, poplars, cramp bark, wintergreen, uva ursi	– May increase plasma levels of methotrexate – Decreased excretion to methotrexate
Quercitin-containing	Quercitin, glucosamine sulfate, apples	– Inhibit topoisomerase 2
Antioxidants	Grape seed extract, bilberry, vitamins C and E, selenium, β-carotene, pycnogenol, quercitin	– May increase or decrease the efficacy of free-radical generating chemotherapy agents and radiation therapy
Immune-enhancing herbal therapies	Astragalus, echinacea, ashwaganda, beta-glucans, cat's claw	– Bone marrow transplantation – Immune-derived malignancies
Anticoagulants/antiplatelets	Arnica, chamomile, gingko, celery, fenugreek, licorice root, passionflower, red clover, evening primrose oil, fish oils, flaxseed, ginger, ginseng, green tea, IP-6, Reishi, vitamin E	– May increase efficacy of these medications
Estrogenic herbs[74]	Clovers, soy sprouts, alfalfa sprouts, red clover, flaxseed, black cohosh, hops, licorice, angelica	– May be contraindicated in survivors at risk for developing breast cancer

Aromatherapy

Aromatherapy is the therapeutic use of essential oils for the improvement of physical, emotional, and spiritual well-being. Essential oils are most commonly inhaled directly from the bottle, dispensed into the air through the use of a diffuser, or applied by topical application in a carrier oil. Essential oils consist of naturally derived steam-distilled material expressed from aromatic plants, each of which retains specific healing properties. The proposed mechanism of action of essential oils begins with the absorption of volatile odor molecules through the nasal mucosa, which initiate chemical signals that affect the olfactory bulb, amygdale, and limbic system, the seats of emotion and memory.[11]

Some aromatic oils may have application in the oncology setting. A review of the history and clinical applications of aromatherapy may be found at the National Cancer Institute's Web site (www.cancer.gov). This review found that ginger (*Zingiber officinale*), spearmint (*Mentha spicata*), and peppermint (*Mentha piperita*) are recommended for antiemetic and antispasmodic effects on the gastric lining and colon. Studies in adults show peppermint's efficacy in reducing postoperative nausea and vomiting[12] and chemotherapy induced-nausea.[13] Lavender (*Lavendula angustifolia*) has sedative effects (increased sleep time and greater drowsiness and relaxation) without toxicity,[14] and citrus oils are mentally stimulating. Tea tree oil and peppermint exert antibacterial properties.[15–18] Aromatherapy is a low-risk CAM modality when used as an inhalant and can be applied in the inpatient or outpatient setting; however, consideration must be taken when using aromatic oils around nearby patients. Increased risk of skin irritation may occur when essential oils are applied topically.

Bioenergy Fields (Reiki, Qi Gong, Therapeutic Touch, Healing Touch)

Bioenergy healing includes a range of therapies (Reiki, Qi Gong, Therapeutic Touch, Healing Touch) that exert their therapeutic effectiveness through the alteration of energy fields (biofields). Each of these modalities is based on a different foundation and varies considerably in the technique employed. For example, Reiki and Therapeutic Touch can be administered without physical contact to the patient, whereas external Qi Gong and Healing Touch include systematic movements to move the energy and unblock areas of stagnated or blocked energy flow. Therapeutic Touch and Healing Touch promote stress reduction and pain relief.[19] In one study of 165 adults with cancer, Healing Touch induced a physiological relaxed state and reduced fatigue and negative mood states.[20] Energy therapies are known to be safe and may promote relaxation and a sense of well-being. There is limited evidence for efficacy and no scientific evidence for the mechanism of action. A thorough review of bioenergy theory and therapies has been published.[21]

Table 41-2

Selected supportive care studies conducted in children with cancer.

Author/Year	CAM Therapy	Type of Study	Diagnosis (Sample Size N=X)	Indication	Results
Biological Therapies					
Anderson et al 1998[64]	Glutamine (1.0 g/m²/dose 4 times/day)	Randomized, double blind, placebo-controlled	Bone marrow transplant (BMT) (N=93)	Mucositis	Autologous BMT patients reported less mouth pain ($p = .005$) and a decrease in the duration of opiate use ($p = .005$) compared with placebo controls. No significant results in patients undergoing allogeneic transplants.
Aquino 2005[72]	Glutamine (2 g/m²/dose, maximum dose 4 grams)	Randomized, double blind, placebo-controlled	Stem cell transplantation (N=120)	Mucositis	↓ mean mucositis score in intervention compared with controls ($p = 0.07$). ↓ in the number of days requiring intravenous narcotics in intervention compared with controls ($p = .03$). ↓ in the number of days requiring total parenteral nutrition in intervention compared with controls ($p = .01$).
Iarussi et al 1994[53]	Coenzyme-Q10 (100 mg 2 times/day)	Randomized, controlled trial	Acute lymphoblastic leukemia (N=20)	Cardiotoxicity	↓ in percentage left ventricular fractional shortening in both intervention and placebo groups ($p < .05$, $p < .002$, respectively). Intraventricular septum wall thickening decreased only in control group ($p < .01$). Septum wall motion abnormalities were observed in 2 out of 10 patients in the placebo; no abnormalities observed in intervention group.
Inoue 1998[71]	Colostrum (20 ml/day)	Case report	Various (N=9)	Gut graft-vs-host disease (GVHD)	Clinical improvement in severe gut GVHD in 6 out of 9 patients. Two patients did not adhere to protocol.
Ladas et al 2008[37]	Milk thistle (5.1 mg/kg per day)	Randomized, double blind, placebo-controlled	Acute lymphoblastic leukemia (N=50)	Hepatotoxicity	↓ mean AST ($p < .05$). Trend toward ↓ ALT ($p = .07$). Greater reduction in total bilirubin in cases vs controls ($p < .0069$).

(continued on next page)

Author/Year	CAM Therapy	Type of Study	Diagnosis (Sample Size)	Indication	Results
Melnick et al 2005[44]	Immunocal® (0.5 g/kg/day vs 1.0 g/kg/day)	Phase 1	Various (12)	Cachexia	8 out of 12 patients gained weight ranging from 7.1% to 26.9% from the pre-study weight. Glutathione (GSH) levels were increased and oxidized glutathione (GSSG) levels decreased in all but 1 patient.
Oberbaum 2001[63]	Traumeel™ (swish and swallow, 5 times/day)	Randomized, double blind, placebo-controlled	Stem cell transplantation (32)	Mucositis	GSH levels were increased and oxidized glutathione (GSSG) levels decreased in all but 1 patient. ↓ incidence and severity of stomatitis in cases vs controls (p < 0.01). No significant differences in incidence of complication in cases compared with controls.
Massage					
Phipps et al 2004[30]	Massage	Randomized, controlled trial	Cancer diagnosis; children undergoing BMT	Anxiety	↓ in days to engraftment in combined massage group (p = .02); ↓ in anxiety (p < .0001) and discomfort (p = .004) in massage group.
Field et al 2001[29]	Massage	Randomized, controlled trial	Acute lymphoblastic leukemia (20)	Anxiety, depression, decreased immune function	↑ in mean white blood cell and neutrophil count (p = .01); ↓ in anxiety (p = .05) and depression (p = .01) in treatment group compared with control.
Acupuncture					
Reindl et al 2006[8]	Acupuncture	Randomized, pilot trial	Solid tumors (11)	Efficacy and acceptance of acupuncture for children with cancer	↓ antiemetics in treatment compared with controls. ↓ nausea and vomiting in treatment compared with controls. No adverse events were observed. Significance not reported.
Taromina et al 2006[9]	Acupuncture	Retrospective review	Various (25)	Feasibility of acupuncture for children with cancer	Authors report that children requested multiple treatments for side effects associated with cancer therapy. Acupuncture was administered to children of varied ages, diagnoses, ethnicity, and sex. Authors conclude that acupuncture is feasible for children with cancer.
Taromina et al 2007[10]	Acupuncture	Retrospective review	Children with various diagnosis with thrombocytopenia (32)	Feasibility of acupuncture in children with cancer with thrombocytopenia	Of the 237 sessions, increased bleeding or bruising complications were not observed in patients with thrombocytopenia.

Massage

Massage is the systematic manipulation of soft tissues in the body,[22] with the intention to promote health and well-being.[23] Table 41-3 describes the different techniques and methodologies of massage.

Massage therapy is one of the most commonly used CAM therapies in adult and pediatric oncology. Several Cochrane databases and meta-analyses support the use of massage in adults and children with cancer for management of anxiety, pain, fatigue, and distress.[24] Studies in adults with cancer have found massage effective for reducing anxiety,[20,25–27] fatigue,[25–27] acute pain,[20,25–28] and nausea[25,26,28] and for improving mood.[20,27]

Although massage is one of the most frequently used CAM therapies for children with cancer, there are few studies testing its effectiveness. Field et al reported that children with leukemia had lower anxiety and depression at 2 time points after a 15-minute massage provided by a parent.[29] In two studies conducted by Phipps et al, children undergoing stem cell transplant had less anxiety after massage, while children undergoing bone marrow transplantation did not show significant changes in anxiety after massage.[30,31] Two studies also reported significant lowering of anxiety[32] and fatigue for parents of children with cancer.[33] Although these studies were small and inconclusive, they support the feasibility of providing therapeutic and parent-delivered massage to children with cancer.

Massage is generally considered safe with little concern for adverse events or interactions with cancer therapies. A recommended practice guideline is to avoid deep and intense pressure and not to massage over topical skin ruptures, radiation burns, and sites of solid tumor or intravenous lines.[5] Practitioners selected should be trained, credentialed, and licensed (if available) and should have experience in treating children.

Table 41-3

Common forms of massage therapy.

Massage Method	Description
Swedish massage	Application of effleurage (long strokes), petrissage (short stokes/kneading), with light to medium pressure to superficial muscles in the direction of venous return. Striping (friction in the direction of muscle fibers) and cross-friction (friction against/across muscle fibers) used to break adhesions in muscle tissue. Tapotement/vibration (percussion-like tapping) and active and passive range of motion (ROM) are used to manipulate the nervous system response to break pain-spasm-pain cycles.
Deep tissue massage	Similar stokes and method as Swedish massage, except pressure is slower with medium to deep contact to affect muscles under the superficial layers.
Medical/orthopedic Massage	Addresses where injury or trauma has occurred. Therapists are usually trained in several bodywork modalities to relieve spasm-pain cycles to restore normal function and structural posture. Techniques may include: muscle testing, heat and/or cryotherapy, deep tissue work, myofascial trigger point release, ROM, stretching and strengthening exercises, and other associated alignment and movement methods.
Sports massage	There are 2 types of sports massage: Pre-event focuses on muscles or muscle groups that are primarily used in a particular sport to prevent cramping, strain, or injury. Post-event includes rigorous to calming compression to muscle bellies, jostling, ROM, and stretching techniques of muscles groups that are most stressed for a specific sport.
Aromatherapy massage	Medicinal-grade essential oils are applied to the human body to restore physical, emotional, and spiritual function. Oils are generally mixed with a carrier oil during the massage session.
Shiatsu	Manipulating acupuncture meridians (energy pathways) and applying gentle to hard palmar compression along meridians and finger pressure to specific acupuncture points. Stretching, rocking and ROM techniques are used to open joints and meridians.
Reflexology	A system that uses finger and thumb pressure to manipulate zones and reflex points in the feet and hands that correspond to areas on the body. The therapist detects blockages or congestion in the zones or reflex area and applies pressure and circular movements to the area breaking the blockage, which restores balance to the body.
Rolfing	Formally known as Rolfing® Structural Integration, this system can be an extremely intense deep tissue therapy involving soft tissue and myofascial manipulation with movement education that organizes the body in gravity to achieve changes in posture and structure of the body. Sessions are progressive.

Overall, massage is considered a safe and potentially therapeutic intervention for reduction of anxiety, perceived stress, and mood disturbance.

Biological Agents

Cytotoxic Effects

Some biologic agents have direct tumor cytotoxicity, but most of the biologic agents promoted as being effective anticancer agents are based on preclinical investigations conducted in cell lines or animal models. Furthermore, much of the preclinical work has been conducted in cell lines that represent malignancies observed in the adult population. Few studies have been investigated in pediatric tumor cell lines. The use of biological agents as a treatment for cancer is uncommon among children. However, children with poor prognosis, children who have a strong family history of CAM use, or children receiving palliative care are more likely to turn to biologic therapies in hopes of obtaining a cure.

Scientific summaries of many of the most popular biological agents may be found at the National Cancer Institute's Website (www.cancer.gov). Biological agents that have shown encouraging results in pediatric tumors should be investigated through Phase 1 studies.[34,35] Although the paucity of data creates challenges in advising pediatric patients about the safety and efficacy of biological agents, these scientific summaries and reviews may provide a platform in which practitioners may discuss the risk and benefits of biological agents with patients.

Most children with cancer combine biological agents with conventional therapy to enhance the effects of chemotherapy or radiation, minimize therapy-related toxicity, improve quality of life, or decrease the risk of developing a late effect. Clinical trials that have been conducted among children with cancer are described in Table 41-3. A brief summary of these therapies is presented below.

Antioxidant Agents

Antioxidants are substances that counteract free radicals and prevent them from causing tissue and organ damage.[36] Antioxidants are frequently cited as one of the most common classes of supplements used by individuals with cancer. Patients use antioxidants for cytotoxic effects, to enhance the anticancer effects of chemotherapy or radiation, or to minimize therapy-induced toxicity. Antioxidants exert free radical activity through a variety of mechanisms, thus a comprehensive assessment of the antioxidant that includes the class and mechanism of antioxidant, the form and dose, and the type of cancer therapy is crucial in determining if a specific antioxidant is contraindicated with chemotherapy or radiation.[37]

Most of the data supporting the use of antioxidants in the oncology setting are derived from cellular and animal research. Observational trials have been conducted in adults and children with cancer.[38] Few case studies have been reported among adults with cancer. Observational trials have consistently reported decreased levels of antioxidants in patients receiving cytotoxic therapy. One of the largest observational trials conducted in children with acute lymphoblastic leukemia found that decreased dietary intake of antioxidants was associated with increased risk of developing therapy-related toxicities.[39] Additional trials are needed to determine if dietary counseling emphasizing increased dietary intake of antioxidants or supplementation with antioxidants could reverse this relationship.

Randomized, controlled clinical trials investigating the use of antioxidant supplements in the oncology setting have been conducted among adults with cancer. Trials have reported mixed results. One of the largest well-designed trials found that the combined use of *dl-a*-tocopherol (400 IU/day) and β-carotene (30 mg/day) antioxidants was associated with adverse outcomes in 540 adults with head and neck cancer receiving radiation treatment.[40] Patients in the intervention arm experienced less severe acute side effects from radiation therapy; however, the local rate of recurrence was greater in patients who received both *dl-a*-tocopheral and β-carotene. Further analyses demonstrated that all-cause mortality was significantly increased in the supplement arm (hazard ratio: 1.38, 95% confidence interval 1.03-1.85). The combination of this antioxidant mixture with chemotherapy or radiation in children with cancer is unknown. Until further research is available, practitioners should caution patients against the combined use of β-carotene and vitamin E with radiation therapy.

Immune-Enhancing Agents

Immune suppression is one of the hallmarks of anticancer therapy. Parents may turn to biological agents based on the theoretical assumption that immune-enhancing biological agents will make their child "stronger" and more able to tolerate the prescribed cancer therapy. The underlying assumption is that immune-enhancing agents will stimulate the immune system, providing an additional tool to fight the cancer. Proponents of immune enhancers also suggest that immune-stimulating therapies will facilitate the recovery of the immune system, thereby decreasing the risk of developing an infection and avoiding interruptions in therapy. Popular immune-enhancing herbal and nutrition therapies are astragalus, echinacea, beta-glucans, and mushroom extracts (Reishi, Maitaki, Shitaki). These agents have activity on different aspects of the immune system; however, no trials with these agents have been conducted among children with cancer.

Although there is little research in the pediatric population, a preliminary pilot study has suggested that immune-supporting therapies may be of benefit. Immunocal® is an un-denatured whey-protein derivative that has been investigated among children with cancer. Immunocal® provides precursors of glutathione in a form that can be utilized by cells. Children with HIV/AIDS or cystic fibrosis have gained weight and had improved immune function and quality of life.[41–43] A small pilot study initiated by the Nutrition Committee of the Children's Oncology Group has also found improvements in clinical status, including weight gain and increased levels of reduced glutathione.[44] These preliminary findings need to be investigated in a larger cohort.

Immune-enhancing agents should be avoided in patients with malignancies that evolve from the immune system, such as leukemia, Hodgkin disease, and non-Hodgkin lymphoma. Immune-enhancing agents are also contraindicated in the setting of stem cell transplantation, as they may increase a patient's risk of graft-vs-host disease.

Cardioprotectants

More than half of survivors of childhood cancer are treated with anthracycline-containing regimens, which increase the risk for developing symptomatic heart disease. Late cardiac death is a significant cause of premature mortality in survivors of childhood cancer.[45] Anthracyclines are a crucial component of many pediatric regimens, motivating parents to look for cardioprotectants as an adjunct to care. Biological agents that are promoted for cardioprotective effects are: l-carnitine, coenzyme Q10 (CoQ10), and vitamin E.

Although clinical trials investigating cardioprotective effects of vitamin E have yielded insignificant results,[46–48] studies investigating CoQ10 and l-carnitine show promising effects. CoQ10 is an endogenous compound that promotes membrane stabilization and acts as a cofactor in many metabolic pathways, including the production of adenosine triphosphate in oxidative respiration. CoQ10 may have a cardioprotectant effect by replenishing or scavenging free radicals in cardiac myocytes.[49] Low plasma CoQ10 levels have been observed in adults with melanoma, breast, and lung cancer.[50–52] Studies in children with ALL and non-Hodgkin lymphoma have found significant improvement in cardiac function when supplemented with coenzyme Q10 while being treated with anthracycline-based therapy.[53] A systematic review of clinical trials investigating the efficacy of CoQ10 reported that CoQ10 may have a beneficial effect in patients receiving cardiotoxic chemotherapy, but additional studies with larger sample sizes in homogenous populations are still needed.[54]

L-carnitine is a nutrition supplement that is often promoted for its cardioprotective properties. L-carnitine is required to transport fatty acids across the inner mitochondrial membrane, where fat oxidation and adenysine triphosphate synthesis take place.[55] Several chemotherapy agents have been found to interfere with this network,[56] resulting in alterations in energy utilization and balance and resulting in skeletal muscle fatigue and cardiac muscle inefficiency. Observational studies found that 67% of adult patients with cancer[57] and 60% of pediatric patients with AIDS and chronic illnesses were carnitine deficient.[58,59] Symptoms of fatigue and functional status improved in those patients supplemented with oral carnitine. A randomized Phase II clinical trial found that supplementation with l-carnitine reduced fatigue and improved functional status in adults with cancer.[60] Carnitine has FDA approval for the treatment of cardiomyopa-

thy in children, although it remains to be studied in children with cancer.

Neuropathy

Vincristine-induced neuropathy is prevalent in children with cancer and is most frequently managed by reducing dosages in chemotherapy or delaying treatment. Progressive neuropathy measured by clinical exam has been observed in 67% of children with cancer.[61]

Preliminary laboratory and human data have suggested that glutamine may have a promising role as a prophylaxis against vincristine-induced neuropathy. In vitro studies have found that glutamine does not effect cell cycle distribution, cellular growth rate, or sensitivity to vincristine or l-asparaginase in the CCRF-CEM human leukemia cell lines.[61] In patients with stage IV breast cancer receiving paclitaxel, supplementation with oral glutamine was found to decrease the incidence of motor weakness ($p = 0.04$) and abnormalities in gait ($p = 0.016$). No toxicities were reported.[62] Trials are currently under way in children with cancer.

Topical applications of gels and creams have also been promoted antidotes for neuropathy. Topical application of capsaicin has been suggested to ease the pain associated with neuropathy, most likely due to its analgesic activity, although the application may be associated with topical irritation or burning.

Mucositis

A number of CAM approaches are used as a preventative or treatment for chemotherapy or radiation-induced mucositis. Clinical trials have been conducted in children with cancer. TRAUMEELS®, a homeopathic remedy, was investigated in 32 children undergoing bone marrow transplants. Significant reductions in the severity and duration of mucositis were observed.[63] Glutamine, an amino acid, has also been found to be effective in the prevention and treatment of mucositis in children and adults undergoing anticancer therapy.[64] Doses range from 1 to 2 g/m² twice daily. Chamomile tea was beneficial in the prevention of oral mucositis in adult patients receiving either radiation or chemotherapy.[65] Patients may also benefit from chamomile's ability to ease anxiety. Pure honey may also play a role in the prevention of mucositis. Forty patients with head and neck cancer were instructed to ingest 20 ml of pure honey by mouth (swish and swallow) before and after radiation therapy. The authors reported a reduction in the severity of mucositis, less weight loss, and excellent compliance with the study.[66]

Biological Agents and Interactions with Cancer Therapy

There is little data available from clinical trials investigating herb-drug interactions. Most of the potential interactions discussed in the published literature are either theoretical in nature or have been observed in the laboratory setting. The doses at which the interactions have been observed in the laboratory setting are frequently not attainable within oral dosing recommendations. A review of literature on herb-drug interactions found that 20% of the research on herb-drug interactions is based on laboratory findings, 19% is theoretical, and 18% is empirically derived; however, certain classes of herbal agents should be avoided during cancer therapy (Table 41-1).[67] The risk of a biological remedy interacting with conventional therapy is much greater when the patient is using the supplement during the entire treatment plan, supplementing with multiple biological agents, or ingesting excessively high doses of biological agents. This use of multiple supplements is commonly observed in patients adhering to protocols derived from alternative medical systems such as Traditional Chinese Medicine, homeopathy, or Ayurvedic medicine. In a review of adverse effects of herbal and nutrition supplements, most adverse events were due to product contamination. Supplements may be contaminated with foreign agents or may not contain the amount of herb or nutrient indicated on the label; however, recent legislature is requiring quality control by manufacturers of biological remedies (www.fda.gov). Contamination of supplements is of serious concern for a child with cancer who may have an already compromised immune system.

A thorough discussion and evaluation of the risks and benefits of combining supplements with cancer care should be held at the onset of therapy; therefore, it is important for the practitioner to maintain a nonjudgmental, open forum with the patient and his or her family so harmful risks may be identified and avoided. The patient should be closely monitored for warning signs of an adverse interaction, which may include increased or decreased rate of expected toxicities, unexpected toxicities, or unexpected refractoriness.[68] Strategies to minimize the risk of an interaction have been thoroughly described in the literature.[69] These strategies can be readily implemented in evaluating risk-benefit interactions.

Advising Patients on Complementary and Alternative Medicine

Parents want to know if CAM is a reasonable addition to their child's treatment plan. It is important for health care practitioners to help parents weigh the risks with the potential benefits, evaluate interactions with treatment and medications, determine recommended doses and frequency, and find qualified licensed or certified practitioners who have experience working with children. It is especially important to keep communication open by assuming a

---

Table 41-4

Resources on complementary/alternative medicine.

Centers/Institutions

National Center for Complementary Alternative Medicine, National Institute of Health: http://nccam.nih.gov/

National Cancer Institute, NIH: www.cancer.gov/CAM/

NCI PDQs: www.cancer.gov/cancertopics/pdq/cam

Integrative Therapies Program for Children with Cancer, Columbia University: www.integrativetherapiesprogram.org

Herb Research Foundation: www.herbs.org/index.html

Memorial Sloan Kettering: www.mskcc.org/mskcc/html/1979.cfm

The Office of Dietary Supplements: http://ods.od.nih.gov

Databases

National Library of Medicine: www4.ncbi.nlm.nih.gov/PubMed/

The Cochrane Library: www3.interscience.wiley.com/cgi-bin/mrwhome/106568753/HOME

The NCI's PDQ Clinical Trials Database: www.cancer.gov/clinicaltrials/search

Book References

Therapeutic Research Faculty. *Natural Medicines: Comprehensive Database*. Stockton, CA: Pharmacists Letter; 2001.

Hendler SS, Rorvik D, eds. *Physicians Desk Reference for Herbal Products*. Montvale, NJ: Thomas Healthcare; 2001.

Gruenwald J, Brendler T, Jaenicke C, eds. *Physicians Desk Reference for Nutritional Supplements*. Montvale, NJ: Thomas Healthcare; 2007.

Mark Blumenthal. *The ABC Clinical Guide to Herbs*. Austin, TX: American Botanical Council; 2003.

Cassileth BR, Lucarelli C. *Herb-Drug Interactions in Oncology*. Lewison, NY: BC Decker; 2003.

Product Information

Consumer Lab: www.consumerlab.com

---

nonjudgmental approach and asking patients and families what CAM they use, if any, documenting what the child uses, including dosages and frequency and reasons for use, and evaluating benefits or effects observed. Consideration should also be given to patient preferences. Individualizing therapies is especially important in determining which CAM therapies are of greatest value and interest for the developmental age and motivation of the child or adolescent. A trial approach is often used to determine which therapies are most appropriate for individual patients.

Health care providers and families can find guidance on evaluating safety and use of CAM therapies from reputable resources (Table 41-4). Guidelines have been developed for health care providers. These guidelines offer specific recommendations based on the strength of evidence and the risk-to-benefit ratio available; however, much of the research supporting these guidelines is based on studies conducted in adults with cancer. A commonly used 2-by-2 grid is used to rank safety and efficacy along separate axes. When safety and efficacy are strong, the therapy can be encouraged. When safety and efficacy are weak, it makes sense to discourage it. When evidence supports safety but efficacy is inconclusive, or when there is evidence of efficacy but not safety, then the therapy should be encouraged with caution and monitored closely for effectiveness or safety.[5,70] A dilemma arises when there is no evidence of either safety or efficacy. Each therapy needs to be considered individually, and more research is needed on the mechanism of action, drug-supplement interactions, and seeking novel therapies for conditions that are not responsive to standard treatment options.[5] Research specific to children is especially indicated, as findings from adult CAM studies cannot be generalized to children.

References

1. Kelly KM. Complementary and alternative medical therapies for children with cancer. *Eur J Cancer.* 2004;40(14):2041–2046.
2. Smith WB. Research methodology: implications for CAM pain research. *Clin J Pain.* 2004;20(1):3–7.
3. Committee on the Use of Complementary and Alternative Medicine by the American Public, Board on Health Promotion and Disease Prevention. *Complementary and Alternative Medicine in the United States.* Washington, DC: National Academies Press; 2005.
4. Sampson M, Campbell K, Ajiferuke I, Moher D. Randomized controlled trials in pediatric complementary and alternative medicine: where can they be found? *BMC Pediatr.* 2003;3:1.
5. Deng GE, Cassileth BR, Cohen L, et al. Integrative oncology practice guidelines. *J Soc Integr Oncol.* 2007;5(2):65–84.
6. NIH Consensus Conference. Acupuncture. *JAMA.* 1998;280(17):1518–1524.
7. Kemper KJ, Sarah R, Silver-Highfield E, Xiarhos E, Barnes L, Berde C. On pins and needles? pediatric pain patients' experience with acupuncture. *Pediatrics.* 2000;105(4 Pt 2):941–947.
8. Reindl TK, Geilen W, Hartmann R, et al. Acupuncture against chemotherapy-induced nausea and vomiting in pediatric oncology: interim results of a multicenter crossover study. *Support Care Cancer.* 2006;14(2):172–176.
9. Taromina K, Ladas E, Rooney D, Hughes D, Kelly K. A retrospective review investigating the feasibility of acupuncture as a supportive care agent in a pediatric oncology service. Society for Integrative Oncology, Annual Meeting, November 9, 2006.
10. Taromina K, Ladas E, Rooney D, Hughes D, Meyer A, Kelly KM. Acupuncture is feasible in children with low platelet counts. Society for Integrative Oncology, Annual Meeting, November 14–17, 2007.
11. Lis-Balchin M. Essential oils and 'aromatherapy': their modern role in healing. *J R Soc Health.* 1997;117(5):324–329.
12. Tate S. Peppermint oil: a treatment for postoperative nausea. *J Adv Nurs.* 1997;26(3):543–549.
13. Buckle J. Nausea and vomiting. In: Buckle J. *Clinical Aromatherapy: Essential Oils in Practice.* Arnold, UK: Churchill Livingstone; 2003:[p 337–338].
14. Hardy M, Kirk-Smith MD, Stretch DD. Replacement of drug treatment for insomnia by ambient odour. *Lancet.* 1995;346(8976):701.
15. Lis-Balchin M, Hart S. Studies on the mode of action of the essential oil of lavender (*Lavandula angustifolia P. Miller*). *Phytother Res.* 1999;13(6):540–542.
16. Masago R, Matsuda T, Kikuchi Y, Miyazaki Y, Iwanaga K, Harada H et al. Effects of inhalation of essential oils on EEG activity and sensory evaluation. *J Physiol Anthropol Appl Human Sci.* 2000;19(1):35–42.
17. Schulz H, Stolz C, Muller J. The effect of valerian extract on sleep polygraphy in poor sleepers: a pilot study. *Pharmacopsychiatry.* 1994;27(4):147–151.
18. Schultz V, Hubner W, Ploch M. Clinical trials with phyto-psychopharmacological agents. *Phytomedicine.* 1997;4:379–387.
19. Wilkinson DS, Knox P, Chatman J, et al. The clinical effectiveness of healing touch. *J Altern Complement Med.* 2002;8(1):33–47.
20. Post-White J, Kinney ME, Savik K, Gau JB, Wilcox C, Lerner I. Therapeutic massage and healing touch improve symptoms in cancer. *Integr Cancer Ther.* 2003;2(4):332–344.
21. Hintz KJ, Yount GL, Kadar I, Schwartz G, Hammerschlag R, Lin S. Bioenergy definitions and research guidelines. Altern Ther Health Med 2003;9(3 Suppl):A13–A30.
22. Ernst E. The safety of massage therapy. *Rheumatology (Oxford).* 2003;42(9):1101–1106.
23. Beider S, Moyer CA. Randomized controlled trials of pediatric massage: a review. *Evid Based Complement Alternat Med.* 2007;4(1):23–34.
24. Ezzo J. What can be learned from Cochrane systematic reviews of massage that can guide future research? *J Altern Complement Med.* 2007;13(2):291–295.
25. Ahles TA, Tope DM, Pinkson B, et al. Massage therapy for patients undergoing autologous bone marrow transplantation. *J Pain Symptom Manage.* 1999;18(3):157–163.
26. Cassileth B, Vickers A. Massage therapy for symptom control: outcome study at a major cancer center. *J Pain Symptom Management.* 2004;28:244–249.
27. Hernandez-Reif M, Field T, Largie S, et al. Childrens' distress during burn treatment is reduced by massage therapy. *J Burn Care Rehabil.* 2001;22(2):191–195.
28. Grealish L, Lomasney A, Whiteman B. Foot massage. A nursing intervention to modify the distressing symptoms of pain and nausea in patients hospitalized with cancer. *Cancer Nurs.* 2000;23(3):237–243.
29. Field T, Cullen C, Diego M, et al. Leukemia immune changes following massage therapy. *J Bodywork Movement Ther.* 2001;5(4):271–274.
30. Phipps S, Dunavant M, Rai S, Deng X, Lensing S. The effects of massage in children undergoing bone marrow transplant. *Massage J Ther.* 2004;43(3):62–71.
31. Phipps S, Dunavant M, Gray E, Rai SN. Massage therapy in children undergoing hematopoietic stem cell transplantation: results of a pilot trial. *J Cancer Int Med.* 2005;2(2):62–70.
32. Post-White J, Fitzgerald M, Savik K, Hooke M, Hannahan A, Sencer S. Massage therapy in childhood cancer. Manuscript in preparation.
33. Iwasaki M. Interventional study on fatigue relief in mothers caring for hospitalized children: effect of massage incorporating techniques from oriental medicine. *Kurume Med J.* 2005;52(1–2):19–27.
34. Melnick SJ. Developmental therapeutics: review of biologically based CAM therapies for potential application in children with cancer: part I. *J Pediatr Hematol Oncol.* 2006;28(4):221–230.
35. Melnick SJ. Developmental therapeutics: review of biologically based complementary and alternative medicine (CAM) therapies for potential application in children with cancer: part II. *J Pediatr Hematol Oncol.* 2006;28(5):271–285.
36. Ratnam DV, Ankola DD, Bhardwaj V, Sahana DK, Kumar MN. Role of antioxidants in prophylaxis and therapy: a pharmaceutical perspective. *J Control Release.* 2006;20;113(3):189–207.
37. Ladas EJ, Kelly KM. The antioxidant debate. In: Abrams D, Weil A, eds. *Integrative Oncology.* New York: Oxford University Press; 2008: in press.
38. Ladas EJ, Jacobson JS, Kennedy DD, Teel K, Fleischauer A, Kelly KM. Antioxidants and cancer therapy: a systematic review. *J Clin Oncol.* 2004;22(3):517–528.
39. Kennedy D, Tucker K, Ladas EJ, et al. Low antioxidant vitamin intakes are associated with increases in adverse effects of chemotherapy in children with acute lymphoblastic leukemia. *Am J Clin Nutr.* 2004;79(6):1029–1036.
40. Bairati I, Meyer F, Gelinas M, et al. Randomized trial of antioxidant vitamins to prevent acute adverse effects of radiation therapy in head and neck cancer patients. *J Clin Oncol.* 2005;20;23(24):5805–5813.
41. Grey V, Mohammed SR, Smountas AA, Bahlool R, Lands LC. Improved glutathione status in young adult patients with cystic fibrosis supplemented with whey protein. *J Cyst Fibros.* 2003;2(4):195–198.
42. Micke P, Beeh KM, Schlaak JF, Buhl R. Oral supplementation with whey proteins increases plasma glutathione levels of HIV-infected patients. *Eur J Clin Invest.* 2001;31(2):171–178.
43. Micke P, Beeh KM, Buhl R. Effects of long-term supplementation with whey proteins on plasma glutathione levels of HIV-infected patients. *Eur J Nutr.* 2002;41(1):12–18.
44. Melnick SJ, Rogers P, Sacks N, et al. A pilot limited institutional study to evaluate the safety and tolerability of Immunocal®, a nutraceutical cysteine delivery agent in the management of wasting in high-risk childhood cancer patients. 1st Annual Chicago Supportive Oncology Conference, October 6th, 2005.

45. Hawkins M. Long-term survivors of childhood cancers: what knowledge have we gained? *Nat Clin Pract Oncol*. 2004;1(1):26–31.
46. Legha S, Wang Y, Mackay B, E et al. Clinical and pharmacologic investigation of the effects of alpha-tocopherol on adriamycin cardiotoxicity. *Ann N Y Acad Sci*. 1982;393:411–418.
47. Wagdi P, Fluri M, Aeschbacher B, Fikrle A, Meier B. Cardioprotection in patients undergoing chemo- and/or radiotherapy for neoplastic disease: a pilot study. *Jpn Heart J*. 1996;37(3):353–359.
48. Weitzman SS, Lorell B, Carey RW, Kaufman S, Stossel TP. Prospective study of tocopherol prophylaxis for anthracycline cardiac toxicity. *Curr Ther Res*. 1980;28(5):682–686.
49. Greenberg S, Frishman WH. Co-enzyme Q10: a new drug for cardiovascular disease. *J Clin Pharmacol*. 1990;30(7):596–608.
50. Folkers K, Osterborg A, Nylander M, Morita M, Mellstedt H. Activities of vitamin Q10 in animal models and a serious deficiency in patients with cancer. *Biochem Biophys Res Commun*. 1997;19;234(2):296–299.
51. Rusciani L, Proietti I, Rusciani A, et al. Low plasma coenzyme Q10 levels as an independent prognostic factor for melanoma progression. *J Am Acad Dermatol*. 2006;54(2):234–241.
52. Shinkai T, Tominaga K, Shimabukuro Z, et al. [Platelet aggregation and coenzyme Q10 content in platelets in cancer patients]. *Gan To Kagaku Ryoho*. 1984;11(1):87–96.
53. Iarussi D, Auricchio U, Agretto A, et al. Protective effect of coenzyme Q10 on anthracyclines cardiotoxicity: control study in children with acute lymphoblastic leukemia and non-Hodgkin lymphoma. *Mol Aspects Med*. 1994;15(Suppl):s207–s212.
54. Roffe L, Schmidt K, Ernst E. Efficacy of coenzyme Q10 for improved tolerability of cancer treatments: a systematic review. *J Clin Oncol*. 2004;22(21):4418–4424.
55. Stipanuk MH. *Biochemical and Physiological Aspects of Human Nutrition*. Philadelphia: W. B. Saunders, 2000.
56. Peluso G, Nicolai R, Reda E, Benatti P, Barbarisi A, Calvani M. Cancer and anticancer therapy-induced modifications on metabolism mediated by carnitine system. *J Cell Physiol*. 2000;182(3):339–350.
57. Cruciani RA, Dvorkin E, Homel P, et al. L-carnitine supplementation for the treatment of fatigue and depressed mood in cancer patients with carnitine deficiency: a preliminary analysis. *Ann N Y Acad Sci*. 2004;1033:168–176.
58. Esteban-Cruciani NV. Severe carnitine deficiency in children with AIDS: improved functional activity status after supplementation. *Pediatr Res*. 2001;49:254.
59. Esteban-Cruciani NV. High prevalence of carnitine deficiency in children with chronic illness. *Pediatr Res*. 2002;51:218.
60. Cruciani RA, Dvorkin E, Homel P, et al. Safety, tolerability and symptom outcomes associated with L-carnitine supplementation in patients with cancer, fatigue, and carnitine deficiency: a phase I/II study. *J Pain Symptom Manage*. 2006;32(6):551–559.
61. Dave A, Ladas E, Hughes D, et al. A pilot study investigating the effects of glutamine and vincristine-induced neuropathy in pediatric patients with cancer. Society for Integrative Oncology Annual Meeting, November 14–17, 2007.
62. Vahdat L, Papadopoulos K, Lange D, et al. Reduction of paclitaxel-induced peripheral neuropathy with glutamine. *Clin Cancer Res*. 2001;7(5):1192–1197.
63. Oberbaum M, Yaniv I, Ben Gal Y, et al. A randomized, controlled clinical trial of the homeopathic medication TRAUMEEL S in the treatment of chemotherapy-induced stomatitis in children undergoing stem cell transplantation. *Cancer*. 2001;92(3):684–690.
64. Anderson PM, Ramsay NK, Shu XO, et al. Effect of low-dose oral glutamine on painful stomatitis during bone marrow transplantation. *Bone Marrow Transplant*. 1998;22(4):339–344.
65. Fidler P, Loprinzi CL, O'Fallon JR, et al. Prospective evaluation of a chamomile mouthwash for prevention of 5-FU-induced oral mucositis. *Cancer*. 1996;77(3):522–525.
66. Biswal BM, Zakaria A, Ahmad NM. Topical application of honey in the management of radiation mucositis: a preliminary study. *Support Care Cancer*. 2003;11(4):242–248.
67. Blumenthal M. Interactions between herbs and conventional drugs: introductory considerations. *HerbalGram*. 2000;(49):52–63.
68. Labriola D, Livingston R. Possible interactions between dietary antioxidants and chemotherapy. *Oncology (Huntingt)*. 1999;13(7):1003–1008.
69. Seely D, Stempak D, Baruchel S. A strategy for controlling potential interactions between natural health products and chemotherapy: a review in pediatric oncology. *J Pediatr Hematol Oncol*. 2007;29(1):32–47.
70. McLean TW, Kemper KJ. Complementary and alternative medicine therapies in pediatric oncology patients. *J Soc Integr Oncol*. 2006;4(1):40–45.
71. Inoue M, Okamura T, Sawada A et al. Colostrum and severe gut GVHD. *Bone Marrow Transplant*. 1998;22:402–03.
72. Ladas E, Cheng B, Hughes D, Kroll D, Graf TN, Oberlies NH et al. Milk Thistle is Associated With Reductions in Liver Function Tests (LFTs) in Children Undergoing Therapy for Acute Lymphoblastic Leukemia (ALL). American Society of Hematology Annual Meeting December 9th, 2006. 2008
73. Aquino VM, Harvey AR, Garvin JH, Godder KT, Nieder ML, Adams RH, Jackson GB, Sandler ES. A double-blind randomized placebo-controlled study of oral glutamine in the prevention of mucositis in children undergoing hematopoietic stem cell transplantation: a pediatric blood and marrow transplant consortium study. Bone Marrow Transplant. 2005 Oct;36(7):611–6
74. Piersen CE. Phytoestrogens in botanical dietary supplements: implications for cancer. Integr Cancer Ther 2003;2(2):120–138.

Late Effects of Childhood Cancer Therapy

Nina S. Kadan-Lottick, Joseph P. Neglia, and Ann C. Mertens

Introduction

Childhood cancer has been transformed from a highly fatal disease 3 decades ago[1] to one currently associated with overall 5-year survival rates of over 75%.[2] This achievement has been accomplished through the development of effective multimodal therapy protocols and better supportive care, largely through cooperative multi-institutional clinical trials. With this success comes the obligation to measure outcomes and maximize the quality of life in the growing number of childhood cancer survivors who enter the general population every year.

Survivors are at increased risk for a range of adverse long-term outcomes, termed *late effects*. Potential late effects include mortality, subsequent malignant neoplasms, endocrinopathies, organ dysfunction, neurocognitive impairment, and psychological disorders, among others (see Table 42-1). Of the approximately 10 000 adult childhood cancer survivors followed in the Childhood Cancer Survivors Study (CCSS), 85% had at least one chronic disease, and 37% had a severe chronic disease such as a subsequent malignant neoplasm or myocardial infarction.[3] Late effects, such as cardiomyopathy and infertility, may present even many years after cessation of therapy. In general, the risk and severity of late outcomes have been associated with gender, age at diagnosis, and cumulative doses of specific therapies.[4] However, further research is needed to identify individual factors, including genetic factors, that explain why certain patients are more vulnerable to adverse sequelae from therapy.

This chapter will highlight some of the common late effects of childhood cancer and discuss follow-up care of survivors.

Mortality

Early investigations with small cohorts have shown an excess in mortality rates in 5-year survivors of childhood cancer.[5–10] Increased mortality rates were due primarily to recurrence of the primary disease, with estimates from to 61% to 75% of deaths, depending on the era of treatment (prior to 1970 vs post 1970) and the distribution of the initial cancers. These studies also noted that deaths due to

recurrence were highest 5 to 9 years post diagnosis. There were suggestions that death rates may also be increased due to other causes, including subsequent malignancies. These increases were associated with the original diagnosis,[6,7] radiation,[5,9] and combination chemotherapy and radiation.[11]

Two recent studies, looking at the risk of mortality in children and adolescents who survived 5 years post cancer diagnosis, were able to confirm and quantify these results. The CCSS is a multi-institutional retrospective study of individuals who were diagnosed with cancer between 1970 and 1986 during childhood or adolescence.[12] The second is a population-based study performed in the Nordic countries, on a similar population of children and adolescents diagnosed with cancer between 1960 and 1989.[11] The two studies showed very similar results.

All-cause mortality experience within CCSS from 5 years after initial cancer diagnosis was compared with age-adjusted expected survival rates for the U.S. population (Figure 42-1A). Overall, cumulative mortality was 6.4% at 10 years, 9.3% at 15 years, 11.4% at 20 years, and 14% at 25 years from diagnosis, and individuals remained at excess risk of death throughout this period. Individuals with an original diagnosis of kidney tumors and neuroblastoma had the best overall survival, with cumulative mortality proportions of about 5% at 20 years. Individuals with an original diagnosis of central nervous system (CNS) tumors had the poorest overall survival, with a cumulative mortality of 16.8% at 20 years. The cumulative cause-specific mortality was highest for cancer recurrence (7% at 25 years from diagnosis). The CCSS, which captured cancer treatment information, found a 19-fold increased risk in deaths due to a second or subsequent cancer (Figure 42-1B) related to radiation, alkylating agents, and epipodophyllotoxins. This study also identified an 8-fold increased risk for cardiac deaths, which was associated with exposure to chest irradiation.

Examining the pattern of deaths in 5-year survivors is helpful in understanding late relapse and the late effects of treatment. Both the CCSS and Nordic studies demonstrate that mortality is significantly lower in patients treated during the most recent treatment era, and that there is no increase in observed rates of deaths due to cancer treat-

Table 42-1

Potential late effects of various types of cancer.

Cancer	Potential Late Effects
Leukemias • Cognitive effects (eg, learning disabilities) • Abnormal growth and maturation • Heart problems • Second cancers • Hepatitis C (effects of blood transfusion) • Weakness, fatigue • Obesity • Osteoporosis • Avascular necrosis of bone • Dental problems	**Bone tumor** • Amputation/disfigurement • Functional, activity limitations • Damage to soft tissues and underlying bones (radiation may cause scarring, swelling, or inhibit growth) • Heart problems (e.g. cardiomyopathy, arrhythmias) • Hearing loss • Kidney damage • Second cancers • Hepatitis C • Fertility problems
Brain cancer • Neurologic and cognitive effects (eg, learning disabilities) • Abnormal growth and maturation • Hearing loss • Kidney damage • Hepatitis C • Infertility • Vision problems • Second cancers	**Wilms tumor** • Heart problems • Kidney damage • Damage to soft tissues and underlying bones (radiation may cause scarring, swelling, or inhibit growth) • Second cancers • Fertility problems • Scoliosis
Hodgkin disease • Adhesions and intestinal obstruction (if spleen removed) • Decreased resistance to infection (potential for life-threatening sepsis) • Abnormal growth and maturation • Hypothyroidism (effect of neck radiation) • Salivary gland malfunctioning (effect of irradiation) • Lung damage • Heart problems • Infertility • Hepatitis C • Second cancers (eg, breast cancer in females)	**Neuroblastoma** • Heart problems • Damage to soft tissues and underlying bones (radiation may cause scarring, swelling, or inhibit growth) • Neurocognitive effects • Hearing loss • Hepatitis C • Second cancers • Kidney damage
Non-Hodgkin lymphoma • Heart problems • Hepatitis C • Cognitive effects • Infertility • Osteopenia/osteoporosis	**Soft tissue sarcoma** • Amputation/disfigurement • Functional, activity limitations • Heart problems • Damage to soft tissues and underlying bones (radiation may cause scarring, swelling, or inhibit growth) • Second cancers • Hepatitis C • Kidney damage • Cataracts • Infertility • Neurocognitive effects

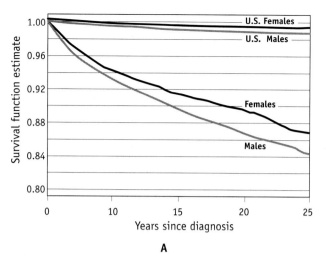

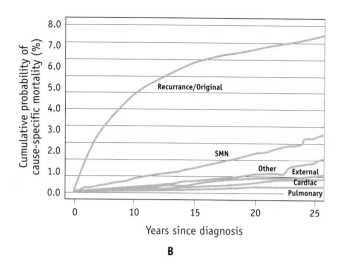

Figure 42-1 (A) All-cause mortality: sex-specific survival in the Childhood Cancer Survivor Study Cohort. (B) All-cause mortality: sex-specific survival in the Childhood Cancer Survivor Study Cohort.

ment. These findings suggest that current therapeutic regimens are successful in improving overall survival while not increasing the likelihood of the late consequences of disease and therapy.

Second Neoplasms

Among the many late effects that occur following the treatment of childhood cancer, few are as severe or disheartening as the occurrence of a new cancer. Second neoplasms (SNs) were first reported in the 1970s.[13] Since then SNs have been investigated in several populations of childhood cancer survivors, resulting in a large body of information describing the frequency of these events and the patient and treatment characteristics associated with an increased risk.

The risk of developing an SN is expressed in several ways, including cumulative risk (the percentage of patients who have developed a new cancer), standardized incidence ratio (SIR; the observed numbers of cancers compared with the expected numbers in a similar population), and annual excess risk (the expected number of excess cancers seen in the group over a specified period of time). Within large cohorts of children treated for cancer, the cumulative risk of cancer is approximately 3% to 5% at 20 to 25 years after primary cancer diagnosis.[14–16] These cumulative risks translate into approximately a 3- to 6-fold elevated risk compared with a non-childhood cancer survivor population. While plainly increased above what is expected, the excess annual risk of cancer among 5-year cancer survivors is only about 1.9 additional cases per 1000 years of follow-up.[14] These risks are higher when neoplasms such as meningioma and nonmelanoma skin cancer are included in the analysis.[17] With extended follow-up, the relative risk declines (as measured by the SIR) but still remains elevated, suggesting that there is an excess risk for life.[18]

Specific diagnostic subgroups have also been examined. The risk of second cancer is most dramatically increased among children with retinoblastoma, particularly those with hereditary retinoblastoma. In a recent study of over 1600 survivors of retinoblastoma, children with hereditary disease had a cumulative risk of a new cancer of 36% by 50 years from diagnosis, compared with 5.7% for children with nonhereditary disease.[19] Risk of a second cancer following therapy for retinoblastoma increases with increasing dose of radiotherapy[20] and alkylating agents.[21]

Patients with Hodgkin disease (HD) are also at particularly high risk of SNs. Among 5-year survivors of childhood cancer in the CCSS cohort (which does not include retinoblastoma cases), children with HD had the highest SIR (9.7), cumulative incidence of a second malignant neoplasm at 20 years (7.6%), and absolute excess risk (5.1 excess cancers/1000 years follow-up).[14] The risk of subsequent breast cancer among women treated for HD as children is strikingly elevated. The Late Effects Study Group estimated the risk of breast cancer at almost 35% by 40 years of age and showed associations with older age at treatment and use of higher doses of radiation.[22] Survivors of HD also appear to be at significant risk of secondary leukemias, thyroid cancers, and nonmelanoma skin cancers.[23,24] The reason for this level of risk among HD patients is unclear but does suggest that these patients require diligent surveillance. It is also important to note that while age may modify risk of subsequent cancer (particularly breast cancer) in this group, any female child treated with radiation to the chest requires close follow-up.[25,26]

Survivors of childhood acute lymphoblastic leukemia (ALL) are at relatively low risk for second cancers. In a study of over 9000 children treated for ALL on Children's Cancer Group (CCG) protocols between 1970 and 1988, the cumulative risk of second cancers was 2.5% at 15 years from diagnosis.[27] Risk was clearly associated with the use of prophylactic cranial radiation in this study and in a very large German study.[28] A more recent sample showed a lower risk, estimated to be 1.18% at 10 years from diagnosis.[29] Survivors of ALL do appear to be at elevated risk for

CNS tumors, both benign (primarily meningiomas) and malignant (often glioblastoma or anaplastic astrocytoma). The earlier CCG study showed a 23-fold excess risk of CNS malignancy among previously irradiated ALL survivors.[27] Among 1612 consecutively treated ALL patients at St Jude Children's Research Hospital, the cumulative risk of CNS tumors (including meningiomas) was 1.4% at 20 years from diagnosis.[30] Children younger than 6 years at diagnosis and who received cranial radiation therapy (CRT) were at greatest risk.

Investigations of specific second cancers have provided information important to the understanding or risk and mechanisms of risk. This is particularly evident in investigations of secondary leukemias, breast cancers, and thyroid cancers. In contrast to secondary solid tumors, secondary leukemias occur earlier after the diagnosis and treatment of the original cancer. Two distinct patterns of secondary acute myeloid leukemias (AML) are evident, one associated with alkylating agent exposure and the other with exposure to epipodophyllotoxins. The elevated risk of AML following alkylating agent exposure typically occurs between 4 and 6 years after exposure and returns to baseline by 15 years from exposure.[31] Risk is associated with increased doses of alkylating agents, and the leukemia cells typically show cytogenetic changes of chromosomes 5, 7, 8, or 9.[32] In contrast, exposure to the topoisomerase II inhibitors (specifically etoposide [VP-16] or teniposide [VM-26]) can result in secondary leukemias with shorter latency and specific abnormalities at the MLL locus on chromosome 11 (11q23). Risk appears to be associated with both the cumulative dose of the epipodophyllotoxin exposure and the timing of those exposures.[33,34]

As noted above, secondary breast cancers are increased among survivors of childhood HD, but any child treated with radiation therapy to the chest for any diagnosis should be considered at risk. The CCSS demonstrated the elevated risk of breast cancer in Wilms tumor patients who received chest radiation.[14] Increased risk has also been found in survivors with a history of childhood sarcomas, a family history of breast cancer, or a family history of thyroid disease. Radiation therapy to the pelvis appeared to reduce later breast cancer risk.[35]

Thyroid cancer risk is elevated after therapy for childhood cancer and is highest among those who received radiation. In contrast to the effect of radiation therapy in other cancers, the risk of thyroid cancer was found to increase with increasing dose of radiation up to 3000 centigray (cGy) but decreased at doses above 3000 cGy.[36] No association was observed with chemotherapy exposure. Children with neuroblastoma may be at greater risk for thyroid cancer[37]; however, this potential association is based on a very small number of cases.

Host modifiers of second cancer risk likely exist. While exposures to radiation and chemotherapy place a child at risk for a second cancer, it is apparent that the majority of children treated for cancer do not develop a subsequent neoplasm. An increasing number of investigators seek to identify factors that will determine which patients will develop SNs. These investigations have focused primarily on polymorphisms of genes that impact tissue repair or metabolism of chemotherapy.

Radiation sensitivity has been investigated through studies of both the ATM and XRCC1 genes. One study suggested that carriers of a mutated ATM gene are at increased risk of radiation-associated breast cancer[38]; however, this finding has not been substantiated in cancer survivors.[39] A study of SNs among radiated patients with a primary diagnosis of HD within the CCSS found an association between polymorphisms of glutathione transferase and risk of subsequent malignancy. Patients with mutations of the XRCC1 DNA repair enzyme gene had a nonstatistically significant increase in breast cancer risk but a decreased risk of thyroid cancer.[40]

Metabolism of chemotherapeutic agents is facilitated by several mechanisms, but investigations of associations between second cancers and drug metabolism have been limited primarily to the thiopurines and methotrexate. One report to date has shown an association between a host polymorphism with impaired thiopurine metabolism and an increased risk of secondary brain tumors.[41] Methylenetetrahydrofolate reductase polymorphisms have not been associated with subsequent cancer risk.[42] Studies of genetic susceptibility to second cancers are still preliminary and require validation by other investigators in other patient populations.

Cardiopulmonary Complications

The cardiotoxic effects of therapeutic radiation to the chest and anthracyclines have been well documented in the literature. These effects may manifest years after therapy and are often progressive in nature. Research has shown that radiation to the chest, mantle, and spine can lead to coronary artery disease, pericarditis, and valvular abnormalities. Those children and adolescents treated for HD who received mediastinal radiation have the highest risk for radiation-associated cardiovascular disease and deaths due to cardiac disease.[43] For HD survivors, radiation-associated coronary artery disease is the most common cardiac outcome.[44,45] Pericardial thickening has been demonstrated in children who received mediastinal irradiation for HD, suggesting that clinically significant constrictive pericarditis will occur with time.[46] Chest radiation is also associated with valvular disease, affecting mostly the left-sided valves.[45,47]

Anthracyclines are commonly used to treat childhood cancer, but their use is limited due to its cardiotoxic effects, particularly dose-related cardiomyopathy.[48] Children treated with anthracyclines may manifest impairment of the left ventricular contractility and increased afterload due to thinning of left ventricular walls, likely progressing to cardiac disease with time. An early case series identified doxorubicin-related congestive heart failure in children 5 to 10 years post diagnosis, an effect that had previously been seen only within the first year after completion of doxorubicin therapy.[49] Subsequent studies have reported subclinical cardiotoxicities, defined as an abnormal systolic function or an increased afterload, in previously healthy survivors of childhood cancer.[123,124] In a systemic review of the literature, Kremer et al found the reported frequency of subclinical cardiotoxicity varied between 0% and 57.4%.[50] When evaluating these studies by mean anthracycline dose, the range of reported frequencies was clearly higher for doses above 300 mg/m^2. One study showed that the incidence of cardiac abnormalities increased in every anthracycline dose level for patients who had also received mediastinal irradiation.[51] The incidence also increased with length of follow-up, suggesting that more time is needed to better estimate the incidence of progressive changes and symptomatic disease in survivors of childhood cancer.

Pulmonary function has also been shown to be compromised by anticancer therapy. The lung is one of the most radiation-sensitive structures in the body, and therapy-related radiation damage to the lung depends on the volume of lung tissue irradiated, total dose received, and the fractionation scheduling.[52] Radiation-induced lung disease involves an acute phase of radiation pneumonitis that occurs 2 to 6 months after exposure. The late phase of this disease is characterized by pulmonary fibrosis, which is usually asymptomatic. However, when the pulmonary fibrosis is symptomatic, it presents with dyspnea and a nonproductive cough.[53,54] Studies of children with cancer who received radiation have shown a significant reduction in lung function and dynamic lung compliance, possibly due to failure of alveolar development resulting from impaired cell proliferation.[53–57] Furthermore, increased occurrence of pulmonary abnormalities has been associated with dose-intensive protocols that include radiation and/or high cumulative doses of chemotherapy in survivors of leukemia,[58–60] rhabdomyosarcoma,[61] and HD[62–64] as well as individuals who received a bone marrow transplant.[65]

Pulmonary toxicity due to chemotherapy, like that associated with radiotherapy, also follows a pattern of an early phase resulting in interstitial lung injury occurring up to several months after treatment and a late phase with pulmonary fibrosis as the most common sequela.[52] Chemotherapy-induced lung fibrosis in childhood may remain asymptomatic for many years. Pulmonary toxicity has been shown to occur after exposure to bleomycin, mitomycin-C, and nitrosoureas, such as BCNU (carmustine) and CCNU (lomustine), busulfan, and cyclophosphamide.[66] Moreover, increased deaths due to pulmonary toxicity have been demonstrated following exposure to bleomycin[12] and BCNU.[67,68]

The CCSS determined the risk of pulmonary complications up to 25 years after diagnosis and treatment.[69] Based on subject self-report, this study identified a high incidence of significant pulmonary pathology, including lung fibrosis, chronic cough, pleurisy, decreased exercise tolerance, recurrent pneumonia, and use of supplemental oxygen among childhood cancer survivors. These adverse pulmonary outcomes were significantly associated with treatment-related factors. This analysis also showed that self-reported pulmonary complications continue to manifest more than 5 years from diagnosis, and the cumulative incidence continues to increase up to 25 years after diag-

nosis for those who received both chest radiation and pulmonary-toxic chemotherapy.

Neurocognitive Outcomes

Treatment for childhood cancer can result in damaging effects to the CNS. The spectrum of potential toxicities includes paralysis, neuropathies, hearing loss, blindness, and seizures. Furthermore, survivors may experience decline in intellectual function, learning problems, behavior disorders, school failure, and impaired employability.[70] Though this phenomenon was originally described for children who underwent CRT, subsequent studies have demonstrated that children treated only with chemotherapy are also at risk for neurobehavioral deficits. Children with leukemia and brain tumors with neoplasms originating in or abutting the CNS are at risk not only because of the primary site of disease but also due to the need to apply CNS-directed therapy.

Children with CNS tumors are uniquely at risk for neurologic late effects. A long-term follow-up study of Nordic children with benign tumors of the CNS found that 69% had at least one deficit and approximately 35% had moderate or severe sequelae, including ataxia, spastic paresis, vision loss, or epilepsy. One study concluded that children with hydrocephalus resulting from their tumor have more severe declines in intelligence quotient (IQ) if they require a ventriculo-peritoneal shunt.[71] A complication unique to children with posterior fossa tumors is the entity of "cerebellar mutism," which is a syndrome of loss of speech, hypotonia, and ataxia that can present in the immediate postoperative period but does not resolve entirely in some instances.[72,73] Relative to a sibling comparison group, a large series of 1607 patients with CNS tumors were at elevated risk for hearing impairments, blindness in one or both eyes, cataracts, and double vision.[74]

The neurotoxic effects of CRT have been well documented and are potentially debilitating. Histological changes associated with CRT consist of subacute leukoencephalopathy, mineralizing microangiopathy, and cortical atrophy, most often becoming apparent several months to years after CRT.[75–77] Figure 42-2 demonstrates some of these findings on magnetic resonance imaging (MRI). White matter seems to be especially vulnerable to CRT exposure.[78]

Domains of neurobehavioral impairment after CRT include impairments in short-term memory impairment, fine motor coordination, visual-spatial ability, and somatosensory functioning as well as easy distractibility.[79–84] These

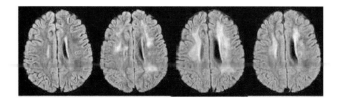

Figure 42-2 Leukoencephalopathy by MRI Fluid Attenuated Inversion Recovery (FLAIR) in patient with ALL at week 132 of therapy who received high-dose intravenous methotrexate.

cognitive impairments have been associated with a significantly reduced IQ and academic failure.[80,85] These deficits sometimes first emerge several years after diagnosis[86–88] and are most severe in those diagnosed at an age younger than 6 years[80,89] and among females.[90,91] Children who received cranial radiation as part of their therapy for ALL are more likely to receive special education services and have lower post-secondary education attainment compared with their siblings.[92] There appears to be a dose-response relationship, with cranial radiation doses of greater than 2400 cGy resulting in greater impairment.[93]

Chemotherapy exposures are also associated with neurobehavioral consequences, although the effects may be less devastating than those produced by CRT. Systemic administration of methotrexate may enhance both the acute and late toxicities of other CNS-directed therapies. Neurobehavioral deficits include decreases in full-scale and verbal IQ as well as in arithmetic achievement.[82] These conclusions were confirmed by Mulhern et al in a longitudinal study that compared children who received 1800 cGy, 2400 cGy, and no CRT.[86] There was no statistically significant difference between these groups, but overall, 22% to 30% of children experienced a clinically apparent deterioration in neurobehavioral function during the period of follow-up. The deficits were most marked among females. Among children with ALL treated on a non-radiation-containing protocol, acute neurotoxic events occurred significantly more often among those children who received intravenous methotrexate in addition to intrathecal methotrexate during consolidation therapy.[94] The presenting acute event was most commonly seizures, which accounted for 80% of the episodes. Computed tomography and MRI findings among those children with acute neurotoxicity were most commonly white-matter changes characterized as hypodense areas with or without microangiopathic calcifications.

Other chemotherapy agents have been associated with neurotoxicity. Patients who receive systemic high-dose cytarabine therapy can develop acute cerebellar syndrome, seizures, and encephalopathy.[95] Systemic and intrathecal cytarabine has also been associated with spinal cord necrosis.[96] The independent effect of glucocorticoids in the pediatric oncology population is less clear because of the confounding neurotoxicities of other concurrent therapies. However, pediatric patients with asthma on long-term steroid therapy experience greater depression, anxiety, and verbal memory deficits.[97] The administration of postnatal dexamethasone to preterm infants results in impaired cerebral cortical gray matter growth[98] and a significantly higher incidence of cerebral palsy and developmental delay.[99]

The intrathecal administration of chemotherapy agents may result in additional toxicity. In a study of patients treated at St Jude Children's Research Hospital, Ochs et al concluded that children who received intravenous methotrexate and intrathecal methotrexate had similar neurotoxicity to those who received 1800 cGy CRT and intrathecal methotrexate. Neurobehavioral deficits included decreases in full-scale and verbal IQ as well as in arithmetic achievement.[82] The effects of intrathecal cytarabine and

hydrocortisone have not been studied extensively as single agents. However, there is biochemical and autoradiographic evidence for glucocorticoid binding sites in the spinal cord.[100]

The clinical presentation of the late effects of CNS-delivered therapies is most evident in the learning difficulties experienced by children treated with combinations of radiation and chemotherapy for ALL, brain tumors, or other conditions requiring CNS-directed therapy. In an excellent recent review of neurocognitive late effects, Mulhern and Palmer described what they termed the "neurocognitive phenotype." This phenotype is characterized by limitations in the age-appropriate activities of daily living, including school performance, independent living, and specific domains of neurocognitive functioning.[101] Of these domains, "executive function," the ability to allocate attentional resources to planning and organization, may be most impacted.

Deficits in neurocognitive functioning often do not present until several years after treatment and can be subtle and/or subclinical. For these reasons, a presymptomatic neuropsychological assessment of intelligence, memory, attention, executive functioning, processing speed, visual motor integration, and math achievement may be beneficial. Patients may demonstrate abnormalities in more than one domain of function, especially as domains of function often show overlap in terms of brain function. The timing of this assessment depends on the individual patient but may be particularly helpful at school reentry to facilitate transition.

The comprehensive neurobehavioral assessment provides valuable data that can be used for educational accommodation and remediation of areas of impairment. An important component of this approach is to communicate test findings directly with teachers and other school staff who can use the information to enhance the child's learning, informally or formally through an individualized educational plan. School education services, such as speech/language therapy and occupational therapy, can help remediate domains of impairment. Other exciting intervention possibilities currently being researched include cognitive rehabilitation and stimulant medications to enhance attention and executive functioning.[102]

Psychological Outcomes

Psychological morbidity associated with CNS treatment has been observed among survivors of childhood ALL and brain tumors. While many studies report rates of psychological disturbance that are only slightly elevated compared with that observed in the general population,[103,104] others demonstrate increased mood disturbance (especially depression), posttraumatic stress symptoms,[105] poor body image, and inadequate coping skills.[104,106,107] Evaluating a patient can be challenging because adjustment problems and mood disorders can manifest as impaired concentration or reduced academic achievement.[103,108,109] Childhood cancer survivors with cognitive deficits may have challenges interpreting nonverbal social cues, which can impact negatively on socialization[110] and lead to feelings of isolation and inadequacy. It is important that evaluation of psychosocial functioning and neurocognitive functioning be done concurrently in distressed childhood cancer survivors to determine the most helpful intervention strategies.

Reproduction

Childhood cancer therapy may adversely affect sexual function and fertility. Disruptions in gonadal function are caused largely by alkylator chemotherapy, radiotherapy, and sometimes surgery. There is limited research on psychosocial aspects of parenthood after childhood cancer, but there is evidence that the illness experience increases the value that survivors place on family ties.[111] Because of gender-specific differences in normal gonadal development, cancer treatment may affect males and females differently.

In females, hormone production and potential for fertility are synchronous.[112] Females are born with their lifetime supply of oocytes, which starts at approximately 1 million to 2 million and decreases to 300 000 at puberty.[113] Therefore, the risk of oligomenorrhea, ovarian failure, and infertility increases with older age at treatment. Ovarian failure is associated with higher doses of alkylator agents, higher doses of radiation to the ovary, and older ages at exposures.[114] Prepubertal females can tolerate cumulative cyclophosphamide agents as high as 25 g/m². Acute loss of ovarian function soon after completing therapy is uncommon in females treated during childhood and adolescence, except in patients who received myeloablative doses of alkylator therapy as part of a stem cell transplant or direct ovarian radiation doses of greater than 1000 cGy.[114] However, even in survivors who initially have preserved ovarian function after therapy, there is an elevated risk of premature menopause later in life. In one series of women who received 2000 to 3000 cGy of whole-body irradiation as children, 26% had premature menopause, and 71% failed to enter puberty.[115] Loss of ovarian function in women is associated with reduced sexual function and libido.[116]

In general, males preserve endocrine function after higher doses of alkylator therapy than females. In contrast, the germinal epithelium is highly susceptible to injury by alkylator agents and radiotherapy because of its high rate of mitotic activity. All alkylating agents are gonadotoxic, while most cisplatin-based regiments cause only temporary interruption of spermatogenesis.[117] Younger prepubertal boys are at lower risk but are not spared.[112] Similarly, even doses of radiation as low as 200 to 700 cGy can cause transient effects on spermatogenesis, with improvement after 12 to 24 months.[117] Radiation doses of above 1200 cGy are more likely to results in permanent sterilization. Compared with the germinal epithelium, Leydig cells are relatively resistant to chemotherapy and radiation, likely due to their slower rate of cell turnover.[118] However, higher doses of alkylator therapy have been associated with failure to progress through puberty in younger patients and loss of libido and erectile dysfunction in adult men.[118] Similarly, higher doses

of radiation of at least 2400 cGy result in Leydig cell dysfunction.[116] Males who undergo bilateral retroperitoneal lymph node dissection frequently experience retrograde ejaculation and impotence.[116]

Long-Term Follow-Up Care

Because of their unique health needs, childhood cancer survivors require risk-based health care that is specific to their individual treatment exposures, genetic predispositions, personal behaviors, and comorbid health conditions.[119] Ideally, this care would be comprehensive and include the following components: (1) surveillance for potential late effects, (2) patient education regarding late outcomes and preventive health practices, (3) psychosocial support for patients and their families, (4) reproductive and sexuality counseling, and (5) genetic counseling, if indicated.[120] Late effects may not manifest until several years after cessation of therapy. Therefore, it is important to maintain active follow-up of childhood cancer survivors as they transition through adolescence and into adulthood.[121] It is not yet clear which health care model (eg, pediatric vs internal medicine vs family practice, physician vs nurse clinician, primary care vs tertiary care setting, etc) would best meet the needs of childhood cancer survivors. This issue is particularly challenging because patients are diagnosed during childhood but require survivorship care throughout adulthood. The Institute of Medicine recommends that cancer survivors be given information about their cancer and its treatment and an individualized plan for follow-up and guidance on preventive health practices at the time of completion of therapy.[120] Efforts are under way to develop ways that this information can be shared such that it remains accessible during adulthood.

In an effort to respond to the lack of consensus regarding the care of survivors, the National Cancer Institute-funded Children's Oncology Group has developed risk-based, exposure-related clinical practice guidelines for screening and management of late effects resulting from previous cancer treatment.[122] These guidelines were formulated by a broad panel of national experts who based their statement of consensus on evidence available in the literature as well as their collective clinical experience. Associated with the guidelines are patient education materials termed "Health Links." The Children's Oncology Group Long Term Follow-Up Guidelines and related Health Links are available at www.survivorshipguidelines.org. Research studies are in progress to determine if adherence to these guidelines impacts morbidity and mortality among childhood cancer survivors.

Summary

All of the therapies necessary to successfully treat a child for cancer carry risk. It is an unfortunate and sometimes very high price paid by these children and their families in exchange for "cure" of the original disease. The evolution of therapy and the information gained by both population and basic investigations of these late effects have allowed us to more accurately predict which patients are at risk and initiate appropriate interventions to allow early identification of late effects and reduce their severity if possible. In some instances primary therapy has been modified to eliminate or reduce exposure to the therapeutic modalities most likely to produce significant late effects. The team caring for each patient must balance the risk of late complications with the treatment needed to cure the primary cancer, knowing that there is risk but also that recurrence of the original disease remains the most likely cause of death in our patients. The knowledge of these outcomes, the need to appropriately screen and counsel patients, and the critical need for research in this area all strongly argue for the continued, thorough follow-up of all children treated for cancer.

References

1. Ries LAG, Smith MA, Gurney JG, et al, eds. Cancer Incidence and Survival Among Children and Adolescents: United States SEER Program 1975–1995. NIH Pub. No. 99-4649. Bethesda, MD: National Cancer Institute SEER Program; 1999.
2. Jemal A, Clegg LX, Ward E, et al. Annual report to the nation on the status of cancer, 1975–2001, with a special feature regarding survival. *Cancer.* 2004; 101(1):3–27.
3. Oeffinger KC, Mertens C, Sklar CA, et al. Prevalence and severity of chronic diseases in adult survivors of childhood cancer: a report from the Childhood Cancer Survivors Study. In Proceedings from the 41st Annual Meeting of the American Society of Clinical Oncology. Orlando, FL. 2005.
4. Hudson MM, Mertens AC, Yasui Y, et al. Health status of adult long-term survivors of childhood cancer: a report from the Childhood Cancer Survivor Study. *JAMA.* 2003;290(12):1583–1592.
5. Li FP, Myers MH, Heise HW, Jaffe N, et al. The course of five-year survivors of cancer in childhood. *J Pediatr.* 1978;93(2):185–187.
6. Hawkins MM, Kingston JE, Kinnier Wilson LM. Late deaths after treatment for childhood cancer. *Arch Dis Child.* 1990;65(12):1356–1363.
7. Robertson CM, Hawkins MM, Kingston JE. Late deaths and survival after childhood cancer: implications for cure. *BMJ* 1994;309(6948):162–166.
8. Nicholson HS, Fears TR, Byrne J. Death during adulthood in survivors of childhood and adolescent cancer. *Cancer.* 1994;73(12):3094–3102.
9. Hudson MM, Jones D, Boyett J, Sharp GB, Pui C-H, et al. Late mortality of long-term survivors of childhood cancer. *J Clin Oncol.* 1997;15(6):2205–2213.
10. Green DM, Reese PA, Michalek AM, Zevon MA, Lowrie GS. Factors that influence the further survival of patients who survive for five years after the diagnosis of cancer in childhood or adolescence. *Med Pediatr Oncol.* 1994; 22(2):91–96.
11. Möller TR, Garwicz S, Barlow L, et al. Decreasing late mortality among five-year survivors of cancer in childhood and adolescence: a population-based study in the Nordic countries. *J Clin Oncol.* 2001;19(13):3173–3181.
12. Mertens AC, Yasui Y, Neglia JP, et al. Late mortality experience in five-year survivors of childhood and adolescent cancer: the Childhood Cancer Survivor Study. *J Clin Oncol.* 2001;19(13):3163–3172.
13. Li FP, Cassady JR, Jaffe N. Risk of second tumors in survivors of childhood cancer. *Cancer.* 1975;35(4):1230–1235.
14. Neglia JP, Friedman DL, Yasui Y, et al. Second malignant neoplasms in five-year survivors of childhood cancer: childhood cancer survivor study. *J Natl Cancer Inst.* 2001;93(8):618–629.
15. Jenkinson HC, Hawkins MM, Stiller CA, et al. Long-term population-based risks of second malignant neoplasms after childhood cancer in Britain. *Br J Cancer.* 2004;91(11):1905–1910.
16. Olsen JH, Garwicz S, Hertz H, et al. Second malignant neoplasms after cancer in childhood or adolescence. Nordic Society of Paediatric Haematology and Oncology Association of the Nordic Cancer Registries. *BMJ.* 1993;307(6911):1030–1036.
17. Jazbec J, Ecimovic P, Jereb B. Second neoplasms after treatment of childhood cancer in Slovenia. *Pediatr Blood Cancer.* 2004;42(7):574–581.
18. Friedman D, Whitton J, Yasui Y, et al. Risk of second malignant neoplasms (SMN) 20 years after childhood cancer: the updated experience of the Childhood Cancer Survivor Study (CCSS). *J Clin Oncol.* 2004 ASCO Annual Meeting Proceedings (Post-Meeting Edition). 2004;22(14S):8509.
19. Kleinerman RA, Tucker MA, Tarone RE, et al. Risk of new cancers after radiotherapy in long-term survivors of retinoblastoma: an extended follow-up. *J Clin Oncol.* 2005;23(10):2272–2279.
20. Wong FL, Boice JD, Abramson DH, et al. Cancer incidence after retinoblastoma. Radiation dose and sarcoma risk. *JAMA.* 1997;278(15):1262–1267.
21. Tucker MA, D'Angio GI, Boice JD, et al. Bone sarcomas linked to radiotherapy and chemotherapy in children. *N Engl J Med.* 1987;317(10):588–593.
22. Bhatia S, Robison LL, Oberlin O, et al. Breast cancer and other second neoplasms after childhood Hodgkin's disease. *N Engl J Med.* 1996;334(12):745–751.
23. Bhatia S, Yasui Y, Robison LL, et al. High risk of subsequent neoplasms continues with extended follow-up of childhood Hodgkin's disease: report from the Late Effects Study Group. *J Clin Oncol.* 2003;21(23):4386–4394.
24. Perkins JL, Liu Y, Mitby PA, et al. Nonmelanoma skin cancer in survivors of childhood and adolescent cancer: a report from the childhood cancer survivor study. *J Clin Oncol.* 2005;23(16):3733–3741.
25. Yasui Y, Liu Y, Neglia JP, et al. A methodological issue in the analysis of second-primary cancer incidence in long-term survivors of childhood cancers. *Am J Epidemiol.* 2003;158(11):1108–1113.
26. Ronckers CM, Land C, Neglia J, Meadows A. Breast cancer. *Lancet.* 2005; 366(9497):1605–1606; author reply 1606.
27. Neglia JP, Meadows AT, Robison LL, et al. Second neoplasms after acute lymphoblastic leukemia in childhood. *N Engl J Med.* 1991;325(19):1330–1336.
28. Loning L, Zimmermann M, Reiter A, et al. Secondary neoplasms subsequent to Berlin-Frankfurt-Munster therapy of acute lymphoblastic leukemia in childhood: significantly lower risk without cranial radiotherapy. *Blood.* 2000; 95(9):2770–2775.
29. Bhatia S, Sather HN, Pabustan OB, et al. Low incidence of second neoplasms among children diagnosed with acute lymphoblastic leukemia after 1983. *Blood.* 2002;99(12):4257–4264.
30. Walter AW, Hancock ML, Pui CH, et al. Secondary brain tumors in children treated for acute lymphoblastic leukemia at St Jude Children's Research Hospital. *J Clin Oncol.* 1998;16(12):3761–3767.
31. Bhatia S, Sklar C. Second cancers in survivors of childhood cancer. *Nat Rev Cancer.* 2002;12(2):124–132.
32. Dann EJ, Rowe JM. Biology and therapy of secondary leukaemias. *Best Pract Res Clin Haematol.* 2001;14(1):119–137.
33. Hawkins MM, Wilson LM, Stovall MA, et al. Epipodophyllotoxins, alkylating agents, and radiation and risk of secondary leukaemia after childhood cancer. *BMJ.* 1992;304(6832):951–958.
34. Pui CH, Ribeiro RC, Hancock ML, et al. Acute myeloid leukemia in children treated with epipodophyllotoxins for acute lymphoblastic leukemia. *N Engl J Med.* 1991;325(24):1682–1687.
35. Kenney LB, Yasui Y, Inskip PD, et al. Breast cancer after childhood cancer: a report from the Childhood Cancer Survivor Study. *Ann Intern Med.* 2004; 141(8):590–597.
36. Sigurdson A, Ronckers C, Mertens A, et al. Primary thyroid cancer after a first tumour in childhood (the Childhood Cancer Survivor Study): a nested case-control study. *Lancet.* 2005;365(9476):2014–2023.
37. de Vathaire, François P, Schweisguth O, Oberlin O, Le MG. Irradiated neuroblastoma in childhood as potential risk factor for subsequent thyroid tumour. *Lancet.* 1988;2(8608):455.
38. Swift M, Morrell D, Massey RB, Chase CL. Incidence of cancer in 161 families affected by ataxia-telangiectasia. *N Engl J Med.* 1991;325(26):1831–1836.
39. Nichols KE, Levitz S, Shannon KE, et al. Heterozygous germline ATM mutations do not contribute to radiation-associated malignancies after Hodgkin's disease. *J Clin Oncol.* 1999;17(4):1259.
40. Mertens AC, Mitby PA, Radloff G, et al. XRCC1 and glutathione-S-transferase gene polymorphisms and susceptibility to radiotherapy-related malignancies in survivors of Hodgkin disease. *Cancer.* 2004;101(6):1463–1472.
41. Relling MV, Rubnitz JE, Rivera GK, et al. High incidence of secondary brain tumours after radiotherapy and antimetabolites [see comment]. *Lancet.* 1999; 354(9172):34–39.
42. Jazbec J, Kitanovski, Aplenc R, Debeljak M, Dolžan V. No evidence of association of methylenetetrahydrofolate reductase polymorphism with occurrence of second neoplasms after treatment of childhood leukemia. *Leuk Lymphoma.* 2005;46(6):893–897.
43. Hancock SL, Donaldson SS, Hoppe RT. Cardiac disease following treatment of Hodgkin's disease in children and adolescents. *J Clin Oncol.* 1993;11(7): 1208–1215.
44. King V, Constine LS, Clark D, et al. Symptomatic coronary artery disease after mantle irradiation for Hodgkin's disease. *Int J Radiat Oncol Biol Phys.* 1996; 36(4):881–889.
45. Hull MC, Morris CG, Pepine CJ, Mendenhall NP. Valvular dysfunction and carotid, subclavian, and coronary artery disease in survivors of Hodgkin lymphoma treated with radiation therapy. *JAMA.* 2003;290(21):2831–2837.
46. Green DM, Gingell RL, Pearce J, Panahon AM, Ghoorah J. The effect of mediastinal irradiation on cardiac function of patients treated during childhood and adolescence for Hodgkin's disease. *J Clin Oncol.* 1987;5(2): 239–245.
47. Lund MB, Ihlen H, Voss BM, et al. Increased risk of heart valve regurgitation after mediastinal radiation for Hodgkin's disease: an echocardiographic study. *Heart.* 1996;75(6):591–595.
48. Adams M, Lipshultz S, Schwartz C, et al. Radiation-associated cardiovascular disease: manifestations and management. *Sem Radiat Oncol.* 2003;13:346–356.
49. Goorin AM, Chauvenet AR, Perez-Atayde AR, et al. Initial congestive heart failure, six to ten years after doxorubicin chemotherapy for childhood cancer. *J Pediatr.* 1990;116(1):144–147.
50. Kremer LC, van Dalen EC, Offringa M, Ottenkamp J, Voûte PA. Anthracycline-induced clinical heart failure in a cohort of 607 children: long-term follow-up study. *J Clin Oncol.* 2001;19(1):191–196.

51. Steinherz LJ, et al. Cardiac toxicity 4 to 20 years after completing anthracycline therapy. *JAMA*. 1991;266(12):1672–1677.
52. Abid SH, Malhotra V, Perry MC. Radiation-induced and chemotherapy-induced pulmonary injury. *Curr Opin Oncol*. 2001;13(4):242–248.
53. Fryer CJ, Fitzpatrick PJ, Rider WD, Poon P. Radiation pneumonitis: experience following a large single dose of radiation. *Int J Radiat Oncol Biol Phys*. 1978;4(11–12):931–936.
54. Jakacki RI, Schramm CM, Donahue BR, Haas F, Allen JC. Restrictive lung disease following treatment for malignant brain tumors: a potential late effect of craniospinal irradiation. *J Clin Oncol*. 1995;13(6):1478–1485.
55. Wohl ME, Griscom NT, Traggis DG, Jaffe N. Effects of therapeutic irradiation delivered in early childhood upon subsequent lung function. *Pediatrics*. 1975;55(4):507–516.
56. Benoist MR, Lemerle J, Jean R, et al. Effects of pulmonary function of whole lung irradiation for Wilm's tumour in children. *Thorax*. 1982;37(3):175–180.
57. Miller RW, Fusner JE, Fink RJ, et al. Pulmonary function abnormalities in long-term survivors of childhood cancer. *Med Pediatr Oncol*. 1986;14(4):202–207.
58. Shaw NJ, Tweeddale PM, Eden OB. Pulmonary function in childhood leukaemia survivors. *Med Pediatr Oncol*. 1989;17(2):149–154.
59. Jenney ME, Faragher EB, Jones PHM, Woodcock A. Lung function and exercise capacity in survivors of childhood leukaemia. *Med Pediatr Oncol*. 1995;24(4):222–230.
60. Nysom K, Holm K, Olsen JH, Hertz H, Hesse B. Pulmonary function after treatment for acute lymphoblastic leukaemia in childhood. *Br J Cancer*. 1998;78(1):21–27.
61. Kaplan E, Sklar C, Wilmott R, Michaels SS, Ghavimi F. Pulmonary function in children treated for rhabdomyosarcoma. *Med Pediatr Oncol*. 1996;27(2):79–84.
62. Mefferd JM, Donaldson SS, Link MP. Pediatric Hodgkin's disease: pulmonary, cardiac, and thyroid function following combined modality therapy. *Int J Radiat Oncol Biol Phys*. 1989;16(3):679–685.
63. Marina NM, Greenwald CA, Fairclough DL, et al. Serial pulmonary function studies in children treated for newly diagnosed Hodgkin's disease with mantle radiotherapy plus cycles of cyclophosphamide, vincristine, and procarbazine alternating with cycles of doxorubicin, bleomycin, vinblastine, and dacarbazine. *Cancer*. 1995;75(7):1706–1711.
64. Bossi G, Cerveri I, Volpini E, et al. Long-term pulmonary sequelae after treatment of childhood Hodgkin's disease. *Ann Oncol*. 1997;8(Suppl 1):19–24.
65. Cerveri I, Zoia MC, Fulgoni P, et al. Late pulmonary sequelae after childhood bone marrow transplantation. *Thorax*. 1999;54(2):131–135.
66. Ginsberg SJ, Comis RL. The pulmonary toxicity of antineoplastic agents. *Semin Oncol*. 1982;9(1):34–51.
67. O'Driscoll BR, Kalra S, Gattamaneni HR, Woodcock AA. Late carmustine lung fibrosis: age at treatment may influence severity and survival. *Chest*. 1995;107(5):1355–1357.
68. O'Driscoll BR, Hasleton PS, Taylor PM, et al. Active lung fibrosis up to 17 years after chemotherapy with carmustine (BCNU) in childhood. *N Engl J Med*. 1990;323(6):378–382.
69. Mertens AC, Yasui Y, Liu Y, et al. Pulmonary complications in survivors of childhood and adolescent cancer: a report from the Childhood Cancer Survivor Study. *Cancer*. 2002;95(11):2431–2441.
70. Stam H, Grootenhuis MA, Last BF. Social and emotional adjustment in young survivors of childhood cancer. *Support Care Cancer*. 2001;9(7):489–513.
71. Packer RJ, Sposto R, Atkins TE, et al. Quality of life in children with primitive neuroectodermal tumors (medulloblastoma) of the posterior fossa. *Pediatr Neurosci*. 1987;13(4):169–175.
72. Gelabert-Gonzalez M, Fernandez-Villa J. Mutism after posterior fossa surgery: review of the literature. *Clin Neurol Neurosurg*. 2001;103(2):111–114.
73. Steinbok P, Cochrane DD, Perrin R, Price A. Mutism after posterior fossa tumour resection in children: incomplete recovery on long-term follow-up. *Pediatr Neurosurg*. 2003;39(4):179–183.
74. Packer RJ, Gurney JG, Punyko JA, et al. Long-term neurologic and neurosensory sequelae in adult survivors of a childhood brain tumor: childhood cancer survivor study. *J Clin Oncol*. 2003;21(17):3255–3261.
75. Riccardi R, Brouwers, Di Chiro G, Poplack DG. Abnormal computed tomography brain scans in children with acute lymphoblastic leukemia: serial long-term follow-up. *J Clin Oncol*. 1985;3(1):12–18.
76. Crosley CJ, Rorke LB, Evans A, Nigro M. Central nervous system lesions in childhood leukemia. *Neurology*. 1978;28(7):678–685.
77. Price R. Therapy related central nervous system diseases in children with acute lymphocytic leukemia. In Mastrangelo R, Poplack D, Riccardi R, eds. *Central Nervous System Leukemia*. Boston: Martimus Nijhoff; 1983.
78. Schultheiss TE, Kun LE, Ang KK, Stephens LC. Radiation response of the central nervous system. *Int J Radiat Oncol Biol Phys*. 1995;31(5):1093–1112.
79. Meadows AT, Gordon J, Massari DJ, et al. Declines in IQ scores and cognitive dysfunctions in children with acute lymphocytic leukaemia treated with cranial irradiation. *Lancet*. 1981;2(8254):1015–1018.
80. Cousens P, Waters B, Said J, Stevens M. Cognitive effects of cranial irradiation in leukaemia: a survey and meta-analysis. *J Child Psychol Psychiatry*. 1988;29(6):839–852.
81. Rodgers J, Britton PG, Morris RG, Kernahan J, Graft AW. Memory after treatment for acute lymphoblastic leukaemia. *Arch Dis Child*. 1992;67:266–268.
82. Ochs J, Mulhern RK, Fairclough D, et al. Comparison of neuropsychologic functioning and clinical indicators of neurotoxicity in long-term survivors of childhood leukemia given cranial radiation or parenteral methotrexate: a prospective study. *J Clin Oncol*. 1991;9(1):145–151.
83. Brown RT, Madan-Swain A. Cognitive, neuropsychological, and academic sequelae in children with leukemia. *J Learn Disabil*. 1993;26(2):74–90.
84. Stehbens JA. CNS prophylaxis of childhood leukemia: what are the long-term neurological, neuropsychological, and behavioral effects? *Neuropsychol Rev*. 1991;2(2):147–177.
85. Radcliffe J, Bunin GR, Sutton LN, Goldwein JW, Phillips PC. Cognitive deficits in long-term survivors of childhood medulloblastoma and other non-cortical tumors: age-dependent effects of whole brain radiation. *Int J Dev Neurosci*. 1994;12(4):327–334.
86. Mulhern RK, Fairclough D, Ochs J. A prospective comparison of neuropsychologic performance of children surviving leukemia who received 18-Gy, 24-Gy, or no cranial irradiation. *J Clin Oncol*. 1991;9(8):1348–1356.
87. Rubenstein CL, Varni JW, Katz ER. Cognitive functioning in long-term survivors of childhood leukemia: a prospective analysis. *J Dev Behav Pediatr*. 1990;11(6):301–305.
88. Jankovic M, Brouwers P, Valsecchi MG, et al. Association of 1800 cGy cranial irradiation with intellectual function in children with acute lymphoblastic leukaemia. ISPACC. International Study Group on Psychosocial Aspects of Childhood Cancer. *Lancet*. 1994;344(8917):224–227.
89. Robison LL, Nesbit ME, Sather HN, et al. Factors associated with IQ scores in long-term survivors of childhood acute lymphoblastic leukemia. *Am J Pediatr Hematol Oncol*. 1984;6(2):115–121.
90. Waber DP, Urion DK, Tarbell NJ, et al. Late effects of central nervous system treatment of acute lymphoblastic leukemia in childhood are sex-dependent. *Dev Med Child Neurol*. 1990;32(3):238–248.
91. Bleyer WA, Fallavollita J, Robison L, et al. Influence of age, sex, and concurrent intrathecal methotrexate therapy on intellectual function after cranial irradiation during childhood: a report from the Children's Cancer Study Group. *Pediatr Hematol Oncol*. 1990;7(4):329–338.
92. Kingma A, Rammeloo LAJ, vander Does-vanden Berg A, Rekers-Mombarg L, Postma A. Academic career after treatment for acute lymphoblastic leukaemia. *Arch Dis Child*. 2000;82(5):353–357.
93. Fuss M, Poljanc K, Hug EB, Full Scale IQ (FSIQ) changes in children treated with whole brain and partial brain irradiation: a review and analysis. *Strahlenther Onkol*. 2000;176(12):573–581.
94. Mahoney DH, Shuster JJ, Nitschke R, et al. Acute neurotoxicity in children with B-precursor acute lymphoid leukemia: an association with intermediate-dose intravenous methotrexate and intrathecal triple therapy—a Pediatric Oncology Group study. *J Clin Oncol*. 1998;16(5):1712–1722.
95. Peylan-Ramu N, Poplack DG, Pizzo PA, Adornato BT, Di Chiro G. Abnormal CT scans of the brain in asymptomatic children with acute lymphocytic leukemia after prophylactic treatment of the central nervous system with radiation and intrathecal chemotherapy. *N Engl J Med*. 1978;298(15):815–818.
96. Watterson J, Toogood I, Nieder M, et al. Excessive spinal cord toxicity from intensive central nervous system-directed therapies. *Cancer*. 1994;74(11):3034–3041.
97. Bender BG, Lerner JA, Poland JE. Association between corticosteroids and psychologic change in hospitalized asthmatic children. *Ann Allergy*. 1991;66(5):414–419.
98. Murphy BP, Inder TE, Huppi PS, et al. Impaired cerebral cortical gray matter growth after treatment with dexamethasone for neonatal chronic lung disease. *Pediatrics*. 2001;107(2):217–221.
99. Shinwell ES, Karplus M, Reich D, et al. Early postnatal dexamethasone treatment and increased incidence of cerebral palsy. *Arch Dis Child Fetal Neonatal Ed*. 2000;83(3):F177–181.
100. Orti E, Tornello S, De Nicola AF. Dynamic aspects of glucocorticoid receptors in the spinal cord of the rat. *J Neurochem*. 1985;45(6):1699–1707.
101. Mulhern RK, Palmer SL. Neurocognitive late effects in pediatric cancer. *Curr Probl Cancer*. 2003;27(4):177–197.
102. Butler RW, Mulhern RK. Neurocognitive interventions for children and adolescents surviving cancer. *J Pediatr Psychol*. 2005;30(1):65–78.
103. Butler RW, Rizzie LP, Bandilla EB. The effects of childhood cancer and its treatment on two objective measures of psychological functioning. *Child Health Care*. 1999;28(4):311–317.
104. Mackie E, Hill J, Kondryn H, McNally R. Adult psychosocial outcomes in long-term survivors of acute lymphoblastic leukaemia and Wilms' tumour: a controlled study. *Lancet*. 2000;355(9212):1310–1314.
105. Langeveld NE, Grootenhuis MA, Voute PA, De Haan RJ. Posttraumatic stress symptoms in adult survivors of childhood cancer. *Pediatr Blood Cancer*. 2004;42(7):604–610.
106. Zeltzer LK, Chen E, Weiss R, et al. Comparison of psychologic outcome in adult survivors of childhood acute lymphoblastic leukemia versus sibling controls: a cooperative Children's Cancer Group and National Institutes of Health study. *J Clin Oncol*. 1997;15(2):547–556.
107. Zebrack BJ, Zeltzer LK, Whitton J, et al. Psychological outcomes in long-term survivors of childhood leukemia, Hodgkin's disease, and non-Hodgkin's lymphoma: a report from the Childhood Cancer Survivor Study. *Pediatrics*. 2002;110(1 Pt 1):42–52.
108. Moore IM, Challinor J, Pasvogel A, et al. Online exclusive: behavioral adjustment of children and adolescents with cancer: teacher, parent, and self-report. *Oncol Nurs Forum*. 2003;30(5):E84–91.

109. Levin Newby W, Brown RT, Pawletko TM, Gold SH, Whitt JK. Social skills and psychological adjustment of child and adolescent cancer survivors. *Psychooncology*. 2000;9(2):113–126.

110. Fossen A, Abrahamsen TG, Storm-Mathisen I. Psychological outcome in children treated for brain tumor. *Pediatr Hematol Oncol*. 1998;15(6):479–488.

111. Schover LR, Motivation for parenthood after cancer: a review. *J Natl Cancer Inst Monogr*. 2005(34):2–5.

112. Friedman DL, Meadows AT. Late effects of childhood cancer therapy. *Pediatr Clin North Am*. 2002;49(5):1083–106, x.

113. Friedman D. The ovary. In: Schwartz D, et al, eds. *Survivors of Childhood and Adolescent Cancer*. Berlin: Springer-Verlag; 2005.

114. Sklar C. Maintenance of ovarian function and risk of premature menopause related to cancer treatment. *J Natl Cancer Inst Monogr*. 2005 (34):25–27.

115. Wallace W, Shalet SM, Crowne EC, Morris-Jones PH, Gattamaneni HR. Ovarian failure following abdominal irradiation in childhood: natural history and prognosis. *Clin Oncol*. 1989;1:75–79.

116. Green DM. Late effects of treatment for cancer during childhood and adolescence. *Curr Probl Cancer*. 2003;27(3):127–142.

117. Howell SJ, Shalet SM. Spermatogenesis after cancer treatment: damage and recovery. *J Natl Cancer Inst Monogr*. 2005(34):12–17.

118. Ginsberg J, Maity A. The testes. In: Schwartz D, et al, eds. *Survivors of Childhood and Adolescent Cancer*. Berlin: Springer-Verlag; 2005.

119. Oeffinger KC, Hudson MM. Long-term complications following childhood and adolescent cancer: foundations for providing risk-based health care for survivors. *CA Cancer J Clin*. 2004;54(4):208–236.

120. Institute of Medicine. *Childhood Cancer Survivorship: Improving Care and Quality of Life*. Washington, DC: National Academies Press; 2004.

121. Oeffinger KC, Eshelman DA, Tomlinson GE, Buchanan GR. Programs for adult survivors of childhood cancer. *J Clin Oncol*. 1998;16(8):2864–2867.

122. Landiér W, Bhatia S, Eshelman DA, et al. Development of risk-based guidelines for pediatric cancer survivors: the Children's Oncology Group Long-Term Follow-Up Guidelines from the Children's Oncology Group Late Effects Committee and Nursing Discipline. *J Clin Oncol*. 2004;22(24):4979–4990.

123. Lipshultz SE, Alvarez JA, Scully RE. Anthracycline associated cardiotoxicity in survivors of childhood cancer. *Heart*. 2008;94:525–533.

124. Silber JH. Role of afterload reduction in the prevention of late anthracycline cardiomyopathy. *Pediatr Blood & Cancer*. 2005:44(7);607–613.

INDEX

A

molecularly targeted therapies for, 26–27, 101
treatment of, 202–204
acyclovir, 229, 492, 494
adaptation, social and behavioral, test battery for, 548, 550, 551
adaptive immune system, 33
ADCC (antibody-dependent cellular cytotoxicity), 38–39, 325
adenoma
  biliary tree, 409
  cystic. See cyst(s)
  hepatic, 409, 416, 417
adjuvant analgesics, 545
adjuvant chemotherapy
  beneficial effects of, 95–96
  for colorectal cancer, 470
  for ependymoma, 274
  for germ cell tumors, 309–310
  for gliomas, 262, 263, 264, 265
  for hepatic tumors, 425–429
  for medulloblastoma, 284
  for melanoma, 473
  for nasopharyngeal carcinoma, 474
  for neuroblastoma, 323
  for osteosarcoma, 389, 391
  for retinoblastoma, 448–449
  for soft-tissue sarcomas, 347, 349
  for systemic germ cell tumors, 370, 374
adjuvant therapies
  for nausea, 537–538
  radioiodine, for thyroid cancer, 462–463
administration routes
  for analgesics, 543–544
  for chemotherapy, 103, 110
adolescents
  astrocytomas in, 291
  social/behavioral adaptations of, 551
adoptive transfer, in immunotherapy, 38
adrenal neuroblastoma, 317, 321
  radiation field planning for, 131, 132
  surgical resection and, 116
adrenalectomy, ipsilateral, in Wilms tumor resection, 117, 118
adrenocortical carcinoma (ACC), 6, 9, 467–468
adrenocorticolytic agents, for adrenocortical carcinoma, 468
adriamycin
  for acute lymphoblastic leukemia, 171, 176
  for hepatic tumors, 426, 429
  for Hodgkin lymphoma, 238, 240
advance directives, 517
advocacy, for global initiatives, 15–16, 17
AF1q gene, 196
afferent signals, in nausea physiology, 531, 532
AFP. See alpha-fetoprotein (AFP)
Africa, cancer care initiatives in, 17
age
  acute myeloid leukemia and, 185, 193
  bone tumor incidence and, 383
  chemotherapy administration and, 103

germ cell tumor incidence and, 304
ionizing radiation risks and, 69
Langerhans cell histiocytosis risk and, 247
nausea and vomiting related to, 532
in nutrition assessment, 525, 526
age at diagnosis
  of acute lymphoblastic leukemia, 166, 167, 177
  neurobehavioral sequelae related to, 548, 549
  of neuroblastoma, 319, 321, 322
  as prognostic factor, 45, 273
  of renal tumors, 329, 332
  of retinoblastoma, 437, 441, 442, 449
  of rhabdomyosarcoma, 345, 346
AHSCT. See autologous hematopoietic stem cell transplantation (AHSCT)
airway compromise
  with rhabdomyosarcoma, 343
  in superior vena cava syndrome, 485–486
AJCC (American Joint Committee on Cancer) staging system, for thyroid cancer, 461, 462
Alagille syndrome, 410, 411
albumin, in nutritional assessment, 525
ALCL. See anaplastic large cell lymphoma (ALCL)
alcohol consumption, hepatic tumors and, 410
alemtuzumab, 39, 256
ALK (anaplastic lymphoma kinase) gene protein, 57, 58, 61, 227, 228, 317
alkaline phosphatase
  in osteosarcoma, 386
  placental, as germ cell tumor marker, 305, 307, 360, 362
alkylating agents
  for acute lymphoblastic leukemia, 172
  acute myeloid leukemia related to, 65, 185, 188
  for Ewing sarcoma, 401–402, 403, 404, 405
  for gliomas, 262, 264
  for Hodgkin lymphoma, 238, 241
  for Langerhans cell histiocytosis, 253
  late effects of, 65, 566, 569
  mechanism of action, 96, 97, 101
  pharmacokinetics of, 104, 105
  for medulloblastoma, 283
  for retinoblastoma, 453
  for rhabdomyosarcoma, 348, 350–351
  for systemic germ cell tumors, 378
ALL. See acute lymphoblastic leukemia (ALL)
alleles
  in immune response, 34
  in tumor suppressor genes, 23, 29
allergic reactions, to transfusions, 506
alloantibody, in transfusion reaction, 506
allogeneic stem cell transplantation, 139, 148

for acute lymphoblastic leukemia, 144–145, 174
for acute myeloid leukemia, 200–201, 203
for hemophagocytic lymphohistiocytosis, 256
for myelodysplastic syndrome/myeloproliferative syndromes, 206, 208
for non-Hodgkin lymphoma, 224, 228
posttransplant lymphoproliferative disease from, 229
allograft rejection, in organ transplant, 229
alloimmunization, with platelet transfusions, 501, 502, 503
allopurinol
  mercaptopurine interactions with, 109
  for non-Hodgkin lymphoma, 218, 219
  for tumor lysis syndrome, 488–489
all-trans retinoic acid (ATRA)
  for acute promyelocytic leukemia, 189, 202
  as molecular therapy, 26, 27
  pharmacology of, 100, 101
alpha particles, in radiation, 124
alpha-fetoprotein (AFP)
  in CNS germ cell tumors, 51, 305–307, 310, 311, 313
  in hepatic tumors, 119, 413, 420, 423, 424, 431
  in systemic germ cell tumors, 358, 359, 362, 363, 366–369, 371
alternative medicine. See complementary and alternative medicine (CAM)
aluminum hydroxide, for tumor lysis syndrome, 489
alveolar rhabdomyosarcoma (ARMS), 26, 51, 342
  risk-directed therapy for, 26, 28, 345, 346
alveolar soft part sarcoma, 343
amantadine, 494
amegakaryocytic thrombocytopenia, congenital, 186, 187
amenorrhea, chemotherapy-induced, 107, 108, 569
American Joint Committee on Cancer (AJCC) staging system, for thyroid cancer, 461, 462
amifostine, 107, 205, 427, 475
AML. See acute myeloid leukemia (AML)
AML1 gene, 186
AML1-ETO fusion gene, 189, 192, 193, 194, 205
amphotericin B, 492, 493, 494, 505
amputation, osteosarcoma resection and, 391, 404
anal abscess, 492
anal manipulation, infection and, 491
analgesics
  adjuvant, 545
  administration routes and methods, 543–544
  non-opioid, 542

opioid, 542–545
prescriptions for, 541–542
analytical epidemiology
environmental, 11
genetic, 9–11
genetic/environmental, 11
anaphylactic reactions, to transfusions, 506
anaplasia
in medulloblastoma, 280, 281
in renal tumors, 330, 332, 334, 336
anaplastic large cell lymphoma (ALCL), 226–228
advanced-disease, 227–228
clinical presentation of, 218
genetics of, 221, 227
histopathology of, 55, 57, 220, 221, 226–227
limited-disease, 227
relapse of, 228
summary of, 217, 230
treatment of, 218–219, 227–228
anaplastic lymphoma kinase (ALK) protein, 57, 58, 61
ANC (absolute neutrophil count), antimicrobials and, 493–494
ancillary techniques, in pathological evaluation, 46–47
androgens, for myelodysplastic syndrome, 205
anemia(s)
in acute lymphoblastic leukemia, 163, 164
cancers associated with, 7, 9, 64, 65, 329
chemotherapy-induced, 107
clinical aspects of, 498, 509
hepatic tumors and, 410, 411
inherited, acute myeloid leukemia and, 186, 187
in Langerhans cell histiocytosis, 251
refractory, with excess blasts in transmission to AML, 206
severe aplastic, 186
transfusion therapy for. See red blood cell (RBC) transfusions
angiogenesis
in cancer pathogenesis, 342
in Ewing sarcoma, 403
in hepatic tumors, 431
in myelodysplastic syndrome, 205
in neuroblastoma, 325
angiography
cerebral, for choroid plexus tumors, 300
magnetic resonance imaging, 71
in surgical planning, for hepatic tumors, 414
angiolipoma, 409
angiosarcoma, 341
hepatic, 409, 421, 422
Ann Arbor staging system, for Hodgkin lymphoma, 238, 239
antenatal exposures, childhood cancers and, 11, 188

anterior segment, retinoblastoma extension into, 444, 445, 446, 447
anthracenediones, 98, 198
anthracyclines
for acute lymphoblastic leukemia, 170, 172, 176
for acute myeloid leukemia, 198, 202, 203, 209
cardiotoxicity of, 105, 107–108, 176, 336, 559, 566–567
for Ewing sarcoma, 401–402, 403, 405
for hepatic tumors, 429
for Hodgkin lymphoma, 238, 241
for Langerhans cell histiocytosis, 253
mechanism of action, 96, 101
myeloid malignancies associated with, 185, 188
for non-Hodgkin lymphoma, 224
pharmacokinetics of, 104, 105, 106
for retinoblastoma, 453
for soft-tissue sarcomas, 350–351
for systemic germ cell tumors, 375
anthropometric measurements, in nutrition assessment, 524, 525, 526, 527
antiangiogenic therapy, 325, 431
antibiotics
for acute myeloid leukemia induction therapy, 198
anemia related to, 498
antitumor. See topoisomerase I/II inhibitors
for infections, 491–492, 493–494
platelet refractoriness and, 503
prophylactic, for myelodysplastic syndrome, 205
antibodies
in immunotherapy, 38–39. See also monoclonal antibodies (mAb)
in pathological evaluation, 46, 47
in posttransplant lymphoproliferative disease, 229
transfusion therapy and, 505, 506, 507, 508
in translational therapy, 25
antibody-dependent cellular cytotoxicity (ADCC), 38–39, 325
anti-CD20–Yttrium-90, for non-Hodgkin lymphoma, 230
anti-CD21/CD24, for posttransplant lymphoproliferative disease, 229
anti-CD52 antibody, therapeutic use of, 39, 256
anticipatory nausea and vomiting (ANV), 532, 533, 537–538
anticoagulants, contraindications for, 554
anticonvulsants, in pain management, 545
antidepressants, in pain management, 545
antiemetic therapy, 107, 532
clinical trials on, 534–536, 537
antifibrinolytic agents, for thrombocytopenia, 504
antifolate agents, 96, 97, 98, 101, 102
antifungal agents, 492, 493, 494

antigen expression patterns. See also CD entries
in acute lymphoblastic leukemia, 164–166
in Ewing sarcoma, 397, 398, 404
in gastrointestinal stromal tumor, 471
in gonadal germ cell tumors, 356
in leukemia, 62, 65, 163, 191–192
in lymphomas, 56, 57, 58, 59, 60, 61
in nasopharyngeal carcinoma, 473
in non-Hodgkin lymphoma, 220, 223, 225, 226–227
in osteosarcoma, 391
in posttransplant lymphoproliferative disease, 228
antigen-presenting cells (APC)
in acute lymphoblastic leukemia, 164–165
dysregulation of, cancers related to, 36–37
in immune response, 33, 34
in immunotherapy, 37–38
in Langerhans cell histiocytosis, 245, 246
antigens
B-lymphocytic, in Hodgkin lymphoma, 235–236
in immune response, 33, 34
in immunotherapy, 35, 36, 37–38, 39
in pathological evaluation, 46, 47
antihistamines
for nausea, 534, 536
in pain management, 545
antimetabolite agents
for acute leukemia, 172, 202
chemical structure of, 96, 102
mechanism of action, 96, 98, 101, 102
pharmacokinetics of, 104, 105
antimicrobials, for infections
as prophylaxis, 491–492
as treatment, 493–494
antioxidant agents, 525–526, 554, 558
antiplatelet therapies, contraindications for, 554
antisense oligonucleotides, in Ewing sarcoma, 396–397, 399, 404
antiseptics, hand, for infection prevention, 491
antithymocyte globulin, 206, 256
α-1 antitrypsin deficiency, in hepatic tumors, 410, 411
antitumor immune response
biological, 33–35
therapy as. See immunotherapy
antiviral agents, 229, 492, 493, 494
ANV (anticipatory nausea and vomiting), 532, 533
anxiety
complementary and alternative therapies for, 556, 559
as late effect, 568
nausea and vomiting related to, 532
pain management and, 541, 544

data analysis, in clinical trials, 156–157
data and safety monitoring committee
    (DSMC), in clinical trials, 154–155,
    157
data monitoring, interim, in clinical trials,
    157
data-capture instrument, for clinical trials,
    156
daunomycin
    for acute leukemia, 171, 198, 204
    for non-Hodgkin lymphoma, 228
    pharmacology of, 98
daunorubicin, 375
DCTER regimen, for acute myeloid
    leukemia, 198
DDAVP (desmopressin acetate), for
    thrombocytopenia, 504
de novo pathway, of gliomas, 262
dead end gene, 358
death and dying
    in palliative care, 515–516, 518, 519
    statistics on. *See* mortality/mortality
        rates
DECAL regimen, for non-Hodgkin
    lymphoma, 222, 224, 225
decision making, for palliative care,
    514–517
    communication approaches to, 514–515
    death and dying issues in, 515–516, 518,
        519
    ethical issues in, 516
    on home *vs.* hospital setting, 516–517
    on resuscitation status, 516
decitabine, 205
decompression surgery, for cord
    compression, 324, 325, 486–487
deletions, of chromosomes, 23–24. *See also*
    chromosomal abnormalities
demethylating agents, for acute myeloid
    leukemia, 205
dendritic cells
    in histiocytic disorders, 245, 246
    in immune response, 33, 34
    in immunotherapy, 37, 38
dental care, infection prophylaxis for, 492
Denys-Drash syndrome, 49, 118
depression
    complementary and alternative therapies
        for, 556
    as late effect, 568
    pain management and, 544, 545
descriptive epidemiology, 3–9
    ICCC groups in, 3–6
    number of cases, 3, 7
    tumor types in, 7–9
desmoplastic nested spindle cell tumor of
    liver, 423
desmoplastic small round cell tumors
    (DSRCTs)
    cytogenetics of, 343
    hematopoietic stem cell transplantation
        for, 148
    hepatic tumors *vs.*, 420, 422, 423
desmopressin acetate (DDAVP), for
    thrombocytopenia, 504

developing world
    global initiatives of, 15–17, 21
    global research for, 16, 20–21, 313
    improved initiatives for, 18–20
    income definitions for, 15, 17–18, 21
    regional initiatives of, 17–18
development organizations, policy
    promulgation by, 16
developmental delay, with
    opsoclonus/myoclonus syndrome,
    324, 325
dexamethasone
    for acute lymphoblastic leukemia, 170,
        171, 173, 176
    for acute myeloid leukemia, 198
    for cord compression, 486
    granulocyte transfusions and, 504
    for hemophagocytic
        lymphohistiocytosis, 256
    for Hodgkin lymphoma, 241
    late effects of, 568
    for nausea, 534, 535, 536, 537
    for non-Hodgkin lymphoma, 220, 222,
        224, 226, 227, 228
    for osteosarcoma, 391
    pharmacology of, 100
dexrazoxane, for cardiotoxicity rescue,
    107, 108, 177, 405
diabetes insipidus (DI)
    germ cell tumors and, 307, 310,
        311
    Langerhans cell histiocytosis and,
        251–252
diagnosis
    global programs for, 18, 19, 20, 21
    pediatric challenges of, 45–46, 66
Diamond-Blackfan anemia, 7, 186, 187
DIC. *See* disseminated intravascular
    coagulation (DIC)
diet factors. *See* nutrition
diethylstilbestrol, 11
"differentiation" syndrome, 202
differentiation-promoting agents, for
    myelodysplastic syndrome, 205,
    206
diffuse large B-cell lymphoma (DLBCL)
    advanced-disease, 225–226
    clinical presentation of, 217–218
    genetics of, 221, 225, 230
    histopathology of, 55, 56–57, 220, 221,
        225
    limited-disease, 225
    staging of, 218, 219
    treatment of, 218–219, 225–226, 230
diffusion tensor imaging, in MRI, 71
diffusion-weighted imaging, in MRI, 71,
    72
diphenhydramine
    for nausea, 534, 536
    for transfusion therapy, 506
directed donors, for transfusion therapy,
    509
disclosure, in clinical trials, 155
disialoganglioside (GD2), for
    neuroblastoma, 325

dissection
    of lymph nodes. *See* retroperitoneal
        lymph node (RPLN)
    neck node, for thyroid cancer, 462
    renal hilar, for upper abdominal
        neuroblastoma, 116
disseminated disease. *See also* metastases
    cord compression related to, 486–487
    with germ cell tumors, 360–364, 367,
        373–374
    in Langerhans cell histiocytosis,
        247–248, 250–252
disseminated intravascular coagulation
    (DIC)
    in acute myeloid leukemia, 189
    anemia and, 498
    platelet count and, 500, 501, 508
    transfusion management of, 503
distribution, of chemotherapy agents,
    104–105
    volume of, 103
diuretics
    for hyperleukocytosis, 487
    for transfusion reaction, 506
    for tumor lysis syndrome, 488
DLBCL. *See* diffuse large B-cell lymphoma
    (DLBCL)
DLI (donor lymphocyte infusion),
    35–36
DLT (dose-limiting toxicity), in clinical
    trials, 152, 153
DNA
    alkylation of, by anticancer drugs, 96,
        101
    pathogen binding to, UV light reduction
        of, 508
    radiation impact on, 124, 125, 137
    synthesis of, retinoblastoma and, 437
DNA chip technology, 28, 170
DNA content analysis, 47
    of leukemia, 62
DNA methylation inhibitors, for
    myelodysplastic syndrome, 205
DNA methyltransferases, for acute myeloid
    leukemia, 205
DNA microarrays, 28, 170, 196
DNA mutations. *See also* gene
    rearrangements
    in acute myeloid leukemia, 193,
        195–196
    in choroid plexus tumors, 299
    in colorectal cancer, 469
    common nonrandom, 24–25
    in gastrointestinal stromal tumor, 471
    in hemophagocytic lymphohistiocytosis,
        254
    in hepatic tumors, 411
    in medulloblastoma, 280–281
    in myeloproliferative syndromes, 207
    in oncogenes, 23–24, 28
    in renal tumors, 329–330, 332
    in retinoblastoma, 10, 48, 437, 438–440,
        441
    in rhabdomyosarcoma, 342
    in systemic germ cell tumors, 358

DNA oligonucleotides
    in Ewing sarcoma, 396
    in immunotherapy, 37
DNA ploidy
    in leukemia, 62, 162–163, 166, 167, 169
    in neuroblastoma, 320, 321, 322
    in non-Hodgkin lymphoma, 223
    in pathological evaluation, 47
    in systemic germ cell tumors, 358
DNA probes, 28, 192
DNA repair mechanism
    gliomas and, 262
    retinoblastoma and, 438
    tumor types and, 7, 9, 11
DNA synthesis inhibitors, 96, 101
    for acute lymphoblastic leukemia, 174, 175
DNR (do-not-resuscitate) status, 516, 517
docetaxel, 99, 404
dolasetron, 534, 535
domperidone, 534, 536
donor lymphocyte infusion (DLI), 35–36
do-not-resuscitate (DNR) status, 516, 517
dopamine, in nausea physiology, 532
dopaminergic receptor antagonists, for nausea, 534–535, 536, 537
Doppler ultrasound
    of hepatic tumors, 119
    technical considerations of, 70
    of venous thrombosis, 89
dose escalation, in clinical trials, 152, 153
dose reduction, in clinical trials, 152
dose response curve, in chemotherapy, 95
dose schedule, for chemotherapy, 103
dose-limiting toxicity (DLT), in clinical trials, 152, 153
dosimetry, of radioiodine, for thyroid cancer, 463
dosing
    of chemotherapy, 95, 103
    optimizing, 111
    of radiotherapy. See radiation therapy
Down syndrome
    acute myeloid leukemia and, 185–186, 193, 201–202
    cancers associated with, 7, 63, 65, 161
doxorubicin
    for acute lymphoblastic leukemia, 177
    for adrenocortical carcinoma, 468
    for Ewing sarcoma, 401–402, 403, 405
    for hepatic tumors, 425, 426, 427, 428, 429, 430
    for nasopharyngeal carcinoma, 474
    for neuroblastoma, 322, 323
    for non-Hodgkin lymphoma, 220, 222, 224, 225, 226, 227, 228
    for osteosarcoma, 389, 390, 391
    pharmacology of, 98, 108, 110
    for renal tumors, 334, 335, 336
    for retinoblastoma, 448, 449, 452, 453
    for soft-tissue sarcomas, 347, 348, 349, 350
    for systemic germ cell tumors, 375, 376, 377
dronabinol, 534, 536, 537

drug interactions, in chemotherapy, 109–110
drug monitoring, therapeutic, 103
drug resistance, to chemotherapy, 108–109, 170
    in acute lymphoblastic leukemia, 170, 171–172
    in acute myeloid leukemia, 196–197
    in ependymoma, 276
    in gastrointestinal stromal tumor, 471
    in myeloproliferative syndromes, 208
    in neuroblastoma, 320, 325
drug use/abuse, malignancies associated with, 188, 356
drugs
    antineoplastic. See chemotherapy
    cancers associated with, 8, 11
    clinical pharmacology of, 96–103, 110–111
    for nausea, 532, 534–536, 537
    for pain management, 542–545
DSMC (data and safety monitoring committee), in clinical trials, 154–155, 157
DSRCTs. See desmoplastic small round cell tumors (DSRCTs)
DTaP vaccine, 491
dysgerminoma, 357, 371–372
dyskeratosis congenita, 186, 187

E

E2A gene, 24
E2A-PBX1 gene, 162
ear disease, in Langerhans cell histiocytosis, 248
EBV. See Epstein-Barr virus (EBV)
EBV lymphoproliferative disease (EBV-LPD), 39, 228–229
echinacea, 558
echocardiogram
    for cardiotoxicities, 108, 176–177
    for osteosarcoma, 386, 388, 391
    for superior vena cava syndrome, 486
education
    on complementary and alternative medicine, 560–561
    on infection prevention, 491, 494
    on late effects, 569
    for obesity management, 528
    on palliative care, 514–515, 518
    regional initiatives for, 20, 21
    on transfusion therapy, 509
educational remediation plan, neurobehavioral test battery for, 549, 550
effector cell activation
    in cancer pathogenesis, 342
    in immune response, 33, 34, 35, 38
    in immunotherapy, 38, 39
EGFR (epidermal growth factor receptor), 27, 262, 274, 391
electrocardiogram, hyperkalemia effects on, 488

electrolyte imbalances
    hematopoietic stem cell transplantation and, 140
    in tumor lysis syndrome, 488–489
electromagnetic fields, 11
electron beams, in radiation therapy, 125–126
electron microscopy, in morphologic analysis, 46
electrons, in radiation, 124
eligibility criteria, for clinical trials, 154, 155
elimination, of chemotherapy agents, 105–106
    route of, 103, 104
embolization
    of choroid plexus tumors, 300
    of hepatic tumors, 430
embryology, of systemic germ cell tumors, 356
    histopathology related to, 360–364
embryonal carcinoma, 304, 305, 307, 312
    biological markers of, 358, 359
    histopathology of, 362–363
    immunohistochemical markers of, 360
embryonal hepatoblastoma, 416–417, 418
embryonal rhabdomyosarcoma (ERMS), 341–342, 345–346
    hepatic, 410, 412, 414, 415, 420, 425, 429
    treatment of, 347, 348, 349
embryonal sarcoma, 5, 9
    hepatic, 409, 410, 412
embryonal tumors, 45
emcitabine, 241
emergencies
    hyperleukocytosis as, 487–488
    spinal cord compression as, 486–487
    superior vena cava syndrome as, 485–486
    tumor lysis syndrome as, 488–489
emetic reflex, 531, 532
emetogenic potential
    of chemotherapy agents, 532, 533
    of radiotherapy, 533–534
EMLA (eutectic mixture of local anesthetics), 544
emotional status
    neurobehavioral test battery for, 548–549, 550, 551
    radiotherapy impact on, 313
en bloc resection, of osteosarcoma, 388, 389
endocarditis, prevention of, 492
endocrine abnormalities
    in adrenocortical carcinoma, 467–468
    hematopoietic stem cell transplantation and, 143–144
    in Langerhans cell histiocytosis, 251
    in long-term acute myeloid leukemia survivors, 209
    post-thyroidectomy, 464
endodermal sinus tumor, 51, 305, 306
    hepatic, 420
end-of-life issues, 513, 515–516, 518

pathogenesis of, 254–255
treatment of, 255–256
hemorrhage. *See* bleeding
hemorrhagic cystitis, from chemotherapy, 106, 107
Hep B vaccine, 491
hepatectomy, total, followed by orthotopic liver transplant, 430–431
hepatic adenoma, 409, 416, 417
hepatic carcinoma, 5, 8, 119
    cellular. *See* hepatocellular carcinoma (HCC)
hepatic function
    in clinical trials, 152
    germ cell tumors and, 364
    graft-versus-host disease and, 141, 143
    hepatic tumors impact on, 413
    in Langerhans cell histiocytosis, 250, 254
    osteosarcoma and, 386, 388
    in transient myeloproliferative disorder, 202
hepatic lobectomy, right *vs.* left, 120
hepatic tumors, 409–432
    biology of, 411–412
    chemoembolization of, 430
    chemotherapy for, 425–430
    clinical presentation of, 412
    cystic, 414, 422–423, 424
    diagnosis by pentad, 45
    diagnostic evaluation of, 413–414
    diagnostic histology of, 416–424
    epidemiology of, 5, 8
    epithelial/epithelioid cell, 416–420
    future plans for, 431–432
    histopathology of, 52–54, 119, 415–416
    incidence of, 46, 409–410
    laboratory investigations for, 413
    liver transplantation for, 430–431
    local control methods for, 430
    metastasis of, 412, 414, 420, 427, 428
    mixed, 422–423, 424
    new therapeutic modalities for, 431
    predisposing risk factors of, 410–411, 431
    radiation therapy for, 430
    radiologic investigations for, 413–414
    small-cell, 420–422
    spindle cell, 421, 422
    staging of, 119–120, 414–415, 432
    surgical management of, 119–120, 423–425
    teratoid, 422–423, 424
    treatment and outcomes of, 423–431
hepatic vessels, in hepatic tumor resection, 119, 120
hepatitis A, 508
hepatitis B/C
    hepatic tumors and, 410, 431
    osteosarcoma and, 386, 388
    transfusion transmission of, 505, 507, 508
hepatoblastoma
    chemotherapy for, 425–427

clinical presentation of, 412
epidemiology of, 5, 8, 10–11, 409, 410
epithelial, 416–417, 418
genetic syndromes associated with, 410–411
histopathology of, 52, 53, 119, 415
liver transplantation for, 431
mixed, 422, 423
radiation therapy for, 430
small-cell, 420, 421
staging system for, 414–415
teratoid, 422
hepatocellular carcinoma (HCC)
    biopsy for, 424
    chemotherapy for, 428–429
    clinical presentation of, 409, 412
    diagnostic evaluation of, 413–414
    fibrolamellar, 409, 417, 419, 420, 429
    genetic syndromes associated with, 410, 411–412
    histopathology of, 52, 415, 417, 419–420
    liver transplantation for, 431
    local control methods for, 430
    radiation therapy for, 430
    staging system for, 415
    tumor resection for, 425
hepatoduodenal ligament, in hepatic tumor, 120
hepatotoxicity, of chemotherapy, 106, 107, 555
HER-2 expression, in osteosarcoma metastasis, 391
herbal therapy
    cancer therapy interactions with, 559–560
    classes to avoid, 553, 554
    effectiveness studies of, 553, 555–556
    immune-enhancing, 554, 556, 558–559
    for nausea, 538
hereditary non-polyposis colorectal cancer (HNPCC), 469
hereditary syndromes. *See* genetic syndromes
herpes simplex virus (HSV), 492, 494
herpes viruses, disorders related to, 8, 247, 255
herpes-zoster virus, 492
HFRT. *See* hyperfractionated radiation therapy (HFRT)
Hib vaccine, 491
Hirschsprung disease, 317
histamine receptors, in nausea physiology, 532
histiocytic disorders, 245–256
    classification of, 245
    hemophagocytic lymphohistiocytosis as, 254–256
    Langerhans cell histiocytosis as, 245–254
    lymphoma and, 60–61, 235, 236–237
    summary of, 245, 256
histone deacetylation, in acute myeloid leukemia, 205

histopathology
    of acute lymphoblastic leukemia, 61–62, 164–165, 169
    of acute myeloid leukemia, 64–65, 163, 192
    of anaplastic large cell lymphoma, 55, 57, 220, 221, 226–227
    ancillary techniques for, 46–47
    of bone tumors, 51–52, 53, 384
    of Burkitt lymphoma, 55–56, 219–220, 221
    of choroid plexus tumors, 299
    of colorectal cancer, 470
    of diffuse large B-cell lymphoma, 55, 56–57, 220, 221, 225
    of ependymoma, 271, 272, 273, 274
    of Ewing sarcoma, 51–52, 53, 397
    of gastrointestinal stromal tumor, 471
    of germ cell tumors, 304, 305–306
    of gliomas, 261, 265
    of hemophagocytic lymphohistiocytosis, 245, 254, 255
    of hepatic tumor types, 416–424
    of hepatic tumors, 52–54, 119, 415–416
    of Hodgkin lymphoma, 59–61, 235–236
    of liquid (hematolymphoid) tumors, 54–62, 63
    of lymphoblastic lymphoma, 55, 57–58, 59, 220, 223
    of medulloblastoma, 47, 48, 279, 280, 281
    of melanoma, 472–473
    of myeloid malignancies, 62–66
    of nasopharyngeal carcinoma, 473–474
    of neuroblastoma, 319, 321, 322
    of non-Hodgkin lymphoma, 55–59, 217
    of osteosarcoma, 51, 52, 384–385
    of pleuropulmonary blastoma, 476
    of renal tumors, 330–331, 332
    of retinoblastoma, 52, 54, 440–441, 447
    of soft-tissue sarcomas, 50–51, 341–342, 343
    of solid (nonhematolymphoid) tumors, 47–51
    of thyroid cancer, 461
history taking
    for extragonadal germ cell tumors, 365
    for infection diagnosis, 492, 493
    in neurobehavioral exam, 549
    in pain assessment, 541
HIT-SKK regimens, for infant brain tumors, 293, 294
HIV. *See* human immunodeficiency virus (HIV)
HLA matching
    for allogeneic hematopoietic stem cell transplantation, 139–140, 206, 208, 229
    for platelet transfusions, 503
HLA-A
    in immune response, 34
    in nasopharyngeal carcinoma, 473–474
HLA-B, in immune response, 34
HLA-C, in immune response, 34

recurrence of, 296
summary of, 291, 297
supratentorial primitive
neuroectodermal, 291, 294
infantile hemangioendothelioma, 421,
422
infants
acute leukemia and, 161, 203
brain tumors in, 291–297
neurobehavioral test battery for,
550–551
retinoblastoma in, 437, 441
transient myeloproliferative disorder in,
202
infections/infectious complications,
491–495. *See also* viral infections
acute lymphoblastic leukemia and, 161
anemia related to, 498
cancers associated with, 7–8, 9, 11
of central venous catheters, 113, 114
diagnosis of, 492–493
future directions for, 494–495
hematopoietic stem cell transplantation
and, 141, 142–143
histiocytic disorders related to, 247,
254–255
nasopharyngeal carcinoma and, 473,
475
platelet refractoriness and, 502–503
prevention of, 491–492
prophylaxis for, 491, 492, 504
retinoblastoma and, 437–438
summary of, 491, 494
transfusion transmission of, 491, 497,
504, 505, 507–509
treatment of, 493–494
inferior vena cava (IVC), renal tumors
and, 331
infertility
chemotherapy-induced, 107, 108, 405,
569
hematopoietic stem cell transplantation
and, 143–144
inflammatory bowel disease, 469
inflammatory cells, in Langerhans cell
histiocytosis, 245–246, 254
inflammatory myofibroblastic tumors
(IMT), 422
infliximab, 256
influenza vaccine, 491
influenzae infections, 494
informed consent
for clinical trials, 155
document for, 155, 156
in palliative care, 515, 516
for transfusion therapy, 497, 509
infrastructure development, for global
initiatives, 16–17
infratentorial gliomas, 262
inguinal canal, Wilms tumor of, 118
inherited syndromes. *See* genetic
syndromes
INI1 gene, 294, 296
innate immune system, 33

Institutional Review Boards, for clinical
trials, 155
insulin-like growth factor (IGF), tumors
associated with, 330, 411
insulin-like growth factor type 1 receptor
(IGF1R), 25, 396, 404
insulin-like growth factor/mammalian
target of rapamycin (IGF/mTOR),
349
intelligence
brain tumors impact on, 293, 567
neurobehavioral test battery for, 548,
549, 550
therapy impact on, 267, 312, 313,
568
intensification therapy
for acute lymphoblastic leukemia,
171–172, 177
for acute myeloid leukemia, 199,
203–204
for Ewing sarcoma, 401, 403
for hepatic tumors, 427, 428
for medulloblastoma, 285
for non-Hodgkin lymphoma, 222, 224,
225–226, 227–228, 230
for osteosarcoma, 390
for retinoblastoma, 451, 452, 453
transfusion therapy with, 499, 502
intensity-modulated radiation therapy
(IMRT), 135–136
for nasopharyngeal carcinoma, 475
for primitive neuroectodermal tumors,
282–283, 287
radiation field planning for, 131, 133,
134
intercellular adhesion molecule 1 (ICAM-
1), 35
interferon
for Langerhans cell histiocytosis, 252
for melanoma, 473
for myeloproliferative syndromes, 207,
208
for nasopharyngeal carcinoma, 475
for osteosarcoma, 390
for posttransplant lymphoproliferative
disease, 229
interim monitoring strategy, in clinical
trials, 154, 157
interleukins (ILs)
in hepatic tumors, 431
in immune response, 34
in immunotherapy, 37, 38, 39
for melanoma, 473
for neuroblastoma, 325
International Acute Lymphoblastic
Leukemia Group, 15
International Classification of Childhood
Cancer (ICCC)
group descriptions in, 4–6
number of cases based on, 3, 7
survival rates in, 11, 12
International Confederation of Childhood
Cancer Parent Organizations
(ICCCPO), 17

International Germ Cell Consensus
Classification (IGCC), of systemic
germ cell tumor risk, 368–369
International Network for Cancer
Treatment and Research, 16
International Outreach Program (IOP), 16,
19
International Society of Pediatric
Oncology (SIOP)
advocacy programs of, 15
chemotherapy protocols of. *See* SIOP
regimen
regional initiatives of, 17
renal tumor staging system of, 332
International Union Against Cancer
(UICC)
advocacy programs of, 16
osteosarcoma staging system of, 388,
389
TNM staging system of, 345
Internet resources
for complementary and alternative
medicine, 553, 558, 560, 561
for global initiatives, 16–17, 19
intervertebral foramina, tumor extension
through, 486–487
intracranial hemorrhage,
hyperleukocytosis and, 487–488
intracranial neoplasms, ICCC description
of, 4, 6. *See also* brain tumors
intramedullary extension, of Ewing
sarcoma, 395
intraocular pressure, in retinoblastoma,
443
intraoperative consultation, on hepatic
tumors, 416
intraspinal neoplasms, ICCC description
of, 4, 6
intrathecal administration, of
chemotherapy, 110
intravenous gamma globulin, 229, 255,
324
intravenous immunoglobulin, 492
intraventricular administration, of
chemotherapy, 110
invasive procedures
infection prophylaxis for, 491, 492
platelet levels needed for, 501
red blood cell transfusions for, 499
investigational therapeutic interventions.
See experimental therapies
involved field radiotherapy (IFRT), for
Hodgkin lymphoma, 238–241
iodine deficiency, thyroid cancer and,
459
IPACTR staging system, for adrenocortical
carcinoma, 468
ipsilateral factors, in Wilms tumor
resection, 117, 118
IPV vaccine, 491
irinotecan
for colorectal cancer, 470
for Ewing sarcoma, 404
for hepatic tumors, 430

molecular oncology, 23–31
  nonrandom mutations in, 24–25
  oncogenes in, 23–24
  overview of, 23, 31
  risk-directed therapy in, 25–26
  subtypes of cancer in, 24–25
  targeted therapies in, 26–31
  translational therapy in, 25–31
  tumor suppressor genes in, 23–24
molecularly targeted therapies, 26–31
  for acute myeloid leukemia, 203–205
  for Ewing sarcoma, 404
  future perspectives for, 111
  for gliomas, 267
  mechanism of action, 100, 101
  for myelodysplastic syndrome, 206
  for myeloproliferative syndromes, 208
  for non-Hodgkin lymphoma, 230
  novel trial designs for, 30–31
  oncogene addiction in, 27–28
  for osteosarcoma, 391
  for retinoblastoma, 451
  for thyroid cancer, 464
monitoring protocols, for clinical trials, 154–155, 156, 157
monoblastic leukemia, acute, 65
monoclonal antibodies (mAb)
  acute lymphoblastic leukemia and, 164–165, 175
  for acute myeloid leukemia, 191, 204
  for colorectal cancer, 470
  Ewing sarcoma and, 397, 404
  for hemophagocytic lymphohistiocytosis, 256
  as immunotherapy, 38–39
  for neuroblastoma, 325
  for non-Hodgkin lymphoma, 230
  for osteosarcoma, 391
  for posttransplant lymphoproliferative disease, 229
monocytes, in hemophagocytic lymphohistiocytosis, 245, 254, 255
monosomy 7
  in acute myeloid leukemia, 186, 188, 195
  in myelodysplastic syndromes, 64, 206
Montevideo Document (SIOP), 15, 18
Monza International School of Pediatric Hematology and Oncology (MISPHO), 17, 18
mood disturbances, therapy-induced, 568
MOPP regimen
  for infant brain tumors, 291, 295
  for lymphomas, 146
morphine, 542–543, 545
morphology
  of acute lymphoblastic leukemia, 164–165, 169
  of acute myeloid leukemia, 191, 194, 197–198
  of hepatic tumors, 415

of non-Hodgkin lymphoma, 219, 220, 223, 225, 226
of pleuropulmonary blastoma, 476
of posttransplant lymphoproliferative disease, 228, 229
of supratentorial primitive neuroectodermal tumors, 287
of tumor types, 3–6, 46
mortality/mortality rates
  age-standardized, 11–12
  all-cause trends in, 563, 565
  factors influencing, 3
  income associated with, 15, 21
motion sickness, 531, 532, 533
motor deficits, therapy-induced, 107, 108, 567
mourning, 519
MPS. See myeloproliferative syndrome (MPS)
MRD. See minimal residual disease (MRD)
MRI. See magnetic resonance imaging (MRI)
MRI cholangiopancreatography (MRCP), for hepatic tumors, 414
MSH genes, 469
MSTS (Musculoskeletal Tumor Society) staging system, for osteosarcoma, 388
MTC (medullary thyroid cancer), 459, 460, 464–465
MTD. See maximally tolerated dose (MTD)
mTOR (mammalian target of rapamycin), 175, 349
mucositis
  as chemotherapy toxicity, 106, 107
  complementary and alternative therapies for, 555, 556, 559
  nasopharyngeal carcinoma and, 475
mucous membranes
  in graft-versus-host disease, 141, 143
  rhabdomyosarcoma of, 342, 344
multicentric hemangioendothelioma, 422
multidisciplinary treatments, in clinical trials, 154, 156
multidrug resistance (MDR)
  in acute myeloid leukemia, 196–197
  in ependymoma, 276
  in neuroblastoma, 320, 325
multidrug resistance-associated protein (MRP), 109, 276, 325
multi-hit concept, of leukemogenesis, 193
multikinase inhibitors, for hepatic tumors, 428, 431
multileaf collimator, in conformal radiation therapy, 135
multimodality approach, to chemotherapy, 95
multiple endocrine neoplasias (MEN) Type 1 and 2
  cancer associated with, 9, 10, 467
  clinical characteristics of, 460
  thyroid cancer and, 459–460, 464

multiple gated acquisition scan, for osteosarcoma, 386
multislicing, in computed tomography, 70–71
Murphy stage, of non-Hodgkin lymphomas, 217, 219, 220, 223, 225
muscarinic receptors, in nausea physiology, 532
muscle wasting, in malnutrition, 525, 526
musculoskeletal system
  in graft-versus-host disease, 143
  rhabdomyosarcoma of, 341, 342–344
Musculoskeletal Tumor Society (MSTS) staging system, for osteosarcoma, 388
mushroom extracts, 558
Mustargen. See nitrogen mustards
MYC gene, 24, 280, 281
MYC-IgH gene, 162
MYCN gene
  in medulloblastoma, 280, 281
  in neuroblastoma, 48, 49, 319–320, 321
  targeted therapies for, 23, 26
myeloablative chemotherapy, hematopoietic cell rescue for, 39, 107, 301
  in acute myeloid leukemia, 200
  in choroid plexus tumors, 301
  in Ewing sarcoma, 403, 404
  in germ cell tumors, 312, 313, 345
  in hospitalized patients, special considerations for, 140, 141
  in infant brain tumors, 147, 293, 294, 295, 296
  in neuroblastoma, 323, 324, 325
  in pleuropulmonary blastoma, 477
  in primitive neuroectodermal tumors, 287
  in retinoblastoma, 452, 453, 454
  in solid tumors, 147–148
myelodysplastic syndrome (MDS), 205
  hematopoietic stem cell transplantation for, 145–146, 206
  histopathology of, 62, 63–64, 205
  risk factors for, 186, 188
  systemic germ cell tumors and, 369
  treatment and outcomes of, 205–206
myelodysplastic/myeloproliferative syndrome (MDS/MPS)
  histopathology of, 62, 64, 206
  treatment and outcomes of, 206–207
myelofibrosis, idiopathic, 207
myelogenous leukemia. See chronic myelogenous leukemia (CML)
myeloid leukemia. See acute myeloid leukemia (AML)
myeloid leukemic lineages
  in acute lymphoblastic leukemia, 165, 166
  in lymphoblastic lymphoma, 57–58, 59
myeloid malignancies
  histopathologic classification of, 62–64

simultaneous integrated boost, in IMRT, 135
  for primitive neuroectodermal tumors, 287, 288
single nucleotide polymorphisms (SNPs)
  in acute lymphoblastic leukemia, 169
  translational therapy and, 29–30
single-photo emission computed tomography (SPECT), 72, 82, 131
SIOP regimen
  for germ cell tumors, 311, 313
  for renal tumors, 334
SIOP staging system, for renal tumors, 332
SIOPEL staging system, for hepatic tumors, 119–120
sirolimus, 175
skeletal muscle, differentiation of, in rhabdomyosarcoma, 341, 342
skeletal muscle relaxants, 545
skeleton. *See* bone *entries*
skin
  acute myeloid leukemia and, 188, 203
  Langerhans cell histiocytosis and, 249–250, 252
  non-Hodgkin lymphoma and, 218, 219, 226, 227, 228
skin carcinoma, 6, 9
skin lesions
  in graft-versus-host disease, 141, 143
  infectious, 492
skin type, melanoma risk related to, 472
skull
  chordoma of, 468–469
  Langerhans cell histiocytosis and, 248, 249, 254
  nasopharyngeal carcinoma and, 474
small blue cell tumors, 45, 47, 53, 54, 279
small round cell tumors, 25, 51
  desmoplastic, 148, 343, 420, 422
  Ewing sarcoma as, 397, 398
  metastasis to liver, 420, 422
small-cell hepatoblastoma (SCHB), 420, 421
small-cell tumors, hepatic, 420–422
smooth muscle tumors, hepatic, 422
SNPs. *See* single nucleotide polymorphisms (SNPs)
SNs. *See* second neoplasms (SNs)
social adaptation
  inadequate, as late effect, 568–569
  neurobehavioral test battery for, 548, 550, 551
social behavioral functioning. *See* neurobehavioral *entries*
socioeconomic status
  cancer outcomes related to, 15, 17–18, 21
  Hodgkin lymphoma and, 237
  retinoblastoma and, 437, 451
sodium bicarbonate, for tumor lysis syndrome, 488, 489
soft-tissue sarcomas, 341–351
  chemotherapy for, 347–348, 349, 350, 351
  classification of, 344–345

clinical presentation of, 342–344
diagnostic evaluation of, 344
epidemiology of, 9, 341
experimental therapies for, 349–350
histopathology of, 50–51, 341–342
ICCC description of, 5
imaging of, 83–87
late effects in, 350–351
long-term outcomes of, 350–351
molecular pathogenesis of, 341–342, 343
radiotherapy for, 348–349, 350, 351
recurrence/relapse of, 349, 350, 351
risk assignment protocol for, 345–346, 351
staging of, 344–345, 347, 350
summary of, 118–119, 341, 351
surgical management of, 118–119, 348, 349
treatment and prognosis of, 347–349
soft-tissue structures, imaging of, 70, 71
soft-tissue tumors
  diagnosis by pentad, 45
  percent incidence of, 46
software packages, for sample size, in clinical trials, 154
solid (nonhematolymphoid) tumors, 45–46
  histopathologic classification of, 47–51
solvents, organic, 11
somatic cell mutation
  in germ cell tumors, 357
  in non-Hodgkin lymphoma, 223
  in retinoblastoma, 437, 454
Sonic hedgehog (SHH) signaling pathway, 280–281
sorafenib, 428, 431
Sotos syndrome, 8
South America, cancer care initiatives in, 18
Southern Blot analysis, in molecular genetic tests, 47
special-interest groups, global initiatives of, 17
SPECT (single-photo emission computed tomography), 72, 82, 131
spectroscopy
  in molecularly targeted therapies, 31
  proton, 71
speech deficits, 567
spermatogenesis, therapy impact on, 107, 405, 569
sphincter incompetence, in cord compression, 486
spinal cord compression, 486–487
  in acute myeloid leukemia, 189
  in neuroblastoma, 318, 324, 325
spindle cell tumors, of liver, 421, 422
  desmoplastic nested, 423
spiritual care, 518–519
spleen
  hematopoietic stem cell transplantation and, 143
  in Langerhans cell histiocytosis, 250

in myelodysplastic syndrome/myeloproliferative syndromes, 206, 207
platelet refractoriness and, 502–503
squamous cell carcinoma, 6, 9
staging by imaging, 70–71, 72
  of central nervous system neoplasms, 72–73
  of Ewing sarcoma, 398, 399, 403
  of lymphoma, 76–79
  of medulloblastoma, 281
  of melanoma, 472, 473
  of neuroblastoma, 82
  of osteosarcoma, 386, 387, 388
  of primitive neuroectodermal tumors, 281, 452
  of sarcomas, 86
  of Wilms tumor, 82
staging systems
  for adrenocortical carcinoma, 468
  for CNS germ cell tumors, 306, 368, 377
  for ependymoma, 276
  for graft-versus-host disease, 141–142
  for hepatic tumors, 119–120, 414–415, 426, 428, 432
  for Hodgkin lymphoma, 238, 239
  for medulloblastoma, 281, 282
  for melanoma, 472
  for nasopharyngeal carcinoma, 474, 475
  for neuroblastoma, 318, 319, 321
  for non-Hodgkin lymphoma, 164, 217, 218, 219, 220, 223, 225
  for osteosarcoma, 386, 387, 388, 389
  for renal tumors, 117, 332, 337
  for retinoblastoma, 444–446, 447
  for rhabdomyosarcoma, 344–345, 347, 350
  for soft-tissue sarcomas, 344–345, 347, 350
  for systemic germ cell tumors, 367–369, 370, 371, 377
  for thyroid cancer, 461, 462
  for Wilms tumor, 117, 332, 337
stains/staining, in pathological evaluation, 46, 47
  for acute myeloid leukemia, 190
  for rhabdomyosarcoma, 341
Stanford-Binet Intelligence Scales, 551
Staphylococcus spp. infections, 493, 508
statins, for osteonecrosis, 177
statistical determination, of sample size, for clinical trials, 154
stem cell factor, in systemic germ cell tumors, 356
stem cell transplantation (SCT)
  complementary and alternative therapies for, 555–556
  hematopoietic. *See* hematopoietic stem cell transplantation (HSCT)
  infection prevention and, 492
  T cell infusions with, 39–40
stem cells
  clonal disorders of, in neoplasms, 63–64
  leukemic, 163, 192, 203–204
  in myeloproliferative syndromes, 207

stereotactic body immobilization system, 130–131
stereotactic radiosurgery, 127
stereotactic radiotherapy, 127
"steroid refractory" graft-versus-host disease, 142
ST-PNET. *See* supratentorial primitive neuroectodermal tumors (ST-PNET)
Streptococcus spp. infections, 494
stress, pain management and, 541
stress-response signaling pathways, radiation therapy impact on, 124
stromal epithelial tumor of liver, nested, 423
stromal tumors
  gastrointestinal, 471–472
  hepatic, 420, 422, 423
subclavian vein, central line placement in, 113
subspecialty institutions, global efforts of, 16–17
subspecialty professionals, training programs for, 20
substance P antagonists, for nausea, 532, 535–536, 537
suicide, physician-assisted, 516
suicide gene therapy, 451
sun exposure, malignancy risk and, 437, 472
sunitinib, 471
superior vena cava syndrome (SVCS), 218, 485–486
supportive care
  for acute myeloid leukemia, 199
  complementary and alternative medicine as, 553–561
  for emergencies, 485–489
  for infectious complications, 491–495
  for late effects, 563–570
  for leukemia, imaging in, 86–88
  for nausea, 531–538
  nutritional, 523–528
  for osteosarcoma, 390–391
  pain management as, 541–545
  palliative care as, 513–520
  psychological, 547–551
  regional initiatives for, 18
  transfusion therapy as, 497–510
supratentorial malignant (high-grade) gliomas, 263–265
supratentorial primitive neuroectodermal tumors (ST-PNET)
  future directions for, 288
  in infants, 291, 294
  pathology of, 279, 285, 287
  radiation field planning for, 131, 133, 134
  relapse of, 287
  treatment of, 287
surgical excision
  of adrenocortical carcinoma, 468
  of Hodgkin lymphoma, 240
  of Langerhans cell histiocytosis, 252

  of medulloblastoma, 282
  of pleuropulmonary blastoma, 476
surgical management, 113–120
  of colorectal cancer, 470
  of Ewing sarcoma, 399–400
  of hepatic tumors, 119–120, 416, 423–425
  of melanoma, 472–473
  of nasopharyngeal carcinoma, 474
  palliative care integration with, 517
  of renal tumors, 117, 332–333, 334, 336
  of retinoblastoma, 446, 448, 449, 450, 452, 454
  second, indications for. *See* second-look surgery
  of soft-tissue sarcomas, 118–119, 344–345, 348, 349
  summary of, 113, 120
  transfusion therapy refusal and, 509
  of vascular access lines, 113–114
surgical margins
  for colorectal cancer, 470
  for hepatic tumors, 416, 424–425
  for melanoma, 472
surgical resection
  of choroid plexus tumors, 300–301
  of ependymoma, 273, 274, 275, 276
  of gastrointestinal stromal tumor, 471
  of germ cell tumors, 308, 310
  of gliomas, 262–263, 265
  of infant brain tumors, 292, 293, 294, 295, 296
  of neuroblastoma, 114–117, 323
  of osteosarcoma, 387, 388–389, 390, 391
  of rhabdomyosarcoma, 119, 344–345, 348, 349
  of systemic germ cell tumors, 369–371, 377
  of thyroid cancer, 462, 464, 465
  of Wilms tumor, 117–118
Surveillance, Epidemiology, and End Results (SEER) Program, in U.S., 3, 151
survival rates
  age-standardized, 11–12
  clinical trials comparison of, 151
  factors influencing, 3
  income associated with, 15, 21
  sex-specific trends in, 563, 565
  undernutrition impact on, 523
survivors
  epidemiology of, 11–12
  long-term effects in, 563–570. *See also* late effects
  long-term monitoring of, 203, 208–209, 569
  neurocognitive impairment in, 547–548
SVCS (superior vena cava syndrome), 218, 485–486
Swyer syndrome, 357
sympathetic nervous system, in nausea physiology, 531

sympathetic nervous system tumors
  epidemiology of, 4, 8
  neuroblastoma as, 115–117, 317
symptom distress, 518
symptom management, in palliative care, 517–518
synovial sarcoma, 341, 343, 349
systemic germ cell tumors, 355–378
  adult therapy for, lessons from, 372–375
  biology of, 356–360
  biomarkers of, 358–360, 366, 367, 368–369
  chemotherapy for, 369, 370, 372–375
  chemotherapy trials on, 375–377, 378
  classification of, 360
  clinical features of, 364–367
  diagnosis by pentad, 45
  differential diagnosis of, 360, 364–365
  embryology of, 356
  epidemiology of, 6, 9, 355–356
  genetics of, 357–358
  histopathology of, 51, 360–364
  initial evaluation of, 365–367
  late effects in, 378
  oncogenesis of, 356–357
  percent incidence of, 46
  prognostic features of, 368–369
  radiotherapy for, 371–372
  refractory/ relapsed, 375, 377
  risk stratification for, 368–369, 377
  risk-adjusted therapy for, 368–369, 377–378
  staging of, 367–369
  surgical management of, 369–371
  treatment and outcomes of, 369–378

T

T cell augmentation, 40
T cell helper 1 (Th1), in immune response, 34
T cell helper 2 (Th2), in immune response, 34, 37
T cell infusions, in stem cell transplantation, 39–40
T cell receptor (TcR), in immune response, 33–34, 35
T cells/lymphocytes
  in acute lymphoblastic leukemia, 162, 163, 164–167, 174, 175, 177
  in graft-versus-host disease, 140, 142
  in hemophagocytic lymphohistiocytosis, 254
  in Hodgkin lymphoma, 237
  in immune response, 33–34, 35
  in immunotherapy, 35–36, 37–38
  in Langerhans cell histiocytosis, 245, 246, 247
  in leukemia, 61, 62, 191
  in lymphomas, 55, 57, 58, 59
  in myeloproliferative syndromes, 208
  in non-Hodgkin lymphoma, 219, 221, 223, 225, 226–227

tumor section samples, hepatic, for intraoperative consultation, 416
tumor suppressor genes (TSGs), 23
    in choroid plexus tumors, 299
    inactivation mechanisms of, 23–24
    in neuroblastoma, 320
    in osteosarcoma, 383–384
    in renal tumors, 329–330
    in retinoblastoma, 437
    in rhabdoid tumors, 294
    in solid (nonhematolymphoid) tumors, 48
    in systemic germ cell tumors, 358
    in thyroid cancer, 459–460
tumor volume
    target, in radiotherapy, 129, 131, 401
    time-decay of, with chemotherapy, 114, 115
Turcot syndrome, 261, 469
twinning programs, 16, 17
twins, leukemia risk and, 186, 192–193
two-dimensional imaging, for radiation planning, 130, 131
two-hit hypothesis
    of acute lymphoblastic leukemia, 161
    of retinoblastoma, 438–439
TYMS gene, 169–170
tyrosine kinases
    in acute lymphoblastic leukemia, 162–163, 167, 175
    in Hodgkin lymphoma, 236
    in leukemia, 63
    in medulloblastoma, 281
    in neuroblastoma, 320, 321
    as therapeutic targets, 28, 471
tyrosinemia, hepatic tumors and, 410, 411

U

UICC. *See* International Union Against Cancer (UICC)
ultrasound
    of abdominal abscess, 88
    of germ cell tumors, 365, 367, 370
    of hepatic tumors, 119, 414
    of neuroblastoma, 79
    in radiation field planning, 131
    of renal tumors, 331, 336
    technical considerations of, 70
    of thyroid cancer, 461, 462
    of venous thrombosis, 89
    of Wilms tumor, 82, 83
ultraviolet (UV) therapy
    for blood product preparation, 502, 508
    psoralen with, for Langerhans cell histiocytosis, 252
undernutrition. *See* malnutrition
undifferentiated embryonal sarcoma (UESL) of the liver
    chemotherapy for, 429
    histopathology of, 415, 420, 421
    imaging of, 414
    pathogenesis of, 409, 410, 412

Unidad Nacional de Oncologia Pediatrica (UNOP), 19, 20
United Nations, programs of, 15
unspecified neoplasms, 6, 9
uracil, 102
urate oxidase enzyme
    recombinant, for non-Hodgkin lymphoma, 218
    for tumor lysis syndrome, 489
uric acid (UA) imbalance
    in non-Hodgkin lymphoma, 218, 219
    in tumor lysis syndrome, 488–489
urinalysis, in renal tumor diagnosis, 331
urinary tract. *See* genitourinary tract

V

VAC regimen
    for Ewing sarcoma, 401–402
    for hepatic tumors, 429
    for melanoma, 473
    for rhabdomyosarcoma, 347, 348, 350
    for systemic germ cell tumors, 372, 373, 375, 376
VACA regimen, for hepatic tumors, 429
vaccines/vaccinations
    in immunotherapy, 38, 39
    recommendations for, 491
VACD regimen, for Ewing sarcoma, 401–402
VACD-IE regimen, for Ewing sarcoma, 401–402
vacuum-molded bag, for radiation therapy, 129, 130
vagus nerve, in nausea, 531, 532
VAI regimen, for rhabdomyosarcoma, 347, 348, 350
VAIA regimen, for hepatic tumors, 429
valproic acid, 205
valvular heart disease, therapy-induced, 566
vancomycin, 493, 494
vanillylmandelic acid (VMA), 318
varicella vaccine, 491
varicella-zoster virus (VZV), 494
varicella-zoster virus (VZV) immune globulin, 492
vascular access
    complications of, 113–114
    surgical principles of, 113
vascular endothelial growth factor (VEGF), 196, 403, 404, 431
vascular occlusive agents, for hepatic tumors, 430
vascular support, for transfusion reaction, 506
vascular system
    anemia impact on, 498
    Ewing sarcoma and, 395
    germ cell tumors invasion of, 369–370
    hyperleukocytosis impact on, 487, 499, 507
    immunotherapy impact on, 204
    non-Hodgkin lymphoma impact on, 218

    in retinoblastoma, 441
    ultrasound of, 70
    Wilms tumor invasion of, 117, 118
vasoactive intestinal peptide, in neuroblastoma, 318
venography, magnetic resonance, 89
veno-occlusive disease (VOD)
    in hyperleukocytosis, 487
    immunotherapy and, 204
    platelets in, 500, 502
venous thromboses
    with central venous catheters, 113, 114
    imaging of, 89
    Wilms tumor and, 331
ventricles, intracranial
    chemotherapy injection into, 110
    choroid plexus tumors in, 299
    ependymoma in, 271, 272
    germ cell tumors in, 308, 309
    medulloblastoma obstruction of, 281
    in nausea physiology, 531
vertebral column, tumor extension into, 486
vesicant chemotherapy agents, extravasation of, 108
vimentin, in lymphomas, 61
vinblastine
    for germ cell tumors, 309, 311
    for Hodgkin lymphoma, 238
    for Langerhans cell histiocytosis, 253
    pharmacology of, 99
    for systemic germ cell tumors, 373, 374, 375, 376, 377
vinc alkaloids
    for Langerhans cell histiocytosis, 253
    mechanism of action, 96, 99, 101, 103
    pharmacokinetics of, 104, 105, 107
    for soft-tissue sarcomas, 348, 349
vincristine
    for acute lymphoblastic leukemia, 170, 171, 172
    for acute myeloid leukemia, 199
    for choroid plexus tumors, 300
    for ependymoma, 274
    for Ewing sarcoma, 401–402, 403, 404
    for gliomas, 263, 264, 266
    for hepatic tumors, 425–426, 428, 429, 430
    for Hodgkin lymphoma, 238, 240
    for infant brain tumors, 291, 292, 293, 295, 296
    for Langerhans cell histiocytosis, 253
    for medulloblastoma, 283, 284, 288
    neuropathy related to, 107, 108, 559
    for non-Hodgkin lymphoma, 220, 222, 224, 225, 226, 227, 228
    pharmacology of, 99, 110
    for renal tumors, 334, 335, 336
    for retinoblastoma, 448, 449, 451, 452, 453
    for rhabdomyosarcoma, 347, 348, 349
    for systemic germ cell tumors, 373, 375, 376
Vineland Adaptive Behavior Scales, 551

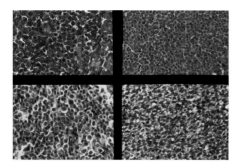

Plate 1
Figure 5-1 Small blue cell tumors of childhood. Note the similar embryonal appearance of four different such tumors (clockwise from upper left: rhabdomyosarcoma, lymphoblastic lymphoma, neuroblastoma, and nephroblastoma, or Wilms tumor). 200X, hematoxylin and eosin stain.

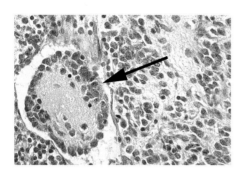

Plate 2
Figure 5-2 (A) Homer Wright rosette (arrow) in neuroblastoma. 400X, hematoxylin and eosin stain.

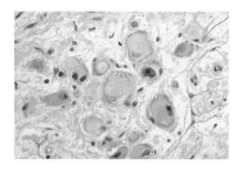

Plate 3
Figure 5-2 (B) Ganglion cell differentiation in neuroblastoma. 400X, hematoxylin and eosin stain.

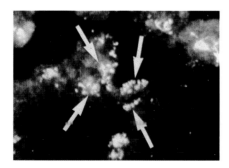

Plate 4
Figure 5-2 (C) Homogenously staining regions with MYCN amplification (arrows) in neuroblastoma. 200X, FISH.

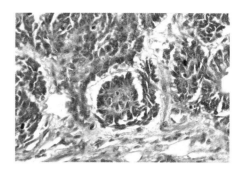

Plate 5
Figure 5-3 (B) Favorable histopathology nephroblastoma or Wilms tumor with triphasic histology, including tubular and glomeruloid structures. 400X hematoxylin and eosin stain.

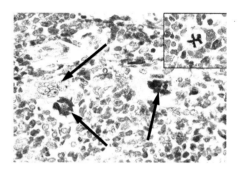

Plate 6
Figure 5-3 (C) Unfavorable histopathology in nephroblastoma or Wilms tumor. Both nuclei (arrows) and mitotic figures (inset) can be three to four times the size of their neighboring cellular counterparts. 200X, hematoxylin and eosin stain.

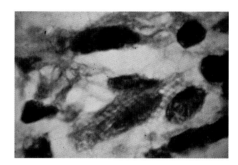

Plate 7
Figure 5-4 (A) Rhabdomyoblast showing skeletal muscle differentiation (contractile elements or cross striations) (arrows) defining the malignancy as rhabdomyosarcoma at the light microscopic level. 630X, hematoxylin and eosin stain.

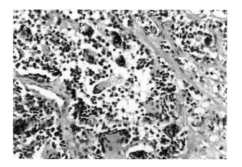

Plate 8
Figure 5-4 (B) Classical alveolar rhabdomyosarcoma (unfavorable histopathology) with cystic, cleft-like (or alveolar) spaces and associated tumor giant cells. 200X, hematoxylin and eosin stain.

Plate   C-1

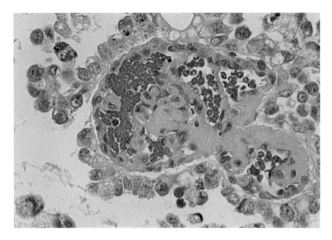

Plate 9

Figure 5-5 (B) Yolk sac carcinoma (with Schiller-Duvall structure), a typical occult malignant germ cell tumor that may be found focally in an otherwise benign cystic teratoma as in 5A. 400X, hematoxylin and eosin stain.

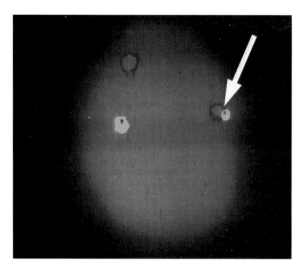

Plate 12

Figure 5-6 (D) Cytoplasmic membranous immunostaining for CD99 in Ewing sarcoma, 200X, hematoxylin counterstain, CD99 immunostaining.

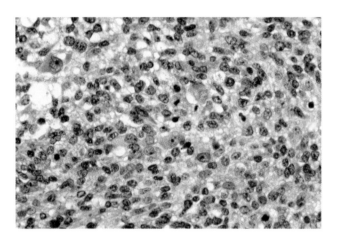

Plate 10

Figure 5-6 (B) Monotonous, uniform small blue cell appearance of Ewing sarcoma. 400X, hematoxylin and eosin stain.

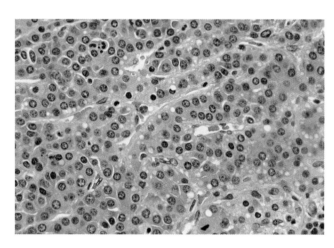

Plate 13

Figure 5-7 (B) Hepatoblastoma, fetal subtype. 400X, hematoxylin and eosin stain.

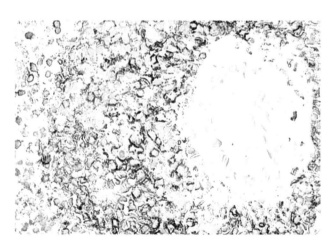

Plate 11

Figure 5-6 (C) Cytoplasmic membranous immunostaining for CD99 in Ewing sarcoma, 200X, hematoxylin counterstain, CD99 immunostaining.

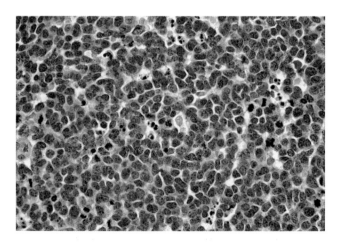

Plate 14

Figure 5-8 (B) Retinoblastoma in many areas can have an embryonal or undifferentiated small blue cell appearance. 400X, hematoxylin and eosin stain.

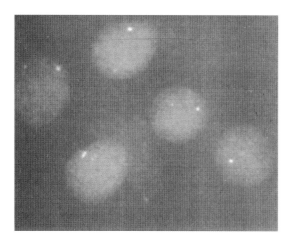

Plate 15

Figure 5-8 (C) In familial cases, rb1 deletions may be seen in associated somatic tissues such as white blood cells. 400x, hematoxylin and eosin stain.

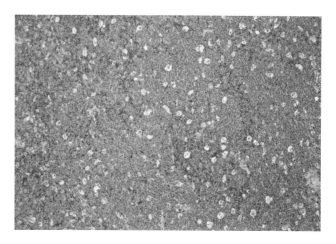

Plate 18

Figure 5-9 (C) Burkitt lymphoma, low power showing multiple tingible body macrophages, giving rise to the starry sky morphology. 100X, hematoxylin and eosin stain.

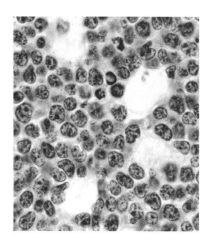

Plate 16

Figure 5-9 (A) Burkitt lymphoma showing relatively monormorphous population with high mitotic rate and tingible body macrophages. 400X, hematoxylin and eosin stain.

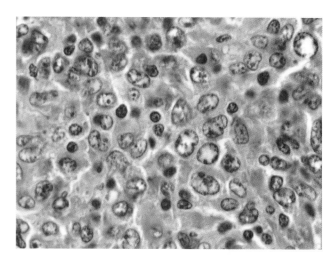

Plate 19

Figure 5-10 Diffuse large B-cell lymphoma showing large neoplastic lymphoid cells with nuclei that are greater than 2 to 3 times the size of a small lymphocyte with relatively abundant eosinophilic cytoplasm. 400X, hematoxylin and eosin stain.

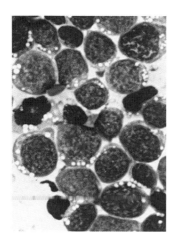

Plate 17

Figure 5-9 (B) Burkitt lymphoma showing vacuolation of the cytoplasm and monomorphic nuclear appearance. 1000X oil, Wright's stain.

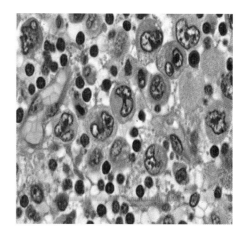

Plate 20

Figure 5-11 (A) Anaplastic large cell lymphoma, classic type, showing a proliferation of large anaplastic cells that are horseshoe-shaped and multinucleated with abundant, slightly basophilic cytoplasm. 400X, H&E.

Plate   C-3

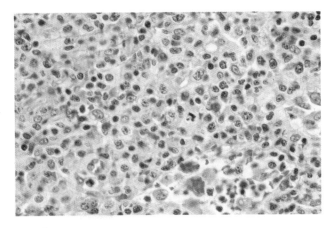

Plate 21
Figure 5-11 (B) Anaplastic large cell lymphoma, small cell variant, showing a smaller atypical neoplastic proliferation of T-cells that are small to intermediate in size and show evidence of vascular invasion. This tumor stained positively with both CD30 and ALK-1. 200X, hematoxylin and eosin stain.

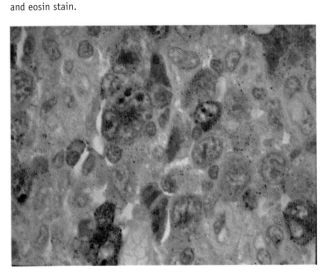

Plate 22
Figure 5-12 (A) CD30 staining in anaplastic large cell lymphoma showing typical strong staining in a cytoplasmic and Golgi pattern in the neoplastic cells. 1000X oil, hematoxylin counterstain, CD30 immunostaining.

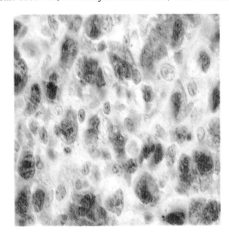

Plate 23
Figure 5-12 (B) ALK-1 in an anaplastic large cell lymphoma that carries the t(2;5) translocation showing the typical nuclear and cytoplasmic staining pattern seen with that translocation. 400X, hematoxylin counterstain ALK-1 immunostaining.

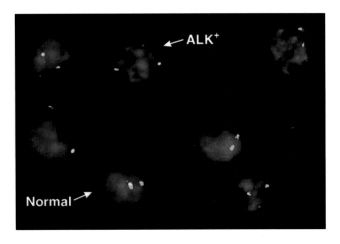

Plate 24
Figure 5-13 FISH analysis for the ALK translocation in anaplastic large cell lymphoma showing breakapart of the yellow fusion signal when a translocation is present giving rise to separate red and green signals. 1000X, FISH.

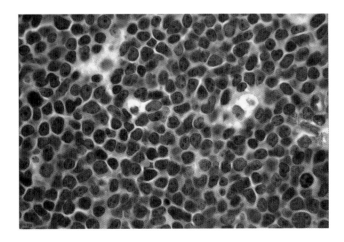

Plate 25
Figure 5-14 Precursor T lymphoblastic lymphoma showing monomorphic infiltrate of neoplastic cells with fine chromatin, minimal cytoplasm and slightly irregular nuclear contours. 400X, hematoxylin and eosin stain.

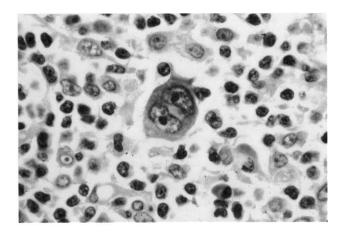

Plate 26
Figure 5-15 Reed-Sternberg cell from classical Hodgkin lymphoma showing the typical binuclear Reed-Sternberg cell with prominent eosinophilic nucleoli that are the neoplastic cell in classical Hodgkin lymphoma. 1000X, hematoxylin and eosin stain.

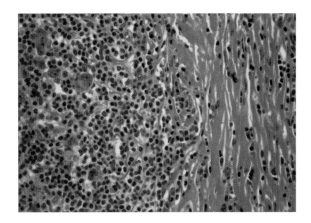

Plate 27

Figure 5-16 Nodular sclerosis classical Hodgkin lymphoma. This shows the nodular appearance of a classical Hodgkin lymphoma of the nodular sclerosis subtype. There are broad bands of collegen fibrosis separating nodules that are composed of a mixture of reactive cells with numerous Reed-Sternberg cells and variants. 200X, hematoxylin and eosin stain.

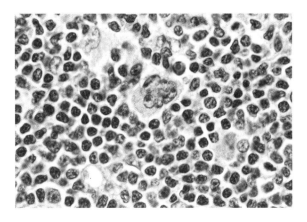

Plate 28

Figure 5-17 L&H Reed-Sternberg cell variant. The Reed-Sternberg cell variant that is seen in nodular lymphocyte predominant Hodgkin lymphoma with the classical multilobated nucleus, giving rise to the "popcorn cell." 1000X, hematoxylin and eosin stain.

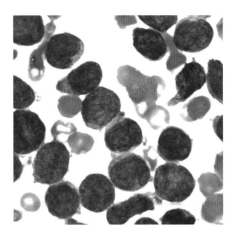

Plate 29

Figure 5-18 (A) L1 lymphoid blast. These lymphoid blasts show relatively little morphologic diversity and have a low nuclear: cytoplasmic ratio with minimal cytoplasm and relatively smooth nuclear contours. 1000X, Wright's stain.

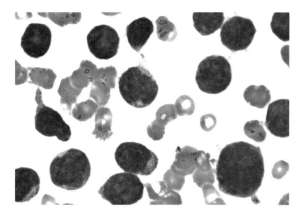

Plate 30

Figure 5-18 (B) L2 lymphoid blast. These lymphoid blasts show more diversity in nuclear size and shape with variation from small L1 type blasts to larger blasts with more abundant cytoplasm and somewhat irregular nuclear contours. 1000X, Wright's stain.

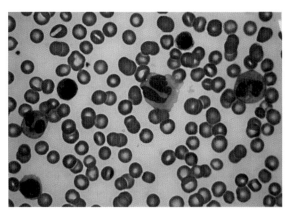

Plate 31

Figure 5-19 Peripheral blood in JMML. The peripheral blood of this child shows a monocytosis with circulating nucleated red blood cells and dyspoietic changes in the neutrophils including abnormal segmentation and granulation of neutrophils. Platelets also appear hypogranular. 1000X, Wright's stain.

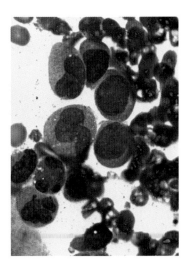

Plate 32

Figure 5-20 AML with monoblastic differentiation and 11q23 abnormality. This AML showed strong NSE positivity and monoblastic markers by flow cytometry. Cytogenetics showed 11q23 abnormality. 1000X, Wright's stain.

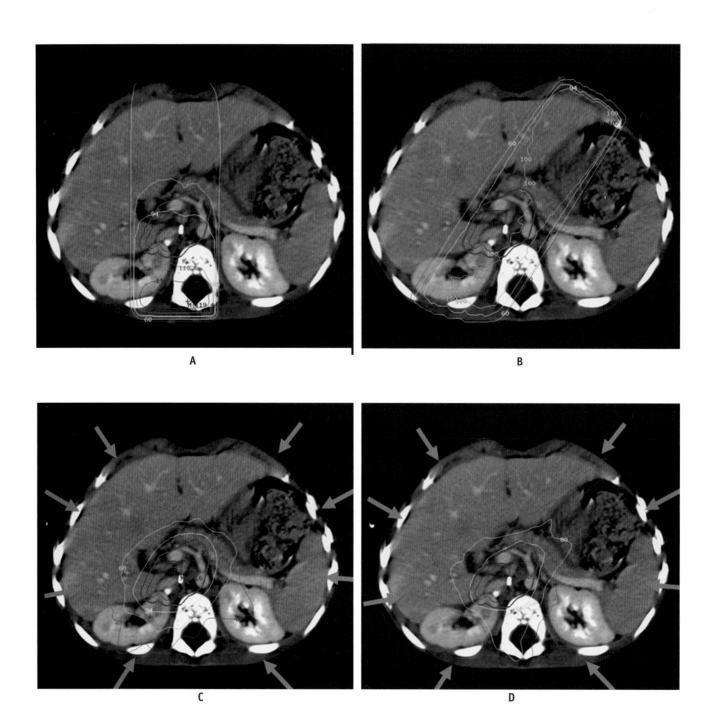

Plate 33

Figure 9-6 Comparison of treatment plans for a right adrenal neuroblastoma. The planning target volume (PTV) is in red. The 94, 60, and 40 isodose surfaces (IDS) are shown in each illustration. (A) Single posterior beam. The dose is highest 1 to 2 cm from the posterior body surface and decreases gradually as the beam travels anteriorly. The PTV is encompassed by the 86 IDS, whereas the spinal cord is encompassed by the 115 IDS. Forty-six percent of the right kidney also receives a higher dose than the PTV and is within the 94 IDS. The maximum dose at this axial level is 119, 38% higher than the minimum dose to the PTV. (B) Two opposing oblique beams. The beams are angled obliquely to reduce the proportion of the liver and left kidney receiving a significant dose compared with what they would receive from straight anterior and posterior beams. The obliquity increases the proportion of the right kidney receiving a high dose, however. The dose is fairly homogeneous throughout the beam path. The 94 IDS encompasses the PTV, 87% of the right kidney, and 14% of the liver. The maximum dose is deposited in normal tissues rather than the PTV, and is 107 at this axial level. (C) Eight coplanar non-IMRT (3-dimensional conformal) beams. The 94 IDS encompasses and conforms to the shape of the PTV. The 60 IDS encompasses 10 to 14 mm of normal tissue surrounding the PTV, including less than 1% of the left kidney, 9% of the liver, and 42% of the right kidney. The 40 IDS encompasses 26% of the left kidney, 20% of the liver, and 89% of the right kidney. Unlike the single-beam and opposing-beam plans, the maximum radiation dose (99 at this axial level) is within the PTV. (D) Eight coplanar IMRT beams. The 94 IDS encompasses the PTV. The liver and right kidney receive lower doses than with the other plans. The 60 IDS encompasses none of the left kidney, 7% of the liver, and 20% of the right kidney. The 40 IDS encompasses 2% of the left kidney, 15% of the liver, and 30% of the right kidney. Typical of IMRT plans, the dose is less homogeneous within the PTV (maximum dose on this axial level 105) than in the 8-beam non-IMRT plan.

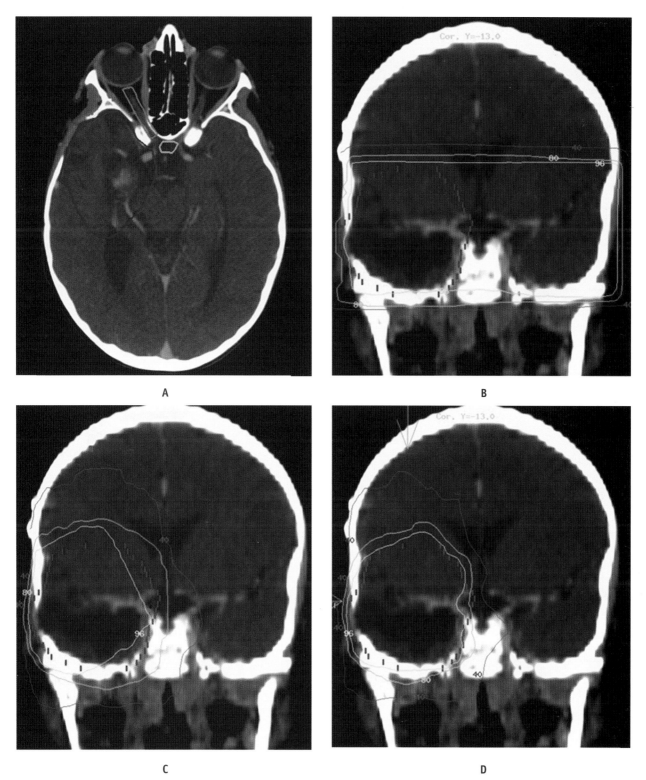

A

B

C

D

Plate 34

Figure 9-7 Comparison of treatment plans for a supratentorial primitive neuroectodermal tumor. (A) The GTV is in close proximity to the right optic nerve (outlined in red) and optic chiasm (outlined in orange). In illustrations B-D, the margins of the PTV are indicated by red dashes and the 96, 80, and 40 IDSs are shown. (B) Two opposing lateral beams. The dose to the contralateral side of the brain, bilateral optic nerves, and optic chiasm is equal to the dose (minimum of 96) to the PTV. Maximum dose is 105. (C) Eight noncoplanar non-IMRT (3-dimensional conformal) beams. To avoid exceeding the tolerance dose of the optic chiasm and right optic nerve, the superior-medial and inferior-medial portions of the PTV must be underdosed and are not encompassed by the 96 IDS. The optic chiasm, right optic nerve, and pituitary gland are within the 80 IDS. In contrast to the opposing lateral beam plan, almost all of the right cerebral hemisphere is spared from receiving high-dose radiation and is outside the 40 IDS. Maximum dose is 104. (D) Eight noncoplanar IMRT beams. The same 8 beams shown in Figure 9-6C produce isodose surfaces that conform to the PTV and exclude the optic chiasm, right optic nerve, and pituitary gland better when IMRT is used. The 96 IDS encompasses the entire PTV except where it overlaps the optic chiasm and distal optic nerve. The optic chiasm, right optic nerve, and pituitary gland are mostly outside the 80 IDS. The volume of normal brain within the 80 and 40 IDSs is smaller than in the non-IMRT plan in Figure 9-6C. Maximum dose is 106.

Plate   C-7

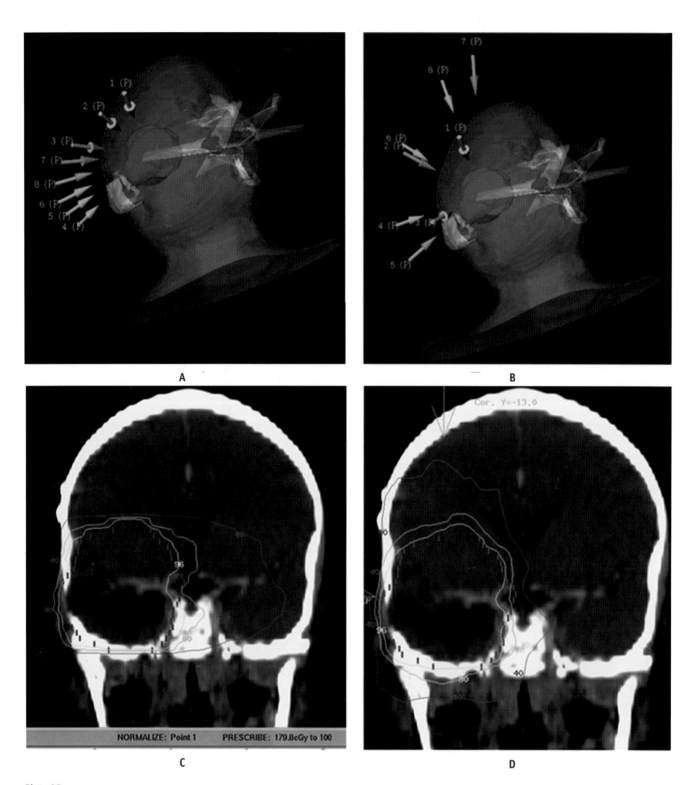

Plate 35

Figure 9-8 Comparison of coplanar and noncoplanar IMRT treatment plans for the supratentorial primitive neuroectodermal tumor in Figure 9-7. A and B show 3-dimensional reconstructions of the PTV in red and the patient's head and neck with the immobilization mouthpiece in place in brown. The green arrows indicate the central axes of the 8 radiation beams in a coplanar (A) and noncoplanar (B) plan. The isodose distribution of the coplanar plan is shown in C, and that of the noncoplanar plan is shown in D. The noncoplanar plan provides equal coverage of the PTV with greater dose homogeneity (maximum dose 106 vs 110) and less dosage to the optic nerves, optic chiasm, pituitary, and contralateral side of the brain.

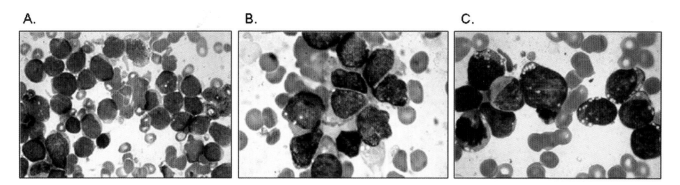

A.   B.   C.

Plate 36
Figure 12-1   Morphological classification of ALL. French American and British (FAB) morphological classification of lymphoblasts. (A) L1 blasts. (B) L2 blasts. (C) L3 blasts.

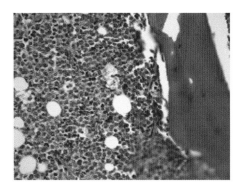

Plate 37
Figure 14-1 (A)   Burkitt leukemia involving the bone marrow with complete effacement of normal bone marrow architecture (H&E section, 400X magnification).

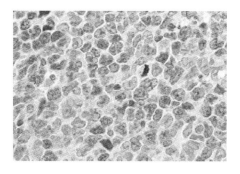

Plate 40
Figure 14-2 (B)   Precursor T-cell lymphoblastic lymphoma/leukemia (H&E stain of lymph node, 400X magnification).

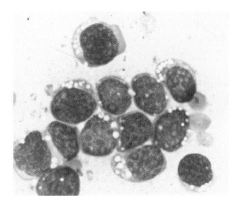

Plate 38
Figure 14-1 (B)   Cytologic preparation demonstrating Burkitt cells in a cerebral spinal fluid preparation (Wrights stain, 1000X magnification).

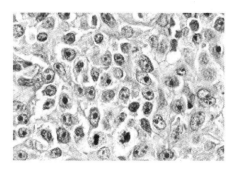

Plate 41
Figure 14-2 (C)   Diffuse large B-cell lymphoma (H&E stain, 400X magnification).

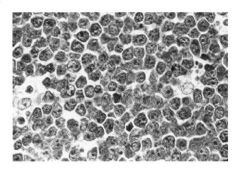

Plate 39
Figure 14-2 (A)   Burkitt lymphoma (H&E stain, 400X magnification).

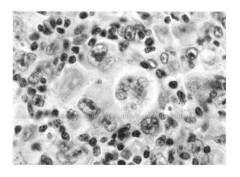

Plate 42
Figure 14-2 (D)   Anaplastic large-cell lymphoma, *CD30* positive and *ALK-1* positive (H&E stain, 400 X magnification).

Plate   C-9

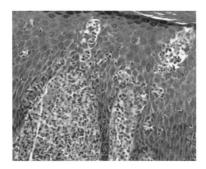

Plate 43

Figure 14-3 (A) Section of the skin (H&E stain, 1000X magnification).

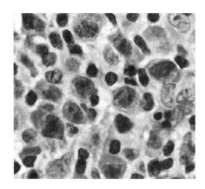

Plate 44

Figure 14-3 (B) Malignant infiltrates from primary cutaneous anaplastic large-cell lymphoma demonstrating large anaplastic cells (H&E stain, 1000X magnification).

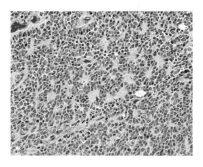

Plate 45

Figure 19-3 Photomicrograph (200x) of classic medulloblastoma with sheets of small primitive tumor cells and numerous Homer Wright (neuroblastic) rosettes, with tumor cells surrounding central collections of neuropil (neuronal processes).

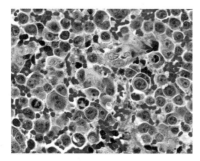

Plate 46

Figure 19-4 Photomicrograph (400x) of large-cell medulloblastoma. The tumor cells are enlarged and the nuclei feature vesicular chromatin and prominent nucleoli. There is also a brisk mitotic index and cell wrapping (tumor cells enveloping one another).

Small volume conformal boost

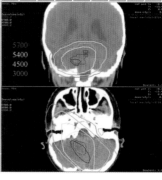

Plate 47

Figure 19-5 Conformal radiation distribution for a patient with medulloblastoma treated with multiple shaped fields to a limited target volume (cyan contour) defined by the tumor bed with a 1.5-cm margin. Note that the prescribed radiation dose volume spares the cerebrum and the contralateral cochlea.

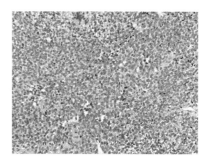

Plate 48

Figure 28-4 (A) Histologic and immunohistochemical features of Ewing sarcoma/pPNET: Classic Ewing sarcoma appears as sheets of monotonous, round cells. (Hematoxylin and eosin, original magnification X200).

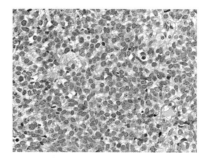

Plate 49

Figure 28-4 (B) Histologic and immunohistochemical features of Ewing sarcoma/pPNET: The cells have scanty cytoplasm and round nuclei with evenly distributed finely granular chromatin and inconspicuous nucleoli. (Hematoxylin and eosin, original magnification X400.)

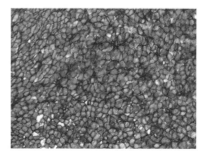

Plate 50

Figure 28-4 (C) Histologic and immunohistochemical features of Ewing sarcoma/pPNET: Strong, diffuse membrane staining is observed with the O13 monoclonal antibody to p30/32MIC2. (Immunoperoxidase, original magnification X400).

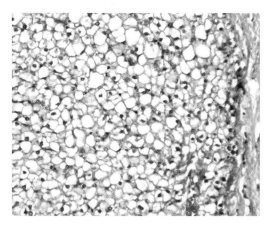

Plate 51

Figure 29-2 (C) Photomicrograph of hepatic adenoma with clear cells due to fatty accumulation.

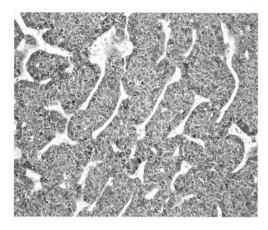

Plate 54

Figure 29-4 (E) Macrotrabecular pattern composed of thick multicellular cords defining sinusoidal spaces.

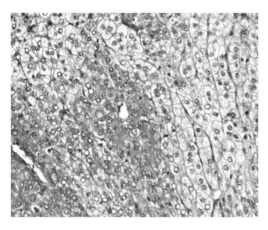

Plate 52

Figure 29-4 (C) Morphology of fetal hepatoblastoma showing uniform population of neoplastic hepatocytes with distinct cell borders. Some have clear cytoplasm; other areas show slight nuclear enlargement.

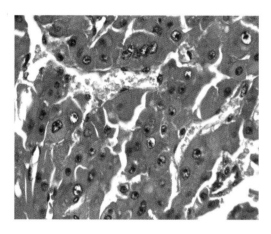

Plate 55

Figure 29-5 (B) Morphology of relatively well differentiated HCC showing large polygonal cells and abundant cytoplasm, large nuclei, and distinct nucleoli, delimiting sinusoidal spaces.

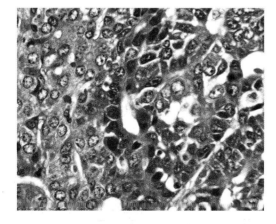

Plate 53

Figure 29-4 (D) Embryonal hepatoblastoma adjacent to fetal component, showing increased nucleo-cytoplasmic ratio and embryonal morphology. The tumor is recognizable as hepatoblastoma, given its recapitulation of trabecular morphology.

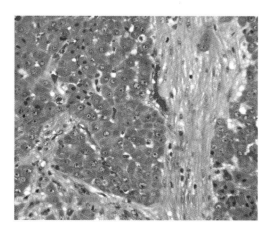

Plate 56

Figure 29-6 (B) Microscopic appearance of fibrolamellar variant, composed of large, brightly eosinophilic cells and distinctive lamellated collagenous stromal response.

Plate C-11

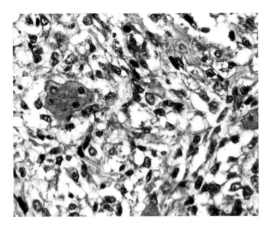

Plate 57
Figure 29-7 (A) Microscopic appearance of undifferentiated embryonal sarcoma showing a spectrum of cells; some appear primitive, other cells are large and pleomorphic.

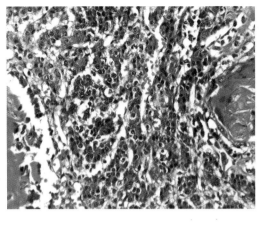

Plate 60
Figure 29-11 (C) Histology of mixed (epithelial / mesenchymal) HBL with primitive appearing mesenchyme and bone production.

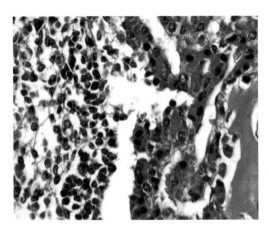

Plate 58
Figure 29-8 Microscopic image of small cell hepatoblastoma component (center) as part of mixed hepatoblastoma showing osteoid (upper right).

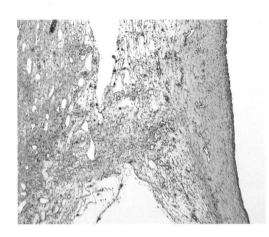

Plate 61
Figure 29-12 (B) Large myxoid degenerative areas with cyst devoid of any lining; other areas show the multifocal, hamartomatous features of bile ducts formation, mesenchyme, and vascular structures amid liver tissue.

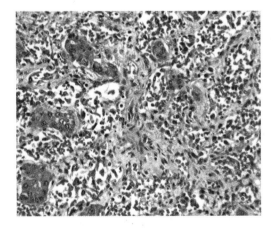

Plate 59
Figure 29-10 (B) Microscopic appearance of hemangioendothelioma composed of solid growth of spindle cells defining occasional inconspicuous vascular structures. There is mild pleomorphism of the endothelial cells but no malignant features. Note entrapped hepatocyte clusters.

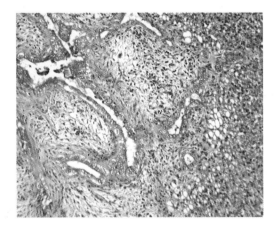

Plate 62
Figure 29-12 (C) Large myxoid degenerative areas with cyst devoid of any lining; other areas show the multifocal, hamartomatous features of bile ducts formation, mesenchyme, and vascular structures amid liver tissue.